# CONTRIBUTING AUTHORS

STANLEY AINSWORTH, Ph.D., Professor and Chairman of Speech Correction, University of Georgia

OLLIE BACKUS, Ph.D., Professor of Speech and Director of the Speech and Hearing Clinic, University of Alabama

H. HARLAN BLOOMER, Ph.D., Professor of Speech and Director of the Speech and Hearing Clinic, University of Michigan

BRUCE P. BOGERT, Ph.D., Member of Technical Staff, Bell Telephone Laboratories

JON EISENSON, Ph.D., Associate Professor of Speech and Director of the Speech and Hearing Clinic, Queens College

VICTOR P. GARWOOD, Ph.D., Associate Professor of Speech and Associate Director of the Speech and Hearing Clinic, University of Southern California

VICTOR GOODHILL, M.D., Associate Clinical Professor of Otolaryngology, University of Southern California School of Medicine; Senior Attending Otolaryngologist, Children's Hospital, Los Angeles County Hospital, and Eye and Ear Hospital; Physician-in-charge of Hearing and Speech Center, Children's Hospital; and Director of Otologic Laboratory, Institute for Medical Research, Cedars of Lebanon Hospital

GILES WILKESON GRAY, Ph.D., Professor of Speech, Louisiana State University

T. D. HANLEY, Ph.D., Associate Professor of Speech, Assistant Director of the Speech and Hearing Clinic, and Associate Director of the Speech Science Laboratory, Purdue University

WENDELL JOHNSON, Ph.D., Professor of Speech Pathology and Psychology, University of Iowa

HERBERT KOEPP-BAKER, Ph.D., Professor of Clinical Speech Pathology and Director of the Cleft Palate Training Program and Center, University of Illinois, College of Medicine

JACK MATTHEWS, Ph.D., Professor and Chairman of the Speech Department and Chairman of the Graduate School Committee for Speech and Hearing Disorders, University of Pittsburgh

ROBERT MILISEN, Ph.D., Professor of Speech and Director of the Speech and Hearing Clinic, University of Indiana

G. PAUL MOORE, Ph.D., Associate Professor of Speech Re-education, Northwestern University

HELMER R. MYKLEBUST, Ed.D., Professor of Audiology and Director of the Institute for Language Disorders in Children, Northwestern University

WILLIAM H. PERKINS, Ph.D., Associate Professor of Speech and Supervisor of Clinical Training, University of Southern California

GORDON E. PETERSON, Ph.D., Associate Professor of Speech and Director of the Speech Research Laboratory, University of Michigan

MARGARET HALL POWERS, Ph.D., Director of the Bureau of Physically Handicapped Children and the Division of Speech Correction, Chicago Public Schools

S. RICHARD SILVERMAN, Ph.D., Director of the Central Institute for the Deaf, St. Louis, and Professor of Audiology, Washington University

CLARENCE T. SIMON, Ph.D., Sc.D., Professor of Psychology of Speech, Northwestern University

M. D. STEER, Ph.D., Professor of Speech, Director of the Speech and Hearing Clinic, and Director of the Speech Science Laboratory, Purdue University

LAVERNE DEEL SUTHERLAND, M.A., Speech Correction Teacher, Los Angeles

LEE EDWARD TRAVIS, Ph.D., Professor of Psychology and Speech and Director of the Speech and Hearing Clinic, University of Southern California

C. VAN RIPER, Ph.D., Director of the Speech Clinic, Western Michigan College

ROBERT WEST, Ph.D., Professor, Brooklyn College and New York Medical Center

ZELDA S. WOLPE, Ph.D., Clinical Psychologist, Beverly Hills, California

KENNETH SCOTT WOOD, Ph.D., Professor of Speech and Director of the Speech and Hearing Clinic, University of Oregon

# HANDBOOK OF
# SPEECH PATHOLOGY

## WITHDRAWN

Edited by

## LEE EDWARD TRAVIS

Professor of Psychology and Speech, and
Director of the Speech and Hearing Clinic
University of Southern California

New York: APPLETON-CENTURY-CROFTS, Inc.

# PREFACE

JUST A QUARTER of a century ago, one man could have reacted intelligently, even authoritatively, to the whole field of communication disorders. In one book of average length he could have presented in relatively complete fashion the findings of the laboratory and the practices of the clinic. The present work, from the standpoint of both size and content, shows that speech pathology has grown away beyond the grasp of any one man. Each contributing author felt that he could have, should have, written more. Each chapter could have been a book. Each of several chapters could have been more than one book. Since this work was not possible from the pen of one man, twenty-seven authorities in the various areas of speech pathology contributed thirty-three chapters. Each author is truly a specialist in his subfield, yet each is keenly sensitive to other subfields and to the field as a whole.

The student of speech and of speech pathology, particularly the beginner, too often feels that he is coping with sounds, speech organs, physiology, and emotional complexes. He gets enmeshed in decibels, vocal folds, phonetic symbols, and proving the proposition. With an air of wisdom he makes phonetic transcriptions of articulation errors, audiometric examinations, voice recordings, and IQ ratings. All of these things are important, and they are discussed in this book. But the point is also made in this volume that in attempting to comprehend the individual's perception and production of speech, one is really trying to comprehend the speaker and/or the listener. We may say with conviction that in order to understand an individual's speech, it is necessary not only to understand his sensory, integrative, and motor communication equipment, but his person as well. A speech disorder is a disorder of the person as well as a disorder in the reception and transmission of spoken language. Yet we must be wary of oversimplifying this proposition. There are those whose right to speak well is baffling. Too, there are those whose right to speak so poorly, if at all, is equally baffling. Some people with considerable organic involvement of the speech apparatus have little associated speech trouble. Others with little organic pathology have great associated speech disorder. In studying the social and personal histories of some individuals, one is amazed that they talk at all, let alone relatively well. In making the same approach with others, one is struck that they have so much speech disturbance. Many and complicated longitudinal and cross-sectional interrelationships function to make dynamic connections between behavioral events and organismic characteristics at any one time very difficult to assay. In speech pathology, as well as in related disciplines, symptom selection offers the greatest research possibilities.

As the editor of this volume, I have been subjected to a very fine education.

I ought to be one of the most widely read speech pathologists in the country. Thanks are due to many publishers, foundations, and associations who granted permission to quote from material previously published under their auspices. I am greatly indebted to my wife, Lysa Virginia Travis, who has compiled the index of authors, edited all of the bibliographies and made them conform to the system of citation used by the *Psychological Abstracts,* and cut, typed, and pasted manuscript. May I take this opportunity to reveal my gratefulness to Chancellor Rufus Bernhard von Kleinsmid, Vice-President Albert Sydney Raubenheimer, and Professor Milton Metfessel for the privilege of serving at the University of Southern California.

If this work helps to disseminate existing knowledge of speech, hearing, and voice disorders, to foster a cross-disciplinary approach in the several related fields of medicine, speech, psychology, and education, and to inspire young clinicians, scholars, and teachers to more creative effort, the authors and editor will have been amply rewarded.

LEE EDWARD TRAVIS

*University of Southern California*

# CONTENTS

## Part III

### SPEECH AND VOICE DISORDERS UNRELATED
### TO ORGANIC ABNORMALITIES

## Part IV

### PSYCHOTHERAPY AND SPEECH THERAPY

# PART I

# Basic Considerations in
# Speech Pathology

# CHAPTER I

# THE DEVELOPMENT OF SPEECH

● *Clarence T. Simon, Ph.D., Sc.D.*

IN THIS MODERN WORLD, some two and a half billion people pour out words in astronomical numbers. Daily they talk to each other in person and, in certain areas of the world, over the telephone, on radio and television. Uncounted trillions of additional words are used in the covert processes of remembering, thinking, and imagining. Civilization and culture, business and commerce, as well as the infinite complexity of personal relationships, all depend on speech.

This prodigious verbal output is characteristically and distinctively human; a unique form of behavior apparently limited to *Homo sapiens*. Although many animals can and do make distinctive noises and convey literal and limited messages, they cannot master the symbolizations and abstractions involved in speech. A pet dog can bark his thanks for the luscious bone, but he cannot discuss dietary problems with other dogs nor advocate Pure Food and Drug laws. A monkey will recognize some hunger satisfaction if he eats two bananas; he will try to get two more and feel greater satisfaction if he gets and eats them. But he cannot know that two plus two equals four, nor can he invoke the aid of mathematical or verbal symbols.

## Definition of Speech

In any study of the phenomenon of speech, certain basic and critical questions demand immediate attention. Specifically, what *is* speech? On what basis is it characterized as a distinctly human behavior? If other animal forms do not possess this accomplishment, where is the dividing line? Of even more importance to studies of learning: Does speech differ from other forms of man's activity? How? From one view, speech is the audible product of muscle action, involving primarily the smaller muscles, and is used, in certain situations, as a substitute for acts of other types. In many instances this substitution seems to accomplish the same sort of results that would be achieved by action of the larger muscles, but more easily and expeditiously. Outside of the size of the muscles and the amplitude of the movements, however, what distinguishes speech from, for example, locomotive and manipulatory patterns? *How* does speech differ from other forms of man's behavior?

In view of these questions, an over-all and not too technical preliminary

3

definition describes *speech,* in its noun form, as an established communicative system of *arbitrary* and *conventionalized* acoustic *symbols,* produced mainly by action of the muscles of the respiratory and upper alimentary tracts.[1] In its verb form, the term implies *communicative* behavior through the use of these conventionalized and arbitrary symbols. Speech thus indicates either a system of abstractions with their appropriate symbols or, as a verb, the use of such system as a substitute for other types of behavior.

### Speech Employs Arbitrary, Self-Initiated Symbols

Inherent in this preliminary definition are several concepts which need to be spelled out in more detail. While the "words" which form the basis of this communicative activity are symbols or signs that conveniently substitute for the objects they represent, this representative role alone does not distinguish words from other stimuli which the organism may produce, or to which it may respond. Over and beyond this substitute and representative status, these words have an *arbitrary* significance; they mean only what the group employing them has learned that they mean. Whether names for objects, actions, or concepts, the "words" may bear little or no literal resemblance to the "things" they represent. This arbitrary and self-initiated symbolism, essential to speech, distinguishes oral communication from other forms of human behavior as well as indicating its restriction to the human level.

To illustrate this distinctive characteristic of speech, use may be made of the three kinds of symbolic, or substitute, behavior listed by Deese (1952). According to this author, the most primitive symbolic behavior, exemplified by the Pavlovian conditioned response, is *simple learned behavior* which serves to lead the animal from place to place. Seemingly this exists throughout the animal scale, for Paramecium and Amoeba have been taught to turn around at an obstruction instead of following their tropistic pattern of backing away at an angle (Day and Bentley, 1911; Mast and Pusch, 1924). A second type of symbolic behavior, appearing in higher animals, consists of a *representational* type of response to cues that are not directly in the environment. Though to the observer the animal may appear to be responding in the absence of cues, this actually is not the case; the cues either exist within the organism itself or are mediated by those that the organism has learned. This type of symbolic response serves to bridge a gap in external stimulation and enables at least the higher animals to "remember," and so respond appropriately even after external stimulation has been removed. In his original studies of the "delayed-reaction test," Hunter (1912) found that rats could delay about 10 seconds, dogs about 5 minutes, while young children could delay almost 30 minutes. Later studies (Harlow, 1932) demonstrated that apes could delay longer than monkeys, but that subnormal human adults (mental age about two years) did only about as well as the apes.

---

[1] For simplicity, this definition neglects the support and amplification of meaning frequently supplied by accompanying nonacoustic gestures. It also omits reference to recorded or otherwise preserved sounds.

Thus, the *simple learning* and *representational* types of symbolic behavior are subhuman as well as human accomplishments. The third form of symbolic behavior, however, consists of the use of learned and self-initiated cues, that is, of "language." So far as is known at present, this third function, the *linguistic,* which enables the organism to manipulate his environment symbolically, is limited to human beings. Double-alternation problems, for instance, are grasped in a few seconds by an adult using verbal symbols, but in contrast are solved by rats only with great difficulty (Hunter and Hull, 1941) and by monkeys only after prolonged training (Gellerman, 1931a). Similarly, children who can verbalize learn this type of problem quite easily, though preverbal children find it quite difficult (Gellerman, 1931b; Hunter and Bartlett, 1948). Successful solution of double alternation problems thus seems to depend on self-initiated symbolic processes, as distinct from cues from the environment or from previous conditioning.

This third type of symbolic behavior, as distinct from simple learned and representational behaviors, characterizes human speech. Employing arbitrary and self-initiated symbols, human speech goes beyond the instinctive outcries and reaction-getting noises of the animals to highly symbolic processes. Speech thus is not only distinctively human but is also set apart from other forms of human behavior.

### Speech Is a "Novel Response"

Included also in the general definition given above is the concept that speech is a *novel* response, a new form of behavior. While the process of speech may occasion an "usurpation of biological mechanisms," it is not a mere compounding of previously existing biological patterns. Neither does speech represent a simple linking of movements or connecting of sounds already in the repertoire of the organism. Although both the higher animals and the preverbal child produce a wide range of vocal sounds, human speech involves more than an accidental, or even intentional, use of sounds already in reflexive use. Whether we think of speech as developed by primitive man or learned by the child, it is more than a linking of previous reflexes or earlier sounds and apparently is not reached solely through the greater complexity of neuromotor equipment. In both the race and the child, speech represents a *novelty,* a "jump" to a symbolic process employing arbitrary and conventionalized cues. It goes beyond the conditioned and representational behavior of the animals, and beyond mere learned response and memory for the human being. Speech is a cultural acquisition rather than a natural function or reflexive motor response.

### Speech Is a Social Phenomenon

For a complete description of this complicated but exceedingly common behavior, mention should be made also of the social nature of speech. The child learns speech in a social situation and fails to learn it in the absence of that environment. Similarly, evidence seems to indicate that primitive man developed his symbolic communication within the framework of his inter-personal relations. Additional emphasis is supplied to this social aspect by Allport's (1924) descriptive term, *circular reaction* and Pronko's (1946) characterization as "bi-stimulational and referential." Speech is both inter-personal and communicative.[2]

In its technical sense, therefore, speech as a form of human behavior in-dicates the use, in interpersonal and bi-stimulational situations, of a socially established system of arbitrary and conventionalized acoustic symbols as a means of response to, or stimulation of, other individuals.

### Speech Is Unique in Nature and Time

Perhaps at the outset of this comprehensive volume—dealing with the deviations and disorders of the process of speech production and reception—the reader may well pause for a moment to consider the miracle of speech: the amazing fact that any of us can talk at all. The regrettable deficiencies and lacks in human speech, to be discussed later, may be seen in truer per-spective after some preliminary reflection on the uniqueness of the develop-ment, by the human race in its infancy, of this efficient substitution of small-muscle for big-muscle behavior.

Although man shares with many of the higher animals a primitive repertoire of vocal sounds and some ability to perform "novel" acts, as well as social organization, no animal has developed the process of symbolization, the "cognitive map," to go beyond the representational production of sounds to true speech. In fact, this great gap between man and even his nearest mammalian relatives—the apes—remains one of the great unsolved mys-teries of comparative psychology. Seemingly, the ape has all the vocal ap-paratus necessary for speech, and some chimpanzees have been able to make all the vowel and consonant sounds. Yet attempts to teach apes to speak have met with only limited success. Gua, the chimpanzee reared by the Kel-logs (1933) in company with an infant child, learned faster than the child to co-operate with her foster parents, to obey simple commands, and to an-ticipate her bowel and bladder needs. Regardless, however, of her maturity, which developed more rapidly than that of the child, speaking—the use of symbols to control others—was impossible. Another chimpanzee reared by human "parents" (K. J. and C. Hayes, 1950) profited from a long period of special training to the extent of seemingly using three words: *cup, mamma, papa*.[3] From his observations, Hayes (1950) thinks this lack of ability to talk is a kind of aphasia rather than a deficiency in intelligence; he believes

---

[2] Although speech most commonly involves a speaker, a hearer, and an object or event, the same symbols may be employed when two or all three of these are com-bined in one individual. With the communicative situation confined within the limits of one organism, however, the essential characteristic of symbolic manipulation of the environment may be absent. Under such circumstances the behavior of the speaker is more commonly and accurately described as thinking, imagining, arguing with him-self, or soliloquizing (Simon, 1951).

[3] Probably as representational rather than symbolic cues.

there is something missing from the nervous system. Whatever the reason for this gap between apes and man, it seemingly cannot be bridged by a favorable environment, by skillful training, or appropriate and constant stimulation. Speech behavior is unique in the animal world.

The extremely late arrival of speech ability in evolutionary history is another indication of its novelty and uniqueness. Sense organs and muscles as well as fairly complicated brains have existed for a long time. The first jointed larynx appeared something like 200 million years ago; true and false vocal bands and a well-developed cochlea have been in use some 55 million years. Speech, however, as a new note in the chorus of animal noises, appeared but yesterday.

A true perspective of the development of speech can be had only with an understanding of its recency in proportion to the infinite reaches of preceding earth-time. Estimates of the age of the earth vary, but recent studies of the ancient rocks indicate that these foundations were laid down not less than two billion nor more than five billion years ago, with the more common estimates varying from two and a half to three billion years.[4] But these rocks were far from ready for life. In fact, such evidence as exists, indicates that approximately half of all earth-time had passed before the appearance of the first living cell; the duration of the Azoic Era seeming at least equal to the total of all subsequent eras. Yet, even though life probably began this billion years ago, change and development were unhurried, and half of this great span carried the complexity of living structures only to the level of the sponges and mollusks (Colton, 1952; Barnett, 1952).

Figures of this magnitude, however, have little tangibility. Perhaps we can sense a bit more clearly the position of man in the diary of the world and its life with a momentary speculative interlude. Suppose we imaginatively start a tiny organism, a blob of peripatetic protoplasm, from San Francisco when life began, to arrive in Chicago today. At this rate, approximately 2,000 miles to represent one billion years, the evolution of the algae and one-celled plants would have found this indestructible traveler about 800 miles from his starting point and in the vicinity of Salt Lake City. Had he kept to his timetable, he would have reached Denver with the advent of hard body parts and the establishment of the major invertebrate forms; the Nebraska border with the first vertebrates—the fish; the middle of that state with the lung fish; and Omaha with the rib-breathing, mammal-like Cynognathus with the first larynx. He would have met the arboreal insectivores (forerunners of the primates)—with their lungs, diaphragm, true and false vocal bands, and well-developed ear—in the hills of Iowa City. Crossing the Mississippi into

[4] Three methods have been used to determine geologic time: chemical analysis of the relative amounts of radioactive materials and lead in the rocks, measurement of the amount of salt in the sea, and studies of stellar combustion. These methods indicate a beginning of the earth not more than four or five billion years ago, nor less than two billion. As judged on the basis of their radioactivity, the oldest rocks yet found seem to be about two and one-half billion years old. If this estimate be correct, it indicates that at least a portion of the earth's crust had solidified by that time.

Illinois would have occurred with the descent of the short-jawed apes from the trees and the beginning of the upright position. *Australopithecus africanus,* an ape man with a somewhat arched forehead and expanded cranium, would have existed well in the western part of the state. About two miles from the end of his journey, this meandering microorganism would have greeted *Pithecanthropus erectus*—probably the earliest known man and the first "talker." The final arrival of "Modern Man," Cro-Magnon, would have left only 500 feet of this supposititious safari to complete by today. Man and his unique and characteristic speech are indeed evolutionary "Johnny come-latelys."

This late arriving, "novel" human behavior, providing for response to and manipulation of the environment through small-muscle activity has given man a tool for knowing, and perhaps ultimately understanding, his world and himself.

## DEVELOPMENT OF SPEECH IN THE RACE

Statements of man's inquiries and speculations concerning the development of his own speech and language are almost as old as written language itself. Beginning with the religious theories—that man acquired speech through divine revelation—first stated in holy writings and continued by theologians and philosophers, many "theories" of the origin of speech have appeared successively in the writings of philosophers, psychologists, and linguists. The literature containing these observations and surmises concerning the origin of language is a voluminous one indeed; the extensive citations and references of such writers as Max Müller (1863 and 1865), Jespersen (1922), Gray and Wise (1946), and Stein (1949) constitute only a representative sample. Confusion and controversy have so marked the language used to "explain" the origin of speech and language that in 1866 the Société de Linguistique of Paris passed a resolution forbidding any further discussion of the subject, apparently believing it unsolvable. In 1930 Paget offered two apologies in his Preface for the publication of his extensive work, and succeeding authors have bemoaned the lack of knowledge and the welter of speculations. As Miller (1951, p. 1) comments, "In some respects the scientific study of communication resembles the task of soaring off the ground with a tug at your own bootstraps." Nevertheless, the relatively recent accumulations of geological, anthropological, and psychological knowledge would seem to warrant yet another listing of the "knows" and "don't knows" of the origin of speech. While there is much that we do not know, and may never know, the painstaking investigations of the recent years have given us many valuable clues.

### Obstacles to Precise Knowledge

Speech, practically alone of all man's activities, has left no record of its origin and development. Ashes of camp fires, abandoned tools and utensils may remain for a future finder. The earliest drawings and writings, valuable as they are for man's history, indicate only that complex symbolic processes already were developed and that the "beginning" of speech had long since passed. Any knowledge concerning the origin of speech, therefore, must be inferred from the structure of primitive men and the records of the lives they lived. There are, however, wide gaps in the basic archeological and anthropological data which depend on remaining and *discoverable* bones, tools, and other evidences of man's nature and activities. Many great areas of the world have not been explored adequately; in few have geological conditions been right for the preservation of the remains of the past; only ideal conditions can hold bones and relics for thousands of years. There is no way of knowing how many, or how ancient, specimens have been destroyed by weathering or buried beyond discovery, washed away by floods or pulverized by glaciers. It may be that the few early bones so far discovered indicate the relative abundance of man rather than his first appearance.

Had time and climate alone, however, been the only destructive factors, more information might be available; certainly the data would be more orderly. Unfortunately for the modern anthropologist, the first known human forms appeared early in the Pleistocene Era, practically simultaneously with the first of the four periods of glaciation marking the Ice Age. Four times great ice sheets moved down over the land, plowing, mixing, breaking, and crushing. The scratches and gouges, as well as the crevasses and moraines left by the retreating ice caps, indicate the probable destruction, displacement, and mixing of various strata and deposits. While the earliest bones of man have been found in the geological deposits of the Pleistocene Era, flints indicating "human" craftsmanship have appeared in the earlier Pliocene. Though the earliest evidences of men seem all about the same age, they come from the far corners of the Old World. Moreover, in China have been found the bones of men and the tools they made, but in Java only the bones; Europe and Africa have yielded only the tools (Braidwood, 1948).

The fluctuating levels of the waters of the earth with the alternate freezing and thawing of the Ice Ages may well be another barrier to our knowledge of ancient human life. With great amounts of water held in the glaciers, the level of all oceans, lakes, and rivers was lowered. There were times in the Ice Age when the whole North Sea was drained of water, England was a part of the mainland, the Rhine River drained the Thames, and land bridges probably divided the Mediterranean. Remains of early man, living where water was available, along the sea coast and on the banks and deltas of great rivers, may long ago have been covered with silt or by the rising waters of the melting glaciers.[5]

Another obstacle to anything like precise dating is interposed by the prob-

[5] The last ice advance ended about 20,000 years ago—a period equaling about half the former interglacial periods. Although approximately half of the ice formed in the last glaciation still remains in Greenland, Antarctica, and scattered glaciers, ocean levels are now some 200 feet higher than at earlier times.

able nature of the developmental process itself. Modern knowledge of the development of complex behaviors would indicate that speech was an evolution rather than a spontaneous or even short-time creation. Certain it is that no prodigy suddenly sat up and said, "Let's talk!" Nor did speech come suddenly because "ideas" needed expressing, for speech symbols are the fabric of ideas. In all probability, primitive man laughed, danced, gestured, sang, and used vocal calls and yells for a long time before he produced *speech* sounds. The transition from the merely representative use of preverbal sounds to the arbitrary symbols of speech may well have been most gradual. Thus, even if we had more extensive knowledge of primitive man and his ways, and some means of recapturing the noises and sounds of a million years ago, it still would be impossible to pinpoint the "beginning of speech."

### Estimated Time of Speech Development

In spite of this limited knowledge of primitive man and his ways, however, there are certain cues or signs in his bones and relics which provide a basis for inference concerning man's developing ability to use the substitute symbols on which speech depends. Knowledge of his posture, physical structure, and skill in tool-making offers more than a mere guess.

**Bases of estimates.** This chattering, featherless, furless, mammalian biped —*Homo sapiens*—physically has much in common with the higher vertebrates, many of his structures being modifications of those which appeared much earlier in the evolutionary scale. He is set apart, however, by the nature and extent of these modifications. He is distinct not only in his posture but also in the development of some of his receptors and effectors—particularly the organs for locomotion and manipulation. The development of the small muscles of the hand and head with their complex innervation and, most marked, the growth of the brain are a unique dimension in the evolution of animal life.

About the middle of the Cenozoic Period, thirty to forty million years ago, most students believe that the primate stock of the vertebrates split in two. One division kept to its home in the trees and evolved into monkeys and apes. The other kept more and more to the ground and evolved into man. With more than figurative meaning, this "descent from the trees" may be regarded as the first start toward speech development—still forty millennia in the future. With increasing terrestrial living and the upright position, and development of new neuromotor mechanisms for equilibrium, the locomotive functions shifted increasingly to the legs and feet, thus freeing the fore paw from responsibility for partial support of body weight and for maintenance of position. Subsequent eons of increasing use of this emancipated member for exploratory and manipulative activities probably encouraged the change from the clumsy paw of the ape to a flexible hand, noticeably different in shape and structure. The thumb of the ape is small and, for the most part, a passive member of the hand; the human thumb is larger and capable of active movement in opposition to the hand as a whole and to each of the fingers separately. Marked as was this growth toward a novel "tool," however, it did not occur alone, but was accompanied by corresponding changes in the afferent and efferent neurons and particularly in the sensory and motor areas of the cerebral cortex. Both hand and brain assumed new complexity and functional adaptability (Hooton, 1931, 1942; Weidenreich, 1946).

During this same period, with the upright posture and development of manual dexterity came freedom of the mouth from crude grasping and manipulative duties. As a result, structures of the throat and mouth were free to evolve into specialized organs, able later to subserve the speech process. Such variations as increased intricacy and flexibility of the larynx, shortening and widening of the tongue, and increased flexibility of the lips were associated with the more obvious changes which have been preserved in bone and from which the record may now be read; widening and shortening of the mandible, gradual appearance of the chin, and a developing brow to elevate the facial plane from its apish slant.[6]

At least as marked as any other change was that of the size and shape of the cranium—evidence of the increasing volume and complexity of the brain, particularly of the cerebrum. The slow cerebral growth shown by the lower animals accelerated with the mammals. In the lower primates the greatest increases occurred in the visual and motor areas, probably concurrently with increasing use of the fore paw as a grasping and manipulative tool. With the first known human, however, there is evidence of a marked development of undifferentiated cerebral cells free from routine sensory, motor, and physiological activities. Although the brain of this early human was inferior to that of modern man, it was distinctly larger than that of any known ape.[7] More significantly, it was not merely an enlarged ape's brain; its pattern must be classed as human (Tinley, 1928, 1930; Keith, 1915). The frontal lobes, associated with the higher mental processes, were enlarged, and there is evidence of a rudimentary motor speech center—Broca's area (Davison, 1934; Childe, 1936, 1944).

These changed structures—a skeleton adapted to erect posture, enlarged thumb, shortened and widened mandible, expanded and heightened cranial vault—are fossil evidence of a physical mechanism seemingly adequate to serve for at least primitive speech. Yet physical structures alone give little more than evidence of equipment that *might* have been used to produce speech. Evidence of the actual *use* must come from indications of the ability to use symbols over and beyond the conditioned responses and memory of

[6] Other changes in ear, palate, muscles of mastication, for example, related to the establishment of a speech-adequate mechanism, accompanied these more obvious changes (Negus, 1929; Hooton, 1931, 1942; Carhart, 1938).

[7] An estimated cranial capacity of 55–73 cubic inches for *Sinanthropus*, for example, is a marked increase over the anthropoid capacity of 24–37 cubic inches, but still short of the 79–98 cubic inches of modern man (De Pradenne, 1940, p. 192). Kroeber gives the following as maximum capacities in cubic centimeters: gorilla, 585–655; *Pithecanthropus*, 775–935; *Sinanthropus*, 915–1225; *Cro-Magnon*, 1500–1880 (1948, p. 122).

the animal intelligence. A monkey can throw a handy coconut or use a convenient stick, but the preparation of a "tool"—even of the crudest sort—implies an independence of merely representational cues through the use of self-initiated symbols.

**Estimated timetable.** The earliest beginnings of the structural developments leading ultimately to a "speech mechanism" appear with the short-jawed apes, of the Pliocene Epoch, perhaps seven million years ago. These earliest terrestrial bipeds that had descended from the trees and were experimenting with the upright position were developing somewhat larger brains. Still later in this Pliocene Epoch, *Australopithecus africanus* made small but definite advances toward human form. The fighting teeth of earlier forms were changed to those of more human type. Though the cranium was but half the size of modern man's, the significant change in the ratio between head and body sizes was under way. In addition, the skull had lost the bisecting anthropoidal ridge and begun the arching of the forehead. These were early and slight changes, however, and provide no suggestion of the ability to use acoustic communication beyond the animal level (Clark, 1934).

The earliest human forms so far discovered, archeologists believe, are indicated by two separate deposits of fossilized bones. Though widely separated geographically, these men are judged to have been approximately contemporaneous in the early Pleistocene Epoch, a million years ago, or slightly less. *Pithecanthropus erectus,* commonly known as "Java man" because of the location of his remains, was discovered by Dr. Eugene Dubois in 1891, twenty years after the publication of Darwin's *Descent of Man.* No objects definitely identifiable as tools have been discovered, nor any indications of the use of fire, in the gravels containing the bones. Tools and evidences of fire, however, have been found with the remains of *Sinanthropus pekinensis* ("Peking man") at Chou Kou Tien in 1929 (Smith, 1932). These bones were not deposited by running water in river gravels but were left by their owners on the floor of a limestone cave, making both age and the manner of life more certain. Peking man used not only fire, but also tools of sandstone and quartz, and sometimes of a poor quality flint. There are also many split pieces of heavy bone (which may have been split for the marrow or perhaps to use as tools), and each one of the skulls had the base broken out of it. Splitting bones lengthwise and carefully removing the base of a skull require tools, and people to make and use them (Braidwood, 1948). Both fire and tools, the relics of Peking man, give evidence of at least primitive cause-to-effect reasoning through the use of symbols.[8]

The bones of these men, indicating usable speech structures and probably just adequate brains, combine with the evidences of symbolic manipulation of the environment to warrant the inference that these primitive men of the Pleistocene Epoch used speech in the human sense (Childe, 1942; Kerr, 1926; Smith, 1932).

[8] The geological deposits of this same epoch, the Pleistocene, have yielded the tools made by as yet unknown men in Africa and Southern Europe.

Even with this naming and approximate dating of some probable "first talkers," anything like a complete and detailed timetable still is impossible. There is some evidence that speech may have developed in several parts of the world, perhaps at different times and rates of accleration.[9] Additional uncertainties rise from subsequent mixings of types of men and their various symbolic codes. The changes in climate, rainfall, lake and river levels, and shifts in plant and animal life occasioned by the four great glaciers, with the intervening long periods of warm weather, would be ample reason for many variations in both form and rate of speech development as a confusing prelude to the startling total of some 1500 languages in the world today.

Even a sketchy timetable, however, should include a few of the better-known examples of early man to indicate the general rate of development. Some improvement in speech equipment was shown by Heidelberg man, presumed to have lived during the second interglacial period, approximately 500,000 years ago. His brain, while smaller than modern man's, was similar in construction and superior to that of his predecessors. One of the better-known forms, and the first human fossil to be recognized as such, Neander-thal man, dates from the third interglacial period, 100,000 to 150,000 years ago. At least a dozen examples have been found, many of them in caves, with consequently more-adequate knowledge concerning their lives and the tools they made. Neanderthal man had greatly improved equipment for speech. His total brain volume, for instance, was about 1500 cc, as contrasted with the 940 cc achieved by the earlier Java man. His mode of living and his manufacture and use of more and better tools show his behavioral gain from his cerebral enlargement in the temporal areas and particularly in the frontal and other association areas.

The slow changes in structure and behavior, sparsely indicated in this sketchy timetable, reached the modern level no more than 50,000 years ago. Far superior to all known forerunners, Cro-Magnon man was similar to modern man in appearance and ability, though somewhat larger in both body and head; and all relics of his mode of living indicate considerable use of his fully developed speech mechanism. These first truly "modern" men reached a relatively high level of cultural development and left behind them carvings, tools, and paintings showing imagination and skill.

Anthropologists believe that these men, carrying their culture and, we would assume, their speech, spread from Asia or Africa to Europe to popu-late and dominate at least the southern portions of that continent. Their descendants likewise reached the American continent by a land bridge be-tween Asia and Alaska, eighteen to twenty thousand years ago, and from Alaska spread out through both North and South America.

Aided by their speech, these modern men and their descendants were able to recognize and utilize the minerals found in the rocks and to replace their

[9] This also happened with the development of tools, and later, with village cultures, food producing, and writing. Weidenreich (1946) believes the ancestors of man were spread out over Europe, Africa, and Asia.

bone and stone tools and weapons with superior implements of copper, bronze, and finally iron, to extend their adaptation to, and control over, their environment.

The use of speech symbols to recall the past and plan for the future likewise fostered the first basic change in human economy, the "food-producing revolution" (Childe, 1942). For nearly a million years man had spent his life following animals to kill and eat, or moving from one berry patch to another; himself living much like an animal. Around 7000 B.C. in the Near East, and somewhat later in other parts of the world, however, he began his first attempts at planned agriculture and animal husbandry. As he learned to plant grain and to raise and herd certain animals, man's living sites became relatively permanent, with the larger and more stable communities forming a basis for a broadening social organization. Partially freed from the hunt by storing food in granaries and "on the hoof," time was available for attention to the arts and crafts, invention, and to tales and ballads of tribal lore. This "talking animal" established the beginnings of civilized cultures.

Under the stimulation of wider interpersonal contacts and with the increased time for stories, ballads, and deliberations, speech undoubtedly received vastly increased developmental impetus. In any event, from this revolution to the bards of 5000 B.C. and the appearance of written language about 4000 B.C.[10] are but short steps in the million-year journey from primitive speech to the number and complexity of modern languages and the media of mass communications (Childe, 1925, 1942; Kroeber, 1948; Herskovits, 1948).

### Estimated Pattern of Speech Development

Difficult as it is to say "when' speech began, the "how" is no more obvious. Not that the world's literatures lack "theories," but so many of them are speculative constructs offering partial and frequently conflicting views. Many, influenced by earlier current psychologies, stress the part for the whole, or emphasize "purpose" or "intent,"[11] or else slip into the "fallacy of the single cause."

**"Theories" of development.** The earliest theories, stated mainly by theologians and philosophers, tended to suggest divine or other supernatural origins, or to depend on such anthropomorphic causes as "forces," "powers," or "faculties." The invention theories of the *Empiricists*—that language was invented by individuals—directly opposed the belief of the Nativists that language was innate with an always-existent correlation between objects and images as one part, and sounds as the other.

The nineteenth century, however, brought considerable change in the

---

10 This date refers to Egyptian letter signs; their hieroglyphics appeared approximately a thousand years earlier.

11 Psychology is moving away from the concept of "elements of behavior" as earlier it abandoned the idea of elements of sensation. With the scientific approach, moreover, the use of purpose or intent as an explanatory principle practically has disappeared.

subsequent formulations. Influenced by the growth of linguistic research and increasing interest in the social studies, more attention was given to the structure of language and its social use as possible causative elements. A limited but suggestive list of typical statements might well include such formulations as the Social Pressure Theory outlined by Adam Smith (1792), the Scottish political economist, based on the previous work of the philosopher John Locke; the briefly held Theory of Roots offered by Bopp (1816) and restated by Müller (1863), the "roots" being neither mere imitations nor interjections but "phonetic types"; and the statements by Geiger (1869), who traced the origin of language to the instinct of imitation. Greater linguistic attention to the individual "words" of language brought other writers to a belief in the "onomatopoetic" source of the words (von Herder, 1772; Key, 1874; Comrie, 1876; Lefèvre, 1894). Other scholars, such as Condillac (1789), stressed "interjections" as the more likely source of language— a view accepted in part by Whitney (1868). Noiré, a philosopher rather than a philologist, stressed the importance of the interjections made by a group of men engaged in a common task to suggest the Work Theory (1877).

These theories were accepted fully by few writers, though each statement had its proponents as at least a partial explanation. Seemingly, the majority of the scholars of that day combined two or more of the suggested origins, or saw each as accounting for some of the words of language. Whitney (1868), for example, and Farrar (1873) combined the onomatopoetic and the interjectional, whereas Sayce, like others, believed "The origin of language, then, is to be sought in *gestures, onomatopoeia,* and to a limited extent *interjectional* cries" (1883, I, p. 110).

Later statements, such as Wundt's Gesture Theory (1897), the Vocal Play Theory by Jespersen (1922), and the Social Control Theory (de Laguna, 1927), reflect the growing store of psychological and anthropological, linguistic and phonetic knowledge. One of the more elaborately documented statements was Paget's Oral Gesture Theory (1930), which was a continuation and development of Wundt's Gesture Theory to include a detailed explanation of the nature of the transition from bodily gestures to oral language.[12]

No less fragmentary, unfortunately, are the more recent views involving Emergence or Reflex theories. Assumed to be supported by the "usurpation" of mechanisms already functioning for biological purposes, these concepts see speech as dependent on, or "caused by," the extensive development of the cerebral cortex and its accompanying complex system. Usually phrased in neurological or physiological terms, these concepts regard speech as a sort of by-product of the brain—the expanded cortex leading to a compounding or linking of previously existing sound-producing neuromotor

---

[12] While the general nature and implications of these theories are suggested by the titles, the interested student will find extensive descriptions of these and many others, with comments and criticisms, in Whitney (1868), Sayce (1883), Sapir (1921), Stein (1949).

patterns; in other words, an adding together of sounds already in reflexive use.

These theories of the origin of speech in the race are true "theories" in the sense that they represent efforts to construct, speculatively, all-inclusive explanations which ignore the gaps in knowledge and, occasionally, the existence of conflicting evidence. Nevertheless, the stated results of this scientifically necessary procedure of theorizing do point out the vast amount of research that has been done. Even more important, perhaps, the student of speech disorders receives an indication of the store of knowledge gained by the sciences dealing with speech and language.

**Descriptive view of speech development.** Scientific knowledge of man and his learning process has grown rapidly in recent years, resulting in at least two marked changes in the attempts to reconstruct a probable pattern of speech development. In the first place, as in other scientific areas, students of language are making ever greater use of descriptive explanations based on observation. Thus the earlier tendency to seek one developmental condition or influence, one "cause," has lessened in favor of the newer view of speech as part of the larger whole of human growth and development. In consequence, the second change has been the disappearance of the view that speech development needed a separate learning process or a special "kind" of learning.

Although speech *is* a "novel" act and more than a chain of reflexes, its development seems part of general human learning, innovation and adaptation. Numerous studies indicate that both men and animals learn "novel" acts, responses not already in their repertoire. Skinner (1938, pp. 339–340), for example, taught a rat to "buy" food by pulling a string to get a marble, carrying this in its fore paws to a tube projecting above the floor, and lifting and dropping the marble down the tube. As the investigator comments, "Every step in the process had to be worked out through a series of approximations, since the component responses were not in the original repertoire of the rat." On the human level, many manual skills, including the acts involved in writing, are novel (Munn, p. 190). There is no need, therefore, to seek a special variety of learning to account for the development of speech.

Over a period of half to three-quarters of a million years, man's hand tools progressed from crude "choppers" to "flakes" and to "blades." Inventive tool makers changed both the materials used and their workmanship, seemingly guided by available stones, the remembered results of experience, and also by some measure of cause-to-effect reasoning and advance planning through the use of self-initiated cues. Thus, the interaction between man and his environment led not only to "novel" skills but also to a definite selection of more appropriate and efficient techniques within the "topographical map" of tool-making and using.

Within this same pattern of learning, speech apparently developed slowly from crude beginnings, with the selection and adoption of appropriate symbols accomplished in the total experience of living. Certainly the efficient combination of larynx and ear, which seems so "natural" today, was not the only possibility. Several other sensory-motor mechanisms, which likely aided man's primitive communicative efforts and are now in use by some animals, might have been usurped to serve the function of human language, except for certain distinct disadvantages of each.

A language of touch, for instance, survives now in lobsters and some insects; gestural communication is used by lower forms,[13] and remains of use to man in spite of his high development of oral language. Odors both inform and signal in the animal world; human odors seem to vary with changing emotional states, as is sometimes noticeable even by dulled human olfactory organs.

The general noise-making, common to nearly all vertebrates, however, provided a basis for communicative efficiency seemingly not obtainable otherwise. Useful in darkness, unobstructed by barriers, variable in intensity for distance, and with no need for physical proximity between the communicants, sound waves carried stimuli and responses under the widest range of natural conditions, as well as serving to transmit information, orders, and ideas while the eyes and hands were occupied watching for danger, or working, fighting, or making love.

Thus the process of communication, developing under the conditions pertaining then, came to depend increasingly on the larynx and ear, with the resultant determination not only of the nature of language but also of later inventions, cultural achievements, and social processes. It is interesting to speculate concerning the form of this book in a language of touch, or the telephone with a language of odors. Because communication by means of sound waves was most useful, we now have radios instead of kineos and teletactors, use audio-visual instead of odio-visual aids in the classroom, and relax at the sound-tracked cinema rather than at the feelies or smellies.

**Motivation or "cause" of speech-learning.** From this descriptive view, in harmony with present biological and psychological knowledge, the development of speech in the race is best understood as "learning" occurring within a total configuration involving an internal energy system and an external energy field—each as a part of a whole. The "cause" or motivation, descriptively rather than speculatively considered, lies in the instability and irritability of living tissue and the biological mechanisms for the maintenance of homeostasis. To say that speech-learning occurred through the dynamics of living tissue explains it just as much—and no more—as applying the terms *release of tension* or *restoration of homeostasis* to the reproductive fission of the Amoeba or the locomotive behavior of the Paramecium.

Throughout evolutionary history, receptors, effectors, and connecting neural tissue have developed together. A hand does not become an instrument of manipulation without a brain and an eye to guide it, nor does a

[13] Von Frisch has shown that bees can communicate such things as location and distance of a food supply by an elaborate series of movements (1950), and Thorpe (1950) takes it almost as established fact that this ability must be learned.

brain develop with static receptors and effectors. Changing function and structure are characteristic of living organisms, with the speed of change seemingly accelerated with the complexity of the forms involved and the degree of disturbance of homeostasis.

It is not beyond the bounds of probability that apes, with their ability to climb as well as run, were better adapted to life and food-getting than was man, and hence had less homeostatic need to develop better terrestrial locomotion, a tool-using hand, a bigger brain and symbolic noise-making. Primitive man's "disturbances of homeostasis" may well have been frequent and marked in view of his vulnerability to larger animals and the forces of nature. Certainly his state was not a comfortable or happy one, particularly during the periods of food shortages probably occurring with the cooling of the tropical and subtropical climates in front of the ice sheets. Hungry or not, however, man developed his hand, and brain, and speech, and did not relearn to swing through the trees for "the more abundant life."

These adaptive changes constituting speech development were facilitated and accelerated by man's expanding brain. Most of the more recent accounts of the origin of speech stress the role of the cerebrum in man's symbolic processes, the necessary arbitrary and self-initiated cues being attainable only with a size and complexity above that of other mammals. From this descriptive view, however, the cerebral cortex assumes an additional and important influence through the inhibitory power of these higher nerve centers. This cortically mediated ability to inhibit impulses and reflexes and to delay immediate and habitual responses brought the beginnings of conscious control and discriminative action. Man, thus freed from the dominance of inherited and stereotyped behaviors, was able to develop symbolic meanings in addition to representative learning, and to vary his responses adaptively through problem-solving by the use of self-initiated cues. This same discriminative action offers a most likely means by which the symbolic and cognitive meanings characteristic of speech were added to the purely emotional and literal meanings of noises. Thus the inhibitory powers of the cortex, as much as its "associative" functions may well have been of service in the substitution of symbolic for literal and representative vocalizations.

**Types of learning.** Learning commonly is defined, on a descriptive or operational basis, as a change in the behavior and perception of an organism as a consequence of its experience, that is, as such change not due to maturation alone. Since speech is a "novel" act, however, there may be some question whether primitive language-learning was identical with the learning exhibited by the present-day human adult, or indeed with language-learning by the modern child. Speech-acquiring *Pithecanthropus* had to learn "what means what"—a significance—rather than neuromotor responses; meanings rather than a chain of habits. Hence, the acquisition of language by primitive man likely resembled more the learning now exhibited by the higher animals and by human children prior to their mastery of language.

Although the transition from learning that is nonverbal to that which uses words has been but slightly explored, there are some studies which suggest very real differences between these areas. For example, Kuenne's study (1946) in transposition (the ability to respond to the relational properties of stimuli rather than to their absolute values) found that children who were too young to have highly developed verbal skills performed much as do animals in this discriminative situation, and hence were unable to master "far-transposition" problems. Older children, however, found these problems quite easy because they spontaneously verbalized the principle necessary to the solution. As another instance, the double-alternation problem of Hunter and Bartlett (1948)[14] can be solved by intelligent animals only after prolonged practice, and preverbal children find it extremely difficult. Older children who can verbalize, however, solve it quite easily.

Seemingly, therefore, the nonverbal or preverbal and the verbal constitute different areas, with the transition from one to the other representing a critical period in the history of the individual or the race. To the extent that this distinction is real, and first speech development corresponds more closely to the preverbal type of learning, some caution should be exercised in attempting to describe primitive language acquisition as analogous to speech development by the modern child. Certainly there is no reason for the student of speech to depend overmuch on the results of the problems involving the use of verbal ability with which modern studies of human learning are so heavily loaded.

Fortunately, however, the experimental work, using higher vertebrates as well as human children on the preverbal level, has been sufficient to warrant the supposition that the *how* of speech learning by primitive man was similar to the preverbal learning exhibited in today's laboratories.

Although students of learning agree reasonably well on a definition of learning as a change in perception and performance not due to maturation, the statements concerning the how or nature of this learning are varied and contradictory. As Miller (1951, p. 160) comments: "It is as difficult for psychologists to agree about learning as it is for a group of theologians to agree on a definition of sin." Actually, at least ten theories of major importance have been stated (Hilgard, 1956) and each of these has been varied and modified by various supporters. For the purpose of this study, however, these formulations may be grouped into two broad categories with little, if any, warping of individual views: "Effect Theory," frequently called Association Theory, and Contiguity Theory or Field Theory.

The older of these views, Effect Theory, says in essence that responses are learned or fixated because of their "effects" or "consequences." This principle, historically related to Darwin's theory of natural selection, carries two centuries of philosophical and psychological speculation. Basically ana-

[14] This type of problem requires the animal or child to learn a sequence of acts rather than a single performance. In the maze type, for example, the animal may be required to circle twice in one direction and then twice in the other before being rewarded.

lytic, it analyzes any behavior into its elements, and studies these elements independently to discover principles or laws governing the combinations of elements. First stated on an experimental basis by Thorndike in 1898, it has been outlined in many different ways, each an attempt to be more precise or more inclusive. In 1942 McGeoch, for example, divided the general principle into three statements to achieve clarity and accuracy. Two of these were purely descriptive or operational statements, but the third offered a reason *why* reinforcing stimuli are reinforcing: they satisfy a motive state. One of the most elaborate and comprehensive statements, made by Hull in 1943, points out that organisms can be regarded, in one sense, as bundles of needs —needs that arise from the continuously active processes of the body and from things and conditions in the environment. Since the function of behavior is to satisfy needs and bring the organism to a state of equilibrium, needs bring responses. Any response that reduces a need therefore is reinforced, with a resulting increased tendency for that response to occur again.

The more recent view, variously labeled as Contiguity or Field or Insight Theory, is essentially a protest against Association Theory. These theorists do not build the action pattern out of its component parts, for the parts have significance only in terms of the total configuration. This organismic view naturally brings a distinctly different concept concerning the nature and place of reinforcement in the learning process. To the theorists of this type, motivation and reward are important because they make responses occur, but that is all that is important about them. To Guthrie (1930, 1935), for example, nothing is necessary to define reinforcement except that stimuli and movements occur together. His Stimulus-Response-Contiguity Theory (1935, p. 26) holds that "A combination of stimuli which has accompanied a movement will on recurrence tend to be followed by that movement."

Similarly, Tolman (1932) believes that the experimental animal learns the *significance* of the stimuli, and that its response is determined by this rather than by the stimuli as such. His Sign-Significate Theory indicates that the repeated contiguous association of stimuli and responses, as with a rat running a maze, is sufficient for acquisition of "what leads to what" and drive reduction is not necessary. Although Tolman denies the necessity for reinforcement for learning, he recognizes that some form of need gratification may be necessary for later utilization of the "cognitive map" which has been learned.

Experiments in latent learning, which provide the strongest support for nonreinforcement, indicate that animals acquire useful information which is not utilized in performance till an incentive is offered at a later time (Buxton, 1940). These data, however, are not accepted as satisfactory evidence that learning takes place without reinforcement of some kind. As Munn (1951, p. 191) comments, "It may well be that stronger or more obvious reinforcement is required for the learning of responses *per se* (as in conditioning experiments) than for the perceptual, incidental, or latent learning which Tolman stresses and which is so evident in human beings."

Whatever these experiments in latent learning may indicate concerning the need for reinforcement, they do support the belief that animals learn meanings as well as responses; learn a significance, "what means what," as well as specific neuromotor reactions to stimuli. Learning by nonverbal forms is not confined to conditioned responses.

Actually, there seems to be no crucial experimental evidence one way or the other, the theories leading to nearly the same predictions. Contiguity Theory predicts that animals will learn when they are rewarded, but for different reasons than those given by Effect Theory. On the other hand, Effect theorists have a ready answer when animals seem to learn when there is no apparent reward in the situation (Deese, 1952, p. 40). Regardless of how it happens, the rat learns to get the food either in Skinner's box with the bar (1938) or the latent-learning maze of Blodgett (1929). Animals learn to make conditioned responses and, equally, they acquire information, a meaning and significance, for later use. Learning on the nonverbal, as well as the verbal level, is a change in both perception and behavior.

**Speech developed as meaning; "What means what."** Obviously from the evidence so briefly suggested here, speech development by primitive man need not be regarded merely as "conditioning" with learning taking place only with immediate reward or reinforcement. With a neurological equipment superior to that of any animal, man was able to learn a meaning and significance, a "what means what"; was able to establish a symbolic vocal code whether rewarded at the time or not. The modern student of the development of speech, therefore, is freed from the necessity of searching for, or postulating, the immediate "causes" or rewarding conditions demanded by older learning theory. Moreover, contiguity theorists, with their interest in concepts and meanings rather than specific "words," have enabled us to view speech as a "novel" response rather than as a mechanical or fortuitous compounding of previously existing reflexes or biological behaviors. From the descriptive point of view, therefore, speech is seen as a "cognitive map," a symbolic significance. Like tool-making, fire-building, and other activities, speech was a means of maintenance of homeostasis in the interaction between the internal energy system and the external energy field.

This estimate of the development of speech in the race has been concerned with its beginning. To the modern child, learning to talk in an environment with an established language, Association or Effect theories of learning may apply, in part at least: "In order to respond correctly to a word it is necessary for another organism to intervene and reward us each time we respond correctly" (Miller, 1951, p. 5). There is slight indication, however, that this association type of learning can describe the "origin" of oral communication. In drawing inferences concerning the time and manner of the nonobservable "first use," therefore, the tenets of Field Theory and the concepts of learning embodied in Contiguity Theory have been illuminating.

**Later reinforcements: Rewards.** With the concept and use of self-initiated and symbolic cues started, however, it seems likely that learning of the conditioned-reflex and immediately-rewarded type added its accelerating influence. With his erect posture, and a mouth freed from grasping and manipulatory demands, and with terrestrial life putting a premium on audible communication, primitive man was in an excellent position to profit from the use of even the most primitive speech. So, while the obvious advantages of vocal communication should not be considered as "causes" of speech as such, they may well have fostered additions of new words and changes in form and meaning of existing symbols, as well as the increasing complexity and meaningfulness of language patterns.

Although primitive man represented the peak of something like a billion years of evolutionary development, he apparently had need of all the survival aids he could muster. His life was not an easy one. Crude in his use of fire, or lacking it entirely, and possessing only the simplest all-purpose tools, he was highly vulnerable to environmental changes and crises. He was a food gatherer, eating such plants and animals as he could find and kill. He may have been the hunted as well as the hunter, for his bones are found mixed with those of animals larger and more powerful than himself. In the one very early cave dwelling that has been discovered, that of Peking man in China, the human bones have been found split lengthwise and the skulls with the base carefully removed—both indications of cannibalism. Apparently primitive man had to be on guard not only against animals but also against his fellows. In this struggle for existence, the possibilities for co-operative effort through small-muscle vocal communciation, while eyes and hands were busy fighting or working, undoubtedly presented immediately rewarding survival value.

To the influence of these physical reinforcements must be added the frequently mentioned gains from thinking, problem-solving, invention, and planning for the future. This ability to analyze and manipulate himself and his environment through the use of symbols helped give man the freedom and challenge of learning and adaptability in place of the supine tropisms of plant life and the stereotyped instincts of the insects and lower animals.

Likewise, the human ability to "tell" instead of "show" the next generation provided considerable reinforcement and acceleration to the development not only of language but also of social patterns, tools, and physical aids to survival. Using short-cut symbolic behavior, the human parent can convey information in terms of cues and general principles, to the accumulating profit of each succeeding generation; the human child is heir to the lore and wisdom of the ages. "Man is the only animal that knows he's an animal," and can do something about it. With developing speech as a "tool," the verbalizing human race has built a sense of the past in folk-tale and saga, in customs, traditions, and laws; has evolved not only an adaptability to the present but a concept of the future as well. Speech and civilization have developed together; each acting as a framework for, and reinforcement of, the other.

## Summary on the Development of Speech in the Race

This descriptive view of the when, why, and how man added the symbolic use of vocal sounds to the reflex cries and reaction-getting noises of the animals clearly indicates the uniqueness, relative recency, and survival and developmental advantages of speech. The history of verbalizing man shows a constantly accelerating rate of accumulation of knowledge, of growth in complexity of social and industrial organizations, and increased efficiency and productivity in agriculture, manufacturing, transportation, and communication. The changes in all these areas occurring in the last century are at least as great as those accumulating throughout all previous time.

If we were to compress the million years of man's existence to one twenty-four-hour day, our total range of written history represents 10 minutes; Christ was born less than 3 minutes ago. With our present time set at noon, David was King of Israel at 11:55; Julius Caesar conquered the then known world at 11:57; Columbus discovered the New World at 11:59, and the United States is 15 seconds old. We have been telephoning for about eight seconds, and turning our radio dials for three. The atom bomb and the end of World War II have occurred in the last second. Modern language, knowledge, and culture are very new. One million years represents approximately forty thousand generations. Eighty generations cover the Christian Era; fewer than three hundred reach back to the ancient civilizations and the beginning of written history, with some 39,700 generations before the existence of written records. Speech, in the modern sense, had indeed a long "beginning."

## SPEECH DEVELOPMENT IN CHILDREN

For technical diagnosis and appropriate therapy, the deviations and disorders of speech should be seen in contrast to so-called "normal" speech and its development. Before hastening to such needed comparisons, however, there should be some concept of the "normal," what is really typical. Thus, accurate work in this field depends on acceptable answers to three basic questions. First, as a needed prelude to the others, can speech development in children be observed with some assurance that the resulting data will be both valid and reliable? Again, can the learning process, and the conditions which act to facilitate or retard it, be described rather than inferred or assumed? Third, are there discoverable patterns of development; are there steps or stages sufficiently constant and typical to serve the purposes of the diagnostician and therapist?

### Studies in Speech-Learning

These questions certainly do not arise from any lack of attention to speech development in children. Actually they come from the very multitude, and confusion, of the reports from observers in many areas. Teachers and parents, physicians and psychologists, linguists and rhetoricians, with various degrees and types of experience and motivation, have contributed their findings and comments;[15] reports have appeared not only in popular literature but in the journals and texts from anthropology, biology, education, linguistics, medicine, philology, phonetics, psychology, and speech.

Fortunately for the reader, however, some bibliographies and reviews provide a representative sampling of the published information. Preyer (1889 and 1898) and Tracy (1893) list numerous references to the work done in earlier years. More readily accessible to the present-day student are such samplings as the review of bibliographies by Allen (1931), the surveys by Anderson (1939), Sanford (1942) and, for the period 1931–43, by Goodenough. McCarthy listed a wide range of studies in 1946, and Leopold provided probably the most comprehensive coverage of all contributing areas in his *Bibliography of Child Language* of 1952. Limited to specific periods are Irwin's review (1941) of the research dealing with speech sounds of the first six months, and the summaries of the studies of the first year by Irwin and Chen in 1943. This last review is particularly useful to the student, not only because it presents data concerning vowel and consonant production for each month but also because of its critical comments on the reliability of these data.

Even with these careful selections and summaries, however, confusion remains. A quick scanning of the reports might seem to indicate that each child studied went his own individual way, with slight regard for so-called sequences or norms. In retrospect, however, this confusion may have been more apparent than real. In the earlier years particularly, few of the investigators were phonetically trained for accurate discrimination and transcription; whereas some transcribed phonetically, others used their own varieties of phonic spelling or diacritical markings. Recording equipment apparently was not widely used, though it is essential for any precise information concerning children's speech. For instance, using phonograph recordings to check the accuracy of four other methods of reporting the speech of children in the fourth through the sixth grades, Betts (1934) found that court reporters made the most complete records, but still missed 20 per cent of the material; shorthand writers missed 47 per cent. Longhand writing caught only 32 per cent of the utterances; phoneticians were able to transcribe a mere 15 per cent. Regardless of the degree of completeness, accuracy by the four methods was about the same: 85 per cent.

With the younger children, the problem is even more acute. McCarthy (1930), for example, reported that only 26 per cent of the speech sounds of 18-month-old children were comprehensible. Fortunately for observers without recorders, this figure rises rapidly to 67 per cent at two years and 93 per cent at three years. Ample reasons for the scientifically necessary "agreement among observers"!

Adding even more to the unreliability of the data, observers frequently differed in their distinctions between crying sounds and speech sounds, dis-

[15] Leopold (1954) lists also philosophers and students of law and astronomy.

agreed in their enumeration of "type" or "frequency" of sounds, and varied in the sizes of the samples used.

Many of the studies were made somewhat casually, without sufficient control, and used as subjects single children, or twins, or larger groups—frequently with unknown backgrounds. Various samples, moreover, were taken under a wide variety of conditions of free play and direct stimulation, and in quite different situations in the home, the nursery, the school. Thus the seeming confusion of earlier studies, while regrettable, is at least understandable.

About the third decade of this century, however, several factors apparently combined to establish better design of observations, increased knowledge and control of conditions, and greater precision of recording. While the importance assigned to the various influences in this development of a more scientific approach may vary with the individual reviewer, undoubtedly many forces were at work. In the preceding years, psychological and educational journals had been reporting an increasing number of behavioral studies with rigorous controls for validity and reliability. In the field of speech, McCarthy's study (1930), using established methods, undoubtedly set a standard for many subsequent investigations.[16]

Increasing accuracy of transcription, so necessary in the complex babbling and early speech of the child, was fostered not only by the increased availability and use of recording equipment but also by the growing work of phoneticians, linguists, and phonetically trained teachers of speech and speech correctionists. Jespersen, for instance, gave major consideration to children's speech in his *Language, Its Nature, Origin and Development* (1922). Jakobson (1941) and Leopold (1937, 1949), both able linguists, applied phonetic analysis to their studies of children's language, adopting the concept of "sound categories" rather than individual sounds as the basis for study of language development.[17] As Leopold comments, "Instead of trying to find the sequence in which children learn sounds, which has proved futile, the attention must be focused on the sequence in the acquisition of sound categories." (1953, 1954, p. 3.)

To Irwin and his co-workers, however, must go the bulk of the credit for the use of sufficient statistical controls to establish estimates of the validity and reliability of data obtained under various conditions of observation and through the use of different items of measurement; estimates so necessary for scientific knowledge and the determination of usable norms of speech development. As summarized by Irwin in 1947 (*a* and *b*), the reliability of discriminations between crying and whining was established by Irwin and Chen (1941) and that between crying and speech sounds by Irwin

[16] Prediction of the wide influence of McCarthy's insistence on control of conditions was made by Allen in 1931 and its actuality confirmed by Goodenough in 1944.

[17] Leopold gives full credit to Jakobson for establishing this concept of "sound categories." Its use, however, is by no means confined to these two, nor to linguists and phoneticians.

and Curry (1941). In 1945, Irwin indicated the optimum size of the sample of sounds, and in other studies determined the differences between measurements taken of "sound type" and of "sound frequency" (Irwin, 1947a), of consonants as compared with vowels (Irwin, 1946), and of the "type-token ratio" (Chen and Irwin, 1946).

Thus in the recent years, with the increasing use of recording equipment under controlled conditions, the application of phonetic analysis and modern statistical techniques, considerable order has emerged from the earlier chaos. There seem to be recognizable patterns which, with some latitude, may be regarded as reliable "norms" for the development of speech in children.

## Conditions of Learning

The modern child, as the descendant of primitive man, possesses substantially the same sensory, neural, and motor equipment. In the earliest months of his life, moreover, the child, like earliest man, uses these structures to produce a wide range of reflexive vocal sounds as a part of the over-all response of the organism to its external and internal environment. Today's child, however, gains a concept of communication within a few short months, whereas primitive man needed an unknown number of centuries to develop even the first glimmer of the symbolic use of vocal sounds as distinct from reflexive and literal signal-making noises.

At all stages, man has learned speech; the ape has not. Obviously the child is dependent, as was primtiive man, on human sensory, motor, and neural mechanisms exhibiting normal maturation. It is in the language-using environment, however, rather than in the organism itself or the nature of the learning process, that the student of speech development sees the forces influencing the child's speedy recapitulation of the learning experience of the race. Such evidence as exists would seem to indicate that a child reared in isolation and deprived of the usual talking environment will fail to develop articulate speech. As indicated by Mason's report of the child imprisoned with a mute and uneducated mother for six and one-half years (1942), normal structures and their growth do not assure any use of conventionalized vocal symbols. Thus in the environment probably lie the differences in speed of language-learning, not only as between the earliest men and the modern child but also between structurally normal children of differing cultural and behavioral backgrounds. The conditions of learning, therefore, include structural equipment, maturation, and environmental influences.

**Maturation sets the pace.** Within the energy field established by the structural equipment of the organism and the environment, maturation probably sets the pace for speech-learning. Maturation, which may be defined as "the growth and development which is necessary before any unlearned behavior can occur, or before the learning of any particular behavior can take place" (Boring, Langfeld, and Weld, 1948), is the evolvement from conception till death of the genetic factors which are present at the time of conception. If inheritance be regarded as the potentialities for development of structures and functions, maturation is the development of these structures and functions under environmental conditions. Some of the changes which occur in the individual from conception to death take place rapidly and the resulting functions are present before or soon after birth; other functions reach their functions only later in life. Ordinarily, the simpler the function the more rapid is its development, whereas the more complex the function usually the slower it is to mature.

Maturation thus seems to determine not only when a behavior may be learned, but even more important for the teacher, the most efficient time for that learning to take place. In other words, maturation apparently establishes various periods in the life of the organism when it is most open to certain kinds of stimulation from the environment, and when it will profit most from that stimulation, that is, a "readiness" to learn a given activity.

Speech, as a relatively complex function, obviously depends on maturation for its development. Normal growth and development of the structures used for speech supply a "readiness" for the birth cry and for the reflexive sounds of the early months of infancy. Not till the time of puberty, however, is the organism "ready" for the changes in pitch and quality to produce the adult voice. Similarly, the transition from prelinguistic to linguistic vocalization occurs only gradually as the organism attains sufficient structural and functional development. The relatively late development of Broca's area, for example, in addition to other structures, would seem to influence the timetable of speech-learning. Not until seventeen months after birth does this significant area of the cortex attain the degree of anatomical differentiation shown by other motor centers some six months earlier (de Crinis, 1932).

With a normal environment, therefore, speech-learning by the child depends on a step-by-step process of maturation; the child learns when he is "ready." Moreover, experiments such as Strayer's (1930), using co-twins, indicate that even intensive instruction will not significantly accelerate speech-learning beyond the level of maturation. While special stimulation may push a child slightly ahead of his normal development, such instruction seems to have little, if any, permanent value.

Speech development thus represents a series of stages remarkably similar in all normal children; each step made possible by the gradual maturation of the organism. Paced by his maturation (Peacher, 1949a), therefore, each child shows a period of "speech readiness," a time at which his organism is most open to language stimulation and his speech development seems to proceed at a maximum rate. During this time, most commonly occurring between 12 and 18 months but which may include the 9 to 24 months span (Stinchfield and Young, 1938), speech is learned most efficiently and thoroughly.[18] While a child may be taught to speak after this time, it is accomplished only with increased difficulty. McCready (1940) believes the difficulty increases each month after the fifteenth; other writers suggest limits to the period of readiness varying between 30 and 42 months. Van Riper

[18] Broca's area reaches its anatomical differentiation only at the seventeenth month.

(1954), for example, is convinced that any child who does not begin to speak intelligible two-word phrases by 30 months should be referred to the physician and the speech correctionist.

**Influences on speech-learning.** Speech-learning results from the growth and development of a human organism in a human environment; from the changes in the structure and functioning of the child's sensory, motor, and neural equipment occurring in the conditions and forces surrounding the organism. In other words, speech-learning occurs within a total energy field of interaction between internal and external energy systems.

Speech-learning, in this total energy field, is thus subject to a multiplicity of factors—both positive and negative—each acting relatively within the total framework; factors more accurately named "influences" than considered as "causes" in the older sense of isolated or independently acting etiological elements. Clinical experience has shown that seldom, if ever, will any influence appear in isolation and act alone either to retard or accelerate speech. Beckey (1942), for example, found no one particular item which seemed to be the only reason for the delay in speech. Even in the cases in which normal speech was interrupted by some inhibiting condition, the history of each child revealed other organic factors which might have made the organism more susceptible. In fact, three or more factors were operative in 84 per cent of the fifty children with delayed speech, but in only 20 per cent of the normal group. Only deafness, paralysis, and marked mental deficiency would seem able to act as solitary negative influences. Yet even with these significant detriments, other influences may exaggerate their effect, or lift speech-learning above the degree of handicap. Each organism matures and learns as a whole, and speech development is determined by the total field.

Even the most elaborate clinical survey, therefore, may not be able to reveal, let alone evaluate, even a major portion of the influences operative in the speech development of a given child. Recent investigations, however, have assigned varying degrees of significance to selected items acting primarily in either the external or the internal energy system, and thereby affecting the interaction between the two. Some of the studies deal with children of two years or older who are in the process of learning language patterns; a few refer to younger children. Unfortunately, however, apparently no horizontal studies show the degree to which those factors that influence the earlier development of a concept of communication and the acquisition of speech sounds as symbols operate also on the later learning of the formal patterns of established language.

In spite of this multiplicity of influences, or even perhaps because of it, this discussion of the learning and development of speech may well confine itself to the brief presentation of a sample list, leaving to the later discussions of etiology and therapy the privilege of extensive clinical diagnosis.

Among the influences operating primarily in the internal energy system, various investigators have listed sex, mental deficiency, hearing loss, and neurological anomalies. It generally is believed that girls develop speech somewhat faster than boys. Yet Irwin (1952b) reports three studies which revealed statistically significant differences favoring the girls only from the twentieth month and when measured on the basis of phoneme type. Phoneme frequency measurements, however, gave no reliable differences at any age.

Schlanger (1954), Irwin (1952), Karlin and Strazzulla (1952), Peacher (1949a), and others agree that mental deficiency may delay or prevent speech. Irwin found that the speech performance of three-year-old imbeciles and idiots was the equivalent of that of normal children in their first year. Karlin and Strazzulla, after defining speech as the symbolic verbal means of communication which may be regarded as a tool and a manifestation of language, conclude that language defects in the mentally retarded children are more striking than speech defects.

Within the more nearly normal range, likewise, it has been generally assumed that a relationship exists between measures of various aspects of language development and the scores obtained on the abilities measured by most intelligence tests. It seems now, however, that this supposed relationship may be limited in area and, to the extent that it exists at all, apply only in the third or later years—after speech-learning is well under way. Williams (1937), for instance, found that size of vocabulary correlated closely with intelligence, but that other measures of speech proficiency did not. While accuracy of articulation, correct usage of words, length, completeness, and complexity of sentences, for example, correlated with one another, they showed little relation either to size of vocabulary or to intelligence scores. These are dubious relationships and cause a real question concerning the feasibility of using intelligence scores as an index of a child's readiness for, or probable proficiency in, speech development—even after he has reached an age to accomplish the comparatively elaborate patterns tested in the Williams study.

The first two years of life, however, are even more critical in the speech development of the child. Irwin and Chen (1945), using 91 infants 24 months of age and under, compared Kuhlman mental-test scores with the scores obtained on a differential speech-development index devised by the latter author. Later (1949), Spiker and Irwin tested 48 infants from 1 to 28 months in age to determine possible relationships between Kulhman test scores and six indices of speech sound development.[19] In both studies, however, the significance and predictive efficiency of the correlations were sufficiently low to provide ample reason for the authors' earlier statement that, "speech sound development for the first two years is independent of intelligence test scores" (Irwin and Chen, 1945, p. 296).

Deafness and neurological pathologies have been considered generally as detrimental to speech development about in proportion to the severity of the disability. In both conditions, however, studies have suggested the modification of their influence by the presence of related factors. Auditory dis-

[19] Type and frequency for vowels, consonants, and phonemes.

crimination, for example, varies considerably from one child to another, and audiologists are well aware of the individual variations among the hard-of-hearing in the relationship between hearing acuity as measured by speech perception and by audiometric curves (Carhart, 1946; Hirsh, 1951, Ch. 5). In the neurological area, Schlanger (1954) found definite differences in speech development occurring between 21 matched pairs of mentally retarded children, one group institutionalized, the other living at home with parents. The suggested causes for the lowered language output for the institutionalized children included the loss of speech motivation, the complete association with peers, the overstimulation of continual contact, and the severance of familial ties.

The influences operative in the external energy system obviously are more numerous and even more highly interrelated, with each varied by its coexistence with others. In general, speech development seems to be influenced by the occupational status of the family, though Irwin (1948a and 1948b) believes this factor becomes operative mainly after the first year and a half of life. The home atmosphere as determined by the personalities of the parents seems to McCarthy (1954) to be the most important single factor influencing the child's acquisition of language. A number of studies have also pointed out the influence of siblings in the home. It appears from these studies that an only child has the advantage because of his association primarily with adults, whereas twins and children born into bilingual homes are at a distinct disadvantage (Day, 1932; Davis, 1937). Emotional conflicts in the home, emotional shocks and illnesses of the child, if severe or prolonged, comprise additional negative influences.

In short, the significant positive influences on speech-learning are those which foster the total energy system of a healthy child, in full possession of all sensory, motor, and neural capacities, living in a happy, cultured home where parental time and interest provide adequate speech stimulation. That this summary fits the "average child" obviously should not be assumed by those who would establish "norms."

**Nature of speech-learning.** Any consideration of the nature of speech-learning must be wary of oversimplification. Because the child produces reflexive sounds, then babbles, and later talks, it is easy to assume that one leads mechanically and inevitably to the other. But this is oversimplification.

Reasonable as it might seem to expect the child to select the sounds he needs from his babbling, he does not seem to do so; he is not able spontaneously to use the phonetic elements of his babbling as the phonemes of his language. In fact, it is not clear just how important early babbling is for the development of words (Miller, 1951, p. 146). The most frequently used language sounds are not those that babies babble earliest and most often. During the first two months the consonants the child produces (outside of crying) are principally glottal, with a few velar k's and g's added. At two months, 87 per cent of the child's consonants are glottal h or the glottal stop (Irwin, 1947a and b; 1948); whereas in adult speech the more forward consonants are preferred—the seven alveolar consonants accounting for over half the consonant sounds used by the adult. A similar progression occurs with the vowel sounds. The most commonly babbled vowel at two months, [ɛ] , represents 43 per cent of all vowel sounds at this age, but supplies only 8 per cent of adult vowel sounds; and [ʌ], which accounts for one-fourth of the infant's vowel production, is used by the adult least of all.

These changes in sound frequency, however, are not the only interruptions of the change from babble to talking. Children in English-speaking homes often babble a wide variety of sounds not usable in English, such as the German umlaut sounds and the French gutteral r. Neither is it uncommon to find that a child has produced l and r during his babbling, but is unable later, at two or three years, to produce these sounds clearly in English words. As Jakobson (1941) observes, the child must tediously relearn his babbled sounds as words and parts of words in connected speech.

Speech, however, is more than a relearning and linking of babbled sounds which are reflexive, associated principally with breathing, swallowing, hiccoughing, and other physiological processes and are not tied to specifically meaningful situations. Parents who claim to derive knowledge of the infant's needs from these sounds likely are reading into the situations to derive meaning (Miller, 1951, p. 143). More objective parents and trained nurses fail to find meaningful distinctions between infantile sounds (Sherman, 1927).

Uncertain as the importance of babbling may be for the development of speech, there seems to be even less certainty concerning the changes from vocal play to the verbal habits of a particular language. For the acquisition of speech, the child must not only link his babbled sounds into connected patterns, relearning many of them in the process, but must also learn meanings and a conventionalized code. Like primitive man, he must learn what means what, and when.

This process, like learning in all areas, represents a change in performance and meaning; a merging of increased sound production and developing perception. Beginning with the birth cry, the earlier sounds appear to be reflexive, stimulated and maintained by varying physiological states. The process of sound production is not regenerative. Very shortly, however, the greater maturation of nerves and muscles seemingly provides for autostimulation, and babbling, as distinct from the purely reflexive sounds, is under way. Figuratively and descriptively speaking, the speech-producing circuit has become regenerative through kinesthetic and auditory feedback.[20]

This tendency to perseveration has long been of interest to psychologists, for it appears in various muscle groups and behavior patterns. Many psychologists have assumed that some kind of circular reaction is set up (Baldwin, 1895), and Allport (1924) gives an extensive discussion of the probable means of establishment of such circular reaction and its role in the

---

[20] One of the first indications of deafness may be the lessening or disappearance of babbling; kinesthesis alone being insufficient to maintain this particular circuit.

development of speech. Other psychologists have used the word *imitation* with various meanings, ranging from instinct to figurative description.[21]

Whatever descriptive terms may be assigned to the process, seemingly it occurs with the maturation of the organism and represents a time of greater differentiation of structure and of increased specificity and precision of behavior. Common to all animal life (Coghill, 1929; Anderson, 1936), it will occur even in a minimal environment, as a characteristic of living tissue.

In the course of speech development, the establishment of this regenerating circuit through maturation, and the resulting babbling, represents the beginning of control of motor development coming from perceptual processes; changes in meaning are soon added to changes in performance for the first stages of learning on the human level.[22] With sufficient maturation the infant can respond to others as well as to himself. By two months, the baby responds to the human voice; by six months he seems able to distinguish, at least in terms of his overt responses, between affectionate and scolding tones. About nine months after birth the normal child begins to pay attention to a few familiar words and can respond to simple commands by the first birthday.[23] Thus merging sound production and perception, motor performance and concepts of meaning, lead to coded vocal communication; through maturation-paced changes in performance and perception, the child learns the conventionalized code of his language and what means what.

Various psychologists have applied different premises to the attempted explanation of this process of learning patterned sound production and conventionalized meanings. The Association theorists, for example, tend to approach the problem of speech development from the view of stimulus-response learning involving the Law of Effect. The speech-learning child is analogous to the lever-pressing rat. This older view, with its emphasis on reinforcement, emphasizes the role of another person. In order to learn to respond correctly to a word, "it is necessary for another organism to intervene and reward us each time we respond correctly" (Miller, 1951, p. 5).

Other psychologists, however, rejecting Association theory, stress the acquisition of meaning and significance through contiguous association of stimuli and responses. Those holding to the Contiguity or Insight theories thus could not accept the view of speech-learning as the establishment of a chain of conditioned reflexes, for the responses have significance only in terms of the total behavior. Hence specific reinforcements are not needed, and motivation and rewards are significant to the learning process only because they make responses occur.[24] Certain typical field-theory experiments,

---

[21] While the child does "imitate"—first himself and then others—terms borrowed from electrical analogues may seem preferable to those which may carry with them a marked tinge of instinct-theory.

[22] The danger of interference with normal maturation through too-frequent interruptions of babbling is a very real one, not only in these earliest stages but throughout the babbling period.

[23] The child understands the speech of others earlier than he uses the same words himself.

[24] See above.

moreover, have shown that if the animal's need is intense, its solution to the experimental problem may be delayed; an indication that strong motivation can sometimes interefere with learning rather than aiding it.

At the present stage of knowledge concerning the learning process, little can be said beyond the objectively demonstrated fact that certain skills or responses are chosen ahead of others for practice and progress toward specificity. This, however, does represent some approach to descriptive accuracy if not to "explanation" in the speculative sense. Wtih the study of infant behavior dominated by an older view that reflexes are specific from the outset and that the development of behavior consisted of tying these discrete reflexes into chains, observers are likely to select from the total behavior of the subject those aspects which fit this structuralistic definition.

In contrast to this, the more recent studies in genetics, physiology, and psychology seem to indicate that the development of behavior proceeds from the generalized, un-co-ordinated responses of the infant to the specific and more highly differentiated behavior of the adult. Paralleling this differentiation, which is a matter of development, there occurs a process of integration or recombination of responses resulting, seemingly, from experience.[25] Since generalized responses as such have little or no adaptive character, the organism maintains homeostasis by developing simpler and more specific responses. As this progressive differentiation proceeds, complexity grows in the stimulus area rather than in response; skill and effectiveness of behavior increase as responses become simpler and more specific, but encompass a wider and more complex range of stimulating situations.

This general description, clearly demonstrated in sensory-motor behavior, applies also with symbolic responses. Language symbols are simple and specific as motor acts; as symbols they become more valuable as they apply to wider areas of experience. In the vocal patterns of the infant, for instance, wide varieties of sounds appear, not all of them by any means utilized in later language. From these, selection must be made, since competing responses are impossible in a unitary organism. Speech necessitates doing a particular thing at a particular time.

The human infant thus appears as an organism with a wide range of abilities and potentiality for an infinite variety of responses, maturing in an environment of multifold possibilities and demands; growing and developing in an external energy system of social pressures which impinge upon the organism with increasing strength as the child grows older. In the interaction, therefore, between the child's potentiality for infinite variety of responses and the pressures, forces, and demands of the environment, both differentiation and selection establish new and adaptive patterns of response. From the generalized, undifferentiated vocal responses of early life, the dynamic interaction between a maturing organism and an external energy field selects and integrates the relatively simple responses of speech sounds to respond sym-

---

[25] This is a theoretical distinction only, since either experience or development without the other is impossible.

bolically to an infinitely complex range of stimuli. The child learns both performance and what means what. The as yet far from completed task of the learning theorist is to explain why or how one response is more likely to appear and more apt to be learned than another. Until that ultimate day, descriptive accounts of the observed dynamics of growing and developing organisms must suffice, for learning and living are one process.

**Stages in speech-learning.** From the time the birth cry announces the presence of a rudimentary human sound generator to the final terminal plateau, speech development is a continuous process. There is no way of knowing when a sound or a series of sounds "begins." Careful testing will reveal that a certain phonetic element does or does not appear today. If it does, there is little guarantee that it will occur again in the immediate future; if it does not, the observer is left with the open question whether it was used yesterday or will be tomorrow. Obviously, therefore, any selected stages or steps in the continuum of speech development must be arbitrary; conveniences, rather than precise realities.

This phrase "continuous process" means only that there are no discoverable gaps or breaks so far as the process itself is concerned. It does not imply that there is a metered or cadenced progression maintaining a constant relationship with time. Not only does each organism grow and develop spasmodically, now here, now there, but each establishes its own timing relative to other children. There is even behavioral evidence of periods of recession within the total pattern of maturation, as when the school child starts making errors in addition when beginning on subtraction or multiplication.

These variations indicate that each child, within the limits set by the genetic factors and environmental forces, is a "law unto himself." They constitute real reason for wide flexibility in the application of estimated stages or norms of development to the individual child.

Varying bases of division have been used by different writers to outline a pattern of speech development. Jespersen (1922, p. 103), for instance, discerns three periods in the child's linguistic development and graphically titles them Screaming Time, Crowing or Babbling Time, and Talking Time. The last division he subdivides into the period of "little language"—the child's own—and "common language"—the language of the community. Other writers have preferred a two-step organization, using such titles as prelingual and lingual, or nonpurposive and purposive.

Without in any way implying discreet categories, the progression from birth cry to established language patterns would seem to include two distinguishable types of verbal behavior; one predominant early and the other later, with considerable coexistence between. Since patterns of behavior are more readily observed and classified than are inferred inner states, larger agreement among observers is promised by the terms *prelinguistic* and *linguistic* than by *nonpurposive* and *purposive*.

The prelinguistic stage of speech development is marked initially by the reflexive sounds associated with physiological states. During the greater part of this period, the vocalization seems to be stimulated mainly by changes in physiological states of the infant or in the surrounding environment but is not differentiated for the nature of the stimulating situation. Most of the vowel-like sounds used at this time are similar to adult front vowels and out-number the consonants 5 to 1. Subsequently the back vowels become more frequent, and more consonant sounds are produced.[26]

During the third month, or shortly thereafter, vocal play, or babbling, appears and increases in the succeeding months; seemingly an indication that the organism has matured sufficiently to establish "feedback" and thus stimulate its own vocal patterns. By the sixth month, the babbling consists of somewhat regular repetitions of similar sounds with a more noticeable rhythm in the patterns. At this time, the speech of another will interrupt this babbling only if the speaker constitutes an effective stimulus within the comprehension of the child; otherwise the babbling will continue or even increase. The speech circuit responds primarily to autostimulation.

These early months represent the infant's establishment of himself as an independent organism, with most of his growth and development directed to the means of satisfying his immediate biological needs. Re-establishment of his growth rate at birth and the beginning of segmental movements of the body are early indications of a successful start. Later, the further-differentiated behaviors of sitting up, first with support and then briefly alone, using the hand to grasp objects and carry them to his mouth, and shifting from the supine position to the side and later to the prone, show normal continuation at the job of staying alive.

With immature equipment, and so much business of his own to attend to, naturally the child's first concern must be with stimuli coming from his own internal energy system. Understandably, he lives and works in a world of his own, and so can well be called, as does Piaget (1926), egocentric.

Following the sixth month, the babbling increases in variety, and later inflectional patterns are added. During the latter part of the eighth month, or slightly beyond, the child begins to repeat the commonly used syllables of the parents (mama, dada, byebye, etc.); seemingly in his babbling and vocal play rather than as an actual response to stimulation by another person.

Through the first nine months, therefore, the child's success in the establishment of his existence as an independent organism may be shown by crawling, sitting without support, and standing by holding to some rigid object. He is ready to develop appropriate responses to others. By the close of this period he will imitate rhythmical activities of adults, show retreat or crying behaviors in the presence of strangers, and variably approach or retreat from other children. Quite likely he will have accomplished a "far-transposition" task by holding out his arms when an adult displays activity

[26] Chen and Irwin (1946) have proposed the vowel-consonant ratio as an index of development during the prelinguistic period.

preparatory to picking him up, thus demonstrating some degree of symbolic behavior.

His sound production, initially reflexive, with self-stimulation added later, is similar to the reflexive and reaction-getting cries of the animals. His level of maturation, however, permits exercise and further differentiation and specificity of acoustic neuromotor patterns, through repetition of a wide variety of sounds and under the stimulation and control of his own auditory and kinesthetic feedback.

The last months of the first year of life constitute a transition period from the egocentric to a social orientation. A developing nervous system apparently enables the child to respond to a range of stimuli outside those arising primarily from his own changing physiological states. As one sign of this, many children show what seems to be an effort to respond to the speech of others by producing similar sounds. This echoic response, generally referred to as "imitation," may more appropriately be described as the addition of outside stimulation to the former self-stimulation or feedback. With this addition, the child increases his echoic response whenever the adult interrupts the vocal play by speaking, with moderate intensity, the sound being babbled, or when the adult uses a sound already practiced by the child. It is thus during this period of transition from the prelinguistic to the linguistic period that the adult can become a factor in the learning process. The growth and development of the child have brought sufficient differentiation and specificity of behavior to permit response to a growing number of outside stimuli.

During this transitional period the child likewise seems to show the first symbolic behavior on the human level. Whatever learning theorists may say about the learning involved, the process of perception develops new meanings, an awareness that certain sounds are meaningfully substituted for things and events. Some children, though far from all, attain the first true word by the close of their first year; true word, that is, in the adult sense of a conventionalized and arbitrary symbol. The child has had the phoneme for a long time in his prelinguistic behavior.

The year-old child thus stands at the threshold of the transition from egocentric to socialized sound usage; the change from prelinguistic vocalization, similar to the reflexive and action-getting cries and calls of the animals, to the linguistic use of the conventionalized and arbitrary symbols of speech. This threshold seems to mark a critical point in the development to the human level. It may be, as the psychiatrist would describe it, that the growing organism must surrender some pleasure to face reality. Or it may be that at this point he needs a considerably increased maturation to establish the needed specificity of response to a wide variety of stimuli. In any event, this seems to be a period at which forces and influences in the external energy system begin their greatest influence to favor or hinder the development of speech.

Growth and development of the organism and a regularly stimulated speech circuit have prepared the child to profit from a talking environment.

So, with favorable influences, linguistic and otherwise, the "speed-up" begins. To this point the child has followed the timetable probably approximated by his most primitive ancestors. Now, with "readiness" established, appropriate environmental factors spark the rapidity of speech-learning which is so in contrast to the slow acquisition of symbolic expression by the race. The child learns to be a human sound generator and receiver; normally he learns it in a hurry. Early in his second year he likely has exceeded the cumulative life-gains of a good many generations of early man, and certainly is beyond the attainable level of any subhuman organism.

The first words used by the child in his linguistic activity may closely resemble those of the adult, but they are likely to have different meanings. Further, some are used as one-word sentences and all are apt to be very general in their reference. In spite of increased use of words, echoic responses comprise a statistically significant portion of his sound production, and continue to do so to about 30 months of age (Zipf, 1949).

By 18 months the average child has acquired some ten to twenty meaningful words. He uses these to respond to and control his environment, along with his echoic responses, and a great deal of incomprehensible mish-mash and jabber, or "jargon." This jargon, the richly varied successor to earlier vocal play and babbling, would appear to be an important part of speech-learning, instead of the unmitigated nuisance it seems to some adults. It is a channeling of the energy of the developing organism into the speech patterns for the development of a wider variety of differentiated responses, not only to persons and things, but also to the child's own variant experiences and emotional tensions. As an apparent means of transition from the simple, monotonous, and frequently laggard speech of childhood to the varied, fluent language flow of the adult, jargon reaches its peak at about 18 months, and then diminishes to negligible amounts by the end of the second year. As a channeler of energy for greater differentiation of vocal behavior and as an attainable self-satisfying response to the verbal world of adults, jargon seems a necessary part of the dynamic process of learning to talk.

During the latter part of his second year, the child begins a more rapid development of his vocabulary, a part of his linguistic attainment that has moved comparatively slowly. At this time, however, with increased differentiation of behavior and developing symbolic skill, the child is ready to form the more complicated patterns of distinct and conventionalized words in their established grammatical relationships. At two years he will be talking—awkwardly, perhaps, and with confusions in meanings and certainly in grammar. But the pattern has been established; human speech is within his grasp.

The debt of this discussion of speech-learning to the concept of the "average child" is obvious; without this shadowy figure few behavioral studies could be written. Like the old psychological construct of the "raw, untutored child of nature," however, this "average child" exists only in theory and in statistical tables. Useful in verbalizing, in neither diagnosis nor therapy should he be substituted for the individual human child.

This description of speech development by the child, largely in behavioral terms, has attempted a dynamic view of speech-learning in terms of its conditions and stages. With an understandable disinclination to use "instinct-theory" as an explanation of the acquisition of language skills, this survey has been equally reluctant to search for a hypothetical "speech motivation" or "drive." The preference has been to follow modern physiological and psychological procedures and recognize the dynamics of living tissues and organisms. Growth and development are observed in all living organisms, with continuous changes in the direction of greater differentiation and specificity of behavior. During this process many behaviors appear and are discarded. Out of the infinity of possible responses, the living organism will select those which favor adaptation, those which maintain the homeostasis of the living organism.

The close of this description at the second birthday does not imply that speech is "learned" by that date. Quite the contrary. Many new words are to be added, at a decreasing rate after three years, but still acquired. Continued differentiation and repetition bring greater precision in articulation, meaning, and linguistic style. Speech-learning is a continuous process, moving slowly for approximately a year and a half after the birth cry, then at an accelerated pace for about a year, to continue at a slower rate to some unpredictable, and probably unrecognized, terminal plateau.

## BIBLIOGRAPHY

ALLEN, C. N. 1931. Bibliographies in child study and developmental psychology. *Psychol. Bull.,* 28, 277–296.

ALLPORT, F. H. 1924. Social psychology. Boston: Houghton Mifflin.

ANDERSON, J. E. 1936. Child development and the interpretation of behavior. *Science,* 83, #2150, 245–252.

———— 1939. The development of spoken language. Yearbook National Society for Study of Education, 38, Part I, 211–224.

BALDWIN, J. M. 1895. Mental development in the child and the race: methods and processes. New York: Macmillan.

BARNETT, L. 1952, 1953. The world we live in. *Life* magazine, XXXIII, #23, Dec. 8, 1952, 85–103; XXXIV, #6, Feb. 9, 1953, 58–82; XXXIV, #15, Apr. 13, 1953, 86–109; XXXIV, #23, June 8, 1953, 74–98; XXXV, #10, Sept. 7, 1953, 54–74; #16, Oct. 19, 1953, 90–109.

BECKEY, R. E. 1942. A study of certain factors related to retardation of speech. *J. Speech Disorders,* 7, 223–250.

BETTS, E. A. 1934. An evaluation of certain techniques for the study of oral composition. *Res. Stud. Elem. Sch. Lang.* No. 1, *Univ. Iowa Stud. Educ.,* 9, No. 2, 7–35.

BLODGETT, H. C. 1929. The effect of the introduction of reward upon maze behavior of rats. Univ. of California publications in psychology, 4, 113–134.

BOPP, F. 1816. Conjugations system. Analytical comparison of the Sanskrit, Greek, Latin, and Teutonic languages. Frankfort am Main: Andreaische. *Cited* by Jespersen, 1922.

———— 1857. Vergleichende Grammatik (2nd ed.). Berlin: Ferdinand Dümmler. *Cited* by Jespersen, 1922.

BORING, E. G., LANGFELD, H. S., and WELD, H. P. 1948. Foundations of psychology. New York: Wiley.

BRAIDWOOD, J. R. 1948. Prehistoric men. Chicago: Chicago Natural History Museum.

BUXTON, C. E. 1940. Latent learning and the goal gradient hypothesis. *Contributions to Psychol. Theory*, 2, #6.

CARHART, R. 1938. Evolution of the speech mechanism. *Quart. J. Speech*, XXIV, 557–568.

———— 1946. Speech reception in relation to pattern of pure tone loss. *J. Speech Disorders*, 11, 97–108.

CHEN, H. P., and IRWIN, O. C. 1946. The type token ratio applied to infant speech sounds. *J. Speech Disorders*, 11, 126–130.

CHILDE, V. G. 1925. The dawn of European civilization. New York: Knopf.

———— 1936. Man makes himself. London: Watts.

———— 1942. What happened in history. Harmondsworth, Middlesex, England: Penguin Books.

———— 1944. Progress and archeology. London: Watts.

CLARK, W. E. L. 1934. Early forerunners of man. Baltimore: W. Wood & Co., 143, 216.

COLTON, F. B. 1952. Our home-town planet, earth. *National Geographic*, CI, #1, 117–138.

COMRIE, P. 1876. *J. Anthropological Institute*, VI, #2, 119.

CONDILLAC, E. B. 1789. Les oeuvres de Condillac, revues et corrigées. Paris. *Cited* by Whitney (1868), 429 f.

DAVIS, E. A. 1937. The development of linguistic skill in twins, singletons with siblings, and only children from age five to ten years. Univ. of Minnesota child welfare monogr., Series No. 14.

DAVISON, D. 1934. Men of the dawn. London: Watts.

DAY, E. J. 1932. The development of language in twins: I, a comparison of twins and single children. *Child Developm.*, 3, 46–52.

DAY, L., and BENTLEY, M. 1911. A note on learning in paramecium. *J. Animal Behavior*, 1, 67–73.

DE CRINIS, M. 1932. Die Entwicklung der Grosshirnrinde nach der Geburt in ihren Beziehungen zur intellektuellen Ausreifung des Kindes. Wein, Klinisch Wochenshrift, 45, 1161–1165.

DE LAGUNA, G. A. 1927. Speech: its function and development. New Haven: Yale Univ. Press. Ch. I.

DEESE, J. 1952. The psychology of learning. New York: McGraw-Hill.

DE PRADENNE, A. V. 1940. Prehistory. London: Harrap.

FARRAR, F. W. 1860. An essay on the origin of language. London: J. Murray. Ch. IV.

———— 1865. Chapters on language. London: Longmans, Green.

GEIGER, L. 1869. Ursprung und Entwickelung der menschlichen sprache und Vernunft. Stuttgart. *Quoted* by Sayce, 1883, I, 81.

GELLERMAN, L. W. 1931*a*. The double alternation problem: I, the behavior of monkeys in a double alternation temporal maze. *J. genet. Psychol.*, 39, 50–72.

———— 1931*b*. The double alternation problem: II, the behavior of children and human adults in a double alternation temporal maze. *J. genet. Psychol.*, 39, 197–226.

GOODENOUGH, F. L. 1944. Bibliographies in child development: 1931–1943. *Psychol. Bull.*, 9, 615–633.

GRAY, G. W., and WISE, C. M. 1946. Bases of speech (rev. ed.). New York: Harper.

GUTHRIE, E. R. 1930. Conditioning as a principle of learning. *Psychol. Rev.*, 37, 412–428.

―――― 1935. The psychology of learning. New York: Harper.

HARLOW, H. F. 1932. Comparative behavior of primates: III, complicated delayed reaction tests on primates. *J. comp. Psychol.*, 14, 241–252.

HAYES, K. J. 1950. Vocalization and speech in chimpanzees. *Amer. Psychologist*, 5, 275–276.

―――― and HAYES, C. 1950. Vocalization and speech in chimpanzees. 16 mm. sound film., Psychological Cinema Register, State College, Pa.

HERSKOVITS, M. J. 1948. Man and his works. New York: Knopf.

HILGARD, E. R. 1956. Theories of learning (2nd ed.). New York: Appleton-Century-Crofts.

HIRSH, I. J. 1951. The measurement of hearing. New York: McGraw-Hill.

HOOTON, E. A. 1931. Up from the apes. New York: Macmillan.

―――― 1942. Man's poor relations. New York: Doubleday, Doran.

HULL, C. L. 1943. The principles of behavior. New York: Appleton-Century-Crofts.

HUNTER, W. S. 1912. The delayed reaction in animals and children. *Behavior Monogr.*, 2, #1.

―――― and BARTLETT, S. C. 1948. Double alternation behavior in young children. *J. exp. Psychol.*, 38, 558–567.

HUNTER, W. S., and HULL, B. E. 1941. Double alternation behavior of the white rat in a spatial maze. *J. comp. Psychol.*, 32, 253–266.

IRWIN, O. C. 1941. Research on speech sounds for the first six months of life. *Psychol. Bull.*, 38, 277–285.

―――― 1945. Reliability of infant speech sound data. *J. Speech Disorders*, 10, 227–235.

―――― 1946. Infant speech equations for consonant-vowel ratios. *J. Speech Disorders*, 11, 177–180.

―――― 1947a. Infant speech: the problem of variability. *J. Speech Disorders*, 12, 173–176.

―――― 1947b. Infant speech: variability and the problem of diagnosis. *J. Speech Disorders*, 12, 287–289.

―――― 1947c. Infant speech: consonantal sounds according to place of articulation. *J. Speech Disorders*, 12, 397–401.

―――― 1947d. Infant speech: consonantal sounds according to manner of articulation. *J. Speech Disorders*, 12, 402–404.

―――― 1948a. Infant speech: development of vowel sounds. *J. Speech Hearing Disorders*, 13, 31–34.

―――― 1948b. Infant speech: the effect of family occupational status and of age on use of sound types. *J. Speech Hearing Disorders*, 13, 224–226.

―――― 1948c. Infant speech: the effect of family occupational status and of age on sound frequency. *J. Speech Hearing Disorders*, 13, 320–323.

―――― 1951. Infant speech: consonantal position. *J. Speech Hearing Disorders*, 16, 159–161.

―――― 1952. Speech development in the young child: II, some factors related to the speech development of the infant and young child. *J. Speech Hearing Disorders*, 17, 269–279.

―――― and CHEN, H. P. 1941. A reliability study of speech sounds observed in the crying of newborn infants. *Child Developm.*, 12, 351–368.

IRWIN, O. C., and CHEN, H. P. 1943. Speech sound elements during the first year of life: review of the literature. *J. Speech Disorders*, 8, #2, 109–121.

—— 1945. Infant speech sounds and intelligence. *J. Speech Disorders*, 10, 293–296.

IRWIN, O. C., and CURRY, T. 1941. Vowel elements in the crying vocalization of infants under ten days of age. *Vowel Developm.*, 12, 99–109.

JAKOBSON, R. 1941. Kindersprache, Aphasie und Allgemeine Laute. Uppsala: Almqvist and Wiksell.

JESPERSEN, O. 1922. Language, its nature, origin and development. New York: Holt.

KARLIN, I. W., and STRAZZULLA, M. 1952. Speech and language problems of mentally deficient children. *J. Speech Hearing Disorders*, 17, 286–294.

KEITH, A. 1915. The antiquity of Man. Philadelphia: Lippincott.

KELLOGG, W. N., and KELLOGG, L. A. 1933. The ape and the child. New York: McGraw-Hill.

KERR, J. G. 1926. Evolution. London: Macmillan.

KEY, T. H. 1874. Language: its origin and development. London: George Bell.

KROEBER, A. L. 1948. Anthropology (rev. ed.). New York: Harcourt, Brace.

KUENNE, M. R. 1946. Experimental investigation of the relation of language to transposition behavior in young children. *J. exp. Psychol.*, 36, 471–490.

LEFÈVRE, A. 1894. Race and language. New York: Appleton. Ch. II, 42–43.

LEOPOLD, W. F. 1937, 1949. Speech development of a bilingual child. Northwestern Univ. Studies, Vols. I–IV.

—— 1952. Bibliography of child language. Evanston: Northwestern Univ. Press.

—— 1953, 1954. Patterning in children's language learning. *Language learning: A J. appl. Linguistics*, 5, Nos. 1 & 2, 1–14.

MCCARTHY, D. A. 1930. Language development of the preschool child. Institution of child welfare monogr. series, #4., Minneapolis: Univ. of Minn. Press, xii & 174.

—— 1946. Language development in children. *In* Carmichael, L. (ed.), Manual of child psychology. New York: Wiley. Pp. 476–581.

—— 1954. Language disorders and parent-child relationships. *J. Speech Hearing Disorders*, 19, 514–523.

MCCREADY, E. B. 1940. The management of defects of speech in children. *Med. Rec.*, 151, 299–303.

MacCURDY, G. G. 1924. Human origins. New York: Appleton.

—— 1932. The coming of man. New York: University Society, Inc.

MCGEOCH, J. A. 1942. The psychology of human learning. New York: Longmans, Green.

MASON, M. K. 1942. Learning to speak after six and one-half years of silence. *J. Speech Disorders*, 7, 295–304.

MAST, S. O., and PUSCH, L. 1924. Modification of response in amoeba. *Biol. Bull.*, 46, 55–59.

MÉTRAUX, R. W. 1950. Speech profiles of the preschool child 18 to 54 months. *J. Speech Hearing Disorders.*, 15, 37–53.

MILLER, G. A. 1951. Language and communication. New York: McGraw-Hill.

MÜLLER, M. 1863 and 1865. Lectures on the science of language. Series I & II. New York: Scribner.

MUNN, N. L. 1946. Learning in children. *In* Carmichael, L. (ed.), Manual of child psychology. New York: Wiley.

—— 1951. Psychology, the fundamentals of human adjustment. Boston: Houghton Mifflin.

NEGUS, V. E. 1929. The mechanism of the larynx. London: Heinemann.

NOIRÉ, L. 1877. Der Ursprung der Sprache. Mainz. *Cited* by Sayce (1883), I, 82.

OGDEN, C. K., and RICHARDS, I. A. 1923. The meaning of meaning. New York: Harcourt, Brace.

PAGET, R. 1930. Human speech. New York: Harcourt, Brace. Ch. 7.

PEACHER, W. G. 1949a. Neurological factors in the etiology of delayed speech. *J. Speech Hearing Disorders*, 14, 147–161.

———— 1949b. The neurological evaluation of delayed speech. *J. Speech Hearing Disorders*, 14, 344–352.

PIAGET, J. 1926. The language and thought of the child. *Translated* by M. Warden. New York: Harcourt, Brace.

PREYER, W. 1889 and 1898. The mind of the child: observations concerning the mental development of the human being in the first years of life. Part II. *Translated* by H. W. Brown. New York: Appleton.

PRONKO, N. H. 1946. Language and psycholinguistics: a review. *Psychol. Bull.*, 43, 226–227.

SANFORD, F. H. 1942. Speech and personality. *Psychol. Bull.*, 39, 811–845.

SAPIR, E. 1921. Language, New York, Harcourt, Brace.

SAYCE, A. H. 1883. Introduction to the science of language (2nd ed.), I. London: Kegan Paul, Trench & Co.

SCHLANGER, B. B. 1954. Environmental influences on the verbal output of mentally retarded children. *J. Speech Hearing Disorders*, 19, 339–343.

SHERMAN, M. 1927. The differentiation of emotional responses in children: II. *J. comp. Psychol.*, 7, 335–351.

SIMON, C. T. 1951. Speech as a science. *Quart. J. Speech*, 37, 283–298.

SKINNER, B. F. 1938. The behavior of organisms. New York: Appleton-Century-Crofts.

SMITH, A. 1792. A dissertation on the origin of language, in the theory of moral sentiments (7th ed.). London: A. Strahan, T. Cadell.

SMITH, G. E. 1932. The discovery of primitive man in China. Annual report of the Smithsonian Institution for 1931. Washington: Government Printing Office.

SPIKER, C. C., and IRWIN, O. C. 1949. The relationship between IQ and indices of infant speech sound development. *J. Speech Hearing Disorders*, 14, 335–343.

STEIN, L. 1949. The infancy of speech and the speech of infancy. London: Methuen.

STINCHFIELD, S. M., and YOUNG, E. H. 1938. Children with delayed or defective speech. Palo Alto, Calif.: Stanford Univ. Press.

STRAYER, L. C. 1930. Language and growth: the relative efficacy of early and deferred vocabulary training studied by the method of co-twin control. *Genet. Psychol. Monogr.*, 8, 209–319.

THORNDIKE, E. L. 1898. Animal intelligence. *Psychol. Rev.*, monogr. suppl., 2, #8.

THORPE, W. H. 1950. The concepts of learning and their relation to those of instinct. *Symposia of the society for experimental biology*. Vol. 4.

TINLEY, F. 1928. The brain from apes to man. New York: Hoeber. Pp. 875–884.

———— 1930. The master of destiny: a biography of the brain. New York: Doubleday, Doran.

TOLMAN, E. C. 1932. Purposive behavior in animals and men. New York: Appleton.

TRACY, F. 1893. The language of childhood. *Amer. J. Psychol.*, 6, 107–138.

VAN RIPER, C. 1954. Speech correction principles and methods (3rd ed.). New York: Prentice-Hall.

VON FRISCH, K. 1950. Bees, their vision, chemical senses and language. Ithaca: Cornell Univ. Press.

VON HERDER, J. G. 1772. Ursprung der Sprache. Prize essay before the Berlin Academy. *Cited* by Jespersen (1922), 26–29.

WEIDENREICH, F. 1945. Giant early man from Java and South China. Anthropological papers of the American Museum of Natural History of New York.

———— 1946. Apes, giants and men. Chicago: Univ. Chicago Press.

WHITNEY, W. D. 1868. Language and the study of languages. Lecture XI. New York: Charles Scribner's.

———— 1875. Life and growth of language. London: Henry S. King & Co.

WILLIAMS, H. M. 1937. An analytical study of language achievement in preschool children. Univ. Iowa studies in child welfare. 13, #2, 35–46.

WUNDT, W. 1897. Outlines of psychology. Leipzig: W. Engelman.

———— 1916. Elements of folk psychology. *Translated* by E. L. Schaub. New York: Macmillan.

YACORZYNSKI, G. 1951. Medical psychology. New York: Ronald Press.

ZIPF, G. K. 1949. Human behavior and the principle of least effort. Cambridge: Addison-Wesley.

CHAPTER 2

# TERMINOLOGY AND NOMENCLATURE

● *Kenneth Scott Wood, Ph.D.*

## GENERAL PROBLEMS

ALL AREAS OF SCIENTIFIC STUDY are afflicted with a certain amount of ambiguity, duplication, inappropriateness, and disagreement in the use of terms.
Like other sciences, speech pathology and the entire cluster of studies associated with the production and perception of speech have been developing
over the years a terminology and nomenclature which leave much to be
desired in the way of logic and stability. Many terms and their meanings are
not well crystallized because the subject matter is ever changing, concepts
themselves are often tentative and fluid, and many writers have liberally
coined new terms whenever they felt a need to do so. The growth of speech
pathology, stimulated as it has been by so many different workers, has generated hundreds of terms, some of which are interchangeable, some of which
have different meanings to different people, some of which are now rare or
obsolete, and some of which for various reasons have had only a short
literary life.

Hammond and Allen (1953) in an exploratory study asked a number of
psychiatric social workers, graduate students in psychology, and practicing
clinical psychologists to define 61 terms which are often used in clinical reports. They found a relatively high percentage of the words inadequately,
vaguely, and even absolutely incorrectly defined.

When the graduate student is required to read a great quantity of technical literature in a limited time, many of the words he encounters at first sight
are unfamiliar to him. He may look these words up, but usually he does not
because his time is limited and the context frequently makes the word intelligible. As he continues his reading, these words are encountered again and
again, and they become familiar to him. Consequently, even though the
words are imperfectly understood, or their meanings only guessed at, the
student uncritically assumes that he knows their full meanings. Thus, he fails
to form habits of verbal accuracy. When the meanings of some technical
words are still not agreed upon and different authorities use the same term to
mean different things, the whole problem of accuracy is aggravated.

To take another example from psychology, Grayson and Tolman (1950) studied the possibility of semantic differences in the use of psychological terms as an obstacle to interprofessional understanding. They selected 50 words appearing with greatest frequency in psychological reports and analyzed the definitions returned by 20 psychologists and 17 psychiatrists together with definitions of the same words appearing in six authoritative sources. The definitions of the first 20 words were analyzed by establishing the number of words used in each definition and by placing each definition in the conceptual response category into which each fell.

In the quantitative analysis, psychologists were found to be more verbose and circuitous in their definitions than were the psychiatrists. This was true whether the terms were psychological, psychiatric, or psychoanalytical ones. Further analysis showed that only rarely did as many as 75 per cent of the definition responses for each term fall into a single category. It was concluded that although a central core of meaning tended to prevail, wide variations occurred. The most striking finding of this study was the looseness and ambiguity of the definitions of most of the terms. It was pointed out that verbalization and conceptualization have clearly lagged behind the useful application of psychological terms and that the lack of verbal precision seems to stem from theoretical confusion in the face of complexity and logical inconsistency of psychological phenomena. Grayson and Tolman (1950, p. 229) state: "Verbal discrepancies can only be reconciled by a deeper understanding of these underlying phenomena which will require many years of careful, penetrating, and analytical psychological experience."

Johnson and Wilson (1945) found a low degree of agreement among 20 psychologists as to the applicability of three words—*hypothesis, theory,* and *law*—to a group of 20 statements each of which had been labeled in one of three ways by the original author of the statement. This study concludes that lack of such basic agreement might well account for a considerable portion of the controversy existing in the field of psychology.

The problems in the terminology of psychology and psychiatry probably apply with equal force to speech pathology, since all deal with aspects of persons and their behavior. When confusions pose a threat to adequate communication among those who are interested in the nature and correction of failures in the communication process itself, it is important to give some direct attention to terminology. The student should keep in mind, however, that there will always be a considerable number of irreducible ambiguities and confusions which he will just have to learn to tolerate. It remains for him to understand in each instance the nature of the ambiguity and the reasons why it exists. Improving terminology is not so simple a task as getting "a definition-cutter with his logical scissors" to straighten matters out once and for all. It is not the function of a glossary or dictionary to create terms or to assign meanings; they should clarify and reflect, insofar as possible, the usages among the professional members of the field.

## LEARNING TERMS AND NAMES

The acquisition of terms and the things, processes, and concepts for which they stand is an important part of securing a working knowledge in speech pathology; but the student entering this field cannot acquire his terminology in advance of his basic knowledge. The real meanings of terms are never learned first. They are acquired simultaneously with concepts, or they come later. In a sense, all speech pathologists are continually enriching, expanding, and qualifying the terms they know. The real meanings and implications of terms are learned not so much from linguistic context or from dictionaries and glossaries as they are learned operationally and empirically. Defining terms by circumlocution with a generic vocabulary may help some, but a term like *aphasia,* for example, can never really be comprehended until the student observes and relates himself to persons with *aphasic* symptoms. There are, on the other hand, things the student can learn about certain terms which will help to clarify his concepts before the relatively slow dawn of term-meaning comes to him from the context itself. For example, if he knows that striated muscles are often named by their points of attachment, the meanings of terms such as *thyroarytenoid* and *cricothyroid* are more readily attainable.

If the student will get acquainted with some of the Greek and Latin roots, prefixes, and suffixes, he may be able to formulate central meanings of many terms even though the current meanings may have twisted away from the significance of the roots. The etymology or history of a term often yields a good beginning clue to its meaning and lends to it semantic reinforcement. For example, if one learns that *thyro* comes from a Greek word meaning "shield" and that *oid* is a suffix meaning "form," he may visualize the *thyroid cartilage* as having the shape of a shield, thus enriching his concept. It is possible to learn terms by rote without ever seeing any logical relationship between the term and its meaning, but they are probably less easily remembered. It is much easier to remember the location of the *adrenal glands* when it is known that *ad* means "near" and *renal* means "kidney." As a further example, it will serve the student to know at the beginning that the prefix *para* carries the meaning of "faulty" and "disordered" and that *dys* means "bad" or "ill." From this he will have a better start on such words as *paralalia, parasigmatism, dyslexia,* and *dysphasia.*

It should, of course, be held in mind that the acquisition of terminology in any field is always related to the general vocabulary of the student. In many cases, when the student has difficulty with the technical vocabulary, his real trouble is traceable to the fact that he does not know the meanings of more commonly used words.

The glossaries of earlier works in speech pathology include terms which properly belong to such fields as anatomy, psychology, orthopedics, neurology, physics, and medicine; but they are included because they are commonly referred to in speech pathology. The name of every muscle, nerve, and sense organ directly related to the speech process is necessarily part of the terminology of this field. The terms speech pathology has borrowed from other fields are evidence that it is closely related to these many fields. They are signs of a natural eclecticism. It makes little difference as to which field a term originally belonged—if there is a need for it in speech pathology, it becomes part of the terminology of this field.

Because there is no limit to the acquisition of terms from other fields, the first and central concern of the student should be to master as soon as possible a core terminology which represents specific speech defects as symptoms, as collections of symptoms, and as having predominating psychological or somatic causes. It should be learned early that some terms designating speech defects refer to symptoms, as in the case of *idiolalia* or *invented language;* others refer to cause, as in the case of *uraniscolalia* or *speech difficulty due to cleft palate;* and still other terms refer to both the symptoms and cause, as in the case of *deaf-mutism.* Meanings of the core terms may often be acquired first from the general definitions; these then become more and more specific in context. Often it will be helpful to have a means of checking back to the general definitions when terms are found in contexts which do not adequately clarify them.

The student or professional worker in speech pathology will be continually involved in three types of communication: He will be reading the literature in the field; he will be talking about speech pathology in various situations; and he will be writing clinical reports for professional purposes or writing for publication. In all of these communication functions, his ability to use and understand appropriate terminology and nomenclature is of signal importance. It is important enough to warrant a direct approach to the development of a technical vocabulary.

## ANATOMICAL TERMS

In 1895 the Anatomical Society, meeting in international convention in Basle, Switzerland, adopted a list of nearly 5,000 anatomical terms which are known today as the B.N.A. (Basle Nomina Anatomica). This is the system of terminology now used in anatomy, although it has been under revision for some time in an attempt to decrease the number of terms and to make them simpler. Many muscles of the body have two names, one in Latin and one in English. Some muscles have more than one Latin name, and some have Anglicized versions of the B.N.A. names.

Muscles are named on the basis of several characteristics: (1) their shape, such as the *orbicularis oris* which is circular; (2) their location, such as the *buccinator* which is situated in the cheek; (3) the direction in which their fibers run, such as the *transversus linguae* with fibers running across the tongue; (4) the number of their divisions, such as the *quadriceps femoris* consisting of four muscles attached to a common tendon; (5) their action, such as the *levator palati* which raises the soft palate; and (6) their points of attachment, such as the *glossopalatinus* with one end attached to the tongue and the other to the soft palate.

Nerves are similarly named according to their locations, the structures they serve, their arrangement, and their functions.

## A GLOSSARY OF TERMS FREQUENTLY USED
## IN SPEECH PATHOLOGY

*abdominal muscles:* rectus abdominis, transversus abdominis, obliquus internus abdominis, and obliquus externus abdominis; muscles in the abdominal wall important in exhalation because they compress the viscera.

*abducent n.:* VIth Cranial nerve; innervates the external rectus muscle of the eye.

*abduct:* to draw away from the axis of the body; to move away from the midline or from a neighboring part or limb; opposite to *adduct.*

*aberration:* deviation from the usual course; a disordered mental state.

*ablate:* to remove, especially by cutting.

*abreaction:* the process of acting off, working off, or discharging original, repressed feelings by living through them again in speech or action, usually in the presence of the psychoanalyst.

*abscissa:* the horizontal axis of reference in a two-dimensional graph. Dist. from *ordinate.*

*acalculia:* inability to do simple arithmetic.

*accent:* an articulative effort giving prominence or stress to one syllable of a word or group of words over adjacent syllables.

*accessory n.:* same as *spinal accessory nerve.*

*acoustic n.:* the sensory nerve for hearing and equilibration; the VIIIth Cranial nerve having two roots, the vestibular branch originating in the vestibule and the semicircular canals and the cochlear branch originating in the cochlea.

*acoustic spectrum:* the distribution of the intensity levels of the various frequency components of a sound.

*acoustics:* the science of sound including the production, transmission, and effects of mechanical vibrations and waves in any medium, whether audible or not.

*adduct:* to draw toward the midline or toward the axis of the body. Opp. to *abduct.*

*adenoids:* a mass of lymphoid tissue located in about the center of the posterior wall of the nasopharynx; the pharyngeal tonsil, but commonly called *adenoids.*

*adiadochokinesis:* inability to perform rapid alternating movements such as opening and closing the jaws or lips, raising and lowering the eyebrows, or tapping the finger.

*aditus laryngis:* that part of the laryngeal cavity above the glottis.

*adrenal gland:* a ductless gland located at the upper end of each kidney. Same as *suprarenal gland.*

*aerophagia:* spasmodic swallowing of air followed by belching.

*affective:* an adjective connoting any variety of feeling, emotional experience, or emotional accompaniment.

*afferent:* conducting toward the brain or spinal cord; refers to nerves which convey sensory impulses from the periphery to the central nervous system. Opp. to *efferent.*

*affricate:* a fricative speech sound initiated by a plosive. Examples are [tʃ] as in *chew* and [dʒ] as in *jam.*

*agitographia:* extremely rapid writing with unconscious omission and distortion of letters, words, or parts of words.

*agitophasia:* extremely rapid speech in which sounds, words, or parts of words are unconsciously omitted or distorted. Same as *agitolalia.*

*agnosia:* loss of the function of recognition of individual sensory stimuli; varieties correspond with the several senses.

*agonist:* a contracting muscle opposed in action by another muscle called the *antagonist.*

*agrammalogia:* inability to produce words in their correct sequence; impairment of the power to speak grammatically and syntactically. Same as *agrammatalogia, agrammatica,* and *agrammatism.*

*agraphia:* inability to express thoughts in writing due to a lesion in the central nervous system.

*air blade:* descriptive of friction sounds emitted through an opening that is wide horizontally and very narrow vertically as in the sound of [f].

*air conduction:* the normal process of conducting sound waves through the ear canal to the drum membrane. Dist. from *bone conduction.*

*alalia:* inability to speak due to impairment or absence of one or more of the peripheral speech organs, that is, impairment of muscles and sense organs involved in speech.

*alexia:* complete inability to read, characterized by an associative learning disability. See *dyslexia.*

*alogia:* inability to speak due to a lesion in the central nervous system or to mental impairment.

*alpha wave:* a type of brain wave registered by an electroencephalograph representing about ten major discharges of cortical cells per second. Alpha rhythm is relatively low in frequency and high in voltage and is associated with reduced levels of consciousness. Dist. from *beta wave.*

*alveolar ridge:* the upper or lower gum ridge containing the row of sockets which enclose the teeth.

*alveolus:* tooth socket; also, an air sac of the lung.

*ambidextrous:* able to use either hand effectively.

*ambivalence:* the simultaneous existence of contradictory and contrasting emotions toward the same person; Bleuler's term for the tendency of some patients to give expression equally to opposing impulses.

*amentia:* a permanent form of mental retardation with a wide variety of clinical manifestations; mental deficiency based on congenital or developmental factors which retard the rate of maturing and reduce the ultimate level of behavior. Dist. from *dementia.*

*amnesia:* a disorder characterized by partial or total inability to recall or to identify past experiences; lack or loss of memory.

*amplitude:* largeness; wideness, breadth of range or extent; the distance through space a vibrating body moves; directly related to intensity of sound and sometimes used synonymously with *intensity* and *volume.*

*amusia:* inability to produce or to comprehend musical sounds.

*anacusis:* total deafness. Same as *anakusis.*

*anesthesia:* loss of feeling or sensation.

*anarthria:* inability to articulate due to brain lesion or damage to peripheral nerves which innervate the articulatory muscles.

*aneurysm:* a sac formed by the dilation of the walls of an artery or vein and filled with blood.

*angular gyrus:* a convolution of the cerebral cortex continuous anteriorly with the supramarginal gyrus; in the left hemisphere a probable center for some of the functions of speech.

*ankylosis:* the stiffening of a joint which impairs articulation of the bones at the joint.

*annular:* shaped like a ring.

*anomaly:* a structure or a function which deviates from the normal.

*anomia:* loss of the power to name objects or to recall and recognize names.

*anorexia:* lack or loss of appetite for food.

*anoxemia:* deficiency in the oxygen content of the blood.

*antagonist:* a muscle which acts in opposition to another muscle. Opp. to *agonist.*

*anterior:* situated in front of or in the forward part of; toward the head end of the body; also, toward the ventral side. Opp. to *posterior.*

*antitropy:* a condition in which an organ forms a symmetrical pair with another; such as the cerebral hemispheres.

*aphasia:* loss of symbolic formulation and expression due to brain lesion. See *dysphasia.*

*aphemia:* inability to speak due to a lesion of the central nervous system; term originally used by Broca and later supplanted by the term *aphasia.*

*aphonia:* loss or absence of voice as a result of the failure of the vocal cords to vibrate properly.

*aphrasia:* inability to speak in phrases or to understand words arranged in phrases.

*aplasia:* incomplete or defective development of tissue.

*apperception:* focused perception, as exhibited in the relative clearness or prominence of certain of the data in perception.

*apraxia:* loss of the ability to execute simple voluntary acts; especially loss of the ability to perform elementary units of action in the expression of language.

*articulation:* literally the state of being united by a joint or joints; in speech, the production of individual sounds in connected discourse; the movement and placement during speech of the organs which serve to interrupt or modify the voiced or unvoiced air stream into meaningful sounds; the speech function performed largely through the movements of the lower jaw, lips, tongue, and soft palate.

*aryepiglottic:* pertaining to the arytenoid cartilage and to the epiglottis.

*arytenoid:* shaped like a pitcher; one of a pair of cartilages mounted on the cricoid cartilage and attached to the vocal band at the posterior end. The movement of the arytenoids approximate the vocal bands.

*aspirate:* a phonetic unit whose identifying characteristic is the sound generated by the passage of air through a relatively open channel; the sound of [h]; a sound followed by or combined with the sound of [h].

*assimilation:* a process of adaptive change in speech sounds uttered in close sequence. When two sounds become contiguous, one or both may undergo changes which make each more like its neighbor.

*atavism:* the reappearance of long-absent or dormant characteristics after one or more generations.

*ataxia:* a disorder characterized by marked disturbance in muscular co-ordination; irregularity of muscular action.

*athetosis:* a recurring series of slow, twisting movements of the skeletal musculature due principally to brain lesion.

*attenuate:* to reduce in intensity or amount.

*atrophy:* a wasting away or diminution in the size of cell, tissue, organ, or part.

*audiogram:* a graphic summary of the measurements of hearing loss showing number of decibels loss at each frequency tested.

*audiology:* the study of the entire field of hearing including the anatomy and function of the ear, impairment of hearing, and the education or re-education of the person with hearing loss.

*audiometer:* a device for the testing of hearing; it is calibrated to register hearing loss in terms of decibels.

*auditory aphasia:* defect, loss, or nondevelopment of the ability to comprehend spoken words, due to disease, injury, or maldevelopment of the hearing centers of the brain; word deafness. Same as *receptive aphasia.*

*auditory discrimination:* ability to discriminate between sounds of different frequency, intensity, and pressure-pattern components; ability to distinguish one speech-sound from another.

*auditory memory span:* the number of related or unrelated items that can be recalled immediately after hearing them presented.

*auditory perception:* mental awareness of sound.

*aural:* pertaining to the ear or to the sensation of hearing. Same as *auditory.*

*auricle:* the portion of the external ear not contained within the head. Same as *pinna.*

*auscultation:* the act of listening for sounds within the body.

*automatic speech:* inappropriate words or phrases produced without voluntary control as characteristic of aphasic adults; also, words such as consecutive numbers, days of the week, expletives, and various kinds of accessory expressions.

*autonomic nervous system:* the efferent system of peripheral nerves, ganglia, and plexuses which innervate smooth muscles, gland cells, and the heart. Same as *visceral system.* Dist. from *central nervous system.*

*azygous:* having no fellow; said of an unpaired muscle.

*babbling:* a stage in the acquisition of speech during which the child carries on vocal play with its random production of different speech sounds.

*baby-talk:* a speech defect characterized by substitution of speech sounds similar to those used by the normal-speaking child in the early stages of speech development. Same as *lalling* and *infantile speech.*

*barbaralalia:* habitual use of the speech sounds and rhythmo-melody of a native language when learning to speak another. Same as *foreign accent.*

*basal ganglia:* the collection or mass of nerve cells below the cortex of the brain connecting the cerebrum with the lower centers and comprising the thalami, corpora striata, corpora quadrigemina, tuber cinerum, and geniculate bodies.

*basilar membrane:* the lower boundary of the scala media or middle passage of the cochlear canal in the internal ear.

*Bell's palsy:* paralysis of the facial muscles due to lesion of the seventh cranial or facial nerve resulting in a characteristic distortion of facial symmetry.

*beta wave:* a type of brain wave registered by an electroencephalograph representing about 20–30 discharges of cortical cells per second. Beta rhythm is relatively high in frequency and low in voltage and is associated with heightened states of attention. Dist. from *alpha wave.*

*bicuspid:* having two cusps or points; one of eight premolar teeth in man, two on each side, upper and lower, located between the cuspid and first molar.

*bifurcation:* divided into two branches like a fork.

*bilabial:* used to describe a consonant sound formed with the aid of both lips as in [p], [b], and [m].

*bilingual:* having two native languages; being reared in a two-language environment.

*binaural:* pertaining to both ears.

*B.N.A.:* the system of scientific anatomical terminology adopted by international convention at Basle, Switzerland, in 1895; Basle Nomina Anatomica.

*bone conduction:* the transmission of sound waves through the head bones to the inner ear. Dist. from *air conduction.*

*Broca's area:* the inferior frontal gyrus in the left cerebral hemisphere of right-handed persons identified by Broca in 1861 as the cortical association center for motor speech. Same as *Broca's convolution* or *center.*

*bronchus:* one of two main branches of the trachea.

*buccal:* pertaining to the mouth cavity and the cheeks.

*buccinator:* the flat muscle of the cheek which controls compression and distention of the cheek wall.

*bulbar:* pertaining to the medulla oblongata, the bulb of nervous tissue continuous above with the pons and below with the spinal cord.

*bulbar paralysis:* paralysis due to changes in the motor centers of the medulla oblongata or bulb usually marked by paralysis and atrophy of the muscles of the lips, tongue, mouth, pharynx, and larynx.

*canine:* the single cuspid tooth between the lateral incisor and the premolar. Same as *cuspid.*

*caninus m.:* a muscle originating in the fossa of the maxilla and inserted in the orbicularis oris; it is innervated by the facial (VIIth Cranial) nerve and acts to raise the corners of the mouth.

*catalogia:* the insane repetition of meaningless words and sentences. Same as *verbigeration.*

*catarrhal deafness:* hearing loss caused by inflammation of the mucous membrane of the air passages in the head and throat with blockage of the Eustachian tube.

*catharsis:* see *psychocatharsis.*

*caudal:* toward the tail; in a posterior direction. Opp. to *cephalic.*

*caudate nucleus:* a pear-shaped mass of nerve cells, the largest component of the corpus striatum in the brain; it lies in contact with the cephalic end of the thalamus and has relation to the production of voluntary activity.

*central nervous system:* the brain and the spinal cord; abbreviated *C.N.S.*

*central tendon:* the heart-shaped fibrous cord of connective tissue in which the muscle fibers of the diaphragm end.

*cephalic:* pertaining to the head or directed toward the head end of the body. Opp. to *caudal.*

*cerebellum:* a main division of the brain situated behind the cerebrum and above the pons; it is concerned with the co-ordination of muscular activity.

*cerebral dominance:* a condition in which one cerebral hemisphere leads the other in the initiation and control of bodily movement.

*cerebral palsy:* paralysis or muscular inco-ordination due to intracranial lesion; the term is applied to a group of cerebral afflictions in children including Little's disease, spastic paralysis, and many others.

*cerebrospinal fluid:* the fluid contained within the cerebral ventricles, subarachnoid sinus, and the central canal of the spinal cord.

*cerebrum:* the main portion of the brain consisting of two equal hemispheres united at the bottom by a band of connective tissue called the corpus callosum.

*cerumen:* wax-like secretion found in the external canal of the ear.

*cervical:* pertaining to the region of the neck; the term is applied to the vertebrae and to the nerves distributed in this region.

*chorditis tuberosa:* a small whitish node on one or both vocal bands.

*chorea:* a convulsive nervous disease characterized by involuntary and irregular jerking movements.

*chronic:* long-continued; not sharp, severe, or acute.

*cleft palate:* congenital fissure of the soft palate and roof of the mouth, sometimes extending through the premaxilla and upper lip.

*clinic:* an establishment where patients are admitted for special study and treatment usually by a group of specialists in different areas.

*clinical:* literally, pertaining to the bedside; pertaining to or founded on actual observation and treatment of cases as distinguished from theoretical or experimental; pertaining to individual diagnosis and treatment on the basis of individual symptoms and not on the basis of membership in a stereotyped group.

*clonus:* muscular spasm in which there is an alternation of rigidity and relaxation.

*cluttering:* rapid, nervous speech marked by omission of sounds or syllables.

*cochlea:* the auditory part of the internal ear; it is shaped like a snail shell and contains the basilar membrane upon which are situated the hair cells or end organs of the cochlear branch of the eighth cranial nerve.

*concha:* a structure resembling a shell in shape as the hollow of the external ear or the turbinate bones in the nose.

*conduction deafness:* an impairment of hearing due to damage or obstruction of the ear canal, drum membrane, or the ossicular chain in the middle ear; a failure of air vibrations to be adequately conducted to the cochlea.

*consonant:* a conventional speech sound produced, with or without laryngeal vibration, by certain successive contractions of the articulatory muscles which modify, interrupt, or obstruct the expired air stream to the extent that its pressure is raised.

*continuant:* a speech sound in which the speech organs are held relatively fixed during the period of production. Examples are [s], [m], [f], and the vowels.

*contralateral:* associated with a part on the opposite side.

*conversion:* a psychoanalytical term referring to the transformation of repressed emotions into a physical manifestation as in hysterical deafness or hysterical aphonia.

*corniculate cartilage:* a small nodule at the apex of each arytenoid cartilage in the larynx.

*corpus callosum:* an arched band of white matter whose transverse fibers connect the two cerebral hemispheres at the bottom below the longitudinal fissure.

*cortex:* the outer layers of an organ as distinguished from its inner substance; the cerebral cortex is the ashen-gray matter making up the outer layers of the cerebrum.

*cranial nerve:* a nerve which originates or terminates within the cranium; there are 12 pairs numbered I–XII. Dist. from *spinal nerve.*

*cretinism:* a congenital condition due to thyroid deficiency and characterized by physical and mental retardation.

*cricoarytenoid m.:* an intrinsic muscle of the larynx originating in the side and back of the cricoid cartilage and inserted at the base of the arytenoid cartilages; the lateral pair closes the glottis and the posterior pair opens the glottis; all are innervated by the recurrent laryngeal nerve.

*cricoid cartilage:* a ring-like cartilage forming the lower and back part of the laryngeal cavity.

*cricothyroid m.:* an intrinsic muscle of the larynx originating on the front side of the cricoid cartilage and inserted at the lower border of the thyroid cartilage; it is innervated by the superior laryngeal nerve and acts to tense the vocal bands.

*cuneiform cartilage:* a wedge-shaped cartilage on either side of the aryepiglottic fold in the larynx.

*cuspid:* a tooth having one cusp or point. Same as *canine.*

*cutaneous:* pertaining to the skin.

*cyanosis:* blueness of the skin due to insufficient oxygenation of the blood; usually the result of heart malformation.

*cybernetics:* studies involving the analogous functioning of the nervous system and electro-mechanical control systems such as computing machines.

*damping effect:* diminution of the amplitude of vibrations because of the absorption of energy by the surrounding medium.

*deaf:* pertains to congenital loss of all usable hearing.

*deafen:* pertains to adventitious loss of all usable hearing.

*deaf mute:* a person who can neither hear nor speak; usually one who is born deaf.

*decibel:* a logarithmic ratio unit indicating by what proportion one intensity level differs from another; the decibel is equal to approximately one just-noticeable-difference of loudness under certain conditions; sometimes inaccurately called a *sensation unit.*

*decussation:* the crossing of nerve tracts in their course to or from lower centers of the central nervous system.

*delayed speech:* failure of speech to develop at the expected age; usually due to slow maturation, hearing impairment, brain injury, mental retardation, or emotional disturbance.

*denasality:* pertains to the quality of the voice when the nasal passages are obstructed to prevent adequate nasal resonance during speech.

*dental:* a speech sound made by tongue or lip contact with the teeth; pertaining to teeth.

*dextral:* pertaining to or located on the right side of the body. Opp. to *sinistral.*

*diadochokinesis:* the performance of repetitive movements such as lowering and raising the mandible, occluding and opening the lips, and tapping with the finger.

*diagnosis:* the study of the nature of a disorder, its origin, development, and symptoms; also the identification of a disorder by such procedure.

*diaphragm:* the muscular and tendonous partition which separates the abdominal and thoracic cavities; the chief muscle in breathing.

*diathesis:* an inherited tendency or predisposition to certain diseases or disorders.

*diphthong:* a speech sound gliding continuously from one vowel to another in the same syllable such as [ɑʊ], [ɔɪ], and [ɑɪ].

*dorsal:* the back side; pertains to any part which corresponds to the back in position. Opp. to *ventral.*

*drum membrane:* the ear drum or membrane which separates the external ear from the middle ear. Same as *tympanic membrane.*

*dyne:* a unit of force; the amount of energy required to move one gram a distance of one centimeter in one second.

*dysarthria:* a disorder of articulation due to impairment of the part of the central nervous system which directly controls the muscles of articulation.

*dyslalia:* defective articulation due to faulty learning or to abnormality of the external speech organs and not due to lesions of the central nervous system.

*dyslexia:* partial inability to read characterized by associative learning difficulty; a form of dysphasia. See *alexia.*

*dyslogia:* defective speech associated with mental impairment.

*dysphasia:* partial or complete loss of the ability to speak or to comprehend the spoken word due to injury, disease, or maldevelopment of the brain. Same as *aphasia*.

*dysphemia:* a nervous disorder of speech arising from psychological disturbance; includes stuttering.

*dysphonia:* a disturbance of vocalization; any defect of phonation.

*dysrhythmia:* abnormality in speech rhythm characterized by defects of stress placement, defects of breath-grouping, or defects of inflection.

*ear canal:* see *external auditory meatus*.

*echolalia:* automatic reiteration of words or phrases, usually those which have just been heard.

*efferent:* conducting from a central region to a peripheral region; refers to nerves which convey motor impulses from the central nervous system to the muscles. Opp. to *afferent*.

*elasticity:* the capacity of a body to return to its original form or position after deformation by some applied force.

*electroencephalograph:* an instrument for graphically recording electrical currents developed in the cerebral cortex during brain functioning; often abbreviated EEG.

*emphasis:* a prominence of utterance given to one or more words or syllables.

*encephalitis:* inflammation of the brain or its membranous envelopes.

*endolymph:* the fluid contained in the labyrinth of the inner ear.

*enuresis:* involuntary discharge of urine.

*epiglottis:* a lid-like cartilage, shaped like a bicycle seat, which covers the entrance to the laryngeal cavity.

*epilepsy:* a chronic functional disease characterized by convulsions and loss of consciousness for short periods; the mild form is called *petit mal* and the severe form *grand mal*.

*epileptiform:* refers to behavior which resembles manifestations of epilepsy.

*esophageal voice:* low-frequency vibrations produced by the upper narrow portion of the esophagus when swallowed air bubbles are belched out.

*ethmoid bone:* the sieve-like bone which forms a roof for the nasal hollows and a portion of the floor of the anterior fossa of the cranium.

*etiology:* the study of causes of a given condition.

*euphoria:* bodily comfort; well-being; sometimes a pathological mental state characterized by unfounded feelings of optimism, strength, or health.

*Eustachian tube:* a channel about 35 mm. long connecting the tympanic cavity with the nasopharynx and serving to adjust air pressure within the tympanic cavity to that of the air on the external side of the drum membrane.

*experimental phonetics:* a laboratory science concerned with measurement, description, and analysis of speech signals, their production, and the processes by which they are perceived and interpreted; sometimes the same as *voice science*.

*expiration:* the act of breathing out and expelling air from the lungs.

*expressive aphasia:* a disturbance of speech due to brain lesion and in which the major difficulty is inability to remember the pattern of movements required to produce words even though the patient knows what he wants to say.

*extensor:* any muscle which functions to extend the organ to which it is attached. Opp. to *flexor*.

*external auditory meatus:* the passage through the temporal bone from the external ear to the tympanic cavity of the middle ear where it is sealed by the drum membrane.

*extrapyramidal tract:* outside the pyramidal tracts.

*extrinsic muscle:* a muscle whose origin and insertion are not in the same organ or part; a muscle which connects an organ to the bony skeleton or to other organs or parts. Dist. from *intrinsic muscle.*

*facial n.:* the VIIth Cranial nerve, motor to the muscles of the face.

*falsetto:* the artificial voice of the male lying above his natural range of pitch.

*fauces:* the passage between the mouth and the pharynx.

*febrile:* pertaining to fever.

*fenestra ovalis:* an oval opening in the inner wall of the middle ear into which the footplate of the stapes is inserted. Same as *oval window.*

*fenestra rotunda:* a round opening in the inner wall of the middle ear below the oval window and covered by a membrane permitting accommodation of pressure on the fluid in the cochlea. Same as *round window.*

*fenestration:* the act of perforation; specifically, the operation for improvement of hearing in otosclerotic conditions in which a substitute "window" is formed in the bony wall of the middle ear and into the horizontal semicircular canal in order to enable sound waves to excite the cochlea.

*finger-spelling:* the use of the manual alphabet to spell out words for the deaf.

*flaccid paralysis:* paralysis with loss of tonus and absence of reflexes in the affected parts producing a weak, flabby, and relaxed condition. Dist. from *spastic paralysis.*

*flexor:* any muscle which flexes or bends a joint. Opp. to *extensor.*

*foreign accent:* the influence of speech sounds of a native language on those of a later learned second language.

*fossa:* a pit, depression, hollow, or trench.

*Fourier analysis:* application of a mathematical principle according to which any complex sound may be represented as the sum of a series of pure tones whose frequencies increase in the ratio of the natural numbers 1, 2, 3, 4, 5, etc.; resolving complex vibrations into single components.

*free field testing:* a method of measuring auditory sensitivity by reducing sound intensity to the threshold of perception and measuring the actual intensity of the sound after the subject has been removed from the field in order to eliminate the effect of absorption, reflection, and diffraction by the body.

*frenum:* a fold of the skin or mucous membrane which checks or limits the movements of an organ or part; usually the lingual frenum under the tongue.

*frequency:* the number of cycles per second of a wave or other periodic phenomenon.

*fricative:* any speech sound produced by forcing an air stream through a narrow opening and resulting in audible high-frequency vibrations. Examples are [f], [ʃ], and [v].

*frontal lobe:* that part of either hemisphere of the cerebrum which lies above the Sylvian fissure and in front of the Rolandic fissure.

*functional defect:* any defect in which structural alteration can be neither demonstrated nor inferred. Dist. from *organic defect.*

*fundamental tone:* the lowest tone in a complex tone. Dist. from *overtone.*

*general semantics:* an adaptation of the science of meaning developed by Alfred Korzybski and applied to human problems; a collection of such doctrines aimed at improving interpersonal adjustment by securing better orientational adequacy of word-fact relationship.

*genioglossus m.:* a muscle originating in the mental spine of the mandible and inserted in the under surface of the tongue and in the hyoid bone; it is innervated by the hypoglossal nerve and acts to depress, retract, and protrude the tongue.

*glossal:* pertaining to the tongue.

*glossopalatinus m.:* a muscle originating in the under surface of the soft palate and inserted in the side of the tongue; it lifts the back of the tongue and narrows the fauces.

*glossopharyngeal n.:* the IXth Cranial nerve; distributed to the middle ear, pharynx, meninges, tonsils, and tongue; serves the taste receptors in the back of the tongue and motor functions of the throat.

*glottis:* the opening between the vocal bands.

*gutturophonia:* a form of dysphonia characterized by a throaty or guttural voice.

*gyrus:* a fold or convolution of the cerebral cortex bounded by fissures and sulci.

*hard-of-hearing:* applied to those whose hearing is impaired but who have enough hearing left for practical use.

*hard palate:* the bony anterior part of the roof of the mouth.

*harelip:* a congenital cleft of one or both of the lips, usually the upper lip.

*harmonic:* a partial tone or overtone whose frequency is an exact multiple of the lowest or fundamental tone.

*hearing aid:* any device which amplifies or focuses sound waves in the listener's ear; usually refers to the various types of wearable amplifiers which operate with miniature loudspeakers in the ear or oscillators on the head.

*heliocotrema:* a small opening in the basilar membrane at the apex of the cochlear canal through which the scala tympani communicates with the scala vestibuli.

*helix:* the margin or curved border of the pinna or outer ear.

*hemiatrophy:* atrophy or wasting away of one side of the body, organ, or part. See *atrophy.*

*hemorrhage:* escape of blood from ruptured vessels.

*hyoglossus m.:* an extrinsic tongue muscle; it is innervated by the hypoglossal nerve and acts to depress the sides of the tongue and retract the tongue.

*hyoid bone:* a horseshoe-shaped bone situated at the base of the tongue and above the thyroid cartilage.

*hypacusis:* same as *hard-of-hearing.*

*hypertonicity:* excessive tonus, tension, or activity. Same as *hypertonia.*

*hypertrophy:* the morbid enlargement or overgrowth of an organ or part due to increase in its tissue elements.

*hypnosis:* an artificially induced state resembling sleep but physiologically distinct from it and characterized by increased suggestibility.

*hypochondria:* morbid anxiety about health and pessimistic interpretation of bodily discomfort.

*hypoglossal n.:* the XIIth Cranial nerve; it innervates the hypoglossus muscle of the tongue.

*hypophonia:* a form of dysphonia characterized by a whispered voice.

*hypoplasia:* defective or incomplete development.

*idioglossia:* omission, substitution, distortion, and transposition of so many sounds that speech is unintelligible and appears to be an invented language; often associated with mental retardation. Same as *idiolalia.*

*idiolalia:* see *idioglossia.*

*idiopathic:* pertains to a pathological condition of spontaneous origin; that is, not the result of some other disorder or injury.

*implosion:* the process of building up internal pressure in the air tract immediately prior to its explosive release in the production of plosive speech sounds.

*incisor:* any one of the four front teeth in either the upper or lower jaw.

*incus:* the anvil-shaped middle bone of the three ossicles in the middle ear.

*infantile speech:* see *baby-talk.*

*inferior:* situated below.

*information theory:* a broad theory of communication which treats quantitatively the probability and accuracy of events in the transmission and translation of messages composed of symbols.

*inner speech:* the mental image of words in terms of visual, auditory, and kinesthetic sensations.

*innervation:* the supplying of any organ with efferent nerve impulses.

*insertion:* the place of attachment of a muscle to the bone it moves.

*insight:* a sudden apprehension of meaning without reference to previous experience.

*intensity:* the magnitude or degree of tension, activity, or energy; refers to the measure of the pressure or energy flow acting to produce a sound wave.

*intercostal:* situated between the ribs.

*interdental sigmatism:* substitution of [θ] and [ð] for [s] and [z]. See *lisping.*

*introjection:* the mental process of absorbing or appropriating the attributes of others into one's own personality system.

*intrinsic muscle:* a muscle whose origin and insertion are in the same organ; any muscle which lies wholly within a given organ. Dist. from *extrinsic muscle.*

*ipsilateral:* situated on the same side. Opp. to *contralateral.*


*kinesthetic:* pertaining to the sense by which muscular motion, position, or weight are perceived.

*kymograph:* an instrument used to record variations in any physiological or muscular process.


*labial:* pertaining to the lips; a speech sound produced with the aid of the lips. Examples are [p], [b], and [m].

*labio-dental:* a speech sound produced by the contact of the lips with the teeth. Examples are [f] and [v].

*labyrinth:* the ramified passages of the internal ear made up of the cochlea, vestibule, and semicircular canals.

*lalling:* a babbling, infantile form of speech.

*lalopathy:* any form of speech disorder.

*language:* any means, vocal or other, of expressing or communicating thought or feeling.

*laryngectomy:* surgical removal of the larynx, usually because of cancer.

*laryngitis:* inflammation of the larynx often resulting in hoarseness or loss of voice.

*laryngology:* the study and treatment of the throat, pharynx, larynx, nasopharynx, trachea, and bronchial tree.

*laryngopharynx:* the lower portion of the pharynx lying between the larynx and the oropharynx.

*laryngoscope:* an apparatus used for visual examination of the larynx.

*larynx:* the cartilaginous and muscular structure situated at the top of the trachea and below the tongue roots and hyoid bone; the organ of voice consisting of nine cartilages connected by ligaments.

*lateral:* pertaining to a side.

*lateral lisping:* defective production of the sibilant sounds due to excessive escape of air over or around the sides of the tongue.

*laterality:* sidedness; handedness.

*lesion:* an injury or wound in any part of the body; deficit of tissue.

*levator:* any muscle concerned with lifting an organ or part.

*levator veli palatini m.:* a muscle which raises the soft palate.

*ligament:* a tough, fibrous band of tissue connecting bones or cartilages.

*ligate:* to tie or bind.

*lingua-dental:* a speech sound produced with the aid of the tongue and teeth. Examples are [θ] and [ð].

*lingual:* pertaining to the tongue.

*linguistics:* the study of the origin, structure, and modifications of speech; it includes phonetics, morphology, and semantics.

*lip-reading:* the art of comprehending the speech of another through the visual interpretation of gestures, facial movements, and especially lip movements. Same as *speech-reading.*

*lisping:* defective production of the sibilant sounds, caused by improper tongue placement or by abnormalities of the articulatory mechanism.

*logopedics:* the study and treatment of speech defects.

*logorrhea:* a mental aberration characterized by continuous, incoherent talking.

*longitudinal:* lengthwise, running in the direction of the long axis of the body, organ, or part.

*longitudinalis inferior m.:* a muscle originating in the under surface of the tongue at its base and inserted in the tip; it is innervated by the *chorda tympani* and acts to shorten the tongue.

*longitudinalis superior m.:* a muscle originating in the submucosa and septum of the tongue and inserted in the edges of the tongue; it is innervated by the hypoglossal (XIIth Cranial) nerve and acts to shorten the tongue and to raise its edges and tip.

*loudness:* the intensity factor in sound.

*lumen:* the area of the interior cross section of a tube.


*macroglossia:* an abnormally large tongue.

*malingering:* the pretending of illness or disability.

*malleus:* the first of the ossicles in the middle ear joining the drum membrane to the incus.

*malocclusion:* a condition in which the teeth do not come together properly due to malformation.

*mandible:* the lower jaw.

*manualism:* a method of instruction for the deaf in which the chief element is communication by means of finger-spelling and sign language.

*masking:* a partial or complete obscuring of a tone by the simultaneous presentation in one or both ears of another sound of different frequency.

*masseter m.:* the large chewing muscle; it originates in the upper maxilla and is inserted in the lower jaw; it is innervated by the mandibular branch of the trigeminal nerve.

*mastoid:* pertaining to the mastoid process located just behind the ear.

*maxilla:* the irregularly shaped bone articulated with the ethmoid bone and forming the upper jaw.

*meatus:* a canal. Same as *external auditory meatus.*

*medial:* pertaining to the middle; near the median plane.

*medulla oblongata:* the portion of the brain which is continuous with the spinal cord below and the pons above; it lies ventral to the cerebellum and its back forms the floor of the fourth ventricle.

*melancholia:* a form of mental disorder marked by depressed and painful emotional states with inhibited mental and bodily activity.

*meninges:* the three membranes which envelop the brain and spinal cord; the *dura mater, pia mater,* and *arachnoid mater.*

*meningitis:* inflammation of the meninges.

*mental:* pertaining to the chin, from *mentum;* also pertaining to the mind, from *mens.*

*mentalis m.:* a muscle originating in the mandible and inserted in the skin of the chin; it is innervated by the facial (VIIth Cranial) nerve and acts to raise the lower lip and wrinkle the skin of the chin.

*microglossia:* an abnormally small tongue.

*mirror writing:* the tendency to write mirrored forms of letters, words, and numbers so that they are read correctly when seen in a mirror.

*modiolus:* the central column or pillar of the cochlea.

*molar:* one of the back grinding teeth of which there are three on each side in both jaws.

*mongolism:* congenital mental defection marked by hyperactivity, imitativeness, malformation of the skull, oblique eye-slits, and shortness of thumbs and little finger.

*motor aphasia:* See *expressive aphasia.*

*moto-kinesthetic method:* a method for developing speech in which the therapist manually manipulates some of the speech muscles of the patient or touches parts to suggest movement at that point.

*mucous membrane:* a membrane which secretes a viscid, watery substance called mucus.

*musculus uvulae:* an unpaired muscle originating in the posterior nasal spine and forming the greater part of the uvula; it acts to raise and shrivel the uvula.

*mutism:* inability to speak due to hysteria, abnormal inhibition, or deafness.

*myotatic reflex:* a reflex contraction of a muscle by suddenly stretching it longitudinally.

*nares:* the nostrils, both anterior and posterior.

*nasal:* pertaining to the nose; also a voiced continuant speech sound having nasal resonance as its distinctive acoustic characteristic. Examples are [m], [n], and [ŋ].

*nasal septum:* the partition in the midplane which separates the two nasal cavities.

*nasality:* the quality of speech sounds when the nasal cavity is used as a resonator; especially when there is too much nasal resonance.

*nasopharynx:* the portion of the pharynx above the level of the soft palate.

*nasoscope:* an instrument used to inspect the nasal cavity.

*negative practice:* the deliberate and voluntary practicing of errors in order to break habits which have become automatic.

*neologism:* a new word; also a meaningless word spoken by a psychotic patient.

*neurasthenia:* nervous exhaustion; a psychoneurosis characterized by abnormal fatigue.

*neurogram:* an automatic response; a habit.

*neurosis:* a relatively minor functional nervous disorder in which the personality system remains for the most part intact.

*nominal aphasia:* aphasia marked by inability to recall names of objects. See *aphasia.*

*obturator:* an artificial disc, plate, or bulb used to partially or completely close an opening; used especially in cleft-palate cases.

*occipital lobe:* a cerebral lobe in the back part of the brain corresponding to the occipital bone.

*occlude:* to close tightly; to fit together.

*occulomotor nerve:* the IIIrd Cranial nerve; it is motor to all muscles of the eye except the external rectus and superior oblique muscles.

*olfactory nerve:* the Ist Cranial nerve; the sensory nerve of smell originating in the olfactory lobe and distributed to the nasal mucous membrane.

*omohyoid m.:* a muscle originating in the border of the scapula and inserted in the hyoid bone; it retracts and depresses the hyoid.

*ontogeny:* the developmental history of the individual.

*optic n.:* the IInd Cranial nerve; the sensory nerve of vision originating in the occipital cortex and distributed to the retina.

*oralism:* a method of instruction for the deaf in which the chief means of communication is lip-reading and talking.

*orbicularis oris m.:* the sphincter muscle which closes the mouth and wrinkles the lips; it is supplied by the seventh cranial or facial nerve.

*ordinate:* the vertical axis of reference in a two-dimensional graph. Dist. from *abscissa.*

*organ of Corti:* the spiral apparatus in the internal ear lying on the basilar membrane in the cochlear canal.

*organic defect:* a defect in which structural alteration is an important contributing cause. Dist. from *functional defect.*

*orifice:* an aperture or opening.

*origin:* the more-fixed end or attachment of a muscle as distinguished from *insertion;* also the point at which a cranial nerve emerges from the brain.

*oropharynx:* that portion of the pharynx extending from the level of the hyoid bone to the soft palate.

*oscillograph:* an instrument for recording oscillations.

*ossicle:* a small bone; one of the three bones in the middle ear.

*otitis media:* inflammation of the middle ear.

*otolaryngology:* the single specialty of *otology* and *laryngology.*

*otology:* the study and treatment of the ear.

*otosclerosis:* the formation of spongy bone in the labyrinth of the ear; especially such growth around the footplate of the stapes impeding its movements in the oval window.

*oval window:* see *fenestra ovalis.*

*overtone:* any partial in a complex tone except the fundamental tone; when the frequency of an overtone is an exact multiple of the fundamental tone, it is called a harmonic. Dist. from *fundamental tone.*

*palatogram:* an imprint on a thin artificial hard palate made by contact of the tongue when a given sound is produced.

*palatopharyngeus m.:* a muscle originating in the soft palate and inserted in the posterior border of the thyroid cartilage and in the pharynx; it acts to narrow the fauces and shut off the nasopharynx. Same as *pharyngopalatinus muscle.*

*palpation:* the act of feeling with the hand or fingers.

*paragrammatism:* see *agrammalogia.*

*paralalia:* the substitution of one speech sound for another; sometimes any speech disturbance.

*paralambdacism:* faulty production of the sound [1].

*pararhoticism:* faulty production of the sound [r].

*parasigmatism:* faulty production of the sounds [s] or [z].

*parasympathetic nervous system:* that part of the autonomic nervous system which is made up of the ocular, bulbar, and sacral divisions.

*parathyroid gland:* any one of the two small glands on each lobe of the thyroid gland.

*parietal lobe:* a cerebral lobe in the upper center of the cerebrum corresponding to the parietal bone.

*partial:* one of the frequency components of a complex tone.

*Passavant's ridge:* a ridge projecting from the posterior and lateral walls of the pharynx at the level of the soft palate; it acts with the palate in closing the opening to the nasopharynx.

*patellar reflex:* the knee jerk elicited by striking the tense patellar tendon and bringing about a contraction of the quadriceps extensors.

*pathology:* the study of the nature of disease and its resulting structural and functional changes.

*PB words:* a phonetically balanced list of words for articulation tests in hearing; so-called because the words include speech sounds in approximately the same relative frequency of occurrence as in the stream of ordinary speech.

*pediatrics:* the study and treatment of children and their care.

*peripheral:* situated more or less in the outward part or surface of the body as distinguished from the central mechanism consisting of the brain and spinal cord; muscles and sense organs.

*pH:* a symbol representing the hydrogen ion concentration in liquids; a low *pH* indicates acidity, and a high *p*H alkalinity.

*pharyngeal constrictors:* three muscles in the pharynx, *superior, middle* and *inferior,* which contract the pharynx as in swallowing.

*pharyngopalatinus m.:* see *palatopharyngeus muscle.*

*pharynx:* the muscular and membranous sac between the mouth and nares and the esophagus; it consists of three main divisions, the laryngopharynx, oropharynx, and the nasopharynx.

*phi phenomenon:* the apparent motion of stationary stimuli when they are presented successively in neighboring positions.

*phobia:* pathological fear of some specific stimulus or situation.

*phonation:* the production of voiced sound by means of vocal cord vibrations.

*phoneme:* a group or family of closely related speech sounds all of which have the same distinctive acoustic characteristics in spite of their differences; often used in place of the term *speech sound.*

*phonetic method:* an approach to the treatment of articulation difficulties in which the therapist directs attention to the specific movements and placements of the articulatory structures.

*phonetics:* the study of the production and perception of speech sounds including individual and group variations as to their use in speech.

*phonics:* the study of speech sounds with special reference to reading.

*phonophobia:* morbid fear of speaking aloud.

*phrase:* a word or group of words uttered without perceptible pause and set aside as a group by pauses of sufficient duration to perform this function.

*physiogenic:* originating from physiological causes. Dist. from *psychogenic.*

*pinna:* same as *auricle.*

*platysma m.:* the platysma myoides, a muscle which depresses the mouth and lower lip.

*play therapy:* a process of examination and treatment by observing the child as he plays freely with a selected inventory; the role of the therapist is usually a passive one.

*plosive:* any speech sound made by creating air pressure in the air tract and suddenly releasing it. Examples are [p], [d], and [t].

*pneumogastric n.:* same as *vagus nerve.*

*pneumograph:* a device for recording the rate and extent of breathing movements.

*pneumophonia:* a form of dysphonia; voice characterized by breathiness.

*polylogia:* same as *logorrhea.*

*pons:* the pons Varolii; a large transverse band of nerve fibers in the hind-brain which forms the cerebellar stem and encircles the medulla oblongata.

*posterior:* pertaining to or located in the rear. Opp. to *anterior.*

*presbycusis:* the diminution of hearing acuity associated with old age.

*primary stuttering:* the neuromuscular spasms in the early speech of children about which there is an absence of awareness and anxiety and an absence of irrelevant movement of distant parts.

*prognathism:* a marked projection of the jaw, usually the upper jaw.

*prognosis:* prediction or judgment concerning the course, duration, termination, and recovery from a pathological condition.

*projection:* the tendency of a person to attribute to the external world repressed mental complexes which are his own.

*pseudobulbar paralysis:* paralysis which appears to be a result of bulbar lesion, but is not.

*psychasthenia:* a neurosis marked by morbid anxiety, obsessions, feelings of inadequacy, self-condemnation, and fixed ideas.

*psychiatry:* that branch of medicine which deals with mental disorders.

*psychoanalysis:* a dynamic system of psychology, developed by Freud, which attributes behavior to repressed factors in the subconscious and which has a specialized technique for the investigation and treatment of such factors.

*psychocatharsis:* Freud's treatment of neurosis in which the patient relates everything that is associated with a given train of thought; it is closely related to *abreaction.* Same as *catharsis.*

*psychogenic:* originating in the mind. Dist. from *physiogenic.*

*psychometry:* the broad field of mental measurement.

*psychotherapy:* the treatment of disorders by any of a wide variety of psychological methods.

*pterygoid m.:* external and internal pterygoid muscles which raise the lower jaw and draw it forward.

*pure tone:* periodic sound waves of the sinusoidal type which have no partials or overtones.


*quadratus labii inferioris m.:* a muscle innervated by the facial (VIIth Cranial) nerve and which acts to depress the lower lip.

*quality:* when applied to *voice,* the acoustic characteristics of vowels resulting from their overtone structure or the relative intensities of their frequency components.


*raphe:* a ridge which marks the line of union between halves of symmetrical parts.

*rapport:* a relationship of ease, harmony, and accord between the subject and examiner or therapist.

*receptive aphasia:* a disturbance of speech due to brain lesion in which the major difficulty is inability to comprehend the meaning of words heard. Same as *auditory aphasia.*

*recurrent laryngeal n.:* the branch of the Vagus (Xth) nerve which innervates all intrinsic muscles of the larynx except the cricothyroid muscle; also called *inferior laryngeal.*

*recruitment:* when applied to hearing, the condition in which the patient cannot hear sounds of moderate intensity but experiences no loss of his sense of loudness for loud tones; it is associated with nerve deafness.

*reflex:* a movement performed involuntarily as a result of the stimulation of a sensory nerve which sends an impulse through a connecting nerve to a nerve center and thence to a motor nerve; this functional unit of the nervous system is called a *reflex arc.*

*relaxed palate:* functional failure of palatal movement, not due to paralysis or muscular weakness.

*resonance:* the vibratory response of a body or air-filled cavity to a frequency imposed upon it.

*retarded speech:* slowness in speech development in which intelligibility is severely impaired; often preceded by late or delayed emergence of speech.

*rhinolalia:* speech characterized by abnormal nasal resonance.

*rhythm:* the serial recurrence of stress, sounds, or organic movement.

*rima glottidis:* see *glottis.*

*Rinné test:* a tuning-fork test used to aid in differentiating conduction from nerve deafness.

*risorius muscle:* a muscle originating in the fascia over the masseter muscle and inserted in the angle of the mouth; it is innervated by the buccal branch of the facial (VIIth) nerve; it acts to draw the angle of the mouth out and to compress the cheeks.

*round window:* see *fenestra rotunda.*

*rugal:* pertaining to a ridge, fold, or furrow; especially the transverse ridges extending outward on both sides of the raphe of the hard palate.


*sagittal:* shaped like an arrow; running in a plane parallel to the long axis of the body.

*salpingopharyngeus m.:* a muscle originating in the Eustachian tube near the nasopharynx and inserted in the posterior part of the palatopharyngeus muscle; it is innervated by the accessory (XIth Cranial) nerve and acts to raise the pharynx.

*scala tympani:* the spiral canal in the cochlea situated below the basilar membrane.

*scala vestibuli:* the spiral canal in the cochlea situated above the basilar membrane.

*secondary stuttering:* neuromuscular spasms of the speech mechanism accompanied by anxiety about nonfluency and accompanied by habitual irrelevant movements used as devices to break up or conceal speech blockages.

*semantics:* the study of the history and evolution of word meanings. Dist. from *general semantics.*

*semicircular canals:* three bony canals lying at right angles to one another at the posterior end of the vestibule of the inner ear; they are filled with a fluid and serve as the sense organs of equilibrium.

*sensorium:* the entire sensory mechanism; sometimes the part of the cerebral cortex concerned with the reception of sensory nerve impulses.

*sibilant:* accompanied by a hissing sound; especially a type of fricative speech sound called a sibilant. Examples are [s], [z], [ʒ], [ʃ], [tʃ], and [dʒ].

*side-tone:* the auditory signal which gives a speaker information concerning his own speech performance.

*sigma:* when spelled out, one-thousandth of a second.

*sign language:* a system of communication among the deaf through conventional hand or body movements which represent ideas, objects, action, etc. Dist. from *finger-spelling.*

*singer's nodule:* see *chorditis tuberosa.*

*sinistral:* pertaining to or located on the left side of the body. Opp. to *dextral.*

*sinus:* a recess, cavity, or hollow space in the bone or other tissue.

*slurring:* passing over speech sounds so lightly during utterance that they are obscured, suppressed, omitted, or only partially produced.

*soft palate:* a fibromuscular, movable curtain which is attached to the posterior margin of the hard palate; it helps to separate the oral cavity from the pharynx and, when elevated, closes off the nasopharynx. Same as *velum.*

*somatic:* pertaining to the body substance in general.

*sonant:* a voiced sound. Opp. to *surd.*

*spasm:* a convulsive involuntary contraction of a muscle or group of muscles.

*spasmophemia:* a disturbance in the rhythm of speech; a blocking or convulsive repetition of sounds. Same as *stuttering.*

*spastic paralysis:* paralysis marked by rigidity and heightened tendon reflexes. Dist. from *flaccid paralysis.*

*speech:* communication through conventional vocal and oral symbols.

*speech audiometry:* the measurement of hearing in terms of the reception of spoken words presented at controlled levels of intensity.

*speech correction:* the professional field which deals with the elimination and alleviation of speech defects or with the development and improvement of speaking intelligibility; sometimes dist. from *speech improvement.*

*speech defect:* any deviation of speech which is outside the range of acceptable variation in a given environment.

*speech disorder:* a deviation of speech together with the underlying conditions causing such a deviation; often the same as *speech defect.*

*speech education:* the broad field dealing with the training of the person to speak and listen more effectively.

*speech improvement:* the betterment of poor or average speech; sometimes distinguished from speech correction.

*speech pathology:* the study and treatment of all aspects of functional and organic speech defects and disorders; often the same as *speech correction.*

*speech-reading:* see *lip-reading.*

*speech re-education:* the process of restoring a lost speech function by means of an appropriate form of training; same as *speech rehabilitation.*

*speech science:* the broad field dealing with the study, analysis, and measurement of all the components of the processes involved in the production and reception of speech; sometimes the same as *voice science.*

*sphincter:* a ring-shaped muscle which, on contracting, wholly or partly closes a natural opening.

*spinal accessory n.:* the XIth Cranial nerve; partly united with the Vagus nerve, it originates in the medulla and spinal cord and is motor to the larynx and pharynx; same as *accessory nerve.*

*spirometer:* an instrument used to measure the air-capacity of the lungs.

*stammering:* same as *stuttering.*

*stapedius m.:* a tiny muscle originating in the inner wall of the middle ear and inserted in the neck of the stapes; it is innervated by the VIIth Cranial nerve (Facial) and acts to retract the stapes.

*stapes:* the stirrup-shaped third bone in the chain of ossicles in the middle ear; its footplate is inserted in the oval window of the cochlea.

*sternohyoid m.:* a muscle originating in the clavicle and inserted in the body of the hyoid bone; it acts to depress the hyoid and the larynx.

*sternothyroid m.:* a muscle originating in the sternum and inserted in the thyroid cartilage; it acts to depress the larynx.

*stimulation method:* an approach to the treatment of speech defects in which major emphasis is placed upon the development of auditory concepts; teaching speech sounds by having the subject listen to them.

*stop:* a speech sound produced when the air stream is blocked and then suddenly released; same as *plosive.*

*stress:* in speech, the relatively increased force of breath in the production of some syllables as compared with others.

*stretch reflex:* see *myotatic reflex.*

*stridor:* a harsh, shrill, high-pitched sound.

*stuttering:* a disturbance of rhythm and fluency of speech by an intermittent blocking, a convulsive repetition, or prolongation of sounds, syllables, words, phrases, or posture of the speech organs.

*styloglossus m.:* a muscle originating in the styloid process and inserted in the side of the tongue; it is innervated by the hypoglossal (XIIth Cranial) nerve and acts to raise and retract the tongue.

*stylopharyngeus m.:* a muscle originating in the styloid process of the temporal bone and inserted in the side of the pharynx; it raises and dilates the pharynx.

*sulcus:* a depression or furrow in the surface of the brain; same as *fissure.*

*superior:* situated above.

*superior laryngeal n.:* the branch of the Xth Cranial nerve (Vagus) which innervates the cricothyroid muscles and supplies sensory fibers to the mucous membrane of the larynx.

*surd:* a voiceless sound. Opp. to *sonant.*

*sweep-check test:* an audiometric method of screening out possible hearing-loss cases by testing for auditory response to different frequencies presented at a constant intensity level.

*sympathetic nervous system:* the system of ganglia lying outside the spinal cord in the lumbar and thoracic regions and the peripheral nerves which serve the viscera. Same as *autonomic nervous system.*

*symptom:* a structural or functional change or peculiarity which indicates the presence of a disease or disorder in a given individual; the answer given by an organism to demands of the environment which it cannot meet.

*symptomatology:* the systematic study of symptoms; the combined symptoms of a disorder.

*synapse:* the region of contact between one nerve cell and another in a neural chain.

*syndrome:* a complex of symptoms; a set of symptoms which occur together.

*synergy:* the combining of elementary motor processes into a complex, coordinate movement.

*tachyphemia:* speech characterized by great rapidity and volubility, especially in nervous patients.

*temporal lobe:* a major division of each cerebral hemisphere; it lies on the undersurface and side of the brain and contains the hearing centers.

*temporalis m.:* a muscle originating in the temporal fossa and side of the head and inserted in the mandibular process; it is innervated by the mandibular branch of the trigeminal (Vth Cranial) nerve and acts to shut the mouth and retract the jaw.

*tendon:* a fibrous cord of nonelastic connective tissue in which muscle fibers end and by which they are attached to a bone.

*tensor tympani:* a muscle originating in the temporal bone and inserted in the handle of the malleus; it is innervated by the otic ganglion and acts to keep the drum membrane taut.

*tensor veli palatini m.:* a muscle which renders the soft palate tense.

*thalamus:* a mass of gray matter situated at the base of the cerebrum projecting into and bounding the third ventricle.

*therapy:* the science which deals with the treatment or application of remedies for the cure, alleviation, or prevention of disorders.

*thoracic cavity:* the chest; the portion of the body between the neck and the abdomen; it contains the bronchi, lungs, and heart; sometimes called the *thoracic cage.*

*thyrohyoid m.:* a muscle originating on the side of the thyroid cartilage and inserted in the greater horn of the hyoid bone; it is innervated by the upper cervical nerves and acts to raise and change the shape of the larynx.

*thyroid cartilage:* the large cartilage of the larynx shaped like a shield in front and forming the eminence known as Adam's apple.

*thyroid gland:* one of a pair of endocrine glands situated on either side of the larynx; it secretes hormones which maintain basal metabolism rate and is important for normal growth and development.

*timbre:* a qualitative aspect of a complex tone dependent upon the number and relative intensities of partial tones present. Same as *quality.*

*tongue-tie:* limited movement of the tongue due to abnormal shortness of the lingual frenum.

*tonsil:* a small, almond-shaped mass between the faucial pillars on either side; it is mainly composed of lymphoid tissue and is covered with a mucous membrane.

*tonus:* a condition of tension in muscles which exists independently of voluntary innervation.

*trachea:* the windpipe; the cartilaginous and membranous tube descending from the larynx to the bronchi.

*tracheotomy:* the formation of an artificial opening in the trachea.

*trachyphonia:* roughness or hoarseness of the voice.

*transference:* development of positive or negative emotional attitudes toward a person, usually the psychoanalyst, when such attitudes are derived from earlier relationships between the patient and his parents.

*transverse:* lying or moving across; crosswise.

*transversus linguae m.:* a muscle originating in the median septum of the tongue and inserted in the edges; it is innervated by the hypoglossal (XIIth Cranial) nerve and acts to narrow and stretch the tongue as well as to raise its edges.

*trauma:* any wound or injury, especially an organic injury.

*triangularis m.:* a muscle originating in the lower border of the mandible and inserted in the lower lip; it is innervated by the facial (VIIth Cranial) nerve and acts to pull down the corners of the mouth.

*trigeminal n.:* the Vth Cranial nerve; it is sensory and motor with three main branches, the *ophthalmic, maxillary,* and *mandibular.*

*trochlear n.:* the IVth Cranial nerve; it is motor to the superior oblique muscle of the eyeball.

*tuning fork:* a two-pronged instrument of highly tempered metal alloy constructed to vibrate at a constant frequency when set into motion.

*turbinate bone:* the *concha nasalis;* one of three small shell-like bones in the nose.

*tympanic cavity:* an air-filled cavity in the temporal bone which communicates with the nasopharynx by means of the Eustachian tube; it is bounded laterally by the tympanic membrane and contains the ossicular chain; known also as the middle ear.

*tympanic membrane:* same as *drum membrane.*

*ulcer:* an open sore other than a wound; loss of substance on a cutaneous surface causing disintegration of tissue.

*unilateral:* pertaining to one side of the body.

*uraniscolalia:* speech difficulty due to a cleft palate.

*uranoschisis:* same as *cleft palate.*

*uvula:* the appendage which hangs from the free margin of the soft palate.

*vagus n.:* the Xth Cranial nerve; it is a motor and sensory nerve sending fibers to the larynx, lungs, heart, esophagus, stomach, and most of the abdominal viscera; sometimes called the *pneumogastric nerve.*

*vegetative:* pertaining to nutrition and growth.

*velum:* same as *soft palate.*

*ventral:* located on the belly side; opp. to *dorsal.*

*ventricle:* one of the cavities in the brain; any cavity or hollow organ of the body.

*verbigeration:* see *catalogia.*

*verticalis linguae m.:* a muscle originating in the upper surface of the tongue near the sides and inserted under the surface; it is innervated by the hypoglossal (XIIth Cranial) nerve and acts to flatten the tip of the tongue.

*vertigo:* a sensation of whirling or dizziness from overstimulation of the semicircular canal receptors; often associated with disease of the ear and deafness.

*vestibule:* a portion of the labyrinth of the inner ear; it is situated between the cochlea and the semicircular canals.

*vibrato:* periodic variations in pitch or loudness of a tone.

*viscera:* the large internal organs of the body.

*visible speech:* audible speech patterns which have been transformed by electronic apparatus into visual patterns which may be read by the deaf.

*vital capacity:* the maximum amount of air which may be exhaled following a maximal inhalation.

*vocal cords:* the thyroarytenoid ligaments which produce sound when set into vibration; same as *vocal bands.*

*vocalization:* same as *phonation.*

*voice:* sound produced primarily by the vibration of the vocal bands.

*voice science:* see *speech science.*

*volume:* the loudness of a tone.

*vowel:* a conventional vocal sound produced by certain positions of the speech organs which offer little obstruction to the air stream and which form a series of resonators above the level of the larynx. Dist. from *consonant.*

*vowel glide:* a speech sound in which the speech mechanism moves from the position for one vowel to that of another without interruption and accompanied by continuous voicing. Examples are [aɪ], [ɪu], and [eɪ].

*Weber test:* a tuning-fork test in cases of unilateral hearing loss to differentiate conduction from nerve deafness.

*Wernicke's area:* a region in the superior convolution of the temporal lobe of the cerebrum identified as the center for understanding speech heard.

*word-deafness:* same as *auditory aphasia.*

*zygomaticus m.:* major and minor zygomaticus muscles innervated by the facial (VIIth Cranial) nerve and which act to draw the upper lip upward, outward, and backward.

## ROOTS, PREFIXES, AND SUFFIXES

*a-, (an-):* Gr. not; without
*ab-:* L. away from
*acro-:* Gr. tip or extremities; highest
*ad-:* L. toward

*ambi-:* L. both
*amphi-:* Gr. both; around
*ana-:* Gr. up; upward
*ante-:* L. before

*antero-:* L. in front
*anthrop-:* Gr. human being; man
*anti-:* Gr. against
*apo-:* Gr. from; away from; off
*arch-:* Gr. first; chief; principal; great
*aryten-:* Gr. pitcher
*auto-:* Gr. self
*bari-:* Gr. heavy
*bene-:* L. well; good
*bi-:* L. two
*biblio-:* Gr. book
*brachy-:* Gr. abnormally short
*brady-:* Gr. slow
*capit-:* L. head
*cardio-:* Gr. heart
*cata-:* Gr. downward
*ced-:* L. move; yield
*centi-:* L. hundred; hundredth
*cephalo-:* Gr. head
*chrom-:* Gr. color
*chron-:* Gr. time
*circum-:* L. round about
*com-:* L. with; together
*contra-:* L. against; in opposition
*corp-:* L. body
*cresc-:* L. rise; grow
*crypto-:* Gr. hidden; covered
*cut-:* L. skin
*cycl-:* Gr. ring; circle; cycle
*de-:* L. reversal; undoing
*dec-:* Gr. ten
*demi-:* L. half
*dent-:* L. tooth
*derm-:* Gr. skin
*di-:* Gr. twice
*dia-:* Gr. through; between; across
*dic-:* L. say
*dis-:* L. apart; separated from
*dolicho-:* Gr. long
*duc-:* L. lead
*dyna-:* Gr. power
*dys-:* Gr. ill; bad; hard
*ec-:* Gr. out of
*ecto-:* Gr. outside; external
*-ectomy:* Gr. surgical removal
*embolo-:* Gr. wedge; stopper
*en-:* Gr. in
*endo-:* Gr. inside
*epi-:* Gr. on; upon
*eso-:* Gr. inner
*eu-:* Gr. good; advantageous
*ex-:* L. out of; from
*extero-:* L. outside
*extra-:* L. beyond; outside of
*fac-:* L. make; do

*fin-:* L. end
*flu-:* L. flow
*fort-:* L. strong
*gastro-:* Gr. stomach
*gen-:* Gr. origin
*glosso-:* Gr. tongue
*-gnosis:* Gr. knowing; recognition
*-gram:* Gr. something drawn or written
*-graph:* Gr. writing
*helio-:* Gr. sun
*hemi-:* Gr. half
*hepta-:* Gr. seven
*hetero-:* Gr. unlike; different
*hexa-:* Gr. six
*histo-:* Gr. tissue
*homo-:* Gr. same; similar
*hydro-:* Gr. water
*hyper-:* Gr. excess; over; superiority
*hypno-:* Gr. sleep
*hypo-:* Gr. under; less than ordinary; inferior
*idio-:* Gr. personal; separate; distinct
*infra-:* L. below; lower
*inter-:* L. among; between; together
*intro-:* L. directed inward
*-ism:* Gr. state; condition
*iso-:* Gr. equal
*-itis:* Gr. inflammatory disease
*juxta-:* L. close to
*kata-:* see *cata-*
*kilo-:* Gr. thousand
*kine-:* Gr. movement
*labio-:* L. lip
*-lalia:* Gr. speech
*lalo-:* Gr. speech
*loc-:* L. place
*log-:* Gr. words; reasoning
*luc-:* L. light
*macro-:* Gr. large
*mal-:* L. defect; bad
*man-:* L. hand
*medio-:* L. middle
*mega-:* Gr. great; powerful
*meningo-:* Gr. membrane
*meso-:* Gr. in the middle
*meta-:* Gr. after; change
*-meter:* Gr. measure
*micro-:* Gr. small
*milli-:* L. one thousandth; thousand
*mis-:* L. and A.S. wrong
*mono-:* Gr. one; single
*-morph:* Gr. characterized by a specific form
*multi-:* L. many
*myo-:* Gr. muscle

*neo-:* Gr. new; recent
*-nomy:* Gr. a system of laws
*non-:* L. absence
*oculo-:* L. eye
*-oid:* Gr. like; resembling
*-oma:* Gr. growth; tumor
*omni-:* L. all
*onto-:* Gr. existing
*-onym:* Gr. name
*-opia:* Gr. related to the eye
*ortho-:* Gr. straight; correct
*-osis:* Gr. diseased condition
*oto-:* Gr. ear
*pan-:* Gr. all
*para-:* Gr. faulty or disordered condition; subsidiary
*path-:* Gr. suffering; disease
*-pathy:* Gr. feeling; disease; treatment
*ped-:* L. foot
*pedo- (ped-):* Gr. child
*penta-:* Gr. five
*peri-:* Gr. around
*phil-:* Gr. love
*-phobia:* Gr. morbid fear
*phon-:* Gr. sound
*photo-:* Gr. light
*phren-:* Gr. diaphragm; mind
*pneumato-:* Gr. air; respiration
*pneumono-:* Gr. lung
*-pod:* Gr. footed
*poly-:* Gr. many; manifold
*post-:* L. later; after
*pre-:* L. before
*pro-:* L. in front of; in place of
*proto-:* Gr. first in time or status
*pseudo-:* Gr. false; erroneous

*psycho-:* Gr. mind
*pyro-:* Gr. fire
*quadr-:* L. four
*quasi-:* L. seemingly
*quinque-:* L. five
*re-:* L. again
*rect-:* L. straight
*ren-:* L. kidney
*retro-:* L. backward; situated behind
*rhino-:* Gr. nose
*-scope:* Gr. instrument for observing
*scoto-:* Gr. darkness
*-sect:* L. cut; divided
*semi-:* L. half
*sept-:* L. seven
*sex-:* L. six
*somno-:* L. sleep
*son-:* L. sound
*sphygmo-:* Gr. pulse
*spiro-:* L. respiration
*stereo-:* Gr. a solid body
*sub-:* L. beneath; of lower order
*super-:* L. above; of higher order
*supra-:* L. above in position
*syn-:* Gr. together
*tachy-:* Gr. quick; swift
*tele-:* Gr. far
*tetra-:* Gr. four
*thermo-:* Gr. heat
*thyro-:* Gr. shield
*-tomy:* Gr. a cutting
*trachy-:* Gr. rough
*trans-:* L. across
*tri-:* L. three
*ultra-:* L. extreme; beyond
*uni-:* L. one
*zo-:* Gr. animal

## BIBLIOGRAPHY

COATES-LONGERICH, M., and LONGERICH, E. B. 1945. German-English speech terminology. *J. Speech Disorders*, 10, 39–46.
DE VRIES, L. 1946. German-English science dictionary. New York: McGraw-Hill.
——— 1951. French-English science dictionary. New York: McGraw-Hill.
DORLAND, W. A. N. 1951. The American illustrated medical dictionary. Philadelphia: Saunders.
DREVER, J. 1952. A dictionary of psychology. Baltimore: Penguin Books.
FAIRCHILD, H. 1944. Dictionary of sociology. New York: Philosophical Library.
FODOR, N., and GAYNOR, F. 1950. Freud: dictionary of psychoanalysis. New York: Philosophical Library.
GOOD, C. V. 1945. Dictionary of education. New York: McGraw-Hill.
GRAYSON. H. M., and TOLMAN, R. S. 1950. A semantic study of clinical concepts. *J. abnorm. soc. Psychol.*, 45, 216–231.

HAMMOND, K. R., and ALLEN, J. M. 1953. Writing clinical reports. New York: Prentice-Hall.

HENDERSON, I. F., and HENDERSON, W. D. 1949. Dictionary of scientific terms: pronunciation, derivation, and definition of terms in biology, botany, zoology, anatomy, cytology, embryology, physiology. New York: Van Nostrand.

HINSIE, L. E., and SHATZKY, J. 1940. Psychiatric dictionary with encyclopedic treatment of modern terms. London: Oxford Univ. Press.

HUTCHINGS, R. H. 1943. A psychiatric word book: a lexicon of terms employed in psychiatry, and psychoanalysis designed for students of medicine and nursing, and psychiatric social workers. Utica, N.Y.: State Hospitals Press.

JOHNSON, W., and WILSON, J. T. 1945. The degree of extensional agreement among twenty psychologists in their use of the labels, hypothesis, theory, and law. Proceedings of the Iowa academy of science, 52, 255–259.

JONES, H. W., HOERR, N. L., and OSOL, A. 1949. Blakiston's new Gould medical dictionary. Philadelphia: Blakiston.

KAHN, S. 1940. Psychological and neurological definitions and the unconscious. Boston: Meador Pub. Co.

LONGERICH, E. B., and LONGERICH, M. C. 1946. French-English speech terminology. *J. Speech Disorders*, 11, 193–196.

OGILVIE, M. 1942. Terminology and definitions of speech defects. New York: Columbia Univ.

ROBBINS, S. D. 1947. Principles of nomenclature and of classification of speech and voice disorders. *J. Speech Disorders*, 12, 17–22.

—— 1951. A dictionary of speech pathology and therapy. Cambridge, Mass.: Sci-Art Publishers.

ROBBINS, S. D., and STINCHFIELD, S. M. 1931. Dictionary of speech terms dealing with disorders of speech. Boston: Expression Co.

STEDMAN, T. L., and STANLEY, T. G. 1946. Stedman's medical dictionary. Baltimore: Williams and Wilkins.

WARREN, H. C. 1934. Dictionary of psychology. Boston: Houghton Mifflin.

WISE, H. S. 1946. A revised classification of disorders of speech. *J. Speech Disorders*, 11, 327–334.

CHAPTER 3

# THE NEUROPHYSIOLOGY OF SPEECH

● *Robert West, Ph.D.*

## INTRODUCTION

THE SUBJECT OF the *neurophysiology of speech* is vast. Directly and indirectly the processes of speech involve the entire body; hence a treatise of the material covered by this ambitious title would not really be complete without including practically all that is known about human physiology and neural anatomy. Therefore the author has decided not to attempt to record those facts that are in the possession of the graduate student of speech science, either in his memory or in his library of human physiology and anatomy; for in the attempt at such a factual recital one would be constantly vexed by the unanswerable question of where to stop. Instead the author has decided (with the editor's approval) to compose an essay on a few of the principles of structure and function that are significant in the understanding of the speech mechanism. Even this limitation of the subject to *principles* rather than *facts* is difficult to rationalize. Principles involve definitions of organs and functions, and definitions lead us into semantics. Again the question, Where do we stop?

Some of the principles selected for discussion have obvious and direct applications to the general field of this textbook. For the inclusion of those we need not apologize. Others, however, have been chosen largely because they are presently much talked about when neurophysiologists meet around the council fires. Where applications of these principles to the practical business of the rehabilitation of speech is not suggested in this chapter, it is hoped that keen-eyed students who read this book will see the significance of what is discussed.

## MULTIPLE USES OF THE SPEECH APPARATUS

Speech is a behavioral reaction that involves the use of the muscular walls of the torso, the muscles of the respiratory tract, the pharynx, the tongue, the lips and face, the nasal passageways, the hands and eyes (to a lesser degree), and those parts of the cerebrospinal nervous system that control and monitor the organs mentioned. Roughly, we can designate these organs and parts as the speech apparatus. Most of these organs and parts, however, have many functions other than speech.

These other-than-speech functions may be classified in the following manner:

A. Those that are *innate,* automatic, vegetative reactions, such as swallowing, gagging, breathing, vomiting, suckling.
B. Those that are *learned,* automatic, vegetative reactions, such as biting, chewing, sucking.
C. Those that are *learned,* automatic, *emotional* reactions, such as grimaces, mannerisms, tics.
D. Those that are *innate,* automatic, *emotional* reactions, such as laughing, sobbing, smiling.
E. Those that are learned, *nonautomatic, discriminatory,* and specially *voluntary* reactions, such as exploratory movements of the tongue, spreading of the lips, kissing, blowing.
F. Those that are learned, automatic, *practical* reactions, such as whistling, playing a wind instrument, humming a tune.

It should be understood that all the learned automatisms—B, C, and F—are, at the beginning of their learning, classifiable under E. They are learned, but not yet automatic. They are voluntarily initiated. They do not arise automatically from promptings of environment or of situation. This difference is well illustrated by the difference between sucking and suckling. The baby does not have to be taught the special milking movements of the tongue and lips involved in suckling; but the child does have to experiment at some length to learn how to suck water through a straw. At first his *sucking* is classifiable under E, later under B. The *suckling* reactions would never be classifiable under any heading but A. These five classes of functions compete with each other for the control of the parts involved. When one automatism clashes with another, one or both of the given functions must be modified or one of them must be suspended.

Now the mechanisms of speech are of two sorts:

G. Those that are learned, nonautomatic, discriminatory, and specially voluntary reactions, such as the beginning of a sentence or phrase after a break in utterance, a clothing of an idea in unique and original phraseology, the translation of an idea from the native language to another.

H. Those that are learned, automatic, practical reactions, such as the oral reading of familiar material, expressing ideas that have been so expressed many times before, reading silently material that, though not necessarily familiar, does not involve an unfamiliar vocabulary. Let us take as an illustration of G and H the utterance of such a statement as: "The Japanese and the German nations had one prompting in common that made them allies, and that was a demand for *Lebensraum.*"

The seven-year-old child could read very little of this sentence. Certainly the meaning of the sentence as a whole would escape him. The parts that he could read would be isolated words such as *one, in, made, for.* The utterance of each of these monosyllables would involve a special act of volition and would entail only the most rudimentary automatisms. The average English-speaking adult, however, would read most of the sentence automatically. Though the particular combination of words involved in the statement is one that the reader may never before have met, he still has the advantage of phrases that "play themselves," such as: *the Japanese, and the German nations, in common, that made them allies,* and so on. These he has run into in so many other contexts that they are well-developed automatisms. But when he comes to the last word, the average adult (with no German background) reacts in one of four ways:

1. He signals unemotionally in one way or another that he cannot complete the sentence.

2. He proceeds to break the word into syllables and to utter them one by one in order. His reactions are without automatic control, as under category G.

3. If the situation is one in which failure to complete the sentence would embarrass him severely, he may find his speech apparatus so preoccupied with innate, automatic, emotional reactions (category C) that he cannot attempt the word.

4. If he is unsure of the word *Lebensraum,* he may select his automatism, or combination of automatisms, that seems to him to be closest to the given word and speak it with a grimace or tic (category C) which, in spite of him, will distort the articulation or distract the attention of the audience from the meaning of the sentence.

### The Automatisms in Conflict

It was stated above that the various uses to which the speech apparatus can be put may conflict with each other. We have listed eight such uses (A to H), the last two (G and H) being speech uses. Let us now examine those conflicts in which speech uses are involved. The conflicts are of two kinds: pre-emptive and associative. It is obvious one cannot speak while drinking a glass of water; but that conflict does not really disturb speech. One merely decides to postpone either the drinking or the talking. That is a simple pre-emptive conflict.

Let the speaker, however, try to express something that has deep emotional significance for him, and the same motive that prompts him to speak also prompts him to engage his speech apparatus in other-than-speech uses. This conflict is not settled by an *either-or* choice. It is not a choice between speech and emotional expression; it is speech and the associated emotional reaction or no speech at all. Suppose, to carry the matter one step farther, the thing he is trying to express by speech is his frustration in communication with others. His very attempt at speech is frustrated by the emotional uses of the speech apparatus, and so the frustration increases in the expression of it. This is an associative conflict.

The important clashes to watch, therefore, are the associative conflicts between speech uses (G and H) and the learned emotional automatisms (C) on the one hand, and the innate emotional automatisms (D) on the other. It is these conflicts that cause a large proportion of speech disorders. We need to examine, therefore, the nervous mechanisms through which C and D are produced and controlled.

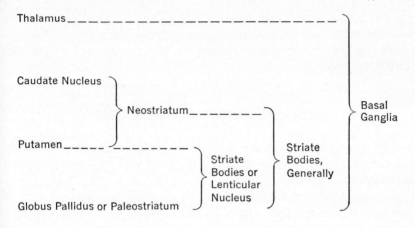

TABLE 1. The relation of the basal ganglia to one another

## THE BASAL GANGLIA

The innate emotional automatisms are controlled by the system of the basal ganglia, in the center of the cranium. Starting first with the individual organs in this system, they can be envisaged as though arranged in line, as are the instruments in an electronic amplifier, from the input to the output end. The first in line is the *thalamus* or *optic thalamus,* a largely sensory organ; next, the *caudate nucleus,* an associative instrument, in which some primitive and unconscious interpretations are made of the sensations that have been received in the thalamus; next in line, the *putamen,* a center where are "stored" innate patterns for motor responses appropriate to the interpretations made by the caudate nucleus. Last, the *globus pallidus,* a body made up largely of efferent neurons that are immediately responsible for activating impulses that will result in behavioral reactions of the body—the reactions in which we are presently interested, being those that are innate emotional automatisms. All of the organs described in this paragraph are usually referred to as the basal ganglia, or basal nuclei. The caudate nucleus, putamen, and globus pallidus are by some referred to as the *corpora striata,* or striate bodies; though some limit this term to the putamen and the globus pallidus. The globus pallidus and the putamen are physically intimately related and are together often referred to as the lenticular nucleus or lentiform body. The globus pallidus alone is called sometimes the paleostriatum in contrast to the neostriatum, consisting of the *putamen and the caudate nucleus*. To help the student to move with ease among the organs and ideas here mentioned the following chart is prepared. (See Table I.)

The basal ganglia are interconnected with many other parts of the central nervous system; those connections most important in speech are: (1) the efferent tracts that lead from the globus pallidus to terminate eventually in the synaptic fields of the peripheral neurons leading to the muscles of phonation and articulation; (2) the nerves that lead from the basal ganglia to the hypothalamus where interconnections are made with the autonomic nervous system; and (3) the fibers that connect the motor cortex of the cerebrum with the basal ganglia.

## EMOTIONAL INTERFERENCE WITH SPEECH

With these essential parts described we are ready to define the sequence of events that take place when speech is interfered with by innate emotional automatisms.

*Situation 1.* The person is speaking. He experiences a sudden twinge of pain from an infected tooth. The pain causes the thalamus to send activating impulses to the caudate nucleus, which prompts the putamen to react; this in turn triggers the reaction of the globus pallidus. The globus sends out impulses which dominate the synapses of those lower motor neurons in the vagus nerves that make up the laryngeal nerves. Up to this moment that synaptic field has been under the uncontested control of the nerves in the pyramidal tracts from the motor cortex of the cerebrum. But now the cerebrum and the basal ganglia compete, resulting in either a cry of pain, instead of phonation for speech, or an alteration of the intensity, quality, or inflections of the voice. This may be regarded as one of the most primitive of the reactions of the basal ganglia. Since vocalization for speech is less primitive, it is difficult for the cortex to maintain its dominance in the face of pallidal demand for control.

*Situation 2.* One is reading aloud from a letter. He comes across a passage conveying to him very painful news. The so-called cortico-thalamic tracts bring to the basal ganglia patterns of impulses—excitations and inhibitions—that start a series of reactions through the ganglia quite parallel to events that took place in situation 1. Thus we have two sources of input to the basal ganglia: (1) the ascending impulses from the sensorium, and (2) the impulses descending from the cerebrum.

In this struggle for the control of the lower motor neurons the cerebrum must, through the cortico-thalamic association pathways, inhibit the functioning of the basal ganglia or lose the dominance of the synaptic field of the lower motor neuron.

This dominance is maintained except under the following conditions:

1. When the direct afferent stimulation of the thalamus is intense.
2. When the cerebrum relays strong emotional patterns to the ganglia.
3. When the cerebrum or its connections with the ganglia are so damaged as to render it powerless to inhibit the activity of the organs of the basal chain.
4. When the pyramidal tracts are so damaged that there is left but a feeble direct control by the cerebral cortex of the lower motor neuron.
5. When the general biochemical status of the body is such that the basal ganglia are hyper-irritable and easily escape from the control of the cerebral cortex.

The learned, emotional automatisms involve the cerebrum principally (as do all learned behavior patterns) and the basal ganglia secondarily. The original learning begins with a conscious, purposive act. The following may illustrate the sorts of behavior with which these automatisms start:

1. A blinking of the eyes, or momentary dropping of the lids, to shut out distracting sights while one is attempting to concentrate on a problem.
2. A drawing downward of the upper lip to cover a dental brace that one feels is too conspicuous.
3. A turning of the head to one side to hide the face from too close scrutiny.
4. The utterance of a meaningless vocal sound intended to convey to one's hearer that he has not yet finished his remark and that, when he gets his thoughts organized, there will be more to follow.

In the first instance, and in the early repetitions of these acts, many association areas of the cerebral cortex take part. Each act is guided and monitored by sensory reports from many sources—auditory, visual, kinesthetic, and tactile tracts. These reports pass through the thalamus without significantly modifying the input of impulses to the caudate nucleus. In the cortex of the cerebrum, auditory, visual, kinesthetic, and tactile areas of association react to the reports as they are received by the primary sensory areas in the temporal lobe, cuneus, and along the posterior bank of the fissure of Rolando. The association areas contiguous to these centers, through cortico-cortico fibers, trigger reactions in motor association areas of the frontal lobe parallel with, and anterior to, the narrow strip of primary motor cortex on the anterior bank of the fissure of Rolando. These motor association areas prompt the motor cortex to the specific patterns of nerve impulses involved in the act to be performed. From here the line of command descends through the pramidal tracts to the lower motor neurones and to the muscles involved. That is a simplified statement of the complex picture of the directing and producing of one of these acts before it has become habitual. The statement does not include the reaction of the subject to the environment that prompted the whole chain of reactions described above; or, in other words, the statement omits those antecedent events in the frontal lobe that we call volition.

Repetition after repetition of the acts mentioned above is accompanied by a short-cutting of the complex pathways described. Instead of involving many sensory association areas, only one may be left in the chain. The pattern of neuromuscular reactions becomes simplified, until that which began with rather general facial activity is reduced to a single pair of muscle antagonists. The volitional activity of the frontal lobe becomes less and less dominant.

Since the acts described above were at first basically purposed to make the subject more comfortable, there was even at the original performance a parallel reaction through the basal ganglia. Each repetition of the act strengthens the association between the cerebral and the basilar activity, until eventually either the cerebral or the associated basilar pattern will automatically elicit the other. When this state has been reached, a full-blown tic has evolved.

The conflict between speech and the tic takes place principally in the motor cortex of the cerebrum. Through the convolution of Broca, patterns of motor association—engrams of words, phrases, and sentences—are being rapidly fed to those parts of the motor cortex that control the muscles of phonation and articulation. Some of these patterns are in conflict with the patterns of the tic. In such a case those reactions that are reinforced by the lenticular activity are likely to be dominant and to pre-empt the neuromuscular systems, so that speech is either blocked or significantly modified.

Thus far we have described relatively simple, emotionally actuated, learned automatisms. In these tics the locus of the interference is chiefly in the roots of the pyramidal tracts. The same mechanism, in general, operates to produce more-complicated automatisms, in which the patterns of reaction are not limited to a single functioning muscular unit or group of muscles, but include complicated serial response patterns. In these the interference with speech processes is not in the motor cortex proper but in the motor association areas anterior to it. As in the case of simple tics, there is an emotional precipitation and reinforcement of these complex automatisms through an associated reaction across the basal ganglia.

These patterns of response are much too complex to be called tics; *mannerisms, stereotypes, idiosyncracies* are better terms to describe them. Examples are: a nervous giggling, a series of sighs, a pet word or phrase, and even a recurrent idea. A person who feels socially inadequate may beg for his hearer's indulgence by stating a sentence, then ending it abruptly by saying, "You know what I mean?" His hearer nods, and the speaker goes on without finishing his original idea. Later the phrase is used in any situation of social stress, whether it is logically apropos or not. Then it becomes corrupted to "know what I mean," then to "what I mean," and to "I mean."

## ALL-OR-NONE REACTIONS

One of the principles important in the understanding of the speech processes is that of the all-or-none law of the functioning of the nerve cell. Because a nerve acts like a stick of dynamite (it completely converts its energy
from a static to a dynamic form if the detonating force be great enough to
upset its electro-chemical equilibrium), the nerve is said to *fire*. The force
of the explosion is not dependent upon the vigor of the detonation. The
nerve, not the stimulus, furnishes the energy for this firing. The measure of
the force necessary to cause a nerve to fire is the threshold of its irritability.

An analogy more modern than that of dynamite is that type of electronic
vacuum tube that withholds its discharge until pressure on the electrostatic
trigger, or grid, reaches a given level, at which point the tube fires to its
maximum capacity. Discharges of this kind make up all of the functioning
of the nerves that control the speech apparatus. A sensory, or afferent, fiber
will not fire until the stimulus upon its end-organ reaches the threshold. This
nerve will not, in turn, trigger the association fiber with which it synapses
unless the original charge of that afferent nerve is strong enough so that,
upon discharging, it can release forces great enough to discharge the association fiber. That fiber, when discharging into the synaptic field of the efferent
neurons, will detonate the field only if the association fiber carries potential
sufficient to overcome and upset the equilibrium of that field.

Having stated the doctrine of the all-or-none character of nerve reaction,
we are now in position to discuss certain reactions of the nerve that apparently deny our doctrine. The practical operating units of the nervous system
are not individual nerve fibers but whole bundles of such cells. The bundles
are usually designated as *nerves*. While an individual fiber follows the all-or-
none law, the bundle does not. All, or part, of the fibers may fire. So,
though the reaction of the fiber may not vary in strength, the reaction of the
nerve may.

The doctrine of the all-or-none reaction does not mean that the reactions
of the nerve fibers of which a nerve bundle is composed are invariable in
intensity from hour to hour and day to day. Both the threshold and intensity
of explosion vary with the factors that alter nerve metabolism. So the "all"
is not constant; and when it is low, it may seem a "part."

After every detonation of a nerve fiber there is a phase of inertia, called
the refractory period, whose duration is remarkably constant for each given
fiber. For a thousandth part of a second or more, the fiber that has just reacted cannot be stimulated to fire. From this axiom three corollaries may be
derived: (1) that nervous discharges are in barrage form, (2) that a muscle
is held in contraction by a series of stimulations rather than by one continuous impulse, and (3) that the stimulation of a muscle by a nerve, or of one
nerve by another, is dependent upon, and varies with, the closeness of the
matching of the refractory periods of the connected units.

To review these corollaries: All stimulation of the nervous system (except for certain conditions of pathology) arises in the end-organs of the afferent fibers. Since these fibers react intermittently, all stimulation passed along from nerve to nerve, and eventually to muscle, is intermittent. Even the fastest movement of the speech articulators involves many separate stimulations from the efferent nerve fibers supplying the acting muscles. These impulses follow each other so closely that the contracting muscles have no time to relax between stimulations. The end-organs of a given afferent nerve react asynchronously, so that, although a given fiber continuously stimulated reacts with precise regularity, the reactions of all the end-organs taken together make up a completely random barrage. This barrage pattern of the incoming stimulation is one that rather generally dominates the reactions of the entire central nervous system.

If, in any serial connection of one nerve fiber with another, the firing and refractory periods of one correspond with those of the other, the two fibers are a virtual continuity; but, if their timings are out of phase, the synapse between them is a place of "resistance" to the passage of the impulse of stimulation from the first to the second. With matched timing the second fiber is stimulated by the first; with asynchronous timing the second is inhibited by the first. This inhibition by asynchronous timing is due to the prolongation of the refractory period of the second fiber. The recovery of the fiber after detonation is delayed by random impulses that impinge upon the fiber at the moment when irritability is about to return. These impulses are not adequate to produce a firing of the second fiber; they merely block its recovery. In general, fibers that make up circuits of a given functional level in the C.N.S. (central nervous system) are "matched" in timing; but those fibers that make up circuits involving two levels are unmatched, the higher tending to inhibit the lower. Thus, if a given lower motor neuron has two connections, one from across the cord at its own level and the other from above in the C.N.S., the descending fiber serves to oppose the across-the-cord neuron. Hence, as one level of the C.N.S. is superimposed on another, the higher is in general inhibitory of the lower.

Other factors than the asynchronisms of firing are doubtless involved in this matter of inhibition of one level by levels superior to it. All the factors, taken together, make up a pattern of inhibition so real and definite that it seems as though the C.N.S. were functionally polarized: the higher, the more inhibitory; the lower, the more stimulatory.

## THE ELECTRONICS OF THE C.N.S.

It is this appearance of polarization that makes the electronic analogy to the C.N.S. so apt. At many points of synaptic connection several fibers are involved in the process of triggering a given neuron arising at the synapse. We can here assume that our synapse (Fig. 1) is like the three-grid vacuum tubes (Fig. 2).

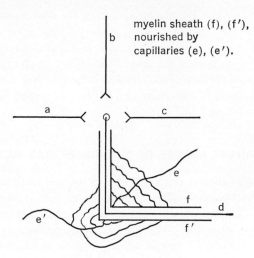

myelin sheath (f), (f'),
b    nourished by
     capillaries (e), (e').

FIG. 1. Neurologic diagram.

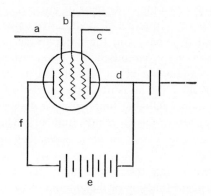

FIG. 2. Electronic diagram.

## An Electronic Analogy to the Nerve Synapse (Fig. 2)

Grid *a* is the association fiber that has been activated by the afferent neuron. Grid *b* is a pyramidal fiber whose function is largely inhibitory. Grid *c* may represent any of several extra pyramidal fibers which are, as often as not, excitatory. Anode *d,* with its continuation in and through the condenser, is the motor neuron. Battery *e* is the source of nourishment and recharge of this motor neuron. The space between cathode *f* and anode *d* is the field of the synapse. Electrons will pass across this gap from cathode to anode only if the grids are sufficiently positive to permit their flow. When grid *a* becomes positive, because of the firing of an input tube just before this one in line, the field next to the cathode is made positive. If this were the only grid in the tube, it would fire. But grids *b* and *c* exert their potentials upon the field. Hence, only when the algebraic sum of the charges upon *b* and *c* is positive, or if negative, is less than the positive charge upon *a*, will the field be in condition to start the flow of electrons and thus discharge the tube and the condenser; or only when the sum of the excitatory charges in a synaptic field is greater than the sum of the inhibitory charges, plus the force required to reach the threshold of irritability of a nerve fiber arising in that field, will such a nerve discharge.

## THE BINARY NATURE OF NEUROMUSCULAR ACTIVITY

Inasmuch as all mental processes are, in the last analysis, the result of activity of nerve fibers, so mental functions, as well as simple muscle responses, follow the law of all-or-none reaction. Since there are only two states of a living nerve fiber—(1) that of activity or discharge, and (2) that of rest and recharge—all mental activity can be reduced to formulas of binary numbers.[1]

| Binary: | 0 | 1 | 10 | 11 | 100 | 101 | 110 | 111 | 1000 | 1001 |
|---|---|---|---|---|---|---|---|---|---|---|
| Decimal: | 0 | 1 | 2 | 3 | 4 | 5 | 6 | 7 | 8 | 9 |

In the body there are two major systems of internal communication, the nervous and the endocrine. In terms of quantitative values, the former may better be represented by binary and the latter by decimal numbers. The strength of contraction of a given muscle at a given instant depends, among other factors, upon the amount of the stimulation by the nerve supplying the muscle. This amount is the measure of the number of nerve fibers firing at the instant in question, each fiber functioning at maximum intensity. The amount is, therefore, expressible in binary numbers. The strength of contraction of a given muscle is also, in part, dependent upon the hormonic conditioning of the muscle by catalysts carried from the endocrine gland, through the blood stream, into the cells of the muscle itself. The amount of hormonic effect is a linear function of the amount of the catalyst brought to the muscle, and can best be represented in degrees, percentage, proportions, or other values expressed decimally. The picture of a functioning motor nerve is like a halftone, its surface being made up of black dots on a white background. None of the dots, even on the areas that seem gray, are any-

[1] The binary number system is one in which there is only one digit (instead of nine) and the zero. In this system every number is an expression of a selection between one value or another, or one series or another, of a series of such selections. In this system 0 (decimal system) = 0 (binary system), and 1 (*d*) = 1 (*b*). The choice here is between whether something *is* or *is not*. 0 (*b*) means *is not*. The number 2 (*d*) is in last analysis two choices as to whether two things are or are not, with the decision being "are" in both cases. This doubling of the positive decision is in the binary system indicated by placing the figure 1 in the first space to the left, as is done in a decimal system to indicate ten. Thus if "one-zero" (10) equals ten in a system of 10 digits, "one-zero" (10) equals two in a system of 2 digits. 3 (*d*) is really the result of the decisions involved in 2 (*d*) with one more decision as to whether an additional thing *is* or *is not*. 4 (*d*) involves two decisions such as in 2 (*d*). 5 (*d*), the same as 4 (*d*), plus the additional decision as to an extra unit, etc. Represented in the binary system the digits of the decimal system are:

thing but black, each as black as the rest. The picture, however, of the hormonic effect of the endocrine gland is like that of a colored photograph in which the color consists of dyes. The color of any one area, no matter how small, can be expressed in shades and tints of primary colors. Thus, we listen, and think, and speak in terms of either-or, plus-minus, 1–0 process; but the thresholds at which these intellectual phenomena appear are determined by more-less, stronger-weaker, acid-basic, combinations and relations.

## CYBERNETIC REACTIONS OF THE C.N.S.[2]

An electronic calculating machine makes use of the all-or-none principle and the binary system of numbers. Such an instrument seems functionally analogous to the human central nervous system. Just as the calculating machine receives and stores information to use later in solving problems, stating over-all values, and making predictions, so the human being receives and stores information and later, sometimes many decades later, makes linguistic pronouncements on the basis of the information received.

Just as the accuracy and validity of the record that issues from the calculating machine are dependent upon the material that was punched upon the tapes making up the creature's experience, so the accuracy and validity of this record that you are now following with your eye are dependent upon the author's experience. What you are now reading is like the tapes that your electronic cousin scans with his electric eye. You can respond to this "tape" by reading it, either silently or aloud, or by copying it in your notebook; or you can respond to it as it becomes one of a great many tapes you have experienced in the past. Just as the reliability of the calculating machine suffers when a condenser is shorted or a tube is blown, so the reliability of your machine is disturbed by defects of structure. A single bullet may destroy either machine, or it may cause either to function erratically.

It is obvious that all automatisms subtended by the central nervous system, both innate and acquired, are developed, stored, and "played back," much as are the routine reactions of any man-made cybernetic device. Following this figure a little further, we can say the C.N.S. is not one cybernetic instrument but several interlocking automatic devices employing many of the same mechanical effectors. It is true that in the cerebellum the vermis is an automatic integrator of the various, often conflicting, machines; yet this clearing-house center leaves unresolved many of the conflicts among the acquired automatisms, and, in clearing the demands of conflicting cybernetic instruments, gives precedence to those whose functions are vital and vegetative, to the detriment of the intellectual and linguistic instrumentalities. In fine, the automatic talking machine often is the last cleared.

Cybernetics helps us to understand not only the acquired automatisms

---

[2] *Cybernetics* (Greek *kubernētēs* = steersman) is a word adapted by Norbert Wiener to generalize his study of communication and control in the theory of messages. Hence *cybernetic,* used adjectivally as here.

already described in this chapter but also most of our intellectual processes. Practically all that we call *mind* can be conceived in part as being the product of an electronic calculating machine or of a binary system or of both.

### Cybernetic Parallels

1. Association of ideas
2. Conditioned reflexes
3. Mathematical processes
4. Prediction of future events
5. Intuition
6. Recall and imagination
7. Rote memory
8. Immediate memory span and positive after-image
9. Hypnosis and suggestion
10. Analogical thinking and figures of speech

### Binary Parallels

1. If a word has both a synonym and an antonym the utterance of that word will by free association call forth the antonym rather than the synonym: *boy-girl,* rather than *boy-lad; bad-good,* rather than *bad-evil; yes-no,* rather than *yes-O.K.*

2. Negative questions and answers. Illustration: Suppose you ask someone about the weather today. If you really want information, you inquire, "*Is it nice today or isn't it?*" In terms of the binary system you are asking for 1 or 0. If you have already discovered the weather to be pleasant you say, "*Isn't it nice?*" You ask for an answer exactly opposite to what you expect. You virtually say "*Is it foul out today?*" The answer to "*Isn't it nice?*" is "*yes.*" The informer is agreeing, not to the question as stated, but as implied. His answer is equivalent to "*Yes, we have no bananas.*" If you have discovered the weather to be unpleasant, you say, "*It isn't nice today, is it?*" Again the answer is illogical, but still clear by negative implication or association. The reply is "*no.*"

3. Antonyms made by change of sign (like changing the 1 to 0): like-dislike, like-unlike, behave-misbehave, polite-impolite, typical-atypical, thing-nothing, encode-decode, can-can't, where-nowhere, body-nobody. We even have double reverses of meaning like: encouraged-discouraged-undiscouraged. One perfect example of the binary system is the antonymous pair *one-none* (*one-no-one* or 1–0).

4. The negative after-image. No doubt the phenomenon of seeing a spot of black after staring at a bright lamp for a moment is based in part upon the phenomenon of fatigue. Fatigue, however, is responsible only for the general pattern of the reaction—that part which is represented by the prefix *after.* The image, and its negativity, are partly products of cerebration—products of the functioning of nerves far removed from those directly exposed to the fatiguing stimulation. We have the same sort of after-image if we stare at a spot of black on a white wall. We now perceive a spot of white in place of the black. This we cannot explain on the basis of fatigue, since black does not stimulate the retina. Now we must explain the after-pattern on the basis of a resting of sensory end-organs. Whether the negative after-image is explainable on the basis of fatigue or rest, or merely difference of intensity of stimulation, the negative aspect demonstrates the great propensity of the C.N.S. to resolve quantitative differences into a polarized system in which there are no midpoints or degrees.

*Examples of Binary Processes*

On a higher level of experience we polarize our reactions to many aspects of an environment. The room is either "hot" or "cold," seldom "just right" (and never "just right" for the whole party). "Love" and "hate" are notoriously identified as related polarizations of romantic attachments. We and our allies are noble: our enemies are evil: and we have no difficulty in switching our opinion from "bad" to "good," when an enemy changes sides and becomes our ally. All the characters in the Western thriller may be placed in two simple categories, the "good ones" and the "bad ones." Most opinions about individuals from social, racial, political, and religious groups other than our own are drawn from generalizations in which various qualities of character and sundry physical aspects are listed as being either present or absent. Hence our first question about such a person, to whom we have just been introduced, is not a decimal calculation of "to what degree?" but a binary question of "is he, or isn't he?" Delusions of persecution are but overextensions, or oversimplifications, of these "black or white" polarizations. The Whigs won the last election. Our party lost. Now we can expect a depression, high taxes, and severe drouth.

Much of our problem-solving, mathematical or otherwise, is by binary processes. "If one dozen oranges costs 30 cents, how much would 18 cost?" The child who first encounters such a problem in his "oral arithmetic" does not move at once to the correct method of solution. He tries many methods, rejecting each in turn until he finds one that satisfies him. He has in this simple problem the numbers, ½, 1, 2, 3, 6, 12, 18, and 30. Shall he add, subtract, multiply, or divide? Several right, and many wrong, combinations are available. The question always comes to him: Is this right or wrong? Seldom does he list all the possibilities and then make a selection. He employs binary judgements of random suggestions. Even an experienced adult employs some binary processes in the solution of this problem. He has several correct methods to try and, if he wishes, reject. For example, he tries the very logical method of finding the cost of one orange, but rejects the method when he discovers that the cost would not be even money. Then, "on second thought," he may see that the cost of one orange could be expressed as 30/12 of one cent; and thus one solution would require the multiplication of 30 by 18, followed by division by 12. This seems too big a project to solve without paper and pencil. Then he starts again and finds that he can easily discover the cost of six oranges, and that 18 is exactly three sixes. This flitting from method to method is done with such great speed that it is only by dint of sharp introspection that one can discover his binary calculator at work.

Another example of perceptive binary processes is that of proofreading. The proofreader makes rapid judgements as to whether what he hears the copyreader say is, or is not, the same as what he sees on the proof sheet. Whenever the general pattern of one agrees with the other, the judgement is "same." His mistakes consist of letting what he sees influence what he hears or vice versa. Advertisers exploit this propensity to binary error by making meaningless claims that seem to have definite meaning. "After a national survey of the dentifrice used by 50,000 dentists it was found that more dentists chose Scratcho than any other dentifrice." What the average reader understands this to say is that "dentists use more Scratcho than any other dentifrice." His error arises from the fact that he tries to fit a meaning to the over-all pattern of the sentence, not noticing that the word *more* modifies *dentists* rather than *Scratcho*. No meaning fits the sentence as a whole, but he accepts his version just as the proofreader accepts *house* for *horse* in the sentence, "He put spurs to his house."

The binary and cybernetic illustrations seem even more cogent when one considers what happens to an individual's mental processes when the machinery back of those processes is damaged. Just as a damaged card-sorting machine will make errors in assembling cards in predetermined categories, so a lesion in the C.N.S. will manifest itself in one or more of the following:

1. Bizarre association of ideas, or a paucity of association.
2. Disturbances of reflexes, conditioned or otherwise, sometimes absence of reflexes.
3. Failure to apply measures consistently in solving problems involving counting or other numerical processes.
4. Failure to employ past experiences in anticipation of future situations.
5. Degeneration of intuition into impulsive, unrealistic rationalization.
6. Inability to construct in imagery that which is not presently sensed.
7. Inability to learn such stereotypes of expression as poems, musical compositions, prayers, and dance routines, or the inability to change a stereotype once learned.
8. A perseveration of pattern of immediate response, such as verbal iterations.
9. Tendency of the patient to respond to conflicting suggestions (ambivalent reactions).
10. Inability of the patient to make any but the most literal interpretations of what he hears or reads; or the tendency to invest literal language with absurd figurative meanings.

Just as a person inexperienced in the manipulations of the binary number system will be slow, clumsy, and inaccurate in his calculations in the 0–1 notation, so will the damaged brain show binary errors. The patient will record 0 instead of 1 for two quite different reasons:

1. The loss of the concept of *opposite*. Associations are all of one sign: *good, evil, bad, kind* are all responses to either of the following questions: what words mean the same as *nice?* What words mean the opposite of *nice?* In spite of this failure the patient usually knows what each of these words means. He has but lost the concept of the relationship between ideas.

2. The uncertainty of response involving words having well-known opposites. He may say *yes* when he means *no*. He knows that *yes* and *no* are opposite, but he is not sure of which is which. He often chooses 1 instead of 0, or vice versa.

## NERVE NETS

One of the all-pervasive mechanisms of the cerebrospinal nervous system is that of the "feedback circuit." Again a close analogy can be drawn from the realm of electronics. If the microphone into which a person is talking— such as the microphone of the hearing aid—be brought too close to the earpiece of the instrument, a squeal results. The electrical output of the amplifier is converted into acoustic energy, a part of which finds its way to the diaphragm of the microphone. This increases the flow of electrons from the cathode of the microphone tube, thus causing an extra discharge across the amplifier with increased output to the ear piece. The frequency, or pitch, of the discharge and the feedback will be that to which the entire circuit is most resonant. The simplest feedback circuits of the cerebrospinal system are much like the circuit described above. A contracting muscle pinches, and thus stimulates, the kinesthetic end-organs in the tendon of the muscle. The afferent fibers thus stimulated start impulses across association neurones of the cord. These neurones synapse with fibers that stimulate the muscle. Hence the muscle by its contraction furnishes its own ever increasing stimulation. A severe muscle cramp results.

To prevent such a neuromuscular feedback, another purely nervous feedback checks it. This circuit is like the automatic volume control (AVC) of the audio amplifier. In such a circuit a small part of the electrical output of one of the tubes in line is fed back into a special grid of the tube. Before it passes to the grid, however, its voltage is reversed from + to —. Thus, when the output of the tube reaches a predetermined level it checks itself through the inhibiting feedback to the AVC grid. In the neuromuscular circuit described above, the cramp is prevented in a similar manner. At the point where the impulses enter the cord, to synapse with the across-the-cord association neurones, synapses are also made with ascending neurones, which carry relatively weak impulses to association fibers on a higher level of the C.N.S. These fibers synapse with descending neurones, which in turn end in the synaptic field of the lower motor neurones supplying the muscle. We thus have two parallel bridges from the primary afferent neurone to the final motor neurone. The upper bridge, however, transmits impulses that, though they may be weaker, are opposite in sign to those from the lower, more direct, bridge. Since the impulses are opposite in sign they serve to check the effects of the neuromuscular feedback.

Another interesting feedback is that which enters the thalamus by way of fibers that originate in the globus pallidus, so that a part of the output of the basal ganglia is fed back into the ganglia at the opposite end of the chain (Fig. 3). Thus when the basal ganglia are allowed to escape from inhibitory control by the cerebrum, a circular reaction is set up, so reinforcing itself that the cerebrum has difficulty in re-establishing its checks. Thus, crying spells occur, and temper tantrums, and hysterical laughter.

The nervous system is made up of a complicated maze of such closed circuits, interconnected and interacting. They are variously designated: feedback circuits, reverberating circuits, nerve nets, resonant circuits. The maintenance of body tonus is largely brought about by such a circular reflex; so is postural balance. Breathing, walking, and suckling and similar reciprocating reactions are negotiated through nerve nets that intermittently restrain other nerve nets.

From the point of view of the student of speech, however, the most interesting of the nerve nets are those in the cerebrum that are involved in the

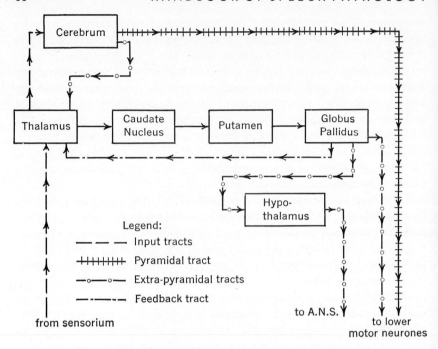

**FIG. 3. The basal ganglia and their connections.**

intellectual activity which (apparently) takes place there. A child is holding a stick of candy to bite off the end of it. Most of the output of the motor cortex is used to effect movements of the muscle systems involved in the complex of reactions. If, however, the child is listening to his mother's pleadings that he should stop eating the candy and drink his glass of milk, a great deal of the output of the motor cortex is fed back into the association areas resulting in increased cerebral activity that has little, if any, muscular or peripheral effect. There is little outward evidence of this activity but, unless we completely discount our introspections, we must accept the reality of this and other hidden mental processes. Worry, recurrent fears, dreams, and so on, are to most of us incontrovertible realities. We know that we have experienced them; and we know that, for the most part, we can conceal these processes from the observer. We assume, however, that others have similar experiences; and that, without a recounting by the dreamer of the plot of his dreams, we can have little, if any, knowledge of what he is dreaming. These inner experiences are processed by feedback mechanisms. All contemplations, imaginings, plannings, calculations, considered decisions, and the like, are similarly processed. Accompanying all speech except the most mechanical processes of reading and reciting is a great deal of reverberating, circular cerebration employing feedback nets.

An illustration: You are asked to introduce one of your friends to another. You look at each to recall his name. Your memory of the name of each is immediate, but you are dismayed to discover that only the first name of each "comes to your mind." The more you struggle to recall the last names, the more you are disconcerted, and the more loudly these first names ring out in your auditory memory. There is no use in struggling with the problem. To wrestle with a reverberating nerve net is futile. All you can say is "If I had not wanted to speak his name, it would have come to me instantly; but never mind, don't tell me; it will come to me later." Then, after a change of association, the "reverberations" will stop and you will interrupt a conversation with, "I have it now: Your name is Williams." If instead of trying to introduce your friends you had sat alone in the quiet of your home and had called each on the telephone, you would have had no difficulty in finding their numbers in an alphabetical listing of their last names. There is probably a good deal of this type of reverberation in stuttering.

It is obvious that many mental fixations, compulsions, and recurring fantasies of psychopathologies are also viewable as the result of complex reverberating circuits. In fact, the rationale frequently offered for electroshock therapy is to break up such nerve nets in which the patient's personality is ensnared. One such resonant circuit is particularly significant in the understanding of the speech failures of young children. Speech depends for its initial motivation upon an instinct, or appetence, for gregarious relations. The child who is completely indifferent to his human environment does not develop speech. Antisocial attitudes are more productive of speech than the asocial. Asocial attitudes in a child potentially normal in intellectual equipment involve preoccupation with his fantasy life. Such a child learns to derive great psychic income from inner experiences unrelated to the social world of reality. The child whose mental mechanisms are prompted by the attitudes, remarks, and deeds of persons around him is not so likely to develop self-stimulating nerve circuits as the one whose promptings are from within his own system. In limiting his reactions to those triggered from within, the variety of response is restricted, until finally the repertoire of these responses is reduced to those few mental mechanisms that characterize his special and particular aberrations. These mechanisms have very aptly been labeled autistic. There is in this label a definitely *double entendre: autistic* signifies, *psychologically,* a preoccupation with self and a rejection of the psycho-social environment, and, physiologically, a lowering of the threshold of stimulation of the nerve nets of the brain by impulses from other nets and a raising of the threshold to stimulations brought over exteroceptor pathways.

In an early section of this chapter we referred to certain classes of automatisms. In a real sense we have now returned to a discussion of some of those automatisms under new names and in new frames of reference. Automatisms are often brought about through resonant circuits or through feedback in interconnecting nerve nets. Similarly, a cybernetic reaction may usually be classified as an automatism. The justification of the concept of the reverberating circuit, in addition to that of the simple automatism, is

that the former involves greater continuity than the latter. The former signifies a control, the latter a mere triggering. The machine gun fires itself and
continues to do so until it is stopped; but the rifle needs to be triggered for
each discharge. Each explosion of the machine gun triggers the next; but
each explosion of the rifle is a single automatic response to a single movement
of the trigger. The machine gun is a reverberating mechanism, the rifle is
automatic only.

The automatisms described in early paragraphs of this chapter can thus
be re-analyzed. Those listed under A—the innate, automatic, vegetative reactions—have in them very little of the element of reverberation. All of the
rest of the automatisms—B to F—are serial, or reverberating, or cybernetic
automatisms. The gag reflex is a simple, uncomplicated automatism; but
an iteration of word or phrase is only partially described by the term *automatism*. It should be noted that, by and large, in the catalogue of disorders of
speech the pure automatisms are arrayed against the more complex mechanisms. Speech lapses are rarely the result of failure of pure automatisms;
rather they come as an effect of a dys-integration of some speech synergy,
or an interference with such a synergy by a simple automatism that obtrudes
itself into the motor outlets and pre-empts the lower motor neurons of the
muscles of articulation.

## BIBLIOGRAPHY

*Concerning the All-or-None Principle:*
BRAZIER, M. A. 1951. The electrical activity of the nervous system. New York:
Macmillan.

*Concerning Physiological Inhibitions:*
GASSER, H. S. 1935. Nerve potentials produced by rapidly repeated stimuli and
their relation to responsiveness of nerve stimulation. *Amer. J. Physiol.,*
III, 35.

*Concerning Cybernetics:*
FAIRBANKS, G. 1954. A theory of the speech mechanism as a servo-system.
*J. Speech Hearing Disorders,* 19, 133.
WIENER, N. 1948. Cybernetics or control and communication in the animal and
in the machine. New York: Wiley.

*Concerning Reverberating Circuits:*
LORENTE, DE NO, R. 1935. Facilitation of motoneurones. *Amer. J. Physiol.,*
113, 505.
Patterns of organization in the central nervous system. 1952. Proceedings of
the Association for Research in Nervous and Mental Diseases (New York
session, 1950). Baltimore: Williams & Wilkins.

# CHAPTER 4

# SPEECH SOUND FORMATION

● *Giles Wilkeson Gray, Ph.D.*

## GENERAL CONSIDERATIONS

ANY ATTEMPT to describe completely the manner in which the sounds of speech are formed must necessarily take into consideration a number of possible contributing factors. For one thing, it is now generally recognized that, contrary to earlier theory, one of the distinguishing characteristics of speech sound formation is that it consists not of fixed, static positions of the organs of articulation, but rather of dynamic, functional activity, of movements of those organs, though generally about some fairly consistent and uniform pattern. Moreover, these movements are themselves highly complicated and extremely variable. They are modified by their phonetic context, that is, by the influence of the preceding and following sounds. They are further modified, in continuous speech, by both the logical content of the utterance and the emotional attitude of the speaker at the moment, by the formality or informality of the speaking situation, by the immediately desired precision of the articulation and, at times, by the demands of utmost intelligibility.

Still further, since the same speaker will not always utter a given sound in the same combination of context, ideational content, and emotional attitude, his articulatory movements will never follow identical successive patterns, a fact which adds to the variability of the formation itself. Added to this basis for individual variation is the fact that no two persons' oral configurations are identical, the differences giving rise to significant differences in the manner in which sounds are formed by different people. These differences are further observable in the ease in which our friends' voices and speech patterns are identified.

At least one further factor will influence a full and complete description of the manner in which speech sounds are formed. That is the use which is to be made of that description. Very few will have use for such minute detail as Jesperson (1889) developed in his Analphabetic system; furthermore, his descriptions were based on a positional rather than a functional theory. Perhaps as an indication of what might be involved in the production of a single sound his analysis might be helpful to the phonologist; but to the teacher in-

terested in helping his students to speak more distinctly it offers little that
is usable. Accurate and detailed descriptions may in some instances be
highly desirable; in other situations they would be so cumbersome as to be
useless. It is to be suspected that most of us, including speech pathologists
and therapists, who are dealing with everyday problems involving articulation and pronunciation, will be interested first of all in developing speech of
acceptable intelligibility, after which it may be possible to add the more delicate shadings which may contribute significantly to speech over and above
bare understanding.

It is not the purpose of the present chapter, therefore, to develop a complete phonetic theory with respect to the formation of the sounds of speech.
It is rather to present as concisely and as directly as possible the minimum
essentials of speech sound formation which will be of value to the therapist
in the developing of a practically functional degree of intelligibility. Further
development of that theory may be found in any of a number of excellent
recent texts on the subject. The criterion is to be, What is required for a
given sound, in context, to contribute to an understanding of the content of
the utterance?

In the production of any sound of speech, whether in isolation or in context, four essentials must be observed.[1] First, the sound must be correctly
formed; second, it must be adequately formed; third, it must be supported
by sufficient breath; and fourth, the "release," or the movement into the next
sound formation, whichever is called for in the context, must be clean, sharp,
and positive.[2]

### Correct Formation

It was pointed out in the first paragraph that although an essential aspect
of sound formation consists of movements, at the same time these movements are generally around some fairly consistent position. Unless there were
some common elements in the production there could be no consistency in
the product, and oral language itself would be impossible. Although it is
true that many factors influence the essential movements, the positions about
which those movements center are what give the sounds their identifying
individuality. An attempted s-sound, for instance, formed with the tip of the
tongue between the teeth, is incorrectly formed; the sound will not be a
characteristic [s]. Whatever the context may be in which a [b] occurs, at
some time in its formation the lips must come together if the [b] is to be
correctly produced. My laryngologist insists on my using the vowel [e] whenever he wants to examine my vocal bands. I tell him, "You can't do that":
the [e], if it is to be a good one, cannot be formed with the tongue held down

---

[1] As an indication that these essentials are also involved in normal speech, see
G. W. Gray and W. W. Braden, 1951, pp. 518 ff.

[2] See also Pierre Jean Rousselot and Fauste Laclotte, 1913, p. 25: Sound formation
consists of three acts: ". . . prendre la position voulue, maintenir celle-ci quelques
instants et ensuite l'abandonner."

far enough for an adequate examination of the larynx. (What he wants, of course, is to get the epiglottis out of the way.) Movement in the articulation of speech sounds is important; but instruction in the production of those sounds will more profitably focus on the positions about which those movements center. The [k] in *beak* and *book* is not the same, it is true; nor in *keel* and *cool*. Nor is the [l] identical in the last two words. But in teaching either the [k] or the [l] in these and other contexts, the emphasis should be laid on the consistency with which the tongue rises to the palate at approximately the same places every time the sounds are produced.

### Adequate Formation

It is not enough that the articulatory organs move about some distinguishing position and do it correctly; the movement must be positive and the position definite. When the tongue is brought to the palate in a [t], the movement and the position which the tongue takes must have adequate strength to produce the sound cleanly and without confusion. A major problem in voice-training consists in strengthening and invigorating the musculature of articulation sufficiently to produce the sounds with adequate distinctness. Inadequacy of formation, whether resulting from careless habit or from pathological conditions, results in indistinct, inarticulate speech which interferes seriously with the effectiveness of the communication. The movements and the positions may be, so far as the general *place* of articulation is concerned, entirely correct; but if they are so indefinite, so weak that many of the sounds themselves are unidentifiable, the inevitable result is unintelligibility, partial or complete.

### Adequate Breath Support

One may close and open one's lips repeatedly without producing a sound. With strong support from the breath, however, creating a pressure against each occlusion, a series of [p]'s will result. Except for certain abnormal or unusual conditions, breath is essential in the production of voice. Even under these extreme conditions, such as esophageal speech, some stream of air must be provided to produce the vibrations necessary for any sound at all. Actually, it takes very little pressure of breath to produce the sounds of speech, and very little breath in the utterance of a single phrase. But unless that adequate little pressure is present, either the sounds will lack positiveness or the utterance will be entirely inaudible. In fact, there may not even be any sounds at all.

### Definite Ending

Sometimes the peculiar nature of the sound itself, or of its phonetic context, calls for a definite finish. In such instances, as in the case of a final vowel or a final continuing consonant, as in *see, will, rare, sing,* the sound is ended either by stopping the flow of breath, or by opening the glottis so that no further vibration is produced. In other instances, the articulatory organs move directly from the characteristic position of the sound being produced to that for the next. In still others the organs move sharply away from the sound position, providing a "release" or a positive ending to the sound itself. In no case, however, should the sound be permitted to fade out indefinitely, or to glide so vaguely into the next that most of the distinctness, and hence the intelligibility, is lost.

The [t] provides a good illustration of the second and third cases. When appearing as a final sound, as in *get,* the tongue pulls sharply away from the palate, so that a slight aspiration, or escape of breath, follows, giving a finish to the sound and to the entire word. Without this "release" *cat* and *cap* may be indistinguishable; the difference in the sound of the aspiration, however, contributes to the difference between the two words as they are heard. In combination, as in *aptly,* the tongue pulls away from the palate only partly (as also in this last word), leaving the tip in position for the following [l]. Two common errors here consist, first, of insisting on the aspiration before forming the [l], and second, of omitting the [t] altogether, taking away part of the word's distinctiveness.

For the maximum correctness and distinctness of utterance, the organs of articulation, especially the tongue and lips, must be exercised to develop precision and strength of movement and definiteness of position. Overprecise, pedantically meticulous articulation is not the goal; but consistent and persistent drill on tongue and lip movements and positions will contribute immeasurably to the effectiveness of communication.

## BASES OF CLASSIFICATION

Speech sounds may be classified on a number of bases. One such basis is the mode of production. According to this classification, the sounds of speech are formed: (1) by the modification of vocal tones in the resonating cavities of the throat, mouth, and nose; (2) by partial or complete obstruction to the emission of breath by the vocal folds, the soft palate, the tongue, or the lips; (3) by a combination of these two.

But they may be classified on bases other than that of the manner of their production. They may be differentiated according to the position around which the movements take place, and the customary designations of the sounds include references to these positions. For example, a sound described in part as bilabial would be produced by specific movement or juxtaposition of the two lips. Similarly, a sound indicated as labiodental would be produced by interaction of the lips and teeth—in all sounds in English the upper teeth and lower lip. An alveolar sound would be one in the formation of which the tongue touches or approximates the ridge of the hard palate just slightly back of the upper teeth. Other sounds are similarly designated.

Speech sounds are further classified according to the degree of obstruction or occlusion set up against the outgoing breath stream. In certain sounds, for instance, the closure is complete; and is usually followed in English speech by a fairly sharp aspiration, as already described, immediately following the "release." Such sounds are quite appropriately called "plosives"; if the fact of the closure rather than of the release is to be emphasized, they may be designated as "stops." They are of necessity of short duration, as contrasted with many other sounds in which the obstruction is only partial (or so slight as hardly to constitute any obstruction at all), and which may be continued for as long as desirable, or as long as the breath holds out. Those sounds which may be held indefinitely are known as "continuants."

Reference to the essential characteristics of the various sounds as they have been classified here and on still other bases will be helpful in identifying the sounds themselves.

## THE VOWELS

Let us first consider those sounds with which most of us are familiar, the vowels. They consist entirely of vocal tones modified by positions and movements of the tongue and lips which cause changes in the resonators and thereby in the harmonic structure of the sounds themselves. Other laryngeal structures, such as the epiglottis, are also involved; but since we have no conscious control over them, they are not included in the present descriptions. Since the actual positions and movements are not readily defined, the descriptions of the formations themselves are therefore less specific and somewhat more difficult than of the consonants. Furthermore, since the formation constantly shifts from the beginning of a vowel to its ending (Black, 1937), any description must take only that portion of the movement, or that position, which seems to be most positively characteristic of that vowel. This shifting varies in degree from the barely perceptible, and that by a trained ear, to the readily identifiable diphthongs.

So far as conscious control is involved, the different vowels are produced chiefly by varying movements and positions of the tongue and lips, together with varying degrees of tenseness of the muscles. Actually, as Heffner points out, none of the so-called organs of articulation are absolutely essential to the production of identifiable sounds (1952, p. 90). In most cases, however, their absence is likely to be the exception and requires highly specialized techniques in order to develop acceptable and intelligible speech. For the most part, the tongue is the most important organ, not excepting the larynx itself.

With respect to the part played by the tongue, therefore, the vowels may be classified as front, central, and back; high, mid, and low; tense and lax; close or open; the lips may be narrow or wide, rounded or unrounded (Heffner, 1952, p. 96).[3]

[3] This classification seems to have been developed by Alexander Melville Bell some ninety years ago. He was able to postulate a total of 72 vowels, some of which, he admitted, were purely theoretical. Of these only from 16 to 20 are used in the English language, depending in part on the particular dialect spoken.

**The Basic Positions**

The four basic positions, as indicated by Heffner (pp. 88 f.), are the high front, the high back, the low front, and low back. If one raises the blade of the tongue, at about C on Fig. 1, so that it is very close to the hard palate at about 5 on the figure, providing a narrow slit between tongue and palate, and then produces a vocal tone, the resulting sound will be the "high front" vowel [i]. The spaces both in front and back of the position of closest approximation form resonance cavities which give the [i] its characteristic timbre. One may get much the same result from raising the tongue to whistle the highest note possible, and then without moving the tongue, producing a vocal tone, which should be close to an [i].

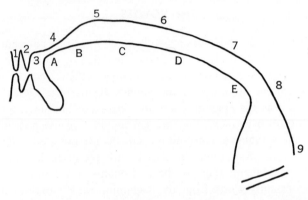

FIG. 1. Relative positions of closest approximations of tongue and palate in the formation of the various sounds of speech. See text for details of descriptions.

If, now, one raises the back of the tongue, at about E, to approximately the point 7 (Fig. 1),[4] where the hard and soft palate are joined, so that a narrow slit is formed between the tongue and palate at that point, and then produces a vocal tone, the resultant sound will be the "high back" vowel [u]. Rounding and protruding the lips slightly at the same time will aid in producing a more definite vowel. Producing a vocal tone with the lips and tongue in position to whistle the lowest tone possible should give much the same effect.

With the tongue lowered as far as it will go without forcing, and drawn slightly back toward the pharynx (Heffner, 1952, p. 104), the sound should be the "low back" [ɑ]. The entire resonating cavity above the larynx, with the exception of the nasal passages, seems to be functioning as a single resonator. In these and all other English vowels the nasal cavities are closed off from the oral by means of the soft palate, which rises to close against the back wall of the oral pharynx, except as hereinafter noted.

The remaining front and back vowels are characteristically produced by

---

[4] All such notations will refer to the tongue and palate positions as indicated in Fig. 1. The former will be indicated by capital letters and the latter by Arabic numerals.

successively lowering the tongue through positions from the high front [i] to the low front [a], and from the high back [u] to the low back [ɑ]. The familiar vowel diagram (Gray and Wise, 1946, p. 223), which represents graphically these positions, will help to clarify these relationships. The left side, indicating the front of the tongue, begins with [i] at the extreme high point, representing the "high front" vowel, then goes downward successively through [ɪ], [e], [ɛ], and [æ], to [a], the "low front" vowel. The right side, indicating the back of the tongue, drops successively from [u] at the extreme high position—the "high back" vowel—through [ʊ], [o], and [ɔ], to [ɑ], the "low back" vowel.

When the lips are brought into play in the formation of these successive vowels they characteristically, though not necessarily, exhibit a fairly definite progression. In producing the [ɑ] the lips are normally open, relaxed, and "unrounded." As one advances through the series of back vowels, from [ɑ] progressively through [ɔ], [o], and [ʊ], to [u], the corners of the mouth draw in, the lips become more and more rounded, and tend to protrude slightly. Because of this progression the back vowels are also classified as "rounded."     •

If, on the other hand, one advances through the front vowels, from [a] successively through [æ], [ɛ], [e], and [ɪ] to [i], the corners of the lips are progressively drawn back fairly widely, so that for [i] the opening between them becomes narrow and elongated. It is difficult to produce an [i] with the teeth as far apart as the width of two fingers. These are the "unrounded" vowels.

These positions of the lips are all relative; and while helpful for instructional purposes, they are not absolutely essential in the formation of the vowels. It is possible to produce readily distinguishable front vowels with only a very slight spreading of the lips, or even with none at all; or one may produce the back vowels with the lips completely relaxed. Labial agility is not a basic requirement in the formation of the vowels.

### The Central Vowels

The central vowels are so called because of the fact that in their formation neither the front nor the back of the tongue is elevated other than as it is influenced by the movement of the central portion. In the lowest of these, [ʌ], the tongue is raised only slightly more than for [ɑ] and is perhaps a bit more forward; it is lax and the lips are unrounded. The vowel occurs in such words as *but, come, tub, enough, mother, touch, bug,* but rarely if ever in unaccented syllables. Closely related to this sound is the [ɜ], which occurs syllabically or in stressed syllables when the "r is dropped," in such words as *her, bird, world, first, colonel.* In this central vowel the midportion of the tongue is elevated slightly higher than for [ʌ], with the sides curving up to touch lightly the molar teeth. Whereas in [ʌ] the tongue is lax, in [ɜ] it is tense. In a third of these central vowels, [ɝ], used characteristically syllabically or in stressed syllables (as in the *her* words listed above in this para-

graph) by those speakers who "retain their r's," the fore part of the tongue is
raised still higher, narrowing the opening between the tongue and the palate
at about D-6 (Fig. 1). According to most descriptions of this sound, the tip
of the tongue tends to curl backward, giving rise to its description as a "retro-
flex" movement. Although it is quite true that an extreme sound can be made
by such curving back, it is doubtful if retroflexion is an essential aspect of
the formation of [ɝ].

The fourth of these central vowels is known as the "schwa," a name said
to be derivative of the Hebrew *sh'wa*. It is represented by the symbol [ə],
and seems to resemble as closely as may be a completely unstressed [ʌ]. The
tongue and lips are completely relaxed, and the sound itself is so short in
duration that it is difficult to identify its characteristic timbre, if indeed it has
one. The sound is used in two ways, both of them in unstressed syllables. It
serves for the "er" syllable (with its various spellings) in such words as
*mother, sailor, forward,* and so on, by speakers who do not use the [ɝ] in
stressed syllables, that is, by those who habitually "drop their r's." Again, it
is used by all speakers in the unstressed syllables of such words as *sofa,
Illinois, Iowa, formative, vowel,* where there is no indication of an *r*-sound
in the spelling. In this connection it has no relation to the *r*-sounds.

The *schwa* [ə], as a substitute for the unstressed "er" syllables, has its
counterpart in [ɚ] for those speakers who commonly retain the r's in these
words, and who use the [ɝ] in stressed syllables. With respect to the use of
the *r*-sounds, the usage of these four central vowels may be shown in the
following:

|  | Stressed Syllables | Unstressed Syllables |
|---|---|---|
| For those who "retain their r's" | ɝ | ɚ |
| For those who "drop their r's" | ɜ | ə |

Further discussion of the consonantal *r*-sounds will be presented in a later
section.

### The Diphthongs

It is well known that none of the vowels remains constant throughout its
duration (Black, 1937; Stetson, 1951, p. 37). Gemelli and Pastori (1934)
point out that there is in every instance a period during which the sound is
being built up, so to speak, either from the initiation of the sound itself or
through a transition from the preceding sound. Following this formative
period come a few waves, the number depending on the duration of the
total vowel, which exhibit the "typical" wave form, and presumably the
characteristic timbre of that particular vowel. Finally comes the ending, occurring either by a "dying-out" of the waves or by a transition into the following sound. These changes are normal; since they are ordinarily imperceptible to the ear, they do not affect the identification of the vowels. They
can be isolated only through the most careful observation by a trained ear

or by instrumental analysis. In some of the vowels, notably [e] and [o], the final shift in characteristic timbre is considered by most phoneticians to be so marked as to warrant identifying the sounds themselves as *diphthongs*, which are defined by Thomas (1947, p. 104) as "a vocalic glide within the limits of a single syllable." According to Heffner (1952, p. 112), they consist of "a syllable element, which begins with one sound and shifts to another. . . ." This shift is exclusive of "those brief building-up and dying-out stages which characterize every speech sound."

The identification of the various diphthongs themselves will serve to indicate the direction and the degree of shifting. In the words *try, fine, sigh, my,* in which the diphthong [aɪ] occurs, the shift is from low front [a] to the high front lax [ɪ]. In words such as *now, house, found, plow,* in which the diphthong [aʊ] is found, the shift is from [a] up and back to the mid back lax [ʊ]. In the diphthong [ɔɪ], as it is heard in *boy, noise, employ,* the shift is from the low back lax [ɔ] forward and up to the high front lax [ɪ].

Theoretically, diphthongs can be formed from almost any combination of two vowels; indeed, when an intermediate vowel is distinctly recognizable or where there is a pronounced glide-consonant mixed in, we may even have a triphthong, as in an occasional southern [hæjənd] for [hænd] *hand.* In the typical diphthong, however, the shift is from one of the lower to one of the higher vowels, with the one exception of [ju], both elements of which are high.

## THE CONSONANTS

The sounds of speech commonly known as consonants are characteristically produced by interposing some sort of partial or complete obstruction to the passage of the breath as it is forced from the lungs. In some of these, the vibrations set up by the passage of the breath as it is forced past the obstruction produces the only sound heard; in others it is the sudden stoppage in the emission by a complete occlusion, followed by a "release," that produces the only sound. In still others it is a combination of the two. To these various ways in which such sounds are formed is, in many instances, added still another element, that from the vibration of the vocal folds; and in some instances it is the sound from this vocal fold vibration which is modified in the oral and nasal cavities, much as are the vowels. In fact, in some instances the obstruction is so slight that the sound itself takes on something of the characteristics of a vowel.

Two other means of identifying the consonants as differentiated from the vowels which may be useful lie, first, in the fact that before words beginning with a consonant we use the article *a,* whereas before words beginning with a vowel we characteristically use *an.* Although this difference does not describe the essential nature of the two classes of sounds, it may serve to distinguish them as they are used. Second, whenever a sound can be used syllabically, that is, without the aid of any other sound to complete the syllable, it has in that situation the characteristics of a vowel rather than a consonant. For instance, in *button* [bʌtn̩], when the [t] explodes directly into the [n] without an intervening [ə], the [n] stands alone, forming a syllable by itself; hence it is syllabic and essentially a vowel. Similarly, when *bottle* is so pronounced that the [t] explodes directly into the [l], the [l] becomes syllabic and vocalic rather than consonantal.

### The Plosives

If a complete obstruction is set up in the oral chambers so that no breath can escape, then additional pressure is built up against this dam; and finally, if this dam is suddenly broken and the breath released, there is created one of a prominent group of consonants known as *plosives*. A further essential aspect of this complete closure is that the velum be pressed firmly against the back wall of the oral pharynx, so that none of the breath escapes through the nasal passages. Like most other consonants, these plosives may be accompanied or unaccompanied by vibration of the vocal folds, the former being "voiced" and the latter "unvoiced."

It should be noted that for the best production of these plosives, to insure that all the conditions mentioned in the early pages of this chapter be met, the obstruction must be in the right place; it must be firm and definite, and the breath pressure must be built up behind it; finally, the "release" must be sharp and positive. If any of these are lacking or inadequately achieved, the sound will be indistinct and some of the intelligibility may be lost.

The first of the positions where these plosives may be produced is at the two lips: hence the term applied to them, *bilabial*. The formation is simple: press the lips firmly together, build up the breath pressure back of them, and suddenly separate them. The only sound that can be produced in this manner is a [p]. If to this sound is added the vibration of the vocal folds, the sound must be a [b]. It is probable that the pressure is greater for a voiceless plosive than for a voiced; the distinction for present purposes is not important. Both [p] and [b], then, are bilabial plosives, unvoiced and voiced respectively.

Neither of these plosives, nor indeed any of the others, ever stands alone in our language. They are not prolonged except very briefly in such expressions as *cap pistol, top pile, tub bath, mad dance, book keeper,* and the like. In such cases, although there are two *letters,* in successive words, suggesting two sounds, actually there is only one plosive. The *stop* phase of the sound, that is, the closure, is merely prolonged and finally released into the following sound.[5] The pronunciation of two separate and successive consonants in such instances—frequently heard in speakers who have been told that they must articulate distinctly—is probably the result of overcompensation. It smacks of highly objectionable pedantry.

[5] For a discussion of "incomplete plosive consonants" see Daniel Jones, 1922, pp. 36 f.

The second place where plosives may be produced is at the alveolar ridge in the hard palate, about 4 on Fig. 1. If you will slide the tip of your tongue back from the base of the upper teeth, you will notice a smooth ridge from a quarter to a half inch back of the teeth. This is called the alveolar ridge. Now if the tip of the tongue is pressed firmly against this ridge, closing off all emission of breath (the velum being closed), and then if the pressure is built up against this occlusion, and finally if the tongue is then pulled sharply down from the palate, the only possible resulting sound is a [t]. When voice is added the result is a [d]. The terms designating these two sounds are derived from the point of occlusion; hence voiceless and voiced alveolar plosives.

A readily identifiable [t] and [d] can be formed at various positions in the general area of the alveolar ridge; but in English the formation of these consonants is characteristically as here described.

A third place where plosives can be formed is at the back of the oral cavity. If the back of the tongue is brought into firm contact with the palate, about where the hard and soft palates are joined, and as before the breath pressure increased, and finally the tongue drawn down from the palate, the resulting sound will be a [k]. If voice is added it will be a [g]. Since these are formed at the soft palate, or the velum, they are called velar plosives, voiceless and voiced respectively.

It was said that lingual agility is not required for the production of adequate vowels. The same cannot be said for the production of most of the consonants, for in these sounds the lips and tongue must move very rapidly and very positively indeed. Drills designed to develop the ability to produce sharp, distinct consonants in rapid succession are of great value in the development of intelligible speech.

### The Fricatives

Many of the sounds of speech are produced not by complete, but by partial obstruction of the breath emission, so that what is heard is the friction or hissing as the breath passes through the narrow opening: hence the term *fricative*. Each sound so produced, with only the friction of the breath, has its counterpart in another sound produced in the same manner, but with the addition of the voice. Like the plosives, the fricatives can be produced at various positions in the oral cavity.

The first pair of these sounds to occur in English speech consists of the *labiodentals,* so called from the fact that they are produced by placing the inner surface of the lower lip lightly against the tip of the upper teeth, forming a narrow slip, and forcing the breath through the opening so provided. The voiceless labiodental fricative is [f], the voiced [v]. Since they can be maintained so long as the breath holds out, they are also designated as continuants.

A second fricative in English is that produced by placing the tip of the tongue against the back of the upper teeth, sometimes even protruding between the upper and lower teeth, and forcing the breath through the narrow slit thus formed. An attempted [s] formed with the tongue too far forward often approaches this sound; when substituted for an [s] the sound is often called a lisp. Because the tongue is so often placed between the teeth, with or without protrusion, these sounds are sometimes designated as *interdentals;* because the tongue is often placed directly behind the teeth, they are sometimes thought of as *postdentals.* Heffner (1952, p. 158) calls them *dental spirants.* The voiced interdental fricative continuant, as in *thin,* is represented by the Greek *theta* [θ], while the voiced counterpart, as in *this,* is represented by a [ð], which was the old "crossed *d*" of Anglo-Saxon.

If the fore surface of the tongue at about B (Fig. 1) is brought into close contact with the alveolar ridge, so that only a narrow opening is left along the median line of the palate and tongue, and the breath is forced through the narrow passage, the friction will produce a hissing sound readily identified as [s]. The correct formation of this fricative does not permit much latitude; if the tongue is too far forward the resulting sound will approach a [θ]; if too far back, or if the opening is too wide, it will take on some of the characteristics of a [ʃ]. If the sound is permitted to escape over one or both sides of the tongue, instead of past the middle, the result will be a particular kind of deviation from the normal known as a *lateral s,* which may be either unilateral or bilateral. The voiced cognate of the [s] is of course [z], incorrect formations of which may produce either [ð] or |ʒ], or a lateral. In the formation of these sounds [s] and [z] it is necessary that the occlusion between the tongue and the palate be complete except for the very narrow opening at the median line of the alveolar ridge.

The sounds formed next to the [s] and [z] are [ʃ] and [ʒ], voiceless and voiced respectively. In these the tongue is brought to the palate just slightly back of the alveolar ridge, and the opening is somewhat wider than for those sounds formed on the ridge. The lips are sometimes slightly protruded, but not always; a slight protrusion seems to help in the production of the sound. Apparently the small space thus provided serves somewhat as a resonator for the characteristic high frequencies present; at any rate, it is difficult if not impossible to produce a good [ʃ] or a [ʒ] with the lips spread widely and drawn back at the corners.

No other fricative continuants produced by linguadental or palatal action at points farther back are heard in English speech. The sound combination [hju], in such words as *Hugh, huge, humor,* and the like, may sometimes be produced as a palatal fricative. This sound, known as the *ich-laut* [ç], is represented in German spelling by *ch* when following a front vowel. In its formation the blade of the tongue at about D is brought close to the hard palate at about 6 (Fig. 1) to form a close, fairly narrow opening. When the breath is forced through the passage a hissing sound of a peculiar character is produced, much as if one were clearing a small bit of mucus from the palate. The result is a pronunciation of the words above represented as [çu], [çudʒ], [çumə].

Just as in the case of the plosives, the fricatives must be made with the articulatory organs in the right places; there must be an adequate firmness in the constriction set-up for the restricted passage of the breath; and there must be an adequate pressure to force the breath through the narrow openings. Finally, the release or the movement into the next sound, whichever is called for in the context, must be positive and clean.

### The Affricates

Partaking somewhat of the nature of both plosives and fricatives are a pair of sounds known as the affricates. These are the sounds represented in English by such spellings as *ch* for the voiceless form, and *j* or *g* (usually before *e* or *i*) for the voiced, and phonetically by [tʃ] and [dʒ] respectively. In these sounds the first element, consisting essentially of an alveolar stop (sometimes postalveolar) very similar to a [t], is generally produced at position 4, but sometimes nearer to 5 (Fig. 1). It releases relatively gradually into [ʃ] rather than suddenly into the aspirate as is usual for the plosives. The formation for [dʒ] is the same, with the addition of voice.

There has been some question as to whether these affricates are to be considered a single sound, or as no more than a [t] plus [ʃ], or [d] plus [ʒ]. There are many instances in our speech of stops followed by fricatives; these two, however, are so often used together phonemically that it seems justifiable to consider them as an integrated unit, at the same time recognizing that, somewhat like the diphthongs, they consist of at least two elements.

It may be well at this point to emphasize the definite distinction that should be made between the voiceless and the voiced consonants. The difference should be stressed in teaching the formation of the sounds of speech, since the meaning often depends on whether the sounds are voiced or not. *Patch, batch,* and *badge* are all different words whatever the context; and their difference lies in the voicing or unvoicing of the consonants. Similarly, *pig, big,* and *pick* depend for their identification on whether the consonants are voiced or unvoiced. Insistence on this difference will result in cleaner, more distinct, more intelligible speech.

### The Nasal Consonants

In English three distinct sounds are used which are generally known as nasals. These are [m], [n], and [ŋ]. In formation they are somewhat similar to the plosives, in that the oral occlusions are in the same places as for the latter, [p], [t], and [k] respectively. They differ in two respects: they are voiced continuants, rather than plosives, and as such have some of the characteristics of the vowels. Moreover, they can be used syllabically; that is, they can form syllables by themselves, without the aid of other sounds, as in [bʌtn̩], [opm̩], [θɪŋkŋ̩] (more often [θɪˈkən]).

The second way in which the nasals differ from the plosives is that whereas in the latter the obstruction to the breath emission is complete, with the velum being closed, in the former the occlusion occurs only in the oral passage. Since the sounds are continuants, there must be some passage for the breath and the voice to escape. This passage is provided by dropping the velum, which ordinarily is pressed against the back wall of the oral pharynx to close off the nasal passages, and forcing the breath or voice through the oral cavities. When the velum is dropped and the oral occlusion maintained, the nasal cavities are opened up so that the breath and voice go out through them. The addition of these cavities to the resonating chambers gives to the nasal sounds their peculiar character.

It is not generally recognized, although it seems quite obvious, that the effect of the nasal consonants on the preceding vowels is to induce nasalization in them, *when occurring in the same syllable*. It is possible to pronounce the vowels in this situation without nasalization; but in ordinary speech nasalization occurs through the process of regressive assimilation (Gray and Wise, 1946, p. 476). In moderation the phenomenon should cause no concern, since it is a normal linguistic phenomenon. Nasality is offensive when excessively strong, when accompanied by much tension of the resonator walls, or when occurring in sounds which neither by assimilation nor otherwise should be nasalized at all. The "nasal" voice is nasal even in the absence of nasal consonants.

## The r-Sounds

It is quite incorrect to speak of the r as if there were but one r-sound, although in the English language most of the sounds of this group center about approximately the same position. There are many variations in other languages, which are described in current texts; but since they are rare in our own language, they need not be discussed here. Perhaps a brief discussion of the various uses of the sound-group may have some significance.

The vocalic r-sounds have been discussed in the section on the Vowels. Consonantal [r] may be found in two basic types of phonetic context: a prevocalic and a postvocalic position, with variants of each of these. The prevocalic [r] occurs in such words as *run, wreck, rare, real, recede;* the postvocalic [r] occurs in *heart, here, horse, their,* and the like. A variant of the former is found in the consonant combination in which [r], as part of the combination (as in *strong, bring, fresh, shred, pride,* and so on), still precedes the vowel. When following the voiceless consonants in such combinations, the [r] is likely to be voiceless through at least the first part of its duration, and to take on something of the character of a fricative. The intervocalic [r] (as in *far away, character*), though it is postvocalic, is at the same time prevocalic, and takes on the character of the latter.

In usage, the prevocalic [r] is—or should be—always pronounced in all American dialects; and since the [r] is influenced more by the following than by the preceding vowel, the intervocalic sound is also, correctly, always pronounced. The postvocalic [r] may or may not be heard, depending on the particular dialect in which it may occur. In General American it is, at least theoretically, heard wherever it is indicated by the spelling. Also theoretically, it is characteristically omitted in Eastern and Southern speech; actually, it is becoming more and more common in all phonetic contexts, in all of the major American dialects.

The central position about which the movements are focused in producing the consonantal [r] in any context is basically similar to that in the formation of the vocalic [r], or the central [ɝ], as it is used in General American speech. That is, the sides of the tongue curve up to touch lightly the molar teeth. The agreeableness or disagreeableness of the sound depends largely on the degree of tenseness in the tongue itself, and perhaps on the nonessential retroflexion of the tongue tip, which demands additional tension. In the initial, or prevocalic [r], the movement of the tongue is away from its characteristic position; in the postvocalic, when the [r] is used at all, the movement is toward it. In the intervocalic position the tongue approaches the palate to form the [r], and then moves quickly into position for the next sound. In these movements the [r] may be thought of as a "glide-consonant."

One more variant may be heard among those speakers who characteristically omit the postvocalic [r]. When used finally, as in *here, bare, fire, door, your, poor,* the vowel often becomes in effect a diphthong, the final element being [ə].

### The *l*-Sounds

In some respects the *l*-sounds resemble in their functioning the *r*-sounds. They may be used syllabically, as in *little, bottle, meddle;* consonantally in initial, medial, or final positions, or in consonant combinations such as in *black, flight, slender,* and so on. The [l] is not heard as a vowel, as are the vocalic *r*-sounds in *were, heard, further,* and the like. When occurring prevocally the organs move away from the *l*-position; when postvocal they move toward it. In the intervocalic [l] the tongue moves first into, and then away from, the characteristic position.

In the normal [l] the tip of the tongue is raised to the roof of the mouth at the alveolar ridge, so that it touches the palate *only* at the median line, the sound going off over the sides. If one simply places the tongue tip against the ridge and utters a vocal sound, the result will be an [l]. This position, however, is not critical; actually, the tip of the tongue can touch the palate at any point from the base of the teeth as far back as it will reach, and a readily recognizable sound will be produced, so long as only the tip is touching, and the sound goes over the sides. As the tongue lies normally in the mouth the tip as it rises will probably touch the palate at or near the alveolar ridge.

The [l] following a voiceless consonant in combination will tend to be voiceless itself, through at least a part of its duration, as in *play, fly, slack, cling* (Jones, 1950, p. 90). Intervocalic [l], like the [r], may also be thought of as a glide-consonant. Syllabic [l] is produced primarily by releasing a plosive directly into the *l*-position without going through an intervening vowel, as in *buckle, bugle, mettle, medal, apple, bubble.* In these the tongue may form an *l*-position even before the release of the plosive, or so close afterward that no vowel can be formed. The syllabic [l] is much less frequent following other consonants.

### The Glide-Consonants

It will be helpful to consider the so-called "glide-consonants" [j] and [w] together, since they follow much the same principles. In their formation they resemble somewhat the diphthongs in that they consist essentially of two elements, an initial, followed by a rapid but smooth glide into the second, or into the following sound. They differ from the diphthongs in at least two respects: first, they are always used consonantally, the consonant itself consisting of the initial element and the glide. Second, whereas the final element of a given diphthong is always the same, or of the same phoneme, the final element of the glide-consonant may be any following vowel or diphthong.

Consider, for instance, the glide [j] in the words *ye, yip, yea, yes, yap, yard, yawl, yo-yo, your, use*. In each case there is a constriction of the tongue close to the palate at about the position for [ɪ] (Jones, 1922, p. 66; Thomas, 1947, pp. 54 f.; Heffner, 1952, p. 154). This constriction may be held for an appreciable time, although such a hold is not essential. In fact, so long as the position is held the [j]-glide cannot be completed. What is important is the release from the constriction to the following sound. Apparently, the higher the vowel into which the glide moves the more tense the constriction. But the release may move into any of the vowel positions, and thence, often, into a diphthong, as in *yipe, yowl, yoicks*—although these are not common words. The initial element is sometimes thought of as a fricative; Heffner (1952, pp. 150 f.) insists that the friction is an essential characteristic of the sound itself. Probably the nearest sound to the voiceless counterpart is heard in certain dialectal pronunciations, at one time advocated by the lexicographer and elocutionist, John Walker, as giving a certain "elegance" to the pronunciation of *card* as *kyard, cow* as *kyow* (*garden* as *gyarden*), in which the [j] follows the plosive, voiced or voiceless. The [ç] described above (the *ich-laut*) as in some pronunciations as *huge, humor, human*, also approaches the voiceless palatal glide-consonant.

The [w] consists of a glide from a lip and tongue position very similar to that for a [u] or [ʊ] into the position for the following vowel or diphthong. It is often called a bilabial semivowel, often a bilabial glide-vowel. It functions as a consonant, however, in somewhat the same manner as does the [j] glide. In such words as *we, will, way, wet, wag, watt, wall, woke, wood, woo*, the tongue tends to take the position for the following vowel while the lips are forming the initial bilabial constriction. The release is into the vowel or diphthong which has been forming. *Wide* and *wound* (pret. of *wind*) represent perhaps the principal diphthongs preceded by the bilabial glide-consonant.

The voiceless counterpart of [w]—[ʍ]—is heard in General American *wheat, which, whey, whet, wham, what, whoa* (often if not usually [wo]), *whup* (an old rustic pronunciation of whip), *whoop* (often simply [hup]), and *whirl*. The formation is essentially the same as for the voiced [w]; voicing, however, does not normally begin until the initiation of the following vowel. The expulsion of breath is considerably stronger than for [w], since the chief audible element is dependent on that expulsion, and not on the following vowel. Like [j] and [w], [ʍ] is a glide-consonant, with as many variations as there are sounds which may follow it.

## The Glottal Fricative

About the only characteristic of [h] is that it consists of a forcible emission of breath through an open or partially open glottis, and through pharyngeal and oral cavities formed to produce a following vowel or diphthong (Jones, 1922, p. 61; Thomas, 1947, p. 101; Heffner, 1952, pp. 150 f.). From another point of view, since the [h] rarely if ever occurs without a following vowel, it may be thought of as a strongly aspirated voiceless vowel immediately preceding the voiced vowel. A still further approach may be to consider the [h] as a particular manner of attacking a vowel. When the articulatory mechanism is in position for the following vowel the friction of breath as it is forced through the glottis and oral passages produces a whispered sound readily identified as the appropriate vowel. It is this sound which in English normally constitutes the [h] in any given phonetic context (Heffner, 1952, p. 151).

The descriptions given above are intended to present only the minimum essentials of speech sound formation for the production of speech of socially adequate intelligibility. They will not, obviously, satisfy the phonetician or the linguist; on the other hand, it is thought that they will be found sufficient for the correction of many if not most of the common articulation errors, for both the therapist and the classroom teacher of "normal" speech. For those who would like to pursue the study still further, a thorough familiarity with the sources listed in the bibliography will give as complete information as is presently available for an understanding of the manner in which the sounds of speech are formed. There still remains much to be discovered; the search for yet more complete understanding is a fruitful field of inquiry.

## BIBLIOGRAPHY

BLACK, J. W. 1937. The quality of a spoken vowel. *Arch. Speech*, 2, 7–27.

GEMELLI, A., and PASTORI, G. 1934. La durata minima di un fonema sufficiente per la sua percezione. *In* L'analisi elettroacustica del linguaggio. Milano: Università Cattolica del Sacro Cuore. I, 149–163.

GRAY, G. W., and BRADEN, W. W. 1951. Public speaking: principles and practice. New York: Harper.

GRAY, G. W., and WISE, C. M. 1946. The bases of speech (rev. ed.). New York: Harper.

HEFFNER, R. M. S. 1952. General phonetics (Students' ed.). Madison: Univ. Wisconsin Press.

JESPERSEN, Otto. 1889. The articulations of speech sounds represented by means of analphabetic symbols. Marburg in Hessen: N. G. Elwert.

JONES, Daniel. 1922. An outline of English phonetics. New York: G. E. Stechert.

———— 1950. The pronunciation of English. Cambridge: University Press.

ROUSSELOT, P. J., and LACLOTTE, F. 1913. Precis de prononciation française. Paris: H. Welter.

STETSON, R. H. 1951. Motor phonetics. Amsterdam: North Holland Publishing Co.

THOMAS, C. K. 1947. An introduction to the phonetics of American English. New York: Ronald Press.

# CHAPTER 5

# THE ACOUSTICS OF SPEECH

• *Bruce P. Bogert, Ph.D., and Gordon E. Peterson, Ph.D.*

## PART I. TECHNICAL ASPECTS OF ACOUSTIC WAVE FORMS*

### PRELIMINARIES AND FUNDAMENTALS

THE SIGNALS USED in communication are varied and complex, and it is helpful in many cases to have ways to analyze them in meaningful terms. To this end, various simple types of wave forms will be discussed and their use as building blocks of signals will be indicated.

### Periodic Wave Forms

A periodic wave form is one which repeats itself after some time interval $T$, called the period:

$$F(t + T) = F(t)$$

In general, we denote as a wave form some single-valued function of time, by which is meant that there is a unique value $F$ of the quantity involved (voltage, sound pressure, displacement) for every instant of time $t$ (Fig. 1).

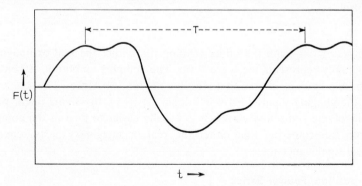

FIG. 1. A periodic function $f(t)$, of period $T$.

* By Bruce P. Bogert.

The simplest periodic wave is the *simple harmonic* or *sinusoidal* wave (Fig. 2):   $a \sin (2\pi f t + \varphi)$.

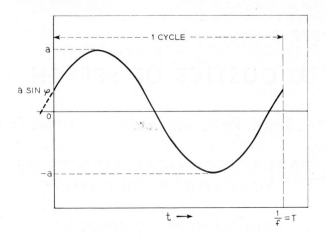

FIG. 2. One cycle of a sine wave of amplitude a, phase $\Psi$, and period T.

The values attained by the sinusoid range between $-a$ and $a$, where $a$ represents the *amplitude*. The quantity $f$ is the *frequency*—measured in cycles per second. The *period* $T$ is $1/f$. The *phase* $\varphi$ determines the point on the sinusoid corresponding to the instant of time $t = 0$. The duration of the wave corresponding to one period $T$ is a cycle. It is common to write $2\pi f$ as $\omega$, the *angular frequency*, measured in radians per second. $2\pi$ radians angle is equal to 360 degrees, which corresponds to one cycle. The r.m.s. (root-mean-square) amplitude of the sinusoid is $a / \sqrt{2}$, and is the quantity for a sine wave analogous to the amplitude of a constant quantity (such as a direct current) in calculations of power, heating effects, etc.

It is often convenient to write the expression for a sinusoidal wave in complex form:

$$A e^{j\omega t}$$

where $j = \sqrt{-1}$, with the understanding that either the real or imaginary part actually represents the wave form. The complex amplitude $A$ contains the phase $\varphi$ as $A = a e^{j\varphi}$ so that $A e^{j\omega t} = a e^{j(\omega t + \varphi)}$. Since $e^{jz} = \cos z + j \sin z$, the imaginary part $\mathrm{Im} A e^{j\omega t} = a \sin (\omega t + \varphi)$. In solving linear problems involving sinusoidal waves, it is usually easier to deal in the complex notation, remembering that either the real or imaginary part alone has physical significance.

### Superposition, Fourier Series

A broad class of physical systems which can be readily treated theoretically has the property of linearity. By linearity is meant that if $A$ is the response to the excitation $a$, $B$ the response to $b$, then the response to $a + b$ is

$A + B$, and the response to $aa$ is $aA$ where $a$ is a constant. Because of this, if elementary solutions to a problem are found, it is possible to construct other solutions by adding multiples of the elementary ones. This property is known as the *principle of superposition*.

Consider a periodic wave form of period $T$ (Fig. 3). It is possible to represent it by means of a series of sinusoids harmonically related:

$$F(t) = \tfrac{1}{2}\, a_0 + a_1 \sin \omega t + a_2 \sin 2\omega t + \cdots + b_1 \cos \omega t + b_2 \cos 2\omega t \cdots$$

$$= C_0 + C_1 \sin (\omega t + \varphi_1) + C_2 \sin (2\omega t + \varphi_2) + \cdots$$

$$+ C_n \sin (n\omega t + \varphi_n) + \cdots$$

$$= 1 + \sum_{k=1}^{\infty} C_k \sin (k\omega t + \varphi_k)$$

where $\omega T = 2\pi$.

The coefficients of amplitude $C_k$ and phase $\varphi_k$ can be computed from the function $F(t)$ over one period. The leading coefficient $C_0$ represents the *aver-*

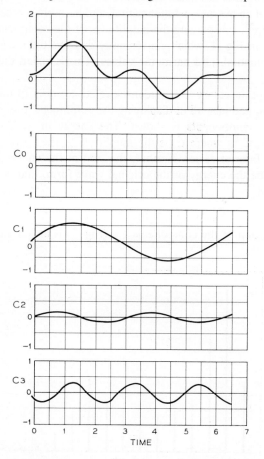

FIG. 3. One cycle of a periodic wave, showing its Fourier decomposition with an average value $C_0$, fundamental $C_1$, and second and third harmonics $C_2$ and $C_3$.

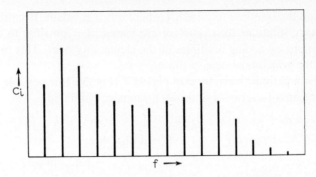

F.G. 4. A representative Fourier amplitude spectrum.

*age* value of the wave form. The next term $C_1 \sin (\omega t + \varphi_1)$ is the *fundamental* of amplitude $C_1$ and phase $\varphi_1$. The terms following have frequencies which are integral multiples of the fundamental frequency $f = \omega/2\pi = 1/T$, and are called harmonics. This representation of an arbitrary periodic wave form in terms of an average, a fundamental, and harmonics is called a *Fourier series*. A method of displaying the amplitudes of the components of a wave form is shown in Fig. 4, which conveniently displays the magnitudes of the average, fundamental, and harmonic values. This is called the *spectrum* of the wave form.

Often it is not necessary to consider the relative phases of the components of a wave form, and instead of displaying the amplitudes, the relative energy in each of the components is shown. The energy in each component is proportional to $C_i^2$, where $C_i$ is the amplitude of the corresponding component of the Fourier series. Further, the sum of the energies in the components must be the energy of the original wave form, that is, $F^2$, averaged over one period.

$$<F^2> = C_0 + C_1{}^2 + \cdots + C_n{}^2 + \cdots$$

The representation of the components $C_i^2$ (Fig. 5) is called an *energy spectrum*.

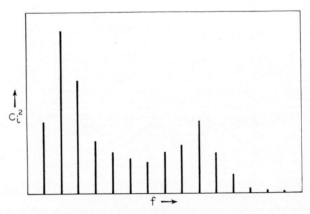

FIG. 5. A representative Fourier energy spectrum.

## Pulses

A train of pulses of unit height, such as is shown in Fig. 6, has the amplitude spectrum shown in Fig. 7. If the length of the pulse is $\tau$ and the period $T$, then

$$f(t) = \frac{\tau}{T} + \frac{2}{\pi} \sin \frac{\pi\tau}{T} \cos \omega t + \frac{2}{2\pi} \sin \frac{2\pi\tau}{T} \cos 2\omega t$$

$$+ \cdots + \frac{2}{n\pi} \sin \frac{\pi n\tau}{T} \cos n\omega t + \cdots$$

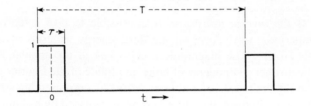

FIG. 6.   Pulses of width $t$, unit height, and period $T$.

The rapidity of fall-off with harmonic number of the harmonic amplitudes is proportional to the ratio $\tau/T$. As the pulse becomes narrower ($\tau \to 0$), the amplitudes of the harmonics become uniform, and their magnitudes decrease toward zero. If the height of the pulse increases proportionately, the pulse becomes a *unit impulse* in the limit of $\tau \to 0$, and the harmonics are of uniform finite amplitude.

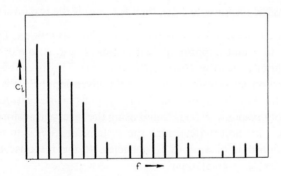

FIG. 7. Amplitude spectrum of the pulses shown in Fig. 6.

## Nonperiodic Wave Forms

A nonperiodic wave is one which does not repeat itself in any finite time It may be regarded as a periodic wave in the limit of $T \to \infty$. If a Fourier series representation is made in $e^{jn\omega t}$, the fundamental angular frequency

$\omega$ approaches zero and the harmonic spacing becomes smaller. In the limit, the series representation becomes the *Fourier Integral Transform:*

$$F(t) = \frac{1}{2\pi} \int_{-\infty}^{\infty} G(\omega)e^{j\omega t}d\omega$$

in which

$$G(\omega) = \int_{-\infty}^{\infty} F(t)e^{-j\omega t}dt$$

is known as the *inverse transform.* It is possible to give a representation of any nonperiodic wave form having finite energy in terms of frequency components $G(\omega)$, whose magnitude is $|G(\omega_1)|d\omega$ at the angular frequency $\omega_1$. Thus the distinct components of finite amplitude of the Fourier series has gone over in the limit as $T \to \infty$ to a quantity $G(\omega)$ representing a frequency component at any frequency $\omega$, the series being replaced by its limiting form, the integral.

It has been shown that under the two broad assumptions listed below, the Fourier transform will provide a means to determine the response of a system to any input. The two assumptions are:

1. Linearity, as has been defined before. This implies the principle of superposition. In addition, the system concerned must have a simple sinusoidal output if its input is sinusoidal.
2. Time invariance. By this is meant that the same input to the system at a later time produces the same response at a later time. Symbolically, if $F_o(t)$ is the response to $F_i(t)$, then $F_o(t-a)$ is the response to $F_i(t-a)$.

The response to a given input signal is determined as follows. The response of the system to a unit impulse applied at time $t = 0$ is found, denoted by $I(t)$. The Fourier transform $H(\omega)$ of $I(t)$ is found. This is called the *system function.* The Fourier transform $G_i(\omega)$ of the given input $F_i(t)$ is also determined. Then the Fourier transform of the output $G_o(\omega) = H(\omega)G_i(\omega)$. From $G_o(\omega)$ the output response $F_o(t)$ is found using the inverse transform. Another and more usual method to determine the system function is to measure the response to sinusoids of various frequencies. If the response to an input $\sin \omega t$ is $A(\omega) \sin [\omega t + \varphi(\omega)]$, then

$$H(\omega) = A(\omega)e^{j\varphi(\omega)}$$

is the system function. Thus measurements of the amplitude and phase response to a sine-wave input take on great importance in the analysis of communication systems.

### Energy and Power Spectrum

In a similar way to that used with Fourier series, the energy spectrum is defined for a nonperiodic function as $E(\omega) = |G(\omega)|^2$, since $E(\omega)\Delta\omega$ represents the energy in a frequency band $\Delta\omega$ [assuming $G(\omega)$ is the transform of the voltage across, or the current passing through, a unit resistance].

When a signal is of infinite duration but of finite average power, a quantity of interest is the *autocorrelation* function

$$\psi(\tau) = \lim_{T \to \infty} \frac{1}{2T} \int_{-T}^{T} f(t)f(t - \tau)dt.$$

The autocorrelation function measures the degree to which $f(t)$ depends on previous and succeeding values. The quantity $\psi(0)$ represents the average power of the quantity $f(t)$. An important relation between the autocorrelation functions $\psi(\omega)$ and the *power spectrum* $S(\omega)$ is that they are Fourier transforms of each other:

$$S(\omega) = \int_{-\infty}^{\infty} \psi(\tau)e^{i\omega\tau}d\tau$$

$$\psi(\tau) = \frac{1}{2\pi} \int_{-\infty}^{\infty} S(\omega)e^{-i\omega\tau}d\omega.$$

The significance of the power spectrum is that $S(\omega_0)\Delta\omega$ represents the average power of the signal in the frequency band $\Delta\omega$ wide, centered at the angular frequency $\omega_0$.

## Noise

Noise is considered to be a wave form which is characterized by a number of frequencies combined in a random manner. A distinction is made between *impulse noise* and resistance or *thermal noise*. Impulse noise may be regarded as a random sequence of distinct wave forms, that is, a train of pulses or clicks with random occurrence. Radio static is a typical example. Acoustic noise of thermal type is characterized by a smoothness in sound, such as one hears in the roar of the sea or the hiss from a jet of air. Thermal electrical noise results from the thermal agitation of electrons in a resistance. Thermal noise may be regarded as a superposition of sinusoids of all frequencies with random phases. It is usually characterized by its autocorrelation function or its power spectrum, as these quantities are independent of a particular sample of the noise wave form. If the power spectrum is uniform over an extended range of frequencies, the noise is called *white noise*. Its autocorrelation is then a spike at $\tau = 0$, and there is no interdependence between separated points of the wave.

**Oscillating Systems**

Fundamental to an analysis of electrical or acoustic signals is the understanding of the properties of oscillating systems. Consider the mechanical system shown in Fig. 8. A mass, $m$, is subject to a restoring force proportional

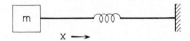

FIG. 8.   A schematic representation of a mass M constrained by a spring.

to its displacement $x$ from an equilibrium position, the proportionality factor being denoted by $k$. Newton's equation of motion for this system is

$$m \frac{d^2x}{dt^2} + kx = 0.$$

The solution to this equation is

$$x = A \sin \sqrt{\frac{k}{m}}\, t + B \cos \sqrt{\frac{k}{m}}\, t,$$

where $A$ and $B$ are constants determined by the velocity and position of the mass point at the time $t = 0$. Entirely analogous to the above mechanical system is the electrical one, shown in Fig. 9, consisting of an inductance $L$ and a capacitance $C$. In this case $M$ is replaced by $L$, $k$ by $1/C$, and the charge $q$ on the condenser is equivalent to $x$:

$$q = A \sin (t/ \sqrt{LC}) + B \cos (t/ \sqrt{LC}).$$

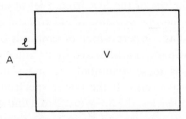

FIG. 9.   An oscillating electric circuit consisting of an inductance L and a capacitance C.

Inspection of the solutions for $x$ and $q$ shows that they are periodic with period $T = 2\pi \sqrt{m/k}$ or $2\pi \sqrt{LC}$, as the case may be. The larger the mass or inductance the larger is the period; and the larger the stiffness $k$ or the smaller the capacitance $C$, the shorter the period.

The acoustical equivalent to the mass and spring mechanical system is the *Helmholtz resonator*, consisting of a cylinder of volume $V$ connected to the atmosphere bv a neck of area $A$ and (effective) length $l'$ (Fig. 10). The

FIG. 10. A Helmholtz resonator consisting of a volume V communicating with the atmosphere by a neck of area A and length l.

mass of air in the neck moves approximately as a rigid plug with inertance $L = \rho_0 l'/A$, where $\rho_0$ is the density of air. The effective length $l'$ is greater than the actual length because of the movement of some of the air beyond the ends of the neck in phase with the air in the neck. Approximately, $l' = l + 0.8\sqrt{A}$. The volume $V$ of air in the bottle acts as a restoring force of value $\rho_0 c^2 V$, where $c$ is the velocity of sound in air. Thus the period of oscillation is

$$T = (2\pi/c)\sqrt{Vl'/A}.$$

## Damped Oscillators

If an oscillating system with a small amount of damping is excited by an impulse, a *damped oscillation* (Fig. 11) will be the result:

$$F(t) = Ae^{-at}\sin\left(\sqrt{\omega_0^2 - a^2}\,t\right).$$

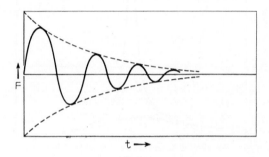

FIG. 11. A damped oscillation.

The damping causes a decay in the amplitude of the oscillation, as can be seen by the $e^{-at}$ term, and its presence also influences the frequency of oscillation, lowering it relative to that of the undamped oscillation $\omega_0$. $a$ is called the damping constant. When $\omega_0 > a$, the oscillations are underdamped, $\omega_0 < a$, the response is overdamped and does not have an oscillatory nature. When $\omega_0 = a$, the system is critically damped, and represents the boundary between oscillating and nonoscillating behavior.

## Resonance

If an oscillating system is excited with a sinusoidally varying force, the response is sinusoidal with the same frequency as that applied. If we have an inertial force $mdv/dt$, a resistive force equal to $-rv$, a spring force $-kx$ and a forcing function $F\sin\omega t$, we have the equation

$$m + r\frac{d^2x}{dt^2}\frac{dx}{dt} + kx = F\sin\omega t, \qquad (m, r, k > 0)$$

whose solution, after all starting transients have died away, is (Fig. 12)

$$\frac{x}{F} = \frac{m\,(\omega_0{}^2 - \omega^2)}{m^2\,(\omega_0{}^2 - \omega^2)^2 + r^2\omega^2}\sin\omega t - \frac{r\omega}{m^2\,(\omega_0{}^2 - \omega^2)^2 + r^2\omega^2}\cos\omega t,$$

where $x$ is the displacement, and $\omega_0 = \sqrt{\dfrac{k}{m} - \dfrac{r^2}{4m^2}}$ is the free resonant angular frequency. The amplitude of the resulting motion depends on the frequency of the applied force and is a maximum when $\omega = \omega_0$. *Resonance* occurs when this condition is satisfied. When the damping (proportional to $r$) is small, the maximum of response is large, and conversely.

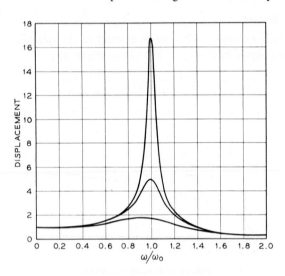

FIG. 12. Resonance curves showing the amplitude of response of a damped oscillating system vs. the frequency of the excitation. The results of three differing values of damping are shown, the maximum amplitude (at the resonant frequency) decreasing as the damping increases.

A convenient measure of the sharpness of resonance is a quantity called "$Q$," or quality factor. This may be written as

$$Q = \frac{f_0}{f_2 - f_1}$$

where $f_0$ is the resonant frequency and $f_2$ and $f_1$ (with $f_2 > f_1$) are those frequencies where the amplitude of vibration is $\sqrt{1/2}$ as great as at $f_0$. Large $Q$ corresponds to sharp resonance and light damping. The $Q$ of a system is related to the mass $m$ and the resistance $r$ and is a measure of the ratio between the kinetic energy stored in the mass and the energy dissipated as heat in the resistance $r$. Analogous relations hold for electric circuit elements. The $Q$'s of electrical circuits range up to about 200–400, and the $Q$'s of piezo-electric crystals used in oscillators and wave filters are as great as 140,000. Measured $Q$'s of vowel resonances range from about 2 to 25.

If periodic impulses are applied to a resonant system, periodic damped oscillations are produced. The exponential decay of a damped oscillation in the system varies inversely with $Q$, through the relation $\alpha = \omega_0/2Q$. The Fourier spectrum of these damped oscillations shows harmonic components accentuated around the frequency of resonance, as shown in Fig. 13. If the wave form has decayed to a low value by the end of the pulsing period $T$, the envelope of the Fourier components $C_i$ is essentially the same as the response to the forcing function as shown in Fig. 12.

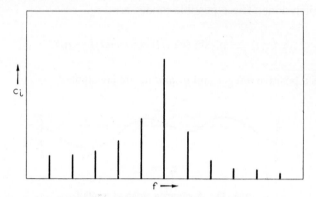

**FIG. 13.** Amplitude spectrum of a recurring damped sinusoid. The spacing between the lines corresponds to the recurrence frequency.

## Vibrating String

We have discussed the sinusoidal motion of a mass point restrained by a spring. Consider now a stretched string which extends indefinitely in both directions. Such a string will support two traveling waves, proceeding in opposite directions (Fig. 14). The equation for the waves is

$$y = f_1(x + ct) + f_2(x - ct),$$

where $y$ is the lateral displacement, $x$ the distance along the string, and $t$ the time. The quantity $c$ is the velocity of propagation of the waves. The functions $f_1$ and $f_2$ are arbitrary (continuous) functions of their arguments. If we consider a hypothetical point moving with velocity $c$ along the string in the

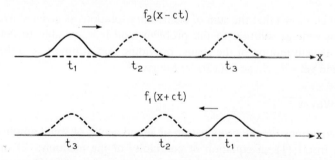

**FIG. 14.** Traveling waves on a string of infinite extent: $f_2(x - ct)$ represents the wave to the right; $f_1(x + ct)$ represents the wave traveling to the left.

direction of increasing $x$, we see that the argument of $f_2$ is a constant, and we see a stationary picture of $f_2$. Similarly, moving backwards along the string with velocity $c$ will enable us to see a stationary picture of $f_1$. Thus $f_1(x + ct)$ represents a traveling wave moving backwards, and $f_2(x - ct)$ represents a forward traveling wave (Fig. 14).

Consider a string of length $l$ fixed at both ends (Fig. 15). The possible motions of a string so constrained are much more limited than if the string were infinitely long. These possible modes are

$$y_n(x, t) = q_n \sin(n\pi x/l) \cos(n\pi ct/l - a_n)$$

where $n$ is a positive integer and $q_n$ and $a_n$ are constants.

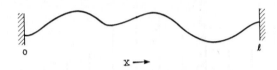

**FIG. 15.   A vibrating string of length $l$.**

Thus the string of length $l$ has an infinite number of possible modes of vibration, and to each there corresponds a particular frequency. All of these frequencies are multiples of the lowest, or fundamental, frequency and are called overtones or harmonics of the fundamental. It is not generally true that the frequencies of the higher modes of a vibrating system are related so simply to the frequency of the lowest mode. If the motion of the string is sufficiently small so that the preceding equation holds, it is possible to superpose linearly any of those solutions given above, and the resultant is also a solution:

$$y(x, t) = \sum_{n=1}^{\infty} a_n \sin(n\pi x/l) \cos(n\pi ct/l - a_n).$$

It can be shown that the sum of elementary solutions as given above forms the most general solution to the problem, and it is possible to determine the subsequent motion of the string, providing that at time $t = 0$ the shape $y(x,0)$ and velocity shape $\partial y(x,0)/\partial t$ are given.

### Sound Waves

The equations for the propagation of sound waves of small amplitude are derived from: (1) an equation of continuity of the medium; (2) the compressibility of the medium; and (3) the equation of motion. From these relations the wave equation is derived, which gives the pressure and particle velocity in the sound wave. The sound pressure $p$ is the difference between the actual pressure $p'$ in the medium and the static pressure $p_0$ (atmospheric pressure)

$$p = p' - p_0.$$

The values of the velocity components $v_x$, $v_y$, $v_z$ of a particle in a sound wave are most readily obtained from a quantity known as the *velocity potential* $\varphi$ by the relations

$$v_x = -\frac{\partial \varphi}{\partial x}, \; v_y = -\frac{\partial \varphi}{\partial y}, \; v_z = -\frac{\partial \varphi}{\partial z}.$$

The pressure can also be expressed in terms of the velocity potential by the equation

$$p = \rho_0 \frac{\partial \varphi}{\partial t}$$

where $\rho_0$ is the static density. The equation for the velocity potential, the *wave equation*, is

$$\frac{\partial^2 \varphi}{\partial x^2} + \frac{\partial^2 \varphi}{\partial y^2} + \frac{\partial^2 \varphi}{\partial z^2} = \frac{1}{c^2} \frac{\partial^2 \varphi}{\partial t^2} ,$$

where $c$ is the velocity of sound. The sound velocity is related to the properties of the gas by

$$c = \sqrt{\gamma p_0 / \rho_0} ,$$

where $\gamma$ is the ratio of the specific heat at constant pressure to the specific heat at constant volume. For air at $20°$ centigrade and $p_0 = 760$ mm of mercury, the velocity of sound is 344 meters per second.

## Plane Waves

The representation of a plane progressive sinusoidal sound wave traveling in the positive $x$ direction is of the form

$$p = P e^{jk(x-ct)},$$

where $P$ is the effective sound pressure. The particle velocity is

$$v_x = V_x e^{jk(x-ct)},$$

where

$$V_x = P/\rho_0 c.$$

The rate at which sound energy is transmitted by the wave per unit area is called the intensity, and is given by

$$I = \frac{p^2}{\rho_0 c} = \rho_0 c V_x^2.$$

## Acoustic Impedance

The ratio of pressure to particle velocity $p/v$ is called the specific acoustic impedance. For a plane progressive wave in air, its value is $\rho_0 c = 42$ acoustic ohms. An analogy can be made between electrical and acoustic systems in which pressure corresponds to voltage and volume velocity to current. *Volume velocity* is defined as $Sv$, where $S$ is the area and $v$ the particle velocity. Similarly the acoustic impedance $Z = p/Sv$ is analogous to the electrical impedance $Z = E/I$. For example, the acoustic impedance of the closed end of an acoustic pipe is very high, and the impedance of the open end is a function of the ratio of wave length of the sound wave to the size of the opening. For small wave lengths compared to the diameter, it is $p_0cS$, where $S$ is the area of the pipe. For very long wave lengths the air at the end acts as a mass plug, as in the Helmholtz resonator.

### Spherical Waves

The general solution of the wave equation for spherical waves emanating from a point is

$$\varphi = \frac{1}{r} f(r - ct), \qquad (r > 0)$$

in which $f$ is an arbitrary continuous function of its argument and $r$ is the distance from the source point. These expressions differ from those for plane waves by the factor $1/r$, which means that $r = 0$ represents a singular point and the sound pressure is infinite there. In reality, the source is of finite size so that the wave starts from a surface with a finite radius.

Since the sound intensity is proportional to the square of the velocity, and thus to the square of the velocity potential, the sound intensity for spherical waves is inversely proportional to the square of the distance $r$ from the source.

### Acoustic Pipes

The acoustic analogy to the finite string is the acoustic pipe. The two boundary conditions for the pipe, corresponding to an open or closed end, are that the sound pressure be zero (approximately) or the particle velocity be zero, respectively. The natural frequencies for a pipe of length $l$ either closed or open at both ends are determined by the fact that the wave length $\lambda_n = c/f_n$ of the $n$th mode must be

$$n\frac{\lambda_n}{2} = l', \qquad \text{or} \qquad \frac{nc}{2l'} = f_n,$$

where $l'$ is the effective length of the pipe, $n$ an integer, and $c$ the velocity of sound (Fig. 16). If the pipe is open at one end and closed at the other, the allowed frequencies are $f_n = \dfrac{(2n - 1)c}{4l}$, as only an odd number of quarter wave lengths can be supported. The effective length $l'$ takes into account the additional equivalent length of an open end, which is approximately $l' = l + 0.8\sqrt{A}$, where $A$ is the area of the end of the pipe.

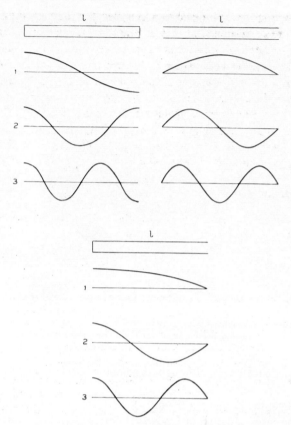

FIG. 16. Pressure distribution for the lowest three modes of acoustic pipes. A pipe closed at both ends, one open at both ends, and one open at one end and closed at the other end are shown.

## The Decibel

The decibel (abbreviated db) is an often used representation for the ratios of quantities used in acoustics and electrical communications. It is a logarithmic unit, with definition based on a power ratio:

$$\text{number of decibels} = 10 \log_{10} \frac{P_2}{P_1}.$$

$P_1$ may represent a unit of power, in which case powers $P_2$ greater than $P_1$ are characterized by positive decibel values, and powers less than $P_1$ by negative decibel values. A power ratio of two amounts to three decibels, of ten to ten decibels, of one hundred to twenty decibels, and so on.

When the impedance level of the points where the power measurements are made is the same, the ratio of voltages or currents (sound pressure or particle velocity) may be used, in which case

$$\text{number of decibels} = 20 \log_{10} \frac{E_2}{E_1}.$$

If there is no possibility for confusion, the latter formula is used without re-

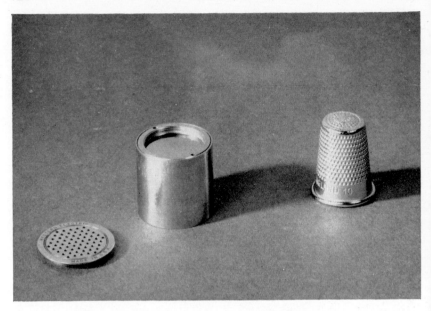

FIG. 17. A condenser microphone with its protective grid removed to show the diaphragm. A
sewing thimble is shown for a size comparison.

gard for impedance levels, although its meaning in reference to power ratios
is then lost.

In acoustics, the datum for sound pressure is generally .0002 dynes per
cm.$^2$ In some cases, a datum of 1 dyne per cm$^2$ is used. For electrical signals,
a datum of .001 watt (1 milliwatt) is often used, in which case the abbrevia-
tion "dbm" is employed instead of "db."

## THE ELECTRICAL ANALYSIS OF WAVE FORMS

### Microphones

Microphones are used to convert acoustical into electrical signals. The
more common types used in the analysis of acoustic wave forms are described below.

**Condenser microphone.** The condenser microphone, shown in Fig. 17,
consists essentially of a taut metal diaphragm, acted on by the incident sound
field, with a metal plate parallel and in close proximity to the diaphragm. The
plate and diaphragm act as an electric capacitor, the spacing between the
"plates," being varied by the sound pressure. If a source of high voltage is
placed across the "plates" through a high resistance, the variation of capacitance will cause a corresponding voltage variation across the high resistance.
This voltage is amplified by a vacuum tube, usually located in the microphone support to avoid the effect of long cables whose fixed capacitance
would otherwise diminish the sensitivity of the microphone.

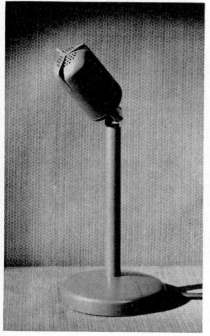

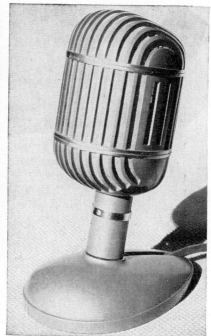

FIG. 18. A dynamic microphone and its stand.     FIG. 19. A cardioid microphone with its table
                                                                                    mounting.

Condenser microphones are small, and they do not unduly distort the sound field. They have a frequency range extending to over 10,000 cps, and maintain accurate pressure calibration.

They are used primarily in broadcasting and recording studios and in laboratories where an accurate and quantitative reproduction of acoustic wave form is desired.

**Dynamic microphone.** The dynamic or moving-coil microphone consists essentially of a coil of wire attached to a diaphragm, the coil placed in a magnetic field. The motion of the diaphragm causes the coil to move in the magnetic field, thereby generating a voltage across the terminals of the coil. The electrical impedance of the moving coil is low—of the order of 25 ohms —so that long cables between the microphone and associated apparatus have little effect on performance. The frequency response of the dynamic microphone illustrated in Fig. 18 is uniform to about 8000 cps, but is more irregular than that of the condenser microphone due to its larger and more complicated structure. The moving-coil microphone is sensibly nondirectional. Its sensitivity is approximately —85db ref 1 volt per dyne/cm² open circuit.

**Ribbon microphone.** The ribbon or velocity microphone consists of a flexible corrugated aluminum ribbon suspended vertically between the pole pieces of a magnetic structure. The pressure gradient of the sound field

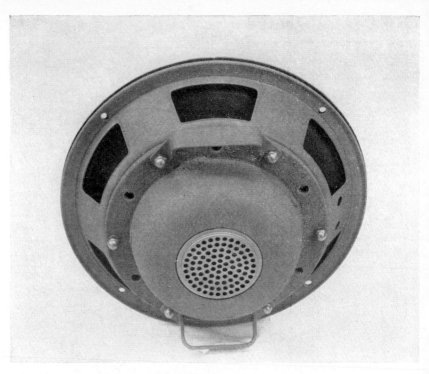

FIG. 20. A moving-coil direct-radiator loudspeaker, rear view. The cone of this loudspeaker is approximately 12 inches in diameter.

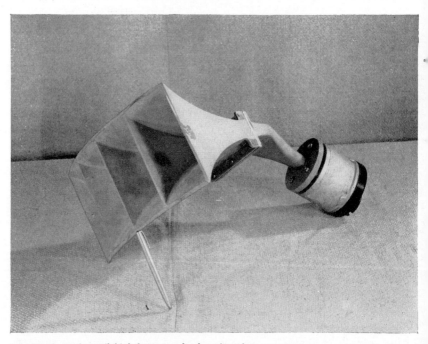

FIG. 21. A moving-coil high-frequency loudspeaker shown coupled to a multicellular horn. A mechanical pencil is shown for size comparison.

causes the ribbon to move in the magnetic field and thereby generate a voltage. The electrical impedance is very low, so that a transformer is provided in the base of the microphone to step up the impedance to about 250 ohms. The frequency response of a typical ribbon microphone (RCA Type 44BX) extends to 15,000 cps and its directionality is bilateral, with a null of sensitivity in the plane of the ribbon. The open circuit sensitivity is about $-85$db ref 1 volt per dyne/cm.$^2$

**Cardioid microphone.** In certain circumstances, it is desirable to have a microphone which is more directional than the ribbon type (Fig. 19). If an undirectional moving coil and a bidirectional ribbon type of microphone are combined, it is possible to obtain a range of directional patterns from nondirectional through the cardioid to the bidirectional (figure-eight) pattern. Such microphones are often used in public-address systems and in broadcasting to avoid pickup of undesired sounds.

**Crystal microphone.** A common type of microphone consists of a diaphragm actuating a piezoelectric crystal. The motion of the diaphragm bends or twists the crystal, generating a voltage between electrodes on the crystal surface. A crystal microphone has a high electrical impedance, but having a capacitance of about .002 microfarad, reasonably long cables may be used without their capacitance affecting the performance. Crystal microphones are approximately nondirectional and have a relatively high output, of the order of $-50$db ref 1 volt per dyne/cm$^2$.

**Carbon microphone.** The carbon microphone has great importance because of its extensive use as a telephone transmitter. It consists of a diaphragm which exerts a variable pressure on a number of small granules of carbon in accordance with the incident sound pressure, thereby varying the resistance to the passage of an otherwise steady electrical current. The resulting alternating current is the desired output. The frequency range of telephone transmitters is restricted to an upper limit of about 5000 cps. By utilization of mechanical and acoustical resonances, the sensitivity can be made high, of the order of $-40$db ref 1 volt per dyne/cm$^2$ for a steady current of 60 milliamperes. The sensitivity depends somewhat on the physical position of the microphone, due to the resulting changes in packing of carbon granules. Carbon microphones are rather nonlinear, and therefore do not lend themselves to accurate determinations of acoustic wave forms.

## Loudspeakers and Receivers

The usual sources of sound used in studies of the acoustics of speech (aside from the human voice itself) are moving-coil loudspeakers for generating large sound fields and electromagnetic, moving-coil and piezoelectric earphones, or receivers.

**Moving-coil loudspeaker.** This loudspeaker consists of a large conical diaphragm with a cylindrical coil of wire (the voice coil), attached to the apex (Fig. 20). The voice coil is placed between the concentric pole pieces of

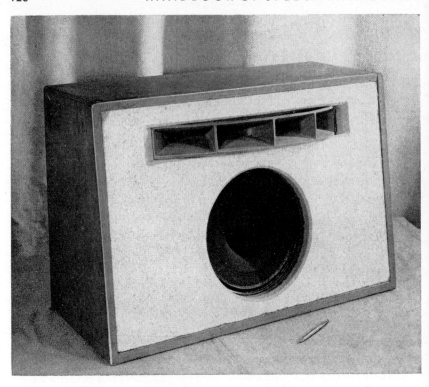

FiG. 22. A high-frequency loudspeaker unit and horn (tweeter) (Fig. 21) and a low frequency direct radiator loudspeaker (Fig. 20) mounted in an enclosure.

the field magnet, which supplies a radial magnetic field of considerable intensity. The interaction between the signal currents in the voice coil and the fixed magnetic field causes the diaphragm to vibrate and to radiate an acoustic signal. Single loudspeakers of this type will radiate more or less uniformly over a frequency range from 60 to 10,000 cycles per second. For larger frequency ranges, several speakers are used, each operating in a restricted frequency range. The low-frequency speakers ("woofers") are of the design described above, whereas the high-frequency units ("tweeters") often use a small spherical diaphragm acoustically coupled to the atmosphere by a horn, which matches the mechanical impedance of the diaphragm to the lower acoustic impedance of the atmosphere (Figs. 21 and 22).

**Electromagnetic receivers.** The electromagnetic receiver is the most common type and is typically used in telephone handsets. It consists of a diaphragm actuated by a polarized electromagnet consisting of a coil of wire wrapped around pole pieces, with a permanent magnet providing a steady biasing force on the diaphragm. The signal current in the windings generates an alternating magnetic field which, by virtue of the polarizing magnet, is biased to be in one direction only. Thus the alternating force on the diaphragm is approximately linear with the current in the winding, so that the sound output is approximately a linear function of the signal current. If no polarizing magnet were used, the sound pressure would be proportional to the square of the signal current and would cause excessive distortion of the sound output.

**Moving-coil receiver.** Except for a smaller diaphragm, the moving-coil receiver is quite similar to the moving-coil loudspeaker (Fig. 23). The frequency range and linearity of the moving-coil receiver is superior to the electromagnetic type, and it is widely used in acoustic studies. Sensitivity is about 50 dynes/cm$^2$ per milliwatt available power per receiver.

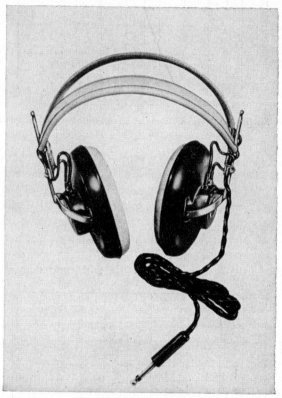

FIG. 23. Moving-coil receivers, shown attached to a headband, and equipped with ear cushions (Permoflux Corporation).

**Piezoelectric or crystal receivers.** The crystal receiver consists of a small diaphragm driven at the center by a piezoelectric crystal. It has a high electrical impedance and a wide frequency range. Sensitivity of the crystal receiver is of the order of 2 to 5 dynes/cm$^2$ per volt at 1000 cps.

## Amplifiers

Amplifiers are electronic circuits used to amplify electrical signals without appreciable distortion. Important characteristics are gain, frequency range, linearity or amount of amplitude distortion (both harmonic distortion and intermodulation), phase shift, noise output, power output, input and output impedance, and stability.

**Gain.** The gain of an amplifier is a measure of the increase in signal magnitude in transmission from the input to the output. It is usually measured in decibels, computed as $10 \log_{10} P_2/P_1$ where $P_2$ is the output power when $P_1$ is the input power. Amplifiers for general use have maximum gains in the range 30 to 70 decibels, and for use with microphones, the gains are usually in the range of 70 to 120 decibels.

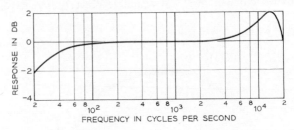

FIG. 24. The frequency response curve of a representative audio amplifier.

**Frequency range.** Amplifiers for general use for speech studies at audio frequencies are satisfactory if they transmit uniformily in the frequency range of 50 to 8000 cps (Fig. 24). Wide-range audio amplifiers may have a range of 20 to 20,000 cps with a variation in gain of ½ to 1 decibel. Special-purpose amplifiers may be had which transmit from direct current (zero frequency) to well over 20,000 cps. Fig. 24 shows a representative gain vs. frequency curve for a typical amplifier.

**Linearity.** Linearity, or constancy of gain with output level changes, is

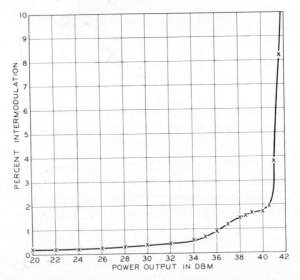

FIG. 25. An intermodulation curve of a representative audio amplifier showing the percentage of intermodulation vs. the power output.

usually expressed in terms of the amount of harmonic distortion or inter-modulation products produced in the output which are not present in the input signal. These products consist of multiples, sum, and difference frequencies of the input. High-quality amplifiers used in speech studies generally have less than 2 per cent harmonic distortion or 5 per cent inter-modulation products at rated power. Fig. 25 shows the manner in which the intermodulation products increase with output power for a typical amplifier with a rated power output of +41 dbm (12 watts).

**Phase shift.** The phase shift between output and input signals is of importance in connection with the reproduction of transient wave forms (pulses, square waves, etc.). A phase shift proportional to the frequency

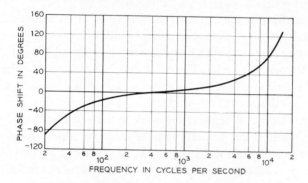

FIG. 26. The phase shift of an amplifier vs. frequency.

represents a delay of all frequency components of the signal, and a departure from linearity of phase shift with frequency will cause a change of shape of the output wave form which is called transient distortion, although there may be no variation of the gain with frequency. A curve of phase shift vs. frequency for a typical amplifier is shown in Fig. 26.

**Noise output.** Undesired signals in the output which are independent of the input signals are called noise. This noise normally falls into two categories; hum and random noise. Hum consists of the power-line frequency and its harmonics and is picked up from the alternating current power lines by induction in magnetic structures, electrostatic pickup, or through the direct-current power supply to the amplifier circuits. Random noise is generated by the thermal agitation of electrons in resistances in the amplifier and by the fluctuation of current leaving the cathodes of the vacuum tubes. The noise generated in the first stage of the amplifier is of the greatest importance, since it is amplified by the succeeding stages. In well-designed amplifiers, the total noise is no more than 3–10 decibels higher than that due to the unavoidable thermal noise in the input impedance of the amplifier.

**Power output.** The maximum power output of an amplifier is limited by the permissible amount of distortion products generated. In general, these products remain at a low level as the power output is increased until a critical point is reached when the amount of distortion products increases rapidly with further increase in power output, as may be seen in Fig. 25.

**Input and output impedance.** The input and output impedances of amplifiers depend on the particular application. For maximum power transfer from a source to its load, the source impedance and load impedance should be complex conjugates. Such a match over a wide band of frequencies would be difficult, so that generally the magnitudes of the impedances are matched. Exceptions to impedance-matching occur when other limitations, such as allowable nonlinear distortion, are factors.

High-impedance input circuits are used with some transducers, such as crystal microphones and phonograph reproducers. Moving-coil and velocity microphones generally operate in the impedance range 50 to 600 ohms, as the shunting effect of the capacitance of long cables is ameliorated by the lower impedance level. A standard impedance of 600 ohms is often employed in voice frequency filters, equalizers, and attenuators, as this value is typical of telephone circuits. The voice-coil impedance of loudspeakers is generally in the range of 2 to 16 ohms, so that power amplifiers for loudspeaker use are designed to operate into such impedances.

**Stability.** The use of negative feedback in the amplifier circuits makes it possible to stabilize the properties of the amplifier which would otherwise change due to aging of the vacuum tubes or other components. By proper application of feedback, the input or output impedances can be stabilized, which is desirable when the amplifier operates into or out of a filter.

### Attenuators

Whereas amplifiers are used to increase the power of a signal, attenuators are used to reduce the power by known amounts. They are usually calibrated in decibels. Adjustable attenuators for laboratory use are often of the decade type, in which several attenuators are used in tandem, each having steps ten times as great as the preceding. In this way, wide ranges of attenuation may be had which can be adjusted in small increments. In some cases, fixed attenuators (pads) are used, which may be equipped for plug-in mounting to facilitate changes.

### The Electrical Analysis of Signals

The electrical analysis of signals is usually carried out in either of the two representations, as functions of time or as functions of frequency. The distinction between the two is not sharp, as the so-called sound translator and sound spectrograph provide a representation in both time and frequency. The frequency analysis of a signal is generally made by means of electric filters or electric or mechanical wave analyzers. These provide a means of determining the frequency spectrum of a signal with varying degrees of precision.

## Filters

Electric wave filters are circuits which transmit with only a small loss certain frequencies or bands of frequencies, called the pass bands, and provide large attenuation for others (stop bands). They fall into classes depending on the position of their pass bands. These are low-pass, high-pass, band-pass, and band-elimination filters. A low-pass filter transmits easily all frequencies below a certain cutoff frequency, and a high-pass filter transmits all frequencies above its cutoff. Band-pass filters transmit and band-elimination filters attenuate frequencies in the interval between a low and a high cutoff frequency. A resonant circuit may be regarded as a form of simple band-pass filter for which the two cutoff frequencies correspond to the points at which the attenuation is 3 decibels greater than at the resonant frequency.

The analysis of steady-state power spectra may be carried out by the use of a group of fixed band-pass filters which span the frequency range of interest. Often these will consist of filters having octave band widths, for example, 250–500 cps, 500–1000 cps, 1000–2000 cps, and so on, or if finer details of the spectrum are wanted, narrower band width may be employed. The output of these filters is time-averaged and this average gives an approximation to the power spectrum of the source being measured.

The heterodyne wave analyzer is used when a more accurate picture of the spectrum is desired (Fig. 27). The frequency range to be analyzed is modulated by a variable frequency oscillator and passed through a fixed narrow band-pass filter (e.g., 4 cps band width). The frequency components of the original wave which pass through the filter depend on the frequency of the variable oscillator, so that the over-all effect is that of a narrow band-pass filter, of adjustable pass-band frequency, in the frequency range of interest. The output of the filter is time-averaged to yield the value of the power spectrum at the frequency selected. The heterodyne wave analyzer is especially useful for determining the amplitudes of single frequencies which are spaced closely, and for measuring the amplitudes of modulation products generated in nonlinear circuits. Because of the narrow pass-band generally used, the stability of the frequencies to be analyzed must be such that they will remain in the pass-band of the analyzing filter during their measurement.

A similar type of wave analyzer has an analyzing band width proportional to the center frequency, so that greater instability of higher frequency components does not affect their measurement any more than that of the lower frequencies.

The analysis of time-variable power spectra is generally carried out by means of a harmonic analyzer which sweeps the frequency range of interest in a time interval sufficiently short that the spectrum has not changed appreciably within the measuring time interval. For slowly changing spectra it is possible to display the output by means of an oscillograph. The rate at which the analyzer may be swept is limited by the transient response of the analyzing filter to a frequency modulated wave. Another method to achieve

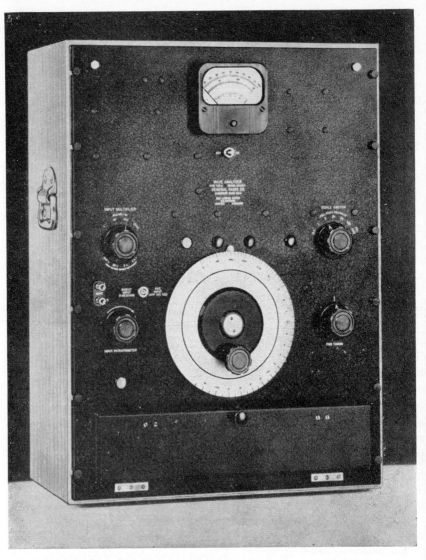

FIG. 27. A heterodyne wave analyzer (General Radio Company, Type 736-A).

the same effect involves the use of fixed narrow-band filters, the outputs of which are scanned by a commutator and displayed successively on a cathode ray oscilloscope.

### Sound Spectrograph

The sound spectrograph provides a convenient and rapid way to display the spectrum of a signal of about 2.4 seconds duration. It was developed by the Bell Telephone Laboratories for use in the study of speech sounds and has proved to be of great importance in speech analysis (Fig. 28).

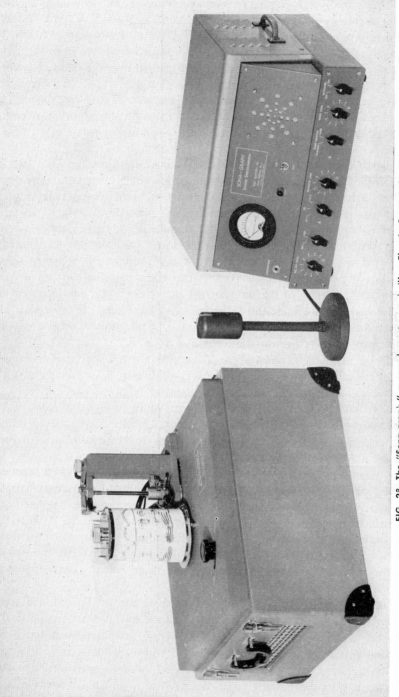

FIG. 28. The "Sona-graph," a sound spectrograph (Kay Electric Company).

The sound spectrograph, commercially known as the "Sona-graph," consists essentially of a means to record magnetically the sample to be analyzed and to reproduce it repeatedly. A heterodyne wave analyzer performs the actual analysis of the sound as it is reproduced from the recording. The frequency region being analyzed is slowly varied over the band of interest as the recording is repeated, and the results are displayed by marking paper on a drum moving in synchronsim with the recording of the sound. The darkness of the marking on the record of the analyzer output indicates the energy level at a particular frequency and at a particular instant of the signal. The vertical position of the marking stylus corresponds to the frequency of analysis; and as the analyzing frequency increases from the lower to the upper part, the position of the stylus moves accordingly. The resulting picture shows a frequency versus time representation, with frequency as ordinate and time as abscissa. In the commercially available instrument, the frequency range portrayed extends to 8000 cycles per second corresponding to a vertical distance on the paper of four inches. The analyzing filter may be selected to have either a 45-cycle or 300-cycle band width. When speech is analyzed, the 45-cycle filter permits the frequency resolution of the individual harmonics of the fundamental pitch. The 300-cycle filter, on the other hand, is not sufficiently discriminating to resolve the harmonics but is rapid enough in its time response to show the pitch rate as time variations, which appear as vertical striations closely spaced.

In the instrument shown in the illustration, the left-hand unit contains a magnetic recording disk under the cover, with the stylus assembly and drum above it. The right-hand unit contains the amplifying and analyzing apparatus. To operate the spectograph, the signal to be analyzed is recorded on the magnetic disk, which rotates at about 24 rpm during the recording process. When the recording process is terminated, the last 2.4 seconds of signal remain recorded on the disk. The analysis of this signal is made with the magnetic disk rotating at 80 rpm. As the signal is reproduced over and over, the signal is scanned by a filter which is shifted in frequency a small amount during each repetition. The analyzing filter output is amplified and recorded on a piece of dry facsimile paper wrapped around the drum on the recording and reproducing unit. The stylus moves vertically along the drum in step with the analyzing filter and the filter output is recorded by changes in the appearance of the facsimile paper, with high-intensity levels appearing as dark regions (Fig. 29).

Since the range of darkening of the marking paper is limited, additional means are available to portray the amplitude versus frequency at a particular instant of the signal. This "section," so-called, permits a quantitative determination of the amplitude spectrum of the signal at a selected time, with a uniform decibel scale of amplitude over a 35 db range covering 1½ inches horizontally on the marking paper. Because the amplitude is portrayed horizontally along the paper, sections cannot be made closer in time than about 0.4 second at any one time.

In order to make a "section," pins are inserted in one or more holes in the top of the drum above the spectrogram of the signal, at points corresponding to the location of the sections desired. These pins actuate a switch associated with the analyzing circuits which indicate the intensity of the frequency components of the signal at that point in time. A black mark on the facsimile paper is made of length proportional to the intensity level in decibels. In this way, a complete plot of the intensity versus frequency spectrum may be obtained for a particular part of the signal.

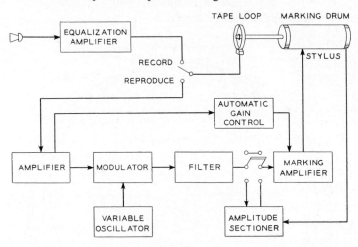

FIG. 29. Block diagram of a sound spectrograph.

In addition to making spectrograms and sections, it is also possible to display the intensity level of the signal as a function of time. An example of this is visible above the narrow-band spectrogram portrayed in the illustration.

# PART II. ACOUSTICAL PROPERTIES OF SPEECH WAVES*

Speech may be considered a multidimensional signal, involving frequency, energy, and time. The experimental study of the acoustical composition of speech extends well into the past century. Early studies were seriously limited, however, because instrumentation did not afford a continuous observation of the energy-frequency composition of the signal as a function of time.

With the development of the sound spectrograph, observation of the time structure of the speech signal became possible. When complete displays are desired, sequences of amplitude sections with the spectrograph may be assembled to form three-dimensional models.

* By Gordon E. Peterson, Ph.D.

## STATISTICAL MEASURES OF SPEECH SPECTRA

The time variations of the frequency composition of the acoustical wave are basic in speech. However, certain engineering interests have led to analyses of the long-time average spectrum of speech. Such information about speech has been determined by a number of investigators, and their results are in substantial agreement. Such information has had various applications, including the specification and measurement of communication equipment, and the calculation of the intelligibility of speech under various conditions of noise and frequency distortion.

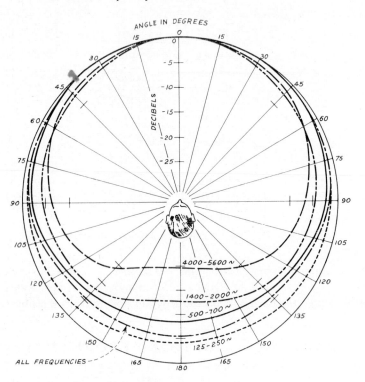

FIG. 30. Contours of equal pressure distribution in various frequency bands about the human head in the horizontal plane (Dunn and Farnsworth).

### Positional Distributions

Dunn and Farnsworth (1939) measured the distribution of sound pressures about the human head in a room which approximated free space. The measurements were in root mean square pressures for 15-second intervals. The data were obtained with a condenser microphone; under close conditions an associated calibrated probe was employed. The rms values were derived from circuits supplying a vacuum thermocouple and Grassot fluxmeter. The study involved only one speaker, but pressures within various

requency bands as well as over-all pressures were determined. The distributions of pressures within a selected set of frequency bands are shown in
Figs. 30 and 31. The scale in decibels shows the variation in front of the
mouth as a function of distance. The contours represent pressures equal to

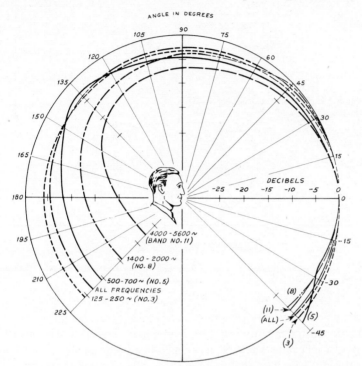

FIG. 31. Contours of equal pressure distribution in various frequency bands about the human
head in the vertical plane (Dunn and Farnsworth).

that for each individual band at a distance of 60 cm directly in front of the
mouth. Fig. 30 shows the distribution of pressures in the horizontal plane,
and Fig. 31 shows the distribution in the vertical plane.

## Long-Time Spectra

Dunn and White (1940) made more extensive studies of speech pressures
at a distance of 30 cm in front of the lips. They determined the peak pressures
in ⅛-second intervals within various frequency bands. The data were
plotted with peak pressures versus frequency. A family of curves was derived which showed the pressures which were exceeded for various percentages of intervals. Similar data were obtained for rms pressures in ⅛-
second intervals. The basic system consisted of a set of parallel channels. In
each channel a filter was followed by a square-law rectifier, integrating circuit, and a thyratron. The thyratron outputs operated mechanical counters.
Dunn and White also integrated short-interval rms values to obtain long-
time averages.

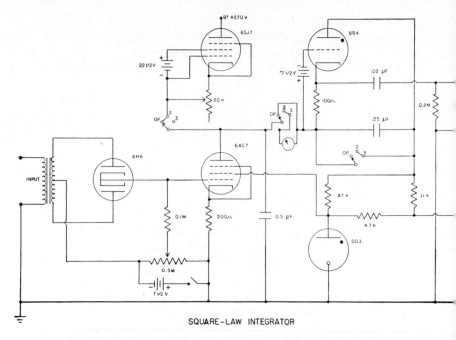

SQUARE-LAW INTEGRATOR

**FIG. 32.** Diagram of the square-law integrating unit of the audio spectrometer (Benson and Hirsh).

At Harvard University (Rudmose, *et al.*, 1948) an Audio Spectrometer was developed for measuring the rms pressures in speech. The instrument employed a mel filter bank, with 13 pass-bands of equal width according to a subjective pitch scale for pure tones. These were sharp filters with relatively flat pass-bands and steep attenuation characteristics. A system was employed so that average rms pressures within the various bands could be determined.

More recently, Benson and Hirsh (1953) have employed an Audio Spectrometer for the measurement of speech spectra. Their system consisted of a magnetic-tape recorder-reproducer, two variable-frequency band-pass filters, a square-law integrator, and a pulse counter. In these systems a square-law characteristic of a vacuum tube is employed. The output is supplied to a condenser which operates a thyratron when a certain voltage is reached. Since the condenser discharges vary rapidly through the tube, it restores promptly to its charging position. The high-speed counters indicate the number of discharges which have occurred, and the pressure values are determined from the counting rates. A diagram of the square-law integrator is shown in Fig. 32.

Benson and Hirsh compared their results with those of the Harvard study and also with the earlier work of Dunn and White. The comparison of the three sets of data is shown in Fig. 33. Less energy is found in the lowest frequency band for women's voices, of course.

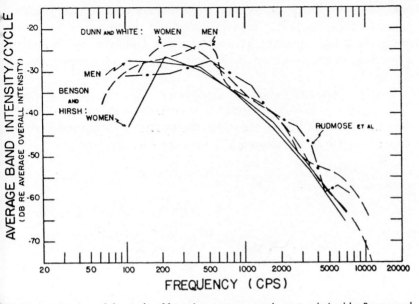

FIG. 33. A comparison of the results of long-time average speech spectra derived by Benson and Hirsh, Rudmose and associates, and Dunn and White. The various curves have been placed on the same graph by the use of a relative intensity scale (Benson and Hirsh).

## PSYCHOPHYSICAL TECHNIQUES IN SPEECH MEASUREMENT

Auditory identification tests have been employed extensively in the study of speech. These tests have included the recognition of vowels and consonants, nonsense syllables, meaningful words of various syllable lengths, phrases, and sentences. The first major quantitative use of such listening tests was developed at the Bell Telephone Laboratories (Fletcher and Steinberg, 1929) during the first quarter of this century. Articulation or intelligibility curves are now widely employed in communication measurements (Egan, 1948; French and Steinberg, 1947). Such curves are shown elsewhere in this book. In general, the dependent variable is the percentage of correct recognitions. The independent variable usually takes some form of over-all gain of the communication channel. Other parameters which may be involved in such tests include frequency band width and location, signal to noise ratio, communication-channel distortions, dialectal differences among speakers and listeners, and hearing acuity.

Such tests are obviously limited to the structure of a particular language unless the speaker and subject are specialized in phonetics. For example, in nonsense-syllable tests, vowel and consonant recognition will normally be based upon the phonemic system of the listener.

In the study of the acoustical characteristics of speech, such intelligibility measures are somewhat limited. This results primarily from the fact that any one language normally involves a rather restricted sample of the various types of sounds which can be made by the human vocal mechanism. Techniques for the evaluation of speech signals which extend beyond the confines of specific dialects, however, have not been well developed. This is primarily a problem in the basic psychophysical evaluation of complex auditory stimuli.

Speech is sufficiently complex that it is not easily specified and defined. Basically, speech may be described by statements about statistical distributions within a given form of the signal, and by statements about the relationships among the various forms in which the signal occurs.

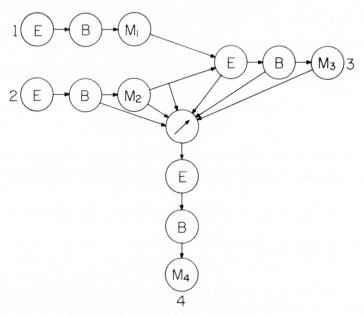

FIG. 34. A schematic representation of the processes involved in the experimental evaluation of speech signals. Four individuals are indicated in the diagram: 1 and 2, speakers; 3, listener; 4, experimenter. E, ear; B, brain; M, motor mechanism; ↗, meter.

Fig. 34 has been drawn to illustrate the nature of the problems involved in the evaluation of speech signals. In this figure are shown the essential communication linkages which are of concern in such an analysis. In a very schematic manner, four separate individuals are represented. $E$ represents a sense organ, as Eye or Ear; $B$ represents Brain, or more generally, the Central Nervous System; $M$ represents a motor organ or mechanism, as Mouth; and ↗ is the conventional representation of a meter.

In the oral communication process, a series of very complicated transformations are involved in transmitting a message from one individual to another. It is the nervous system, of course, which controls the musculature of speech production. The neural impulses are converted to positions and movements of the mechanism. These movements in turn produce complex acoustical oscillations within the vocal cavities. These oscillations are transmitted through a medium to the ear of the listener. Here they are transformed to a sequence of mechanical vibrations; and the mechanical oscillations, in turn, generate neural impulses within the Central Nervous System of the listener.

Depending upon certain philosophical concepts, either the Central Nervous System or the Vocal Organs of the speaker may be considered as the source of the transmitted message. Once the source has been specified, however, it is fundamental in Communication Theory that no further *source* information is added to the message along the transmission path (Shannon, 1948). In fact, due to noise and distortion, the information content generally degenerates as one proceeds away from the source. When the message is received by the listener, however, he brings his own background of experience and information to the interpretation of the message. He may miss information which was there; he may add or infer information which was not intended, and thereby arrive at false conclusions. Thus, because of noise in channel transmission and because of the specialized nature of human perception, there may be marked distinctions and even contradictions between information sent and information received.

The two individuals (1 and 2) at the left of the diagram are shown as originators of the speech signal; the individual (3) at the right is the recipient of the message; and the individual (4) at the bottom may be considered as an experimenter. This latter individual may be equipped with measuring instruments of various types for the careful analysis of the various processes involved in oral communication. At the present time relatively exact observations on the structure of the acoustical wave are possible; somewhat less complete observations on the physiological behavior of the vocal mechanism and the auditory apparatus are possible; and present descriptions of the neural processes involved in speech production and reception are markedly limited in scope.

We take a position such as that occupied by individual 4 in Fig. 34 in attempting the specification or description of speech. As indicated above, this individual may attempt to derive the structure of speech from statistical studies of one of the processes or forms of the signal. Secondly, he may seek to define the relationships among the various processes or signal forms.

In order to derive the physiological or acoustical parameters which are of significance in speech, it is desirable to compare signals produced by different speakers, as by individuals 1 and 2 of Fig. 34.

Two speech samples are functionally similar if they produce the same motor response in the listener. That is, utterances by individuals 1 and 2 may be considered functionally similar if they produce the same responses by individual 3 at some $M_3$.

Since two utterances cannot simultaneously occupy the same space and time, they are never truly indistinguishable. They may be indistinguishable in certain attributes, however. Thus, two speech samples are perceptually similar or equivalent in certain properties when individual 3 cannot produce responses at some $M_3$ which are distinct for these particular properties of the utterances.

## THE ACOUSTICAL CHARACTERISTICS OF SPEECH STRUCTURE

The essential nature of the acoustical form of speech was not generally understood nor easily portrayed in visual form until the development of the sound spectrograph. The almost continuously changing nature of the spectrum of the speech signal and the important interrelationships between vowels and consonants are well represented in the sound spectrograms which are made with this instrument. An extensive set of carefully made spectrograms and the details of the consonant-vowel influences in American speech were first described in *Visible Speech* (Potter, Kopp, and Green, 1947). A discussion of the dynamical aspects of sound spectrograms, and of the implications of such analyses for linguistic theory, has been presented by Joos (1948). The modern tools of acoustical analysis have clarified many former issues regarding the nature of speech; they have also directed attention to certain very basic problems in theory and experiment which were not previously clearly defined.

### The Human Vocal System

In the past, the research and writings of phoneticians and speech pathologists have placed great emphasis upon the generating mechanisms of speech. According to the considerations of the previous section, this emphasis appears to be considerably justified. Thus it seems reasonable that those interested in the nature of the acoustical waves of speech have also shown considerable interest in the physical behavior of the vocal mechanism.

We may first consider the sublaryngeal breath supply for speech. Unfortunately, the acoustical properties of this system have received relatively little experimental or theoretical analysis according to physical principles. Gray and his associates (1936) have studied the relationships among types of respiratory movements and certain characteristics of speech production, such as intensity of voice. They found no clearly defined correspondences between speech waves and respiratory function. Experimenters have found the specification of respiratory structures and functions to be a very complex matter. It is obvious, of course, that most of normal speech requires a sublaryngeal source of breath supply. Clearly a general co-ordination is required between exhalation and speech production. Any further close relationships among respiratory functions and the acoustical properties of speech waves, however, are yet to be demonstrated experimentally.

Stetson (1951) has made certain observations concerning thoracic and abdominal pressures and movements in speech production. He found sublaryngeal pressure fluctuations which occurred at what he called syllable rates. It is yet to be determined whether these pressure variations are developed from systematic neural innervations, or whether they are secondary effects which simply result from the articulatory constrictions along the path of the breath stream during speech production.

Carhart (1938) studied certain subglottal effects by means of a mechanical model related to that previously developed by Ewald. Carhart did not attach supraglottal resonators, but studied the effects of infraglottal tube length and breath pressure supply upon the frequency of response of the model. He found that the frequency of response of the artificial vocal cords had a certain dependence upon the length of the supply tube; for given conditions of the model larynx the response was not facilitated at certain supply-tube lengths. In general, when the cushions (simulating the vocal cords) responded at a particular frequency, another response could be obtained by increasing the supply-tube length by one-half the wave length of the frequency involved. If the behavior of the human laryngeal system is interpreted in terms of the results of the experiments, then: (1) increased breath pressure produces a rise in laryngeal frequency; (2) increased tension on the vocal cords produces a rise in laryngeal frequency; (3) a controlled balance between breath-supply pressure and laryngeal tension is required to produce continuous and smooth phonation over a broad range of frequencies.

In order to obtain a better understanding of the behavior of the human larynx, various stroboscopic and motion-picture studies have been made. Considerable valuable descriptive information has been obtained from the high-speed motion picture film produced by Farnsworth (1940) at the Bell Telephone Laboratories. This film shows the operation of the larynx under a variety of conditions and has had a rather wide distribution among scientists in the field.

The larynx is essentially a nonlinear device, and an exact physical description of its operation is somewhat difficult. Wegel (1930) has developed a mathematical analysis of its behavior. Also, Olson (1947) has suggested an electrical analog to the larynx. The model involves a triode and associated circuit elements which produce an output having a sawtooth wave form.

Most of the recent acoustical analyses of the behavior of the vocal mechanism have treated the larynx as a high-impedance generator. The laryngeal or generating tone is complex in its frequency composition and has a fundamental frequency which corresponds to the rate at which the glottis opens and closes.

Within the vocal tract, oscillations are established by the driving bursts of air which escape periodically through the glottis. The burst rate determines the fundamental frequency of the sound, and it is well known that the oscillations within the resonators above need have no integral relationship to the vocal-cord rates. The resonant frequencies are known as formant frequencies.

For the lower formant frequencies, the wave lengths are sufficiently long that the resonances are largely independent of the details of cavity shape. Thus lumped values of the cavity and constriction sizes adequately specify the formant frequencies. Wegel, Olson, and others have described lumped-constant electrical analogs of the human vocal tract. A simple analog composed of resistances (dissipations), inductances (constrictions), and capacitances (cavities) is shown in Fig. 35. This model does not have a nasal resonator. Actually, of course, the components all vary in magnitude according to the cavity formations.

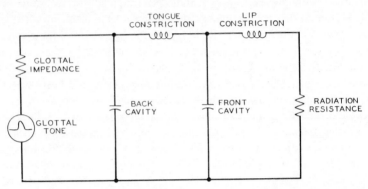

FIG. 35. A simple lumped-constant electral analog to the human vocal tract. Cavities are represented by capacitances and constrictions are represented by inductances.

In this model the resonance oscillations are excited by the driving function of the larynx. Damped or decaying waves occur at the resonator frequencies. These oscillations are regenerated at the basic vocal-cord rate. Thus the output wave may be considered as sequences of sets of damped oscillations. Such a wave is periodic. When analyzed with a narrow filter, the overtones occur in integral multiples of the fundamental laryngeal frequency; if a frequency of resonance differs appreciably from the harmonic values, no response will be found at the resonant frequency. However, when such a wave is measured with filter widths which approximate the fundamental frequency of the vocal cords, then peak energies are observed at the resonant frequencies and the individual harmonic frequencies are not resolved. The periodic laryngeal source appears at the output of such a wide-filter analysis as the excitation of the recurrent decaying wave patterns.

When the higher frequencies of the audible spectrum are considered, then the details of cavity shapes have considerable importance in determining the resonant frequencies of the upper formants. In order to obtain a more complete understanding of the acoustical properties of the vocal system, Dunn (1950) made a theoretical analysis of the vocal tract which takes into account the details of cavity shapes. He developed a distributed constant or transmission line analysis of the supralaryngeal cavities as a series of short cylinders of different cross-sectional areas along the tract. An actual electrical analog to the vocal cavities was constructed by Dunn and Schott (1950). A schematic of the device is shown in Fig. 36, and a picture of the instrument is shown in Fig. 37. The various controls make it possible to adjust the cavity

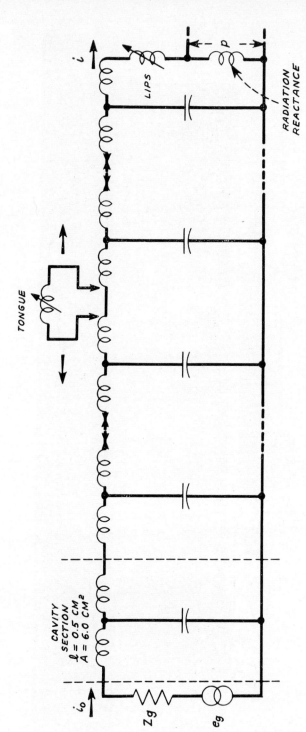

FIG. 36. Schematic of the electrical vocal tract developed by Dunn and Schott (Dunn).

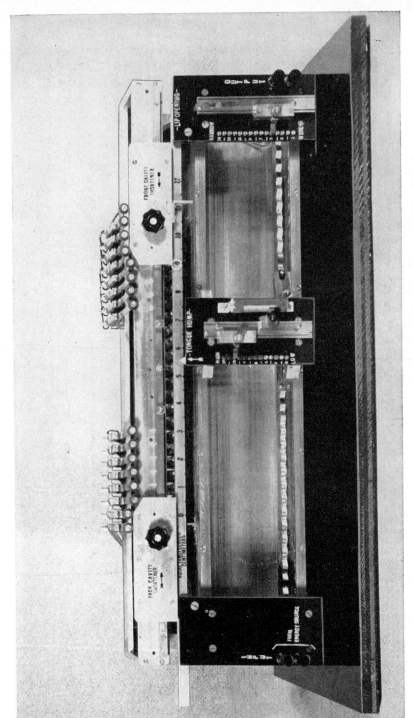

FIG. 37. The construction of the electrical vocal tract developed by Dunn and Schott (Dunn).

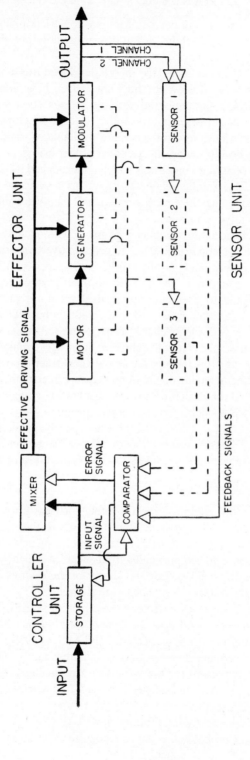

FIG. 38. A theoretical model of the speech mechanism as a closed-cycle control system (Fairbanks).

length, the tongue position and degree of tongue constriction, and degree of lip constriction. Dunn and Schott also added an analog, not shown in the figure, for the nasal passageways.

More recently Fant has extended the theory developed by Dunn to include dissipation, and Stevens, Kasowski, and Fant (1953) have constructed an electrical analog which simulates the variable cross-sectional area of the vocal tract. The electrical sections are similar to those employed by Dunn, but several different values of inductance are available at each section and the dissipation may be adjusted by means of variable resistors.

The sustained vowels and semivowels which are produced by these systems have a quality which is authentic. Also, by means of various connections along the transmission line, Stevens, Kasowski, and Fant were able to synthesize plosive and fricative consonants.

Although some hand adjustments can be made with such systems, these devices are essentially static in character. In order to overcome this difficulty, certain studies have been made on the synthesis of speech with independent parallel electrical resonators to generate the formant frequencies. These can be adjusted according to previously prescribed temporal patterns, based upon analyses of actual utterances. It would obviously be difficult, however, to equip such devices with the mechanisms necessary to predict the transient properties of an utterance. Neural delays and muscle dynamics are both fundamental in the time functions of the actual vocal tract. In order to better simulate the dynamic behavior of the human speech mechanism, Fairbanks (1954) has suggested the design of a speech generating system with a feedback control. This proposal has considerable promise in electrical speech synthesis, since much of the time pattern of the speech signal is determined by the prominent auditory feedback path. The basic model proposed by Fairbanks for the speech mechanism as a servo-system is shown in Fig. 38.

### Acoustical Properties of Vowels

The pharynx, mouth, and nose form a rather tortuous transmission path for the laryngeal tone. The cross-sectional area along the pharyngeal and oral cavities is variable. A whole series of resonant frequencies occur in such an acoustical system, and the particular frequencies at which resonance occurs depends upon the specific sizes and shapes of the cavities; by adjusting the cavity shapes, the resonant frequencies are altered.

These resonant frequencies have long been identified with vowel values. They have been specified and described previously by such men as Helmholtz (1895), Stumpf (1926), Paget (1930), and Miller (1926). Much of the early analysis involved men's voices, and specific resonant frequency values have usually been expressed for the vowels of a particular language. These resonant frequencies have been called *formant* frequencies, and they are numbered according to their order along the frequency scale from low to high; that is, first formant, second formant, and so on.

Lloyd (1890) was probably the first to recognize that at least certain types of vowels are not well defined by absolute magnitudes of resonant frequency. It is fairly easy to anticipate this fact when it is recognized that men, women, and children do not have vocal cavities of the same size; yet all three types of speakers are quite capable of producing highly intelligible speech. In general, when such acoustical structures have similar shapes, the resonances of the smaller structures will be higher in frequency. This is illustrated by reference to the equations for tubes and Helmholtz resonators in an earlier section of this chapter. An examination of these equations will show that if all linear dimensions of the system are divided by some constant $k$, then the resonant frequencies will all be multiplied by the same constant $k$. Advantage is often taken of this proportionality in the use of scale models to study the behavior of various acoustical systems.

As indicated earlier, the lower formant frequencies depend more upon gross cavity sizes and constrictions than upon exact shapes. The adjustment of the higher formant frequencies in general depends progressively more upon specific cavity sizes and shapes. There are certain physiological constraints, of course, in the possible adjustments of the vocal cavities. Thus, there is a definite limitation in the degree to which one speaker with a mechanism of given dimensions can match the physical magnitudes within vowels produced by another speaker whose vocal cavities differ markedly in over-all size. Essentially, matches in absolute magnitude can be made only over a limited range of frequencies; as the difference in dimensions increases, the frequency range over which exact formant matching is possible is decreased.

Lloyd, and more recently Potter and Peterson (1948), developed the hypothesis that vowel sounds are determined in part by the relative values of the formant frequencies, rather than by the absolute magnitudes of these frequencies. Thus the relationships among formant frequencies are considered of significance in determining vowel values. Because of the nature of human perception, however, there is little reason to anticipate that the above principle will hold far beyond the range of normal voice production. These limitations should apply to formant frequency values, damping constants, and fundamental voice frequencies. For example, it is well known that vowel intelligibility degenerates when spectral multiplication or division is obtained by extensive speed change in reproducing recorded speech.

Joos (1948) and Potter and Peterson (1948) have noted the relationship of acoustical charts of the formant frequencies to the conventional vowel diagram. Such an acoustical chart is obtained, for example, when the frequency of the second formant is plotted against the frequency of the first formant. The conventional vowel diagram has been employed for many years and has been drawn in several different forms; it is presumed to represent physiological dimensions. However, as previously noted (Peterson, 1951), numerous physiological dimensions would actually be required to specify vowels. Such specifications, even then, would be only approximate. They might include such factors as: position of the hump of the tongue along the vocal tract, degree of constriction between the tongue hump and the pharyngeal wall or the palate, length of the tongue constriction, magnitude of spacing between the lips, length of the lip constriction or rounding, and so on.

It should be observed that disturbing noise, distortion, and other factors may affect the correspondence between the physiological formations and the acoustical speech waves. However, there is no reason to assume an inconsistency between these two forms of the signal. The acoustical signal simply represents a somewhat degraded condition of the information initiated by the vocal mechanism. The acoustical signal represents a rather com-

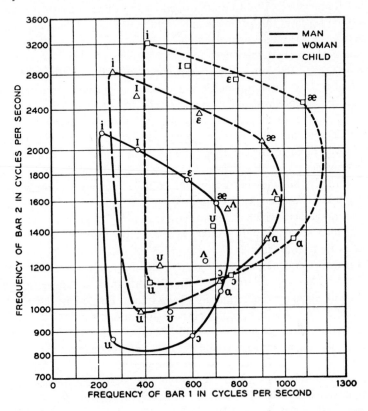

FIG. 39. Loops constructed with the frequency of the second formant plotted against the frequency of the first formant for vowels produced by a man, a woman, and a child (Peterson).

plicated transformation of the physiological movements, however, and it appears that in the acoustical form the vowel waves are much more readily specified and described; that is, it is operationally practical to specify vowels in terms of acoustical data.

Fig. 39 shows the frequency of the second formant plotted against the frequency of the first formant for similar vowels produced by a man, a woman, and a child (Peterson, 1951b). The displacement in frequency of these vowel loops is obvious. The frequency scale employed in this plot is

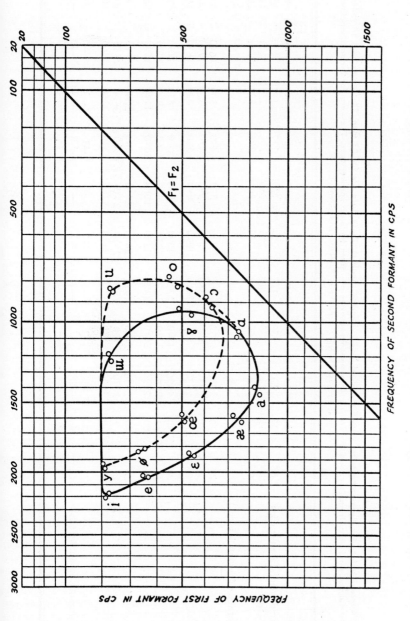

FIG. 40. Loops for the frequency of the second formant plotted against the frequency of the first formant for sustained vowels by one speaker. Each vowel was spoken twice, and the points are plotted along a mel scale. The solid line represents unrounded vowels, and the dashed line represents rounded vowels (Peterson).

TABLE 1. Average values for measurements on vowels produced by 76 different speakers. These data are for 33 men, 28 women, and 15 children. Values for the fundamental voice frequency, and the first three formant frequencies are given for each speaker type. The data for formant amplitudes have been combined for all 76 speakers (Peterson and Barney).

| | | i | ɪ | ε | æ | ɑ | ɔ | ʊ | u | ʌ | ɝ |
|---|---|---|---|---|---|---|---|---|---|---|---|
| Fundamental frequencies (cps) | M | 136 | 135 | 130 | 127 | 124 | 129 | 137 | 141 | 130 | 133 |
| | W | 235 | 232 | 223 | 210 | 212 | 216 | 232 | 231 | 221 | 218 |
| | Ch | 272 | 269 | 260 | 251 | 256 | 263 | 276 | 274 | 261 | 261 |
| Formant frequencies (cps) | | | | | | | | | | | |
| $F_1$ | M | 270 | 390 | 530 | 660 | 730 | 570 | 440 | 300 | 640 | 490 |
| | W | 310 | 430 | 610 | 860 | 850 | 590 | 470 | 370 | 760 | 500 |
| | Ch | 370 | 530 | 690 | 1010 | 1030 | 680 | 560 | 430 | 850 | 560 |
| $F_2$ | M | 2290 | 1990 | 1840 | 1720 | 1090 | 840 | 1020 | 870 | 1190 | 1350 |
| | W | 2790 | 2480 | 2330 | 2050 | 1220 | 920 | 1160 | 950 | 1400 | 1640 |
| | Ch | 3200 | 2730 | 2610 | 2320 | 1370 | 1060 | 1410 | 1170 | 1590 | 1820 |
| $F_3$ | M | 3010 | 2550 | 2480 | 2410 | 2440 | 2410 | 2240 | 2240 | 2390 | 1690 |
| | W | 3310 | 3070 | 2990 | 2850 | 2810 | 2710 | 2680 | 2670 | 2780 | 1960 |
| | Ch | 3730 | 3600 | 3570 | 3320 | 3170 | 3180 | 3310 | 3260 | 3360 | 2160 |
| Formant amplitudes (db) | $L_1$ | −4 | −3 | −2 | −1 | −1 | 0 | −1 | −3 | −1 | −5 |
| | $L_2$ | −24 | −23 | −17 | −12 | −5 | −7 | −12 | −19 | −10 | −15 |
| | $L_3$ | −28 | −27 | −24 | −22 | −28 | −34 | −34 | −43 | −27 | −20 |

that developed by Koenig (1949) as an approximate pitch scale, linear below 1000 cps and logarithmic above.

When the origin is placed at the upper right in such a plot, the loop takes the form of the traditional vowel diagram. Separate loops for rounded and unrounded vowels are shown in Fig. 40. The co-ordinates on this graph are constructed with a frequency spacing according to the mel or pitch scale of Stevens (1940). It is of interest that the unrounded and rounded vowel loops markedly overlap. This indicates the necessity of additional acoustical dimensions for the exact phonetic specification of vowels, even when produced by a single speaker.

Various facts suggest that the lower formant frequencies are of primary importance in determining vowel value. As indicated above, exactness of cavity size and shape is less important in determining the lower resonance frequencies of the vocal tract; also, the transmission of these lower formant frequencies is less affected by the details of the acoustical environment. Other considerations are that in general the second formant lies within the most sensitive range of human hearing, and that the range of the second formant roughly corresponds to the range of the frequency spectrum which makes the greatest contribution to speech intelligibility. These and other considerations suggest that the higher formants are of somewhat less importance than the first two in determining the phonetic quality of vowel sounds. In gen-

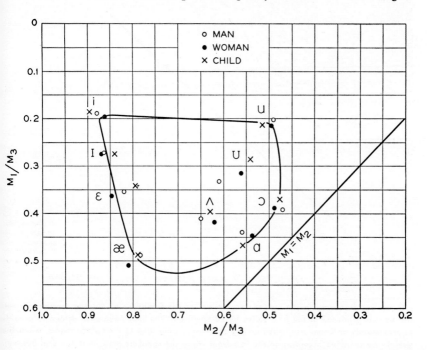

FIG. 41. A loop of the mel ratios of vowel formants. The vowels were produced in sustained form by a man, a woman, and a child; the points are based on mel values for the first three formants (Peterson).

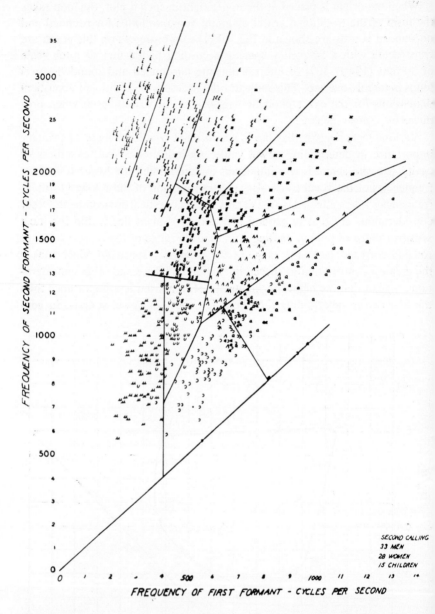

**FIG. 42.** The frequency of the second formant versus the frequency of the first formant for the ten vowels produced in the *h*V*d* series by 76 speakers. The lines have been drawn to provide approximately optimum separation among the vowels according to the two formants, when the vowels are classified according to the lists from which the speakers read (Peterson and Barney).

eral, it appears that the higher formant frequencies primarily contribute to increased definition or exactness of vowel quality. However, a suitable multi-dimensional portrayal of the vowel formants is not easily constructed. Some three-dimensional models have been developed by Peterson (1954). Within such models, lines of equal formant ratio may be constructed. The paths of such lines will depend, of course, upon the particular scales employed in the model. Fig. 41 has been prepared as a plot of specific formant ratios to show the nature of the relationships. The plot is for a set of similar vowels produced by a man, a woman, and a child. It is likely that the nonlinear characteristics of audition do affect the judgment of vowel quality, and so, for the purpose of illustration, the ratios in Fig. 41 have been based upon mel or pitch values (Stevens and Volkmann, 1940).

Peterson and Barney (1952) made measurements of the fundamental voice frequency and the formant frequencies of a series of vowels produced by 76 different speakers; these included 33 men, 28 women, and 15 children. The vowels were located in an $hVd$ combination. The speakers represented various dialects throughout the United States, but were predominately General American; a limited number of persons with foreign dialect were included. Table I above shows the average values for the various measurements, according to speaker type: men, women, and children. In the amplitude data it was assumed that the amplitudes of the first formants are related approximately according to the relation of over-all powers, as previously given by Fletcher (1929). The amplitude of the first formant in [ɔ] was used as a reference for the remaining vowels.

The individual values for the frequencies of the first two formants are plotted in Fig. 42. The co-ordinates in this chart are linear below 1000 cps and logarithmic above. The boundary lines are drawn to provide an optimum discrimination or separation among the vowels. The vowels were also classified by means of a series of listening tests, but the separating lines in Fig. 42 are according to speaker classification; that is, the symbol representing each vowel on the chart is determined by the spelling in the $hVd$ list which the speaker originally read. From this chart, a table was constructed showing the percentage correct identification for each vowel. The average correct recognition according to speaker classification for the ten vowels is 79 per cent. The overlapping points in part illustrate the inadequacy of two formant values for complete vowel specification. Also, considerable formant movement was actually involved in the utterances, since the vowels were formed in a consonant environment. An experimental determination of the manner in which these movements affect vowel evaluation has not yet been made. Thus the overlapping of points in Fig. 42 doubtless in part results from difficulties in evaluating the changing formant patterns.

The formant band widths for the vowels by the speakers in the above set of data were studied by Bogert (1953). He found that the formant widths at the half power (3 db down) points are relatively independent of frequency; thus the $Q$'s of the resonances tend to increase for the higher formant fre-

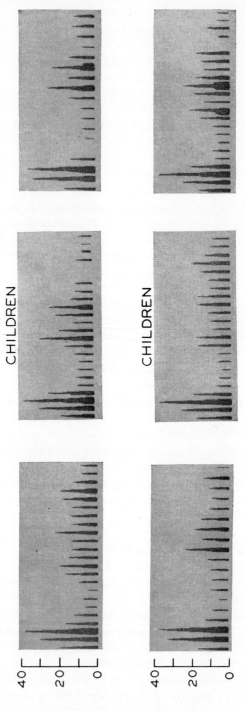

CHILDREN

CHILDREN

FREQUENCY IN KILOCYCLES

AMPLITUDE IN DECIBELS

40

20

0

40

20

0

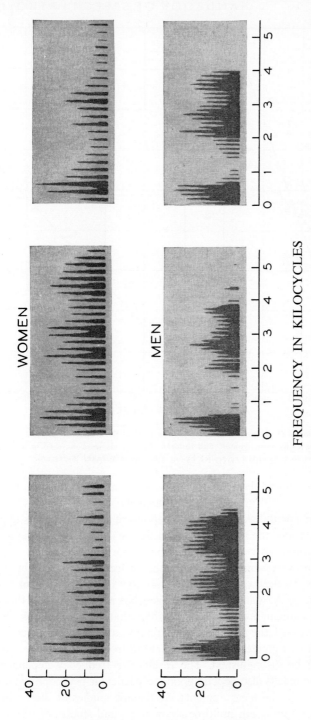

WOMEN

MEN

AMPLITUDE IN DECIBELS

40 20 0

40 20 0

FREQUENCY IN KILOCYCLES

0 1 2 3 4 5

FIG. 43. Amplitude sections with the sound spectrograph for the vowel [I]. The vowels were all matches to a single recorded reference, and the sections are for men, women, and children, as indicated (Peterson).

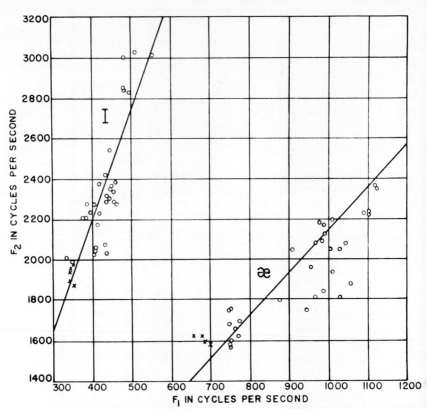

FIG. 44. The frequency of the second formant plotted against the frequency of the first formant for a series of vowels by men, women, and children. The vowels were matched in a free-space room to a recorded reference by an adult male speaker (Peterson).

quencies. Bogert found the average widths for formants 1, 2, and 3 for male speakers to be 130, 150, and 185 cps, respectively.

Further fundamental work on the perception of speech signals is required in order to determine the manner in which the various acoustical parameters of vowels contribute to vowel identification. Some progress in this direction has been made by Stevens (1952) who studied frequency discrimination of damped waves. In the extreme, with a very low damping constant (a very sharp resonance), the damped wave approaches a pure tone. In this case, ability to discriminate frequencies resembles that for sine waves. As the damping is increased, the ability to discriminate waves of various frequencies decreases; that is, a greater difference in central frequency is required before two tones can be distinguished. The results are frequency dependent, of course; and the results also depend upon the particular psychophysical technique employed in the measurements. Systematic studies of discrimination among complex tones with multiple resonances, and studies of discrimination among tones with changing resonant frequencies should be of considerable aid to a further understanding of the basis of vowel perception.

Peterson (1952) studied the relationships among the vowel formants and the fundamental voice frequency when speakers matched vowel sounds under carefully controlled conditions. In these experiments, subjects imitated recorded vowel references. It should be observed, however, that techniques of just noticeable differences have not yet been generally applied to the study of the acoustical properties of actual speech, and the above method probably does not approach the precision possible with JND techniques.

Fig. 43 shows a set of amplitude sections for the vowel [ɪ], as obtained with the above matching technique. These spectra show harmonics for the voices of various men, women, and children. Fig. 44 shows a plot of the frequency of the second formant versus the frequency of the first formant for two sets of vowel data obtained with this method. The diagonal lines are lines of constant frequency ratio which pass through the origin.

The patterns produced by the sound spectrograph have emphasized the kinetic nature of speech. The speech organs are in an almost continuous movement as phonemic sequences are produced, and these movements are reflected in the changing acoustical structure of the speech wave. The manner in which the changing formant frequencies determine vowel value is a matter of considerable interest, and there is much research yet to be carried out on this subject. In a preliminary study (1952), it has been observed for individual speakers that the sustained vowel formant values of the phoneme are often approximated where the rates of formant change are slowest within the utterance. This relationship is illustrated in Fig. 45, which is for relatively rapid speech. The horizontal lines connect formants of immediately preceding and following isolated vowels.

An interesting problem in the acoustical description of vowels is the effect of nasalization. Some speculations have been presented concerning the relationship between nasal resonance in vowel formation and the spectral structure of vowels. However, preliminary investigations indicate that this subject is rather complex, and thus far no systematic study of the acoustical properties of nasal vowels has been carried out. Some of the effects which may occur are illustrated in Fig. 46. This figure shows broad-band spectrograms and amplitude sections for a sequence of vowels. The upper chart is for an oral series and the lower chart is for a similar nasal series. The frequency scales extend to 3500 cps in both the spectrograms and the sections. These charts should be considered only as qualitative illustrations of acoustical effects which occurred in vowel nasalization by one speaker.

Fairbanks and House (1953) have studied the effects of consonants upon the associated or secondary acoustical characteristics of vowels. They observed the effects of consonant environment upon the fundamental frequency, the duration, and the intensity of vowels. The data were obtained for a set of systematically constructed syllables. Six vowels and twelve consonants of General American speech were employed; the consonants included the plosives, nasals, and fricatives which normally occur in both initial and final positions. A set of 72 syllables was constructed with these sounds. In

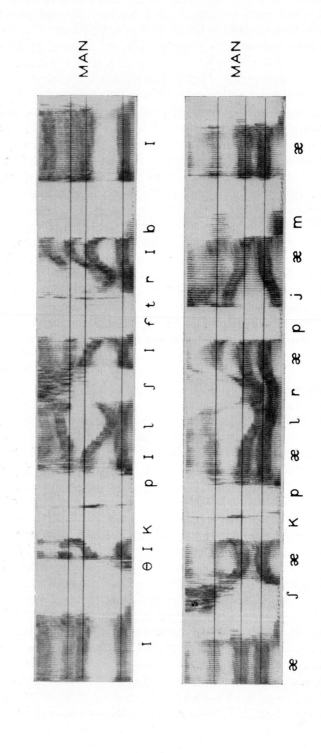

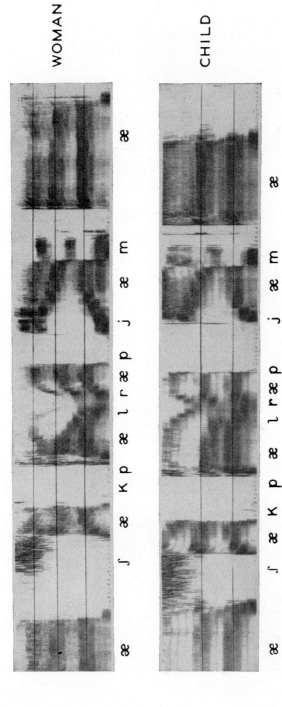

FIG. 45. Wide-band, 3500-cps spectrograms of syllable sequences by a man, a woman, and a child. The lines connect formants of corresponding vowels which immediately preceded and followed each syllable sequence (Peterson).

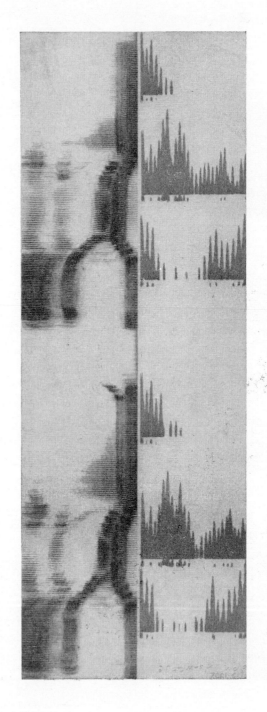

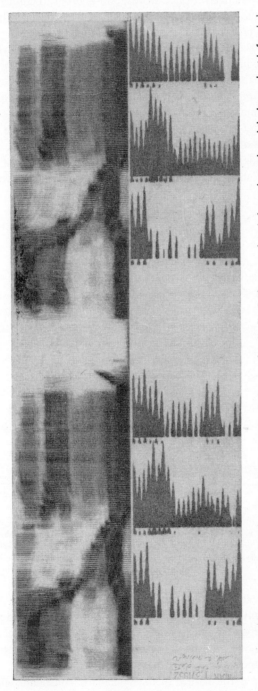

FIG. 46. Broad-band spectrograms and amplitude sections of the vowel series [iau]. The upper chart is for oral vowels and the lower chart is for similar nasal vowels.

each syllable the vowel was preceded and followed by the same consonant. Some of these combinations formed words, and in order to eliminate semantic influences, each syllable was preceded with unstressed [hə]. The syllables were recorded by a group of 10 General American speakers.

Vocal durations were measured from sound spectrograms. Measurements of fundamental frequency were derived from oscillograms of the syllables. The total length of the vowel was divided by the total number of cycles, and the film speed was then divided by this value to obtain the mean voice period. Relative intensity measurements were obtained from a high-speed-level recorder. It was found practical to base the measurements on the maximum level marked by the recorder within each syllable.

The results of this study are shown in Fig. 47. In the graph at the left of the figure, the variables are plotted according to the various vowels. The

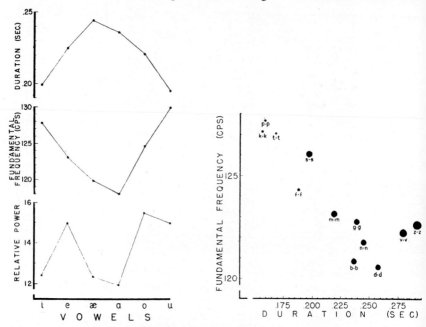

FIG. 47. Mean duration, fundamental frequency, and relative power of vowels as influenced by consonant environment. In the left chart consonant environments have been combined to show the effects according to vowels. In the right chart the data for the various vowels have been combined to show the effects according to the various consonants employed in the study (House and Fairbanks).

points represent mean values for each of the six vowels when the data for all twelve consonant environments are combined. The points in the right-hand graph of Fig. 47 represent means when the data for all six vowels are combined. This chart shows the effects of the various consonants upon duration, fundamental frequency, and relative intensity.

These graphs show the nature of the systematic consonant effects upon vowels which were observed. Although the data were obtained within the phonemic framework of General American speech, there is reason to expect that similar effects may extend to other languages, at least where the language structure does not involve specific contrasts to the above indicated principles.

## Consonants

Various types of acoustical consonant structure are shown in Fig. 45. These include regular striated, vowel-like patterns of voiced energy for sounds such as semivowels, glides, and nasals. The random-like energy normally represents some type of frictional or sibilant formation. Voiced fricatives, of course, involve combinations of voiced and voiceless energy structure. Whenever a silent interruption occurs, as during the closure for a voiceless plosive or a click, a blank space appears on the spectrogram; the burst, explosion or implosion, which follows is usually shown by some sort of vertical line through the spectrum of the visible speech pattern.

It will be noted that the various types of consonants have markedly different types of boundary or transition patterns. It is also immediately obvious that the consonant formations have considerable effect upon the formant frequency movements to and from the vowel positions. These movements have been called *influences,* and are described in detail in *Visible Speech* (Potter, Kopp, and Green, 1947).

The influence effects appear to be most pronounced on the second formant; and in the interpretation of visible speech patterns a major emphasis is placed upon the movements of this formant in frequency. For any given speaker, each of the speech sounds appears to have a potential or characteristic frequency position for the second formant. This characteristic frequency position has been called the *hub* of the sound. Fig. 48, from *Visible Speech,* shows a chart of the hubs for a General American speaker. It is evident in this chart that those sounds which have the greatest variation in physiological formation, according to phonemic environment, also have the greatest variation in the frequency position of the second formant.

A study of the effects of the transitional patterns of the second formant upon consonant recognition in English has been made by Cooper and his associates (1952). For this work, a Pattern Playback was employed as a speech synthesizer. The Pattern Playback reproduces a harmonic series of sustained tones which have been recorded optically. The control unit of the instrument is a screen onto which patterns resembling sound spectrograms may be painted. The tones are integral multiples of a fundamental, but are not variable in frequency, so that the speech is reproduced at a constant fundamental voice frequency.

The study concerned the effects of the shape of the second formant upon plosive recognition. The signals were presented without the other elements which normally accompany plosive formations in English. That is, in the case of voiced plosives there was no preceding low frequency resonance or voice bar and no spike or burst; in the case of the voiceless plosives there

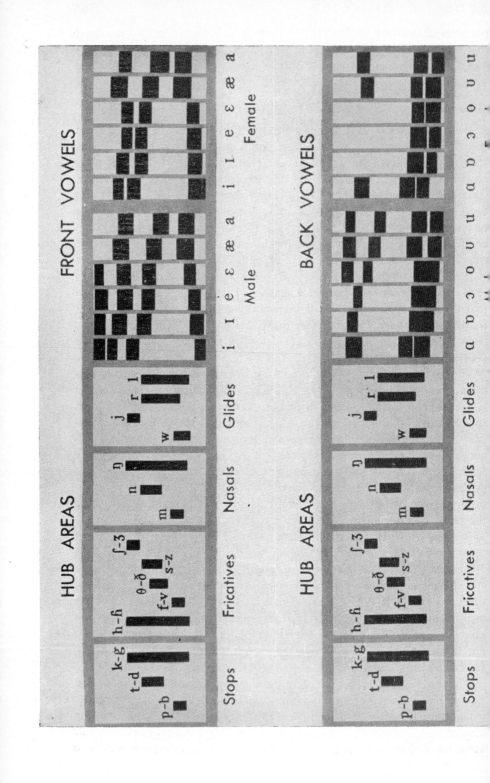

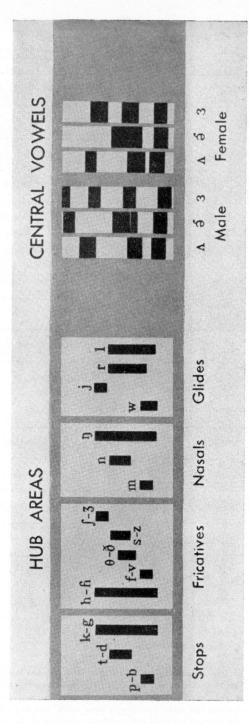

FIG. 48. Summary charts of spectrographic analyses of speech for a man and a woman. The hub areas show the frequency regions in which the second formant appears for the consonants indicated when preceding the various vowels (Potʻer, Kopp, and Green).

# FIRST FORMANT SHAPE

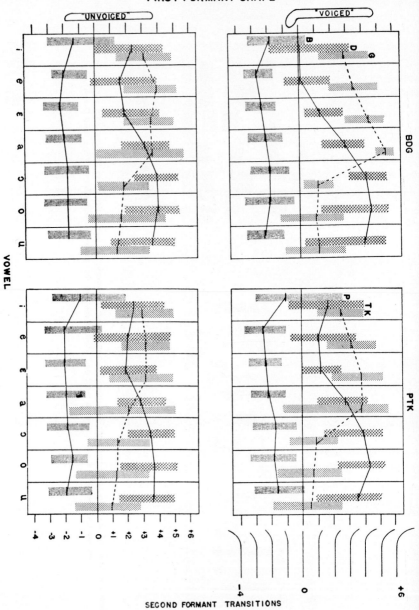

FIG. 49. The identification of stop consonants according to second formant influence. In the charts at the left, a group of 33 subjects were asked to limit their responses to the voiced plosives; in the charts at the right, a similar group of subjects were instructed to limit their responses to the voiceless plosives. The upper two charts were made with the indicated first formant transition, and the two lower charts were made without a transitional movement on the first formant (Cooper and associates).

was no spike and no transitional aspiration. Also, third and higher formants were not present in the tests.

The first and second formants were located according to the various sustained vowel values. Eleven different conditions of initial second formant transition were employed in the tests. A summary of the results is shown in Fig. 49. Two different shapes for the first formant were employed in the experiment, as indicated at the left in the figure. The various shapes employed for the second formant are shown at the right, and the pattern shapes are designated according to the numbers shown at the right. In the experiments for the two charts at the left, the subjects were asked to select for each test item one of the three voiced plosives of English. For the two charts at the right the subjects were asked to indicate whether each vowel appeared to be preceded by [p], [t], or [k]. The lines have been drawn through the median judgments; the ends of the areas indicate the quartile values.

Quantitative data on the acoustical characteristics of consonants in actual speech are limited. There is an increasing interest in this subject, however. As ever, there is need for care in experimental design, so that the measurements may provide more exact data and also increased insight into the structure of oral language.

## BIBLIOGRAPHY

### Part I

This is a collection of books and papers dealing with selected subjects as follows:

*General Acoustics*

BERANEK, L. L. 1954. Acoustics. New York: McGraw-Hill.

MORSE, P. M. 1948. Vibration and sound (2nd ed.). New York: McGraw-Hill.

OLSON, H. F. 1947. Elements of acoustical engineering (2nd ed.). New York: Van Nostrand.

———— and MASSA, F. 1949. Applied acoustics (2nd ed.). Philadelphia: Blakiston.

RAYLEIGH, LORD. 1894. Theory of sound (2nd ed.). London: Macmillan.

RICHARDSON, E. G., ed. 1953. Technical aspects of sound. Vol. 1. Amsterdam: Elsevier Publishing Co.

*Acoustic Measurements*

BERANEK, L. L. 1949. Acoustic measurements. New York: Wiley.

*Sound Spectrograph*

KOENIG, W., DUNN, H. K., and LACY, L. Y. 1946. The sound spectrograph. *J. acoust. Soc. Amer.*, 18, 19.

POTTER, R. K., KOPP, G. A., and GREEN, H. C. 1943. Visible speech. New York: Van Nostrand.

RIESZ, R. R., and SCHOTT, L. 1946. Visible speech cathode-ray translator. *J. acoust. Soc. Amer.*, 18, 50.

*Electrical Circuits and Measurements*

LANGFORD-SMITH, F., ed. 1952. Radiotron Designers Handbook (4th ed.). Sydney, Australia: Wireless Press. (Reproduced and distributed by R. C. A., Harrison, N.J.)

Research Council of the Academy of Motion Picture Arts and Sciences, Motion Picture Sound Engineering. 1938. New York: Van Nostrand.

TERMAN, F. E. 1943. Radio Engineers' Handbook (1st ed.). New York: McGraw-Hill.


PART II

BENSON, R. W., and HIRSCH, I. J. 1953. Some variables in audio spectrometry. *J. acoust. Soc. Amer.,* 25, 499–505.

BOGERT, B. P. 1953. On the band width of vowel formants. *J. acoust. Soc. Amer.,* 25, 791–792.

CARHART, R. T. 1938. Infra-glottal resonance and a cushion-pipe. *Speech Monogr.,* 5, 65–96.

COOPER, F. S., DELATTRE, P. C., LIBERMAN, A. M., BORST, J. M., and GERSTMAN, L. J. 1952. Some experiments on the perception of synthetic speech sounds. *J. acoust. Soc. Amer.,* 24, 597–606.

DUNN, H. K. 1950. The calculation of vowel resonances, and an electrical vocal tract. *J. acoust. Soc. Amer.,* 22, 740–753.

———— and FARNSWORTH, D. W. 1939. Exploration of pressure field around the human head during speech. *J. acoust. Soc. Amer.,* 10, 184–199.

DUNN, H. K., and WHITE, S. D. 1940. Statistical measurements on conversational speech. *J. acoust. Soc. Amer.,* 11, 278–288.

EGAN, J. M. 1948. Articulation testing methods. *Laryngoscope,* 58, 955–991.

FAIRBANKS, G. 1954. A theory of the speech mechanism as a servosystem. *J. Speech Hearing Disorders,* 19, 133–139.

FARNSWORTH, D. W. 1940. High-speed motion pictures of the human vocal cords. *Bell Laboratories Record,* 18, 203–208.

FLETCHER, H. 1929. Speech and hearing. New York: Van Nostrand.

———— and STEINBERG, J. C. 1929. Articulation testing methods. *Bell System Technical J.,* 8, 806–854.

FRENCH, N. R., and STEINBERG, J. C. 1947. Factors governing the intelligibility of speech sounds. *J. acoust. Soc. Amer.,* 19, 90–119.

GRAY, G. W. 1936. Studies in experimental phonetics. Baton Rouge: Louisiana State Univ. Press.

HELMHOLTZ, H. L. F. 1895. On the sensations of tone (3rd ed.). *Translated* by A. J. Ellis. New York: Longmans, Green.

HOUSE, A. S., and FAIRBANKS, G. 1953. The influence of consonant environment upon the secondary acoustical characteristics of vowels. *J. acoust. Soc. Amer.,* 25, 105–113.

JOOS, M. 1948. Acoustic Phonetics. *Monogr. Suppl. to Language,* Vol. 24.

KOENIG, W. 1949. A new frequency scale for acoustic measurements. *Bell Laboratories Record,* 27, 299–301.

LLOYD, R. J. 1890. Vowel-Sound. London: Turner and Dunnett.

MILLER, D. C. 1926. The science of musical sounds. New York: Macmillan.

OLSON, H. F. 1947. Elements of acoustical engineering (2nd ed.). New York: Van Nostrand.

PAGET, R. 1930. Human speech. New York: Harcourt, Brace.

PETERSON, G. E. 1954. Acoustical vowel relationships. *Georgetown Monogr. Series on Languages and Linguistics,* 7, 62–73.

———— 1951*a.* The phonetic value of vowels. *Language,* 27, 541–553.

———— 1951*b.* Vocal gestures. *Bell Laboratories Record,* 29, 500–503.

———— 1952. The information-bearing elements of speech. *J. acoust. Soc. Amer.,* 24, 629–637.

————— and BARNEY, H. L. 1952. Control methods used in a study of the vowels. *J. acoust. Soc. Amer.*, 24, 175–184.

POTTER, R. K., KOPP, G., and GREEN, H. 1947. Visible speech. New York: Van Nostrand.

POTTER, R. K., and PETERSON, G. E. 1948. The representation of vowels and their movements. *J. acoust. Soc. Amer.*, 20, 528–535.

RUDMOSE, H. W., CLARK, K. C., CARLSON, F. D., EISENSTEIN, J. C., and WALKER, R. A. 1948. Voice measurements with an audio spectrometer. *J. acoust. Soc. Amer.*, 20, 503–512.

SCHOTT, L. O. 1950. An electrical vocal system. *Bell Laboratories Record*, 28, 549–555.

SHANNON, C. E. 1948. A mathematical theory of communication. *Bell System Technical J.*, 27, 379–423, 623–656.

STETSON, R. H. 1951. Motor phonetics. Amsterdam: North-Holland Pub. Co.

STEVENS, K. N. 1952. Frequency discrimination for damped waves. *J. acoust. Soc. Amer.*, 24, 76–79.

—————, KASOWSKI, S., and FANT, C. G. M. 1953. An electrical analog of the vocal tract. *J. acoust. Soc. Amer.*, 25, 734–742.

STEVENS, S. S., and VOLKMANN, J. 1940. The relation of pitch to frequency: A revised scale. *Amer. J. Psychol.*, 53, 329–353.

STUMPF, C. 1926. Die Sprachlaute. Berlin: J. Springer.

WEGEL, R. L. 1930. Theory of vibration of the larynx. *Bell System Technical J.* 9, 207–227.

# CHAPTER 6

# INSTRUMENTS OF DIAGNOSIS, THERAPY, AND RESEARCH

● M. D. Steer, Ph.D., and T. D. Hanley, Ph.D.

FEW SCIENTIFIC INSTALLATIONS are as difficult to generalize about as the speech laboratory. They vary in size and the modernity of their construction, in the quantity and quality of their instruments, and in the number and training of the personnel who run them. One university speech laboratory boasts a multithousand dollar anechoic chamber; another, a custom tape recorder-reproducer. A hospital speech laboratory has the latest thing in versatile audiometric equipment, while a rehabilitation center shares with another service a remarkably intricate recording device for brain waves. In contrast, many speech departments and clinics have no space at all set aside for a laboratory and virtually no equipment, yet the laboratory approach is strongly present in teaching, research, and clinical practice.

This laboratory approach, the scientific method, an attitude of mind, is perhaps the most important contribution made by the speech laboratory. The sound-treated rooms and expensive instruments merely facilitate the basic aims of the therapist or researcher: to form and test and verify or reject hypotheses. In the speech laboratory, these hypotheses have to do with auditory symbols of communication, with the persons who form them, and the persons who perceive them. The laboratory provides a more or less complete medium for system display of these auditory symbols, producers, and perceivers on dynamic bases for inspection and evaluation or on static bases for recording and measurement.

In the laboratory, or by means of laboratory techniques, clinical diagnoses of speech disorders are made. The simple act of examining an individual's dental structure for proper occlusion is a laboratory method; the tongue depressor is a laboratory tool.

Clinical speech therapy, like diagnosis, may rely heavily on laboratory methods and instruments. The tape recorder is an aid in the teaching of sound discrimination by auditory means, while the cathode ray oscilloscope may fill the same function as a visual aid in the course of therapy.

Most at home in the laboratory setting, no doubt, is the voice scientist or experimental phonetician, the person who conducts research in speech. By means of his observations and measurements, he attempts to derive generalizations or laws about superior, normal, and aberrant speech. He attempts to find explanations for phenomena of normal and deviate sound production and reception. One of his basic aims is to provide the therapist with all the information possible about the anatomy and physiology of the vocal mechanism and the acoustics of sound production and transmission.

The purpose of this chapter is to acquaint the reader with some common and special instruments and methods employed in the speech laboratory. No single laboratory now in existence serves as a model for the chapter. Rather, information has been assembled from many sources and a composite laboratory is described. Of necessity, selection and exclusion have taken place. Some important tools and methods are dealt with cursorily or omitted entirely. Since it is not possible to describe in detail all of the adjuncts of the laboratory, selection has been on the bases of most common use, most significant, and most general interest.

## DISC- AND TAPE-RECORDING

A basic tool in the speech laboratory, and among the most common of the instruments to be found there, is some device for the recording and reproduction of speech and other sounds. Two major types of recording device, acetate disc and paper- or plastic-tape recorders, are in most general use. Both types are to be found in a wide range of cost and quality. Each has some advantages and disadvantages not shared by the other. The basic function of both, however, is the same: the retention, or storage, of auditory events for future subjective evaluation or objective measurement.

**Disc-recording.** In his excellent brief history of the disc recorder, Windesheim (1938) gives credit for its invention to Thomas Edison in 1877. From its crude beginnings as a sound-powered engraver of tin foil, many improvements have been made. The names of Bell and Tainter, Berliner, and Masfield and Harrison are associated, respectively, with the substitution of stylus-cutting for stylus indentation, the substitution of the lateral for the vertical cut, and the introduction of microphone, amplifier, and electrically activated cutting stylus.

Today, phonograph disc-recording is obtained by converting sound to electricity and back to sound again. This is accomplished by transforming mechanical energy into electrical energy (microphone), then using an amplifier to enlarge the small electrical variations from the microphone and a device for transforming electrical energy back into mechanical vibrations (recording head). Typical types of microphones are indicated in Fig. 1. The mechanical action of the recording head and stylus results in an engraving process applied to a rotating disc. Reproduction is accomplished by converting the sound wave patterns on the acetate disc into mechanical vibrations (pick-up needle). The mechanical vibrations are converted into electrical impulses (pick-up head), magnified into useful proportions (amplifier), and then transformed into mechanical vibrations (loudspeaker) as sound. Graphically, the recording processes are represented in Fig. 2 and typical

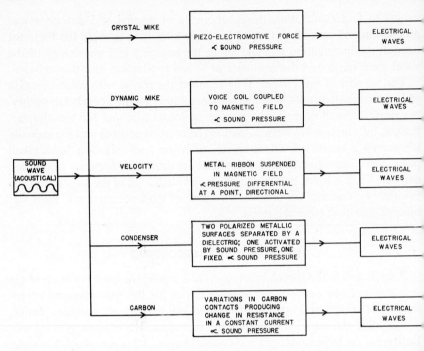

FIG. 1. Functional characteristics of microphones.

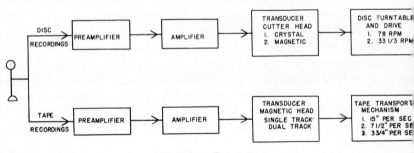

FIG. 2. Recording systems.

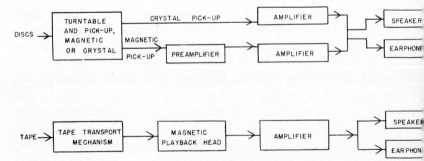

FIG. 3. Reproducer systems.

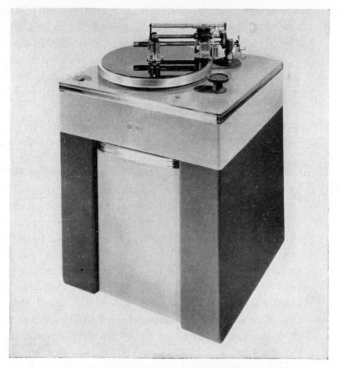

**FIG. 4. Representative disc recorder (Presto 8-D).**

reproducer systems are shown in Fig. 3. A representative high-fidelity recording system is pictured in Fig. 4.

Fidelity of recording and reproduction is a function of the acoustics of the recording studio, the disc employed, and the frequency-response characteristics of the recording and reproducing apparatus. The recording chamber should be free from excessive reverberation and peculiarities of resonance. The room should not be too "dead," or brilliance of tonal quality will be lost. Rooms constructed with no two walls parallel are desirable but infrequently found. Square rooms are usually bad for recording purposes unless acoustic treatment affords compensation. Reverberant rooms, having poor acoustical qualities, can be improved by placing monk's cloth or other sound-absorbing material on three or more walls and ceiling, and a heavy carpet on the floor. Commercial acoustical materials are available and should be used for permanent installations. Frequency-response characteristics of the apparatus are determined by the nature of the component elements of the equipment and the proper matching of the components to each other. A high-quality amplifier will not yield high-fidelity recordings if the microphone and/or the recording head is of poor quality. Likewise, when all the components are of high quality, recordings may still lack fidelity if the elements are mismatched.

In making a laboratory disc-recording, microphone technique is important.

Usually adequate results may be obtained by facing the microphone at a distance of 18 to 24 inches. Speaking into a microphone from a distance of 6 inches or less often increases the bass response of the instrument and causes distortion. Lip and tongue noises and breathing noises are usually objectionable at close operating distances. Greater distances usually result in too weak a voice signal in relation to room noises. A "conversational level" of voice should be adequate in all but unusual circumstances.

Before the actual cutting of the disc, the operator should check the cutting action of the stylus on a practice disc. The chip (portion of the disc removed by the stylus) should be about the diameter of a coarse human hair, and should fall away from the stylus. The groove should be shiny and a little more than twice as wide as the uncut portion between grooves, the land (ratio 70/30). Adjustments for depth of groove can be made on the tension of the spring supporting the cutting head during this checking operation.

Another preliminary checking operation which should be performed is a testing of the electrical components: responsiveness of the instrument to microphone-channel gain controls and of the stylus to an input signal. The former is observed by inspection of the VU meter (or other volume indicator) when the gain control is manipulated with a constant signal entering the microphone. The presence of stylus action is verified by a finger touch on the stylus when a signal is transmitted to it; the stylus should be felt to vibrate.

The uses to which the disc recorder may be put are many and varied. The discs provide, for the clinician, excellent evidence of the results of therapy. For the client they provide both opportunity for learning sound discrimination and a strong motivating influence for improvement (Henrikson and Irwin, 1949; Williamson, 1935). The researcher finds the disc a most convenient means of preserving, presenting, and re-presenting auditory stimuli to the subjects of his investigations (Henrikson, 1943) or to analyzing instruments. Many other uses of disc recorders undoubtedly will suggest themselves to the reader.

**Tape-recording.** A more recent development than the disc recorder, the magnetic tape (or wire) recorder probably dates back to the Telegraphone of Poulsen of Denmark, developed in 1898. Even earlier, Marconi is reported to have experimented with this type of recording in his investigations of electromagnetic radiation. The evolution of the primitive wire recorder was slow until World War II, when the demands of the military brought about rapid advances in mechanical and electronic perfection of this type of recording instrument (LeBel, 1951).

The principle of magnetic recording is simple: it depends on inducing a magnetic pattern in a semipermanent magnet (wire or tape treated with a metal oxide) (Shaney, 1947). For reproduction, the magnet (wire or tape), with its varying degrees of magnetic-field strength, is moved through a coil. This motion results in a series of electrical impulses which, when amplified, may be converted into sound by a loudspeaker.

A block diagram of the magnetic recorder would appear similar to that

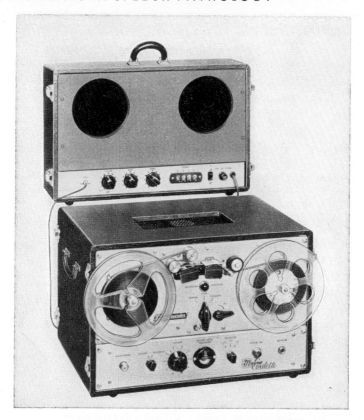

FIG. 5. Portable tape recorder (Magnecorder PT6-GAHP).

for a disc recorder (Fig. 2) with the principal exceptions that wire or tape replaces disc, stationary coil of wire and magnet replace stylus, and an "erase" coil is added immediately preceding the "record" coil. The microphone, amplifier, and speaker are similar or identical to those used for disc-recording. Most commonly the material on which the recording is made is paper or plastic tape, impregnated with a ferrous ink. Typical high-fidelity portable and laboratory tape recorders are illustrated in Figs. 5 and 6.

The uses and techniques of tape-recording are much the same as those of disc-recording. Advantages include greater simplicity of operation, greater facility in word- or sound-spotting, higher fidelity, and greater versatility (Sherman, 1954). Among the comparative disadvantages are bulkiness in the storage of tapes and the possibility of the accidental erasure.

## PERIPHERAL SPEECH MECHANISM: INSTRUMENTATION

Within the restrictions of ethical practice (American Speech and Hearing Association, 1943), it is standard practice to conduct a thorough examination of the major organs of speech in many types of speech disorder. Such examination is performed not for purposes of medical diagnosis but to reveal

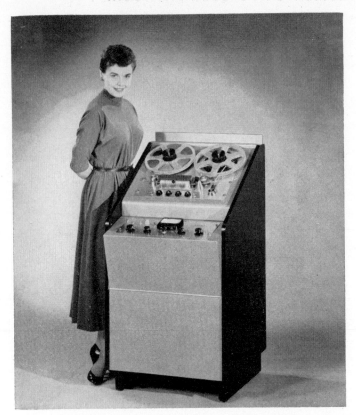

FIG 6. Laboratory tape recorder installation (Ampex 350-C).

the normal or abnormal functioning of such organs as tongue, lips, velum. When abnormalities or apparent pathologies are observed, prompt referral of the client is made to a member of the medical profession.

The routine of the examination is described elsewhere in this book (Ch. 8), and in most standard textbooks of speech pathology (Ainsworth, 1948; Bender and Kleinfeld, 1938; Berry and Eisenson, 1942, 1956; Borden and Busse, 1925; Johnson, *et al.*, 1948; Koepp-Baker, 1936; Van Riper, 1954; West, 1936).

In the following paragraphs will be found only a brief description of some of the instruments most commonly used by the examiner (Fig. 7).

**Tongue blade or tongue depressor.** This is a flat, smooth-surfaced wooden blade, 6 inches long, rounded at both ends. As its name implies, the tongue depressor is used to depress the client's tongue in his mouth, to afford a better view of the oral structures. It may also be used to stimulate such structures as the posterior pharyngeal wall, so that the examiner may observe muscular activity. Once used, the tongue blade is discarded.

**Dental and guttural mirrors.** These are small, round, undistorted mirrors, ranging in diameter from approximately ½ inch to 1 1/16 inches. The mirrors

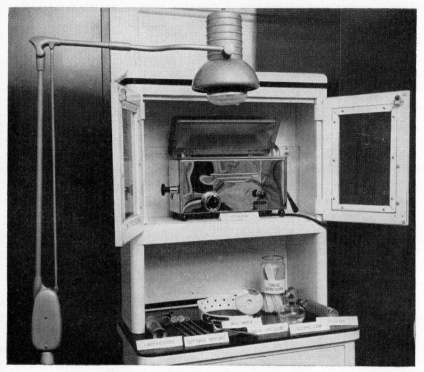

FIG. 7. Instruments for physical examination.

are attached at an angle of 45° to nickel-plated handles, 8 inches long. The mirrors are used to reflect to the examiner's view structures not directly observable, such as the glottis or naso-pharynx. Usually a strong light source is employed with such mirrors to illuminate the structures under study. Before and after use, the mirrors are sterilized. During use, the mirrors are heated to body temperature to prevent fogging.

**Laryngoscope.** This is a combination laryngeal mirror and light source, with wheat grain bulb affixed to the mirror handle for more efficient direction of the light. The use is the same as described above for laryngeal (guttural) mirrors. The laryngoscope is sterilized before and after use.

**Nasal speculum.** This is a device consisting of a pair of smooth, rounded, convex metal wedges, attached to pincers-like gripping handles. In the closed position, the wedges may easily be inserted in one of the anterior nares (nostrils) of the client. Slight pressure on the handles forces the wedges gently apart, widening the nostril for inspection. Used in conjunction with a strong light source, the speculum affords a better view of the anterior nasal passages.

**Stethoscope.** This standard medical instrument consists of a flat, round diaphragm of hard rubber or plastic mounted in a slightly larger hollow metal head. Rubber tubes lead from the head to ear pieces, spring-mounted so that they may be inserted in the examiner's external auditory canals and remain there, freeing the examiner's hands for placement of the diaphragm. The instrument is used for auditory examination of surface vibrations from the speech mechanism (West, 1936).

**Otoscope.** This is a viewing tube with built-in light source for examining the external auditory canal and tympanic membrane. Plastic tubes of varying sizes are supplied with the otoscope, permitting examination of auditory canals differing widely in diameter. These plastic inserts should be sterilized before and after use.

As previously mentioned, the speech therapist examines ears, nasal passages, lips, tongue, teeth, hard and soft palate, pharynx, and larynx of many of his clients. The purpose, of course, is to detect any abnormality possibly related to manifested speech disorder. The speech researcher also has occasional recourse to the instruments just described. Usually, as in a series of studies directed by Fairbanks (Fairbanks and Spriestersbach, 1950; Fairbanks and Green, 1950; Fairbanks and Bebout, 1950; Fairbanks and Lintner, 1951), the purpose is to detect the presence of structural abnormalities in the subjects under investigation. The limited discussion of the instruments used in examining the peripheral speech mechanism does not imply limited usefulness of these instruments. Although they are simple, uncomplicated tools in the hands of the expert, their skillful management requires extensive practice, which is thoroughly justified by the importance of the examinations for which they are intended.

## EXAMINATION OF OTHER PHYSIOLOGICAL ATTRIBUTES

It is recognized that more structures than the vocal folds, resonators, tongue, teeth, and lips share the overlaid functions which contribute to the formation of speech sounds. In a broad sense, almost every biological function and anatomical entity can be shown to be related, however indirectly, to the act of communication. In a narrower and more restricted sense, however, certain functions are inextricably interrelated with the immediate or long-term capacity of the individual to utter intelligible symbols.

The necessity for respiration to take place, providing a breath stream upon which vibrator, resonators, and articulators may act, is obvious. In turn, it is recognized that the nervous system must energize the respiratory musculature, as well as the muscles of such organs as the larynx and pharynx. Less obviously, it appears that cardiological and serological systems may influence the speech act and be related to certain vocal anomalies. Accordingly some hospital and university speech laboratories are equipped with instruments and techniques for extensive physiological examination. Some of these techniques are described in the following paragraphs.

### Respiration

Physiologists and speech scientists jointly are interested in two principal aspects of respiration: breathing capacity and bodily movements associated with inspiration and expiration. The basic instrumentation and techniques

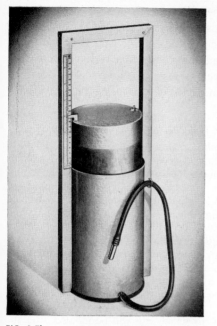

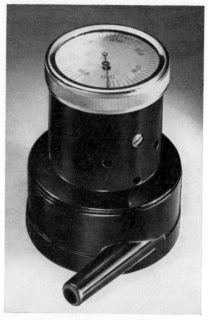

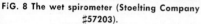

FIG. 8 The wet spirometer (Stoelting Company #57203).

FIG. 9. The dry spirometer (Stoelting Company #57220).

of measurement have grown out of experimental physiology. These scientific techniques are now standard in the modern speech laboratory.

**Spirometer.** A pioneer in the study of breathing capacity was John Hutchison (1852), who in 1846 built an apparatus for measuring the amount of air an individual could exhale after a full inspiration. The general design of the wet spirometer (Fig. 8) has not changed since it was introduced by Hutchison, who described it in these words:

> The Spirometer is merely a vessel or receiver, inverted in another vessel, which contains water, like an inverted wine glass in a tumbler of water; by means of a flexible tube, communication is made with the inverted receiver, and air is blown into it. The receiver then rises, assisted by counterbalance weights; the degree of ascent being according to the volume of air introduced. Such instruments have been known as Pulmometers.

Later modifications of the wet spirometer have been primarily in the method of recording. Smoked-drum kymographs and reflected light-beam recording devices have been designed and used successfully, making possible the determination of the amount of air exhaled per unit of time.

A more recent modification has been the design of a dry spirometer (Fig. 9), a miniature anemometer contained within a bakelite case. The volume of air exhaled, causing the vanes of the device to rotate, is registered by a needle on a calibrated dial. While much less cumbersome and space-consuming than the wet spirometer, the dry model appears to be less reliable and more dependent upon the force with which the breath is exhaled.

From an operational standpoint, the spirometer is one of the simplest of speech laboratory devices. As previously described, the wet spirometer is a type of gasometer which is used for measuring certain aspects of breathing. The device consists of a metal tank containing a movable piston with a water seal, input line for air, exhaust valve for resetting, and scale. Breathing functions concerned in speech and methods of measuring them are indicated below.

*Vital capacity* is the total volume of air which the individual can expel from his lungs after they have been filled to the greatest extent possible. To measure this quantity, the subject inhales as deeply as possible, then expels as much air as possible into the spirometer. The volume measured on the scale is known as *vital capacity*.

*Tidal air* is the quantity of air which is inhaled or exhaled in normal relaxed breathing. This quantity can be approximated by having the subject inhale and exhale normally for a time, then at the peak of an inspiration, the subject exhales "normally" into the spirometer. This quantity shown on the scale is *tidal air*.

*Supplemental air* is the quantity of air which can be expelled from the lungs after the tidal air has been expelled. This quantity can be approximated by having the subject breathe "normally" for a time, then at the trough of an exhalation, the subject expels as much air as possible into the spirometer. This quantity is *supplemental air*.

*Complemental air* is that quantity of air which can still be inhaled after the peak of a normal relaxed inhalation. This quantity should be calculated by subtracting from the vital capacity the total of tidal air and supplemental air combined. This quantity is known as *complemental air*.

The quantity of air used for a specified phrase can be calculated by measuring the speech "set" for the phrase and then measuring the quantity remaining after the phrase has been spoken. The speech set may be defined as the preparedness for utterance in terms of air capacity.

Apparatus for the study of respiratory movements has been developed along two lines: a complete, airtight chamber enclosing the body from abdomen to neck, an application of the "plethysmograph" approach (Wiksell, 1936), and direct measurements taken from devices attached to abdominal and thoracic regions. The latter technique with associated instruments has been employed often in speech investigations. Direct mechanical transmission of movement by means of plates and levers from subject to recorder or indirect transmission involving changes in air pressure in closed tubes (pneumographs) are the two common methods associated with graphing respiratory activity.

**Kymograph and polygraph.** The kymograph, a multipurpose recording unit, is employed to provide objective tracings of respiratory activity. Early kymographs were revolving drums around which recording paper was placed. The instruments received motive power either from spring-driven gearwork, weight-driven mechanisms, or later from electric motor drives. Stylus movement was obtained by mechanical lever action. One end of the stylus was attached to a tambour, a hollow drum-like cylinder with one flexible end composed of a rubber dam. A rigid link glued to the rubber dam con-

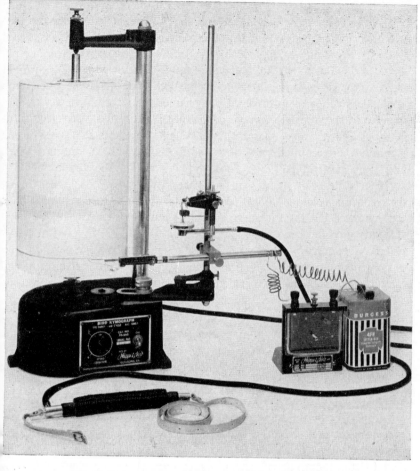

FIG. 10. Modern kymograph with pneumograph (Phipps & Bird).

nected the tambour to the stylus. If air pressure in the tambour was increased, the rubber dam assumed a convex shape and moved the stylus by an amount proportional to the degree of compression. If internal pressure was reduced, the rubber dam assumed a concave shape, and the stylus was moved in the opposite direction by the proper amount. The action was recorded by pointed styli which scratched off the carbon deposit on a smoked paper surface. Other recording media, designed to overcome the limitations of the smoked paper, included plain paper marked by pencil or pen styli, red or blue paper coated with a very thin layer of a white wax-like mixture marked by the scratching of a stylus, and photographic paper on which the movement of a beam of light was recorded (Wendt, 1938). Fig. 10 illustrates a modern kymograph with pneumograph.

Various pneumographs capable of registering the extent, speed, and direction of movement have been used in association with the kymograph in many experiments. Constans (1936) and Sallee (1936) used an instrument which consisted of two tambours attached to a metal plate, adjustable to any part of the chest. This type had many disadvantages, however, and was useful mostly for recording small movements. In another type of pneumograph, employed by Glogau (1916), Gutzmann (1928), and Ray (1932), a rubber bladder was used under a belt encircling the body. The pressure exerted upon the bladder by the expansion of the body caused the recording device to fluctuate. To combat the disadvantage of the tube flattening out, electrical pneumographs which would record all of the inflations and deflations during respiration were reported by Grubbs and Ruckmick (1932), Judson (1932), and Judson and Griffith (1930). These were intended for the measurements of very fine bodily movements and not necessarily gross movements. Many other refinements and modifications of pneumographic instrumentation have been reported, but the foregoing is a representative sampling of the most frequently used devices.

The conventional pneumograph, in use today with kymographs and with the polygraph, consists of a helical spring and rubber tube attached to end plates. Straps or chains from the end plates permit the pneumograph to be held taut around the chest or abdomen. A second, smaller, rubber tube leads from one of the end plates to the recording tambour of the kymograph or bellows of the polygraph, thus completing an airtight system. When the pneumograph is stretched by expansion of the area which it encircles, a partial vacuum is created. This vacuum is communicated by means of the recording tambour to the writing stylus of the kymograph.

In many laboratories the kymograph has been replaced by the polygraph, which operates on the same principle but which has a more efficient pneumatic transmission system, a more convenient recording arrangement, and greater portability. The latest development in the polygraph is optional equipment for the recording of galvanic skin response, pulse rate, and blood pressure. Fig. 11 is a display of a modern, multipurpose polygraph, and Fig 12 is a block diagram of a typical pneumograph-polygraph system.

In later-model polygraphs, a tambour or bellows composes one part of a sealed elastic chamber. This portion of the chamber is connected by means of rubber tubing to the pneumograph. It responds to pressure changes in the sealed system by expanding and contracting, and these movements are transmitted by mechanical linkages to the stylus.

A review of the essential components and operating characteristics of the polygraph will serve to clarify the procedures involved in its use. The principal components of the polygraph are:

1. A motor drive system for moving recording paper at a constant speed
2. Styli for simultaneous recording of each activity to be measured
3. Tambours (or bellows) for each stylus
4. Pneumograph to be connected to each tambour (or bellows) by pneumatic coupling

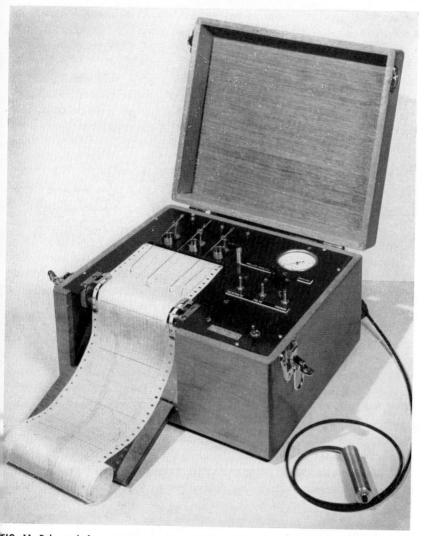

FIG. 11. Polygraph for measurement of respiration, pulse, and tremor rates (Lafayette Instrument Company).

The motor drive system of the polygraph involves a constant-speed motor, coupled to positive-drive wheels which move the recording paper. The constant-speed characteristic of paper travel affords the measurement of the periodicity of breathing activities without inclusion of a separate time line. As the paper moves past the styli, each stylus is activated laterally to make displacement records on either side of a normal line. The displacement from normal is roughly proportional to the magnitude of the activity, and the time involved can be calculated by referring to the constant linear speed of the paper, or by counting the deflections of a time-line stylus.

In use, the pneumographs (thoracic and abdominal) are strapped on the subject while the instrument warms up; then the drive motor is turned on. Records of vegetative breathing are obtained while the subject sits quietly, and records of breathing for speech are obtained while the subject reads aloud or engages in conversation.

The respiratory trace revealed by the polygraph is analyzed for number and relative extent of thoracic and abdominal inhalations and exhalations. A method for objective analysis of polygraph recording is described by Starbuck and Steer (1951). Inspection for abnormalities of pattern also is a part of the analysis made by investigator or clinician.

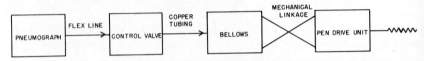

FIG. 12. Pneumograph recording unit with associated polygraph.

In the clinical frame of reference, respiratory apparatus has been found useful both in diagnosis and therapy. Vital capacity may be a related factor in the speech disorder of the cerebral-palsied or post-polio individual, for example, and a test for this and other breathing characteristics should be administered in the diagnostic evaluation. Opposition breathing of thorax and abdomen, revealed by the polygraph trace, sometimes is characteristic of the stutterer (Steer, 1935) and the cerebral-palsied person (Hull and Bryngelson, 1941); hence, the respiratory examination is a normal part of the speech diagnosis for these patients. Both the spirometer and the polygraph have been found useful as motivational devices in therapy and as indicators of the results of therapy. One example of such a therapeutic application is the use of the spirometer in training the cleft-palate patient to direct the breath stream through the oral cavity.

In the research setting, these two instruments have been used in attempts to relate physiological activity and speech proficiency (Wiksell, 1936; Sallee, 1936; Idol, 1936; Barnes, 1926; Lindsley, 1929) and in studies concerned with cerebral palsy and stuttering, such as those of Steer (stuttering) and Hull and Bryngelson (cerebral palsy) mentioned above.

One more instrumental technique is worthy of mention under the heading of respiration. This is the x-ray technique, which may range in complexity from the tracing of organ positions on a fluoroscope screen (Bloomer, 1936) to the recent developments in motion-picture fluoroscopy. The method is not unique to respiratory functions; it has been used in articulation studies, particularly of cleft palate, as well.

### Blood-Pressure Measurements

According to Zoethout and Tuttle (1948), the first blood-pressure measurements were made by Stephen Hales in 1733. In current clinical practice the mercury manometer coupled to a pneumatic arm cuff is employed to measure the amount of blood pressure. This instrument is known as sphygmomanometer. Oscillations correlated to the rhythmical action of the heart are indicated by variations in the level of mercury in the manometer. The blood pressure is increased and a corresponding rise in the mercury column is noted for each *systole* (contraction of the walls of the heart cavity) of the left ventricle. The blood pressure falls and is reflected by a corresponding lowering in the mercury column during the *diastole* (relaxation of the walls of the heart cavity). In the upper arm of adult males, the systolic pressure in the brachial artery is about 120 mm; and the diastolic pressure is about 80 mm. *Pulse pressure* is the difference between these two pressures (40 mm). The *mean pressure* is indicated as the diastolic pressure plus from one-third to one-half of the pulse pressure (Zoethout and Tuttle, 1948).

The usual technique for measuring systolic and diastolic pressure is the ausculatory method of Korotkow. After inflating a pneumatic cuff around the arm, the clinician applies a stethoscope over an artery below the blood-pressure cuff. The pressure in the cuff is raised to the point that circulation is stopped and the stethoscope no longer transmits heart sounds. Gradually the cuff pressure is released and systolic pressure can be obtained from the mercury level of the manometer at the point when the first pulse sounds are again heard in the stethoscope. The diastolic pressure reading is obtained by further releasing the cuff pressure until the pulse sounds are muffled or disappear. The continuous recording of systolic pressure, although often desired for clinical and research purposes, is very difficult to achieve. The common blood-pressure recorder is a compromise which yields *relative blood pressure* only. In this technique, the cuff is inflated above the diastolic pressure level but only to a comfortable point where circulation is not stopped. Although absolute pressures are not indicated, the relative pressure recordings can be correlated with other events (Stevens, 1951). Fig. 13 illustrates a typical relative blood-pressure recorder.

**Electrocardiology**

The electrocardiograph works on the same principle as the galvanometer. Current flow will cause a galvanometer to note the action by appropriate needle or recording indication. If the direction of current flow is reversed through the galvanometer, the indicator will swing in the opposite direction. Thus a galvanometer will reveal the presence of electric current, the direction the current is flowing, and if calibrated, the voltage strength of the current (Zoethout and Tuttle, p. 126, 1948). The activity of the heart is correlated with associated electrical action currents. From specified regions of the body surface, the cardiac action current is detected by suitable electrodes and fed to a continuous recording electrocardiograph. The electrodes are usually placed as follows: lead I, right hand and left hand; lead II, right hand and left foot; lead III, left hand and left foot; lead IV, left leg and chest (Behrendt, 1949). The resulting trace, the electrocardiogram (EKG), shows distinct, identifiable patterns correlating with phases of the heart beat. The electrical deflections appear in regular groups of five waves, each group

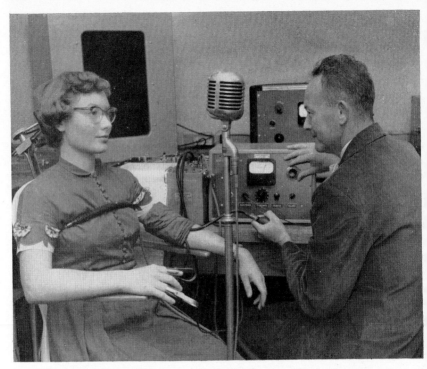

FiG. 13. Typical blood-pressure recording system (Lafayette Instrument Company).

representing one cardiac cycle. The five waves are labeled $P$, $Q$, $R$, $S$, and $T$. Ventricular action produces the $P$ wave and is regarded as the wave of excitation. The electrocardiogram has medical diagnostic value since the various waves may reflect abnormality of cardiac function. Insofar as pathological speech may be related to cardiac disturbance, this laboratory technique may be of importance (Ritzman, 1942; Travis, Tuttle, and Cowan, 1936; Palmer, 1937).

### Galvanic Skin Response

The galvanic skin response (GSR), often referred to as the psychogalvanic reflex (PGSR), is an electrodermal response associated with sweating. It is assumed that the response reflects autonomic activity associated with emotional states (Stevens, 1951). In clinical practice, techniques designed to measure the GSR are sometimes employed to explore internal and environmentally oriented factors related to anxiety, apprehension, and depression. In recent years the conditioned galvanic skin response has been used to assist in the determination of auditory thresholds of infants and adults who are difficult subjects when conventional audiometric techniques are employed (Doerfler and McClure, 1954; Meritser and Doerfler, 1954; Girden, 1952; Hardy and Bordley, 1951; Hardy and Pauls, 1952; Stewart, 1954).

The two basic techniques for investigating the galvanic response related to sweating are the Féré method and the Tarchanoff method. Féré developed

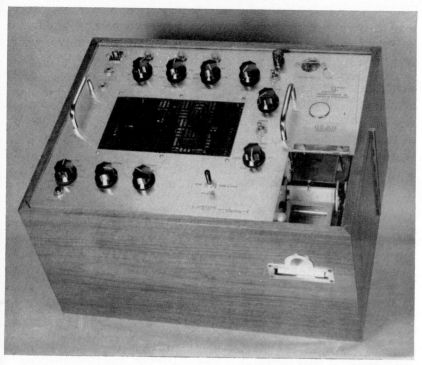

FIG. 14. Typical modern psychogalvanometer (Grason-Stadler Company, Model E664).

the method of measuring skin resistance when an external current is applied; Tarchanoff discovered the skin potential change which arises from currents in the skin. It is believed that the *skin resistance* is a function of the polarization-capacity effect related to sweat secretion and the *skin potential* is associated with smooth-muscle contraction in the sweat glands (Stevens, 1951). Most investigators employ instruments using "resistance" method rather than the "potential" method. Suitable high gain, sensitive d-c amplifiers are not yet available for effective recording of the skin potential.

In recording galvanic response, skin electrodes are usually fastened to the fingers, palm of the hand, or legs and then coupled to a resistance recorder, often known as a psychogalvanometer. When the indicating meter reveals that a steady state balance has been achieved between the skin resistance of the subject and the electronic measuring device, the tracing mechanism is then turned on. The resulting trace is a line showing stabilized activity until the individual is subjected to a stimulating or conditioning experience. Since the GSR is very sensitive to sensory stimuli, factors related to alertness, attention, apprehension, and arousal (Stevens, 1951) result in corresponding changes in skin resistance. The magnitude of psychobiological arousal is related, therefore, to the lowering of skin resistance level and the correlated magnitude of change in the psychogalvanic tracing. Fig. 14 illustrates a modern psychogalvanometer.

## Action Currents and Brain Waves

Of primary usefulness to scientists within or associated with the medical profession, instruments which record electrical discharges from the brain or from specific muscles and muscle groups have been used successfully and importantly by speech scientists. Detailed descriptions of electroencephalographic (brain wave) and electromyograph (action potential) recorders and techniques are available in numerous publications (Garceau and Davis, 1935; Jasper and Andrews, 1936; Davis, R. C., 1948; Davis, J. F., 1952). Only a brief general review of the technique is appropriate here.

Electrical discharges from the brain or from specific muscles are picked up by means of surface electrodes or needle electrodes. After suitable amplification, the form, amplitude, and frequency of these electrical impulses may be graphed on an ink-writing oscillographic recorder, or they may be revealed on the screen of a cathode ray oscillograph and photographed.

As research tools, both electroencephalography and electromyography have been used by investigators interested in the syndrome of stuttering. Freestone (1942), for example, studied the brain waves from adult normal speakers and stutterers, comparing functional conditions of silence, fluent speech, and stuttering. He found that the stutterers had larger waves than normals, and that during moments of stuttering, the waves were larger than during silence and free speech. Travis and Knott (1937) found stutterers during silence to have dissimilar potentials from the two hemispheres, and during speech efforts less dissimilar bilateral brain potential patterns. Using the electromyographic technique, Travis (1934) reported the existence of dissociation of homologous muscle functioning in stuttering. More recently, Williams (1952) used electromyography to study masseter-muscle action potentials of stutterers and nonstutterers, finding slight differences between the two groups.

## PARAMETERS OF SOUND: INSTRUMENTATION

Meaningful auditory symbols achieve their communicative quality by virtue of their unique acoustic characteristics. Were it not for the fact that the speech sound attributes—frequency, intensity, wave form, and time—are manipulatable and under neurological and physiological control by the individual, oral communication would be very different. Conceivably, if man were a unisound producing agent, speech would consist of a conventionalized sequence of bursts of sound, not unlike telegraphy. Fortunately, man developed the capacity to produce an almost infinite number of acoustic symbols, and over many thousands of years a large number of these various combinations have come to achieve meaning.

One of the most challenging tasks confronting the speech scientist is the analysis of the acoustic phenomena of oral communication. Instruments have been developed to make possible measurement and scaling of the sound attributes which contribute to the intelligibility, flexibility, and virtuosity of vocal expression. In the following paragraphs the more important of these laboratory devices, and the uses to which they are put, are described.

## Frequency (Pitch) Measurement

Within the past one hundred years a remarkable series of instruments has been developed by scientists interested in the investigation of the fundamental frequency characteristic of vocal and auditory signals. Fundamental frequency is significant, of course, because it is the component of the complex auditory stimulus which is identified by the listener as the pitch of the sound. The fundamental frequency of the human voice is determined by and is, in fact, identical with the rate of vibration of the vocal cords, measured and reported in cycles per second.

Two aspects of frequency have contributed to the difficulties encountered in devising instruments for its measurement. First, voice frequency and the frequencies of other stimuli within the auditory range are, compared with many other physiological phenomena (respiration, pulse rate), quite high. Hence a fast-acting instrument is required to follow the signal. Second, the fundamental frequency in most acoustic signals is but one component in a complex wave. Therefore, the instrument must be capable of responding only to the fundamental, or of making a response in which the fundamental is clearly to be distinguished from the other components in the sound.

As mentioned earlier, many ingenious devices, dating back to the mid-nineteenth century, have been designed and constructed for frequency measurement. Detailed descriptions of all of these, while of historical interest, would not contribute very much to an understanding of the instruments and techniques in use today. Accordingly, brief mention of the major developments in this field of instrumentation will be made in the following paragraphs.

The earliest method of frequency analysis was achieved by comparison of the unknown frequency with a known frequency. The number of beats (rising and falling pulsations of sound) between the known and unknown frequencies was counted with a known time interval, and thus the frequency of the tone in question was determined by adding or subtracting beats per second to the known frequency.

**Phonautograph.** The phonautograph was an early method utilizing the forced vibrations of a diaphragm, mechanically transmitted to recording paper, as a means of measuring frequency. The instrument was developed by Scott and Koenig in 1859 (in Miller, 1916).

**Manometric flame.** Another development of Koenig was the use of the manometric flame in measuring frequency. First described in 1862 (Miller, 1916), the device consisted of a small acetylene gas flame, the height of which varied in response to pressure variations induced by successive sound waves. Major refinements of the technique utilized with the Koenig manometric-flame capsule resulted in the *Phono-Projectoscope* (Miller, 1937) and

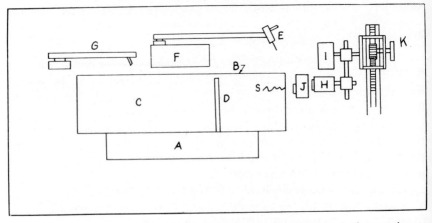

FIG. 15. Schematic drawing of the vibrograph. A, Saga dual speed motor; B, phonograph turntable; C, film drum; D, clamp to fasten film; E, phonograph recording head; F, mechanism to drive recording arm; G, phonograph pick-up; H, phoneloscope optical system; I, light housing; J, lens; K, screw for lowering and elevating optical system; S, sound wave as photographed.

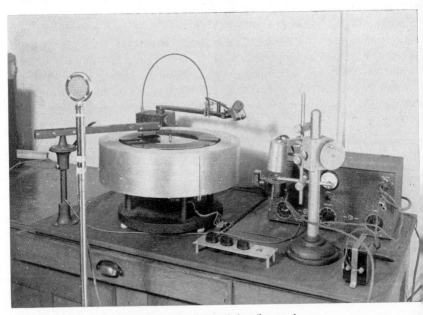

FIG. 16. Illustration of the vibrograph.

*Tonoscope* (Metfessel, 1926) of Seashore. Metfessel (1928) was successful in applying photography to an instrument which evolved from the tonoscope. He used the glow from a neon lamp, flashing with each major fluctuation in the sound wave, as the visual representation of frequency. Metfessel photographed these flashes of light as they were seen through a stroboscopic disc, containing 66 concentric rows of holes spaced at precise distances calculated to correspond to specific frequencies of illumination. With speed of disc rotation, number of holes per row, and speed of film movement as known variables, calculation of frequency became possible.

**Tonometer.** The early tonometer of Scheibler (1834) consisted of a series of tuning forks spread over an exact octave and ascending by equal increments of frequency from the lowest to highest. Any source of sound within the range of the tonometer could be determined by counting the beats with the two forks nearest to it in pitch. In the later Koenig tonometer, there were 154 forks ranging from 16 cps to 21,845 cps. These forks were provided with adjustable resonators and with sliding weights so that the frequencies could be varied within certain limits.

**The vibrograph and its forerunners.** The *Oscillograph* of Blondell and Dubbell, described by them in 1893 (Miller, 1916), the *Sprachseiche* of Scripture (1906), the *Phonodeik* of Miller (1909), and the *Photophono-phonelescope,* originated by Metfessel (1926) and modified by Simon (1926), by Lewis and Tiffin (1933), and by Cowan (1936), all contributed to the final design of the *Vibrograph,* described by Tiffin and Steer (1939).

The vibrograph or its immediate forerunner, the photophonophonele-scope, is today found in many speech laboratories. As revealed in the schematic drawing, Fig. 15, and illustrated in Fig. 16, the apparatus consists of a combination motor-driven phonograph turntable-film drum, phonograph recording and pick-up heads, amplifier, and a phonelescope optical system on a worm gear for controlled elevation and depression.

Standard procedures for making and analyzing phonelegrams, so that pitch measurement is achieved, are described by Tiffin and Steer (1939) as follows:

The function of the wide drum is to hold the film in making photographs of sound waves. With the room darkened, a piece of film, preferably Kodak Lina-graph No. 1127, four-inch recording paper, is wrapped around the drum and held in position by means of a spring clamp. A Dorsey phonelescope serving as an optical lever is mounted on a carriage and may be elevated or lowered by means of a hand crank. The light beam from the phonelescope is focused on the film. The sound wave is picked up from the phonograph record, amplified, and sent into one unit of a standard headset which is fitted and fastened against the diaphragm of the phonelescope. In this manner, . . . the sound waves occurring in one revolution of the phonograph record are recorded on one circumference of the film. As the photograph is made, the phonelescope carriage is slowly lowered so that each succeeding revolution of the record is recorded on a fresh part of the film. Approximately 20 revolutions of the record can be recorded legibly on one circumference of film. . . . A measure of the average wave length over short intervals of time is obtained. . . . The 132 cm film is divided for convenience into 10 equal sections by lines drawn perpendicular to the edge of the recording paper. If the phonograph record is recorded at 78 rpm., the amount of time elapsing in one revolution of the record is given in seconds by the relation

$$\frac{60}{78} = .769 \text{ sec.}$$

This time value, divided by 10, the number of the sections into which the film was divided, yields the amount of time represented by each section of the record:

$$\frac{.769}{10} \text{ sec.} = .077 = \frac{1}{13} \text{ sec. per section.}$$

The periodic recurrence of similar wave forms is measured in cm. The average wave length of the waves in each of the 1/13-sec. intervals is determined. . . .

*Conversion into Frequency.* This may be done by using the formula

$$f = \frac{V}{l}$$

where $f$ equals frequency, $V$ equals velocity, and $l$ equals wave length. The following is obtained by inserting the known values:

$$f = \frac{\dfrac{78}{60} \times \text{film length}}{\text{wave length in cm}}$$

$$= \frac{1.3\,(132\text{ cm})}{\text{wave length in cm}}$$

$$= \frac{171.6\text{ cm}}{\text{wave length in cm}}$$

A typical segment of a phonelegram is illustrated in Fig. 17.

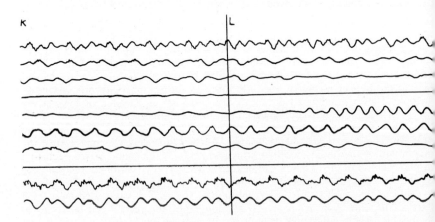

FIG. 17. Segment from vibrograph record (phonelegram).

The projector is adjusted so that the zero-frequency and full-scale reference lines in the projected image coincide with the equivalent reference lines on the ruled grid. This projection results in a 6.16:1 enlargement of the original image. The time scale in the projected image thus becomes 6.16 inches per second for material photographed at 1 inch per second. If fundamental-frequency measurements are taken at intervals of 1/26 second, vertical lines approximately ¼ inch apart on the ruled grid may be used to mark sampling intervals. Fig. 20 is an example of continuous speech photographed in the manner just described.

**Other methods of measuring frequency.** A considerable number of other techniques and devices have been and are being employed in the measurement of fundamental frequency. When the signal to be analyzed is steady state with respect to frequency, unlike continuously variable speech signals, the *Stroboconn* (Fig. 21), a commercial instrument, provides an accurate, instantaneous frequency analysis. A series of 12 scanning windows, each provided with a neon tube and a calibrated stroboscopic disc, is employed by the operator in making frequency analyses. The rate of flash of the neon tube is dependent upon the frequency of the input signal and one ring of the stroboscopic disc appears to stand still if its frequency (number of spokes times revolutions of the disc per second) corresponds to the frequency of the flashing neon bulb. Although there is limited applicability of the Stroboconn to the phenomena most frequently analyzed in speech laboratories, it is, nonetheless, an instrument occasionally found in such laboratories.

The sound spectrograph (Sona-Graph), described in some detail on page 209, is another instrument from which frequency analysis may be made. The resonance bars, or bands of energy, in the sonagram made with a 300-cps filter in the frequency scanning circuit are made up of vertical striations. According to Koenig, Dunn, and Lacy (1946), three of the scientists who worked on the development of the sound spectrograph, "Each vertical striation represents the crest of a beat, and the separation between crests can be seen to vary as the pitch changes." Peterson (1952) has developed a set of equations by means of which frequency analysis of spectrograms may be accomplished.

Last among the fundamental-frequency analysis techniques to be described is one reported by Black (1949), who capitalized upon the magnetic properties of tape-recordings. He found that such tapes, when immersed in iron filings, emerged with striations of filings transversely across the tapes. Each striation represented one cycle of the fundamental frequency. Since tape-speed past the recording head was known, and since number of striations per inch could be counted, calculation of fundamental frequency could be accomplished. For example, if 10 striations were observed in 1 inch of tape originally recorded at 15 inches per second, then the fundamental frequency for that segment was 150 cps (10 cycles per 1/15 sec. = 150 cps).

A great many noteworthy experiments have been performed in investigation of the fundamental-frequency attribute of the human voice. Pronovost

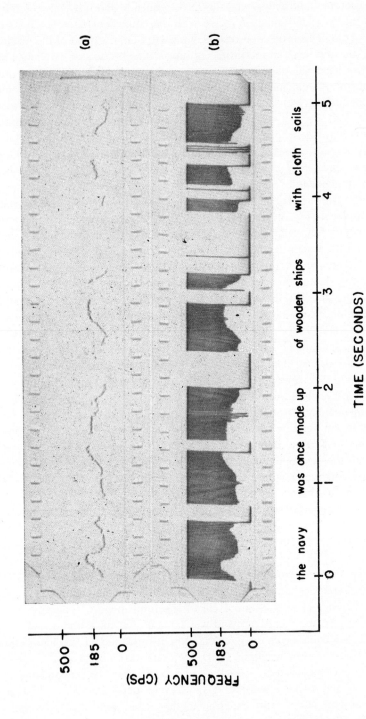

FIG. 20. Sample of continuous speech from the fundamental-frequency recorder (Dempsey).

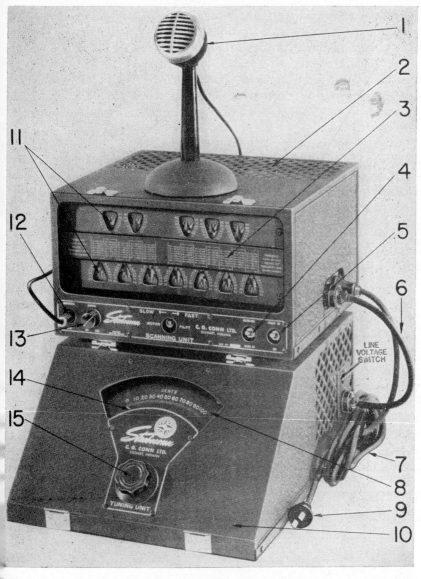

FIG. 21. The Stroboconn. 1, microphone; 2, scanning unit; 3, calibration strip; 4, motor switch; 5, power switch; 6, interconnection cable; 7, AC power cable; 8, tuning unit scale; 9, AC plug; 10, tuning unit; 11, scanning windows; 12, microphone plug; 13, volume control; 14, tuning unit scale pointer; 15, tuning knob.

(1942) and Snidecor (1951), using the phonophonelescope, established pitch norms for superior adult male and female speakers, respectively. Fairbanks and his associates (1949) did the same for children. Fairbanks (1940) also reported the results of a number of doctoral dissertations, completed under his direction, dealing with such aspects of pitch as its relation to simulated emotional status, its contribution to vocal flexibility, and voice breaks in male adolescents. Lewis and Tiffin (1934), employing strobo-photography, investigated relationships between speaking effectiveness and certain pitch measures. Hanley (1951) described pitch characteristics of regional dialects, based on phonelegraphic analysis. Duffey (1954) was able to detect pitch characteristics which appeared to relate to types of cerebral-palsy speech; his analysis was by means of the instantaneous fundamental-frequency recorder.

Although the instruments for frequency measurement until fairly recently have been much more useful to the investigator than the speech therapist, the Purdue Pitch Meter developed by Dempsey is rapidly gaining favor as a clinical instrument. It is a rapid and reliable diagnostic tool, as well as an excellent training device for individuals with faulty pitch levels or restricted pitch ranges. The ability to monitor pitch visually enhances the auditory monitoring conventionally stimulated in voice therapy.

### Measurement of Speech Intensity[1]

According to Fletcher (1953), it was the minuteness of speech power that made measurement of this voice variable very difficult until the discovery of the vacuum tube. Now modern speech laboratories are equipped with cali-brated microphones, vacuum tube amplifiers, and voltmeters. Dunn (1930) and Sivian, Dunn, and White (1931) reported an electrical circuit for meas-uring the average power-frequency distribution of speech sounds. One of the early intensity recorders to be employed by speech scientists was de-scribed by Tiffin (1932). In this technique, a vacuum tube voltmeter was used as a high-speed output-level indicator. A photographic record was ob-tained by means of a Westinghouse supersensitive oscillograph element. The deflections of the oscillograph were photographed on moving film on which decibel lines were automatically traced. A voice was considered variable or

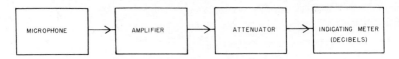

FIG. 22. Sound-level meter components.

[1] Intensity conventionally is listed as one of the four sound and vocal attributes. Under many conditions it is the physical correlative of the sensation of loudness. In the physical sense, the term refers to the work done by a sound wave acting within a specifically defined area. To the acoustician, intensity is a term which must be con-fined to the results of measurements involving definite power units and areas. Broadly speaking, sound power and sound pressure are terms analogous to sound intensity, since the sound wave is evaluated within the same general frame of reference for all. How-ever, different methods and units of measurement are required for each.

Since proportionality exists among all these terms, permitting conversion from one to another, and since intensity is the most frequently used of them (though often incor-rectly), that term will be used consistently within this section. The reader is advised that "sound pressure level," operationally speaking, is the value most often revealed by the instruments in the speech laboratory.

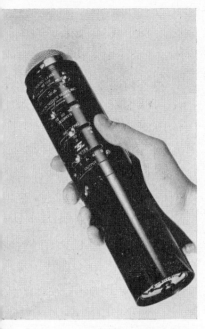

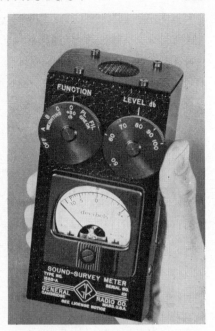

FIG. 23 The H. H. Scott Sound-Level Meter, Type 410-B.

FIG. 24. The General Radio Company Sound-Survey Meter, Type 1555-A.

flexible in intensity to the extent that the maximum excursions of the curves for different syllables spread over a wide range. The average deviation of amplitude values from the mean was used to indicate mean deviation in syllabic power. Typical of published research studies employing this technique were those of Murray and Tiffin (1933), Lewis and Tiffin (1934), and Steer and Tiffin (1934).

In the modern speech and hearing clinic and in most well-equipped speech science laboratories, various instrumental techniques are available for the display of speech intensity. Some of the apparatus are suited for diagnosis and therapy; some are best suited for research. Nearly all of the instruments described below are available commercially.

**VU meter.** The simplest method of inspecting sound levels and variations is afforded by a circuit consisting of a signal (from microphone or a recording) directed to an amplifier with an associated volume level (VU) meter either across the output of the amplifier or bridged within the amplifier. Visual inspection of the meter indicates the relative rather than the absolute intensity. In circuits provided with calibrated reference levels, absolute intensity levels may be noted.

**Sound-level meter.** This instrument, although not originally intended for speech and hearing clinics or speech laboratories, is a valuable diagnostic and therapeutic aid. It also is of importance in the research programs of speech scientists and audiologists. Fig. 22 is a block diagram indicating the basic components of a sound-level meter circuit.

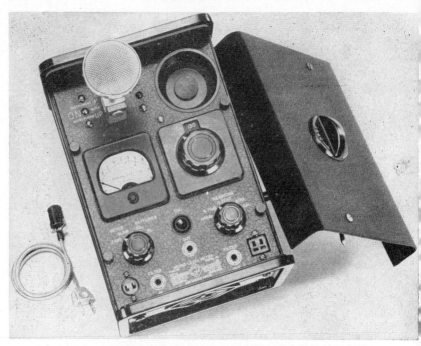

FIG. 25. The General Radio Company Sound-Level Meter, Type 1551-A.

The sound-level meter usually includes a microphone, an amplifier, a calibrated attenuator, an output meter, and frequency-weighting networks for the measurement of noise and sound. The apparent loudness attributed to sounds varies not only with sound pressure but also with the frequency of the sounds. The way it varies with frequency depends on the sound pressure and to some extent provision is made for this phenomenon by the inclusion of the weighting networks (Peterson and Beranek, 1953). Some sound-level meters are designed specifically for portability, as illustrated in Figs. 23 and 24. A popular sound-level meter is the General Radio Company Type 759-B, and its successor, Type 1551-A, which is illustrated in Fig. 25. These instruments are especially useful to the clinician when the maintenance of steady-state vocal intensity levels is an important aspect of the therapeutic

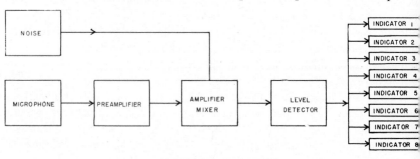

FIG. 26. Speech Intensity Demonstrator diagram.

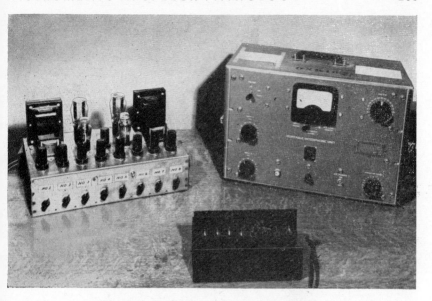

FIG. 27. The Purdue Speech Intensity Demonstrator.

method or when range of speech intensity is required to satisfy a differential diagnosis. To the speech scientist, these instruments provide a means of visual metering of the pressure level of speech stimuli and the sound level in the research environment.

**SID.** This instrument is the Speech Intensity Demonstrator developed at Purdue University (Nordyke, Draegert, and Steer, 1948). The SID consists of an arrangement whereby a signal from microphone or recorded source is fed through appropiate amplifiers to a specially-designed voltage-level selector, capable of detecting eight previously determined voltage levels. The signal from the voltage selector is directed to a bank of eight neon lights. The number of lights activated is a function of the speech signal level converted to voltage. A noise circuit is included to serve as a reference sound level or as a masking signal. A block diagram of the circuit is shown in Fig. 26 and an illustration of the instrument is found in Fig. 27.

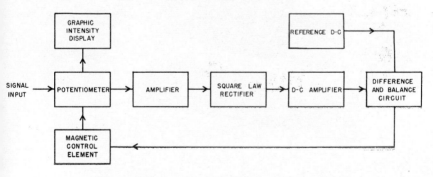

FIG. 28. Block diagram of sound-level recording system.

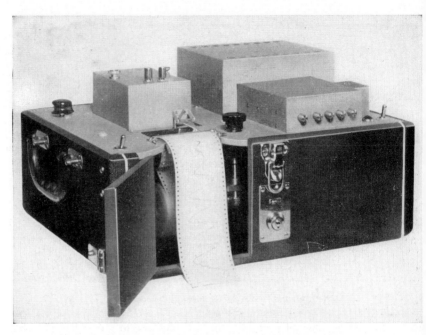

FIG. 29. Illustration of sound-level recorder (Sound Apparatus Company, SL-2).

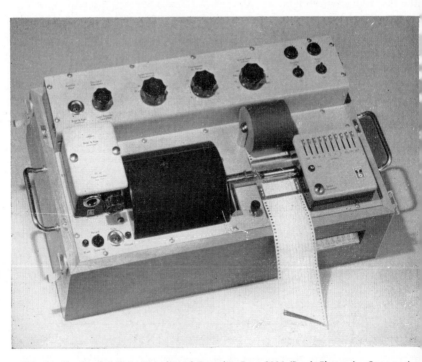

FIG. 30. The Bruel & Kjaer Sound-Level Recorder, Type 2304 (Brush Electronics Company).

The SID represents an effective visual aid when the therapeutic requirement is modification of the speech-intensity variable (Hanley and Steer, 1948).

**Level recorders.** Graphic level recorders are designed to convert sound signal inputs to permanent sound-pressure indications on a time basis. The final record is in the form of tracings plotted on a calibrated decibel scale. Basically, the modern sound-level recorder consists of an electromechanical feedback system in which the signal to be measured is amplified and then coupled to a square-law rectifier, where the intensity of the signal is converted to a d-c signal. The d-c output is balanced against a reference d-c voltage. Differences in these two voltages reflect known amounts of variation in the signal being measured. This is achieved by coupling the difference voltage through a feedback circuit to an electromechanical recording element. Circuits are available to have the indication reflect logarithmic or linear measurements. Fig. 28 is a block diagram of the Sound Apparatus Company Sound Level Recorder (HPL-E) and Fig. 29 illustrates the Model SL-2. Another sound-level recorder often found in speech laboratories is the Bruel and Kjaer level recorder, type 2304, which is distributed in the United States by the Brush Electronics Company. This recorder is illustrated in Fig. 30. Insofar as speech-intensity level is one of the basic voice variables, the sound-level recorder has high priority among instruments required in a well-equipped speech laboratory.

**Amplitude display.** The Amplitude Display Unit is an accessory to the Kay Sona-Graph or Sound Spectrograph. This device is used to provide graphic records in db versus time of the speech sound. When the unit is used as an adjunct to the Sona-Graph, the decibel level of the speech signal is used to control the frequency of a constant-amplitude oscillator. The analyzing section of the Sona-Graph then produces a record of oscillator frequency versus time. This record, thus, indicates graphically the decibel level of the speech signal. A block diagram of this instrument is shown in Fig. 31. The

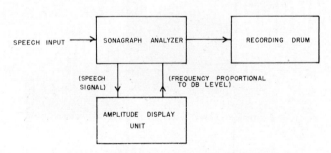

FIG. 31. Block diagram of amplitude display unit.

device appears suited for research purposes and is being installed by those laboratories possessing the Kay Sona-Graph. The value of the equipment has not yet been demonstrated in published research.

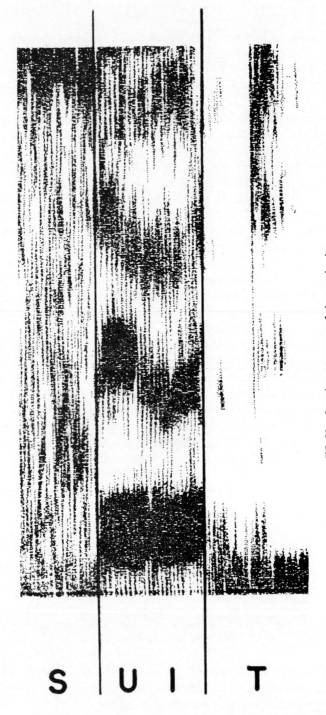

FIG. 32. Sound spectrogram of the word suit.

S U I T

## Voice Quality: Spectrum Analysis

The analysis of voice quality by mechanical and electro-acoustic techniques is accomplished in various ways. The principal task of the investigator is to secure a valid representation of speech signals in terms of frequency composition and relative amplitude of the partials. To the speech scientist, this means the transformation of speech sound waves into representative acoustic spectra. In early studies of vowel spectra, the technique included the preparation of suitable oscillograms of vowel wave forms and the determination of the number and the relative intensity of the partials by means of the Henrici harmonic analyzer (Kelley, 1934; Lewis and Tiffin, 1934; Black, 1937). The development of new electronic analyzers has facilitated the investigation of steady-state and transient sound waves. Benson and Hirsh (1953) have summarized important variables related to modern audio spectrometry.

## Analysis of Wave Composition

**Oscilloscopic inspection.** A cathode ray oscilloscope is used for very simple or very complex electrical measurements; consequently very simple and highly complex oscilloscopes are available. The more numerous the variables to be studied or controlled, the more complex the oscilloscope circuit. Reduced to minimum consideration, an oscilloscope consists of a device to portray voltage or current wave forms on a fluorescent screen. Usually, the vertical dimension is used to portray the wave-form amplitude; the horizontal dimension portrays time. By use of microphone or recorded sound signals, directed to the vertical amplifier, and with an appropriate horizontal time-base, the speech signals can be depicted as visible wave forms.

A sound signal displayed on an oscilloscope appears in the form of simple or complex wave patterns. The greater the amount and amplitude of the harmonics, the more complex the wave form. The relative harmonic complexity thus may be observed by inspection. Objective quantification of harmonic components requires wave analyzers appropriate for the task.

**The Sona-Graph (sound spectrograph).** One of the most versatile instruments to be found in the speech laboratory is the sound spectrograph, developed by Bell Telephone Laboratory engineers and described by them in 1946 (Koenig, Dunn, and Lacy). Its versatility is evidenced by the fact that the spectrograph has been the analytical instrument of choice in research investigations involving frequency, time, and wave composition. An accessory device, the amplitude display unit, also makes possible analyses of sound signals for amplitude values.

The spectrograph, or Sona-Graph, as the commercial instrument is called, is "... a wave analyzer which produces a permanent visual record (spectrogram or sonagram) showing the distribution of energy in both frequency and time" (Koenig, Dunn, and Lacy, 1946). On a conventional sonagram (see Fig. 32 for a small segment cut from a sonagram), time, up to 2.4 seconds, is a

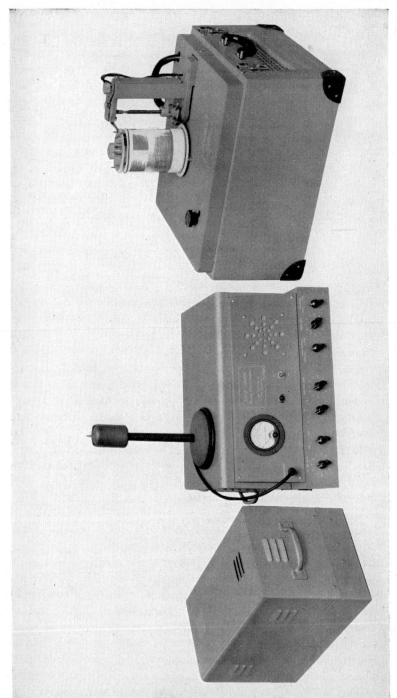

FIG. 33. Illustration of the Sona-Graph (Kay Electric Company).

near value along the horizontal axis; frequency from 85 to 8000 cps is nearly portrayed on the vertical axis. Relative intensity is revealed by the lackness of the sound pattern. Fig. 33 is a picture of the Sona-Graph show-ng power supply, amplifier-analyzer, and recording units.

Speech or other sound signals recorded on magnetic tape within the in-trument are scanned by either a 45-cps or 300-cps band-pass filter, which asses progressively upwards over the 8000-cps range of the Sona-Graph. Vhen energy is detected in the signal, by means of this scanning process, the ecording stylus is caused to fire, and a resulting fine black line appears on he electrostatic recording paper on the drum of the recorder unit.

Since speech sounds are acoustically unique and harmonically individual, ach is revealed in a unique visual pattern on the sonagram and may be Jentified by the trained individual. Analysis of time and frequency charac-eristics of the sounds may be made, as described elsewhere in this chapter. Also, the frequency regions where energy is concentrated may be located. Vhere desired, a "section" or instantaneous harmonic analysis of sound may e made, so that not only the locations of energy regions (formants) may be etermined, but the relative amplitudes of the formants as well. Peterson 1953) has described parameter relationships in the portrayal of signals with ound-spectrograph techniques and Peterson and Raisbeck (1953) have dis-ussed the measurement of noise with the instrument.

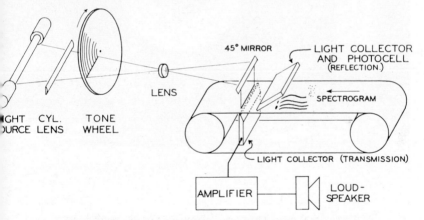

FIG. 34. Block diagram of the Pattern-Playback instrument (Haskins Laboratories).

It may be noted that the approach utilized in the Sona-Graph for analysis f sound waves has been reversed in the synthesis of speech. Liberman, Delattre, Cooper, and Gerstman (1954), among others, have published re-orts describing the preparation of hand-drawn spectrograms which pass hrough visual scanners associated with sound generators. Considerable uccess in sound synthesis has been reported. A block diagram of the Pattern-Playback is shown in Fig. 34. Attempts to produce speech sounds by arti-cial means, of course, are not new. Dudley (1936) described an elaborate lectronic array, assembled to produce speech, and Dudley, Riesz, and

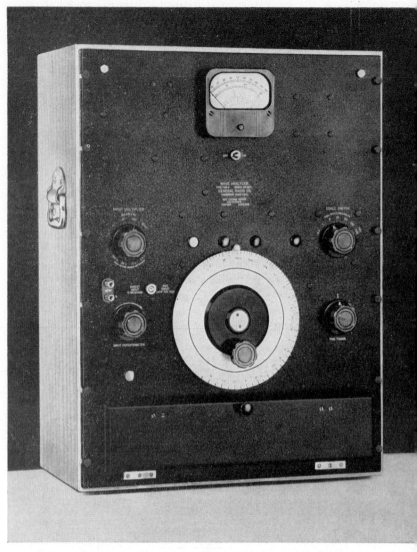

FIG. 35A. General Radio Company Wave Analyzer, Type 736-A.

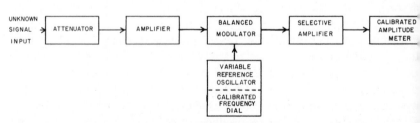

FIG. 35B. Steady-state wave analyzer: constant band-width filter.

Watkins (1939) published a description of an effective synthesizer, the *voder*. Many other such devices have been constructed and reported in technical journals.

For clinical application, an instantaneous, nonrecording sound analyzer, similar in basic design to the Sona-Graph, is the Kay Electric *Sonalator*. In this instrument, the recording circuit of the Sona-Graph is replaced by a long-persistence screen of a cathode ray tube on which the sound patterns appear. Hearing therapists have found the Sonalator useful in working with the deaf, since it provides visual display of speech signals.

**Wave analyzer.** In cases in which steady-state sound signals are to be analyzed, commercial harmonic-wave analyzers are available. Typical of these instruments are the General Radio Wave Analyzer, Type 736-A, shown in Fig. 35A, and the Hewlett-Packard Harmonic Wave Analyzer, Model 300-A. Basically these instruments are frequency-selective, calibrated voltmeters as indicated in Fig. 35B. They usually employ a variable reference oscillator, a balanced modulator, a selective amplifier, and a calibrated indicating meter. The unknown signal to be analyzed is electronically compared with the output of the variable reference oscillator. The constant-difference frequency is obtained and amplified by selective circuits. This signal is then fed to a calibrated voltmeter measurement of amplitude. The relative amplitude of the individual frequency components is indicated on the meter. The frequency of the component is noted on a calibrated dial. It is important to note that these instruments are valid for the measurement of steady-state sound signals and should not be employed in the analysis of transient speech waves. These analyzers are also useful in the measurement of distortion in other audio-frequency instruments used in the speech laboratory where precise calibration is required.

**Variable-filter wave analyzer.** In the steady-state analyzing circuits previously described, the theory involved constant-frequency filters. Unknown sound sources, however, may be analyzed employing variable filter circuits. These filters may be variable continuously or in discrete steps. Typical of the continuously-variable filter system is the Spencer-Kennedy Laboratory Variable Electronic Filter, Model 302; and the General Radio Company Sound Analyzer, Type 760-B, illustrated in Fig. 36. The discrete filter analyzer is being employed currently in the measurement of noise levels where octave-band increments appear suitable. Typical of such instruments are the General Radio Company Octave-Band Noise Analyzer, Type 1550-A, and the Western Electric Company RA-362 Amplifier Filter Set.

*Continuously Variable.* Unknown steady-state sound signals may be analyzed conveniently through the use of continuously-variable electronic filters. By employing two section filters (see Fig. 37), low-pass, high-pass, or narrow and wide-band circuits may be obtained. This is essentially the process employed in the Spencer-Kennedy Laboratory Model 302 Filter.

*Constant Percentage Band-Width Filters.* Steady-state signals may be analyzed also by means of constant percentage band-width filters in which the

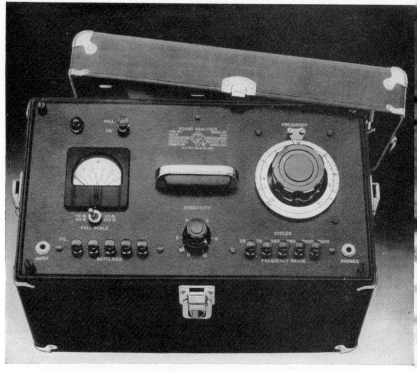

FIG. 36. General Radio Company Sound Analyzer, Type 760-B.

band width is a fixed percentage of the operating frequency. Fig. 38 is a block diagram of such circuits. This is the technique employed in the General Radio Company Sound Analyzer, Type 760-B (see Fig. 36).

*Discrete Band-Width Filters.* In the analysis of noise, octave–band-width measurements are frequently required. Circuits containing fixed filter increments provide immediate indications of intensity levels on an appropriate sound-level meter. These instruments usually provide octave-band, low-pass,

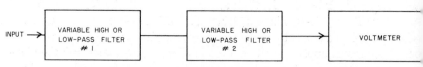

FIG. 37. Steady-state wave analyzer: continuously variable filter.

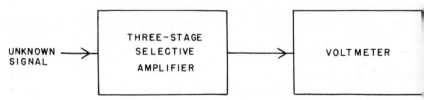

FIG. 38. Constant percentage band-width filter.

or high-pass filtering. The Western Electric Amplifier-Filter Set, RA-362 (see Fig. 39), and the H. H. Scott Sound Analyzer, Type 420-A (see Fig. 40), represent the typical discrete band-width filter. The General Radio Octave Band Noise Analyzer, Type 1550-A, is illustrated in Fig. 41.

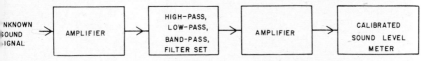

FIG. 39. Block diagram of Western Electric RA-362 Noise Analyzer.

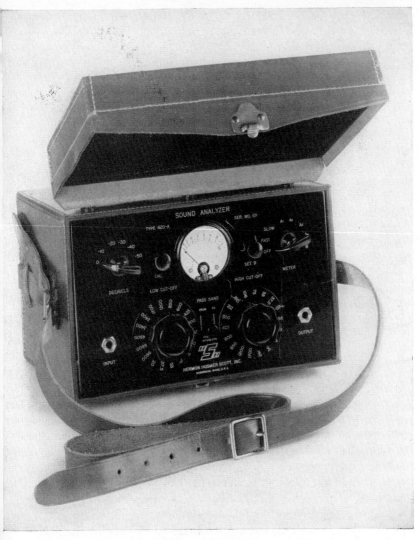

FIG. 40. H. H. Scott Sound Analyzer, Type 420-A.

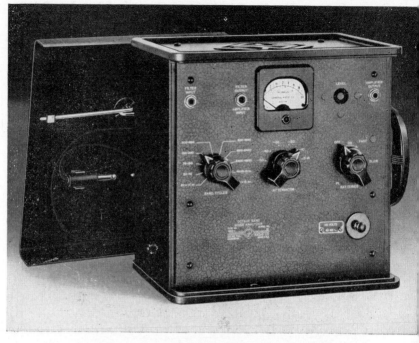

FIG. 41. General Radio Company Noise Analyzer, Type 1550-A.

## TIME MEASUREMENT

The phenomena of speech and hearing are observed and analyzed almost always with time as one axis or dimension. We attend to the variations of pitch with time, to the rapidly changing sequences of harmonic spectra with time and to the fluctuations in sound-pressure level with time. Under some conditions, time itself becomes an object of investigation, as it is related to the production or reception of some auditory signal. The application of instrumental techniques to time measurements, therefore, may be an important ability of the worker in a speech laboratory. Fortunately, time data often are available in the records and analyses collected for measurement of other sound attributes. Not many laboratory instruments have been developed for measurement of time alone.

**The stop watch.** One of the simplest of the conventional methods for making time analyses is the use of the stop watch. By depressing the starting lever at the onset and termination of a given speech sample or auditory phenomenon, the operator collects a record of its duration. Knowledge of the number of words in the sample permits calculation of the rate of speech in words per minute. Obviously the technique is subject to a considerable amount of human error, its reliability being dependent, to a large extent, upon the reaction time of the investigator and upon the size of the sample of speech being analyzed. The error introduced by delayed reaction of the investigator becomes relatively small when spread over the duration of a

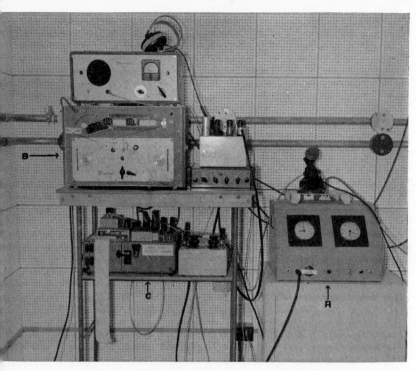

FIG. 42. Instrumental array: (A), Purdue Speech Sound Timer; (B) delayed feedback recorder; (C) High-speed graphic sound level recorder.

500-word reading passage, for example. On the other hand, the error intro-duced in an attempt to measure the duration of a single vowel in a sample of connected discourse undoubtedly would be larger than the phenomenon itself.

**The phonation timer.** An instrument which offers considerably more in the way of versatility and reliability is one of the few electronic devices con-ceived specifically for measurements along the time axis. This is the Purdue Speech Sound Timer (Tyler, Draegert, Hanley, and Steer, 1948), shown in Fig. 42. A schematic block diagram of the instrument is shown in Fig. 43. It consists of two electrically operated clocks. When the operating switch is thrown, one of the clocks begins immediately to record time in hundredths of a second. The other clock, however, is caused to operate only by means of a voice-activated electronic relay, associated with a microphone or the out-put of a tape or disc reproducer. This means that the "phonation speech time clock" will accumulate time units only during such time as voice signals of a predetermined and preset magnitude activate the switching mechanism of the clock. By means of the "total time dial," the investigator may calculate words per minute just as may be done with the stop watch. Through use of the phonation time clock, further calculations may be made, such as phona-tion time ratio, with duration of voicing as the numerator in the fraction and

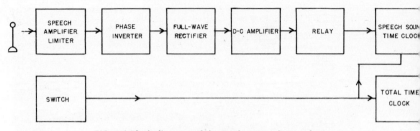

FiG. 43. Block diagram of the Purdue Speech Sound Timer.

total time of speech sample as the denominator. Words per minute exclusiv of pause time and mean word and syllable durations are calculations whicl may be made from the phonation time dial alone.

**Power-level recorder.** One of many instruments which may provide tim data, incidental to its prime function, is the power-level recorder, previousl described. The recording tape (see Fig. 44) of this device passes the record ing stylus at a known, constant rate. Each time the stylus departs from th base line, the existence of sound in time is recorded on the tape. Each tim the stylus returns to the base line, a silence period is recorded. Since linea distance on the recording tape may be converted into time units, such value as phonation time ratio, words per minute, and even duration of individua speech units (words or syllables) may also be computed.

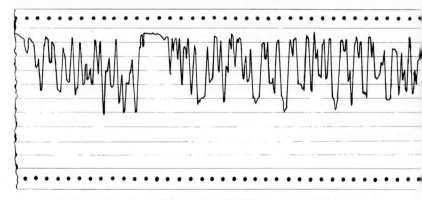

FIG. 44. Section of recorded tape from the high-speed graphic-level recorder.

**Vibrograph (phonelescope).** Another indirect source of time data is th vocal-frequency record produced by the vibrograph or phonelescope. I these frequency records (see Fig. 17), the presence of sound is revealed b the regular succession of waves on the photosensitive paper. Silence is ir dicated by straight lines. On these records, as on power level records, relationship between linear distance and time is established, and the sam calculations of time values can be made.

**Fundamental-frequency recorder.** Pitch records taken from the face c an oscillograph (see Fig. 20), as previously described, may also be used t provide time values. As in the two instruments just described, film spee past the camera lens is known and constant. Therefore, the speech signal identified on the record can be measured for duration as a function of linear distance.

**Sona-Graph.** The visible speech device, discussed in an earlier section, yields very precise information about temporal aspects of speech signals. On he sonagram (see Fig. 32), time again is a known, constant value on the horizontal axis of the record. Moreover, since individual phonemes are uniquely portrayed on the sonagram, onset and termination points may be identified, and duration as a function of distance may be measured. Some of the most exact information now available about the duration of individual speech sounds has been collected from analyses of sonagrams.

**The sylrater.** While not specifically an instrument for time measurement, he sylrater devised by Irwin and Becklund (1953) is significantly associated with one aspect of time. The device is a "sound-pulse rate meter," by means of which the recurrences of pulses of sound energy (syllables) per unit of ime are counted and metered. The sylrater is a direct-reading instrument not equipped with an accessory recorder. It has found its chief usefulness in he determination of diadochokinetic rates for various samples of subjects engaged in a variety of repetitive tasks.

**The voice-rate analyzer.** The Purdue Voice Rate Analyzer is an electronic instrument designed to record the rate of phonation for a spoken passage. The instrument amplifies, rectifies, and filters the signal, leaving only the speech envelope (Fig. 45). Each envelope is then counted, either on a series

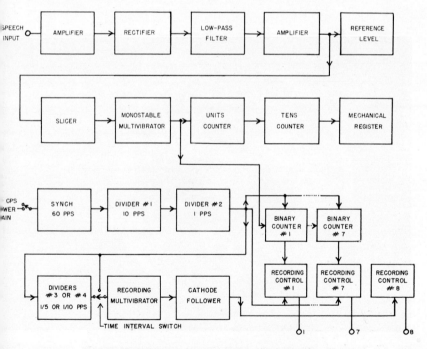

FIG. 45. Block diagram for Purdue Voice Rate Analyzer.

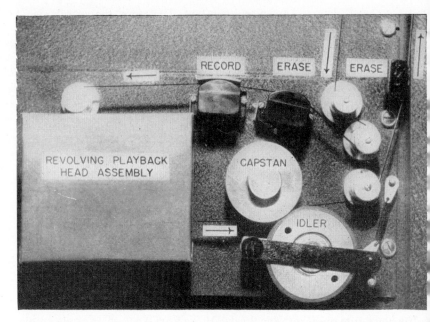

FiG. 46. Portion of the speech compression-expansion instrument (Fairbanks, Everett, and Jaeger).

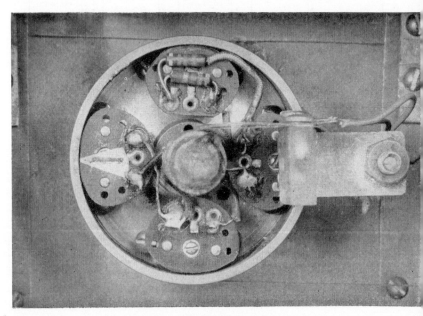

FIG. 47. Revolving four magnetic heads on the compression-expansion apparatus (Fairbanks et al.).

of decade counters for visual indication of the total phonation count, or in a series of binary counters and recording elements for permanent rate recordings. In the latter case the instrument uses the 60-cps line voltage as a time base. A series of dividers is used to obtain one-, five-, or ten-second record intervals during which binary counting of the speech phonations occurs. At the end of the selected time interval, the instrument records the count in binary form on electrographic paper. A dot is recorded or marked simultaneously on an eight-element recorder to indicate timing intervals. This counting and marking sequence continues during the entire speech passage until terminated by the operator. Thus, a record of the variation in phonation rate with time is obtained for subsequent analysis.

**Time compressor-expander.** It has long been observed that compression and expansion of signals along a time axis, with accompanying rise or fall of frequency, may be accomplished by means of accelerating or retarding playback speeds on a tape or disc reproducer. Fairbanks, Everett, and Jaeger (1953) described an important instrument which makes possible the compression-expansion of either time or frequency, with the alternate variable held constant. This device (see Fig. 46) opens up a large area of perceptual phenomenology for controlled investigation. In presenting the operational characteristics of the compressor-expander, the writers acknowledged the similarity in theory and design of their method of approach to the same problem made independently by other investigators. Several of these are summarized by Gabor (1946, 1947, 1948).

Essentially, the method of Fairbanks, Everett, and Jaeger consists of a continuous-loop magnetic tape recorder (Figs. 48, 49, 50). The tape direction and the tape speed are indicated in the block diagrams as $V_T$. Signals recorded on the tape loop are scanned by a revolving four-head playback assembly (see Fig. 47), and the samplings from this unit are recorded (stored) in a conventional tape recorder-reproducer, $V_R$. Since speed and the direction of rotation of the four-head assembly are under the control of the operator, the samplings may consist of successive fractions of the original, total signal (compression) or successive multiples of the original signal (expansion). By adjusting playback speed of the stored samplings in a manner appropriate to the earlier compression or expansion, the operator is able to duplicate the original frequency and also to modify the time aspect in the fractional or multiplicative manner. Conversely, he may play back the modified signal so that the original time values are retained, but frequency is fractionated or multiplied. Control of record and reproduced speeds being continuous, rather than in discrete steps, the operator may elect to compress original signals by any desired fraction. Similarly, expansion is under a wide range of continuous control.

Many voice scientists have engaged in research problems involving temporal aspects of speech. Basic among these studies are those of Darley (1940) and Franke (1939) which provided normative information about oral reading rate, and an investigation by Kelly and Steer (1949) which revealed im-

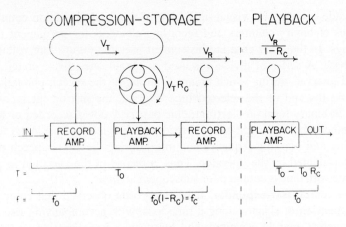

**FIG. 48.  Method of time compression (Fairbanks et al.).**

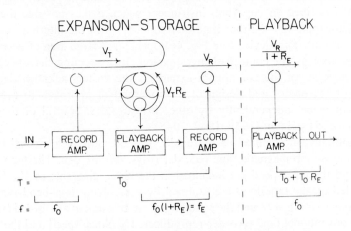

**FIG. 49.  Method of time expansion (Fairbanks et al.).**

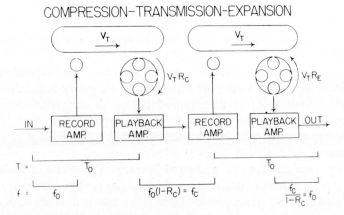

**FIG. 50.  Method of frequency compression-transmission-expansion (Fairbanks et al.).**

portant relationships between perception of speaking rate and various methods of expressing rate. Relations between time measures and speech skills have been reported by Murray and Tiffin (1933), and durational characteristics of voice during emotional expression have been reported by Fairbanks and Hoaglin (1941). Irwin (1953) has published some preliminary findings with respect to diadochokinetic rate revealed by the sylrater. Tiffany (1953), in a study involving arbitrary compression and expansion of vowel sounds, has presented evidence of the importance of duration for phonemic identification. Duration also is a significant contributor to emphasis, according to the findings of Tiffin and Steer (1937). The duration of individual phonemes, measured sonagraphically, appears to be related to regional dialect, according to evidence presented by Hanley (1951). Draegert's (1951) findings indicate that of all voice variables tested, syllable duration was most highly related to speech intelligibility in high-level noise.

The use of instrumentation for time measurment in the speech clinic, in contrast to the laboratory, has been relatively restricted. However, there is some evidence of increased attention being paid by clinicians to the time variable. The significance of rate and duration, revealed in the studies noted above and in many others, has impressed many clinicians with the desirability of teaching control over time values to some of the clients of the clinic. Among those who have received benefit from this type of therapy have been stutterers, cerebral-palsied individuals, and clients with foreign-language speech backgrounds.

## MISCELLANEOUS INSTRUMENTATION

A review of modern instrumentation would not be complete without the inclusion of some additional basic electronic devices important either to the clinician, researcher, or both. Included in this equipment are representative instruments employed in the study of delayed feedback (sidetone), pure tone and speech audiometry, auditory difference limen, nasal pressure, and sound wave generation. Some of these instruments are found in many clinics and laboratories, others are identified only with certain institutions. Nevertheless, all of this equipment is of importance to the clinician and research investigator.

### Delayed Feedback (Sidetone)

The disturbing influence of reverberations in large auditoria upon public speakers has been rather casually observed, over hundreds of years, by the individuals affected. However, not until this century have there been formal attempts to identify the mechanism or mechanisms involved in partial speech breakdown under these conditions—when the speaker's voice is returned to his ear an appreciable time after the sounds have been produced. A name —delayed feedback or delayed sidetone—has been given to the precipitating phenomenon; instruments have been developed or modified in order to induce

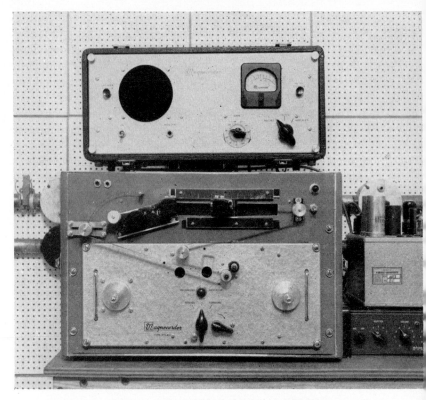

FIG. 51. Delayed feedback system (Magnecorder, Type PT6-AH, custom modified).

and control it, and many investigations have been performed to test its effects under various conditions. Perhaps more importantly, the results of sidetone research have been incorporated into, and in some cases have formed, the basis for theoretical formulations concerning initiation, control, and break-down in speech.

Typical of the instruments developed or modified to provide for a con-trolled delay in returning a subject's speech signals to his auditory mecha-nism is the delayed-feedback tape recorder-reproducer illustrated in Fig. 51. The recorder is equipped with a continuous tape loop, 42 inches in length. In the revolution, the tape passes first over an erase-head, which removes all previous signals, then over a record-head which impresses on the tape the voice signals from the subject. This much of the unit is conventional tape recorder operation. A departure from the conventional recorder, the heart of the delay mechanism, is the playback head, mounted on a slotted track which permits the head to be displaced from the recording head from .9 to 6.10 inches, providing for continuous delay from .062 to .406 seconds. The signals picked up by the playback head, amplified to the level desired by the experimenter, are returned to the subject's ears by means of ear phones.

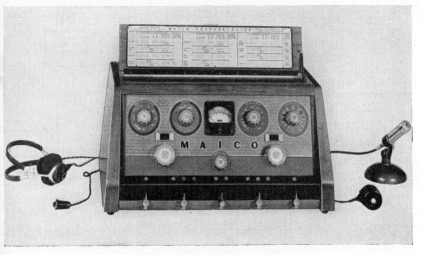

FIG. 52. Maico Clinical Audiometer, Model MA-1.

Early investigations making use of delayed sidetone were designed to establish critical delay times related to maximum disruption of the subjects' normal speech patterns. Lee (1951) and Black (1951) contributed basic information on this point. Spilka (1952) investigated relationships between measured personality traits and degree of speech breakdown under delay conditions, and Atkinson (1953) tested for adaptation to delay. Tiffany and C. N. Hanley (1952) have used delayed feedback as an adjunct to conventional audiometry, finding it a useful technique for the detection of malingering and hysterical deafness. Fairbanks (1954) has incorporated feedback implications into an operational theory of the speech mechanism. He, with many of the other writers on speech theory, acknowledges the important contributions made by Wiener (1950) in *Cybernetics*.

## Conventional Audiometry

Over the years methodologies for investigating auditory acuity have included whisper tests, tuning forks, watch-tick tests, Galton whistles, phonograph speech, and conventional pure-tone audiometers. In recent years we have witnessed the development of the modern speech-reception audiometer, new clinical pure-tone instruments with circuits to facilitate noise-masking, loudness balance, and difference limen tests, and the automatic pure-tone audiometer of Békésy. Note should also be made of electroencephalographic and psychogalvanic applications in recent audiometric measurement.

Typical of modern clinical pure-tone audiometers is the Maico MA-1 illustrated in Fig. 52. This instrument provides two matched dynamic air receivers, bone conductor, choice of white noise or sawtooth masking, reversible time interrupter, Luscher test accessory, automatic output limiter, microphone speech circuit with VU meter, and loudness balance control. Similar instruments also are manufactured by other companies.

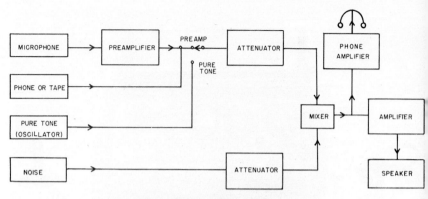

FIG. 53. Speech-reception audiometer.

Calibrated commercial speech-reception audiometers, standard or custom designed, are produced by several companies. These instruments usually provide for live-voice, phonograph, or magnetic tape-recording inputs. Test signals can be directed to either or both calibrated earphones for monaural or binaural testing, or to a high-fidelity loudspeaker. A calibrated pure-tone oscillator is included in the circuit. Provision also is made for the mixing of calibrated levels of masking noise. The attenuators in these circuits are usually calibrated in 1- and 10-decibel steps. A typical custom-designed

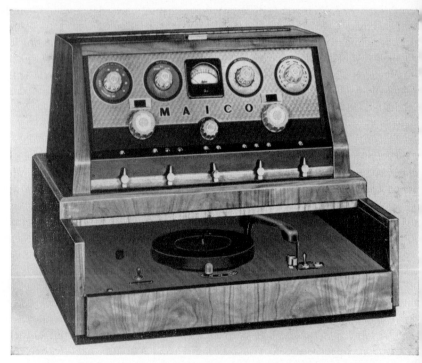

FIG. 54. Maico Clinical Audiometer, Model MA-1, with pedestal phonograph.

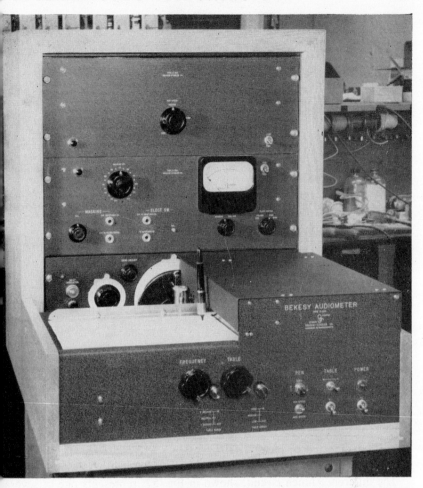

FIG. 55. Over-all view of Békésy Audiometer, Type E524 (Grason-Stadler Company).

speech-reception audiometer is indicated in Fig. 53. Since such equipment is relatively expensive, audiometer companies have made available, as an accessory to the pure-tone clinical audiometer, phonographs which are coupled to the instruments (see Fig. 54). This permits the examiner to administer recorded-speech tests.

The Békésy automatic-recording pure-tone audiometer is now produced by several companies. This instrument currently is being used principally by audiologists engaged in basic military and industrial research. The Békésy Audiometer manufactured by the Grason-Stadler Company is shown in Figs. 55 and 56.

### Difference Limen (DL)

Difference limen (DL) testing is employed in clinical audiology as one of the techniques for measuring auditory recruitment. Difference limen tests

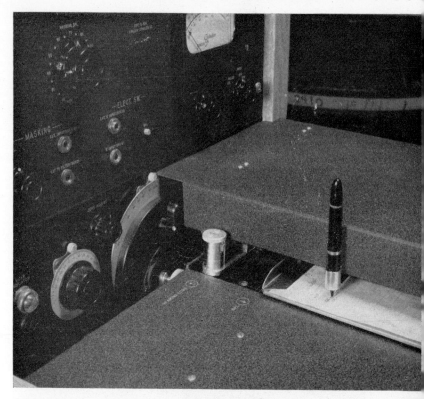

FIG. 56. View of recording table in retracted position, Békésy Audiometer, Type E524 (Grason-Stadler Company).

have been reported by Békésy (1947), Denes and Naunton (1950), Jerger (1952, 1953), Luscher and Zwislocki (1949) and Spuehler (1955).

The difference limen circuit, shown in Fig. 57, represents one of several instrumental techniques which may be employed for difference limen testing. This technique was developed at Purdue by Dempsey for H. Spuehler (1955). An audio-oscillator is used to supply a reference tone through an adjustable attenuator and a mixer-amplifier. The output of the oscillator is

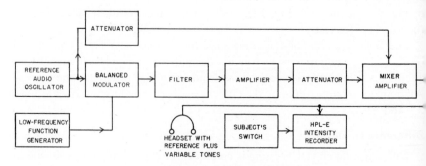

FIG. 57. Block diagram of a difference limen circuit.

also coupled to a specially constructed, balanced modulator. The pure-tone audio signal is amplitude-modulated by the triangular output of a low-frequency function generator. The resulting modulation produces an audio signal which varies in amplitude linearly with time from a minimum to a maximum value. A ± 5 db variation in signal level has been used in the difference limen testing conducted with this equipment. The maximum available change in signal level is 50 db.

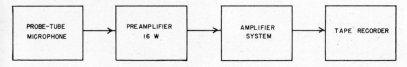

FIG. 58. Block diagram of equipment employed in probe-tube microphone recording.

The modulated signal is passed through a filter to remove any undesirable modulation products. The filter output is coupled through an amplifier and attenuator and mixed in the amplifier-mixer with the unmodulated reference tone. The mixed signals are then coupled to the subject's headset and to a graphic level recorder. The subject is furnished with a switch for indicating when the loudness of the two signals appears equal or different. The indication appears as a momentary break in the graphic record of the mixed signals.

### Probe-Tube Microphone Array

The probe-tube microphone has been used to determine sound pressures in the human ear canal. Its use for this purpose was described by Beranek (1949) and Wiener (1948). Benson (1953) studied the calibration of several probe-tubes of different dimensions. Weiss (1954) employed the probe-tube technique to investigate nasal sound-pressure levels related to judged severity of nasality. Summers (1955) used the same probe-tube assembly to investigate nasal sound-pressure levels of vowels. A block diagram showing the probe-tube-recording system appears in Fig. 58 and the probe-tube assembly used by Weiss is illustrated in Fig. 59.

### Wave-Form Generators

A wide variety of wave-form generators is employed for various psychoacoustic tasks. Those used most frequently in speech laboratories include audio-oscillators for the presentation of sine waves, random-noise generators, sawtooth generators, square-wave generators, and low-frequency function generators.

**Audio-oscillators.** The two basic types of audio-oscillators are the resistance-tuned and the beat-frequency type.

*Resistance-Tuned.* A basic commercial resistance-tuned audio-oscillator consists of a resistance-tuned or R-C oscillator, an amplifier, and a matching transformer. For laboratory work and precise measurements, more elaborate

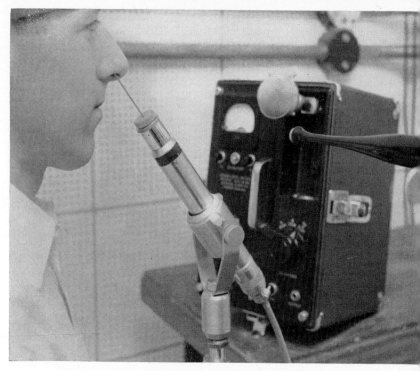

FIG. 59. Probe-tube assembly for measurement of nasal pressure (Purdue).

instruments are available. A typical laboratory audio-signal generator using a resistance-tuned oscillator is the Hewlett-Packard, Model 205AG (see Fig. 60). This device contains in addition to the resistance-tuned oscillator, a 5-watt amplifier, two vacuum tube voltmeters, 110-db attenuator in 1-db steps and a matching transformer-impedance selector. The range of this generator is 20 to 20,000 cps.

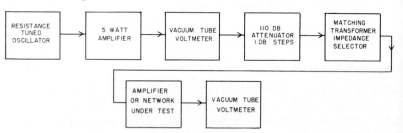

FIG. 60. Block diagram of the Hewlett-Packard Model 205AG Audio Signal Generator.

*Beat-Frequency Oscillator.* Signal generators of this type employ two radio-frequency oscillators and a circuit to detect the difference frequency. An example of this type is the General Radio Company, Type 1304, Beat-Frequency Audio Generator (see Fig. 61). This oscillator uses one fixed and one variable radio-frequency oscillator (see Fig. 62). The two oscillators

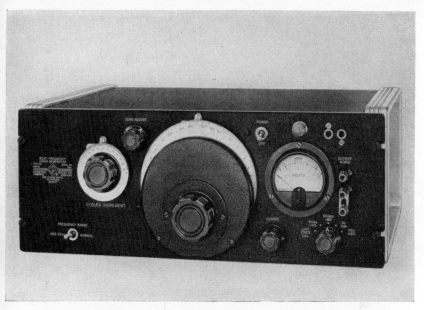

FIG. 61. General Radio Company Beat-Frequency Audio Generator, Type 1304-B.

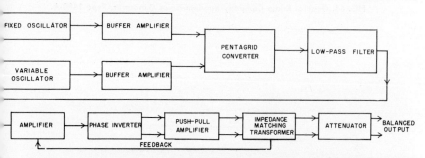

F.G. 62. Block diagram of General Radio Company Beat-Frequency Oscillator, Type 1304-A.

feed a pentagrid converter through buffer amplifiers. The resulting difference frequency, after passing through a low-pass filter, is amplified in a balanced feedback amplifier. The output level is controlled by a constant-impedance attenuator, calibrated in decibels with respect to an output of 1 milliwatt into 600-ohm load. With this type of circuit, a logarithmic frequency scale is used. The frequency range is 20 to 20,000 cps. The output level is

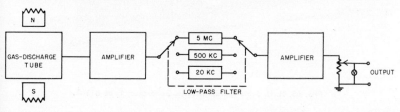

FIG. 63. Block diagram of General Radio Company Random-Noise Generator, Type 1390-A.

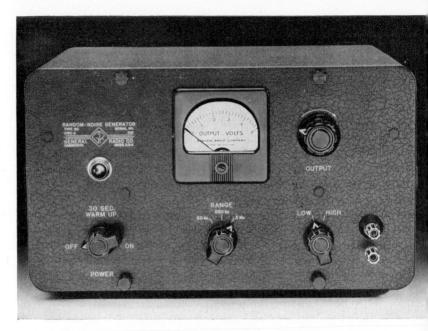

FIG. 64. General Radio Company Random-Noise Generator, Type 1390-A.

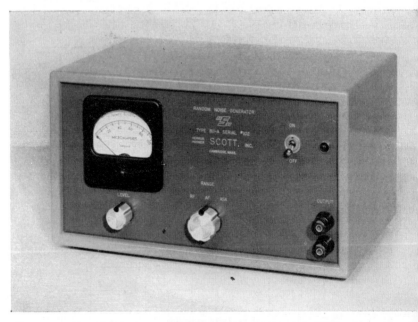

FIG. 65. H. H. Scott Random-Noise Generator, Type 811-A.

within $\pm$ 0.25 db throughout this range. A neon-lamp beat indicator is provided for standardizing the frequency calibration against the power-line frequency or against zero beat.

**Random-noise generator.** Random-noise generators may be used to provide a signal source for acoustical measurements in psycho-acoustical tests, filter tests, and in a variety of other electronic measurement applications.

A typical random-noise generator uses a gas-discharge tube as a noise source (see Fig. 63). A magnetic field is applied to the tube to suppress oscillations usually associated with a gas discharge. The noise output is amplified and passed through spectrum-shaping circuits. The noise is then amplified and coupled to the output potentiometer. A meter is provided across the output for setting the noise level to a desired value. The General Radio Company, Type 1390-A, Random-Noise Generator and the H. H. Scott Random-Noise Generator, Type 811-A are representative of this type of noise generator (see Figs. 64 and 65). Its spectrum-shaping circuits provide noise with uniform spectrum level out to 20 kc, 500 kc, or 5 mc.

**Sawtooth generator.** Sawtooth generators may be used as a source of low-frequency noise in noise generators supplying both low-frequency "line" noise and random noise and as a complex source. Sawtooth-type circuits are also used in oscilloscopes to provide linear sweep-voltages for time-base indication.

A very simple form of sawtooth generator employs a gas thyratron tube and R-C charging circuits. Other more elaborate circuits are often used where highly linear or special wave forms are desired. A basic sawtooth generator is symbolized in Fig. 66.

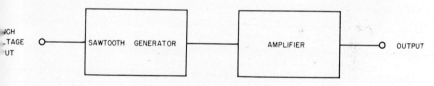

FIG. 66. Basic sawtooth generator.

**Square-wave generator.** Square waves may be produced by various techniques. In some circuits, square waves are obtained by clipping and "infinite" amplification of sine waves. In others, flip-flop circuits or multivibrators are used. These circuits are composed of two triodes with various interconnections depending upon the use for the multivibrator. The astable, or free-running, multivibrator is suited to square-wave generation. The astable multivibrator is a two-stage R-C coupled oscillator with alternately conducting and cutoff tubes. The output occurs as a rectangular or square-wave voltage. The circuits are commonly constructed so that the frequency of the square-wave generator may be synchronized to an external frequency source or standard.

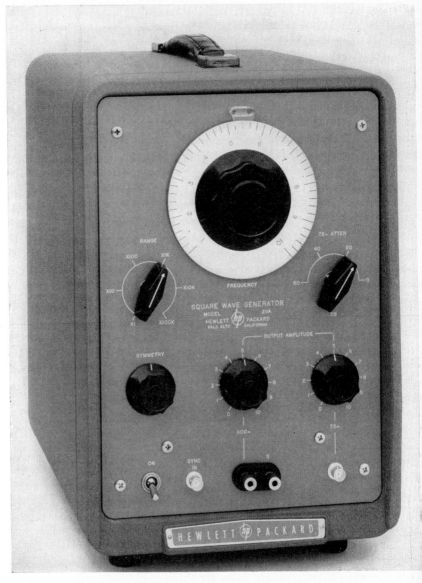

FIG. 67. Basic square-wave generator, Hewlett-Packard Model 211A.

Square-wave generators are used extensively in a great variety of electronic circuits. They may be used also as electronic switches and to provide complex signals rich in harmonics.

**Low-frequency function generator.** The Hewlett-Packard, Model 202-A Low Frequency Function Generator, is a highly versatile and useful laboratory type of wave-form generator. It generates square, triangular, and sine waves from 0.01 to 100 cps. The production of square waves at frequencies as low as 0.01 cps is achieved through the use of a special, highly stable, flip-flop, or bi-stable circuit. The triangular waves are produced by shaping the triangular wave voltage, using a series of amplitude-selective diodes. This

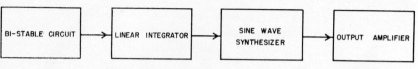

FIG. 68. Low-frequency function generator.

device may be used either as a versatile source of complex wave forms at extremely low frequencies or as a testing device for servo-systems, electro-medical equipment, or any general purpose low-frequency testing application.

## INSTRUMENT CALIBRATION

In concluding this chapter, special attention must be directed to the importance of equipment calibration. Electronic instruments and mechanical devices are expected to comply with predetermined specifications. The degree to which such instruments consistently meet established calibration values is of paramount importance in clinical and research application.

Microphones, earphones, amplifiers, filters, speakers, audiometers, galvanometers, recording and transcription machines, kymographs, polygraphs, and similar equipment justifiably employed in clinics and laboratories should be checked upon arrival and during scheduled time intervals.

Among the frequent causes of instrument failure are inherent faults in design, laxity in quality control during manufacturing, mishandling during shipment, incorrect assembly and usage, accidental injury, deterioration, improper maintenance, and faulty repair. Therefore, it is important that appropriate calibration procedures should be instituted to reflect instrument stability, reliability, and validity.

Illustrative of calibration techniques are the following descriptions concerning earphones, microphones, amplifiers and associated equipment, and speakers. These instruments are component parts of many electronic systems. Also listed are the steps in conducting a quantitative calibration for standard pure-tone audiometers.

**Earphone calibration.** Earphones are usually calibrated by checking the frequency response, electromechanical sensitivity, distortion characteristics, and "maximum undistorted" output. In order to accomplish this an artificial ear, consisting of a headset coupler, a calibrated condenser microphone, preamplifier, and power supply, is usually employed (see Fig. 69). A block diagram of an earphone calibration circuit is given in Fig. 70. (Subjective loudness balance tests may be used to supplement objective laboratory measurements.) In addition to the artificial ear, one or two vacuum tube volt-

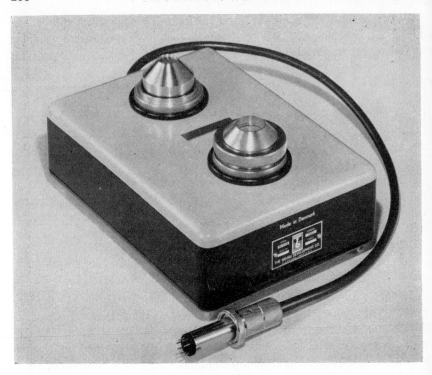

FIG. 69. Artificial Ear, Model 4109, Bruel & Kjaer (Brush Development Company).

meters, a calibrated audio-signal generator, attenuator, cathode ray oscillograph, and a wave analyzer are necessary for the complete calibration of
the earphone.

**Microphone calibration.** Microphones may be calibrated either under
free-field or closed-coupler conditions, depending upon the application of
the microphone. The latter method would be employed for a condenser
microphone used in an artificial ear. The technique employs a calibrated
earphone acting as a standard and the microphone under test as the un-

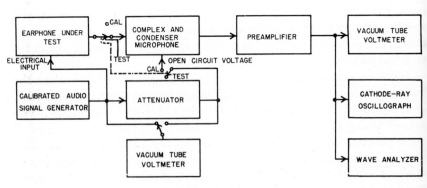

FIG. 70. Earphone calibration circuit.

known. The microphone's response would be compared to that of a known or previously calibrated microphone.

For free-field calibration, reciprocity methods may be employed to give absolute measurements of microphone sensitivity and frequency response. Test circuits similar to those employed in testing speakers may be utilized also. The response of the unknown microphone may be obtained by comparing its performance with that of a calibrated standard microphone.

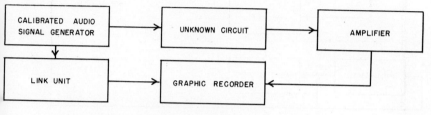

FIG. 71. Amplifier filter, equalizer, etc., test circuit.

**Amplifier, filter, equalizer, etc., calibration.** Tests of amplifier, filter, and equalizer performance will vary with the application and the degree of precision in testing required. Customarily, gain, frequency response, harmonic distortion, intermodulation distortion, and signal-to-noise-ratio tests may be employed in part or in total for the various circuits. Harmonic and intermodulation distortion may be measured by a variety of techniques. Harmonic distortion can be tested using a conventional wave analyzer. Special circuits are available for determining intermodulation distortion.

Frequency response, gain, and signal-to-noise-ratio measurements may be obtained using a mechanically-linked oscillator and graphic recorder test circuit as indicated in Fig. 71.

**Speaker testing.** The results of speaker tests depend both upon the acoustic test environment and the testing technique. Speakers may be tested in anechoic or in "normal" rooms, using frequency-modulated or warbled tones, band-pass noise, and sweep-frequency oscillators mechanically linked to graphic recorders. Testers are not in complete agreement as to the best testing methods. However, the method selected should give reproducible results. A widely used method of testing speaker frequency response employs a test oscillator whose frequency dial is mechanically linked to the carriage of a graphic recorder (see Fig. 72). The continuously-variable frequency, constant-amplitude output of the oscillator is amplified and coupled to the test speaker. The speaker and a calibrated microphone are placed in an anechoic room. The microphone output is amplified and coupled to the graphic recorder. Thus, a graphic record of the amplitude response versus frequency is obtained. This equipment may be provided with accessory devices for testing speaker directivity. The relative efficiency of speakers may be tested using the above equipment. Wave analyzers may be added to obtain measures of harmonic distortion.

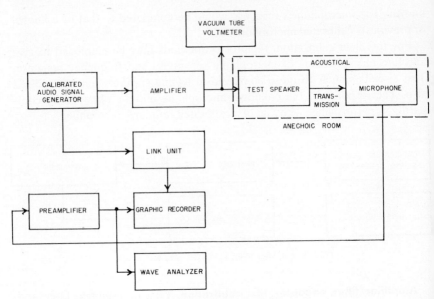

FIG. 72. Speaker test circuit.

**Audiometer calibration (pure tone).** Qualitative calibration of audiometers is conducted by testing the hearing of six to ten subjects of known hearing acuity. Usually subjects are chosen who have no history of previously known ear disease and who are reported to have normal hearing. The audiometer should verify the absence of auditory impairment. This procedure should be used at all clinics not equipped to make quantitative electro-acoustic tests.

The quantitative electro-acoustic calibration procedure for standard pure-tone audiometers (air conduction only) includes the following tests:

1. *Frequency*—Signals from a calibrated audio-signal generator and from the audiometer are coupled to a cathode ray oscillograph (see Fig. 73).

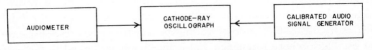

FIG. 73. Lissajous frequency calibration of audiometer.

The resulting Lissajous patterns indicate the comparison of the known frequency (audio-oscillator) with the frequency produced by the audiometer. A typical high-quality cathode ray oscilloscope is shown in Fig. 74.

2. *Linearity of "Loss Dial"*—To check the accuracy of the Hearing Loss Dial (attenuator) readings, the audiometer output is measured at the terminals of the headset with a vacuum tube voltmeter calibrated in decibels (see Fig. 75).

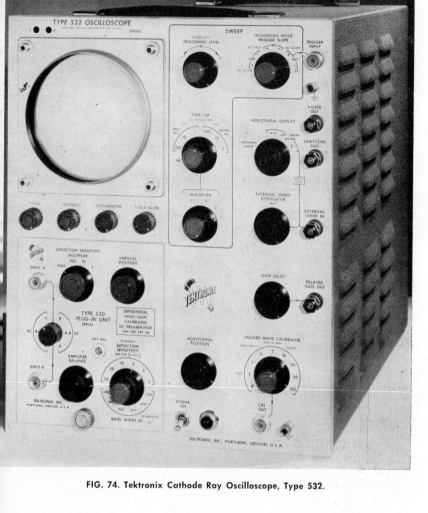

FIG. 74. Tektronix Cathode Ray Oscilloscope, Type 532.

3. *"Loss Dial"—Accumulative Error*—The accumulative error in the readings from the Hearing Loss Dial is calculated from the linearity of "loss dial" measurements.

4. *Acoustic Calibration*—The acoustic calibration is made by using the maximum permissible output level per frequency of the audiometer and then expressing the result in terms of the audiometer zero-reference level (see Fig. 76).

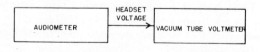

FIG. 75. Electrical calibration of loss dial.

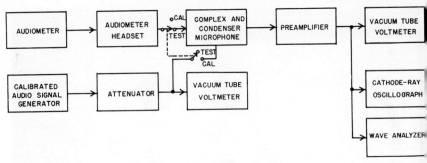

**FIG. 76. Acoustic calibration of audiometer.**

5. *Harmonic Distortion*—Measurement of harmonic distortion is achieved by analyzing the audiometer's acoustic output at the earphone through the use of an artificial ear and a wave analyzer. (A cathode ray oscillograph may be used to provide a general estimate of harmonic distortion.)

The results of the above tests and AMA specifications for audiometers are then compared to determine if the audiometer's performance is within specified limits.

## BIBLIOGRAPHY

AINSWORTH, S. 1948. Speech correction methods. New York: Prentice-Hall. Pp. 36–37, 135.

American Speech and Hearing Association. 1943. Constitution. Principles of ethics.

ATKINSON, C. 1953. Adaptation to delayed side-tone. *J. Speech Hearing Disorders*, 18, 386–391.

BARNES, J. 1926. Vital capacity and ability in oral reading. *Quart. J. Speech Educ.*, 12, No. 3, 176–182.

BEHRENDT, H. 1949. Diagnostic tests for infants and children. New York: Interscience Pub. P. 297.

BÉKÉSY, G. VON. 1947. The recruitment phenomenon and difference limen in hearing and vibration sense. *Laryngoscope*, 57, 765–777.

BENDER, J. F., and KLEINFELD, V. M. 1938. Principles and practices of speech correction. New York: Pitman. Pp. 41–44.

BENSON, R. W. 1953. The calibration and use of probe-tube microphone. *J. acoust. Soc. Amer.*, 25, 128–134.

———— and HIRSH, I. J. 1953. Some variables in audio spectrometry. *J. acoust. Soc. Amer.*, 25, 499–505.

BERANEK, L. L. 1949. Acoustic measurement. New York: Wiley. Pp. 731–735.

BERRY, M., and EISENSON, J. 1942. The defective in speech. New York: Crofts. Pp. 76–79.

———— 1956. Speech disorders. New York: Appleton-Century-Crofts.

BLACK, J. W. 1949. Natural frequency, duration, and intensity of vowels in reading. *J. Speech Hearing Disorders*, 14, 216–221.

———— 1951. The effects of delayed side-tone upon vocal rate and intensity. *J. Speech Hearing Disorders*, 16, 56–60.

———— 1937. The quality of a spoken vowel. *Arch. Speech*, 1, 7–27.

BLOOMER, H. 1936. A roentgenographic study of the mechanics of respiration. *Speech Monogr.*, 3, 118–124.

BORDEN, R. C., and BUSSE, A. C. 1925. Speech correction. New York: Crofts. Pp. 146–147, 233–277.

CONSTANS, H. P. 1936. An objective analysis of the three forms of force in speech. La. State Univ. Studies, No. 27, pp. 7–36. Baton Rouge.

COWAN, M. 1936. Pitch and intensity characteristics of stage speech. *Arch. Speech,* Supplement.

DARLEY, F. L. 1940. A normative study of oral reading rate. Unpublished Master's Thesis. State Univ. Iowa.

DAVIS, J. F. 1952. Manual of surface electromyography. Lab. for Psychol. Studies, Allen Memorial Institute of Psychiatry. McGill Univ., Montreal.

DAVIS, R. D. 1948. An integrator and accessory apparatus for recording action potential. *Amer. J. Psychol.*, 61, 100.

DEMPSEY, M. E. 1955. Design and evaluation of a fundamental frequency recorder for complex sounds. Unpublished Doctor's Dissertation. Purdue Univ.

———— 1949. The Purdue pitch meter: a direct-reading fundamental frequency analyzer. Unpublished Master's Thesis. Purdue Univ. Also, with Draegert, G. L., Siskind, R. P., and Steer, M. D. 1950. Same title in the *J. Speech Hearing Disorders,* 15, 135–141.

————, SISKIND, R. P., HANLEY, T. D., and STEER, M. D. 1953. A fundamental frequency recorder for complex sounds. Technical Report No. SpecDevCen 104–2–34 by the Purdue Univ. Voice Communications Lab. for the Special Devices Center of the Office of Naval Research on SpecDevCen Contract N6 ori-104, T.O. II, Project 20–F–8.

DENES, P., and NAUNTON, R. F. 1950. The clinical detection of auditory recruitment. *J. Laryng., Lond.,* 64, 375–398.

DOERFLER, L. G., and McCLURE, C. T. 1954. The measurement of hearing loss in adults by the galvanic skin response. *J. Speech Hearing Disorders,* 19, 184–189.

DRAEGERT, G. L. 1951. Relationships between voice variables and speech intelligibility in high level noise. *Speech Monogr.,* 18, 272–278.

DUDLEY, H. 1936. Synthesizing speech. *Bell Laboratories Record,* 15, 98–102.

————, RIESZ, R. R., and WATKINS, R. 1939. A synthetic speaker. *Bell Tel. Laboratories Monogr.* B-1148.

DUFFEY, R. F. 1954. An analysis of the pitch and duration characteristics of the speech of cerebral palsied individuals. Unpublished Doctor's Dissertation. Purdue Univ.

DUNN, H. K. 1930. A new analyzer of speech and music. *Bell Laboratories Record,* 9, 118–123.

FAIRBANKS, G. 1954. A theory of the speech mechanism as a servo-system. *J. Speech Hearing Disorders,* 19, 133–139.

———— 1940. Recent experimental investigations of vocal pitch in speech. *J. acoust. Soc. Amer.,* 11, 457–466.

———— and BEBOUT, B. 1950. A study of minor organic deviations in 'functional' disorders of articulation: 3. the tongue. *J. Speech Hearing Disorders,* 15, 348–352.

FAIRBANKS, G., EVERETT, W. L., and JAEGER, R. D. 1954. Method for time or frequency compression of speech. *Trans. Inst. Radio Engineers,* AU2, 7–12.

FAIRBANKS, G., and GREEN, E. 1950. A study of minor organic deviations in 'functional' disorders of articulation: 2. dimensions and relationships of the lips. *J. Speech Hearing Disorders,* 15, 165–168.

FAIRBANKS, G., HERBERT, E. L., and HAMMOND, J. M. 1949. An acoustical study of vocal pitch in seven- and eight-year-old girls. *Child Developm.*, 20, 71–78.

FAIRBANKS, G., and HOAGLIN, L. 1941. An experimental study of the durational characteristics of the voice during the expression of emotion. *Speech Monogr.*, 8, 85–90.

FAIRBANKS, G., and LINTNER, M. 1951. A study of minor organic deviations in 'functional' disorders of articulation: 4. the teeth and hard palate. *J. Speech Hearing Disorders*, 16, 273–279.

FAIRBANKS, G., and SPRIESTERSBACH, D. C. 1950. A study of minor organic deviations in 'functional' disorders of articulation: 1. rate of movement of oral structures. *J. Speech Hearing Disorders*, 15, 60–69.

FAIRBANKS, G., WILEY, J. H., and LASSMAN, F. M. 1949. An acoustical study of vocal pitch in seven- and eight-year-old boys. *Child Developm.*, 20, 63–69.

FLETCHER, H. 1953. Speech and hearing in communication. New York: Van Nostrand. Ch. 4.

FRANKE, P. 1939. A preliminary study validating the measurement of oral reading rate in words per minute. Unpublished Master's Thesis. State Univ. Iowa.

FREESTONE, N. 1942. Brain wave interpretation of stuttering. *Quart. J. Speech*, 28, 466–468.

GABOR, D., the following references in *J. Inst. Electr. Engineers:* 1946, 93, Part III, 427–429; 1947, 94, Part III, 369–386; 1948, 95, Part III, 39, 411–412.

GARCEAU, E. L., and DAVIS, H. 1935. An ink-writing electroencephalograph. *Arch. Neurol. Psychiat.*, 34, 1292–1294.

GIRDEN, E. 1952. The galvanic skin response 'set' and the acoustical threshold. *Amer. J. Psychol.*, 65, 233–243.

GLOGAU, O. 1916. The diagnostic value of records of breathing and of speech. *N.Y. Med. J.*, 103, 108–111.

GRUBBS, W. H., and RUCKMICK, C. 1932. An electric pneumograph. *Amer. J. Psychol.*, 44, 180–181.

GRUENZ, O. O., and SCHOTT, L. O. 1949. Extraction and portrayal of pitch of speech sounds. *J. acoust. Soc. Amer.*, 21, 487–495.

GUTZMANN, H. 1928. Physiologie der stimme und sprache. Berlin: Friedrich Vieweg and Son.

HANLEY, T. D. 1951. An analysis of vocal frequency and duration characteristics of selected samples of speech from three American dialect regions. *Speech Monogr.*, 18, 78–93.

——— and STEER, M. D. 1948. Voice communication: intelligibility training with Purdue speech intensity demonstrator. Technical Report No. SpecDevCen 104–2–8 by the Purdue Voice Communications Lab. for the Special Devices Center of the Office of Naval Research on SpecDevCen Contract N6 ori–104, T.O. II, Project 20–K–1.

HARDY, W. G., and BORDLEY, J. E. 1951. Special techniques in testing the hearing of children. *J. Speech Hearing Disorders*, 16, 122–131.

HARDY, W. G., and PAULS, M. D. 1952. The test situation in PGSR audiometry. *J. Speech Hearing Disorders*, 17, 125–148.

HENRIKSON, E. 1943. Note on voice recordings. *J. Speech Hearing Disorders*, 8, 133–135.

——— and IRWIN, J. 1949. Voice recording—some findings and some problems. *J. Speech Hearing Disorders*, 14, 227–233.

HULL, H., and BRYNGELSON, B. 1941. A study of respiration of fourteen spastic paralysis cases during silence and speech. *Speech Monogr.*, 8, 114–121.

HUNT, F. V. 1935. Direct-reading frequency meter. *Rev. sci. Instrum.*, 6, 43.

HUTCHINSON, J. 1852. The spirometer, the stethescope, and scale-balance; their uses in discriminating disease of the chest, and their value in life offices. London: John Churchill.

IDOL, H. R. 1936. A statistical study of respiration in relation to speech characteristics. La. State Univ. Studies, No. 27, pp. 79–96, Baton Rouge.

IRWIN, J. V., and BECKLUND, O. 1953. Norms for maximum repetitive rates for certain sounds established with the sylrater. *J. Speech Hearing Disorders,* 18, 149–160.

JASPER, H. H., and ANDREWS, H. L. 1936. Human brain rhythms: I. recording techniques and preliminary results. *J. gen. Psychol.,* 14, 98–126.

JERGER, J. F. 1952. A difference limen recruitment test and its diagnostic significance. *Laryngoscope,* 62, 1316–1332.

——— 1953. DL difference test: an improved method for the clinical measurement of recruitment. *A.M.A. Arch. Otolaryng.,* 57, 490–500.

JOHNSON, W., BROWN, S., CURTIS, J. F., EDNEY, C., and KEASTER, J. 1948. Speech handicapped school children. New York: Harper. Pp. 436–438.

JUDSON, L. S. 1932. Combining the breathing undae of speaker and listener with the dictaphone record of the speech. *Amer. J. Psychol.,* 44, 183–184.

——— and GRIFFITH, P. 1930. A variable resistance pneumograph and an electromagnetic tambour. *Science,* 72, 369–370.

KELLY, J. C., and STEER, M. D. 1949. Revised concept of rate. *J. Speech Hearing Disorders,* 14, 222–226.

KELLY, J. P. 1934. Studies in nasality. *Arch. Speech,* 1, 26–42.

KOENIG, W., DUNN, H. K., and LACY, L. Y. 1946. The sound spectrograph. *J. acoust. Soc. Amer.,* 18, 19–49.

KOEPP-BAKER, H. 1936. Handbook of clinical speech. Ann Arbor: Edwards Bros., Vol. 2. Pp. 214–222.

LeBEL, C. J. 1951. Fundamentals of magnetic recording. New York: Audio Devices Co.

LEE, B. S. 1951. Artificial stutter. *J. Speech Hearing Disorders,* 16, 53–55.

LEWIS, D., and TIFFIN, J. 1934. A psychophysical study of individual differences in speaking ability. *Arch. Speech,* 1, 43–60.

LIBERMAN, A. M., DELATTRE, P. C., COOPER, F. S., and GERSTMAN, L. J. 1954. The role of consonant-vowel transitions in the perception of the stop and nasal consonants. *Psychol. Monogr.,* 68, 1–13.

LINDSLEY, C. F. 1929. An objective study of the respiratory processes accompanying speech. *Quart. J. Speech,* 15, 42–58.

LUSCHER, E., and ZWISLOCKI, J. 1949. A simple method for indirect monaural determination of the recruitment phenomenon (difference limen in intensity in different types of deafness). *Acta Oto-Laryngologica,* Supp. 78, 156–168.

MERITSER, C. L., and DOERFLER, L. G. 1954. The conditioned galvanic skin response under two modes of reinforcement. *J. Speech Hearing Disorders,* 19, 350–359.

METFESSEL, M. 1928. A photographic method of measuring pitch. *Science,* 68, 430–432.

——— 1926. Techniques for objective studies of the vocal art. *Psychol. Monogr.,* 36, 1–40.

MILLER, D. C. 1937. Sound waves, their shape and speed. New York: Macmillan. Ch. 2.

——— 1916. The science of musical sounds. New York: Macmillan. Pp. 70–91.

MURRAY, E., and TIFFIN, J. 1933. An analysis of some basic aspects of effective speech. *Arch. Speech,* 1, 61–83.

NORDYKE, H. W., DRAEGERT, G. L., and STEER, M. D. 1948. Purdue speech intensity demonstrator. Technical Report No. SpecDevCen 104–2–6 by the

Purdue Voice Communications Lab. for the Special Devices Center of the Office of Naval Research on SpecDevCen Contract N6 ori–104, T.O. II, Project 20–K–1.

OBATA, J., and KOBAYASHI, R. 1937. A direct reading pitch recorder and its application to music and speech. *J. acoust. Soc. Amer.*, 9, 247–250.

———— 1938. Apparatus for direct-reading the pitch and intensity of sound. *J. acoust. Soc. Amer.*, 10, 147.

———— 1940. Further applications of our direct-reading pitch and intensity recorder. *J. acoust. Soc. Amer.*, 12, 188–192.

PALMER, M. F. 1937. The cardiac cycle as a physiological determinant of energy distribution in speech. *Speech Monogr.*, 4, 110–126.

PETERSON, A. P., and BERANEK, L. L. 1953. Handbook of noise measurement. Cambridge: General Radio Co. P. 6.

PETERSON, G. E. 1952. Parameter relationships in the portrayal of signals with sound spectrographic techniques. *J. Speech Hearing Disorders*, 17, 427–432.

———— and RAISBECK, G. 1953. The measurement of noise with the sound spectrograph. *J. acoust. Soc. Amer.*, 25, 1157–1162.

PRONOVOST, W. 1942. An experimental study of methods for determining natural and habitual pitch. *Speech Monogr.*, 9, 111–123.

RAY, W. S. 1932. A study of the emotions of children with particular reference to circulatory and respiratory changes. *J. genet. Psychol.*, 40, 109–117.

RITZMAN, C. H. 1942, 1943. A comparative cardiovascular and metabolic study of stutterers and non-stutterers. *J. Speech Disorders*, 7, 367–373; 8, 161–182.

SALLEE, W. 1936. An objective study of respiration in relation to audibility in connected speech. La. State Univ. Studies, No. 27, pp. 52–58, Baton Rouge.

SCRIPTURE, E. W. 1906. Researches in experimental phonetics. The study of speech curves. Washington, D. C., The Carnegie Foundation.

SHANEY, A. C. 1947. Elements of magnetic recording—and 999 applications. New York: Amplifier Corp. of Amer.

SHERMAN, D. 1954. The merits of backward playing of connected speech in the scaling of voice quality disorders. *J. Speech Hearing Disorders*, 19, 312–321.

SIMON, C. F. 1926. The variability of consecutive wave lengths in vocal and instrumental sounds. *Psychol. Monogr.*, 36, 41–83.

SIVIAN, L. J., DUNN, H. K., and WHITE, S. D. 1931. Absolute amplitudes and spectra of certain musical instruments and orchestras. *J. acoust. Soc. Amer.*, 2, 330–371.

SNIDECOR, J. C. 1951. The pitch and duration characteristics of superior female speakers during oral reading. *J. Speech Hearing Disorders*, 16, 44–53.

SPILKA, B. 1952. A study of relationships existing between certain aspects of personality and some vocal effects of delayed speech feedback. Unpublished Doctor's Dissertation. Purdue Univ.

SPUEHLER, H. E. 1955. An auditory loudness recruitment test battery: analysis and comparison of sub tests. Unpublished Master's Thesis. Purdue Univ.

STARBUCK, H. B., and STEER, M. D. 1954. The adaptation effect in stuttering and its relation to thoracic and abdominal breathing. *J. Speech Hearing Disorders*, 19, 440–449.

STEER, M. D. 1935. A qualitative study of breathing in young stutterers. *Speech Monogr.*, 2, 152–156.

———— and TIFFIN, J. 1934. A photographic study of the use of intensity by superior speakers. *Speech Monogr.*, 1, 72–78.

STEVENS, S. S., ed. 1951. Handbook of experimental psychology. New York: Wiley. Pp. 474–476.

STEWART, K. C. 1954. A new instrument for detecting the galvanic skin response. *J. Speech Hearing Disorders*, 19, 169–173.

SUMMERS, R. R. 1955. The nasal sound pressure levels of vowels produced at specific intensities. Unpublished Doctor's Dissertation. Purdue Univ.

The Telegraphone. 1901. *Nature*, 64, 183–186.

TIFFANY, W. R. 1953. Vowel recognition as a function of duration, frequency modulation and phonetic context. *J. Speech Hearing Disorders*, 18, 289–301.

——— and HANLEY, C. N. 1952. Delayed speech feedback as a test for auditory malingering. *Science*, 115, 59–60.

TIFFIN, J. 1932. Phonophotographic apparatus. Univ. Iowa Studies in the Psychology of Music, 1, 118–133.

——— and STEER, M. D. 1937. An experimental analysis of emphasis. *Speech Monogr.*, 4, 69–74.

——— 1939. The vibrograph: a combination apparatus for the speech laboratory. *Quart. J. Speech*, 25, 272–278.

TRAVIS, L. E. 1934. Dissociation of homologous muscle functioning in stuttering. *Arch. Neurol. Psychiat.*, 31, 127–133.

——— and KNOTT, J. R. 1937. Bilaterally recorded brain potentials from normal speakers and stutterers. *J. Speech Disorders*, 2, 239–241.

TRAVIS, L. E., TUTTLE, W. W., and COWAN, D. W. 1936. A study of the heart rate during stuttering. *J. Speech Disorders*, 1, 21–26.

TYLER, H. J., DRAEGERT, G. L., HANLEY, T. D., and STEER, M. D. 1948. Purdue speech sound timer. Technical Report No. SpecDevCen 104–2–7 by Purdue Voice Communications Lab. for the Special Devices Center of the Office of Naval Research under Contract N6 ori–104, T.O. II, Project 20–K–1.

VAN RIPER, C. 1954. Speech correction. New York: Prentice-Hall. Pp. 192–195.

WEISS, A. I. 1954. Oral and nasal sound pressure levels as related to judged severity of nasality. Unpublished Doctor's Dissertation. Purdue Univ.

WENDT, G. 1938. Methods of recording action. *Arch. Psychol.*, No. 228, 7–21.

WEST, R. 1936. Diagnosis of disorders of speech. Madison: Coll. Typing Co. Pp. 4–46.

WIENER, F. M. 1948. Equipment for measuring sound pressures in the auditory canal. *Bell Laboratories Record*, 26, 261–264.

WIENER, N. 1950. Cybernetics. New York: Wiley.

WIKSELL, W. 1936. An experimental study of controlled and uncontrolled types of breathing. La. State Univ. Studies, No. 27, pp. 99–164, Baton Rouge.

WILLIAMS, D. 1953. An evaluation of masseter muscle action potentials in stuttered and non-stuttered speech. (Abstract.) *Speech Monogr.*, 29, 190–191.

WILLIAMSON, A. B. 1935. Two years' experience with recording equipment. *Quart. J. Speech*, 21, 195–224.

WINDESHEIM, K. A. 1938. The evolution of speech recording machines. *Quart. J. Speech*, 24, 257–264.

WOOD, A. 1940. Acoustics. New York: Interscience Pub. Ch. 12.

ZOETHOUT, W. D., and TUTTLE, W. W. 1948. Textbook of physiology (9th ed.). St. Louis: C. V. Mosby. P. 186.

# CHAPTER 7

# THE INCIDENCE OF SPEECH DISORDERS

● *Robert Milisen, Ph.D.*

KNOWLEDGE OF THE INCIDENCE of speech disorders is of great importance to therapists as well as experimenters. It acquaints the therapist with the number and kind of defective speakers he will find in a given population and it provides the experimenter with one measure of the importance of each type of disorder, the frequency with which it occurs.

Determining the incidence of speech disorders is not, unfortunately, a simple matter of counting those who are defective. Speech may be defective in many and complex ways. Nevertheless, speech disorders must be classified if the data are to be presented meaningfully. No system of classification has proved completely satisfactory, however, since speech deviations are distributed on a continuum of severity and more than one type of defect may be present in a single individual. Each class is really only one point on the continuum and therefore the variations on the continuum between classes are not properly represented. Some of the variables complicating speech-disorder classification are as follows:

1. Speech is a dynamic process which makes impossible the establishment of any *standard* of speech. No sound is made exactly the same way twice even by the same person. The variability increases as the speech pattern becomes more complex and as the situation becomes more difficult. The speech pattern of each individual goes through a constant change from birth to death.

2. Speech may be defective because of the overemphasis or underemphasis of any element of the speech act. Any effort to analyze the speech act into its component elements is bound to lead to a number of artificial divisions which do not really represent the *whole* of speech. Because the behavior is really on a continuum, the discrete classes provided by a system force the examiner to make arbitrary judgments regarding responses which fall between two classes. The more widely the classes are separated on the continuum, the less descriptive will any class be of the response assigned to it.

3. Speech is a medium of communication and as such it involves both speaker and an audience. In order for speech to be defective, either the

246

audience, the speaker, or both must be reacting to the process of speech in such a way as to interfere with the communication of the content. This interference is frequently unintended and unpleasant.

The amount of attention directed by either the speaker or the listener to speech deviations, which are an aspect of the process of speech, changes constantly. The total changes in listener or speaker responses may take place gradually. Each speech act at any moment is likely to present an either-or condition for each person involved in the act. That is, at any moment each person is reacting either to *how* one speaks or to *what* is said. The person is speaking "defectively" at the moment when attention is directed to how he is speaking, whereas he is speaking "normally" when attention is directed to what he is saying. This complete switch may occur many times during a short conversation. The listener or speaker reactions range on a continuum from complete acceptance to complete rejection. A listener or a speaker may be disturbed by speech deviations at the beginning of a speaking situation and then become unaware of them later on, or vice versa. Thus, a type of deviating speech may be considered defective at one time by the listener and/or the speaker; however, if adaptation has taken place the deviation may not be reacted to at all. These changes in reaction may occur even though the nature and extent of the deviations may remain relatively constant. Thus a measurement of the extent of a deviation (even if this could be done accurately) would not necessarily indicate the extent of the speech defect, because the deviation is important only as it interferes with communication and is reacted to by the speaker or the listener.

4. The judgments used in determining the incidence of speech disorders have a low reliability and validity. Frequently the judgments have been made by persons who have no training in the scientific method and, what is worse, have little interest in the accuracy of the judgments they are making. This is especially true of questionnaire studies. The investigator is faced with the dilemma of whether to use trained or untrained examiners in determining which deviations may be classified as speech disorders. If only trained examiners are used, the reliability of the judgments will be greater but the validity will be more questionable. If untrained observers are used, just the opposite may be true. This is because the trained observer may report accurately many minor deviations which would seldom attract anyone else's attention and therefore should not be classified as speech defects; whereas the untrained observer may classify incorrectly many of the deviations he observes, but for the most part he will report only those deviations which are severe enough to be classified as speech defects. Pronovost (1951) has pointed to wide variations in percentages, according to the type of person making the survey, such as nurse or speech teacher.

No experimental work on the incidence of speech defects has been done which has successfully controlled all of the above variables, simply because the task is impossible. One cannot analyze a dynamic whole into a series of parts and then synthesize those parts back into a whole. In spite of these limitations, the incidence of speech disorders can be reported if the reader will use his own common sense and experiential background to modify reports which do not precisely fit his situation. The only alternative is for each person to satisfy his own professional needs by using his own definitions, classifications, and testing methods when studying incidence.

All good therapists will, to some extent, investigate speech conditions in their own communities but few will have the time to carry on extensive investigations. Furthermore, if they did, they would be confronted with the same difficult problems which have confronted all previous investigators.

Definition of terms may eliminate at least one source of error. As much as possible, the discussion by the writer will be couched in the terms which follow. A *speech deviation* refers to any demarcation from the *assumed* "normal or standard speech pattern." A *speech defect* refers to a deviation which at any moment is sufficiently extreme to attract attention to the process of speech, to interfere with communication or affect adversely either the speaker or listener. A *speech defective* is one who frequently demonstrates a speech defect.

Deviations in speech may involve: (1) articulation—the way a sound is formed; (2) rhythm—the time relationship between sounds in a word and words in a sentence; (3) voice—the sounds produced by the vibrating vocal folds and modified by the resonators and articulators; (4) language usage—difficulty in comprehending speech of others or in projecting one's own ideas through the medium of speech.

## INCIDENCE OF SPEECH DEFECTS IN GENERAL

Estimates of the incidence of speech defects in the general population are few and probably not too reliable. Estimates of the incidence in the school population are more readily available. The White House Conference (1931) reported that 7 per cent of 10,033 school children in Madison, Wis., who were carefully examined by speech pathologists had defective speech, compared to a median percentage of 6.9 in their questionnaire survey which covered 48 cities. However, the results reported from these cities varied from 21.4 per cent (Fresno, Cal.) to 1.0 per cent (Philadelphia). Hawk (1945) reported that individual diagnosis of elementary school children in Ohio showed 9.5 per cent with defects. Johnson (1942) stated that 10 per cent of 30,000 individually tested Iowa school children were judged to have defective speech. Irwin (1948) reported 10 per cent of Cleveland children between kindergarten and grade six were defective in speech. Only 7.7 per cent of the children above kindergarten were defective. Mills and Streit (1942) reported 33.4 per cent of 1196 individually tested children in the first three grades of Holyoke, Mass., had speech defects, 12.6 per cent of them serious. In the first six grades, 10.1 per cent of 4685 children had speech defects, 4.5 per cent of them serious. Blanton (1916) in a personal survey of 4862 school children in Madison, Wis., and including only those serious enough to be evident to the casual observer, reported that 5.69 per cent had speech defects with a gradual decrease from lower to higher grades. He reported a pronounced leveling off at the fourth grade and a sharp decline between the seventh and eighth grades, ascribed to large numbers of children with defective speech leaving school at that time.

The relative number of males and females with speech disorders varies according to the age of the subjects and too often from one study to another. The White House Conference (1931) reported 1.9 males to one female for the entire school population. Mills and Streit (1942) found 1.8 boys to one girl in the first three grades and 3.3 boys to one girl above the third grade. In an early study, Blanton (1916) found 1.7 males to one female for an entire school population. All workers report more males than females for all age levels, and more speech defectives, both male and female, in the first three grades of school.

Surveys of speech defects in high school and college populations show wider discrepancies, probably because of more varying standards of what constitutes a speech defect at these ages. Carhart (1939) in a questionnaire survey of 405 Illinois high schools listed as speech defective 23.3 per cent of freshmen, 21.0 per cent of sophomores, 20.0 per cent of juniors, and 17.8 per cent of seniors, with a sex ratio of 1.3 to 1. Evans (1938) found three students or 1.3 per cent of 224 grade 9A students defective in speech, with 92 or 43 per cent showing slovenly and inaccurate pronunciation and enunciation. Morris (1939) reported speech defects in 16.8 per cent of a random sample of 178 high school sophomores in Kansas City.

Blanton (1921) reported that personal examination showed that 18.13 per cent of 2240 members of the freshman class at the University of Wisconsin "were found to be unable to meet the necessities of English Speech." Six per cent of these stuttered, while the remainder exhibited foreign accent, oral inactivity, mispronunciation of *s* or *z,* abnormally rapid or slow speech, or severe vocal defects. In contrast to this, Morley (1952) reported an incidence over a ten-year period at the University of Michigan of 3.85 per cent of speech disorders. The number screened out decreased over the years. Half the cases had articulation defects and one-fourth stuttering defects. There was a sex ratio of 2.1 to 1. Partridge (1945) described 47 per cent of students at Ohio University as having speech defects, but localisms in pronunciation apparently accounted for the bulk of the cases.

It is certain that a college population is highly selected and not representative of the population as a whole, and since the definition of a speech defect in these studies obviously is as individual as the examiner, it would seem desirable to attempt to study speech defects in a more random sample of the adult population. Carhart (1943) reported that 0.1 per cent of draftees in World War I were reported as having defective speech. This varied from 0.23 per cent in the longer-settled states to 0.02 per cent in the recently settled Western states. Of the 0.1 per cent, well over half were rejected for military service. In World War II, Peacher (1945a) has reported that 0.04

per cent of men examined between November, 1940, and February, 1941, were rejected for speech defects. Johnson (1943) estimated that there were five to eight stutterers alone per thousand of the draft-age population, so the percentage of draft rejections cannot be considered indicative of speech defects in the general population.

It is obvious that reports of speech disorders in the general population vary so much that it is necessary to attempt a summary statement which may estimate a median incidence. From kindergarten through fourth-grade level, roughly 12 to 15 per cent of the children have seriously defective speech. In the next four grades, between 4 and 5 per cent are seriously defective. General estimates above the eighth grade are based on highly selected samples and therefore the best guess as to the incidence of speech disorders in persons over 14 years of age would be about the same as for the upper elementary grades—4 to 5 per cent. This statement is justified by studies of specific disorders which show that little or no change takes place in the speech condition after the child has reached 10 to 14 years of age, unless special therapy is offered.

## INCIDENCE OF SPEECH SOUND DEVIATIONS IN INFANTS

Before presenting information about speech defects and speech defectives one should study deviations in the child who does not talk or who is in the early stages of developing speech. These deviations are important because they may be the precursors of speech defects to follow. Many deviations— voice quality, pitch, loudness, duration, body movement, and others—have been studied. However, the ones most extensively studied and the ones probably most highly correlated with speech development are the frequency and variety of production of speech sounds, particularly as they are reported by Irwin and his co-workers.

Deviations of this sort can be measured in infants by counting the number of times sounds are made during any unit of time and also counting the number of different sounds or phonemes produced during the same period. These results can be placed in distributions; the results farthest from the mean being the significant deviations.

Irwin (1946), in studying the oral behavior of infants, has shown that the frequency of production of sounds increased until 30 months of age. Irwin and Chen (1946) found that the variety of phoneme types produced also increased until 30 months of age, at which time the average child presented a speech-sound behavior pattern similar to that of the adult.

In both studies, at each month the frequency of production as well as the variety of phonemes differed considerably from one child to another.

The variations in infant speech sounds indicate that retardation in frequency of production of speech sounds as well as a reduction in the variety probably are related to retarded speech development and perhaps to the emergence of defective speech. Boys are slower to develop speech and have

ABLE 1. Deviant Speech Sound Development Showing Inferior and Median Responses up to 30 Months of Age.*†

| I-MONTHLY AGE GROUP | PHONEME TYPE VARIABILITY AMONG INFANTS | | PHONEME FREQUENCY VARIABILITY AMONG INFANTS | |
|---|---|---|---|---|
| | 10th Percentile | 50th Percentile | 10th Percentile | 50th Percentile |
| 1–2 | 4.8 | 6.9 | 49.9 | 57.7 |
| 3–4 | 6.9 | 10.7 | 53.7 | 66.4 |
| 5–6 | 7.4 | 12.4 | 60.6 | 72.5 |
| 7–8 | 10.9 | 14.4 | 60.4 | 75.1 |
| 9–10 | 10.6 | 15.5 | 65.0 | 76.0 |
| 11–12 | 11.2 | 18.5 | 68.0 | 90.2 |
| 13–14 | 11.9 | 17.8 | 62.9 | 85.9 |
| 15–16 | 14.3 | 19.4 | 68.0 | 91.3 |
| 17–18 | 15.2 | 21.2 | 76.0 | 97.4 |
| 19–20 | 15.9 | 23.0 | 76.3 | 94.1 |
| 21–22 | 16.2 | 23.3 | 77.4 | 102.6 |
| 23–24 | 20.1 | 24.6 | 84.8 | 110.8 |
| 25–26 | 20.6 | 26.6 | 94.8 | 129.5 |
| 27–28 | 18.9 | 26.9 | 103.0 | 132.0 |
| 29–30 | 23.5 | 27.0 | 107.7 | 148.3 |

* Extracted from O. C. Irwin (1947).
† Any child who performs in the region of the 10th percentile may be retarded in speech sound velopment.

greater percentage of speech defects than girls. Irwin and Chen (1946) reorted that boys tended to be inferior to girls after the second year in the riety of speech sounds produced. Spiker (1951) found girls to be significntly superior to boys from the twentieth to thirtieth month in the variety speech sounds produced. Mentally defective children also develop speech ore slowly and have more speech defects than do normal children. Irwin 942) found mental defectives to be inferior in the frequency of production d the variety of speech sounds produced.

Cerebral-palsied children also learn to speak more slowly and have more eech deficiencies. They too were found by Irwin (1952) to be retarded in fancy.

Orphaned children who received a reduced amount of speech stimulation re definitely inferior in both frequency and type of phoneme produced to infants living in their own homes. Thus infants' speech-sound responses ay be highly related to the age at which speech develops as well as to the equacy of the speech which does develop.

Speech pathologists, ever alert to materials of use in making an early agnosis, may find Table 1 helpful. Only the score results of children funcning in the tenth and fiftieth percentiles are presented here. The data, orted by Irwin and Chen (1946), were gathered in the following manner: total of 1622 records was transcribed in the International Phonetic Albet from the spontaneous speech of 95 infants throughout a period of years. Each record consisted of the sounds uttered on 30 breaths.

To use these for diagnostic purposes (see Irwin, 1947), sounds tran-

TABLE 2. Articulation Defects by Grade in School

| Grade | Root (1925)* Questionnaire Per Cents | Reid (1947) (Francis) Personal Survey Per Cents | Mills and Streit (1942) Personal Survey Per Cents | White House Con ference (1931) Questionnaire Number of cases |
|---|---|---|---|---|
| K |      | 27.8 |      |        |
| 1 | 5.70 | 19.3 | 28.9 | 10,217 |
| 2 | 3.60 | 11.5 | 22.2 | 7,745  |
| 3 | 2.50 | 9.0  | 22.1 | 5,745  |
| 4 | 1.04 | 3.1  | 2.1† | 4,375  |
| 5 | 2.70 | 3.6  | 2.1† | 3,364  |
| 6 | 1.01 | 2.1  | 2.1† | 2,612  |
| 7 | .60  | 2.6  |      | 1,241  |
| 8 | 1.00 | 4.7  |      | 839    |
| 9 |      | 2.6  |      |        |
| 10 |     | 6.7  |      |        |
| 11 |     | 2.1  |      |        |
| 12 |     | 4.7  |      |        |

* Lispers and lallers.
† Average for the three grades combined.

scribed from each of 30 breaths should constitute the sample at a given vis
and at least two such visits should be at hand before a diagnosis is made.

The developmental pattern presented in Table 1 can be extended int
the upper age levels, at least for articulation skills, by using the Templi
(1953) and Roe and Milisen (1942) studies.

## INCIDENCE OF ARTICULATION DISORDERS

It is difficult to assess the incidence of articulation disorders. There is
great variation from child to child, from age to age, and from situation
situation. Evaluations may vary from day to day and from examiner
examiner. Errors in articulation may vary from complete omission to su
stitutions to distortions. Reports on incidence, even when they are the res⸣
of carefully planned studies, must be recognized as being subject to co⸣
siderable error.

All children who learn to speak will produce some sounds defectively
the beginning. Speech has not been "learned" when the first word or se⸣
tence is forthcoming. This is just a midpoint in a long process. Templin a⸣
Steer (1939), reporting on nursery school children, said that none of the ⸣
children tested made all sounds correctly in all positions. Roe and Milis⸣
(1942), in a study of the articulation of elementary school children fou⸣
that all of 772 first- and second-grade children tested made at least one err⸣
Not until the third grade were children tested who did not make a sin⸣
error. These studies show the tendency of most people to accept son⸣
speech-sound errors in young children, since no experimenter or clinici⸣
has diagnosed all first- and second-grade children as speech defectives.

In the first grade, from 15 to 20 per cent of the children are likely to lescribed as having defective articulation. There is a marked decrease (Mills nd Streit, 1942; Reid, 1947) in the percentages reported through the first hree or four grades, after which the decline is likely to become small or onexistent. Table 2 illustrates this trend in the columns in which the inci- lence is given in percentages. Apparently, articulation is likely to improve ntil the age of 9 or 10; but after that age, for the most part, misarticulated ounds remain defective unless therapy is provided. The defect is not only kely to remain, but it is also likely to appear to be a more serious handicap; ince most people of the same age will have normal articulation, and better erformance is expected as the child grows older. Thus the high school tudent or the adult who has defective articulation has an entirely different /pe of problem of adjustment from that faced by the first-grader.

The decrease in the percentage of children who are reported as having efective articulation with increase in grade level is strikingly paralleled by ιe decrease in the number of defective sounds per child. According to Roe nd Milisen (1942), the mean number of defective sounds per child (all ιildren in the grades, not just "defective speakers") decreased from 13.30 ι grade one to 9.99 in grade two, 8.85 in grade three, 7.62 in grade four, ,61 in grade five, and 8.01 in grade six. A similar study by Sayler (1949) ιowed only a very small and inconsistent decrease in the mean number of rors per child in grades seven through twelve. In short, there is marked ιprovement in articulatory skills up to and through the fourth grade, at hich time the average child has achieved much of his adult articulatory ιill. In the absence of speech therapy as such, there is likely to be little im- ovement in articulation after the fourth grade.

Age, as indicated by grade in school, is only one of many factors which ust be taken into consideration in the study of defective articulation. Boys nd to develop articulatory skill more slowly than girls. The White House onference report (1931) covering 31 cities showed a sex ratio of 1.58 to 1 county schools and 1.44 to 1 in city schools. Mills and Streit (1942) gave ;ures which showed a sex ratio for the first six grades of 1.9 to 1. Root 925) gave figures for various types of articulation defects which average 7 to 1. Young (1940) gave figures which show a sex ratio of 1.4 to 1. udies by Roe and Milisen (1942) and Saylor (1949) showed a slight but ι statistically significant difference in the mean number of errors per child, ι boys making more errors.

Other factors, such as intelligence, influence the incidence of articulation fects; Loutitt and Halls (1936) found 2.5 times as many children in classes ι subnormals with articulation defects as in the total school population. allin (1926) stated that defects of articulation were "distinctly more preva- ιt among mental defectives." However, as Van Riper (1954) pointed out, e speech problem may contribute to the apparent subnormality. Lima 927) reported that Binet tests of 402 childern wth speech defects (type t specified) in the St. Paul, Minn., schools showed a median I.Q. of 97.7, ll within the normal range. This sample, however, must not be considered random, since it was a school population from which the "uneducable" would have been excluded.

Certain organic disorders, particularly cleft palate and cerebral palsy are frequently associated with articulation disorders. Wolfe (1950) reported that 30 per cent of 50 cases (a random sample from 746 cases between ages of 5 and 20) of cerebral palsy had normal articulation and that of the 70 per cent with inadequate articulation, 40 per cent were due to the cerebral palsy, 4 per cent to other organic causes and 26 per cent were functional Shover (1945) reported that 50 per cent of 3000 cerebral-palsied children were in need of speech therapy. She also reported that in 1000 cleft-palate cleft-lip cases, surgery was in 90 per cent only a partial rehabilitation and speech therapy was necessary.

In the report of the White House Conference (1931) the largest group of the paralytic articulatory cases can probably be ascribed to cerebral palsy They constituted less than 1 per cent of the population of speech defectives The structural articulatory defects, many of which can probably be ascribed to cleft palate, constituted 8.6 per cent of the total speech defects. Pronovost (1951) said that 11.0 per cent of total speech defects were due to cerebral palsy and 1.2 per cent due to cleft palate. Young (1942) reported that of 788 cases of defective speech, 2 per cent were spastic. Johnson and Gardner (1944) estimated that 5000 school children in the United States had defective speech caused by cleft palate and 65,000 caused by cerebral palsy.

Other organic conditions may cause or complicate speech defects, but they are present in much smaller percentages.

## INCIDENCE OF STUTTERING

Definitions of stuttering vary widely, and figures on incidence will vary with the definition used and the method of survey. The question of differentiating between (1) speech deviations involving rhythm and (2) the speech defect of stuttering is beyond the scope of this chapter. However, it is interesting to note that Davis (1939) in a study of repetitions in the speech of 62 young (24 to 62 months) children, found that 16 did not present any syllable repetitions and one boy who was judged a "stutterer" by parents and teacher alike was 12.4 standard deviations beyond the mean of four syllable repetitions per thousand words, with 66 syllable repetitions per thousand word The child (a boy) with next most frequent repetitions of syllables, 3.6 standard deviation from the mean, was considered a "stutterer" by one teacher and was later voluntarily taken to a speech clinic as a stutterer by the mother Templin and Steer (1939), in a study of growth of speech in preschool children, described two boys out of a group of 27 the first semester and two boys out of a group of 24 the second semester as having severe disturbance of rhythm. However, they emphasized that most of the children repeated sounds, syllables, or words, but the frequency and severity of repetition and blocks varied greatly.

TABLE 3. Incidence of Stuttering for the First Eight Grades

| Grade | MILLS AND STREIT (1942) Personal Survey | BURDIN (1940) Questionnaire | ROOT (1916) Questionnaire | BLANTON (1916) Personal Survey Cases | | | WHITE HOUSE CONFERENCE (1931) Questionnaire Cases | | |
|---|---|---|---|---|---|---|---|---|---|
| | % | % | % | BOYS | GIRLS | TOTAL | BOYS | GIRLS | TOTAL |
| K | | | | 1 | 0 | 1 | | | |
| I | 1.5 | .48 | 1.10 | 2 | 0 | 2 | 623 | 203 | 826 |
| II | 4.3 | 1.66 | .70 | 4 | 0 | 4 | 829 | 244 | 1073 |
| III | 2.5 | 1.13 | .60 | 1 | 1 | 2 | 966 | 265 | 1231 |
| IV | 1.1* | 1.59 | 1.80 | 3 | 1 | 4 | 1052 | 253 | 1305 |
| V | 1.1* | | 2.10 | 5 | 2 | 7 | 1172 | 271 | 1443 |
| VI | 1.1* | | 1.60 | 5 | 1 | 6 | 1095 | 255 | 1350 |
| VII | | | 1.30 | 3 | 2 | 5 | 842 | 178 | 1020 |
| VIII | | | .60 | 2 | 1 | 3 | 678 | 177 | 855 |

* Average for the three grades combined.

According to Van Riper (1954), the vast majority of cases of stuttering begin in early childhood, usually between the ages of two and four years.

As shown in Table 3, there seems to be a marked tendency for stuttering to increase between the second and fifth grades and then to decrease again. Note that the columns headed Mills and Streit, Burdin, and Root are percentages of the total enrollment, whereas those headed Blanton and White House Conference are number of cases reported. There is an interesting parallelism in the small group studied personally by Blanton in 1916 and the large number studied by questionnaire by the White House Conference in 1930. The marked increase in cases of stuttering in the middle elementary grades in both reports was largely due to the great increase in incidence of stuttering among boys. The incidence among girls remained relatively constant.

Statistics on the incidence of stuttering among high school students are very inadequate. Morris (1939) reported five boys and one girl in a random sample of 178 sophomores. This would be an incidence of 3 per cent and a sex ratio of 5 to 1. Louttit and Halls (1936) show an incidence in grade nine of .69 per cent, in grade ten of .66 per cent, in grade eleven of .39 per cent and in grade twelve of .41 per cent, with a sex ratio for these grades of 3.3 to 1.

In college students, Blanton (1921) found that 6 per cent of members of the freshman class at the University of Wisconsin stuttered, while Morley (1952) reported figures indicating that approximately 1 per cent of 33,339 students examined at the University of Michigan were stutterers and that boys outnumbered girls 4.3 to 1.

Peacher (1946) reported seeing 77 pre-induction and 37 post-induction stutterers at Brooke and McGuire General Hospitals but gave no figures on actual incidence in the army in World War II. However, Johnson (1943) estimated that there are five to eight stutterers per thousand draft-age men.

Although the ratio of boys to girls always points to more speech defects in boys, this is nowhere more apparent than in stuttering. While the ratio for articulation defects is something less than 2 to 1, for stuttering it varies from 2.2 to 1 (Root, 1925) through 3.9 to 1 (White House Conference, 1931) to 5.3 to 1 (Mills and Streit, 1942). Travis (1931) has reported a range of from 2 to 1 to 10 to 1. In considering these figures, it must be kept in mind that there is a possibility of various factors influencing these ratios Perhaps girls with defective speech are more likely to drop out of school, perhaps they make themselves less conspicuous, perhaps a speech defect in a girl is considered less important. At least until the sex ratios can be more carefully studied, we should consider the possibility of other factors affecting or exaggerating the ratios as reported.

Another factor possibly influencing the incidence of stuttering is intelligence. Lima (1927) reported on the results of Binet testing of 402 children with speech defects. A median I.Q. of 97.7 was found for this group, 122 of whom were stutterers, but no separate figures were given for stutterers Wallin (1926) reported that "stuttering is more prevalent among normal, retarded and backward children than among mental defectives . . . only one of our morons stuttered, while none of the imbeciles stuttered." Travis (1931) gave the following I.Q. distribution of 73 public-school stutterers in Madison, Wis.:

| I. Q.: | 60–69 | 70–79 | 80–89 | 90–99 | 100–109 | 110–119 | 120–129 | 130–139 |
|--------|-------|-------|-------|-------|---------|---------|---------|---------|
| Per Cent: | 1.4 | 2.7 | 12.0 | 19.0 | 37.0 | 16.4 | 8.2 | 1.4 |

However, Louttit (1936) described 3.22 per cent of subnormals as stuttering compared to 0.77 per cent of stutterers in the total school population Williams (1954) reported at a meeting at Indiana University on the results of tests thus far completed on mentally defective persons at the State School for the Retarded at Butlerville, Ind. Twenty-seven of 1700 tested who ranged in age from 14 to 64 years presented severe rhythm problems Seventeen of the 27 persons were definitely diagnosed as stutterers. Root (1925) found a retardation in school progress of 20.65 months for children with thick speech compared with 8.55 months for stutterers. The average for all speech defects was a retardation of 10.49 months. Whether the retardation was caused by the stuttering, by lower intelligence, or whether there was some other relationship is impossible to say on the basis of the available data.

Fruewald (1936) reported that the incoming stutterers at the Ohio State University ranked definitely higher than the general freshman college population Travis (1931) said that "stutterers in the University of Iowa have been distinctly superior to the average college student in intelligence," but attributed this to a selective factor which may keep the less intelligent stutterer from attempting college.

Numerous other factors have been related to the incidence of stuttering Laterality, especially handedness and change of handedness, has been considered (Bryngelson, 1939; Milisen and Johnson, 1936; Orton, 1937; Travis

931; Van Riper, 1954) to have an important relationship to at least some ases of stuttering. However, emphasis on this area has decreased with re-orts (Daniels, 1940; Heltman, 1940; Van Dusen, 1939; Williams, 1952) which presented contrary evidence.

Birth conditions (Milisen and Johnson, 1936), allergy (Card, 1939), bi-ngualism and race (Travis, Johnson, and Shover, 1937), position in family Rotter, 1939), familial incidence (Wepman, 1939), and many other physi-al and environmental conditions can be related to the incidence of stutter-g, but in most cases the relationships are not entirely clear or have limited pplication. The annotated bibliography can be used by the reader who wishes to explore further the relationships of these factors with the inci-ence of stuttering.

## INCIDENCE OF VOICE DISORDERS

Defects of voice were reported in 1.5 per cent of the total group of 4685 lementary-school children studied by Mills and Streit (1942). In the Madi-on, Wis., personal survey (White House Conference, 1931), out of a total f 10,033 children examined, 69 or 0.7 per cent were classified as functional oice cases, 30 or 0.3 per cent as structural voice cases, and one or .01 per ent as paralytic voice cases, giving a total of 1.0 per cent of voice defects the population studied. Pronovost (1951) reported speech defects in 7.8 er cent of the 87,288 individuals tested. Of those having speech defects, .6 per cent were defective in voice; thus about 0.5 per cent of the popula-on tested had voice defects.

Evans (1938) found no cases of defective phonation in 224 students in rade 9A. Morris (1939) reported four boys and one girl with voice defects, n incidence of 2.8 per cent, in a random sample of 178 high school sopho-ores.

Morley (1952) in an examination of 33,339 university students found at 15.04 per cent of the speech defects were in voice, which is an incidence the total number of students of .58 per cent. However, Blanton (1921) und an incidence of voice defects of 4.5 per cent of 2240 members of a reshman university class.

These figures would seem to indicate that approximately 1 per cent of e total population of this country is hampered by defects of voice and at they constitute between 5 and 15 per cent of the defective speech popu-tion.

## INCIDENCE OF LANGUAGE DISTURBANCE INVOLVING
## COMPREHENSION AND EXPRESSION

Speech as a means of communication is used insufficiently or not at all y people who have delayed speech. In addition to the paucity of expression ome persons, such as the deaf, aphasic, mentally defective, and others also have difficulty in comprehending speech. Before the incidence of delayed speech can be studied and reported reliably, it would be necessary to establish norms of language development for children up to eight years of age. Language retardation could then be determined by comparing a child's language development with the norm. The establishment of such a norm would involve many complications which would be most difficult to control, such as (1) obtaining a random sample of children; and (2) obtaining a random sample of speech behavior of each child which would be representative of his over-all language behavior. This would involve creating a natural situation involving parents and other members of an audience in a strictly laboratory type of experiment. As of the present time, no such study has been reported. However, a few studies have been made relating delayed speech to various organic and environmental factors.

Beckey (1942) found retardation in speech to be more common in children with histories of abnormal conditions during pregnancy and birth, in children with poor motor control, in children who had had two or more severe infectious diseases, especially measles, and in children who were in poor physical condition. Boys tended to outnumber girls. From an environmental standpoint, retardation in speech was more common among more isolated children, in children from lower socioeconomic levels, in children who had had severe frights, in children who had had their wants anticipated, and in children with inferior ratings in intelligence. Children with retarded speech tended to substitute gestures for speech. It should be noted that the incidence of delayed speech is 100 per cent among preschool deaf children. Furthermore, it should be noted that large numbers of mentally defective children have delayed speech, although no reliable data can be cited.

Persons studying incidence of aphasia in young children are subject to even more problems than are those who are studying delayed speech. A major stumbling block is the establishment of a criterion which will separate aphasic from nonaphasic language behavior. Without such a criterion, data on incidence of the disorder are quite meaningless. The examiner of these children receives little language behavior upon which to make judgment and little opportunity to compare the child's speech at the time of examination with his speech at other times.

Reports of incidence of aphasia in adults might be more meaningful, since most adults had adequate speech and comprehension before the brain damage which usually preceded their aphasic behavior. However, most groups available for study are not randomly selected. They are usually hospitalized patients. Many aphasics may not have had brain damage and may not, therefore, have needed hospitalization. Furthermore, the individual symptoms which are seemingly so clear-cut in the textbooks can be duplicated thousands of times in the speech of the so-called normal speaker.

With all these reservations, the following data are presented. The enormity of the uncharted field may explain in part the wide variation in the results reported by various experimenters. Young (1942) reported 18 cases

phasia in a total grade and high school enrollment of 9,448, or an incidence
of 0.2 per cent. Morris (1939) reported one case of aphasia in a random
ample of 178 high school sophomores, or an incidence of 0.6 per cent.
Mills and Streit (1942) in their breakdown into type of defect did not men-
ion aphasia. Blanton (1916) included aphasia in the 1.71 per cent of mis-
ellaneous defects. Pronovost (1951) recorded 0.5 per cent incidence of
phasia in the total cases of *speech defects,* which would be about 0.04 per
ent incidence in the total population studied. Childhood aphasia, then, may
e found in between zero per cent and 0.6 per cent of a school population.
since, by its very nature, aphasia is likely to make success in school very
difficult, it is probable that a sizable proportion of "child aphasics" are not
ncluded in the school population.

At upper age limits, there are few figures available on incidence of apha-
ia. Surveys of speech defects on the college level rarely if ever mention
phasia, probably due to the difficulty the aphasic would have with college
vork. Since brain tumors and cerebral hemorrhages may be more common
1 older people and aphasia is not often completely "cured," there are almost
ertainly more aphasics with an increase in age.

Cerebral trauma as a cause of aphasia has received the most attention,
ince such trauma may be caused by injuries in war. Frazier and Ingham
1927) reported that of 200 head-injury cases at a general hospital in World
Var I, language involvement lasting six months or more was seen in 16 cases.

Peacher (1945) described patients seen at Brooke General Hospital from
May 7, 1943, to September 1, 1944. Admission was not on the basis of
anguage difficulties alone, but for medical or surgical reasons. Of 120 pa-
ents with speech problems, 32 were dysphasic; 18 from craniocerebral
raumata, seven from cerebrovascular disease, six in association with brain
amor, and one following acute meningo-encephalitis.

A summary statement of the incidence of language disturbances, espe-
ially involving delayed speech and aphasia, would be quite meaningless.
his area of defective communication must be more carefully described
nd studied before incidence reports will be more than "best guesses."

The incidence of communication problems involving speech deviations,
efects, and defectives needs to be more carefully studied. At present, better
sting methods are available, more people are well trained, and therapy pro-
rams are well established, all of which should permit the establishment of
ong-term studies which could control more of the variables. Until these
udies are completed, we must continue to quote incidence data as "ap-
roximations."

## BIBLIOGRAPHY

ACKUS, O. L. 1938. Incidence of stuttering among the deaf. *Ann. Otol.,* etc.,
St. Louis, 47, 632–635. Study found 55 stutterers in schools for the deaf,
six of them congenitally deaf.
ECKEY, R. E. 1942. A study of certain factors related to retardation of speech.
*J. Speech Disorders,* 7, 223–249. A clinical analysis of 50 delayed speech

cases, compared with 50 control cases, showed birth complications, infec
tious diseases (especially measles), slow physical growth, inferior ratings i
intelligence, lower socioeconomic status, anticipation of wants of child
substitution of gestures for speech, were all related to retardation of speech

BENDER, J. F. 1939. The organization and guiding principles of the New Yor
City survey of the speech handicapped child conducted Oct., 1939-June
1940. *J. Speech Disorders*, 5, 357–362. Summarized 13 other surveys, bu
gave no results for the New York survey.

BERRY, M. F. 1939. A study of the medical histories of stuttering children. *Speec
Monogr.*, 5, 97–114.

———— 1949. Lingual anomalies associated with palatal clefts. *J. Speech Hear
ing Disorders*, 14, 359–362. Examination showed 65 per cent of cleft
palate children referred to a college speech center lacked requisite mobilit
and muscular co-ordination of the tongue.

———— and EISENSON, J. 1942. The defective in speech. New York: F. S. Crofts

———— 1956. Speech disorders. New York: Appleton-Century-Crofts.

BILTO, E. W. 1941. A comparative study of certain physical abilities of childre
with speech defects and children with normal speech. *J. Speech Disorders*
6, 187–203. Critical analysis of 90 children with stuttering and defectiv
articulation showed them to be inferior as a group in certain large-muscl
abilities.

BLANTON, S. 1916. A survey of speech defects. *J. educ. Psychol.*, 7, 581–592
Examination of 4862 Wisconsin school children showed that 5.69 per cen
had speech defects serious enough to be evident to a casual observer. Tabu
lations given by sex, grade, and type of defect.

———— 1921. Speech defects in school children. *Ment. Hyg.*, 5, 820–827. Ex
amination of 1400 members of the freshman class at the University o
Wisconsin showed that 18.13 per cent were ". . . unable to meet the neces
sities of English Speech." The number with various types of defects wa
given.

BRYNGELSON, B. 1939. A study of laterality of stutterers and normal speaker
*J. Speech Disorders*, 4, 231–234. A comparison of 152 stutterers and 15
normal speakers showed much more ambidexterity and shift of handednes
among the stutterers.

BULLEN, A. K. 1945. A cross-cultural approach to the problem of stuttering
*Child Develm.*, 16, 1–88.

BURDIN, L. G. 1940. A survey of speech defectives in the Indianapolis primar
grades. *J. Speech Disorders*, 5, 247–258. Survey indicated that 2.94 per cei
of the children in the first four grades had serious speech defects.

CAMP, P. B. 1923. Survey of speech defects. *J. Speech Educ.*, 11, 280–283.

CARD, R. E. 1939. A study of allergy in relation to stuttering. *J. Speech Di
orders*, 4, 223–230. Case histories in this study showed all of 40 stuttere
tested gave positive reactions to intradermal tests. Severity of stuttering wa
in direct proportion to percentage of reactions and/or their severity.

CARHART, R. 1939. A survey of speech defects in Illinois high schools. *J. Speec
Disorders*, 4, 61–70. High school teachers judged 20.8 per cent of 144,57
students as in need of speech rehabilitation.

———— 1943. Some notes on official statistics of speech disorders encountere
during World War I. *J. Speech Disorders*, 8, 97–107. Only 0.1 per cent
draftees were reported as having defective speech. This varied from 0.2
per cent in the longer settled states to 0.02 per cent in the recently settle
western states.

CARRELL, J. A. 1936. A comparative study of speech defective children. *Arc
Speech*, 1 (3), 179–203.

CHEN, H. P., and IRWIN, O. C. 1946. Infant speech vowel and consonant types. *J. Speech Disorders*, 11, 27–29. During the first year the mean number of vowels exceeded the consonants, then consonants began to exceed vowels. At 2.5 years, infants exhibited practically the full complement of vowel sounds, but only two-thirds of the consonants.

DANIELS, E. M. 1940. An analysis of the relation between handedness and stuttering with special reference to the Orton-Travis theory of cerebral dominance. *J. Speech Disorders*, 5, 309–326. A survey of 1594 university students and interview and further testing of 154 stutterers, left-handed persons, ambidextrous persons, and persons whose handedness had been shifted, showed little or no relationship between handedness and stuttering.

DAVIS, D. M. 1939. The relation of repetitions in the speech of young children to certain measures of language maturity and situational factors. *J. Speech Disorders*, 4, 303–318. Of a group of 62 preschool children, one boy was considered a stutterer by parents and teachers alike, and another boy who was called a stutterer by one teacher was later taken to a speech clinic as a stutterer by the mother.

DAVIS, I. P. 1937. A survey of speech defects in Akron Public Schools. Unpublished report to Board of Education, Akron, Ohio. Six per cent of the children were definitely handicapped, and only 4 per cent had perfect speech.

EVANS, D. R. 1938. Report of a survey in grade 9A. *Quart. J. Speech*, 24, 83–90. Personal examination of 224 students disclosed three with defective speech, none with defective phonation, and 92 students or 41 per cent with slovenly and inaccurate pronunciation and enunciation.

EVANS, M. F. 1947. Problems in cerebral palsy. *J. Speech Disorders*, 12, 87–103. Different kinds of speech defects are associated with the three general types of cerebral palsy. The ataxic are not likely to have speech disturbances, the athetoid has no consistent pattern of defect, and the spastic has consistent errors due to spastic muscles in the speech mechanism.

FRAZIER, C. H., and INGHAM, S. D. 1927. Neurological aspects of gunshot wounds of the head. Medical department of the U. S. Army in World War I. Washington, D. C., Government Printing Office. 11, 795–803. In 200 head-injury cases in World War I, residual language involvement remaining six months or more, post-injury, was seen in 16 cases.

GRUEWALD, E. 1936. Intelligence rating of severe college stutterers compared with that of others entering universities. *J. Speech Disorders*, 1, 47–52. The stutterers studied ranked higher in intelligence than the incoming freshman population.

GRATKE, J. M. 1947. Speech problems of the cerebral-palsied. *J. Speech Disorders*, 12, 129–134. Describes five levels of speech problems, those entirely apart from the physical handicap of cerebral palsy, those associated with spasticity, the athetoid and ataxic which are inconsistent, children with lack of cerebral dominance and aphasia, and the feebleminded.

HAWK, E. A. 1945. A survey and critical analysis of speech needs in the elementary schools of an Ohio city of 15,000 population with a suggested remedial program in speech. Unpublished Doctor's Thesis. Ohio State Univ. Individual diagnosis of 1200 children showed that 114 or 9.5 per cent had speech defects. Of these, 44 might have been helped by a classroom teacher who had some training in remedial work.

HAWK, S. S. 1936. Speech defects in handicapped children. *J. Speech Disorders*, 1, 101–106. The median I.Q. of orthopedically handicapped speech defectives was between 87 and 100.

HELTMAN, H. J. 1940. Contradictory evidence in handedness and stuttering. *J.*

*Speech Disorders*, 5, 327–331. Little evidence relating laterality to stuttering.

HENDERSON, F. 1940. The incidence of cleft palate in Hawaii. *J. Speech Disorders*, 5, 285–287. Compares incidence in Hawaii—1.98, Wisconsin—1.09
New Jersey—0.48 per thousand live births.

HENDERSON, P. 1947. The incidence of stammering and speech defects in schoo
children. *Monogr. Bull., Minn. Hlth. and Emerg. Publ. Hlth. Lab. Serv.*, 6
102–105. A study of a partly industrial and partly residential county
borough, with a school population of between 13,000 and 14,000, of whom
77 were stammerers, 175 had defective articulation, and 13 had cleft-palate
speech.

HENRIKSON, E. 1945. A semantic study of identification of speech defects. *J
Speech Disorders*, 10, 169–172. Beginning students recognized defects or
different levels (semantically speaking).

HILL, H. 1944a. Stuttering: I. A critical review and evaluation of biochemica
investigations. *J. Speech Disorders*, 9, 245–261. "No findings warrant any
assumption of special metabolic or chemical agents which are causal."

———— 1944b. Stuttering: II. A review and integration of physiological data. *J
Speech Disorders*, 9, 289–324. The basic mechanism of stuttering was considered to be the contraction pattern of shock, startle, or surprise, a universa
emotional reaction.

HOOD, P. N., SHANK, K. H., and WILLIAMSON, D. B. 1948. Environmental fac
tors in relation to the speech of cerebral-palsied children. *J. Speech Hearing
Disorders*, 13, 325–331. A discrepancy has been noted by many worker
between the extent and severity of the cerebral palsy and the severity of the
speech problem.

INGRAM, C. P., PINTNER, R., and STINCHFIELD-HAWK, S. 1941. The auditorially
and the speech handicapped. *Rev. educ. Res.*, 11, 297–314.

IRWIN, O. C. 1942. Developmental status of speech sounds in ten feebleminded
children. *Child Develpm.*, 13, 22–39.

———— 1946. Development of speech during infancy: curve of phonemic fre
quencies. *J. exp. Psychol.*, 37, 187–193.

———— 1947. Infant speech variability and the problem of diagnosis. *J. Speec
Disorders*, 12, 287–289.

———— 1952. Speech development in the young child: 2. Some factors related t
the speech development of the infant and young child. *J. Speech Hearin
Disorders*, 17, 269–279.

———— and CHEN, H. P. 1946. Development of speech during infancy: curv
of phonemic types. *J. exp. Psychol.*, 36, 431–436.

IRWIN, R. B. 1948. Ohio looks ahead in speech and hearing therapy. *J. Speec
Hearing Disorders*, 13, 55–60. Approximately 6000 Cleveland childre
from kindergarten to grade six were tested individually by speech therapist
Ten per cent were found to be defective in speech—stuttering, articulatior
aphasia, or voice. This did not include those who could make sounds cor
rectly after a few stimulations. Only 7.7 per cent of the children abov
kindergarten had speech defects.

———— 1949. Speech and hearing therapy in the public schools of Ohio. *J. Speec
Hearing Disorders*, 14, 63–68. Four per cent of the school population c
certain areas were receiving speech therapy.

JOHNSON, W. 1942. The Iowa remedial education program: summary repor
Iowa City, Iowa: Child Welfare Research Station. About 10 per cent c
approximately 30,000 individually tested school children were judged t
have defective speech. Articulation defects were found in 5.7 per cen
stuttering in 0.7 per cent and voice problems in 3.6 per cent.

———— 1943. The status of speech defectives in military service. *Quart. J. Speech,* 29, 131–136. From November, 1940, to February, 1941, .04 per thousand men were rejected by induction boards for speech defects. An estimate of five to eight stutterers, alone, per thousand of the draft-age population would indicate that the rate of rejections is not a good measure of the incidence of speech defects in that population.

JOHNSON, W., BROWN, S., CURTIS, J., EDNEY, C., and KEASTER, J. 1948. Speech handicapped school children. New York: Harper.

JOHNSON, W., and GARDNER, W. 1944. The auditorially and speech handicapped. *Rev. educ. Res.,* 14, 241–248. A review of surveys with a good bibliography.

KRANTZ, H. C., and HENDERSON, F. M. 1947. Relationship between maternal ancestry and incidence of cleft palate. *J. Speech Disorders,* 12, 267–278. A tendency toward production of cleft-palate children was positively correlated with the number and recency of fusion of color fractions in the maternal ancestry.

KREBIEL, T. E. 1941. Speech sounds of infants in the fourth, fifth and sixth months. Unpublished Master's Thesis. State University of Iowa. Includes frequency and percentage of frequency of each element, and age and sex differences.

LARR, A. 1944. A county speech and hearing conservation program. *J. Speech Disorders,* 9, 147–151. A description of speech survey.

LIMA, M. 1927. Speech defects in school children. *Ment. Hyg.,* 11, 795–803. Binet tests of Minnesota school children with speech defects showed a median I.Q. for 402 pupils of 97.7.

LOUTTIT, C. M. 1936. Clinical pyschology. New York: Harper.

———— and HALLS, E. C. 1936. Survey of speech defects among public school children of Indiana. *J. Speech Disorders,* 1, 73–80. A questionnaire study covering 199,839 children, 3.7 per cent of whom were reported to be defective in speech. Figures were given by grade, sex, type of defect, city-county schools, race, and for subnormals.

McCURRY, W. H., and IRWIN, O. C. 1953. A study of word approximations in the spontaneous speech of infants. *J. Speech Hearing Disorders,* 18, 133–139. There was a significant increase in the number of approximations between the tenth age level (19 and 20 months) and the eleventh age level (21 and 22 months), but no increase in the number of correct pronunciations, and no significant sex differences.

McDOWELL, E. D. 1928. Educational and emotional adjustments of stuttering children. *Teach. Coll. Contr. Educ.,* No. 314. New York: Teachers College, Columbia Univ.

METRAUX, R. W. 1950. Speech profiles of the preschool child 18 to 54 months. *J. Speech Hearing Disorders,* 15, 37–53. A composite view of the speech of the child at seven age levels based on observation of 207 children.

MIDCENTURY WHITE HOUSE CONFERENCE. 1952. Speech disorders and speech correction. *J. Speech Hearing Disorders,* 17, 129–137. Estimated incidence of speech defects among children between 5 and 21 years as 5.0 per cent: functional articulatory—3.0 per cent; stuttering—0.7 per cent; voice—0.2 per cent; retarded speech—0.3 per cent; impaired hearing (with speech defect)—0.5 per cent.

MILISEN, R., and JOHNSON, W. 1936. A comparative study of stutterers, former stutterers and normal speakers whose handedness has been changed. *Arch. Speech,* 1, 61–86.

MILLS, A., and STREIT, H. 1942. Report of a speech survey, Holyoke, Massachusetts. *J. Speech Disorders,* 7, 161–167. Individual testing of all children in the first three grades, with referrals from other grades and some general classroom checks, showed that 4.5 per cent of the total school enrollment had serious speech defects. Data given by sex, grade, and type of defect

MONCUR, J. P. 1950. Environmental factors differentiating stuttering children from nonstuttering children. *Speech Monogr.*, 18, 131–132.

MORLEY, D. E. 1952. A ten-year survey of speech disorders among university students. *J. Speech Hearing Disorders*, 17, 25–31.

MORRIS, D. W. 1939a. A survey of speech defects in Central High School, Kansas City, Missouri. *Quart. J. Speech*, 25, 262–269. Out of a random sample of 178 sophomores, 30 or 17 per cent were reported as defective in speech

——— 1939b. The speech survey. *J. Speech Disorders*, 4, 195–198. A description of methods (questionnaire and personal survey) and discussion of results of earlier surveys.

MORRISON, C. 1914. Speech defects in young children. *Psychol. Clinic*, 8, 138–142.

ORTON, S. 1937. Reading, writing and speech problems in children. New York: Norton.

PALMER, M. F., and GILLETT, A. M. 1938. Sex differences in the cardiac rhythms of stutterers. *J. Speech Disorders*, 3, 3–12.

PARTRIDGE, L. 1945. Dyslalias of Southern Ohio. *J. Speech Disorders*, 10, 249–250. Speech defects were found in 47 per cent of students at Ohio University, but were mostly localisms in pronunciation.

PEACHER, W. G. 1945a. Speech disorders in World War II. *J. Speech Disorders* 10, 155–161. Between November, 1940, and February, 1941, 0.04 per cent of men examined were rejected by draft boards for speech defects.

——— 1945b. Speech disorders in World War II: III. Dysarthria. *J. Speech Disorders*, 10, 287–291. Dysarthria constituted 25.31 per cent of all patients with speech defects studied at Brooke General Hospital.

——— 1945c. Speech disorders in World War II: II. *J. nerv. ment. Dis.*, 102 165–171.

——— 1946. Speech disorders in World War II: VIII. Stuttering. *J. Speech Disorders*, 11, 303–308. At Brooke and McGuire General Hospitals, 77 pre induction and 37 post-induction stutterers were seen.

PHAIR, G. M. 1947. The Wisconsin cleft palate program. *J. Speech Disorders*, 21 410–414.

PINTNER, R., EISENSON, J., and STANTON, M. 1941. Psychology of the physically handicapped. New York: Appleton-Century-Crofts.

POOLE, I. 1934. Genetic development of consonant sounds in speech. *Elem Eng. Rev.*, 2, 159–161.

PRONOVOST, W. 1951. A survey of services for the speech and hearing handicapped in New England. *J. Speech Hearing Disorders*, 16, 148–156. A questionnaire survey of 631 institutions in New England. Tables show type of institutions, types of services, training of therapists, distribution of speech and hearing handicaps, etc.

REID, G. 1947. The efficacy of speech re-education of functional articulatory defectives in the elementary school. *J. Speech Disorders*, 12, 301–313. Reviews studies of articulation defects and gives results of a survey of Iowa City, Iowa, by J. T. Francis, in percentage of cases of functional oral inaccuracy from grade 1 to grade 12.

ROE, V., and MILISEN, R. 1942. The effect of maturation upon defective articulation in the elementary grades. *J. Speech Disorders*, 7, 37–56.

ROGERS, J. F. 1931. The speech-defective school child. Bulletin No. 7. Office of Education, Washington, D. C.

ROOT, A. R. 1925. A survey of speech defectives in the public elementary schools of South Dakota. *Elem. Sch. J.*, 26, 531–541. A questionnaire study cover ing 14,072 pupils which gives information by grade, sex, type of defect, and extent of school retardation. Speech defects were reported for 6.3 per cent.

ROTTER, J. 1939. Studies in the psychology of stuttering, XI. Stuttering in relation to position in the family. *J. Speech Disorders*, 4, 143–148. Significantly more *only* and fewer *middle* children were found among 522 cases of stuttering as compared with a presumably nonstuttering population.

RUTHERFORD, B. 1938. Speech re-education for the birth injured. *J. Speech Disorders*, 3, 199–206. A comparison of spastics with and without speech defects.

——— 1944. A comparative study of loudness, pitch, rate, rhythm, and quality of the speech of children handicapped by cerebral palsy. *J. Speech Disorders*, 9, 263–271. There is no sharply defined "spastic speech," although the range of individual differences is wider and there are more extremes in the cerebral-palsied than in the noncerebral-palsied group.

SAYLER, H. K. 1949. The effect of maturation upon defective articulation in grades seven through twelve. *J. Speech Hearing Disorders*, 14, 202–207. Showed only a slight reduction in sound errors from grade six through grade twelve, in the 1998 pupils tested.

SCHUELL, H. M. 1946. Sex differences in relation to stuttering: Part I. *J. Speech Disorders*, 11, 277–298. The male child, whose physical, social and language development proceeds at a slower rate than that of the female, encounters more unequal competition and consequently more frustrations.

——— 1947. Sex differences in relation to stuttering: Part II. *J. Speech Disorders*, 12, 23–38. Boys encounter more conflict and experience more insecurity than girls.

SHOVER, J. 1945. Illinois program for speech and hearing. *J. Speech Disorders*, 10, 117–122. Of 1000 cleft-palate, cleft-lip cases, surgery was in 90 per cent only a partial rehabilitation and speech therapy was necessary. Of 3000 cerebral-palsied children, 50 per cent were in need of speech therapy.

SNIDECOR, J. C. 1948. The speech correctionist on the cerebral-palsy team. *J. Speech Hearing Disorders*, 13, 67–70. Speech re-education is needed by 60 to 70 per cent.

SPADINO, E. J. 1941. Writing and laterality characteristics of stuttering children. *Teach. Coll. Contr. Educ.*, No. 837. New York: Teachers College, Columbia Univ. There were few, if any, differences between stutterers and nonstutterers.

SPIKER, C. C. 1951. An empirical study of factors associated with certain indices of speech sounds of young children. Unpublished Doctor's Dissertation. State University of Iowa.

STINCHFIELD, S. 1925. The speech of 500 freshman college women. *J. appl. Psychol.*, 9, 109–121.

SULLIVAN, E. M. 1944. Auditory acuity and its relation to defective speech. *J. Speech Disorders*, 9, 127–130. Hearing loss was found in 26 per cent of stutterers and 21 per cent of articulatory cases, in a Minnesota school population of 25,708.

SUYDAM, V. 1948. Speech survey methods in public schools. *J. Speech Disorders*, 13, 51–54. Questionnaire sent to correctionists in eight Midwestern states showed that 75 per cent used speech surveys either alone or in combination with teacher referrals, and 24 per cent used teacher referrals. Criteria were variable and subjective.

TEMPLIN, M. 1947. Spontaneous versus imitated verbalization in testing articulation in preschool children. *J. Speech Disorders*, 12, 293–300.

——— 1953. Norms on a screening test of articulation for ages three through eight. *J. Speech Hearing Disorders*, 18, 323–331.

———— and STEER, M. 1939. Studies of growth of speech in pre-school children. *J. Speech Disorders*, 4, 71–77. In none of 93 tests were all sounds correct in all positions, but a few had all vowels and diphthongs correct.

TRAVIS, L. 1931. Speech pathology. New York: D. Appleton.

————, JOHNSON, W., and SHOVER, J. 1937. The relation of bilingualism to stuttering. *J. Speech Disorders*, 2, 185–189. Significantly more stutterers were found among the bilinguals, but such factors as economic insecurity and emotional instability in many foreign homes must be considered.

VAN DUSEN, C. 1939. A laterality study of nonstutterers and stutterers. *J. Speech Disorders*, 4, 261–265. Little significant difference was found in this questionnaire study of 40 stutterers and 40 nonstutterers.

VAN RIPER, C. 1954. Speech correction: principles and methods (3rd ed.). New York: Prentice-Hall.

VOELKER, C. H. 1944. A preliminary investigation for a normative study of fluency; a clinical index to the severity of stuttering. *Amer. J. Orthopsychiat.*, 14, 285–294.

WALLIN, J. E. W. 1916. A census of speech defectives among 89,057 public school pupils. *Sch. and Soc.*, 3, 213–216. Speech defects were found in 2.8 per cent of the total enrollment and in 9.4 per cent of the dextrosinistrals.

———— 1926. Speech defective children in a large school. *Bull.* XXV, No. 4, Miami Univ., Oxford, Ohio. Stuttering was ". . . more prevalent among normal, retarded and backward children than among mental defectives. . . . only one of our morons stuttered, while none of the imbeciles stuttered." Defects of articulation were ". . . distinctly more prevalent among mental defectives."

WEISS, D. A. 1948. Organic lesions leading to speech disorders. *Nerv. Child*, 7, 29–37.

WELLS, C. G. 1945. Expanding state speech correction services. *J. Speech Disorders*, 10, 123–128.

WEPMAN, J. 1939. Familial incidence in stammering. *J. Speech Disorders*, 4, 199–204. Stammerers do tend to appear more frequently in the families of stammerers.

WEST, N. B. 1939. The heredity of stuttering. *Quart. J. Speech*, 25, 23–30.

WEST, R., KENNEDY, L., and CARR, A. 1947. The rehabilitation of speech (rev. ed.). New York: Harper.

White House Conference on Child Health and Protection. Special education. 1931. New York: Century.

WILLIAMS, D. 1952. An evaluation of masseter muscle action potentials in stuttering and non-stuttered speech. Unpublished Doctor's Dissertation. State University of Iowa.

WOLFE, W. G. 1950. A comprehensive evaluation of fifty cases of cerebral palsy. *J. Speech Hearing Disorders*, 15, 234–251. In a random sample of 50 cases from a group of 746 cases, 30 per cent had normal articulation and 70 per cent inadequate articulation. Of this 70 per cent, 40 per cent were due to cerebral palsy, four per cent to other organic factors, and 26 per cent were functional.

YOUNG, J. A. 1940. Speech rehabilitation in rural schools of Waukesha County, Wisconsin. *J. Speech Disorders*, 5, 25–28. Out of an enrollment of 9553 there were 488 speech cases, or an incidence of 5 per cent.

———— 1942. A city and county speech re-education program. *J. Speech Disorders*, 7, 51–56. Out of a total enrollment of 9448 in the public and parochial schools, 788 or 8.3 per cent were voice cases.

CHAPTER 8

# METHODS OF EVALUATION AND DIAGNOSIS OF SPEECH DISORDERS

● *Robert Milisen, Ph.D.*

A CHAPTER PRESENTING METHODS of examination to use in diagnosing speech disorders might ideally treat the diagnostic methods designed for each therapeutic approach to each speech disorder. Sources describing such detailed testing procedures will be given, but the methods will not be described in this chapter since they have been adequately reported elsewhere in this book. Also, only those testing methods will be described which are directly related to speech therapy.

The classification of speech disorders in this chapter is based entirely upon a description of oral communication behavior, the dysfunctions of which involve (1) comprehension of speech, and (2) expression through speech. The latter may be defective due to (*a*) unavailability of language as a tool of communication, and (*b*) unacceptable pattern of speech used in oral communication.

Many speech disorders seem to be unrelated because each has a separate name and usually a separate examination and diagnostic procedure. In this chapter, the major disorders of speech and the methods of examination and diagnosis are found in a descriptive framework of communication in which the skills of language as well as the limitations are represented. The classifications are as follows:

1. Communication which involves no comprehension of, or expression through, oral language.

2. Communication which involves comprehension of, but little or no expression through, oral language.

3. Communication which involves deteriorated comprehension and/or expression through oral language.

4. Communication which involves comprehension of, and expression

though, oral language with the pattern of expression being unacceptable to the listener and/or the speaker.

The speech examiner should observe speech behavior and report it accurately. In order to do this, he needs a classification of speech disorders which will enable him to record his observations in an unbiased manner without reading into the observations conditions that are not present. The above classification of speech disorders is designed for this purpose.

Once the examiner has determined the nature of the disorder, he should seek to describe it more thoroughly, to determine the conditions which brought about the disorder as well as those which may cause it to be maintained.

Many factors may precipitate these dysfunctions of oral language. A single dysfunction is likely to involve not one but a number of precipitating factors. This is important in diagnosis, since to oversimplify the condition and to see it through too narrow a perspective can only result in defective therapy.

The precipitating factors can be divided into two groups—those involving the participation of the environment, and those involving the physical inadequacy of the client. Many persons have language disorders which have no apparent physical basis, but one seldom if ever finds a person who has a language disorder which has persisted over a period of time and which is *entirely* a function of the physical disability. (Exceptions are the very few persons who are totally paralyzed or who are brain-damaged to the extent of practical decortication.)

In order to understand the subdivisions of environmental behavior which help to precipitate oral language disorders, language must be accepted as a form of learned behavior. As such, it is obviously necessary that the child have the co-operation of the environment if he is to become capable of comprehending and using speech. Environment can adversely affect the development of the skill or interfere with the language skill after it has been established.

The following are some of the *environmental precipitants* which contribute to the development of language dysfunction:

1. Failure to associate the care of the infant with the noises and movements which he makes during early infancy. This slows down the development of a communication attitude.

2. Failure to reinforce the infant's vocal play sounds. This results in a reduction in the number and skill of oral movements developed by the infant.

3. Failure to accompany care of the infant with verbal output. This failure to talk to the infant reduces its comprehension of speech, since comprehension will come only through the association of speech with meaningful behavior.

4. Failure to provide, for imitation, sounds which are new to the infant. Thus, a skill in producing new sounds is not developed and practice in making sounds is reduced.

5. Failure to comprehend, accept, and positively reinforce the first speech attempts. This is likely to result in a refusal of the infant to use speech as a medium of expression.

6. Overacceptance and encouragement of pantomime as a tool of expression. This encourages the substitution of gestures as a means of communication for speech since in the beginning gestures and pantomime are easier for the infant to use.

7. Acceptance and reinforcement of infantile speech behavior, which will result in the maintenance of this type of behavior.

8. Undue positive reinforcement of irrelevant conditions associated by chance with the speech act. This results in the maintenance of this undesirable behavior.

9. Undue penalty associated with the speech act. This may cause the individual to withdraw from oral communication even though the medium is well established.

10. In addition, in some cases there may be a generalized dearth of reinforcement of communication and other learned behavior. There may be so little motivation to learn and so little reinforcement of success that the child, in addition to being seriously deficient in language, is seriously deficient in most other skills and has in fact a "learned mental deficiency."

The physical condition of the child also presents many limitations, hereafter called physical precipitants, to the acquisition of oral language; first, because comprehension and/or movements of expression may be more difficult and, second, because of the effect these limitations may have on the environment which may not try to stimulate the development of oral language for the child.

1. Physical-precipitant sensory disabilities, such as audition, are likely to implement the emergence of environmental precipitants 2–6 which limit the development of language. Other sensory disturbances, visual, tactile, and so on, may reduce the effectiveness of stimulation of the infant by the environment during the language-learning period.

2. Physical-precipitant motor disabilities limiting the co-ordination of movement and also the ability to achieve precise postures of the "speech mechanism" may implement the emergence of environmental precipitants 2, 4, and 5.

3. Physical precipitant involving damage to the brain, especially the association areas, may be an important deterrent to language development in infants. However, the relationship, insofar as infants are concerned, has not been well established and can therefore only be included in a most hypothetical manner. On the other hand, brain damage in adults who have acquired speech is frequently followed by partial or complete language deterioration. Clinical evidence indicates, however, that the deterioration is not purely a function of the brain damage but is also contributed to by environmental precipitants 5, 6, and 9.

4. Physical precipitants involving ill-health during infancy and childhood

may not only reduce the child's physical ability to perform communication acts but also may elicit environmental precipitants 1–7 and 10, which affect adversely the environment's efforts to teach communication.

In order to make the act of distinguishing one precipitating factor from another simpler, the terms *environmental precipitant 1, environmental precipitant 2,* and so on to 10; and *physical precipitant 1, physical precipitant 2, physical precipitant 3,* and *physical precipitant 4* will be used.

## THE EXAMINATION

When a client is admitted for examination, the first problem is to determine in general the type of disorder so that appropriate diagnostic tests can be administered. As a rule, the type of speech disorder can be quickly identified by the skilled examiner, especially if the case history verifies his observations.

Frequently only one member of the family in addition to the child is present during the first interview; therefore, it is essential that efforts be made to obtain through correspondence and other means additional information about the client. A simple way of obtaining this information is by sending brief mimeographed forms to the family, the physician, and the school to be returned before the first interview. These three sources are among the most valuable, but information from other sources such as hospitals, social agencies, guidance centers, churches, should be utilized whenever available. Sample forms which can be used are shown at the end of this chapter. Another valuable source of information is the autobiography, which can be used as a supplement to the case history when dealing with older persons, especially those who have severe disorders and must anticipate a prolonged period of therapy. Usually, the examiner must give some supervision, but he must be careful that the supervision is suggestive in a way that stimulates the person to write expansively. Such suggestions as the following may create a permissive situation which will enable the person to write his thoughts without fear of penalty.

"We need to know as much about you as possible because the better we know you the better we can help you. If you will just think of your life as a story and begin to write about it, you will find it interesting and so will we. Don't feel that you must tell us what caused your difficulty; simply tell us what you know about yourself. No detail in your life is too small or uninteresting for us. You have lived a number of years and had a lot of experiences and thought a lot of thoughts; so, you will probably find that fifty pages is none too much. Don't worry about your writing, grammar, or spelling; we are interested in you—not how pretty the paper looks."

Occasionally, the autobiography will be written in a brief outline form and must be filled in; however, most people enjoy writing about their lives if they believe the examiner is really interested and friendly. Once the autobiography has been finished, the examiner can always ask for additional information if some area of the person's life has been excluded.

When beginning the study of a child, one may observe him first as he interrelates with other members of his family. The tester should direct attention briefly to the adults but should not talk about the child. Some friendly reference should then be directed toward the child, by reacting to his clothes or a new toy, or mentioning what a strong boy he is. An effort must be made to direct his attention to pleasant, real-life activities. Under no circumstances should attention be directed to his speech, mouth, or ears, or any other structure or bodily action which may have been a source of punishment, shame, or anxiety.

If, after a reasonable period of time, the child does not attend to the examiner, it may be wise to turn from the child to others in the room so as to give the child no attention. Presently, the child may insert himself into the situation and demand some attention. Attention should be given the child only after he shows some desire to co-operate. If the child withdraws from the examiner and from the situation, it may be necessary to transfer him to another examiner in another room (play room if available) and, if possible, without the presence of the parents.

Observations made of the child in his home are of course most desirable but are usually impracticable. Observation on a playground or in a room with other children will be most instructive.

During these first observations, information should be gained about the following:

1. General physical behavior and maturity.
2. General physical appearance and his reaction and the reaction of the parents to his appearance.
3. Adjustment of the child in the presence of parents, friends, and strangers when no speech is required.
4. Adjustment of the child while performing guided speech activities in the presence of the same people.
5. Adjustment and general behavior of the parents or others who care for the child while the child is the center of attention and while he is not the center of attention, while he is talking and while he is performing tests. Adjustmental behavior of the parent should also be observed while the child is not in the room.
6. The kinds of interrelationships between the child and his parents.
   *a.* Attitude of parents toward child.
   *b.* Attitude of child toward parents.
   *c.* Methods of control and discipline.
   *d.* Child's reaction to control and discipline.

Observations of this sort should provide a descriptive picture of the child and his behavior which is far superior to one gained through either the "mail-order history" or the personal-interview history. Actually, the personal interview should provide reasons for behavior which was observed, and it is well to put off the history-taking until some observations have been completed.

The "mail-order histories" should be studied before the child is observed, since they prepare the examiner, to some degree, before he meets the child and the parents; but the history obtained by personal interview is in most respects far superior. An excellent example of such a psychodiagnostic blank is reported by Louttit (1947). The personal interview allows the examiner to:

1. Evaluate responses immediately for important clues which should be followed up.
2. Help ease the pain when unpleasant personal matters are discussed.
3. Check answers which are unclear, incomplete, or of doubtful accuracy.
4. Relieve the parents of some anxiety or guilt feelings about some of their past behavior toward the child. At the same time the examiner is able to observe and record the nature of the parental reactions.
5. Establish a friendly rapport between the clinic, school, or agency, and the family.
6. Above all, to follow up the leads which come from the observation period. In this regard, the case history should be considered an extension of the observation period as far back as the birth of the child. (These "observations," however, would not have been made and reported by a clinically trained person.)

By this time the examiner should have gained enough information from the histories and his observations of the child's spontaneous speech to classify, roughly, the speech problem. He can then begin with specific speech or hearing tests which will provide the detailed diagnostic information.

However, a small number of children will remain whose disorders are still a mystery to the examiner and the parents. The best way to tackle their problems is to inveigle the children into doing something—as a matter of fact, almost anything—since it is through the child's behavior and not by his physical characteristics, as measured by wastefully expensive examinations, that we will learn to understand him, recognize his speech disorder, and devise a therapy adapted to his particular needs. The only kind of behavior which will not be helpful is the complete withdrawal when he refuses to participate. This kind of behavior forces the examiner to lean heavily upon the case history and reports of physical and other examinations which are not measures of communication behavior. The case-history information should always be viewed with some skepticism, since it is dependent upon the *memory* of the person being interviewed as well as upon his *objectivity*.

The examiner must also remember that the more deviant or withdrawn the child's behavior, the more apt is the parent's behavior to be affected by guilt. The more guilty the feeling, the less likelihood that objectivity will occur during the case-history interview. Therefore, the speech examiner is confronted with the need to obtain a variety of reactive behavior from the child which he can observe. Some ways of eliciting useful behavior from the child are:

1. Remove the child from environmental contacts which may be restrictive or punitive.
2. Place the child in an environment with interesting objects or toys and friendly people.

3. Build upon any kind of behavior the child demonstrates, even if it is no more than commenting on how well the child walks, sits, or what not. Reinforcement of the child should not only be oral but also pantomimed, and sometimes reinforcement through use of tiny bits of candy is helpful as a conditioner.
4. Place the child in a situation with other children who will include him in their activities.

Over a period of time, all but the most autistic child will begin to participate. Even the autistic child will reveal himself by numerous egocentric activities which exclude other people from his world.

Once the child begins to interact with objects, conditions, and other people, the examiner must keep careful records of his observations. Since these children are functioning in a much more limited manner than most who come for examination, numerous small evidences of behavior may give clues of latent ability as well as focal points for reinforcement which will lead to the development of learned behavior. Such behavior as the following may be valuable:

1. To what kind of stimuli does he respond and how?
   a. Noises, sounds, voices, speech.
   b. Visually to speech, pantomime, colors, toys, people, objects.
   c. Tactile, pressure—being touched, touching, licking, tasting.
   d. Directed activity—play, discipline, punishment.
   e. Food.
2. To what kinds of stimuli does he not respond?
   a. Audible.
   b. Visual.
   c. Tactile.
3. How does he respond?
   a. Sounds—produced under what conditions.
   b. Speech—produced under what conditions.
   c. Movements he makes with special reference to chewing, licking, swallowing, walking, climbing, and hand co-ordination.
   d. How does he attempt to communicate his needs? Sentences, words, sounds, pantomime, crying, whining, temper outbursts.
   e. How does he respond when his efforts to communicate are not understood?
   f. What kinds of behavior does his environment show when he tries to communicate?
   g. If he doesn't respond to ordinary stimuli, does he entertain himself while being oblivious to conditions around him? If so how?

After the histories and physical examinations have been completed, the autobiography written (if indicated), and the observations well on the way to completion, a number of standard tests should be administered which measure intelligence, social maturity, school achievement, and personality.

Both performance and verbal types of intelligence tests should be used. Some satisfactory tests are the Stanford-Binet (1937), the Wechsler Adult Intelligence Scale (1955), the Wechsler Intelligence Scale for Children (1949) and a paper-and-pencil test, the California Test of Mental Maturity (1937).

INDIANA UNIVERSITY SPEECH AND HEARING CLINIC
DATA SHEET (DELAYED LANGUAGE--DELAYED SPEECH)

NAME _____ SEX M F RACE W C AGE ____ GRADE ____ DATE _____

ADDRESS _____ PHONE _____ SCHOOL _____ EXAMINER _____

RECEPTION
    Audiometric test _____
    Reaction to sounds _____
    Comprehension--
      Speech when face is seen _____
    Comprehension--
      Speech when face not seen _____
    Comprehension of
      Pantomime _____
    Behavior _____
EXPRESSION
    Noises _____
    Words _____
    Pantomime _____
    Behavior _____
GENERAL BEHAVIOR
    Interaction with people _____
    Interaction with animals--objects _____

    Environmental method of projecting to child _____

TEST RESULTS
    1.  Intelligence Test:
      Performance _____

      Verbal _____
      Others _____
    2.  Social maturity _____

    3.  Speech Sound development scale (From O.P. Irwin) _____

PHYSICAL DEFECTS
    1.  Sensory defects _____
    2.  Motor defects _____
    3.  Brain injuries _____
    4.  Serious and/or prolonged illnesses _____

ENVIRONMENTAL FACTORS
    1.  Responses to early noise _____
    2.  Responses to vocal play _____
    3.  Verbal output while caring for infant _____
    4.  Stimulation of infant with new sounds _____
    5.  Responses to first word attempts _____
    6.  Response to pantomimic communication _____
    7.  Response to infantile speech behavior _____
    8.  Response to irrelevant behavior during speech _____
    9.  Response to unacceptable speech _____
    10.  Response to learning behavior _____

274

INDIANA UNIVERSITY SPEECH AND HEARING CLINIC
DATA SHEET (DELAYED LANGUAGE—DELAYED SPEECH)
(continued)

COMMENTS:

------------------------------------ EVALUATIONS ---------------------------------

NATURE OF DISORDER _____

_____

PRECIPITANTS _____

_____

RECOMMENDATIONS _____

_____

_____

Some intelligence tests that can be used for persons who are extremely limited in comprehension and/or expression are the Goodenough Draw-a-Man Test (1926), the Grace Arthur Point Scale of Performance (1930), and the Van Alstyne Picture Vocabulary Test. The Nebraska Test of Learning Aptitude for Young Deaf Children (1941) is not an intelligence test but compares a deaf child's performance with that of other deaf children.

Social maturity tests are valuable, and the Vineland Social Maturity Scale (1947) is most satisfactory.

A large variety of school-achievement tests are available. The Stanford Achievement Test series is one of the best because of its choice of subject matter and because it allows for comparisons between grades. The Metropolitan Achievement Tests are also good. The Durrell Analysis of Reading Difficulty and the Iowa and Gates tests provide information about reading disabilities.

Pencil-and-paper personality tests have a questionable value unless each item is studied separately. The Minnesota Multiphasic Personality Inventory is a commonly used paper-and-pencil test. The Children's Apperception Test for children, the Thematic Apperception Test, and the Rorschach Test for adolescents and adults are more desirable because of the evaluations made of each case by the examiner.

The physical examination should follow the direction indicated by the physician; however, the extent of the examination should be related to the nature and severity of the speech disorder. A child with a minor disorder in articulation should not require as extensive an examination as might be anticipated for one who cannot communicate orally.

After the completion of the histories, observations and testing the diagnostician is ready to evaluate the most primitive of the speech disorders.

I. *Communication which involves no comprehension of, or expression through, oral language.*

II. *Communication which involves comprehension of, but little or no expression through, oral language.*

These two classifications of disorders can be dealt with jointly, since they really involve two levels of achievement and usage of language. The test procedures and data sheet for one will suffice for the other.

Whenever possible, a study should be made of the speech-sound development, using the procedure and scale described by Irwin (1947). The Gesell and Amatruda developmental examination of behavior (1941) may also prove useful.

With the use of the information from the case histories, the observations, and the test results, the diagnostician is ready to evaluate the language disorder in relation to the precipitants in an effort to design a therapeutic procedure for those children who do not comprehend or express themselves through oral language.

The case history and observations of the child's behavior will provide the chief sources of evidence indicating the presence of environmental precipitants. The case histories, observations, and test results will provide the sources of information about the presence of physical precipitants.

By correlating the symptoms of the disorder with the precipitants, one may be able to determine which precipitants may be removed or corrected most easily. The success of therapy will depend largely upon the removal of precipitants and/or compensation for those which cannot be removed.

Obviously, if the precipitants cannot be eliminated or compensated for, a poor prognosis must be expected.

Superficially, the symptoms of all children who do not understand or express themselves through speech appear much the same. As a result, chance diagnosis of deafness or mental retardation is often made. Hence, deaf schools have children who are not deaf and schools for retarded children have some children who are not retarded.

In order to avoid such errors, the symptoms of language deficiency must be carefully studied in relation to test results and other evidence of precipitant conditions.

The child not using oral communication as a medium for comprehension or expression, who is not mentally defective but has a severe hearing loss accompanied with environmental precipitants 2–7, is likely to demonstrate the following symptoms:

RECEPTION

| | |
|---|---|
| 1. Auditory acuity | Very little or no evidence of hearing through audiometric testing. |

2. Reaction to sounds — Little or no startle to loud noises or reaction to doorbells etc.
3. Comprehending speech when face is seen — Little or no comprehension.
4. Comprehending speech when face is not seen — No comprehension.
5. Comprehending pantomime — Remarkable ability.
6. Behavior — Numerous temper outbursts when he cannot understand.

### EXPRESSION

1. Noises — Cries and whines often, but cry is of poor resonance. Makes few play noises.
2. Words — Never forms words.
3. Pantomime — Remarkably descriptive.
4. Behavior — Numerous temper outbursts when he cannot make himself understood.

### GENERAL BEHAVIOR

1. Interaction with people — Understands his place in the group most of the time and behaves acceptably when he understands.
2. Interaction with animals, objects, and tests — Understands play with animals and objects. Performance tests higher than verbal tests. Likely to be interested in mechanical things.
3. Environmental method of projecting to child — Most people project their ideas through pantomime or just plain showing.

The child using oral communication as a medium of comprehension but little or none for expression, who is not mentally deficient or psychologically disturbed but has a severe hearing loss and has environmental precipitants 2, 4, and 5, is likely to demonstrate the following symptoms:

### RECEPTION

1. Auditory acuity — Very little or no evidence of hearing through audiometric tests.
2. Reaction to sounds — Very little or no startle effect and little or no understanding of sounds.
3. Comprehending speech when face is seen — Comparatively good understanding.
4. Comprehending speech when face is not seen — Little or no understanding.
5. Understanding of pantomime — Remarkable ability.
6. Behavior — Temper outbursts when he cannot understand speech or pantomime.

### EXPRESSION

1. Noises — Cries often in an unresonant voice. Doesn't make many play sounds.

2. Words — May make a poorly articulated word occasionally and usually will try to repeat if asked. Doesn't like to talk however.

3. Pantomime — He is still the master of pantomimic expression.

4. Behavior — Great unhappiness involving temper tantrums when his pantomime and/or noisy crying are not understood or reacted to as expected.

## GENERAL BEHAVIOR

1. Interaction with people — Usually is oriented and comparatively easy to get along with as long as he understands and is understood.

2. Interactions with animals, objects, and tests — Understands play with animals and objects. Responds consistently to tests.

3. Environmental method of projecting to child — Consistently tries to project through speech and not pantomime.

The child not using oral communication as a medium for comprehension or expression, who is not necessarily mentally defective or severely handicapped in auditory acuity, may present the following symptoms if precipitants 5, 7, and 9 were present in his background as well as additional psychological disturbances:

## RECEPTION

1. Auditory acuity — Probably will not respond to audiometric testing or will respond erratically.

2. Reaction to sounds — Will show erratic behavior. Sometimes shows startle to loud sounds.

3. Comprehending speech when face is seen — Erratic. Understands sometimes. Is partly a function of contact.

4. Comprehending speech when face is not seen — Erratic. Understands sometimes. Is partly a function of contact.

5. Comprehending pantomime — Erratic. Better than understanding of speech but it is primarily a function of contact.

6. Behavior — Makes little effort to comprehend but may throw a terrible tantrum which often involves beating of head when he wants to understand and cannot.

## EXPRESSION

1. Noises — Cries some. Makes many stereotyped noises most of which are not directed toward people or objects. Gives the impression some sounds mean something to the child but chances are they are an extension of self-reinforced vocal play.

| | |
|---|---|
| 2. Words | May say a word or even a sentence occasionally but *will not repeat* when asked. |
| 3. Pantomime | Not very often or very descriptive. Does a lot of leading however. |
| 4. Behavior | Usually waits to be taken care of, doesn't make too many demands, likely to wander off if not watched. When, however, the child wants something very badly and cannot make people understand, he usually throws a terrific temper tantrum involving destructiveness and vicious self-punishment, or he may end up in complete withdrawal. |

### GENERAL BEHAVIOR

| | |
|---|---|
| 1. Interaction with people | Is frequently disoriented, follows in a docile manner much of the time if nothing much is expected. |
| 2. Interaction with animals, objects, and tests | Usually ignores animals, objects, and tests; however, may become completely attached to an object or animal. Test results are erratic and extremely difficult to evaluate. |
| 3. Environmental method used in projecting to child | No consistent method. Parents and others try what seems best to them and usually change frequently from talking to shouting to pantomiming to leading around. |

The child not using oral communication as a medium for comprehension or expression who is not psychologically disturbed, not defective in auditory acuity, but may be mentally defective, may show some of the following symptoms if environmental precipitants 1–5 and 10 are found in his background along with or without any of the physical precipitants.

### RECEPTION

| | |
|---|---|
| 1. Auditory acuity | Extremely difficult to obtain consistent response but usually responds to sounds well above his threshold. |
| 2. Reaction to sounds | Usually startles when hearing unexpected loud noises. Can be trained to avoid danger when warned by sounds. |
| 3. Comprehending speech when face is seen | Usually doesn't understand, but doesn't fight to look away from face. |
| 4. Comprehending speech when face is not seen | Usually doesn't understand, but will do as well as when looking at face of speaker. |
| 5. Comprehending pantomime | More than speech but still not sharp. |
| 6. Behavior | Cries and whines for attention but usually not very extreme in behavior if he doesn't get what he wants. |

EXPRESSION

1. Noises — Usually doesn't make too many sound although he may continually jabbe meaninglessly.
2. Words — Usually none, although if a few ar produced they will be used often an repeated on request.
3. Pantomime — Does more leading around and show ing than descriptive pantomime.
4. Behavior — Complains by crying or whining whe not understood, but accepts his condi tion without much resentment, resist ance, or withdrawal.

GENERAL BEHAVIOR

1. Interaction with people — Usually follows the lead of others with out adding much or demanding much
2. Interaction with animals, objects, and tests — Pays fleeting attention as a rule bu may attend for long periods to a condi tion which is simple and well rein forced. Does poorly on tests and is con sistent from day to day.
3. Environmental method of projecting to child — Usually talks or shows.

The child using oral communication as a medium of comprehension bu not for expression, who is neither psychologically disturbed nor defective ir auditory acuity but may be mentally defective, may show some of the fol lowing symptoms if environmental precipitants 2–6 and 10 are found in hi background along with or without any of the physical precipitants.

RECEPTION

1. Auditory acuity — Responds to audiometric test after he understands.
2. Reaction to sounds — Startle to loud noises and slow but adequate conditioning to sounds.
3. Comprehending speech when face is seen — Adequate.
4. Comprehending speech when face is not seen — Same.
5. Comprehending pantomime — Fairly adequate.
6. Behavior — Usually quiet and unassuming.

EXPRESSION

1. Noises — Usually doesn't make too many sounds, although some jabber continuously.
2. Words — Produces a few words and repeats them willingly.
3. Pantomime — Pantomime isn't too descriptive, does more leading around.
4. Behavior — Cries and whines when people don't understand his wants, but doesn't rebel too much.

## GENERAL BEHAVIOR

| | |
|---|---|
| 1. Interaction with people | Fits into other people's patterns. Demands little. |
| 2. Interaction with animals, objects, and tests | Usually flits from one to another, but may persist on a simple activity for a long time. Does poorly on mental tests both in verbal and performance items. |
| 3. Environmental method of projecting to the child | Talks mostly. |

The child not using oral communication for comprehension or for expression, who is neither defective auditorily nor mentally and is not psychologically disturbed, may show the following symptoms if environmental precipitants 2–6 are found. Any of the physical precipitants may or may not be present.

## RECEPTION

| | |
|---|---|
| 1. Auditory acuity | May or may not respond to audiometric test. |
| 2. Reaction to sounds | Usually startles when hearing unexpected loud noises. Can be trained to avoid danger when warned by sounds. Usually responds to simple conditioning using sounds as the stimulus. |
| 3. Comprehending speech when face is seen | Usually doesn't comprehend. May or may not refuse to look at speaker. |
| 4. Comprehending speech when face is not seen | Usually doesn't comprehend. |
| 5. Comprehending pantomime | Comprehends pantomime. |
| 6. Behavior | Cries and whines for attention. Has many temper outbursts. |

## EXPRESSION

| | |
|---|---|
| 1. Noises | Makes quite a few sounds while playing. Frequently has good inflection and voice quality. |
| 2. Words | Usually none. |
| 3. Pantomime | Uses some pantomime but not too descriptively. |
| 4. Behavior | Complains by crying and whining. Shows resentment with some temper outbursts. |

## GENERAL BEHAVIOR

| | |
|---|---|
| 1. Interaction with people | Is well oriented. Usually fits into situation if conditions are known. |
| 2. Interaction with animals, objects, and tests | Plays well with animals and objects. Responds reasonably well to performance tests. |
| 3. Environmental method of projecting to child | Talks, pantomimes, and shows. |

The child using oral communication for comprehension but little or none for expression, who is neither defective auditorily nor mentally and is not psychologically disturbed, may show the following symptoms if environmental precipitants 2–6 and 9 are found. Any of the physical precipitants may or may not be present.

### RECEPTION

| | |
|---|---|
| 1. Auditory acuity | Will probably respond to the audiometer, although the testing will not measure the threshold accurately. |
| 2. Reaction to sounds | Usually startles when hearing unexpected loud noises. Conditions readily to sound stimuli. |
| 3. Comprehending speech when face is seen | Comprehends very readily when paying attention. |
| 4. Comprehending speech when face is not seen | Same. |
| 5. Comprehending pantomime | Adequate but not used. |
| 6. Behavior | Much like any other child in situations where comprehension is involved. |

### EXPRESSION

| | |
|---|---|
| 1. Noises | Cries and makes vocal play noises of adequate voice quality. May pretend to talk. |
| 2. Words | Will speak a few automatically. May or may not repeat them on request. |
| 3. Pantomime | Can describe needs fairly well with pantomime. |
| 4. Behavior | Angry when needs are not fulfilled. Will turn away when told to say what he wants. |

### GENERAL BEHAVIOR

| | |
|---|---|
| 1. Interaction with people | Is well adjusted to the group unless asked to talk, or unless he needs something which he cannot explain. |
| 2. Interactions with animals, objects, and tests | Plays well with animals and objects. He performs adequately on tests, provided they do not require verbal expression. |
| 3. Environmental method of projecting to the child | Speech. |

Facts about these communication disabilities are little known and the methods of diagnosis have not been experimentally investigated, let alone standardized. One of the best sources at present is Myklebust's book (1954) dealing with problems of children with auditory disorders.

The examiner of delayed-language cases must depend upon ingenuity and observations when making evaluations. He must be careful not to be lured into making judgments based on "known causes." For instance, since aphasia frequently follows brain damage in adults, the assumption is made by many people that brain damage is *the* cause of aphasia. Once having accepted this premise, it is easy to believe that brain-damaged children will have aphasia. Diagnoses of this sort are made frequently even though the child cannot and never has been able to communicate orally. To prove or disprove the presence of aphasia in such a child is impossible with the testing tools that are available at present. On the other hand, a positive diagnosis of aphasia may create problems for the child which would not have occurred if the disorder had only been described as observed. For the most part, good therapy is not dependent upon a name but rather upon careful descriptions of the disorder and of the person having the disorder.

III. *Communication which involves deteriorated comprehension and/or expression through oral language.*

There are actually two quite different groups that can be included under this category. One group, which can involve both children and adults at all levels, is composed of individuals who stop talking primarily because of psychological problems. Many mental patients and some so-called delayed-speech cases belong in this group and are not primarily speech problems but fall in the realm of the psychiatrist or psychotherapist.

The other group comprises the aphasics, whose speech has deteriorated after brain damage. Although the condition follows brain damage, there are undoubtedly both physical and learning factors involved. Environmental precipitants 6, 7, 8, and 9 are likely to be present. Procedures for examination of this group, the aphasics, are described in this section.

## APHASIA

In examining for aphasia, it must always be kept in mind that it is as important, perhaps more important, to know the upper limits of behavior as it is to know what the patient cannot do. For this reason, the examiner must be prepared to use some ingenuity in eliciting the best possible performance, but at the same time must record any helps (such as having the patient indicate an object or use, or select from a multiple-choice) that become necessary in discovering the capacity to perform.

In an informal testing situation, oral-language comprehension can be tested by asking the client his name, occupation, and other data. If he is unable to answer, he can be asked to point to objects in the room or to indicate one of a group of three or more objects or pictures.

He can then be given a simple paragraph to read silently and asked questions to determine his comprehension. If he is unable to respond verbally, he can be asked such questions as: "Point to the name of the boy" or "Show me where it tells about so and so." Another way of testing reading comprehension is by written questions at the end of the selection with multiple-choice answers from which the client may choose.

# INDIANA UNIVERSITY SPEECH AND HEARING CLINIC
## DATA SHEET (APHASIA)

NAME_____ SEX M F  RACE W C  AGE___  GRADE___  DATE_____

ADDRESS_____ PHONE_____  SCHOOL_____  EXAMINER_____

| RECEPTION | G | F | P | NO. R. | EXPRESSION | G | F | P | N |
|---|---|---|---|---|---|---|---|---|---|
| Oral language Comprehension-------- | | | | | Conversational Speech----- | | | | |
| Silent reading Comprehension-------- | | | | | Simple statements--------- | | | | |
| | | | | | Expresses ideas with speech plus pantomime | | | | |
| Visual Recognition | | | | | Naming------------------- | | | | |
| Objects------------- | | | | | Can he repeat?----------- | | | | |
| Pictures------------ | | | | | Words----------------- | | | | |
| Colors------------- | | | | | Sounds---------------- | | | | |
| Forms------------- | | | | | Automatic Speech--------- | | | | |
| Numbers------------ | | | | | Oral Reading------------- | | | | |
| Letters------------ | | | | | Articulation------------- | | | | |
| Words------------- | | | | | Writing | | | | |
| | | | | | Numbers----------------- | | | | |
| Auditory Recognition | | | | | Letters----------------- | | | | |
| Words-------------- | | | | | Spelling----------------- | | | | |
| Sounds------------- | | | | | Arithmetic--------------- | | | | |
| | | | | | Simple skills such as | | | | |
| Tactile Recognition | | | | | Stick out tongue-------- | | | | |
| Objects------------- | | | | | Light a cigarette------- | | | | |
| | | | | | Cut with scissors------- | | | | |

Nature of Injury_____
Date of Injury_____  Location_____
Resulting symptoms (physical)_____
Improvement (physical)_____
Premorbid language skills: Good____  Fair____  Poor____  Explain_____
Nature of language immediately after injury_____
Improvement_____
Education: Grade____  High____  College____  Handedness: R  L  A
Occupation: Unskilled_____  Skilled_____  Business or Profession_____
Vocational prognosis_____
Mental attitude: Patient_____
                 Family_____
-----------------------------------EVALUATIONS-----------------------------------
Nature of language disorder_____

Recommendations_____

Evaluated by_____

284

Visual recognition of objects, colors, forms, and so on can be assessed by having him name them or indicate their use, by matching, or by indicating objects or places as named by the examiner.

Auditory recognition can be determined by naming objects in the room and having the patient point to them and by making noises such as coughing or crumpling paper behind his back and having him indicate the source of the sound. Tactile recognition can similarly be tested by having him hold small common objects, such as a pencil or scissors, in his hand while his eyes are closed and instructing him to name or indicate the object.

Expressive speech can be evaluated on several different levels. The quality of conversational speech can be determined. If it is limited to simple statements or consists largely of single words, this should be noted. It is most important to determine whether the client is able to project his ideas. Can he name objects and repeat words or sounds after the examiner? Does he have any automatic speech, such as that used in counting, at his command?

The patient can then be asked to read a simple selection orally. The quality of this skill can be judged and an evaluation of articulation in all speech activities can then be made.

Writing of numbers and letters read by the examiner can then be tried; and if this should be impossible, the client can attempt to copy them. Similarly, spelling of words can be tested.

The patient can be given simple written problems in addition, subtraction, multiplication, and division. If he seems not to know which process to use, the examiner can work a similar example first. The problem here is to find out how much as well as how little the aphasic individual is able to do.

This type of examination will give a good over-all picture of the aphasic behavior and is readily adaptable to individual problems. It may also be desirable to use standard tests such as the Halstead-Wepman Screening Test or Aphasia or Examining for Aphasia by Eisenson (1954). The Wechsler Adult Intelligence Scale (1955) and the Wechsler Intelligence Scale for Children (WISC) (1949) may also prove valuable, particularly since they allow a comparison between verbal and performance behavior. Standard achievement tests such as the Metropolitan or Stanford may be useful in establishing levels of skills and also as a gauge of progress.[1]

IV. *Communication which involves comprehension of, and expression through, oral language with the pattern of expression being unacceptable to the listener and/or to the speaker.*

## ARTICULATION

It is most important that an adequate phonetic analysis be made of the speech of the individual with an articulation defect. At the very least, it is essential to have an accurate record of the sounds in error. To make a

[1] See Chapters 12, 13, 14, 15, and 16, for a more complete discussion of aphasia.

competent diagnosis and set up an adequate outline of therapy, there should also be a record of the type of error made—omission, substitution, or distortion, including the sound used as a substitute and the degree of distortion; of the consistency of the error, either in different phonetic contexts or from time to time in the same context; and of the degree of improvement, if any, following visual and auditory stimulation.

Ready-made picture articulation tests for commonly missed consonant sounds are available (Bryngelson and Glaspey, 1941, and Anderson, 1953, pp. 54–57). Directions for constructing a picture test are available in Backus (1945, pp. 61–65), Johnson, Darley, and Spriestersbach (1952, pp. 35–36), Irwin (1953, pp. 31–32), Van Riper (1954, pp. 172–177). Suggestions for tests using pictures or objects to elicit the sounds can be found in Berry and Eisenson (1942, pp. 376–379; 1956, pp. 492–522), West, Kennedy, and Carr (1947, pp. 570–571), and Irwin (1953, p. 79).

Words and sentences planned for articulation-testing can be found in Fairbanks (1940, pp. xii–xx), Templin (1947, pp. 392–396), West, Kennedy, and Carr (1947, pp. 565–570), and Van Riper (1954, pp. 176–179).

Test words for all common consonants and vowels in American speech are given below. They may be used equally effectively in constructing a picture, word, or sentence test, in order to adjust to the performance level of the person to be tested.

## ARTICULATION TEST WORDS

CONSONANTS

| | Initial | Medial | Final |
|---|---|---|---|
| [r] | rake, rabbit | carrot | door |
| [l] | lamp | telephone | ball |
| [s] | saw | glasses | house |
| [z] | zipper | scissors | nose |
| [k] | cat | cookies | book |
| [g] | gun | wagon | flag |
| [w] | window | sandwich | |
| [θ] | thumb | birthday cake | mouth |
| [ð] | that | feather | smooth |
| [j] | yellow | onion | |
| [f] | fork | elephant | knife |
| [v] | vase | shovel | stove |
| [ŋ] | | monkey | swing |
| [ʃ] | shoe | dishes | fish |
| [ʒ] | | measure | garage |
| [ʌ] | wheel | | |
| [tʃ] | chair | matches | watch |
| [dʒ] | jelly | soldier | orange |
| [t] | table | letter | boat |
| [d] | dog | ladder | bed |
| [p] | pencil | apple | cup |
| [b] | bus | baby | tub |
| [m] | mouse | hammer | drum |
| [n] | nose | banana | train |
| [h] | hat | | |

VOWELS

| [i] | tree |
| [ɪ] | pig |
| [ɛ] | bell |
| [e] [eɪ] | cake |
| [æ] | hat |
| [ʌ] | gun |
| [ɑ] | car |
| [o] [oʊ] | comb |
| [ɔ] | ball |
| [ʊ] | book |
| [u] | shoe |

DIPHTHONGS

| [ɑʊ] | cow |
| [ɑɪ] | pie |
| [ɔɪ] | boy |

CONSONANT
BLENDS

| [dr] [pt] | dripped |
| [kr] [dl] | cradle |
| [sm] [ʃt] | smashed |
| [tw] [lv] | twelve |
| [θr] | three |
| [br] [ðð] | brother |
| [ldʒɜ·] | soldier |
| [gr] [vz] | groves |
| [rtʃ] | church |
| [sn] [fl] | snuffle |

On the whole, the picture test is likely to be the most desirable for younger children because it will interest the child, is easy to handle, and does not give any unnecessary assistance in making the sounds. For older children or adults, a reading test with words containing the sounds in the desired positions may be more satisfactory. Whatever type of test is used, a record should be kept of the type of error, omission, substitution, or distortion. Then an effort should be made to stimulate the child to improve on the sounds in error. Travis (1931, p. 230) and Johnson, Brown, Curtis, Edney, and Keaster (1948, pp. 108–109) refer to the desirability of giving the child strong stimulation with the correct sound and then getting him to attempt it.

The precise effect of speed of jaw, tongue and lip movements, and of speech sound discrimination on the accuracy of articulation have not been established. Children with slow movements or poor discrimination may have adequate articulation, while children with fast movements and good discrimination may have poor speech. It is only the extremes that are likely to be strongly related, making a fine measurement of these factors of questionable value in most cases. However, if an examiner needs a measurement of these abilities he can refer, in the case of speed of movement, to West, Kennedy, and Carr (1947, pp. 49–50, 87–88), Johnson, Darley, and Spriestersbach (1952, pp. 53–59), and Van Riper (1954, pp. 188–190).

Travis and Rasmus (1931) describe a test of speech sound discrimination. Templin (1943) used a modification of this test, which is also described by Van Riper (1954, pp. 198–199).

Much of the following material on articulation-testing and diagnosis has been taken from Milisen (1954).[2]

First, it is desirable to attempt to assess the general nature of the misarticulations without trying to record them. *A Conversation-Articulation Test* involving pictorial material, toys, pets, and so forth may be used. Conversation directed toward the parents is sometimes helpful in precipitating

[2] *Rationale on Articulation,* Monograph Supplement No. 4.

# INDIANA UNIVERSITY SPEECH AND HEARING CLINIC
## BASIC DATA SHEET

NAME_____  SEX <u>M</u> F   RACE <u>W</u> C   AGE____ GRADE____ DATE____

ADDRESS_____  PHONE_____ SCHOOL_____ EXAMINER____

Understanding of spoken language  Good_____ Fair_____ Poor_____
Use of language (as a medium)     Good_____ Fair_____ Poor_____
Skill in expression in:           Articulation    Rhythm        Voice
  Conversation speech   G  F  P    G  F  P    G  F  P
  Oral reading          G  F  P    G  F  P    G  F  P

| Freq | Sound | ISOLATED-WORD ARTICULATION TEST Words | | | Sound Isol. | STIMULABILITY TEST Non.Syl. | | | Words | | |
|---|---|---|---|---|---|---|---|---|---|---|---|
| | | I | M | F | | I | M | F | I | M | F |
| 3 | r | | | | | | | | | | |
| 5 | l | | | | | | | | | | |
| 4 | s | | | | | | | | | | |
| 9 | z | | | | | | | | | | |
| 8 | k | | | | | | | | | | |
| 15 | g | | | | | | | | | | |
| 10 | w | | | | | | | | | | |
| 21 | θ | | | | | | | | | | |
| 11 | ʒ | | | | | | | | | | |
| 19 | j | | | | | | | | | | |
| 16 | f | | | | | | | | | | |
| 17 | v | | | | | | | | | | |
| 18 | ŋ | | | | | | | | | | |
| 20 | ʃ | | | | | | | | | | |
| 24 | ʒ | | | | | | | | | | |
| 23 | ʒ | | | | | | | | | | |
| 21 | tʃ | | | | | | | | | | |
| 22 | dʒ | | | | | | | | | | |
| 1 | t | | | | | | | | | | |
| 6 | d | | | | | | | | | | |
| 14 | p | | | | | | | | | | |
| 13 | b | | | | | | | | | | |
| 7 | m | | | | | | | | | | |
| 2 | n | | | | | | | | | | |
| 12 | h | | | | | | | | | | |

Speech Mechanism
1. Lips: OK____
  cleft___ repai_
  paralyzed_____
2. Teeth: OK____
  malformed_____
  missing_____
  false_____
3. Jaw: OK____
  ●verbite_____
  underbite_____
  openbite_____
4. Tongue: OK____
  tied____ large_
  small_____
  paralyzed_____
5. Palate: OK____
  high___ narro_
  cleft___ repai_
  hard p._ soft_
6. Larynx: OK____
  V.F.paralyzed_
  infected_____
  growths_____
7. Nasal cavity:_
  occluded_____

Hearing
1. Rt.ear—Good___
2. Lt.ear—Good___

- - - - - - - - EVALUATIONS - - - - - - - -

Nature of disorder_____.

Precipitating conditions_____

Recommendations_____

Evaluated by_____

Brain Injury
  Nature of_____

Coordination
1. Lips      G  F
2. Tongue    G  F
3. Jaw       G  F
4. Breathing G  F
5. General   G  F

288

| Freq | Sound | ISOLATED-WORD ARTICULATION TEST | | | STIMULABILITY TEST | | | | | | |
|---|---|---|---|---|---|---|---|---|---|---|---|
| | | Words | | | Sound Isol. | Non.Syl. | | | Words | | |
| | | I | M | F | | I | M | F | I | M | F |
| | i | | | | | | | | | | |
| | I | | | | | | | | | | |
| | ɛ | | | | | | | | | | |
| | e | | | | | | | | | | |
| | æ | | | | | | | | | | |
| | ɑ | | | | | | | | | | |
| | ʌ | | | | | | | | | | |
| | ɔ | | | | | | | | | | |
| | o | | | | | | | | | | |
| | U | | | | | | | | | | |
| | u | | | | | | | | | | |
| | aI | | | | | | | | | | |
| | ɔI | | | | | | | | | | |
| | aU | | | | | | | | | | |
| | dr | | | | | | | | | | |
| | pt | | | | | | | | | | |
| | kr | | | | | | | | | | |
| | dl | | | | | | | | | | |
| | sm | | | | | | | | | | |
| | tʃ | | | | | | | | | | |
| | tw | | | | | | | | | | |
| | lv | | | | | | | | | | |
| | θr | | | | | | | | | | |
| | br | | | | | | | | | | |
| | ʒ ð | | | | | | | | | | |
| | ld ɔr | | | | | | | | | | |
| | gr | | | | | | | | | | |
| | vz | | | | | | | | | | |
| | ʃtʃ | | | | | | | | | | |
| | sn | | | | | | | | | | |
| | fl | | | | | | | | | | |

omments:

289

speech from the child. This makes it possible to determine whether the chil comprehends speech, whether he can speak understandably, and what h attitude and that of his parents is toward his speech.

Easy and interesting material for an *Oral Reading-Articulation Test* wi allow comparisons between articulation while conversing and reading an may allow observation of sounds not heard during the conversation test.

Material which the child has memorized, such as poems and songs, ca sometimes be used as a *Memory Material-Articulation Test,* particularl when parents are present and can help to get the child started. Songs may b useful as a testing device with the very timid child if the parents will join i

The chief examination, the *Isolated Word-Articulation Test,* permits th examiner to record the nature of the speech responses for each sound in eac position, under constant conditions. The sound in a spoken word should b elicited with pictures for young children and word lists or sentences for olde children and adults. It is important that the sounds be testable in each pos tion in which they occur, that the errors be recorded in sufficient detail to b useful to the therapist, that the evaluations of a given defective sound b consistent among examiners, that the words used be in the vocabulary of th child, and that consonant sounds tested be adjacent to vowels except whe blends are intentionally used for testing purposes.

The method of recording errors differs from the traditional pattern e pecially for indistinct sounds. A recording is made for every sound teste as follows: Omission—"om"; substitution—the phonetic symbol for th sound produced; a severely distorted sound which would attract the atte tion of most untrained observers and frequently make the sound difficult recognize—"3"; a mildly distorted sound which would attract the attentic of many untrained listeners but would not make it difficult to recognize-"2"; and a sound produced correctly—"1."

The data sheet used in the *Isolated Word-Articulation Test* is much th same as the traditional ones with the following exceptions: (1) The soun in the left column are represented by phonetic symbols which are arrange so the most commonly misarticulated ones are listed toward the top. (2) number representing the frequency with which each sound occurs in th language is placed next to each phonetic symbol. (3) Seven additional cc umns are added for the Stimulation Test. A sample of the data sheet appea on page 288.

The administration of the test requires the examiner to keep the child interested that speech responses are made *spontaneously.* For the most pa he should not talk about "testing" the child. He should not administer th entire battery of sounds to all children, since the great majority of cases w not misarticulate sounds past the first 15 on the data sheet. The inform tests mentioned earlier involving conversation, oral reading, and memo should provide the cues as to the consistency and severity of the misartic lations.

## imulability Test

After the articulation tests are completed, all misarticulated sounds are bjected to Integral Stimulation and at varying degrees of complexity of e speech configuration, that is, the sound in isolation, in nonsense syllables, d in words. Articulation responses following stimulation are recorded the same manner as on the *Isolated Word-Articulation Test*. The examiner compares these results of the *Stimulability Test* with those obtained the four articulation tests and thereby determines the effect of stimulation on the misarticulated sounds. Children are able to improve as many as per cent of their misarticulated sounds after receiving only a *few* integral imulations. Any test which measures this ability would be invaluable to erapy.

The *Stimulability Test* was designed to provide an index to such an ability developing a means of testing, evaluating, and recording the quantitative d qualitative changes in articulation which follow a few Integral Stimulations. This index records the changes occurring in response to stimulation r each misarticulated sound in each position and on three levels of speech nfiguration—isolation, nonsense syllables, and words. This index provides ncrete evidence as to which sounds respond immediately and well to tegral Stimulation, which ones are only modified, and which ones are t changed at all. Therefore, the results from this test will pinpoint the unds on which the therapy should begin as well as those on which Integral imulation will obviously precipitate improvement.

The administration of the test involves directing the child's attention to e examiner's face by saying, "I am going to make some noises. You *watch* e and *listen* and do what I do." The examiner makes the sound, syllable, or rd two or three times before signaling the child to imitate. This procedure repeated twice and the best of the child's responses is recorded. The nician must use Integral Stimulation by making the focal articulation int more visible, by giving clues as to the movement of breath stream, by ging the child to "watch" or "listen" carefully if the child's attention is aying and by a wise use of *praise*. The examiner should always begin by mulating a sound which the child can produce correctly in order that he n praise the success and thereby reduce the threat of the testing situation. the beginning the examiner should always praise the response if the child s shown improvement. He may make qualified statements of praise, such "That is better," if the imitation is better than the child's previous one. He ould never say, "That is wrong," even though the imitation was completely correct. Instead, he should say nothing or casually say, "Let's try it again."

After the *Stimulability Test* is completed, the examiner should list each isarticulated sound in each of two columns. The sounds in the first column ould be in such an order that those most distracting to the audience are ward the top. The same sounds would be listed in the second column with ose most stimulable toward the top. The obvious goal of therapy would be,

as much as possible, to work first with those sounds which are toward tl
top in both columns, because they would be the sounds which were mo
easily stimulated yet at the same time the ones most distracting to the listene

In the first column, the sounds which are most distracting to the listen
are listed toward the top. The degree of distraction is determined by con
bining quantitative and qualitative factors of each defective sound. That i
the frequency with which a misarticulated sound occurs (numerical rating
given in the first column of the *Isolated Word-Articulation Test* sheet)
combined with the severity of the misarticulation occurring each time tl
sound is produced. Thus, a sound which occurs frequently and is misarticu
lated badly each time it is produced would be placed toward the top of tl
column. A sound which does not occur frequently and/or is misarticulate
mildly would be placed toward the bottom of the column.

The primary factors determining the order in the second column (Ease ₑ
Stimulation) are the responses on the *Stimulability Test* compared with tl
responses to the *Isolated Word-Articulation Test*. Sounds are considere
more stimulable if they are imitated better in words than in nonsense sy
lables, or in nonsense syllables than in isolation. Another factor is the rel₂
tive quality of the response after stimulation. The quality of this respons
may range from correct, to a mild distortion, to a severe distortion, to
substitution, to a complete omission of the sound. Other factors to be co
sidered are the ease or struggle of the child during the attempted respon
and whether the stimulation produces some change even if not a correct on

The secondary factors involved in estimating the effectiveness of Integr
Stimulation Therapy are visibility of the focal articulation point, audito
acuity, general speech environment, organic conditions, and motivation
factors. Since the child is more likely to respond to stimulation that he c₂
see and hear, the therapist should use every device to make all sounds hea
and all focal articulation points visible. The latter is especially importa
with those sounds which when produced in the ordinary way are only pa
tially visible or are not visible at all.

Sounds made defectively by family, friends, or teachers may be mo
difficult to correct, since the child is exposed to a lot of faulty stimulatio
There may also be resentment by parents or teacher who assume that tl
child is being taught *fancy* speech. Sounds not involving structural a
normalities or poorly co-ordinated muscles may be more easily correcte
Motivation may be more important in correcting some sounds than othe₁
since the importance of a misarticulation to a child frequently determin
how hard he will try. He may, for instance, be more willing to work on a mi
articulated sound in his name than on any other misarticulated sound.

By proper integration of the primary factors with the secondary facto₁
the diagnostician can list the misarticulated sounds in order with the mc
stimulable sounds on top.

After the two lists are completed, the diagnostician is in a position etermine which sounds should be given therapy first and the methods to be sed. The ultimate outcome of articulation therapy is often determined by 1e results which are obtained when treating the first sounds. The correc- on of a misarticulated sound not only improves the quality of the speech, ut it also produces constructive changes in attitude in the child and his 1vironment. This facilitates the therapist's efforts when dealing with the :maining sounds. Hence, one sees the vital importance of treating a sound 1at can be easily corrected, thereby establishing for the child and his en- ironment a learning pattern as well as the motivation to follow it until >eech is "normal."

The obligation of the diagnostician is to furnish methods of therapy which ill produce normal speech in the shortest period of time without creating notional problems in the child or in his parents. By beginning therapy with 1e most distracting sound which is readily stimulated and building a stimu- tion therapy around the three previously mentioned variables, it should be >ssible to produce enough improvement in almost all cases to keep the 1ild and the parents motivated until the speech is normal.

Many children having misarticulations also have maladjustments which ay or may not arise from the defective speech. If the adjustment problem ·ose from the defective speech, it may implement or depress the child's forts to achieve better speech. If it implements therapy, the child will, al- 1ough bothered by his disorder, want to *try hard* to correct it.

The first sound to be corrected for such a child should be the one most stracting which is also stimulable. The continuance of the high motivation ' the child will depend on his awareness of speech improvement. The malad- stment will usually disappear as soon as the speech becomes adequate.

If the maladjustment results in a withdrawal from speech therapy, the agnostician must choose the misarticulated sounds most easily corrected, ·gardless of how much or how little it distracts the listener. The goal at the 1tset is to build confidence for the child in his ability to improve his articu- tion and in the method of therapy. Success on the first sound leads to a illingness to "try" the others.

If the maladjustment has not arisen from the defective speech, the diag- >stician should provide for psychotherapy as well as articulation therapy. psychotherapy is not available, articulation therapy can be started, pro- ding Integral Stimulation produces improvement and provided the child >es not use his defective speech as an attention-seeking device to compen- te for his other maladjustments. Speech improvement in a maladjusted 1ild, like improvement in any other skill, will produce some self-confidence hich may help to compensate for the nonspeech maladjustments. Therapy hich in a natural manner produces improvements will not create new aladjustments or cause old ones to get worse.[3]

[3] For a more complete coverage of disorders of articulation, see Chapters 23 and 24.

INDIANA UNIVERSITY SPEECH AND HEARING CLINIC
DATA SHEET (CLEFT PALATE)

NAME_____ SEX M F  RACE W C  AGE____  GRADE____  DATE_____

ADDRESS_____ PHONE_____ SCHOOL_____ EXAMINER____

CLOSED NOSE TEST
(Fill in sounds reported defective on the Basic Data Sheet)

| SOUND | ISOLATED-WORD ARTICULATION TEST | | | STIMULABILITY TEST | | | | | | | GRIMACES |
|---|---|---|---|---|---|---|---|---|---|---|---|
| | | | | Sound Isol. | Non.Syl. | | | Words | | | |
| | I | M | F | | I | M | F | I | M | F | |
| | | | | | | | | | | | |
| | | | | | | | | | | | |
| | | | | | | | | | | | |
| | | | | | | | | | | | |
| | | | | | | | | | | | |
| | | | | | | | | | | | |
| | | | | | | | | | | | |
| | | | | | | | | | | | |
| | | | | | | | | | | | |
| | | | | | | | | | | | |
| | | | | | | | | | | | |
| | | | | | | | | | | | |
| | | | | | | | | | | | |
| | | | | | | | | | | | |
| | | | | | | | | | | | |
| | | | | | | | | | | | |

Sounds formed correctly_____
Sounds formed correctly but with nasal noise_____
Sounds formed correctly only after stimulation_____
Sounds formed correctly only with nose closed_____
Sounds formed correctly only with nose closed and stimulation_____
Sounds not formed correctly at any time_____
Mouth opening during speech: Little____ Average____ Wide____
Velopharyngeal port: Closure_____ Partial Closure_____ No Closure_____
Nasal drip during inverted drinking: None____ Little____ Some____ Much____
Description of lips_____
Description of hard palate_____
Description of soft palate_____
Description of teeth_____
Medical-surgical recommendations_____
Dental-orthodontal recommendations_____
--------------------------------EVALUATIONS-------------------------------
Nature of disorder_____

Nature of organic disorder_____

Recommendations_____

Evaluated by_____

294

## Cleft Palate

The child with a cleft palate, repaired or otherwise, should be subjected to the same principles involved in general articulation diagnosis, except that in differentiating the sounds to work with first, the effect of the structural abnormality must be measured as it influences the production of sounds under various conditions.

The client should receive the Isolated Word-Articulation Test and Stimulation Test like any other articulation case, with the following changes in procedure: The evaluation of the sound should be based on the quality of the oral sound irrespective of the nasal noise. Each evaluation of each speech sound should be encircled if the client made a nasal noise while making the sound. The examiner should also record the nature of extraneous facial movements used while articulating.

At the completion of the Isolated Word-Articulation and Stimulation Tests, the same procedure would be repeated for the sounds found defective, except that the nose would be held closed in order to prevent the escaping of air. By closing the nose the examiner has, to some degree, artificially counteracted the basic defect of the cleft palate. As soon as the results are recorded on the Data Sheet (Cleft Palate), the examiner should transcribe in red pencil the results from the Isolated Word-Articulation and Stimulability Tests recorded on the Basic Data Sheet.

Sounds can be placed in different groupings as described below to help in predicting the ease of correction. It should also be possible to determine which sounds are affected by air escaping through the nose.

Sounds formed defectively on the Isolated Word-Articulation Test but formed correctly following stimulation could be considered easiest to correct.

The organic condition is primarily involved in sounds formed defectively on the Isolated Word-Articulation Test and on the Stimulability Test but formed correctly on the Closed Nose Isolated Word-Articulation Test. Sounds formed defectively in the Isolated Word Test, the Stimulability Test, and the Closed Nose Isolated Word Test, but correctly in the Closed Nose Stimulability Test, may be presumed to be defective because of a combination of organic and learning deficiencies.

The Articulation Test and Stimulation Test results give no clues to precipitant conditions if defective sounds do not improve either with stimulation, closed nose, or a combination of the two.

The speech pathologist is frequently called upon to determine the effects of the organic structure upon speech. In addition to the above tests of articulation, a test of velopharyngeal closure may be desired. Although fluoroscopic pictures are helpful, a simple method of measuring the degree of closure can be obtained by actual movements of the palate and pharyngeal muscles under stress conditions. Reflex contractions can be initiated by asking the client to swallow water while his head and neck are pointed downward and perpendicular to the floor. If the velopharyngeal port is open water

INDIANA UNIVERSITY SPEECH AND HEARING CLINIC
DATA SHEET (CEREBRAL PALSY)

NAME_____ SEX M F  RACE W C  AGE____ GRADE____ DATE_____

ADDRESS_____ PHONE_____ SCHOOL_____ EXAMINER_____

Sounds from Isolated Word Articulation Test which were produced correctly with

GOOD COORDINATION_____ POOR COORDINATION_____

Defective sounds on test which were improved after stimulation with:

GOOD COORDINATION_____ POOR COORDINATION_____

Defective sounds which did not improve with stimulation. Circle unintelligibl

GOOD COORDINATION_____ POOR COORDINATION_____

Conversational Speech:
  Nature of voice condition_____
  Nature of speech rhythm_____
  Nature of breathing behavior_____

Description of physical behavior_____

Medical diagnosis_____

Medical care up to date_____

Recommendations_____

Developmental behavior: Supporting of head____ Sitting: With support___ Alone
  Grasping successfully with right hand_____ left hand_____
  Talking--Words_____ Short sentences_____
  Crawling_____ Walking with support_____ Walking without support_

Attitude toward disorder:
  Parents_____
  Teachers_____
  Others_____
  The case himself_____
Speech therapy up to date_____

- - - - - - - - - - - - - - - EVALUATIONS - - - - - - - - - - - - - - -
Description of speech disorder_____

Recommendations_____

Evaluated by_____

296

gushes from the nose. This is sufficiently unpleasant to create defensive reflex contractions for each succeeding swallow. If enough tissue is available and if the muscle contractions are sufficiently strong, the water will be forced up past the nasal port and into the esophagus.

Even though the nasal port is never completely closed, the approximations can be estimated by the amount of water which escapes into the nasal cavity.[4]

## Cerebral Palsy

The examination of a child with cerebral palsy must begin with a thorough medical examination by the family doctor and also an orthopedist. Their recommendations should not only provide information about the physical disability and methods of physical restoration but also should indicate limitations in activity determined by the child's health. The speech examiner and diagnostician must stay within those bounds.

The chief function of the speech examination is to describe the nature of the speech condition. It is as important to identify speech movements and behavior which are good as to describe those which are defective. In describing either good or poor speech, the examiner must learn to differentiate the auditory aspect of speech from the visual aspect; otherwise he will frequently mark a correct speech response as defective when it was really the physical co-ordination which was defective.

The chief function of the speech diagnostician in evaluating articulation in cerebral-palsied children is to locate and describe misarticulations, to isolate those sounds which will respond to therapy, and to recommend a workable therapy based on examination results. He must establish an order of articulation habilitation beginning with sounds easily produced and ending with sounds less easily produced.

Voice and rhythm problems, if present, would be studied in the manner recommended in the latter part of this chapter.[5]

## RHYTHM AND STUTTERING

The methods used in examining the stutterer vary from measuring his blood chemistry to evaluating his emotional stability. The methods of therapy range over as wide a territory. It becomes obvious, therefore, that a statement on examination and diagnosis for stuttering would please only the person who wrote it. On the other hand, all therapists whether of one school of stuttering or another must be interested in observations of the person who stutters, observations which when tabulated will provide a better over-all picture of the speech behavior than is gained from the average case report. These observations, however, need not involve highly accurate measurements of overt symptoms or attitudes, because the conditions change so markedly from one period to another and from one situation to another.

---

[4] A more complete discussion of the speech of a person with cleft palate is given in Chapters 19 and 20.

[5] See Chapter 18.

INDIANA UNIVERSITY SPEECH AND HEARING CLINIC
DATA SHEET (RHYTHM-STUTTERING)

NAME_____ SEX M F RACE W C AGE___ GRADE___ DATE___

ADDRESS_____ PHONE____ SCHOOL_____ EXAMINER____

| Symptoms of rhythm disorders during speech reading both | | | | Check Withdrawal behavior of symptoms on continuum | Description of bizarre symptoms |
|---|---|---|---|---|---|
| | | | | Withdrawal | |
| Repetitions | Few | Some | Many | None ←————————→ Much | |
| Phrases-- | | | | | |
| Words--- | | | | | |
| Syllables | | | | | |
| Sounds--- | | | | | |
| Prolonged sounds-- | | | | | |
| Pauses Filled--- | | | | | |
| Silent--- | | | | | |

Stuttering?___ Staccato rhythm___ Drawl___ Estimate of severity_____
Severity in home_____ school_____ work_____ social situations_____

Previous therapy_____

Attitude of parents and teachers toward disorder_____
_____

Behavior of parents and teachers_____
_____

Attitude of the person toward his defect_____
_____

Motivation to improve_____
-----------------------------------EVALUATIONS-----------------------------------

Nature of disorder_____

Precipitating conditions_____

Maintaining conditions_____

Recommendations_____
_____
_____

Evaluated by_____

298

Nevertheless, each therapist needs information regarding the nature and frequency of the overt stuttering symptoms, as well as other types of speech interruptions. He needs information about the withdrawal behavior which occurs in relation to each type of interruption. It is important that he have some measure of the severity of the disorder in different situations, as well as of the attitudes toward the disorder.

A data sheet similar to that on page 298 provides a simple way of evaluating and recording many of the conditions mentioned above. The symptoms of rhythm disorders are descriptive except for "filled" and "silent" pauses. A filled pause refers to any interruption in the forward movement of speech which is filled with body movements, sounds, syllables, words, or phrases which are not an integral part of the language used in expressing the idea. For instance, in the sentence, "The boy a-a-a-a went downtown" a-a-a-a is a filled pause; whereas if the sentence were "I sent a-a-a-a boy downtown" the a-a-a-a would be a repetition of a word.

The term *withdrawal behavior* refers to any act of avoiding a "normal" forward movement during speech. The so-called "conscious" level at which withdrawal may take place usually involves anticipation; however, much withdrawal behavior may be present which is not anticipated.

Many other factors about the stuttering may be measured and recorded. Whether the examiner uses one type of examination or another depends upon the kind of therapy he wishes to offer. If the symptoms of stuttering are to be considered from a neurophysiological standpoint as signs of lack of a dominant gradient in the central nervous system, then motor lead or laterality tests should be added to the more general examinations previously described.

Travis (1931, p. 176) discusses tests of eyedness, mirror-tracing, and writing with both hands simultaneously. Berry and Eisenson (1942, pp. 82–84, 412–415; 1956, pp. 509–514) describe tests of handedness, footedness, and eyedness. Ainsworth (1948, pp. 143–146) gives sample laterality and handedness usage record forms. Johnson, Darley, and Spriestersbach (1952, pp. 155–166) give the Iowa Unimanual Hand Usage Questionnaire and the Iowa Performance Test of Selected Manual Activities. Irwin (1953, pp. 207–287) presents Hull's Hand-Preference Questionnaire. Van Riper (1954, pp. 386–390) discusses tests of eyedness, convergence, strength, thumbedness, footedness, and vertical board or critical-angle board tests of handedness.

If the therapy for stuttering is to include specific work on handling the stuttering blocks or spasms, a detailed analysis of the overt symptoms should be made. West, Kennedy, and Carr (1947, pp. 85–86) give a description of various types of stuttering spasms. Johnson, Brown, Curtis, Edney, and Keaster (1948, p. 442) and Johnson, Darley, and Spriestersbach (1952, pp. 117–120) present a Check List of Stuttering Phenomena. Anderson (1953, pp. 250–251) describes symptoms of stuttering. Van Riper (1954, 393–398) gives a comprehensive section on symptom analysis.

If a primarily learning-therapy approach is to be made in the therapy for

INDIANA UNIVERSITY SPEECH AND HEARING CLINIC
DATA SHEET (VOICE)

NAME_____ SEX M F  RACE W C  AGE___ GRADE___ DATE_____

ADDRESS_____ PHONE_____ SCHOOL_____ EXAMINER____

Check ✓ once if defective
Check ✓✓ twice if severely defective

| | Speech | Reading | Singing | | Speech | Reading | Sin |
|---|---|---|---|---|---|---|---|
| **Pitch** | | | | **Loudness** | | | |
| High---------- | | | | Loud---------- | | | |
| Low----------- | | | | Soft---------- | | | |
| Inflection: | | | | Variation: | | | |
| Narrow------- | | | | Insufficient-- | | | |
| Excessive---- | | | | Excessive---- | | | |
| Pattern------ | | | | Pattern------ | | | |
| **Duration** | | | | **Quality** | | | |
| Fast---------- | | | | Nasal---------- | | | |
| Slow---------- | | | | Denasal-------- | | | |
| Staccato------- | | | | Metallic-------- | | | |
| Variation: | | | | Muffled-------- | | | |
| Insufficient-- | | | | Harsh---------- | | | |
| Excessive---- | | | | Breathy-------- | | | |
| Pattern------ | | | | Hoarse--------- | | | |

Pitch range: no. full notes____ From____ To____ Median pitch_____
Number good quality notes____ From____ To____ Median pitch during speech_____
Effect of pitch on loudness  High P._____ Middle P._____ Low P._____
Effect of pitch on quality   High P._____ Middle P._____ Low P._____
Contribution of voice to personality:  Good_____ Fair_____ Poor_____

Vocal Mechanism
 Nasal---Occlusions?____ Where____ Infection?____ Chronic?____ Origin?____
 Oral----Mouth breather?____ Clefts?____ Velopharyngeal port?____ Always Open____ Clos
        Paralysis or mal function of lips____ Tongue____ Soft Palate____
 Laryngeal--------Infection?____ Chronic?____ Origin?____
        Vocal Folds: Nodes?____ Scar?____ Paralysis____ Short?____ Long?____
 Breathing--------High (chest)____ Middle____ Low (abdomen)____

-------------------------------------EVALUATIONS----------------------------------

Nature of disorder_____

Precipitants_____

Conditions maintaining disorder_____

Recommendations_____
_____
_____

                              Evaluations by_____

300

stuttering, another type of examination may be indicated. Johnson, Darley, and Spriestersbach (1952, pp. 137–152) give the Iowa Scale of Attitude Toward Stuttering and a test for Stutterers Self-Rating of Reactions to Speech Situations.[6]

## VOICE

Effectiveness of voice-testing is determined to a large extent by the representativeness of the voice sample used and the reliability of the examiner. The sample of voice should include speech behavior elicited when the client is just talking and not aware that he is being tested. (This can be done while rapport is being established or while taking the history.) It should also include speech responses occurring when he is aware of the test, as well as samples of oral reading and singing.

The consistency of voice performance helps to determine the nature of precipitating and/or maintaining conditions. For instance, a voice-quality defect present in the speaking voice and not present in the singing voice should not be attributed to an organic disorder; whereas one which is constantly present is more likely to be correlated with an organic condition.

Most of the terms on the data sheet are sufficiently descriptive. However, the following definitions may make some terms more meaningful: *Pitch-inflection pattern* is a stereotyped change in pitch which occurs over and over; *Duration-variation pattern* is a stereotyped change in timing which occurs over and over; *Loudness-variation pattern* is a stereotyped change in loudness which is repeated; *Nasal* refers to excessive resonance in the nasal cavity; *Denasal* refers to absence of nasal resonance; *Metallic* refers to a sharp piercing voice ordinarily associated with tension of the sidewalls of the oral and pharyngeal cavities; *Muffled* is a diffused voice not projected from the mouth and frequently associated with excessive relaxation of the oral and pharyngeal cavities; *Harsh* refers to a rasping sound associated with excessive approximation of vocal folds; *Breathy* involves a whispered quality associated with insufficient approximation of the vocal folds; *Hoarse* is a combination of harsh and breathy.

In addition to an over-all evaluation of vocal behavior involving speech, reading, and singing, the examiner should measure performances of a number of isolated vocal skills.

Pitch range can be measured best in the singing voice. Equipment needed is a pitch pipe and a knowledge of the musical scale. By listening to the speaking voice, the tester can subjectively evaluate the median pitch. The client should sing the scale in both directions until the examiner has a fair sample of the number of full notes in the pitch range as well as the highest and lowest notes. The examiner can also record a subjective judgment of the pitch level of the median pitch.

[6] In speech pathology, stuttering remains a challenging problem to both the clinician and the researcher. The student may find stimulation to his thinking by careful study of Chapters 27, 28, 29, and 30. (*Editor*)

The relation between voice quality and pitch should also be measured. This again can be accomplished by singing of the scale. Each vocal response on each note should be noted as good, fair, poor, or very poor and from a composite of such judgments is determined the pitch range of "good" voice. The median pitch may be determined by isolating the most frequently used pitch. The procedure is extremely subjective.

The effect of pitch upon loudness can be measured as follows: By use of the pitch pipe, high, middle, and low notes can be given to the client who is instructed to sing them loudly. The loudness for each pitch should be evaluated as very loud, loud, moderate, soft, very soft.

In the same manner the effect of pitch upon quality can be evaluated, except that this time the client is instructed to sing at a comfortable loudness. The examiner should evaluate on the basis of good, fair, poor, very poor; defective equality, if present, should be reported.

The evaluation of voice as related to personality is important even though it is extremely subjective. Weak, whiny voices, or high-pitched voices associated with large persons, or deep loud-booming voices with small people, can be important clinically, since so many voice problems are no more than the vocal projection of personality problems.

The examination of the vocal mechanism should be a joint effort dependent upon the physical examination and re-evaluation by the speech examiner of such factors as are most related to vocal function and not pathology.

Evaluations of voice problems must always consider the importance of infections, organic malformations, personality deviations, and environmental stimulation since any or all may be involved in precipitating and/or maintaining voice disorders.

For detailed methods of studying quality of voice, including nasality, hoarseness, harshness and breathiness, see Fairbanks (1940, pp. 201–216), West, Kennedy, and Carr (1947, pp. 571–572), and Johnson, Darley, and Spriestersbach (1952, pp. 71–94). Methods of analysis of habitual and natural pitch level are described in Fairbanks (1940, pp. 165–171), West, Kennedy, and Carr (1947, pp. 544–545) and Van Riper (1954, pp. 287–289).

For suggestions on examining the intensity or loudness of the voice, see Fairbanks (1940, p. 191) and Van Riper (1954, pp. 300–301).[7]

## CONCLUSION

The therapy for most speech disorders varies so much from therapist to therapist that no set of examination methods will be completely suitable. Perhaps as precipitating conditions become better known and universally accepted, more standardized testing procedures can be recommended. In the meantime, the greatest tool of the examiner is *observation*. He must never sacrifice this tool in favor of the standardized testing procedure.

[7] See Chapters 22 and 26 for more detailed presentations of voice problems.

Parents or Guardians: This case history may seem unnecessarily comprehensive. You may think that many of the questions have nothing to do with your child's handicap. However, you cannot be sure which factors are important until the examinations are completed. The form should be filled out IN FULL to the best of your ability and sent to the Clinic before the child is examined so the child may receive the most adequate service. (If more space is needed, write on the back of these sheets.)

## CASE HISTORY

GENERAL:
Child' Name_____ Sex____ Race____ Age____ Grade____
Street or RR_____ City_____ State_____ .

Father's Name_____ Occupation_____ Age_____
Present Address_____ Birthplace_____

Mother's Name_____ Occupation_____ Age_____
Present Address_____ Birthplace_____
Telephone_____ Who cares for child if mother is employed_____

Brothers and Sisters:
Name_____ Age____ Name_____ Age_____
Name_____ Age____ Name_____ Age_____

Relatives or roomers living in the home:
Name_____ Relationship_____
Name_____ Relationship_____

DEVELOPMENT:
Date of child's birth_____ Birthplace_____
Mother's age at child's birth_____ Father's age at child's birth_____
Injury or disease during pregnancy (describe)_____
_____

Birth condition: Normal_____ Premature_____ Prolonged Delivery_____
Nature of delivery_____ Birth injury_____ ' Birth weight_____
What age did child: Tooth_____ Sit up_____ Walk_____ Talk: words____
sentences_____ Control bladder_____ bowels_____ Feed self_____ Dress self____
What diseases, sicknesses, operations, or injuries has child had and at what age?
_____
Which were serious_____ If so, how long did they last_____
Was high fever present_____ At what age_____
How was general physical growth of child: Slow_____ Average_____ Fast____
Physical abnormalities: Cleft palate_____ Was it operated_____
Paralysis_____ Was it treated_____ Hearing_____
Others_____
Level of intelligence: Slow_____ Average_____ Fast_____

EDUCATIONAL:
At what age did child enter school_____ Number of schools attended_____
Which grades were repeated_____ Why_____
Subjects child likes_____ Dislikes_____
Does he like his teachers_____ Do they like him_____
Does he like his classmates_____ Do they like him_____
Explain_____
_____
_____

IV. HABITS AND PERSONALITY
    Child's Sleeping Habits: Regular_____ Alone_____ If not, with whom_____
                             Dreams_____ Wets Bed_____ If so, how is problem
    handled at home_____
    What is child's reaction to trouble_____
    When does child go to bed at night_____ Does he have to be coaxed_____
    Does he go to sleep right away_____ Does child normally take a nap__
    If so, at what time_____ Thumb sucking_____
    When did he stop_____ What did you do to stop the habit_____


    Child's Eating Habits: During infancy how long was he breast fed_____
    Bottle fed_____ Did he have trouble learning to suckle_____
    Explain_____
    Did he have trouble swallowing_____ Explain_____
    At what age did he use a spoon_____ Did he have trouble eating at any time__
    Explain_____
    Foods he does not like_____
    What attempts have been made to get him to eat these_____


    Are there any foods to which he is allergic or which make him ill_____
    What are they_____


    Fears: Is the child afraid___If so, of what_____

    What brought about this fear_____


    Play Activities: Age of playmates_____ About how many_____
    If child plays alone, what attempts have been made to have child play with
    others_____ Is child a leader_____
    What games and activities does child enjoy_____
    Will child willingly share toys with other children_____
    Any particular hobbies_____

    Church Activities: Church preference: child_____
    father_____ mother_____
    Does child attend_____ Does child enjoy it_____ Do parents attend_____

    Check all of the following which describe your child:
    Friendly_____ Unresponsive_____ Temper outbursts_____ Bites Nails_____ Happy_____
    Sullen_____ Aggressive_____ Retiring_____ Quiet_____ Explosive_____ Stubborn__
    Suggestible_____ "Inferiority Complex"_____

    Training of Child: How does he behave when you want him to do something new

    If he resists, do you know why_____
    What do you do_____
    Who disciplines the child_____
    Methods of discipline_____

304

BEHAVIOR DURING SPEECH
Does he understand what you say to him_____If not, describe in some detail_____
_____
Do you know why he doesn't understand_____
Does he have the same trouble with other people_____Explain_____

If you don't understand him, how does he behave_____

If you can't understand his speech, what does he do to express his wants_____

Do you understand then_____How does he behave when you don't understand at all_

If he does talk, does he say as <u>much</u> as most children of his age_____
If not, explain_____

If he does talk as much as other children his age does he talk as well_____
If he has trouble saying sounds please list them_____

If he has trouble saying words please list some_____
_____

Does he repeat sounds or words_____Does it happen often_____When did you first
notice this behavior_____What have you done about it_____
_____

Does he have trouble with his voice_____If so, what_____
When did you first notice it_____Do you know why he had the trouble
_____

What has been done to help him correct his trouble in talking or understanding
at home_____
at school_____
at physician's office_____

SPEECH BACKGROUND
Did he cry much during the first month_____If so, was there much reason_____
_____What was done when he cried_____

Did he make many "play" noises as a baby_____Do you remember when he began_____
If so, when_____Did they stop_____When_____
As a baby, did he imitate sounds made by cows, cats, etc._____
Did he imitate sounds made by adults_____If so, explain_____

When did he say his first word_____Could you understand_____
Explain how his speech developed after the first word_____
_____
_____
_____
_____

# INDIANA UNIVERSITY SPEECH AND HEARING CLINIC

To the Parent: To assure the best service for your child, please have this form filled out at your child's school.

To the Teacher or Principal: In order that we may have complete information about this child, we ask you to complete this form and return it to the parent or send directly to: Speech and Hearing Clinic, Indiana University, Bloomington, Indiana

## EDUCATIONAL HISTORY

Name_____ Age_____ Grade_____ Date_____

Name of town_____ Name of school_____

Did he attend nursery school_____ Kindergarten_____ What grades were repeated_____

Age of entering school_____ Number of schools attended_____ Why were grades repe

Which grades were skipped_____ Why

Does he like his teachers_____ Do the teachers like him_____ Does he like the other

_____ Do the other pupils like him_____ Child's interests_____

Does child play well with other children_____ Does child cooperate with other chi

in school_____ Is child habitually attentive_____ Inattentive_____ Does the child li

to go to school_____ Is attendance regular_____ If irregular, why_____

Achievement in school subjects:

A. Elementary

| | Poor | Average | Good |
|---|---|---|---|
| Reading | ___ | ___ | ___ |
| Spelling | ___ | ___ | ___ |
| Arithmetic | ___ | ___ | ___ |
| Writing | ___ | ___ | ___ |
| Language | ___ | ___ | ___ |
| Art | ___ | ___ | ___ |
| Citizenship | ___ | ___ | ___ |

B. High School

| | Poor | Average | Good |
|---|---|---|---|
| English | ___ | ___ | ___ |
| Mathematics | ___ | ___ | ___ |
| Science | ___ | ___ | ___ |
| Social | ___ | ___ | ___ |
| Foreign Language | ___ | ___ | ___ |
| Industrial arts | ___ | ___ | ___ |
| Other subjects | ___ | ___ | ___ |
| Citizenship | ___ | ___ | ___ |

Which subjects does pupil like_____

Which subjects does he dislike_____

Has any remedial work been done in academic subjects_____ If so, what_____

For how long_____

Success of remedial work_____

Tests that have been administered at school:

Intelligence: Name of_____ C.A._____ M.A._____ I.Q._____

Name of_____ C.A._____ M.A._____ I.Q._____

Achievement: Name of_____ Results_____

Name of_____ Results_____

Does child have a speech defect_____ Describe difficulty_____

Has any remedial work been done_____

Has the child had ear trouble_____ To your knowledge, does he have a hearing loss

What if anything has been done to correct this_____

COMMENTS: (Write on back if you wish)_____

Signature of Principal or Teacher_____

306

e Parent: In order that the Clinic may have a better understanding of your
, we are asking that you take your child to your family physician for a com-
physical examination. Ask him to fill out the following questions and to add
additional information regarding the child.
e Physician: If you would like to receive a copy of our report, please PRINT
name and address:

_____     _____
Name                                 Address

## HEALTH EXAMINATION

_____
Address
_____
e examined the above child and find the following:
Lips_____ Teeth_____ Tongue_____
Palate_____ Throat_____ Nose_____
Tonsils: Small_____ Medium____ Large____ Cut: Well_____ Tags_____ Septic_____
Adenoids: Yes_____ No_____
Recommendation_____

General Condition_____ Hearing: Left_____ Right_____
Recommendation_____

Right: General condition_____
       Vision_____ With lens_____
Left : General condition_____
       Vision_____ With lens_____
       Gross imbalance_____ Color vision_____
       Pupil reflexes_____
Recommendation_____

ITIES AND SURGERY: Deformities (kind):_____
Has any correction been made_____
Surgery (kind):_____ Success_____
Recommendation_____

AL PHYSICAL:
Chest:_____ Lungs_____
Respiratory disorders_____
X-Ray: result_____ Tuberculin test: Pos._____ Neg._____
Heart:_____
       Pulse_____ Blood Pressure_____
Nutrition:_____
Posture:_____
Skin:_____ Athletes foot_____
Urinalysis: albumin_____ Sugar_____
Immunization: Whooping Cough (date)_____
              Diphtheria (date)_____
              Smallpox (date)_____
Other findings:_____

Recommendations:_____

H AND HEARING: Does he need speech therapy_____ Hearing Therapy_____

                                                                    _____M.D.
_____     _____
(Date)                      (Examining Physician)

## BIBLIOGRAPHY

AINSWORTH, Stanley. 1948. Speech correction methods. New York: Prentic Hall.

ANDERSON, V. A. 1953. Improving the child's speech. New York: Oxford Uni Press.

ARTHUR, Grace. Point scale of performance tests. 1930. Chicago: C. H. Stoel ing Co.

BACKUS, Ollie. 1945. Speech in education. New York: Longmans, Green.

BERRY, M., and EISENSON, J. 1942. The defective in speech. New York: Croft

———. 1956. Speech disorders. New York: Appleton-Century-Crofts.

BRYNGELSON, B., and GLASPEY, E. 1941. Speech improvement cards. Chicago Scott, Foresman.

California test of mental maturity. 1937. Sullivan, E. T., Clark, W. W., and Tieg W. E. Los Angeles: Southern California Book Depository.

Children's Apperception Test. 1949. Bellak, L., and Bellak, S. New Yor C. P. S. Co.

Durrell analysis of reading difficulty. Yonkers-on-Hudson, New York: Wor Book Co.

EISENSON, J. 1954. Examining for aphasia. New York: Psychological Corpor tion.

FAIRBANKS, Grant. 1940. Voice and articulation drillbook. New York: Harpe

Gates basic reading tests. New York: Bureau of Publications, Teachers Colleg Columbia Univ.

Gates reading survey tests. New York: Bureau of Publications, Teachers Colleg Columbia Univ.

GESELL, A., and AMATRUDA, C. 1941. Developmental diagnosis. New Yor Hoeber.

GOODENOUGH, F. L. 1926. Measurement of intelligence by drawings. Yonke on-Hudson, New York: World Book Co.

HALSTEAD-WEPMAN aphasia screening test. Chicago: Department of Medici Univ. of Chicago.

Iowa silent reading tests. Yonkers-on-Hudson, New York: World Book Co.

IRWIN, O. C. 1947. Infant speech: variability and the problem of diagnosis. *Speech Disorders,* 12, 287–289.

IRWIN, R. B. 1953. Speech and hearing therapy. New York: Prentice-Hall.

JOHNSON, W., BROWN, S., CURTIS, J., EDNEY, C., and KEASTER, J. 1948. Spee handicapped school children. New York: Harper.

JOHNSON, W., DARLEY, F., and SPRIESTERSBACH, D. 1952. Diagnostic manual speech correction. New York: Harper.

LOUTTIT, C. M. 1947. Clinical psychology (rev. ed.). New York: Harper.

Metropolitan achievement test. Yonkers-on-Hudson, New York. World Book C

MILISEN, R. 1954. Rationale on articulation. Monograph supplement number *J. Speech Hearing Disorders.*

Minnesota multiphasic personality inventory. 1951. Hathaway, S. R., and M Kinley, J. C. New York: Psychological Corporation.

MYKLEBUST, H. R. 1954. Auditory disorders in children. New York: Grune a Stratton.

Nebraska test of learning aptitude for young deaf children. 1941. Hiskey, M. New York: Psychological Corporation.

Rorschach test. Chicago: C. H. Stoelting Co.

Stanford achievement test. Yonkers-on-Hudson, New York: World Book Co.

Stanford-Binet Scale (rev.). 1937. Terman, L. M., and Merrill, M. Bost Houghton Mifflin.

EMPLIN, M. 1943. A study of sound discrimination ability of elementary school pupils. *J. Speech Disorders,* 8, 127–132.

—— 1947. A non-diagnostic articulation test. *J. Speech Disorders,* 12, 392–396.

hematic apperception test. Murry, H. A. Cambridge, Mass.: Harvard Univ. Press.

RAVIS, L. E. 1931. Speech pathology. New York: D. Appleton.

—— and RASMUS, B. J. 1931. The speech sound discrimination ability of cases with functional disorders of articulation. *Quart. J. Speech Educ.,* 17, 217–226.

an Alstyne picture vocabulary test for preschool children. Bloomington, Illinois: Public School Publishing Co.

AN RIPER, C. 1954. Speech correction, principles and methods, (3rd ed.). New York: Prentice-Hall.

ineland social maturity scale. 1947. Doll, E. A. Minneapolis: The Educational Test Bureau.

Wechsler adult intelligence scale. 1955. New York: Psychological Corporation.

Wechsler intelligence scale for children (WISC). 1949. New York: Psychological Corporation.

EST, R., KENNEDY, L., and CARR, A. 1947. The rehabilitation of speech (rev. ed.). New York: Harper.

# PART II

# Speech and Voice Disorders
# Associated with Organic Abnormalities

# CHAPTER 9

# PATHOLOGY, DIAGNOSIS, AND THERAPY OF DEAFNESS

*Victor Goodhill, M.D.*

## QUANTITATIVE AND QUALITATIVE DISTINCTIONS

### The Word *Deafness*

BECAUSE OF LOOSE CONNOTATION, the word *deafness* creates some misunderstandings in otologic literature. As used at the present time, it may describe quantitative speech-threshold shifts of any degree from the relatively minor 15 db deficit to profound or total loss of hearing in the 80 to 100 db range. It may also be used to describe specific qualitative communication deficits such as the high-tone specific-threshold shift in acoustic trauma which is called "high-tone nerve deafness." These quantitatively and qualitatively loose definitions allow confusion that ought to be avoided in order to effect clearer understanding among workers. In the following otologic discussion of hearing losses, more specific terms will be employed.

The term *hypacusis* is used to describe any threshold shift which is potentially correctible by either medical or prosthetic techniques to a practical hearing level.

The term *anacusis* is used to describe either profound threshold shifts or so-neural dysfunctions which cannot be corrected by medical or prosthetic techniques to a practical hearing level. (Occasional cases will fit neither the hypacusis nor anacusis category strictly. Such cases will require special descriptions and classifications.)

The term *dysacusis* is used to describe a defect in audition which is usually central and on an integrative or interpretive level.

These terms may be modified by qualitative and anatomic terms to describe a large variety of threshold shifts or auditory pathway dysfunctions. They further offer the convenience of being used in adjective form to describe psychophysiologic states heretofore described with difficulty in the English language. The term *hard of hearing* is used to describe a large variety of mild or moderate hypacuses. Thus, such a patient may be termed *hypa-*

313

*custic.* This will release the word *deaf* to truly describe the person with non-amplifiable major threshold shifts who might then be described as "ana-custic" or "deaf" in the educational frame of reference.

The term *dysacusis* could then be reserved as a general heading for many varieties of central communication defects including aphasia, psychogenic deafness, "mind" deafness, "word" deafness, and so on, and it might even be used to describe certain aspects of malingering as well as hysterical deafness This controversial subject is more completely covered in other chapters.

### Anatomico-Physiologic Types

For purposes of simplicity, all "deafness" in the past was subdivided into two main groups: "conductive" and "nerve."

**Conductive.** The term *conductive* is still a useful one and will be retained in this discussion. It will be used to describe lesions in the conductive path way of the hearing organ, namely, the external auditory canal, tympanic membrane, tympanic cavity, ossicular chain, Eustachian tube, otic capsule labyrinthine fenestrae, and perilymph space. In other words, any disturbance peripheral to the basilar membrane may be classified within the conductive pathway.

**Neural.** The term *nerve deafness* has been useful but is ambiguous and has led to oversimplification of lesions in the neural auditory pathway. In recent years, the term *perceptive* was acquired from psychologic usage and almost displaced the earlier term, *nerve* deafness. This term, *perceptive* has a useful place, but it is too specific a term for the entire group of lesion in the neural auditory pathway. In the present discussion the author will employ the general term *neural* to describe lesions in the neural auditor pathway. These will be further divided into three anatomic subdivisions namely, receptive, transmissive, and perceptive.

Lesions in the receptor organ (the organ of Corti) may be termed *recepto lesions.*

Lesions in the neural auditory pathway, central to the organ of Corti and including the cochlear ganglion, the dorsal and ventral cochlear nuclei, and the ascending tracts, will be grouped under the heading of "transmissive neural lesions."

Lesions in the subcortical and cortical auditory areas will be termed *pe ceptive neural lesions,* inasmuch as true perception of auditory sensation probably does not occur distal to the auditory cortex and associated subcorti cal integrative areas. It will be difficult to distinguish between *perceptive neural hypacuses* and *dysacuses* in many cases.

### Classifications

ANATOMIC CLASSIFICATION
1. Conduction hypacusis

2. Neural hypacusis or anacusis
   a. Reception
   b. Transmission
   c. Perception
3. Dysacusis

Because time relations in regard to onset have profound significance in neural hypacuses and anacuses, a time or chronological classification will be used in the discussion of these lesions.

CHRONOLOGICAL CLASSIFICATION OF NEURAL HYPACUSES AND ANACUSES
1. Hereditary—genetic
2. Acquired—nongenetic
   a. Infantile
      (1) prenatal
      (2) natal
      (3) postnatal
   b. Childhood
   c. Adult

## OTOLOGIC DIAGNOSTIC TECHNIQUES

The techniques employed by the otologist in the diagnosis and differential diagnosis of deafness comprise: complete chronological otologic history; pertinent medical history; physical examination of the ears, nose, and throat; general medical survey; differential audiologic studies; laboratory procedures.

**Complete chronological otologic history.** The otologic history should be very complete and should be obtained in chronologic fashion. The patient's own descriptions are important; not only all details pertaining to the hearing loss but also in regard to tinnitus, vertigo, otorrhea, and otalgia.

**Pertinent medical history.** Inventories of the respiratory, skeletal, gastrointestinal, neurological, genito-urinary, and other systems are mandatory in any medical survey.

**Physical examination of the ears, nose, and throat.** The physical examination should include a complete inspection of the ears, the nose and paranasal sinuses, the nasopharynx, the pharynx and larynx, as well as the external head and neck. The patency of the Eustachian tubes should be determined by appropriate methods, including visual examination of the orifices by nasopharyngeal mirror, transnasal examination, and nasopharyngoscopic examination, as well as by politzerization and, if indicated, by tubal catheterization and inflation.

Otoscopic examination of the ears should include visualization with magnification (Fig. 1) and diagnostic compression and rarefaction of auditory canal pressures to determine mobility of tympanic membrane (pneumatic or Seigle otoscopy). Diagnostic aspiration, either by needle puncture or diagnostic paracentesis, is indicated in questionable middle-ear effusions.

Examination of the vestibular apparatus begins with observation for spon-

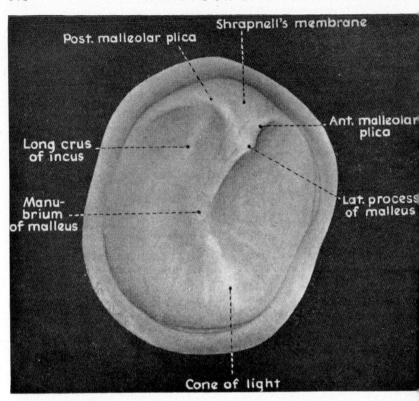

FIG. 1. Illustration of lateral aspect of normal right tympanic membrane. (From Boies, L. R. 1949 Fundamentals of otolaryngology. New York: Saunders. Fig. 3, p. 12.)

taneous nystagmus with or without positional change. It is indicated in al cases of neural deafness and in selected varieties of conduction hypacusis Induced vestibular responses are valuable in differential diagnosis. Such information may be obtained by the Bárány rotation technique, but is mor commonly obtained from the caloric labyrinthine excitation technique, us ing ice water or warm water, or both.

**General medical survey.** The otologist is first a physician and secondl a specialist in ear diseases. His responsibility is to the entire patient, not jus to his ears. Accordingly, he will investigate either personally or through consultant any special medical problems which may co-exist. He must re main constantly alert to the otologic manifestations of systemic disease: His survey will certainly pay attention to such problems as anemia, hype tension, and other vascular diseases, neurological problems, endocrinop athies, and all other systemic problems which the true physician will alway keep in mind regardless of his specialty.

**Differential audiologic studies.** Whereas audiologists, educators of th deaf, speech therapists, and ancillary specialists are all interested in the er tire field of audiometry, the otologist is specifically concerned with *diffe* *ential audiometric diagnosis.* This may be described as audiometric meth-odology in anatomic localization of auditory pathway lesions. It is concerned with differentiation of conductive from neural lesions, and receptor from transmissive or perceptive lesions.

It will utilize bone- and air-conduction differences, masking phenomena, speech-reception and speech-discrimination studies, and tests for recruitment of loudness. The recently suggested psychogalvanic skin resistance technique (Bordley and Hardy, 1949; Goodhill, *et al.,* 1954) is also of value.

No otologic examination is complete without a tuning-fork test confirmation of audiometric findings. Of greatest value are the Rinné and Weber tests using at least the 512 and 1024 tuning-forks. With the Rinné test, masking is just as important as it is with bone-conduction audiometry by conventional techniques.

The Rinné test is undoubtedly the most important fork test. Its precise technique will depend upon the type of fork and the individual practice of the examiner. It is usually a simple practice to test bone conduction first and then air conduction. A significantly better bone-conduction response in terms of intensity and duration usually points to a conduction hypacusis.

Current bone-conduction audiometric techniques require much improvement. Bone-conduction transducers should be designed specifically for testing and should not be ordinary hearing-aid types (a round-faced applicator which would approach a point contact would be preferable). The force of application of the transducer should be at least 400 grams. In future bone-conduction techniques (Goodhill and Holcomb, 1955a), computation of compliance variations due to subcutaneous tissues will possibly add accuracy to bone-conduction threshold studies. The use of the forehead instead of the mastoid area might also yield more consistently valid responses.

In the presence of tinnitus, a *tinnitus identification test* is indicated to attempt to define the precise subjective characteristics of the tinnitus. This may be done by tinnitus-matching records (Goodhill, 1950a, 1952b, and 1952c) as well as by pure-tone sweep audiometry presented to the patient for frequency and intensity characteristic comparison.

**Laboratory procedures.** Otorrhea calls for appropriate bacteriologic as well as cytologic studies and may call for sensitivity tests by in-vitro techniques.

Roentgen studies of the mastoid require special techniques for the visualiation of pneumatization of the mastoid process, for ossicular details in the tympanic cavity, and for information regarding the otic capsule of both vestibular and cochlear labyrinths. Such information requires a number of special views of the skull base including the Schuller, Stenver, Towne, and the very excellent Owen position. Laminography, or body-section radiography, is also useful in roentgen diagnosis of otologic lesions.

In selected cases where some central nervous system diseases may co-exist, examination of the cerebrospinal fluid pressure and chemistry is necessary. The Queckenstedt or Tobey-Ayer test is frequently informative and requires compression of the jugular system to rule out thrombosis of the sigmoid sinus. In some types of neural hypacusis, serologic study of the spinal fluid to rule out syphilis is necessary.

Examination of the blood and urine are of paramount importance in all constitutional medical lesions. Serologic examination of the blood to rule out syphilis is required frequently. Leukemia, anemia, and polycythemia may produce otologic disturbances.

## CONDUCTION LESIONS

### Diagnostic Aspects of Conduction Lesions

*Unless otherwise specified in the ensuing descriptions, the term A.C. will be used for air-conduction threshold, and B.C. for bone-conduction threshold. Unless otherwise stated these thresholds will be described within the speech range.*

Hearing losses of conduction type are always hypacuses and never anacuses, and are characterized by well-defined criteria. These include the following:

*Threshold Losses.* Threshold losses by pure-tone audiometry do not exceed 55 to 60 db in the speech range. Any threshold loss in excess of this is undoubtedly due to a co-existent neural loss.

*Significant B.C.–A.C. Differential.* The B.C.–A.C. "gap" will give a quantitative measure of the extent of the conduction deficit. This deficit cannot be gauged by A.C. comparison with the zero audiometric reference level for "normal." For example: a patient with co-existent presbycusis and otosclerosis may have an A.C. of 70 db and a B.C. of 30 db; his conduction deficit would be roughly 40 db and not 70 db. This differential will be confirmed usually by the negative Rinné test when performed with a 512-cycle or 1024-cycle fork. Major discrepancy between this test and audiometric B.C. and A.C. tests will call for very careful review of B.C. tests with and without masking.

*Close Correlation Between Pure-Tone A.C. Threshold and SRT.* The SRT or speech reception threshold, is the speech audiogram utilizing spondee words. Such correlation is the rule in conduction lesions but is not so uniform in neural lesions.

*Speech Discrimination Normal.* Speech discrimination score within normal limits, according to the supra-threshold speech discrimination tests with PB words.

*Response to Amplification.* Excellent response to amplification with little or no recruitment, and excellent amplification of whispered voice with th classical speaking tube.

Conduction losses may vary from minor 5 to 10 db losses to the 55 to 60 db losses mentioned above. In all such threshold estimations, it must be remembered that the zero level used in conventional audiometry is an ar

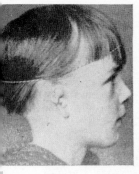 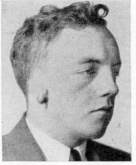 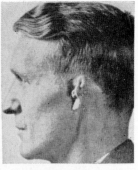

FIG. 2. Congenital types of external ear deformity (microtia). (From Lederer, F. L. 1952. Diseases of the ear, nose, and throat (6th ed.). Philadelphia: Davis. Fig. 1, p. 105.)

bitrary level and may not represent the true predisease threshold of the individual patient.

The patient with an uncomplicated conduction hypacusis can never be described as being profoundly deaf. If he has significant difficulty in understanding speech with adequate amplification, it must be assumed, audiometric findings to the contrary, that he has a neural loss in addition to his conduction loss.

## Lesions of the Auricle and External Auditory Canal

**Congenital malformations (atresias and aplasias).** Congenital malformations of the auricle and external auditory canal are characterized by pleomorphism. They are primarily defects in branchial cleft development. Such lesions are usually not associated with cochlear lesions but are commonly associated with lesions of the tympanic cavity. Thus, normal B.C. thresholds (indicating normal cochlear function) will be found in most cases of microtia (small ear) (Fig. 2) and congenital defects of the auricle and external auditory canal.

Malformations of the auricle alone are of no great significance to the otologist, being primarily cosmetic problems. Atresias of the external auditory canal (Fig. 3), however, are of profound importance, inasmuch as they usually produce a major conduction hypacusis, either alone or in association with tympanic aplasia.

Congenital atresias (imperforations) of the external auditory canal may range from partial lateral atresias (pinpoint openings) to complete medial atresias of the cartilaginous and/or bony canal. In the rare lateral types, it is not unusual to find a normal bony canal and a normal tympanic membrane. In most instances, the atresia is associated with an absence of the tympanic membrane and a congenitally abnormal tympanic cavity. In these cases, as in the auricular aplasias, the cochlea is usually normal. The tympanic membrane is replaced by the primitive tympanic plate and one, two, or all three ossicles may be absent or deformed in a multiplicity of variations.

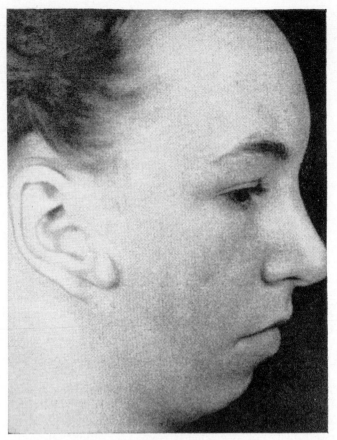

FIG. 3. Photograph of congenital atresia of external auditory meatus with cosmetic deformi
of auricular lobe. (From Lederer, F. L. 1952. Diseases of the ear, nose, and throat (6th ed.
Philadelphia: Davis. Fig. 8, p. 109.)

The surgical treatment of these defects will be discussed later with congen
tal lesions of the tympanic cavity.

   **Acquired lesions (atresias, tumors, exostoses).** Acquired lesions of th
auricle and the external auditory canal are of great importance in conductio
hypacuses.

   The atresia which occasionally follows chronic external otitis can produc
a major conduction loss simply by complete occlusion of the external aud
tory canal. No hearing loss will occur as long as even a microscopic openin
is present in the external auditory canal. In many instances, conductio
hypacuses will occur before such a complete closure because of accumula
tions of cerumen, dead epithelium, or exudate which will close the sma
opening. Such atresias require surgical correction by endaural technique
which involve resection of edematous skin, subcutaneous tissue, thickene
periosteum, and bone. The surgically-widened ear canal is usually covere
with a split-thickness skin graft.

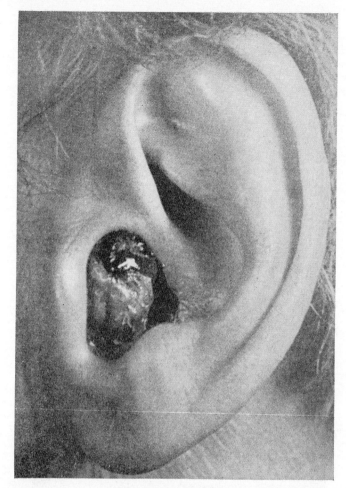

FIG. 4. Epidermoid carcinoma of the external auditory canal, accompanied by facial paralysis. (From Lederer, F. L. 1952. Diseases of the ear, nose, and throat (6th ed.), Philadelphia: Davis. Fig. 43, p. 146.)

Tumors of the external auditory canal may occlude the air conduction pathway completely and produce a conduction hypacusis. Tumors of the external auditory canal may be benign or malignant (Fig. 4). All common types of tumors are found in the external auditory canal, including those of skin as well as of cartilage and bone. The only safe treatment for such tumors is surgical excision. In some instances, radiation may be required in addition.

Bony growths due to exostoses and osteomata are not infrequently found in the external auditory canal. They may not only occlude the canal completely as in atresia, but they may extend to the tympanic annulus and into the tympanic cavity, producing tympanic, as well as canal, conduction hypacuses. Most of these bony tumors are benign. Exostoses are very com-

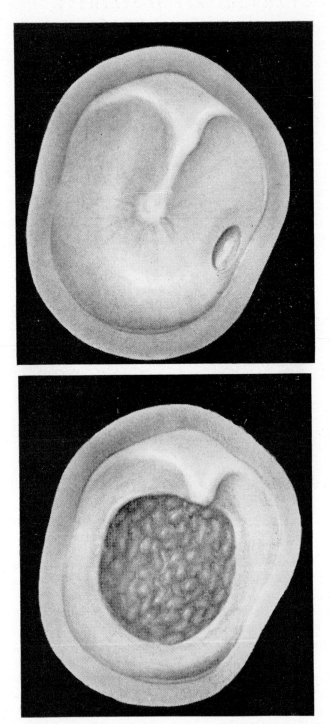

FIG. 5. Illustration of small *central* perforation (top) and large *central* perforation (bottom) i
chronic otitis media. (From Boies, L. R. 1954. Fundamentals of otolaryngology (2nd ed.). Ne
York: Saunders. Fig. 45, p. 85.)

monly found in swimmers, the reason for this being unknown. The proper treatment of exostoses and osteomata is surgical excision by endaural techniques. In most instances, such removal can be accomplished without damage to the tympanic membrane or cavity.

## Lesions of the Tympanic Cavity (Including Ossicular Chain and Eustachian Tube)

**Congenital lesions.** Congenital lesions of the tympanic cavity will frequently accompany congenital atresia of the external auditory canal. In most instances, the tympanic membrane is absent and is represented by a primitive tympanic bony plate, called the "atresia plate." There are also varying degrees of aplasia and deformation of the ossicular chain. Any or all of the ossicles may be deformed or absent. In most instances, the stapes footplate is intact even though the crura may be deformed. In some instances, all three ossicles are present in normal relationship except that the malleus is crowded into an atypically located epitympanic space and, of course, is not attached to a tympanic membrane. In some instances, the malleus is an integral part of the tympanic bony plate and completely fixed. The incus may be fixed to the bone of the fossa incudis. In some instances, the stapes is fixed in the oval window and the findings are identical with those of stapes fixation in otosclerosis.

All of these congenital lesions in the tympanic cavity and external auditory canal can be treated today quite successfully by endaural surgical techniques. Such techniques may include plastic reconstruction of a patent external auditory canal, mobilization of the ossicular chain, and anchorage of the malleus or incus to a new "tympanic membrane" formed by a skin graft. They include, in some instances, a fenestration of the horizontal semicircular canal, where there is evidence of a fixed stapes footplate. Stapedolysis techniques now being employed with success in otosclerosis might find application in atresia cases. Surgical reconstruction of these deformities frequently requires several stages.

### Acquired lesions

*Tympanic Membrane.* Perforations of the tympanic membrane are extremely common as spontaneous or operative sequellae of the acute otitis media secondary to upper respiratory infections. They are more common in children but may occur with great frequency in adults as well. Most permanent tympanic perforations are spontaneous in origin, although occasionally they may result from the surgical procedures of myringotomy or paracentesis. Physical trauma by blasts, burns, foreign bodies, and chemical injuries may also produce perforations.

The conduction hypacusis associated with a tympanic membrane perforation depends upon the size of the perforation (Fig. 5), its location, whether it is dry or wet, scarring in the membrane, and the presence of other lesions within the tympanic conduction apparatus. It is not unusual to find perfora-

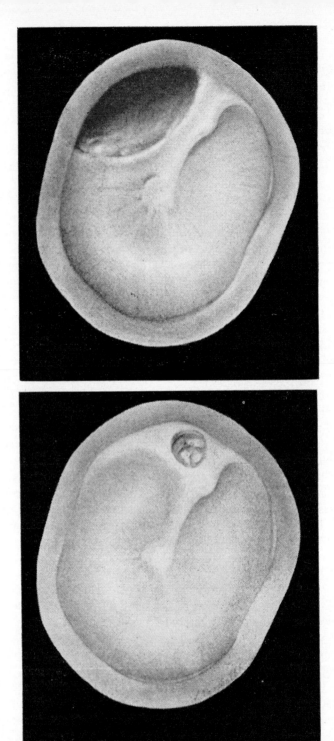

FIG. 6. Marginal perforation due to bone disease is shown at top. Pars flaccida perforation due to attic cholesteatoma is shown below. Both of these perforations represent potentially serious varieties of otitis media. (From Boies, L. R. 1954. Fundamentals of otolaryngology (2nd ed.). New York: Saunders. Fig. 45, p. 85.)

tions occupying one-fourth the square area of the tympanic membrane, with only slight conduction losses. Larger perforations always cause significant conduction losses.

The treatment of a wet perforation depends upon the underlying tympanic or associated tubal or mastoid disease.

The treatment of a dry perforation will depend upon several factors. Smaller "central" perforations may be frequently induced to heal by cauterization of the margins and "patching" with paper or plastic material. Large "central" perforations are difficult to close and may require surgical skin grafting. In some instances, hearing may be significantly improved by placing a bit of moistened cotton, or a small plastic tube or capsule through the perforation in contact either with the stapes or the round-window niche. Gains of 10 to 40 db in the speech range are not uncommon with such simple prosthetic devices. "Marginal perforations" (Fig. 6) involving the bony or annular margin of the tympanic membrane usually indicate serious bony disease in the epitympanic or mastoid regions and may frequently be associated with other findings calling for operative mastoid intervention.

Calcareous deposits in the tympanic membrane usually do not impede its acoustic properties significantly, but marked hypertrophy of the epithelial, muscular, or mucosal layers will produce a conduction hypacusis. The greatest degree of loss occurs in tympanic mucosal hyperplasia, inasmuch as it is usually associated wtih tubal lesions, fibrosis, and some degree of ossicular fixation. Major losses equal to those in otosclerotic stapedial fixation may be encountered in tympanic fibrosis, or in tympanic membrane stiffening. Some of these cases may be helped by fenestration surgery, but stapedolysis is usually of slight value.

*Ossicular Lesions.* Isolated lesions of the *malleus* and *incus* are quite rare unless they are the sequellae of some constitutional bone disease, such as fragilitas ossium (brittle bones), Paget's disease, or syphilis. These two ossicles are rarely involved grossly by otosclerosis, although microscopic evidence of the disease has been reported in them. Specific diseases of the malleus and incus contribute very little to conduction hypacusis, except when their associated motion is inhibited by stiffness or deformation of the incudomalleolar or incudostapedial articulations by fibrosis or arthritis. (True "arthritis" of these joints is rare and is usually not associated with arthritis in other parts of the body.)

Fibrosis of these two joints is not uncommon and is usually accompanied by perforations or other deformations of the tympanic membrane and thickened mucosa in the middle ear. This syndrome of "tympanic fibrosis" is usually a sequel of repeated attacks of otitis media with or without mastoiditis. It usually produces a conduction hypacusis. The severity increases if the fibrosis immobilizes the stapediovestibular joint and/or the round-window membrane.

Treatment of tympanic fibrosis is not completely satisfactory at the present time. Reconstructive surgical procedures of the "tympanoplasty" type are

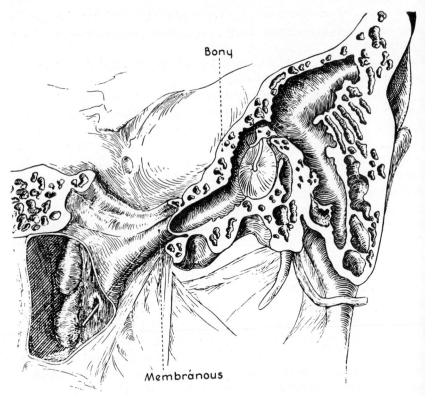

Bony

Membranous

FIG. 7. The Eustachian tube. A drawing from a dissection of the Eustachian tube showing its relationship to the middle-ear space on one end and the nasopharynx on the other end. (From Boies, L. R. 1954. Fundamentals of otolaryngology (2nd ed.). New York: Saunders. Fig. 6, p. 15.)

being studied and offer hope of future progress. Medical measures and local therapy are usually inadequate. Fenestration of the horizontal semicircular canal with special modification, including use of skin grafts, has been an encouraging approach in some cases of tympanic fibrosis with stapedial fixation.

The stapes is the primary ossicle involved in conduction hypacusis. The most common disease involving the stapes is otosclerosis (which is truly a disease of the otic capsule), and the stapes involvement is primarily through the footplate; although in fulminating "juvenile" or "malignant" otosclerosis, gross evidence of the otosclerotic disease may be found in the crura and capitulum of the stapes. The problem of otosclerosis will be covered in greater detail in the section on oval-window lesions.

*Tympanic Cavity.* The tympanic air space is an important physiological factor in auditory function. The regulation of air pressure within this space is a complex function depending primarily upon the activities of the auditory (Eustachian) tube which connects the tympanic cavity with the lateral recess of the nasopharynx. This tube (Fig. 7), lined by respiratory mucous membrane, has bony, cartilaginous, and muscular walls. It is thus rigid in part and flexible in part. It is equipped with both voluntary and involuntary neural and muscular control.

The tympanic-cavity air space is also continuous with the air spaces of the many bony cells of the mastoid process. This relationship does not have the physiological implications of the Eustachian tube but has equally profound pathological implications.

The air pressure in this air space is normally maintained in a dynamic equilibrium with the barometric pressure outside the eardrum, largely by the involuntary regular dilations of the tubal lumen to constantly readjust intra-tympanic air pressure to that of nasopharynx (and presumably of the outside world if the nasopharynx is normal). Voluntary efforts to regulate the tubal lumen are frequently necessary. Our new "civilization," which forces us into the heights of the sky and the depths of the sea and earth, is making greater and greater demands upon this muscular mechanism.

Both negative and positive tympanic air pressure changes may produce conductive hypacuses. The former is the most common sequel of "tympanic barotrauma." Negative tympanic air pressure, with rarefaction of tympanic air, may follow a number of disturbances, including simple occlusion of Eustachian tubal lumen by disease or by too rapid descent in flying, preventing the normal regulatory function of Eustachian-tube muscles.

Otoscopic examination will usually reveal a "retracted" eardrum in such negative pressure conditions. The malleus handle will be pulled up into a nearly horizontal position and other aspects of the tympanic membrane will present an "indrawing" toward the middle ear.

Audiometric studies in these cases will usually reveal a mild conductive hypacusis with relatively normal bone conduction. The air-conduction level may slope either towards high or low frequencies. There is no "classic" audiometric picture, because these cases almost invariably are accompanied by other tympanic deformations including fluid collections, hemorrhage, and so on, and the audiometric picture will represent a summation of several tympanic lesions.

Treatment of this group of cases will depend upon associated findings, but will primarily be directed toward re-establishment of normal Eustachian tubal function. This may involve both local and constitutional mucosa-shrinking measures, insufflation of air through the nasopharynx, and treatment of contiguous areas.

*Tympanic effusion* or *serous otitis media* is a very common disease and a major cause of conduction hypacusis in many children and adults. In its temporary form, it is present for a day or two with many simple colds, allergic attacks, and as the result of atmospheric pressure changes. However, it frequently may be prolonged into a subacute stage lasting two to four weeks or to a chronic stage lasting months and years.

Serous effusion is primarily a collection of serum or clear fluid, usually light lemon in color, which may either partially or completely fill the tympanic cavity (Fig. 8). It is a painless state and carries no constitutional

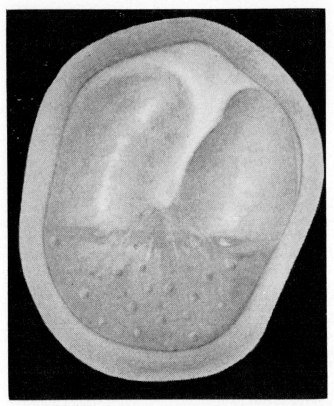

FIG. 8. A serous exudate into the middle ear may occur in an initial stage of an acute inflammatory middle-ear infection or as secretion which is non-inflammatory in origin such as occurs from an allergic change or from the effect of physical factors, such as a rapid change of altitude in flying (otitic barotrauma, aero-otitis media). (From Boies, L. R. 1954. Fundamentals of otolaryngology (2nd ed.). New York: Saunders. Fig. 41a, p. 72.)

symptoms with it, in contrast to *purulent otitis*. It produces a number of clinical otoscopic and audiometric pictures. Unfortunately, it is frequently missed on examination because the otoscopic changes may be very subtle. Whenever suspected, the diagnosis may be confirmed by needle aspiration through the tympanic membrane.

Diseases of the Eustachian tube and its environs are the main contributory etiologic factors. Adenoid tissue blocking the pharyngeal orifice of the tube is the most common cause. Such tissue may be primary or secondary due to regrowth. Surgical removal by "direct adenoidectomy" under direct visual control is the preferred method of treatment. Small lymphoid tissue remnants may require postoperative eradication either by deep x-ray therapy through the neck tissues, or by direct treatment with a radium applicator inserted through the nostril.

Successful treatment to eradicate tympanic effusion must consist of persistent removal of tympanic fluid repeatedly in addition to treatment of the nasopharynx and nasal sinus area. This may require a number of "para-centeses" or incisions of the tympanic membrane followed by suction re-moval of the serous fluid. The prognosis for recovery is usually excellent and complete return of hearing to normal is the rule, provided treatment is prompt and persistent.

*Mucous catarrh of the tympanic cavity,* or "glue ear," is a more serious form of tympanic effusion and is characterized by a filling of the middle ear with a thick glue-like exudate which usually produces a more profound con-duction hypacusis. Pathologically, it is usually due to marked proliferation of mucus-secreting cells of the goblet cell type within the middle-ear mu-cosa. The Eustachian tube is not usually found diseased. Mastoid air cells, however, may represent similar reservoirs of glue-like fluid in these cases. Treatment of the "glue ear" is more difficult and may involve more exten-sive paracenteses and suction procedures and in some cases mastoidectomy as well.

Allergy of the upper respiratory tract is a common causative or contrib-utory factor in middle-ear fluid diseases. True allergic tympanic disease may exist with little evidence of allergy elsewhere. Such cases will require vigor-ous antiallergic management, including dietary elimination, contact sub-stance removal, specific hypo-sensitization by injection, and medication by antihistaminic, sympathicomimetic, and cortico-steroid drugs.

*Hemorrhage* within the tympanic cavity may result from either infection within the middle ear, acute skull trauma with rupture of small tympanic capillaries, fracture of the temporal bone, or physical trauma to the external ear. If hemorrhage is unaccompanied by internal ear trauma, the resultant hypacusis will be simply conduction in type and will usually subside as the blood leaves the tympanic cavity. In most cases, spontaneous absorption occurs; occasionally aspiration is necessary.

If the tympanic hemorrhage is secondary to temporal bone fracture, the resultant hypacusis will have both conduction and neural components. In severe neural damage by cochlear hemorrhage, anacusis may result.

Hemorrhage due to external ear trauma may be accompanied by a major tympanic membrane perforation which may heal only partially or not at all.

*Acute otitis media* is the most common cause of temporary conduction hypacusis of tympanic origin. This is a disease which few humans escape. It is present in some degree with every "cold," every "sinus" attack, and every attack of "hay fever" or "allergy." It may vary greatly in severity depending both upon the host and the invading organisms or toxic agent. The anatomic relations of the Eustachian tube make infants and children particularly sus-ceptible. As the tube changes from a near horizontal to a near vertical posi-tion in adult development, this vulnerability lessens.

Otitis media, or "middle-ear inflammation" is, in the acute stage, a diffuse swelling of all of the tissues of the tympanic cavity (Fig. 9). The exudation of serum soon changes to pus and the contained pus produces pressure phe-nomena within the middle ear. Symptoms of pain, pressure, and conduction

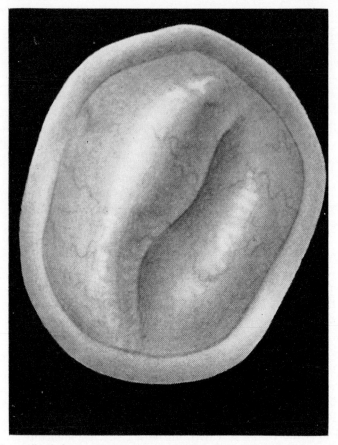

FIG. 9. The swollen bulging eardrum results from inflammatory exudate under pressure in the middle ear. (From Boies, L. R. 1954. Fundamentals of otolaryngology (2nd ed.). New York, Saunders. Fig. 41c, p. 72.)

hypacusis are accompanied by constitutional changes including fever, leucocytosis, and general malaise and toxemia.

Treatment of acute otitis media will depend upon severity and associated clinical findings. Antibiotics, antihistaminics, and surgical release of pus by *myringotomy* (incision of the eardrum) are frequently necessary. Recent developments in antibiotic therapy and precise otologic surgery have lessened the terrors and complications of this disease tremendously.

Inadequate resolution of acute otitis media, persistent subacute otitis media due to tubal disease, and invasion of mastoid air cells by infection are common causes of chronic otitis media.

*Chronic otitis media* is most commonly manifested by continuous or intermittent otorrhea (ear discharge) associated with a tympanic perforation. If the perforation is central and the discharge is entirely nonpurulent and tubal in origin, the chronic otitis may usually be considered nonserious from the viewpoint of danger to life. Nevertheless, such a disease may still produce

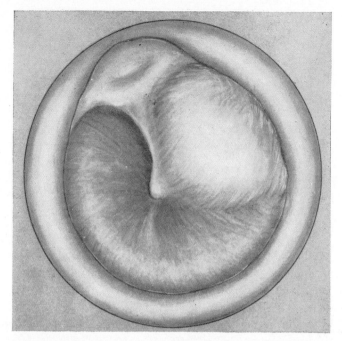

G. 10. Otoscopic appearance of primary cholesteatoma in a five-year-old child. This rare
mpanic neoplasm was diagnosed because of the audiometric discovery of a unilateral 50
decibel conduction hypacusis during routine screening school audiometry.

very major conduction hypacusis. If the perforation is marginal, there
ill usually be other signs of bone destruction both in the annulus and in
1e mastoid process. Such otorrhea is more commonly due to bone disease
nd may signify a distinctly dangerous process with potential intracranial
xtension. (Some central perforations may also fall in this category.)

Cholesteatoma is a fairly common cause of chronic otitis media. Cho-
steatosis of the tympanum, mastoid process, and petrous pyramid is usually
illed a "secondary cholesteatoma" (Fig. 6). Histologically, this is a benign
ɔidermoid cyst which invades the temporal bone as the sequel of an in-
rowth of epithelium from the tympanic membrane through a tympanic
erforation. Such ingrowth may represent an aberrant attempt at healing
f a perforation within the middle ear and mastoid. (Primary or "true"
holesteatoma (Fig. 10) is a congenital epidermoid cyst which may occur
ithin any part of the cranial cavity including the ear, but it is a rare lesion.)

Chronic otitis media due to cholesteatoma will present varying degrees
f conduction hypacusis. A cholesteatoma confined to the "attic" or epitym-
anum may not contact any major segment of the conduction mechanism
nd cause no hearing loss at all. If the cholesteatoma invades the mesotym-
anum, it will usually destroy the incus and part of the malleus and produce
major conduction hypacusis.

The treatment of chronic otitis media is primarily surgical, although

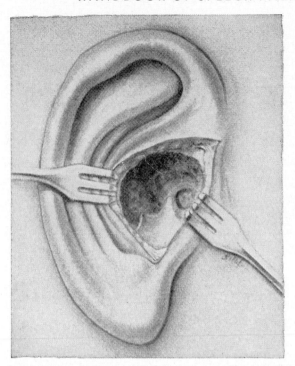

FIG. 11. Illustration of endaural complete radical mastoidectomy with removal of irreversibl
diseased tympanic structures accompanied by slight deterioration in hearing threshold. (Fro
Boies, L. R. 1954. Fundamentals of otolaryngology (2nd ed.). New York: Saunders. Fig. 48, p. 91

medical measures may suffice in the case of tubal origin. Surgical treatmen
of chronic otitis media has been recently improved by the endaural tech
niques of Lempert and others (1950). The endaural surgical approach i
preferred to the older post-auricular incision, not primarily for its obviou
cosmetic advantages, but because endaural incisions allow more direct ana
tomical attack upon tympanic disease with the possibility of more conserva
tive reconstruction of middle ear and ear canal.

Otologic surgeons are now quite conscious of the desirability of preserva
tion of functional tympanic structures in their attack on chronic otitis medi
Such conservatism was not practiced too widely several decades ago. Thu
the complete "radical mastoidectomy" which was almost routine in chroni
otitis media is being replaced frequently by some type of "modified radica
mastoidectomy" and "tympanoplasty."

The term *mastoidectomy* does not mean complete removal of the mastoi
process of the temporal bone, a virtually impossible anatomic feat. It refer
to the surgical exenteration of diseased mastoid cells, the number and ex
tent depending upon the judgment of the surgeon. A "simple mastoidec
tomy" refers to removal of mastoid cells only, with preservation of tympani
and peritympanic structures. A "radical mastoidectomy" (Fig. 11) may b
called an "attico-tympano-mastoidectomy" or "mastoido-tympanectomy

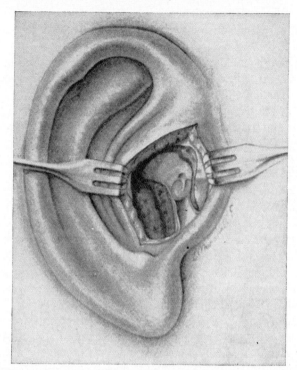

FIG. 12. Illustration of endaural modified radical mastoidectomy with preservation of tympanic structures and preservation of hearing. (From Boies, L. R. 1954. Fundamentals of otolaryngology (2nd ed.). New York: Saunders. Fig. 47, p. 91.)

and refers to a simple mastoidectomy plus removal of the bony canal wall, tympanic membrane remnant, ossicular and muscular contents of tympanic cavity, and final conversion of mastoid and tympanic cavity into one common cavity, as visualized through the auditory meatus. A *modified radical mastoidectomy* (Fig. 12) is the term reserved for any mastoidectomy where some degree of canal and tympanic cavity removal short of complete exenteration is practiced.

The philosophy of surgical conservatism is one of conservation of tissue designed to minimize the degree of conduction hypacusis already present, or to prevent any significant increase in hearing loss. Other objectives may include such techniques as would allow more successful uses of tympanic prostheses or utilization of a hearing aid. Tympanoplasty involves surgical reconstruction of conduction pathways in the middle ear.

*Tumors of the tympanic cavity* other than cholesteatoma may be benign or malignant but are usually serious regardless of histologic type. Hearing losses are primarily conduction hypacusis in nature but may show evidence of superimposed neural hypacusis if the tumor invades the cochlear windows or the cochlea per se.

Glomus jugulare tumor is being recognized more frequently—sometimes referred to as a nonchromaffin paraganglioma or a tympanic carotid body tumor. This tumor starts in the hypotympanum and may produce a pulsatir tinnitus and a conduction hypacusis. Its treatment is largely surgical, a though radiation may help in some cases.

Carcinoma of the middle ear is a very serious disease with a high mortali rate. Its treatment is best carried out through radical surgical excision an postoperative radiation, but the prognosis is poor.

Osteoma of the tympanum may accompany osteoma of the canal. It is benign lesion but may produce irreversible tympanic destruction and cor duction hypacusis.

## Lesions of the Labyrinth, Its Fluids and Windows

Diseases of the bony labyrinth, labyrinthine fluids, and labyrinthine wir dows are border-line lesions from the point of view of conduction and neur hearing losses. Since oval and round windows separate the middle from th inner ear, it is difficult to be very dogmatic about classification, althoug from the physical standpoint one must consider the transmission of sour through labyrinthine fluids as a conduction phenomenon. According to th concept, the conduction of sound remains purely mechanical until the di placement of the basilar membrane produces an electrical change in the res ing potential in the organ of Corti. Lesions which occur within the orga of Corti itself, or central to it, are lesions in the neural apparatus and migl properly be classified as neural losses.

The bony capsule of the labyrinth is composed of very dense bone, b nevertheless may be the site of invasion by almost any constitutional bor disease. Some of the invading diseases are rare and will not be discussed this chapter. There are a few fairly common diseases which invade tl otic capsule and produce significant hearing losses by virtue of the invasio The most common disease in this category is otosclerosis. Less commc bone diseases that may mimic otosclerosis include syphilis, Paget's diseas fragilitas ossium, and osteitis fibrosa cystica.

All of these diseases may invade various parts of the otic capsule and i contents. That there are predilections is known, but random and haphazai distribution of lesions is quite frequently encountered in temporal bor pathologic studies. It is startling to realize how little information we ha on many of these diseases, primarily because of the lack of temporal bor pathologic information. The temporal bone has been tragically ignore throughout the decades of the systematic study of pathology. No area in tl human body has been accorded so little study, from the point of view pathology, as the human temporal bone. This is indeed a great void otologic and audiologic knowledge. It can only be filled by a determined a tempt by physicians and ancillary scientists who would make a concerte effort to study the temporal bones of individuals upon whom there is ava able adequate premortem audiologic data. Only by such co-ordinated studi will we be able to answer many of the unknown oto-audiologic questions today.

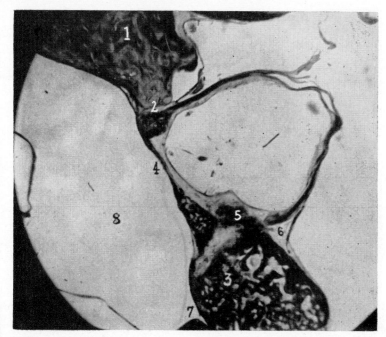

. 13. Otosclerosis. Autopsy No. 4960 (left ear). Oscar Johnson Institute: (1) Normal capsule. Annular ligament, posteriorly, normal. (3) Focus at site of predilection, obliterating annular ament and involving anterior half of footplate. (4) Footplate of stapes. (5) Dystrophic bone volving anterior crus of stapes. (6) Fibrous web extending to anterior crus. (7) Fissula ante testram almost obliterated by focus. (8) Cisterna periotica. X20. B. & L. obj. 32mm. E. P. . 2. (From Guggenheim, L. 1935. Otosclerosis. St. Louis: Zimmerman & Petty. Fig. 101, p. 175.)

**Otosclerosis.** Otosclerosis, or "hardening of the ear," has been known for long time to physicians. It is probably the most common cause of deafness adults. It is primarily a disease of the otic capsule and is represented stologically by a number of pleomorphic forms. According to some in- stigators, the earliest stage of otosclerosis is truly a spongy condition of one sometimes called "oto-spongiosis." Instances of this disease have been escribed in fetuses and children, as well as in adults of all ages. It is con- dered by many that typical histologic otosclerosis represents the healing age in the primary oto-spongiosis, and that otosclerotic bone represents e healed sclerotic and quiescent lesion of the preliminary active oto- ongiotic bone.

The disease occurs bilaterally in most individuals, and it is present in mporal bones in a very large percentage of the population; perhaps as gh as 8 to 10 per cent. But in most of these individuals, the otosclerosis is urely a histological curiosity and does not produce deafness (Guild, 1944). earing losses are produced only when the otosclerotic lesion involves a itical area within the labyrinth (2 per cent). Thus it may very well be that stances of unilateral otosclerosis encountered clinically are still bilateral stologically; in which the lesion has not involved a critical area in one ear.

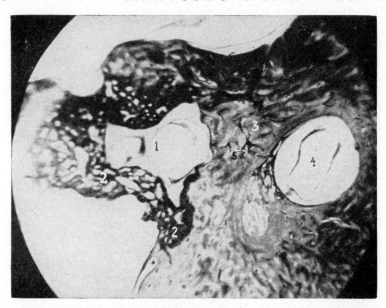

FIG. 14. Otosclerosis. Focus at round window. Left ear. Autopsy No. 4960. Oscar Johnson Institut (1) Niche of round window. (2) Dystrophic bone closing window. (3) Normal capsule. ( Posterior canal. (5) Fracture from niche to posterior canal. X20. B. & L. obj. 32 mm. E. P. No. (From Guggenheim, L. 1935. Otosclerosis. St. Louis: Zimmerman & Petty. Fig. 105, p. 18C

The bony lesion of otosclerosis is not a tumor, but a change in the cor sistency of the bony cellular structure. Its growth may be very rapid or ver slow. It is more commonly seen in its growth form during the postpuber years and in the early twenties. In the thirties and forties it appears to ur dergo a quiescent stage. Marked exceptions in activity, however, do occu The disease is more common in women, perhaps in a ratio of 3 to 1. frequently becomes worse during pregnancy and during lactation. It frequently associated with calcium deficiencies in teeth, and occasionall in other bones. No systematic pattern of calcium disease, however, is foun in all patients. Heredity appears to be a factor in a very large number ( patients, but certainly not in the majority. The genetic aspect of otoscleros is primarily that of a recessive trait.

The disease is limited entirely to the temporal bone and has not yet bee discovered in any other part of the body. It produces no known system effects, and its only symptoms are those confined to the auditory and vestil ular sensory organs.

It more commonly invades the anterior aspect of the oval window (Fi 13) and will slowly involve the ligament of the stapes footplate and er croach upon the anterior aspect of the footplate, as well as upon the anterio crus. When such encroachment occurs, the stapes footplate becomes pro gressively fixed and unable to transmit acoustic energy to the labyrinthir fluids. When complete fixation occurs, as it does in many otosclerotic pa

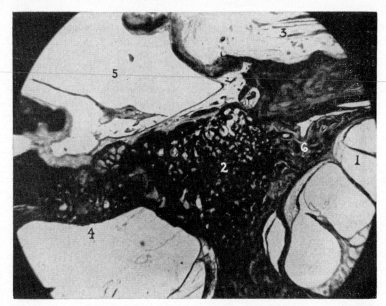

FIG. 15. Otosclerosis. Focus in relation to cochlea. Autopsy No. 4960. Left ear: (1) Cochlea. (2) focus. (3) Tensor tympani muscle. (4) Vestibule. (5) Tympanum. (6) Capsule. X50. B. & L. obj. 6 mm. E. P. No. 2. (From Guggenheim, L. 1935. Otosclerosis. St. Louis: Zimmerman & Petty. Fig. 106, p. 181.)

patients, the complete impedance-matching mechanism of the tympanic membrane and ossicular chain is lost as a functioning unit.

In about one-third of cases, the otosclerotic process may also involve the region of the round-window niche (Fig. 14) and may immobilize the round window. In some instances, it may invade the region of the internal auditory meatus (Fig. 15) and produce pressure phenomena on the auditory nerve or cochlear ganglion.

Although the otosclerotic histologic picture is a reasonably classical one, its counterpart has never been found in other parts of the body, and it has been thought by some that the lesion is not a single disease but the histologic sequel of other disease processes affecting the otic capsule. Thus there may not be just one type of otosclerosis, but several diseases (Figs. 16, 17, 18, 19) which may have separate etiologic origins. The disease may involve any portion of the vestibular as well as cochlear labyrinth, and in such involvement vertigo is not at all uncommon. In fact, some instances of otosclerosis very closely mimic Meniere's disease, with vertigo, tinnitus, and deafness. It is not unusual to find in a family "riddled" with "classical otosclerosis," an occasional instance of progressive deafness which is entirely neural with no conductive component. This is probably due to otosclerotic invasion of neural components of the labyrinth without involvement of the site of predilection, namely, the oval window. Thus "nerve deafness" may be otosclerotic in etiology in some patients.

*The Treatment of Otosclerosis.* There is no known treatment for the dis-

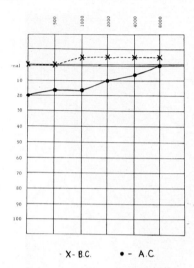

FIG. 16. Early otosclerosis. Slight threshold deficit, especially in lower frequencies A.C./B.C. gap.

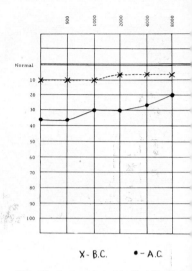

FIG. 17. Progressive otosclerosis. Maintenance of A.C./B.C. gap and increase threshold deficit.

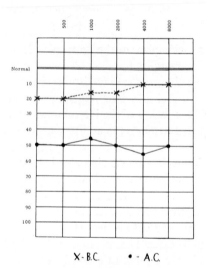

FIG. 18. Advanced otosclerosis with complete stapedial fixation. Persistent A.C./B.C. gap.

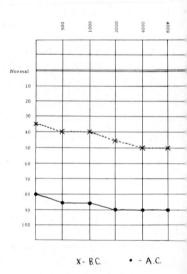

FIG. 19. Markedly advanced otosclerosis with "neural degeneration". This probably involves stapedial fixation and cochlea invasion by otosclerosis. It is possible the round-window fixation may also exist such cases.

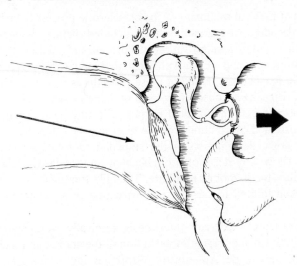

G. 20A. Schematic representation of normal transmission of acoustic energy to perilimph via mobile stapedial footplate.

se which is called otosclerosis *histologically*. The disease which is called osclerosis *clinically* may or may not be the histologic condition itself but ay represent a number of diseases involving the oval window and the ligament of the stapedial footplate, producing the otologic and audiologic picture of stapedial fixation. For the purposes of simplicity, all cases presenting evidence of stapedial fixation, with little or no evidence of associated middle-ear disease, are called "clinical otosclerosis," and most of the treatment described surgically for otosclerosis is really surgical treatment of clinical otosclerosis."

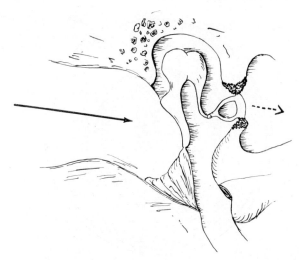

G. 20B. Schematic representation of blocked transmission of acoustic energy to perilymph by ankylosed stapedial footplate in otosclerosis.

Attempts at medical treatment of the otosclerotic process have been mad for several decades. Such attempts have included dietary changes, low an high calcium regimes, administration of hormones (Goodhill, 1952a), vita mins, and minerals, and various physical therapeutic techniques designe to loosen the fixed stapes. None of these procedures or treatments or com binations of drugs have consistently been of value in any significant numbe of otosclerotic cases. For practical purposes, it may be stated that there no satisfactory medical treatment of the disease called otosclerosis. A stud of the pathologic deformation of the stapedial footplate (Figs. 13, 20A will readily show why it is not probable that any medical modality woul ever remobilize the immobile footplate. The only treatment that has been ( value has been limited to surgical reconstruction of a functioning acousti pathway.

The first attempts to treat otosclerosis surgically were made betwee 1875 and 1900, when efforts at mobilization of the stapes, and later remova of the stapes, were made. Attempts to restore hearing by operations directe through the eardrum at the stapedial footplate were made by Kessel (1876 Blake (1892), Jack (1891–92), Miot (1890), Siebenmann (1900), an others. The consensus of opinion, however, at the end of the century wa that stapedial surgery by the techniques then in use was not of significar value; and there is very little in the literature relating to stapedial surger following 1896.

At the beginning of the present century, attempts were made to restor hearing by creating a new window in some portion of the vestibular laby rinth to bypass the blocked fenestra ovalis pathway. It is from these at tempts, principally started by Holmgren (1923), modified by Sourdill (1929), and finally perfected by Lempert (1938), that the fenestration oper

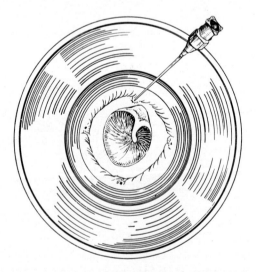

FIG. 21A. Local anesthetic infiltration preliminary to stapedolysis operation.

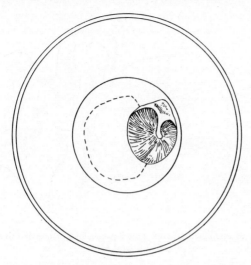

G. 21B. Line of incision (omega shaped) posterior canal wall in stapedolysis operation. Entire operation is performed through an ear speculum.

tion was brought to its present universally accepted position as a practical method for the restoration of hearing in otosclerotic stapedial fixation.

Since 1954, renewed interest in the direct approach to the stapedial foot-late has been created by Rosen (1955) and other investigators, who advise apes mobilization as a precursor to fenestration. The writer (Goodhill, 955a, 1955b, and 1955c) has modified the stapes mobilization operation in veral respects. His technique of "stapedolysis" has been shown to be ffective in the restoration of hearing to a practical level in at least 60 to 70

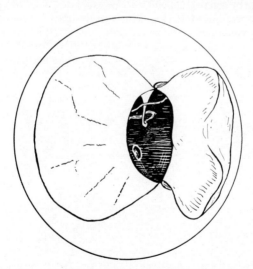

G. 22. Excellent exposure of incudo-stapedial joint in stapedolysis. Skin-drum flap is reflected teriorly, exposing the lenticular process of the incus and the stapes. The chorda tympani nerve is crossing over the incus. The round-window niche may be seen below.

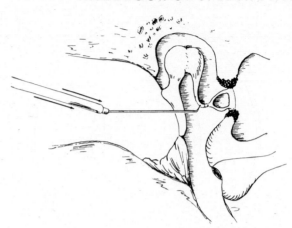

**FIG. 23. Illustration of attempted lysis of stapedial ankylosis in otosclerosis via trans-tympar transincudal force.**

per cent of patients who have good preoperative cochlear function.

*The stapes-mobilization approach of "stapedolysis"* consists of a procedure und local anesthesia (Fig. 21A), in which no external incisions are made. A small i cision (Fig. 21B) is made within the ear canal on the posterior bony canal wa with reflection of skin and tympanic membrane anteriorly to expose the midd ear.

The incudo-stapedial joint is visualized (Fig. 22), if necessary, by removal some bone in the posterior bony segment of the annulus. An attempt is mac (Fig. 23) to produce lysis of the stapedial footplate fixation by application force through the incudo-stapedial mass with an instrument engaged within t incudal periosteum. It is possible to create this remobilization, or lysis, by eith digital pressure or by mechanical vibratory pressure (Fig. 24). Surgical audiomet is done on the operating table (Fig. 25) with the patient under light sedatio Any acceptable calibrated discrete-frequency air-conduction audiometer w

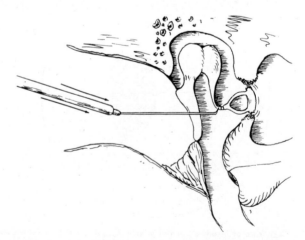

**FIG. 24. Illustration of transincudal force via tympanic cavity producing successful lysis stapedial ankylosis and mobilization of fixed stapes in otosclerosis.**

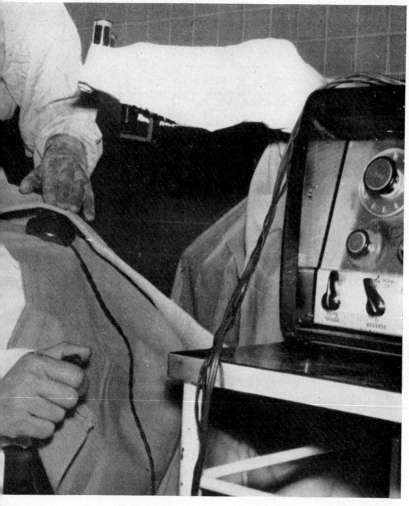

. 25. Illustration of surgical audiometric set-up in the operating room. Air-conduction receiver
placed over auricular region on a sterile sheet and held in place by sterile towel. Patient uses
push-button signal device.

satisfactory. No special equipment is necessary. A sterile sheet is placed over
e patient's auricle and threshold estimations are done at three critical fre-
encies of 500 cycles, 1000 cycles and 2000 cycles. Four minimum steps are
ilized in the audiometric study.

The initial technique of force application is transincudal, in which digital or
echanical vibration is transmitted through the lenticular process of the incus.
the incudo stapedial joint is anatomically loose, force is transmitted through
 capitulum of the stapes, marginally. If the crura are weak or elastic and
nnot transmit force safely, force is transmitted through the footplate directly.
rious fine instruments and techniques may be needed for footplate approaches.
ch approaches involve penetration of the vestibule with occasional postoperative
mporary utricular vertigo (Goodhill, 1956a and 1956b). The surgical progress

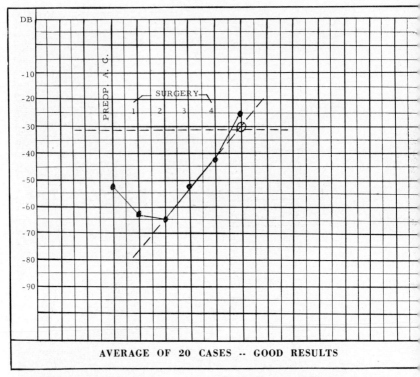

AVERAGE OF 20 CASES -- GOOD RESULTS

FIG. 26. Average nomographic plot of surgical audiometry in 20 successful cases.

is guided throughout its entirety by the procedure of "surgical audiometry"
which has been an indispensable tool.

Step 1. *Preliminary Closed Middle Ear*
    Baseline threshold estimation, after preliminary elevation of the skin
    flap and tympanic membrane, and repositioning of these structures
    prior to any lysis attempt.

Step 2. *Open Middle Ear*
    Opening of middle ear by reflection anteriorly of the skin flap-tym-
    panic membrane segment, with exposure of the incudo-stapedial joint
    —but prior to mobilization or lysis.

Step 3. *Post-Lysis*
    The first post-lysis or post-mobilization threshold estimation, to be
    compared with Step 2 for evidence of significant threshold shift. Sev-
    eral post-lysis studies may be made until definitive conclusions are
    reached regarding the success or failure of lysis of footplate ankylosis.
    Thus there may be Steps 3*a*, 3*b*, 3*c*, etc.

Step 4. *Final Closed Middle Ear*
    Repositioning of tympanic membrane skin flap, as in Step 1, for direct
    comparison with Step 1 for significant threshold shift.

From examinations of our data, it seems that discrete frequency characteristics in surgical audiometry are not as important in guidance as the
average amplitude of response (threshold). We have therefore decided to

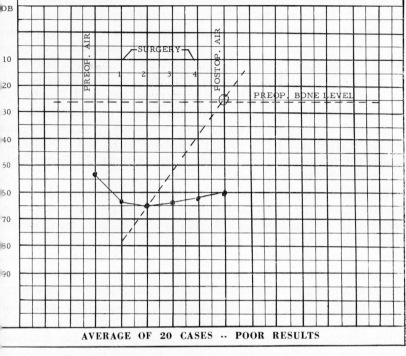

AVERAGE OF 20 CASES -- POOR RESULTS

FIG. 27. Average nomographic plot of surgical audiometry in 20 unsuccessful cases.

ilize an equivalent speech reception threshold in surgical audiometry and ve adopted the Fletcher (1953) formula for conversion of pure-tone thresh-ds to an equivalent speech reception threshold. This technique consists of lecting the two best responses at 500, 1000, or 2000 cycles and averaging ese two responses. This gives us an equivalent SRT, or single "figure of erit," for easy comparison of the different surgical steps. The Fletcher ethod has given us results that are quite comparable with SRT's obtained conventional spondee list methods.

In our attempt, therefore, to obtain a useful and informative method for rgical guidance, we have devised a surgical audiometric nomograph* in nich the Fletcher equivalent SRT technique is used to obtain a single gure of merit" for bone conduction, for preoperative air conduction, and r each surgical audiometric step. These SRT values are then plotted in omographic fashion to indicate to the surgeon the desired objectives for resholds of Steps 3 and 4.

This nomograph is constructed as illustrated in Figures 26 and 27. The dinates (vertical axis) of the graph are in the familiar decibel ratio with spect to the normal audiometric zero level. The abscissa (horizontal axis)

* From the Greek root word "nomos," meaning "law"; thus, a nomograph is literally graphic law or rule.

divisions are made equal to the ordinate even though they represent on
the discrete steps in audiometry. The preoperative bone conduction is show
by a dashed horizontal line at the proper ordinate value, using the one equiv
lent SRT figure of merit. This establishes the surgical objective, or the e·
pected air-conduction level, if the operation is to be an unqualified succe
by our proposed standards. The abscissas consist basically of six positio·
which are used to indicate, first, the preoperative A.C. level, then the fo·
surgical audiometric steps, and, finally, the position of postoperative A.(
level, which is to be charted two weeks following surgery. Where more tha
one test is made at Step 3 the results are shown on the same abscissa li·
labeled (a), (b), (c), etc., the last one being the significant figure. Step
may be treated in the same manner when necessary.

The crucial stage in this operative approach is Step 3, where the surgec
has already produced some degree of force application and perhaps son
degree of lysis of the footplate ankylosis. It is at this point that a decisic
must be made as to whether to terminate the procedure or continue furthe
Thus, a minimal improvement in hearing might erroneously lead the surgec
to consider that his efforts have been adequate and he may conclude th
procedure without attaining the ideal gain which could have been expecte
in this particular patient. On the other hand, excessive force applicatior
at this point without adequate audiometric control may be disastrous t
either destruction of one or both crura or dislocation of the incudostapedi·
joint.

It seems important to us, therefore, that at the critical Step 3 some pr·
dictive reasoning be employed to ascertain the adequacy of the lysis forc
exerted. Obviously, this cannot be measured in any set number of decibel
since the threshold change following complete lysis will depend upon th
degree of stapes fixation in the particular case. Thus a bone-air gap of 20 d
in the patient with a bone-conduction level of 20 db and an air-conductio
level of 40 db is a vastly different problem from the bone-air gap of 50 d
in the patient with a bone-conduction level of 15 db and an air-conductio
level of 65 db. Both of these examples do occur in otosclerosis, and so
simple decibel shift cannot be effectively used in one case and again in th
other case. Thus, a nomographic display becomes desirable for surgic·
guidance.

As the average graph of 20 successful cases shows in Figure 26, the ave.
age gain to be expected from Step 2 to the ideal postoperative air-conductio
level can be roughly divided into three parts. This is in general true wheth·
the required total improvement is 15 or 45 db or any step in between. Th·
where the co-ordinates are equally spaced, a straight diagonal line draw
from the intersection of the preoperative bone-conduction level (and th
expected postoperative air-conduction level) to Step 2 of surgery will b
divided into three equal parts by the intersection of the abscissas of surgic·
Steps 3 and 4. Therefore, regardless of whether the bone-conduction thre·
hold is high or low, and regardless of the threshold of Step 2, this straig·

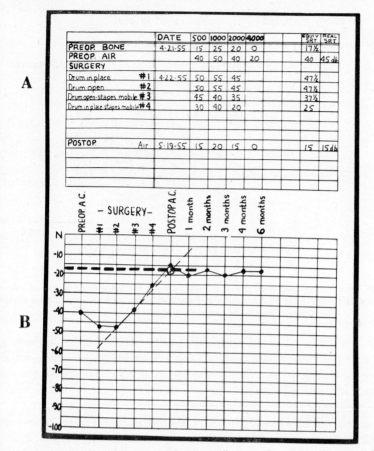

**A**

| | DATE | 500 | 1000 | 2000 | 4000 | | | EQUIV SRT | REAL SRT |
|---|---|---|---|---|---|---|---|---|---|
| PREOP. BONE | 4-21-55 | 15 | 25 | 20 | 0 | | | 17½ | |
| PREOP. AIR | | 40 | 50 | 40 | 20 | | | 40 | 45 db |
| SURGERY | | | | | | | | | |
| Drum in place #1 | 4-22-55 | 50 | 55 | 45 | | | | 47½ | |
| Drum open #2 | | 50 | 55 | 45 | | | | 47½ | |
| Drum open-stapes mobile #3 | | 45 | 40 | 35 | | | | 37½ | |
| Drum in place stapes mobile #4 | | 30 | 40 | 20 | | | | 25 | |
| | | | | | | | | | |
| | | | | | | | | | |
| POSTOP. Air | 5-19-55 | 15 | 20 | 15 | 0 | | | 15 | 15 db |
| | | | | | | | | | |
| | | | | | | | | | |
| | | | | | | | | | |

**B**

. 28. Example of surgical audiometric technique: A illustrates the preoperative, surgical, and
stoperative thresholds; B gives the nomographic representation during and after successful
stapedolysis surgery.

agonal line, which can be dotted in as in Figure 28, is an excellent indica-
n of where surgical Steps 3 and 4 should appear. Thus, after lysis ma-
uvers, if Step 3 falls near or above the line (that is, to its left), it is probable
at Step 4 and the postoperative air conduction will follow suit, provided
ere are no operative or postoperative complications. That the expected
ins between Steps 3 and 4 and between Step 4 and the postoperative A.C.
vel are roughly equal to the gain between Steps 2 and 3 is due to the fact
at the efficiency of the eardrum-ossicular chain mechanism as an acoustic
ansducer is greatest when working into the load of a normally mobile
apes. Thus the impedance mismatch between the drum and stapes foot-
ate is an approximate function of the degree of fixation of the latter. The
vel of Step 4 is materially influenced by the precision with which the middle
r is closed and the drum reapproximated to its sulcus attachment. If the
reshold at Step 4 falls on or above the straight diagonal guide line, the
obability of postoperative success is great.

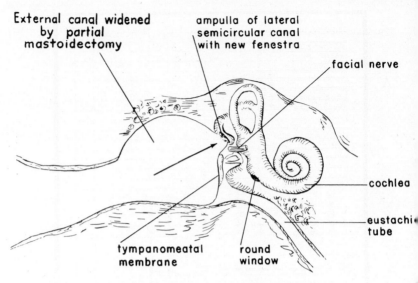

External canal widened by partial mastoidectomy

ampulla of lateral semicircular canal with new fenestra

facial nerve

cochlea

eustachia tube

tympanomeatal membrane

round window

**FIG. 29.** Schematic representation of new acoustic pathway via fenestration in case of staped footplate rigidly ankylosed by otosclerosis and not mobilizable by stapedolysis. Note deform tympanic membrane and absent incus and malleus head.

We have observed in individual cases that where the initial air-bone ga is great Step 3 in successful cases will fall well above the guide line, while narrow air-bone gap cases Step 3 may fall as much as 5 db below the guid line and still prove successful. Step 4, however, is nearly always near above the line in successful cases whether the bone-air gap is large or sma

Inspection of 20 unsuccessful cases when charted in Figure 27 by nom graphic technique reveals no indication that stapes mobilization has o curred. The threshold with the eardrum in place in Step 4 is practical identical with Step 1. The two-week postoperative air-conduction level is or below the preoperative level, the latter indicating probably that surgic edema or other postoperative complications have not completely subside

Following the completion of the procedure, the canal is gently packed wi rayon gauze and cellulose sponge, and the patient is usually able to leave th hospital the following morning. There is very little vertigo or pain attach to this procedure, and the hearing improvement is quite excellent in view the fact that the surgical deficit found in fenestration surgery does not nece sarily exist in this procedure. No ossicular chain removal is necessary in th procedure, and in general the operation is tolerated much better than fene tration surgery. There is usually complete healing within ten days, and the is no necessity for after-care of the operative field.

In 20 per cent of cases, at the time of present writing, there is no improv ment following stapedolysis surgery. This is primarily due to the nature the disease process in which the stapedial footplate has been complete destroyed as a functioning entity. It is physically impossible to restore m tion to a nonexistent anatomic structure. In some cases, there may be path

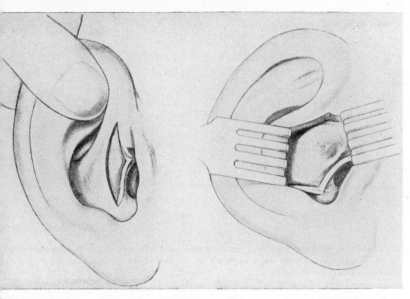

3. 30. Left, incisions; right, endaural antauricular exposure of the mastoid portion of the nporal bone. (From Jackson, C., and Jackson, C. L. 1945. Diseases of the nose, throat, and ear. New York: Saunders. Figs. 300 A and B, p. 381.)

gical atrophy of the stapedial crura, making it impossible to transmit force the footplate. In some cases, the crura are surgically fractured because of sistance by a rigid footplate. Occasionally, visible mobilization or lysis is t followed by a hearing improvement. This is probably due to pathologi- l otosclerotic bone medial to the pathological footplate which still ob- ructs acoustic transmission to the perilymph space. Occasionally, visible sis is followed only by a slight improvement in hearing. This also is prob-

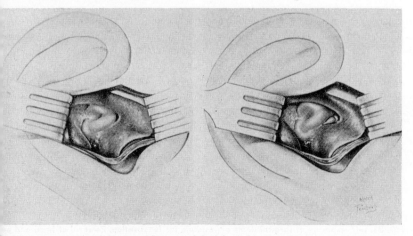

3. 31. Left, exposure of the mastoid aspect of the labyrinthine base; right, transantral opening the epitympanum and exposure of the incudomalleal joint. (From Jackson, C., and Jackson, C. L. 45. Diseases of the nose, throat, and ear. New York: Saunders. Fig. 301 A & B, p. 382.)

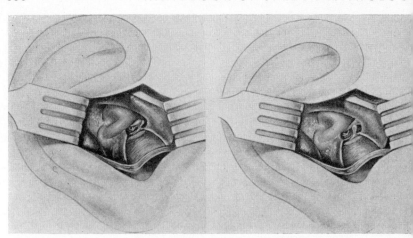

FIG. 32. Left, retrotympanic openings of tympanum and exposure of the incudostapedial joi and chorda tympani nerve; right, exposure of surgical dome of vestibule for fenestratio Removal of incus. (From Jackson, C., and Jackson, C. L. 1945. Diseases of the nose, throat, ar ear. New York: Saunders. Fig. 302 A & B, p. 383.)

ably due to persistence of some pathologic bone which prevents complet acoustic transmission to perilymph space. In other instances, a poor resu may be due to otosclerotic involvement of the round-window membrane. R gardless of cause, a lack of threshold shift in stapedolysis may not be the fin element in the solution of the problem. The patient in most circumstanc is still a good candidate for fenestration surgery.

*The fenestration operation* is a more complex procedure, but in certain respec it does not carry with it the extreme delicacy of technique necessary in the stap operation. The fenestration procedure is basically the creation of a new fenestr

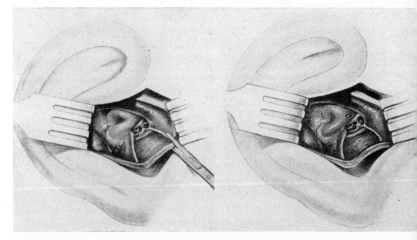

FIG. 33. Left, exposure of surgical dome of vestibule for fenestration. Removal of head and ne of the malleus. Right, creation of the fenestra nov-ovalis in the surgical dome of the vestibu (After Jackson, C., and Jackson, C. L. 1945. Diseases of the nose, throat, and ear. New Yo Saunders. Figs. 303 A and B, p. 384.)

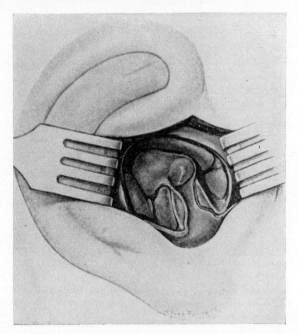

G. 34. Plastic tympanomeatal membrane in position and skin-grafted wound. (From Jackson, , and Jackson, C. L. 1945. Diseases of the nose, throat, and ear. New York: Saunders. Fig. 306, p. 386.)

window (Fig.29), in the ampulla of the horizontal semicircular canal to take e place of the closed oval window. The new window is thus frequently called e fenestra nov-ovalis.

The fenestration operation requires the precise execution of a number of surgi-l steps in order to reach the ampulla of the horizontal semicircular canal. It is st necessary to make a fairly extensive endaural incision (Fig. 30) in which a nall portion of the conchal cartilage may be sacrificed. The cortex of the mastoid ocess is exposed and a modified radical mastoidectomy operation performed ig. 31) in sufficient extent to gain access to the medial aspect of the mastoid trum and the horizontal semicircular canal (Fig. 32). The incus is removed om the fossa incudis. The posterior bony canal wall is removed almost com-etely—converting the epitympanum, external canal, and the mastoid bowl into e cavity. The skin of the posterior canal wall and its continuity with the tym-anic membrane is reflected anteriorly, and the head of the malleus brought into ew and amputated (Fig. 33). The tympanic membrane is reflected sufficiently teriorly to expose the ampulla of the horizontal semicircular canal, the under-ing genu of the facial nerve, and the stapes in the oval window. Under micro-opic control, a new window is placed within the ampulla of the horizontal semi-rcular canal by removing bone with a very fine surgical burr, driven by a ental engine. Otic capsular bone is removed down to the level of the endosteum. he latter is gently removed, thus opening the perilymph space. There will be an nmediate slight exudation of perilymph. The membraneous labyrinth will be en within the lumen of the ampulla. A plastic skin flap created from posterior anal wall skin and contiguous tympanic membrane is then mobilized and re-djusted so that it will cover the newly created fenestra with its thinnest portion ig. 34), which is usually that portion commonly known as pars flaccida of the ympanic membrane. The closure of the fenestra is accomplished by tucking this

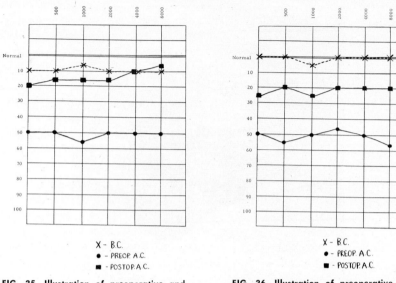

X - B.C.
● - PREOP. A.C.
■ - POSTOP. A.C.

**FIG. 35.** Illustration of preoperative and postoperative A.C. thresholds in a successful stapedolysis procedure.

X - B.C.
● - PREOP. A.C.
■ - POSTOP. A.C.

**FIG. 36.** Illustration of preoperative a postoperative A.C. thresholds in a succe ful fenestration operation.

very delicate epithelium into the newly created opening and packing it gen with cotton to keep it in position. This invagination technique is important create an adherence of the new epithelium to the underlying endosteum at t margins of the fenestra. It is also necessary to cover the fenestra to prevent t further escape of perilymph and the possibility of labyrinthine infection.

When the skin flap has been replaced, the operative cavity is packed and t initial incision sutured. The patient experiences moderate vertigo for several da but is able to be ambulatory within 48 hours after the procedure. The avera patient requires about five to seven days hospitalization, and is able to resur normal activity within two and a half to three weeks.

Although this is a more major surgical procedure than stapedolysis, it not a very traumatic experience and many thousands of patients have h successful fenestration operations, with little or no postoperative discor fort. They have been able to acquire adequate communication function the result of such surgery, in spite of the surgical deficit that is incurred the sacrifice of part of the ossicular chain and remobilization of the tympan membrane.

The evidence to date seems to show somewhat better postoperative hea ing as the result of successful stapedolysis surgery (Fig. 35) as compared successful fenestration surgery (Fig. 36). This would be expected in view the fact that, in stapedolysis, one maintains the normal impedance-matc ing mechanism of the tympanic membrane and ossicular chain, but sac fices most of this mechanism in fenestration surgery. The better hearing a the relatively easier operative and postoperative course for the patient mak stapedolysis the first choice in the surgical treatment of otosclerosis.

Thus, the otologic surgeon may proceed with a stapedolysis operation he first choice, and resort to the fenestration procedure later, if necessary. Obviously, adequate otologic surgical reconstruction of a functioning acoustic pathway demands the skill of a trained otologic surgeon who is capable of doing either or both of these procedures and can thus offer the patient a complete surgical rehabilitation program. Postoperative *closures* may occur either following stapedolysis or fenestration surgery. Such closures may occur either early or late and may call for surgical revision, which is possible with either operation.

At the present time, the stapedolysis procedure offers the possibility of restoration of hearing in about 70 per cent of patients with excellent bone conduction, in about 60 per cent of patients who have fairly good bone conduction, and in about 50 per cent of patients whose bone conduction is in the 35 to 40 db range. The fenestration procedure, in well-selected cases, offers the possibility of good results in 70 per cent to 80 per cent of patients. There still remains therefore a group of patients averaging approximately 20 per cent who cannot be adequately helped surgically by either or both procedures. These patients can still expect useful rehabilitation through the use of a hearing aid. It is only a very rare occurrence for labyrinthitis to occur as the result of otologic surgery, which might make the use of a hearing aid less satisfactory.

### Diseases simulating otosclerosis

*Paget's Disease.* "Paget's disease of bone" is a systemic disease involving a number of the long bones, but particularly the bones of the skull. It is a slowly progressive deformation of calvarial bones with pathologic sequellae produced by encroachment upon vital structures such as blood vessels, nerves, and portions of the central nervous system. Consequently, Paget's disease may involve the temporal bone and mimic almost any aspect of otosclerosis (Fig. 37). It may produce fixation of the stapes, closure of the round window, pressure degeneration of the auditory nerve, and involvement of the vestibular labyrinth as well.

There is no satisfactory systemic treatment for Paget's disease, and there is no surgical treatment for it. In the rare instance where Paget's disease will produce stapedial fixation, fenestration surgery may be considered; but prognosis is not good inasmuch as closure of the fenestra is quite frequently produced by the inevitable progression of the basic systemic bone disease.

*Fragilitas Ossium, or "Brittle Bones."* Fragilitas ossium, or "brittle bones," is a rare disease usually hereditary in nature, characterized by marked fragility of all of the bones in the body and a peculiarity of the sclerae which robs them of pigment and is described as "blue sclerae." In this disease, multiple fractures occur; and it is not unusual for a patient to have as many as 40 to 50 fractures during a ten- or fifteen-year period—resulting in many deformations. Similar lesions may occur in the ossicular chain, in the tegmen mastoidei, tegmen tympani, and in the otic capsule. Lesions which simulate otosclerosis have occurred in this area, thus having given

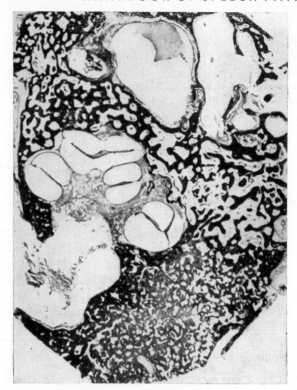

**FIG. 37.** Photomicrograph of case of Paget's disease. (From Fischer, J., and Wolfson, L. E. 1943. Inner ear. New York: Grune and Stratton. Fig. 34, p. 184.)

rise to the erroneous conception that "otosclerosis" is part of fragilitas os-sium. The stapedial fixation produced by this disease physiologically mimics that seen in otosclerosis. Here again, surgical treatment through fenestration is not too satisfactory because of the inevitable systemic bony degenerative changes.

*Osteitis Fibrosa Cystica.* Osteitis fibrosa cystica, or von Recklinghausen's disease of bone, is a disease characterized by cystic formations within the long bones as well as within the skull. It is most usually an accompaniment of hyperparathyroidism, in which there is an intense decalcification of the skeletal system. Lesions may occur in the temporal bone and the functional sequellae will depend entirely upon the random occurrence of these lesions. There is no classical picture, and here again stapedial fixation may occur but the treatment by surgery is usually unsatisfactory.

*Syphilis.* Syphilis, "the great imitator," is fortunately becoming a less common disease in civilized areas since the advent of penicillin and other antibiotics. Nevertheless, its ravages of previous years and the lesions produced through congenital transmission of the disease still make syphilis an important public health problem, and a significant etiologic factor in otologic disease.

Syphilis has been known for years to be a serious invader of the temporal bone. It produces a number of lesions (Goodhill, 1939), including periostitis, gumma formation, and sclerosing lesions in various parts of the skull. It may involve any portion of the temporal bone, and not infrequently produces sclerosis of the stapes with fixation of the footplate, as well as infiltration of the labyrinth and complete obliteration of the perilymph spaces as well as endolymph spaces. Thus, the syphilitic ear picture may present audiometric evidence of conduction hypacusis at times, with superimposed and fluctuating varieties of neural hypacusis, resulting frequently in neural anacusis as a terminal state. Involvement of the vestibular apparatus is just as common, and Meniere's disease may be imitated by syphilis.

The treatment of early syphilis is quite satisfactory today through the use of penicillin. Late syphilis, however, still remains a problem but can be attacked through combinations of heavy metals and fever therapy. Fortunately, the otologic sequellae of the disease are becoming less frequent and constitute a diminishing problem in deafness.

*Meniere's Disease—Labyrinthine Hydrops—Endolymphatic Hydrops.* Eponymic designations in medicine probably do more harm than good. Thus, the term *Meniere's disease* has acquired wide usage in otology but undoubtedly is used to describe a number of related and unrelated diseases of the labyrinth. To most otologists, the true Meniere's disease or syndrome is synonymous with what has been described as endolymphatic labyrinthine hydrops. The designation "Pseudo-Meniere's" syndrome has been applied to other diseases which are characterized by vertigo, with or without tinnitus and deafness.

True Meniere's disease or endolymphatic hydrops is presumed to be a disease of the endolymphatic labyrinth of unknown etiology, in which there occurs a chemical change in the endolymph resulting in hydropic distension of the membranous labyrinth both in the vestibular and cochlear divisions. Within the cochlea it produces a distension of the scala media (cochlear duct) in which Reissner's membrane becomes displaced away from the basilar membrane (Fig. 38). Prolonged hydrops produces varying degrees of damage to the organ of Corti and eventually the spiral ganglion as well. This pathologic picture is characterized clinically by the famous triad of vertigo, tinnitus, and deafness.

The term *vertigo* refers to a subjective false sensation of rotation, occasionally acceleration. This illusion may involve either the subject or his environment. Unfortunately, the word *dizziness* which is frequently used as a synonym for *vertigo* is used in many other ways. The "dizzy" spell of which a patient complains may really be *syncope* or momentary loss of consciousness (fainting); it may represent a transient visual scotoma; it may be used to describe a psychogenic feeling of unreality, headache, or momentary "daydream." All of these confusions in terminology have filled the medical literature with distortions of the place of *vertigo* in disease.

The vertigo of true Meniere's disease is a sudden onset of true rotatory illusion with sufficient severity to produce a major equilibrium disturbance.

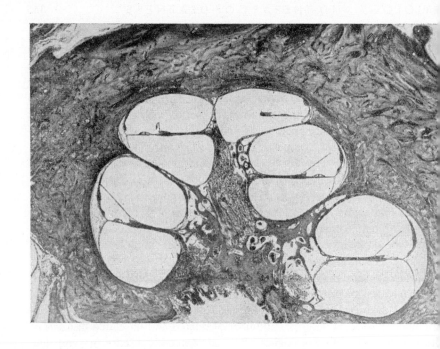

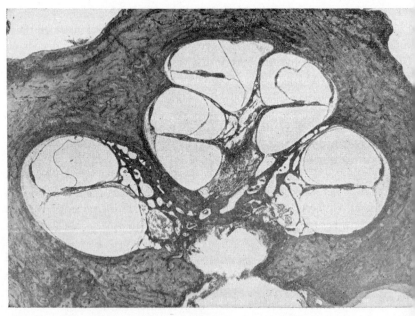

FIG. 38

The patient may feel propelled or pulled to one side and will frequently fall down. The sudden attack is frequently accompanied by nausea and vomiting, perspiration, and even mild shock. The sudden attack will usually require a day or two of complete bed rest with use of sedatives before equilibrium returns. It may then be followed by a prolonged chronic state of dysequilibrium aptly called "giddiness." The mild chronic "giddy" state may be punctuated by recurrent acute severe attacks. Great variation exists in the clinical picture. The severity and side effects will vary from attack to attack.

The deafness of Meniere's disease is usually a neural hypacusis, although in early stages it may appear to be a mixed conductive and neural hypacusis (Fig. 39). This is to be expected in view of the probable conductive block, which, early in the disease, may occur due to the endolymphatic distension alone. When organ of Corti degeneration supervenes, a truly neural audiometric picture is obtained. Thus what starts out as an early mixed lesion with low-frequency predominance will later become a straight-line purely neural lesion (Fig. 40): with chronicity, high-frequency losses will become more evident (Fig. 41). In the case of long duration, this neural hypacusis with greater high frequency involvement will be accompanied by progressive discrimination loss, so that a discrimination score of 50 per cent or less is not unusual with PB word lists. It will also be characterized by evidence of increased recruitment of loudness. Fortunately, the average case of true Meniere's is unilateral, so that the hearing disability is not a serious one.

Tinnitus in Meniere's disease, the third member of the triad, is a very annoying symptom in some patients. The tinnitus is usually amorphous and mixed in tonal qualities, usually in a continuous sustained amplitude. It is variously described as a roaring, ocean-wave sound with occasional bell-like qualities. The tinnitus will vary in intensity and annoyance and will be subject to emotional and nervous excitation. A sudden loud environmental sound may accentuate the tinnitus intensity for hours.

The course of the untreated disease is usually progressive, interspersed with plateau periods of latency. Thus, the hearing loss increases and the tinnitus may also increase in annoyance. The vertigo may become so severe

FIG. 38. Midmodiolar sections of both cochlea in a case of unilateral Menier's disease in a man, aged forty-seven. Death from subdural hematoma resulting from a fall during an attack of vertigo.

Top, horizontal section of right cochlea showing a normal cochlear duct. (The defects in Reissner's membrane in the apical coil are artifacts.) The number of ganglion cells and nerve fibers in the spiral ganglion of the basal coil is reduced. Extravasated red blood cells are present in the internal meatus and modiolus, the result of the head injury.

Bottom, vertical section of the left cochlea. The cochlear duct is moderately dilated throughout, almost filling the vestibular scala and extending into the helicotrema. The spiral ganglion of the basal coil shows a reduction from the normal in number of nerve cells and fibers.

The organ of Corti shows moderate postmortem degeneration in both ears but is sufficiently well preserved to indicate that the antemortem condition was approximately the same histologically in both ears. Remnants of the hair cells are seen throughout all coils in both ears and the stria vascularis is similar in both. (From Lindsay, J. R. 1939. Monograph on Meniere's disease. Chicago: Amer. Acad. Ophthal. Otolaryng.)

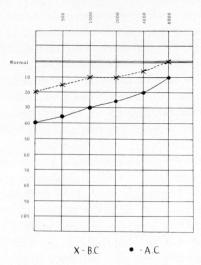

X - B.C      • - A.C.

**FIG. 39.** Audiometric threshold in a case of early endolymphatic hydrops (Meniere's disease). It is fairly typical of a conductive hypacusis.

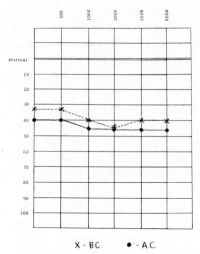

X - B.C.      • - A.C.

**FIG. 40.** Audiometric thresholds in a case of moderately alvanced endolymphatic hydrops (Meniere's disease). The picture is now typical of a neural hypacusis.

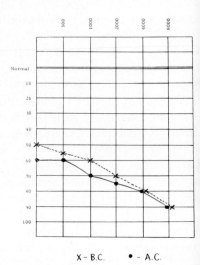

X – B.C.      • - A.C.

**FIG. 41.** Audiometric threshold in advanced endolymphatic hydrops. This is a severe neural hypacusis and is usually accompanied by marked vestibular hypoactivity, poor speech discrimination, and definite recruitment of loudness.

that the patient is in constant anxiety, never knowing when the next attack will occur. Some patients are confined to bed most of the time in the severe stage. The deafness may proceed from a mild or moderate neural hypacusis to a neural anacusis with no practical hearing at all.

The treatment of true Meniere's disease is largely empirical at the present time, although productive research is being carried on along allergic, biochemical, and psychosomatic avenues of investigation. Medical treatment is valuable in most patients and does result in palliation of symptoms and apparent cessation of progression in many instances. Such treatment may consist of a dehydration regime, including the low sodium diet, with administration of such drugs as ammonium chloride, potassium chloride, and Diamox. In other patients a vigorous antiallergic program with desensitization to histamine, pollens, and dust may be valuable. Emotional factors are undoubtedly etiologic in some patients and psychosomatic approaches are essential with them. Dramamine, Bonamine, Benadryl, and Merazine are drugs which have valuable sedative and antivertigo effects.

When medical therapy has been thoroughly tried and the patient is still incapacitated by violent vertigo episodes, surgical labyrinthine destruction becomes necessary, as an antivertigo measure. This may be accomplished with little operative risk via the labyrinthine route, in preference to intracranial section of the N. vestibularis. If there is suspicion of an internal auditory meatus lesion, such intracranial exploration is justified. Surgical interruption of vestibular sensations, either by translabyrinthine or intracranial routes, is usually very effective in controlling the vertigo. Such surgical treatment usually results in anacusis because of destruction of either the cochlear end organ in the translabyrinthine route or the N. cochlearis in the intracranial route.

The Day operation, or its modification, via the labyrinthine approach is a relatively safe procedure. The Dandy intracranial approach carried with it a minor though significant mortality rate. With the latter procedure, it is sometimes possible to preserve cochlear function, but it is also possible for facial nerve damage to occur as a sequel.

### NEURAL LESIONS ("NERVE" DEAFNESS)

#### Diagnostic Aspects of Entire Group

Neural deafness (neural hypacusis, nerve deafness, or perceptive deafness) is characterized by certain typical audiometric and otologic findings. These may be summarized as follows:

*Pure-Tone Audiometric Characteristics.* In neural deafness, pure-tone audiometric threshold losses may vary from a very mild hypacusis to profound hypacusis and anacusis. Bone-conduction threshold losses are usually equal to air-conduction threshold losses. There is no B.C.—A.C. gap in neural losses.

*Tuning-Fork Tests.* In neural lesions the Rinné test is invariably positive.

*Speech-Reception Threshold Correlations.* In contrast with conduction lesions, neural lesions do not always show close correlation between pure-tone air-conduction threshold losses and speech-reception threshold studies with spondee word lists. In some types of neural hypacusis the correlation may be very close, and in other types the correlation may be very poor.

*Speech Discrimination Score.* Intelligibility for speech as determined by speech discrimination scores is quite variable in neural lesions, in contrast with conduction lesions. Speech discrimination may be good in some types but may be very poor or even completely absent in other types of neural lesions. Phonemic regression frequently occurs in neural hypacuses.

*Recruitment of Loudness.* Recruitment of loudness is frequently found in neural hypacuses; particularly in peripheral or organ of Corti lesions.

*Response to Amplification.* In neural hypacuses, amplification of speech will yield variable results with frequent examples of poor response to amplification, occasionally accompanied by distortion.

### Classification of Neural Lesions (Fig. 42).

Neural lesions may be classified by two methods. They may be classified anatomically into reception, transmission, and perception lesions; and they may be classified chronologically in a more systematic etiologic manner.

| | Conduction Lesion | Neural Lesion |
|---|---|---|
| Threshold losses .............. | Hypacuses only | Hypacuses and anacuses |
| B.C./A.C. relations ............ | B.C./A.C. gap | No B.C./A.C. gap |
| Rinné fork test ................ | Negative | Positive |
| SRT (speech reception threshold) and pure-tone air-conduction correlation ................... | Excellent correlation | Variable correlation |
| S.D.S. (speech discrimination score) | Excellent | Variable |
| Recruitment of loudness ......... | None | Variable |
| Response to amplification ....... | Excellent | Variable |

FIG. 42. Conduction and neural "deafness." Basic audiologic differential diagnosis table.

### Anatomic classification

*Reception Lesions.* Neural receptive hypacuses or anacuses usually involve the organ of Corti and the basilar membrane proper, and probably represent the majority of neural lesions encountered in clinical practice. They may be due to degenerative, vascular, and other factors.

*Transmission Lesions.* Neural transmissive hypacuses or anacuses involve the auditory nerve and/or the central auditory pathways. Examples of this type of deafness are seen in acoustic neuroma, in nuclear deafness following erythroblastotic kernicterus, and in other lesions of the neural auditory pathways.

*Perception Lesions.* True neural "perceptive" hypacuses or anacuses are rare and involve the auditory cortex and subcortical integrative areas. They are frequently associated with neural dysacuses.

**Chronological classification.** The term *congenital deafness* has been applied to a large number of types of infantile neural deafness. The term *congenital* most properly should be reserved for genetic lesions, or those transnitted by genes, but is frequently used in the sense of "being present at birth" or "with birth." In order to avoid ambiguity, the term *congenital* will be liminated entirely from this classification and the terms *hereditary* and *acquired* will be used for distinctive purposes.

HEREDITARY NEURAL LESIONS

1. Cochlear Aplasia
2. Heredodegenerative Hypacuses
   a. Infantile heredodegenerative neural hypacusis
   b. Neural hypacuses of childhood and adult life
3. Otosclerotic Neural Hypacusis
   a. Infantile variety
   b. Childhood and adult otosclerotic neural hypacusis

ACQUIRED NEURAL LESIONS

1. Prenatal
   a. Toxic factors
   b. Infections
      maternal rubella
      congenital syphilis
2. Natal
   a. Trauma
   b. Hypoxia and anoxia
   c. Rh factor
3. Postnatal and Infantile Hypacuses and Anacuses
4. Childhood Neural Hypacuses
   a. Viral infections
   b. Mumps
   c. Bacterial diseases
5. Adult Neural Hypacuses
   a. Physical trauma
   b. Acoustic trauma
   c. Acquired syphilis
   d. Presbycusis
   e. Intracranial tumors
   f. Toxins—including streptomycin and other drugs

## A. HEREDITARY NEURAL LESIONS

### Cochlear Aplasia

Genetic aplasia, or developmental arrest of the cochlea, spiral-ganglion, and/or neural auditory pathway has been described histologically and encountered clinically very frequently. Microscopic studies have shown in such cases examples where all turns of the cochlea are completely devoid of organ of Corti formation. In contrast to the extreme examples cited, there are innumerable variables with partial aplasias of various elements of the neural auditory system. Thus both hypacuses and anacuses may be found in this group. The hypacuses may be quite variable in threshold

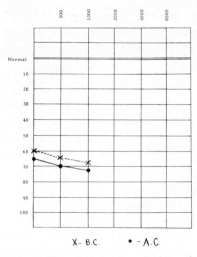

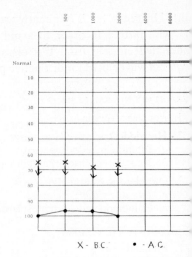

**FIG. 43. Illustration of a type of advanced neural hypacusis of hereditary etiology.**

**FIG. 44. Illustration of a type of neur< anacusis of hereditary etiology.**

losses and in qualitative differentials within the frequency spectrum. Thu all degrees of hearing disability may be found within this group (Figs. 43 an 44). This is undoubtedly a major cause of infantile neural deafness, and major etiologic factor in any survey of the population of schools for the dea Estimates of this factor in the over-all infantile neural deafness picture rang from 20 per cent to 50 per cent of the entire population of profoundly de< infants. Genetic studies have shown both recessive and dominant trends i this defect.

For many decades geneticists have called attention to the prevalence < this defect and have advised against procreation in such families to prevei further dissemination of the genetic trait. There is no satisfactory treatmei medically or surgically for this problem.

## 2. Heredodegenerative Hypacuses

**a. Infantile heredodegenerative neural hypacusis.** There are numerou clinical examples of this peculiar variety of hereditary deafness. In this un usual type there is evidence that the organ of Corti and the neural auditoi pathway are functioning to some degree at birth; perhaps even normally some instances. Atrophy or degeneration begins to occur somewhere arour the twelfth to fifteenth month of life. The resultant neural hypacusis ma extend to an unpredictable threshold loss by the twentieth month of life; most instances, to a profound degree of loss. There is no medical or surgic treatment of value in this variety.

**b. Neural hypacuses of childhood and adult life.** This entity, which sometimes referred to as familial nerve deafness, is another example of genetic degenerative cochlear lesion which may come on at any time in lif Instances have been observed in early and late childhood, in adolescence, arly as well as in late adult life. All quantitative and qualitative varieties of eural hypacuses may occur within this category. In most instances the losses re bilateral; and in most instances the losses are symmetrical and slowly rogressive. The common lesion is that of a predominantly high-frequency ⊃ss with slow involvement of the lower frequencies until major losses in the ⊃eech spectrum are encountered. Once the onset is recognized, progression ⊃pears to be usually fairly regular (Fig. 45), although there are instances

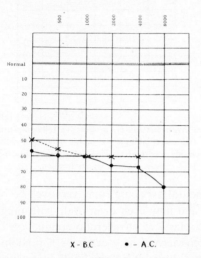

G. 45. Audiometric example of progressive bilateral neural hypacusis of heredodegenerative type with onset in adolescence.

here plateau quiescent states may be observed followed by precipitous ecrements in threshold at unpredictable intervals. There is no satisfactory ⍩edical or surgical treatment.

### Otosclerotic Neural Hypacusis

Otosclerosis, that major cause of adult conductive hypacusis, may occur ⍩ any part of the temporal bone as previously described. In many instances, strong hereditary tendency has been established for the disease. This is by ⍩ means universal, however. Instances have been shown of otosclerosis ⨍ccurring in fetal life in the child of an otosclerotic woman.

**a. Infantile variety.** It is theoretically conceivable that some cases of rofound infantile neural hypacusis may be due to familial otosclerosis in hich the otosclerotic lesion present at birth has involved either the internal ⍩ditory meatus region or the ductus cochlearis per se, with or without tapedial involvement. Such a lesion will present the audiologic picture of a eural hypacusis and possibly even a neural anacusis with all of the educa-onal and rehabilitation problems posed by that group of diseases.

**b. Childhood and adult otosclerotic neural hypacusis.** It is not unusual ⊃ find a neural hypacusis in the child of an otosclerotic conduction hypa-

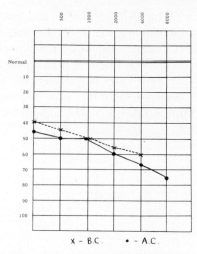

**FIG. 46.** Example of neural hypacusis rapidly progressive following pregnancy in a 25-year-old female in whose family there are multiple examples of typical otosclerosis with conduction hypacuses only. This is probably a case of otosclerotic neural hypacusis, due to cochlear invasion only, without stapes fixation.

cusis patient. Such neural hypacuses may very well be bilaterally symmetrical and progressive and may even deteriorate with pregnancy—a state frequently noticed in a classical otosclerotic conduction hypacusis. Knowing that histologically otosclerosis may occur as a random occurrence in any portion of the temporal bone, it is quite likely that neural hypacusis in such instances (Fig. 46) may be due to the basic otosclerotic lesion which affected the cochlear and spiral-ganglion regions rather than the classical limitation to the stapedio-vestibular articulation. Furthermore, well-defined otosclerotic conduction hypacusis may suddenly show evidence (Fig. 47) of super-

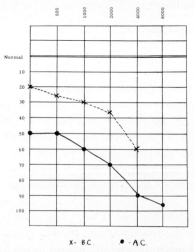

**FIG. 47.** Example of otosclerosis (juvenile type) with marked superimposed neural hypacusis probably due to cochlear otosclerotic invasion.

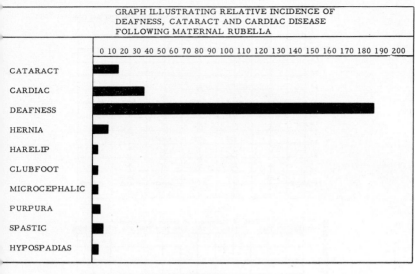

GRAPH ILLUSTRATING RELATIVE INCIDENCE OF
DEAFNESS, CATARACT AND CARDIAC DISEASE
FOLLOWING MATERNAL RUBELLA

**FIG. 48**

mposed neural hypacusis not easily explained by other etiologic factors. It s quite likely that in these patients the otosclerotic process invades cochlear nd spiral-ganglion structures and produces a superimposed neural hypacu- is so that we virtually then have two separate diseases to deal with from he point of view of auditory organ function.

Since there is no satisfactory medical treatment for otosclerosis, there is 10 definite therapy for otosclerotic neural hypacusis. Thus stapedolysis or enestration surgery are of no value in these cases, inasmuch as their indi- ation is purely mechanistic and designed to re-establish a functioning coustic perilymphatic pathway. Neither of these surgical procedures has ny specific effect upon the basic etiologic nature of the disease itself.

## B. ACQUIRED NEURAL LESIONS

. Prenatal

Under the prenatal acquired category may be included a number of dis- ases that are due to prenatal factors, traumatic to the development or mat- ration of the organ of hearing. These may include both toxic and infectious actors.

**a. Toxic factors.** A number of toxic factors present during the period of estation may have an adverse effect on the developing organ of hearing. The xic effects of certain drugs are considered possible etiologic agents in such evelopmental trauma. Quinine taken in the early months of pregnancy may ave an adverse effect upon the developing cochlea; particularly if there is a pecific sensitivity to quinine in the mother. Streptomycin in large doses may imilarly produce damage to the developing organ of hearing, again if there a special susceptibility to streptomycin damage. Alcohol and tobacco have

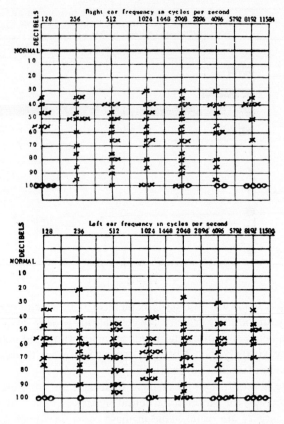

FIG. 49. Scattergram of A.C.-threshold audiograms of 16 patients with neural hypacusis due to maternal rubella.

both been mentioned as possible etiologic factors under this category, but definitive proof of their toxic action is lacking.

**b. Infections.** *Maternal Rubella.* Rubella, one of the mild communicable exanthemata, has been shown to be an exceptionally virulent destructive agent to the fetal organs when it occurs in the mother during the first tri mester of pregnancy. When this effect of rubella was first noticed, it was thought that the primary destruction occurred within the infantile ocular and cardiac systems. It was recognized later (Goodhill, 1950c), however, that the primary site of damage is in the developing cochlea, and that far more deaf ness (Fig. 48) results from maternal rubella than either ocular disease or con genital cardiac disease. In some patients all three defects may co-exist.

The damage to the organ of hearing has not been clearly established ana tomically. Destructive areas have been found not only in the cochlea but in the central auditory pathway. The audiometric picture in rubella deafness is pleomorphic (Fig. 49), and losses varying from 20 to 100 db have been en countered in many studies. The predominating loss is usually in the 50 to 7

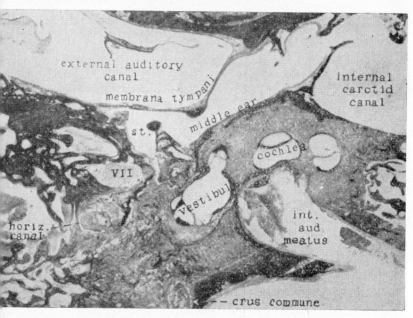

FIG. 50. Syphilis. Horizontal section. Note complete cast of new bone filling crus commune, horizontal canal and part of vestibule. Suppurative labyrinthitis. Marked deformity of stapes.

range, and in most of these instances the patients can be helped by amplification. In most instances, the losses are bilaterally symmetrical and there no satisfactory medical or surgical treatment.

In a number of recent studies, it has been shown that rubella is one of the major causes of infantile neural deafness, and a great factor in the overall etiologic study of infantile deaf populations. In one study (Goodhill, 1950b), rubella appeared to account for at least 20 per cent of the population of a school for the deaf.

Because of increased recognition of the hazard of rubella, some pediatricians and obstetricians have considered the advisability of interruption of pregnancy in instances of maternal rubella during the first trimester. Some public health authorities have urged that all growing girls be intentionally exposed to rubella so that immunity may be developed prior to marriage and pregnancy. No satisfactory method of immunization against this disease is available at the present time. Thus maternal rubella poses an extremely vital public health and preventive medicine question, primarily because of the subsequent fetal deafness.

*Congenital Syphilis.* Syphilis, the great imitator, produced many very serious diseases as the result of "congenital" transmission of the disease. "Congenital" syphilis is still with us, even though syphilis as a whole has been drastically reduced as a public health menace since the advent of antibiotic therapy and better public health control. Congenital syphilis (Good-

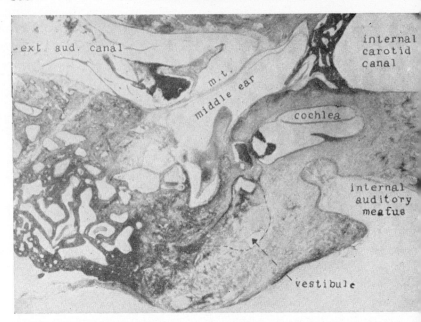

FIG. 51. Syphilis. Horizontal section at level of basal turn of cochlea. Purulent invasion
labyrinth occurs via round window. New bone is seen in vestibule here also.

hill, 1939) may produce primarily a neural hypacusis (Figs. 50, 51, 52)
either unilaterally or bilaterally, which may come on any time in life.
not infrequently will become manifest during the second decade of life, an
progression may be very major or extremely mild. Variable results are bein
obtained with antibiotic, heavy metal, and other antiluetic therapy; and i
general the prognosis today is far better than it was a decade ago. Neverthe
less, permanent hypacuses and even anacuses may result and may defy a
medical therapy attempts. Frequently, congenital syphilitic deafness is ac
companied by other easily recognizable stigmata such as keratitis, denta
defects, and orthopedic defects. The diagnosis is made on the basis of histor
physical findings, and serologic evidence in both blood and the cerebro
spinal fluid.

## 2. Natal

At birth a number of untoward occurrences may adversely influence th
organ of hearing. Trauma, anoxia, and serologic incompatibilities are th
chief factors of such natal damage to the cochlea and neural auditory path
ways.

**a. Trauma.** Physical trauma to the skull during birth occurs infrequentl
It may be due to a faulty pelvic outlet, close approximation of forceps, or
difficult breech or posterior presentation. In current obstetrical practic
such trauma is becoming increasingly rare; and unless an intracranial hemo
rhage has occurred, it is unlikely that cephalic trauma is at the present tim
a major cause of natal ear damage.

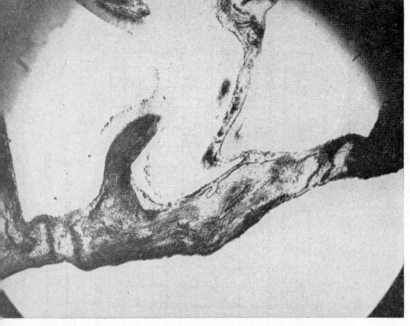

FIG. 52. Syphilis. Marked deformity of crura and foot-plate of stapes.

**b. Hypoxia and anoxia.** Probably the most important cause of natal ear
jury is prolonged hypoxia or anoxia of the infant. Any disturbance in res-
iration or circulation will bring with it the possibility of diminished oxygen
nsion in the circulating blood. Any significant deprivation of oxygen is a
vere nutritional blow to the delicate neural epithelium of the organ of
orti and produces rapid degeneration and atrophy. Many factors may
redispose to hypoxia and anoxia, including long labors, heavy maternal
dation, obstruction of the respiratory passages with mucus, incomplete
evelopment of the lungs, and congenital circulatory and cardiac defects.
noxic sequellae may affect any of the sensory organs and the central
ervous system as well. Thus, cerebral palsy is frequently seen in association
ith anoxic neural hypacusis.

The only treatment for hypoxia and anoxia is preventive. The sequellae
re unfortunately final and irreversible, and are not helped by any type of
edical or surgical therapy. Any quantitative or qualitative variety of neural
ypacusis may be seen as the sequel of natal hypoxia or anoxia.

**c. Rh factor.** Serologic incompatability between the fetus and the mother
responsible for a variety of hemolytic diseases in which red blood cells are
estroyed and the toxic pigment allowed to circulate freely within the fetal
rculation. Such circulation of pigment produces a large number of sequel-
e, principally those due to deposition of pigment in various areas within
e central nervous system and in sensory organs as well.

The prime example of serologic incompatability is erythroblastotic ker-

Patient: G W

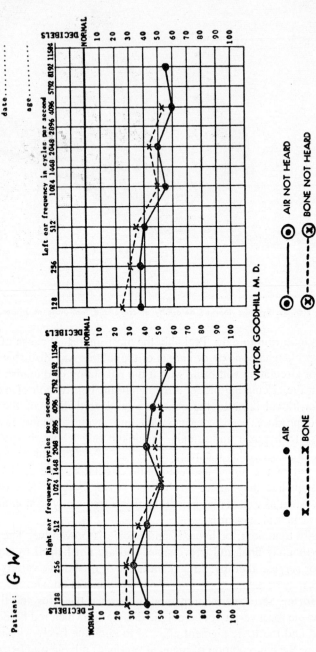

VICTOR GOODHILL M. D.

●────● AIR          ⊙────⊙ AIR NOT HEARD

X------X BONE       ⊗------⊗ BONE NOT HEARD

FIG. 53. Bilaterally symetrical neural hypacusis (transmissive) due to kernicterus.

nicterus. The union of an Rh negative female with an Rh positive male in which the fetus is Rh negative produces no unfavorable sequellae. If the fetus, however, is Rh positive in blood type, the possibility of serious incompatibility due to circulating antibodies will develop. If such incompatibility assumes major proportions due to high titer of maternal antibody, infantile erythroblastosis will occur, reaching its peak at birth. Circulating pigment would be deposited in the skin, in the liver, in the central nervous system, and in many other vital organs. The deposition of pigment in the pons and medulla will produce the neural pathologic state called "kernicterus" or icterus of the cranial nuclei. Among the sequellae of kernicterus are athetoid cerebral palsy due to involvement of the extrapyramidal tracts and a specific type of central deafness due to involvement of the dorsal and ventral cochlear nuclei (which has been termed "nuclear deafness" by the author) (Goodhill, 1950b). There is evidence (Fig. 53) also that some deposition of pigment may occur within the spiral-ganglion and ductus cochlearis as well. At any rate, a very diffuse type of transmissive and possibly receptive neural hypacusis and occasionally anacusis may occur as the sequel of erythroblastotic kernicterus due to Rh factor incompatibility.

Erythroblastosis is usually characterized by progressive increase in serologic incompatibility with successive pregnancies. Thus the first pregnancy with an Rh positive baby is usually uneventful, but subsequent pregnancies may carry greater concentrations of maternal antibodies and greater risk of icteric deposition with neurologic sequellae. The only treatment is prevention, and preventive measures are based upon careful maternal antibody determinations during pregnancy and special measures at birth to prevent kernicterus. These special measures may include blood replacement, transfusions, and the use of some of the newer steroid hormonal drugs. Once the kernicterus lesion has occurred, however, there is no satisfactory medical or surgical therapy at the present time.

The hearing loss is always neural in character and usually indicative of a transmissive rather than a receptive lesion.

Recent studies have shown that incompatibilities within the basic A, B, O blood classifications may also cause erythroblastotic sequellae with kernicterus. Thus it is quite likely that the nuclear deafness previously attributed only to Rh factor incompatibility may conceivably occasionally be due to A, B, O incompatibility and further studies along serologic lines may reveal other types of incompatibilities productive of the same sequellae.

### 3. Postnatal and Infantile Neural Hypacuses and Anacuses

A number of the viral exanthemata may occur during the first year of life. Certain bacterial infections of the central nervous system, including encephalitis and meningitis, are also found fairly frequently during this vulnerable period. All major causes of neural hypacusis at this period produce auditory sensory defects which are educationally identical with prenatal and natal lesions. This is the reason for the common usage of the term *congenital* in categorizing all of these diseases together.

Inasmuch as language acquisition during the first year of life is so vitally dependent upon communication input through hearing, any neural hypacusis sufficiently severe to interfere with language development will concomitantly interfere with the development of speech or communication output. Thus an infant who is born with perfectly normal hearing but who loses most of his hearing as a result of meningococcic meningitis, or measles encephalitis, or mumps meningitis, or tuberculous meningitis will pose the identical educational problem of a child who has congenital cochlear aplasia or maternal rubella deafness or Rh factor central nuclear deafness. These children will have interference with language development and will require the same educational approach as those children with prenatal or natal lesions.

### 4. Childhood Neural Hypacuses

**a. Viral infections.** Almost all of the viral exenthemata may produce serious neurological sequellae. These may be limited to one or another of the sense organs, or may involve the central nervous system proper. Thus neural hypacuses and anacuses may follow measles, mumps, chicken pox, whooping cough, rubella, and members of the so-called virus influenza group. All of these diseases may attack the organ of hearing. Such invasion may be unilateral or bilateral, and partial or complete. In general, cochlear involvement by viruses is relatively infrequent except in mumps.

**b. Mumps.** Mumps or epidemic parotitis may involve one or both parotid glands, and one or both submaxillary salivary glands. It is a highly communicable contagious disease of childhood, and occasionally of adults. Not infrequently mumps will produce marked otalgia and tinnitus during the acute course of the disease. Examination of the ears at this time will usually reveal no significant changes in the tympanic membranes. Nevertheless, the patient may complain of a hearing loss during the actual gland swelling which will become more marked when the swelling disappears. Otologic examination will reveal no changes in the middle ears, but will usually reveal very profound neural hypacusis, usually unilateral, frequently profound and to the anacusis degree. Occasionally such cochlear destruction will be accompanied by vestibular destruction as well, and caloric vestibular studies may reveal total lack of vestibular response on the affected side.

The exact mechanism of invasion of the mumps virus is unknown, as is the percentile incidence of the disease. It is very difficult to evaluate auditory sequellae of an epidemic or communicable disease because of the wide disparity of medical care and the fact that most patients are not hospitalized. Nevertheless, it is well recognized that mumps is a major cause of unilateral neural hypacusis and anacusis, and undoubtedly is the major offender among the viral group from the point of view of acquired lesions. Such deafness may occur in adults as well as in children, and is usually irreversible and

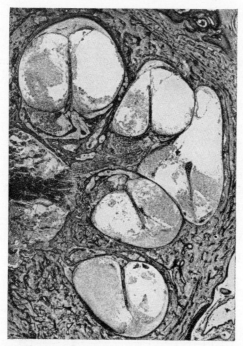

FIG. 54. Microphotograph showing the diffuse purulent stage of meningitic labyrinthitis. Pus cells are diffusely distributed throughout the cochlear spaces and the modiolus. Destruction of the cochlear duct has already occurred in the basal coil. (From Jackson, C., and Jackson, C. L. 1945. Disease of the nose, throat, and ear. New York: Saunders. Fig. 319, p. 396.)

does not respond to any type of therapy.

**c. Bacterial diseases.** Bacterial diseases of childhood which invade the central nervous system may also invade the cochlear and central neural auditory pathways with resultant neural hypacuses and anacuses. Meningitis and encephalitis are the two chief examples of this group, with meningitis being the major offender. Any type of meningitis may affect the auditory organ (Fig. 54). Epidemic or meningococcic meningitis is just as important a cause of such involvement as the coccal meningitis following either streptococcal, pneumococcal, or staphylococcal respiratory infections. Tuberculous meningitis may also produce the same type of invasion with the same sequellae.

Most meningitic neural hypacuses and anacuses are bilateral and most of them result in profound losses; primarily in the anacusis category. In some instances there is also evidence of vestibular disturbance, but this is not a universal finding.

There is no satisfactory treatment for the sequellae of meningitic deafness, but meningitis per se can now be treated far more satisfactorily than it was treated one or two decades ago. Consequently more survivals are reported than ever before. Naturally, many of these survivors will be left with neurologic sequellae, one of which very well may be neural hypacusis.

When the meningitis therapy is started very early in the course of the disease, and where the organism is particularly responsive to the antibiotic agent, avoidance of sensory defects may be expected. It is not too much to hope that early thorough treatment of meningitis may result in the virtual elimination of postmeningitic neural hypacusis as a major cause of deafness.

### 5. Adult Neural Hypacuses

**a. Physical trauma.** Physical trauma to the head may produce varying degrees of damage to the auditory organ. A sharp blow on the auricle with resultant compression of air within the external auditory canal may produce a tympanic membrane rupture and in some instances labyrinthine disturbances. The resultant hearing loss may show evidence of a combined conductive and neural hypacusis—the extent depending upon the degree of damage to each compartment of the auditory organ. Physical trauma to the head itself may result in concussive damage to the labyrinth (Fig. 55) or to an actual fracture of the temporal bone.

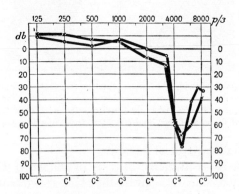

FIG. 55. Blunt head injury without fracture of skull. (From Fowler, E. P. 1947. Loose-leaf medicine of the ear. Baltimore: Williams & Wilkins. Fig. 10, p. 355.)

Concussion of the labyrinth may produce findings similar to those seen in labyrinthine hemorrhage, or in endolymphatic hydrops. Thus they may include tinnitus, vertigo, and varying degrees of neural hypacusis. Such damage may be temporary or permanent, depending upon the degree of disruption of neural epithelial elements and the degree of disturbance of labyrinthine fluids. Treatment of such conditions is rarely surgical but may include such medical techniques as dehydration therapy and prophylactic antibiotic therapy.

Actual temporal bone fractures (Figs. 56, 57, 58) may result in variable sequellae, depending upon extent of fracture and location of fracture line. A temporal bone fracture is usually part of a basal skull fracture and sequellae of major importance may occur. If the fracture carries with it a laceration of the dura, there may be an escape of cerebrospinal fluid as well as of blood through the external auditory canal, and this may carry with it the very grave

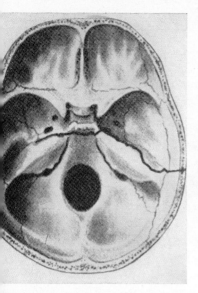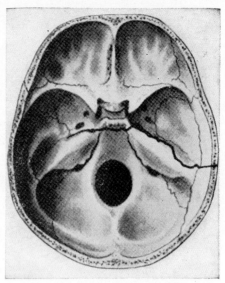

6. Longitudinal fracture of right petrous From Fowler, E. P. 1947. Loose-leaf medi- the ear. Baltimore: Williams & Wilkins. Fig. 1, p. 349).

FIG. 57. Transverse fracture of right petrous bone. (From Fowler, E. P. 1947. Loose-Leaf medicine of the ear. Baltimore: Williams & Wilkins. Fig. 8, p. 353.)

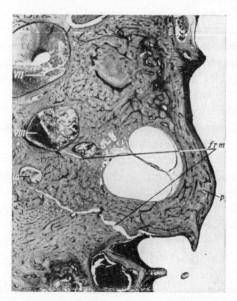

58. Microphotograph of case of longitudinal fracture of temporal bone. (From Fischer, J., and Wolfson, L. E. 1943. Inner ear. New York: Grune and Stratton. Fig. 74, p. 348.)

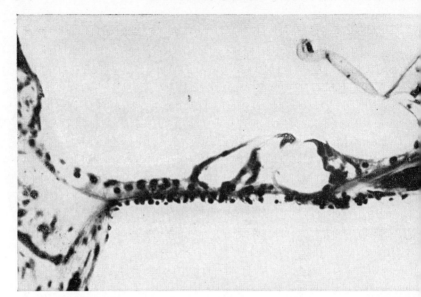

FIG. 59. Effect of noise trauma in the guinea pig. The outer hair cells and some of Deite supporting cells have disappeared at the beginning of the second cochlear turn. (From Fowl E. P. 1947. Loose-Leaf medicine of the ear. Baltimore: Williams & Wilkins. 35, p. 367G.)

prognosis for life itself. In such instances, there are usually resultant perm nent and severe neural hypacuses, along with major vestibular disturbance Therapy is usually directed along preventive lines and may include antibio and other types of supportive therapy.

**b. Acoustic trauma.** A subject of major interest to otologists, audiol gists, and industrial physicians has been that of increased incidence of acou tic injury to the cochlea. It has been known for years that high-intensity no had adverse effects upon the inner ear. Thus "boiler makers'" deafness w described half a century ago, and its high tone loss characteristic was know to otologists of that era. During the past few decades, the increased mechar zation of civilized life and the increased part played by noise in military a tivities have brought with them the inevitable damage to the auditory e organ that one would expect. Thus, neural hypacusis of a number of varieti is being encountered more and more commonly in clinical practice and is n just as serious a civilian problem as it was a military problem in the last w. The human auditory organ was not created to withstand exposure to hig intensity sounds of the nature encountered in today's mechanization.

Pathologically, selective damage occurs within the epithelial elements the organ of Corti, the location and extent depending upon the basic i tensity and frequency characteristics of the offending noise source (Fi 59 and 60). Thus more and more adult neural hypacusis is being encou tered and much of it assumes serious degrees, so that major speech recepti threshold losses occur. No longer are we concerned about the classi high tone dip, or 4096 notch, which was of audiometric interest but whi

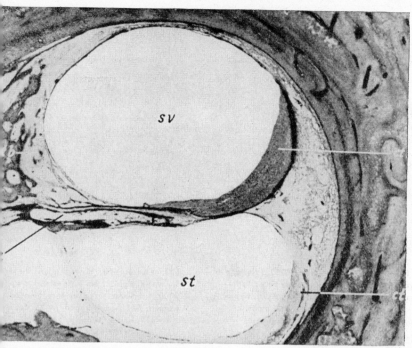

FIG. 60. Microphotograph of case of traumatic deafness. Section through basal turn of cochlea, showing organ of Corti destroyed and replaced by connective tissue filling entire scala media (m); scala tympani (st) also containing connective tissue (ct); network of connective tissue bone (ct b) in scala vestibuli (sv); complete atrophy (a) of spiral nerve. from Fischer, J., and Wolfson, L. E. 1943. Inner ear. New York: Grune and Stratton. Fig. 77, p. 357.)

itself carried few practical implications for the patient. We now find that prolonged acoustic trauma produces deficits in the entire auditory spectrum, and frequently these deficits assume major degrees in the 1000 and 2000 cycle range where they decidedly interfere with the hearing for speech.

The jet age will undoubtedly bring with it further instances of such damage, and the entire problem has reached such magnitude that innumerable agencies are devoted to research in this field. The problem of noise has become so acute in many areas that an entire journal devoted to "noise control" has recently been put into publication.

The treatment of acoustic trauma begins and ends with prevention. There is no treatment for the demonstrable hearing loss which has occurred as the result of such exposure. The efforts of physicians and audiologists must be devoted to (a) prevention of contact of humans with such high-intensity sound areas, (b) selection of adequate sound protective devices, and (c) screening of individuals to eliminate those whose cochleas show susceptibility to noise damage in industries where noise is a major problem.

Undoubtedly, there is a difference in susceptibility to noise trauma. Many anatomic and physiologic reasons could be offered to explain the reason for such variation in susceptibility. An adequate method for rapid screening

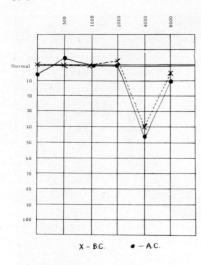

X - B.C.        • - A.C.

**FIG. 61. Classic example of 4000 cycle tone dip (A.C. and B.C.) in traumatic or "stimulation" deafness (high-tone neural hypacusis). SRT within normal limits.**

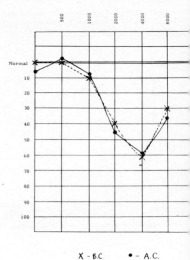

X - B.C.        • - A.C.

**FIG. 62. Further deterioration in case shown in Fig. 61. Note threshold drop 2000 cycles due to persistence of acoustic trauma. SRT has dropped to 25 decibel below acoustic zero.**

techniques to find such susceptible individuals is imperative in an attempt to meet this problem in industry and in military life today.

Individuals who show a characteristic 4000 cycle dip (Fig. 61) bilaterally by both air and bone conduction, and who have a history of known tinnitus upon exposure to high-intensity noise, should be warned against continued exposure to such noise. Exposure to gun fire in such individuals may possibly cause degenerative changes in the lower parts of the spectrum (Fig. 62) particularly at 2000 and 1000 cycles, thus rendering that individual a candidate for serious speech-threshold disturbances as well as speech-discrimination losses. Thus, prevention is the chief responsibility of the otologist meeting the problem of acoustic trauma clinically.

**c. Acquired syphilis.** Syphilis as a public health problem is rapidly diminishing in importance. Acquired syphilis is becoming a fairly rare disease in medical practice today, and when it occurs it can be rapidly controlled by adequate antibiotic therapy. Consequently, syphilitic deafness, which used to be a major problem otologically, has become a rarity and one requiring little stress from the point of view of therapy. Syphilis has always been known as the "great imitator" and as such, in the temporal bone (as well elsewhere in the body), it may imitate any disease, including otosclerosis, Meniere's disease, toxic labyrinthitis, as well as intracranial tumors. By forming large space-occupying gummata and by creating periostitis (Figs. 50, 51 and 52), it may produce all varieties of both conductive and neural hypacuses. Treatment must be directed to the basic problem, and syphilis today usually responds to treatment in the majority of cases.

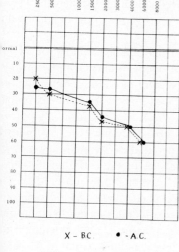

FIG. 63. Typical neural hypacusis due to presbycusis, probably of epithelial atrophy type.

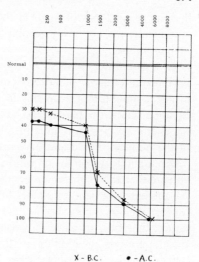

FIG. 64. Neural hypacusis due to presbycusis with evidence of neural atrophy and high-frequency damage.

**d. Presbycusis.** Presbycusis has been used to designate the deterioration hearing commonly seen in older age groups. Recent studies by Schuknecht 955) have done much to clarify the clinical and histopathologic aspects this type of neural hypacusis. His studies have shown evidence of two ajor types of presbycusis: (1) characterized by epithelial atrophy (Figs. 63 d 64) and (2) characterized by neural atrophy.

The epithelial atrophy type is the most common type and is the otological anifestation of an aging process affecting primarily epithelial tissues. It characterized by degeneration which begins at the basal end of the cochar duct and proceeds towards the apex, with involvement of all of the ructures within this area about equally and almost simultaneously.

The second, or neural atrophy type, is characterized by primary degenation of spiral-ganglion cells at the basal end of the cochlea, as well as euron elements in the central neural auditory pathway. This neural atrophy pe is usually superimposed upon the more common epithelial atrophy type d occurs later in life. It is characterized by major high-tone deafness with sproportionately severe discrimination losses.

In general, presbycusis occurs in most adults, but its rate will vary nsiderably. It rarely becomes manifest until the sixth or seventh decades the majority of the population. Premature presbycusis, however, may be monstrated audiometrically in the fourth decade not infrequently. Recuitment of loudness is not always found in presbycusis, although it may cur in some cases. Premature presbycusis may very well be a concomitant a familial or hereditary predisposition and thus may actually represent a ase of heredodegenerative neural hypacusis of the adult type.

There is no satisfactory treatment for presbycusis. Its progress continues in spite of all types of medical therapy. Rehabilitation through the use c amplification is not easily accomplished in presbycusis but is of some valu in many cases.

**e. Intracranial tumors.** Two varieties of intracranial tumors are of im portance in otologic practice. Acoustic neuroma is a fairly common variet of intracranial tumor occurring in 1 to 2 per cent of all intracranial tumor In some series, the percentage has been placed higher. Acoustic neuromal in general are benign tumors histologically which may occur on any portio of the auditory nerve and may reach any size. They may occur within th internal auditory meatus or within the intracranial cavity, and they may ir volve either the cochlear or vestibular branches or the entire eighth nerv All of these are benign humors histologically, though they do produce se ious sequellae purely because of pressure phenomena. As they becom larger, they may produce impairment of facial-nerve function with ensuir facial paralysis in addition to the tinnitus, deafness, and dysequilibriu which usually are present earlier in the clinical picture. Continued growt may involve the fifth nerve with typical trigeminal pain, and eventual obstructive hydrocephalus may occur with visual disturbances and oth evidences of increased intracranial pressure.

Cerebello-pontile angle tumors may be of any histologic type, either b nign or malignant, although most of these are also benign. Such tumors w compress the auditory nerve secondarily and will produce many of the abo symptoms, but in a variable order. Here again, increased intracranial pre sure may result with the classical symptoms of such pressure.

The treatment of these tumors is usually surgical, although complete r moval is virtually impossible. The surgical approach is directed at decom pression and at removal of as much of the tumor as is possible, with prese vation of vital organs. In general, these are slow-growing tumors and the first symptoms may be limited to a unilateral neural hypacusis with mi tinnitus and momentary episodes of vertigo. They may be easily confus with unilateral Meniere's disease and with other lesions of the cochlea a vestibule, particularly in the early stages. Repeated neurological examin tions and careful otologic studies are necessary in order to make an ea diagnosis of such a tumor. Early diagnosis is imperative, inasmuch as ea surgery carries with it a higher degree of safety and a lower mortality.

One characteristic finding in tumors of the internal auditory meatus a vicinity is the rather marked loss of discrimination which is in contrast w the relatively small threshold loss. Recruitment (Fig. 65) is usually r present in the majority of these tumors, thus affording another different diagnostic tool in the evaluation of the problem.

**f. Toxins—including streptomycin and other drugs.** A number of to substances, including drugs, may result in irreversible damage to the neu auditory organ. Quinine, in susceptible individuals, may produce such da age in varying degrees of neural hypacusis, usually bilateral and usua permanent. Of the drugs in common usage, dihydrostreptomycin is the m

mportant potential cause of drug damage to the cochlea. In the earlier years
of its purification, streptomycin caused cochlear damage in a number of
eported instances, along with disturbances of vestibular apparatus. The
estibular disturbance was the primary reason for the search for another
drug and for this reason dihydrostreptomycin was developed to minimize
he possibility of vestibular paralysis.

Unfortunately, dihydrostreptomycin, which was very effective in the
reatment of tuberculosis and which carried with it very little toxicity to the
estibular apparatus, showed very definite predilection for the cochlea, and
dihydrostreptomycin in susceptible individuals may produce neural hypa-
usis because of cochlear degeneration. For this reason, dihydrostreptomy-
in is not being used in large doses, and is being combined with other drugs
n an attempt to minimize its cochlear toxic effect. Susceptible individuals
hould avoid long-term administration of dihydrostreptomycin, inasmuch
s the cochlear hypacusis resulting is irreversible and almost always bilateral.

## TINNITUS

Tinnitus is an otologic symptom. It has many characteristics and can oc-
ur as the result of many causes. It is not a disease or syndrome, but a sub-
ective phenomenon common to many diseases and should be viewed in the
ght of subjective symptomatology in differential otologic diagnosis.

Webster defines tinnitus as a ringing, whistling, or other sensation of
noise which is purely subjective. The word is derived from the Latin, *tinnire*,
meaning "to jingle."

Basically, two types of tinnitus must be distinguished; tinnitus aurium,
nd tinnitus cranii (tinnitus cerebri).

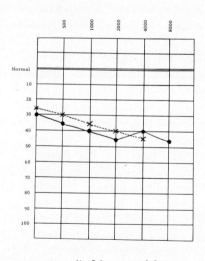

X - B.C.        • - A.C.

Fig. 65. Threshold audiogram of patient with acoustic neauroma. This moderate threshold loss
was accompanied by a speech discrimination score of less than 25 per cent (PB word list).
Recruitment was absent.

Tinnitus cranii is frequently confused with tinnitus aurium and may actually co-exist with it. Tinnitus cranii is a nonlocalized subjective sensation of sound which is usually diffusely in the head and has a nonspecific quality. It is frequently described as a roaring or rushing sound not directed to the ear region. Its diffuse character may be confused with somatic sensations of the neck and upper thorax and, indeed, may be due to vascular phenomena in these areas as well as intracranially. Most usually, tinnitus cranii is due to organic or functional intracranial vascular disease and is a medical neurological problem, one which does not participate significantly in otologic diagnosis.

Tinnitus aurium, on the other hand, is usually localized to one or both ears and is subjectively described with some specificity by the patient.

Tinnitus aurium must be subdivided into two subtypes each of which has been given a number of names. These two principal subtypes and their synonyms may be described as follows:

1. Subjective tinnitus (static-nonvibratory, true, intrinsic). Subjective tinnitus is the subjective cortical perception of auditory sensations inaudible to anyone but the patient. These sensations are most usually due to auditory paresthesia from any location within the auditory pathway.

2. Objective tinnitus (dynamic, vibratory, false, extrinsic). Objective tinnitus may be defined as the subjective cortical perception of auditory sensations, potentially audible to an examiner as well as to the patient.

Inasmuch as objective tinnitus is a relatively rare phenomenon, its characteristics and significance in otologic diagnosis will be briefly surveyed in order to limit the remainder of the discussion to the principal type of tinnitus encountered in otologic practice, namely, subjective tinnitus.

Objective tinnitus is either vascular or muscular in origin. The vascular type of objective tinnitus is usually due to some type of arterio-venous communication producing an audible bruit or murmur which can be heard with or without amplification. The muscular types of objective tinnitus are due to contractions of tympanic or tubal muscles, usually in bizarre or atypical rhythm. The mechanism for such contractions is exceedingly complex in etiology. Muscle spasms, functional tics, and other neuromuscular phenomena related to metabolic and psychosomatic states play a part in this relatively rare group of cases.

The etiology of subjective tinnitus can be discussed from the standpoint of anatomic location and pathologic change. Subjective tinnitus may arise from any location within auditory pathway from the external ear to the auditory cortex. The pathologic state responsible for the genesis of the tinnitus may be any histopathologic abnormality in the auditory pathway. Consequently, the potential causes for tinnitus are innumerable and defy simplification. Tinnitus is a common symptom of many otologic diseases.

In the consideration of subjective tinnitus, it is helpful to differentiate two basic physiologic subdivisions which are quite different anatomically and functionally.

The first subdivision may be described as *unmasked visceral tinnitus*. This tinnitus usually originates in the tympanic region and is usually the sequel of a conduction or impedance lesion. It is caused by the removal of the normal masking effect of surrounding ambient noise and is usually produced by subaudible tympanic and peritympanic vascular and muscular noises. This is the type of tinnitus one meets most commonly in uncomplicated otosclerosis, tympanic fibrosis, and chronic catarrhal otitis with or without perforation. It is also frequently found in glomus jugulare and other tympanic tumors.

The second physiologic type of tinnitus is more common and might be described as *neural discharge tinnitus* of either cochlear or central origin. This is a supra-threshold auditory paresthesia. In this type there is cerebral recognition of auditory stimuli produced by mechanical cochlear deformation or electrochemical neural hyper-irritability in the auditory pathways. This is the type seen in stimulation (traumatic) deafness, some types of presbycusis, Meniere's disease (labyrinthine hydrops), acoustic neuroma, and in many other lesions involving either the cochlea or any of the neural elements of the auditory pathways.

In addition to the above differentiation, which is important from a localization and management point of view, we must also differentiate tinnitus clinically into compensated and decompensated forms. *Compensated* tinnitus is present in much of the population. It accompanies the high incidence of minimal cochlear lesions due to various etiologic factors which are productive of neural discharge tinnitus. In most of these instances the tinnitus is not even noticeable to the patient, except under extremely quiet circumstances. It is not a clinical problem but merely a curiosity.

*Decompensated* tinnitus may be used as a term to describe tinnitus that is recognized as a problem by the patient. There are two types of otologic problems that will produce decompensated tinnitus. The first is tinnitus of low acoustic intensity accompanied by some type of psychosomatic stress. The second is tinnitus of actually high acoustic intensity as measured by comparative methods in a tinnitus analysis study. It is the patient with decompensated tinnitus who is really the subject of our discussions. He is the one who comes for help primarily because of the tinnitus. His other otologic symptoms are frequently subdued and minimized in the history. The tinnitus itself looms as the chief complaint and is the subjective symptom requiring specific otologic management.

As in other medical problems, but especially true in subjective phenomena, a double diagnosis must always be considered: (*a*) the actual organic etiologic otologic lesion, and (*b*) the psychosomatic status of the patient. The latter must take into consideration both the emotional threshold of the patient and specific anxiety states and phobias. This double diagnostic attack is distinctly the responsibility of the otologist and cannot be shifted to another physician.

The fallacy that tinnitus is a specific otologic disease has been strength-

ened and amplified by the numerous papers relating to treatment of tinnitus
in which the therapy, be it surgical or medical, is directed to the general
subject of tinnitus as a pathologic entity. The clinical retention of such a
concept will do nothing to advance our knowledge in this field but will deter
and retard scientific investigations and logical evaluation of therapeutic
techniques. Almost any otologic disease can be accompanied by tinnitus
It is necessary to evaluate the position of tinnitus as a component of that
specific disease.

It may be interesting to review briefly some typical organic otologic lesions which may cause tinnitus:

1. *Middle Ear.*
   Membrana tympani—perforation, adhesive fibrosis, flaccidity
   Fluid collections—hemotympanum, serous effusion, purulent exudate
   　mucoid exudate
   Muscular—spasms, tics
   Vascular—anomalies, anemia, polycythemia
   Ossicular—joint disturbances, fixation (otosclerosis)
   Tumors—glomus jugulare, hemangioma, carcinoma
   Cholesteatomas—several types

2. *Inner Ear.*
   Bony labyrinth—Paget's disease, otosclerosis, fragilitas ossium
   Perilymph diseases—inflammatory, chemical, edema
   Endolymphatic diseases—hydrops, collapse
   Organ of Corti—peripheral neuritis, atrophy, edema, allergy
   Cochlear ganglion—ganglionitis, allergy, atrophy
   Eighth nerve—tumors, inflammation, vascular anomalies

3. *Central Auditory Pathway.*
   Second order neurons—
   Third order neurons—
   Ventral and dorsal cochlear nuclei—　}　Tumors, vascular and
   Lateral lemniscus tract—　　　　　　circulatory anomalies,
   Medial geniculate body—　　　　　　focal inflammatory
   Auditory cortex—　　　　　　　　　lesions

### The Significance of Tinnitus in the Differential Diagnosis of Otologic Disea

In that vast unknown called "nerve deafness," which comprises man
diseases occurring in the intricate neural pathway from the endolymphat
labyrinth to and including the auditory cortex, we have few localizing o
portunities in differential diagnosis. The threshold audiogram, recruitme
tests, speech audiometry, and correlated vestibular studies have given
some insight into "nerve deafness." Tinnitus is an important symptom
lesions of the neural auditory pathway. The identification, accumulatio
and classification of discrete characteristics of tinnitus in these cases, wh
correlated with other otologic data and later with pathologic findings, m
shed much light on the differential diagnosis of "nerve deafness." Rece
studies have shown that much nerve deafness originates not only in t
organ of Corti and in the cochlear ganglion, but in the nuclei, ascendi
pathways, and possibly in the thalamus and cortex. Present audiomet

techniques do not suffice in the segregation of anatomic locations in patients with nerve deafness. It is conceivable that correlation of audiometric data with tinnitus analysis data may yield such localizing information.

## Methodical Analysis of Tinnitus

A methodical analysis of tinnitus should be an integral part of the otologic examination, particularly in clinical research. The following method of analysis is suggested as a somewhat orderly technique in an attempt to obtain useful data.

**Subjective statement of patient.** The patient is requested to describe his tinnitus in his own words to the best of his ability without any specific questions.

**Subjective analysis.** The patient is then questioned for the following specific data:

*The general location of the tinnitus.* Is the tinnitus *within* the patient or does it seem to be somewhere in the room? Occasionally the patients will insist that the tinnitus is not in the head, not in the ear, but to the right or to the left of the head and apparently projected several inches or feet away.

*The somatic location of the tinnitus.* Is it in one or both ears and if so, superficially or deeply; or is it in the head, and if so in what part of the head?

*The specificity in regard to loudness.* If the somatic location is somewhat diffuse and variable, the patient is asked to relate the specificity in regard to loudness. If the tinnitus is stated to be in the head and ear, the predominant intensity is elicited.

*Time relations of tinnitus.* Is the tinnitus louder during certain times of the day? Is it louder at work or at home? Is it louder at certain times of the week? In women, does it vary with menses?

*Positional relations of tinnitus.* Does the tinnitus vary with positions of the head or body? Does it increase on stooping? Is it relieved by any specific position of the body or head?

*Characteristics of the tinnitus—acoustic analysis.* If the tinnitus is a pure tone, it may be identified on the audiometer. For these purposes, the ordinary fixed-frequency audiometer is inadequate. The sweep-frequency audiometer is necessary to accomplish such specific tone localization. By this same technique, the intensity and the masking intensity required to mask the tinnitus can be determined.

If the tone is complex, an attempt is made at audiometric analysis, in terms of dominant and accessory tones. Admittedly, in most patients this is a difficult if not impossible task, but in musically articulate patients it can frequently be accomplished.

*Tinnitus identification test-recording.*[1] In all cases where tinnitus is com-

[1] A number of patients with varying otologic diagnoses, who had either sufficient musical or acoustic experience were able to give data useful for the construction of tinnitus identification recording. This recording was artificially created by sound technicians to mimic as closely as possible the acoustic components described by patients with tinnitus.

plex in nature, the patient is requested to listen to the tinnitus identification recording in an attempt to locate an acoustic component which might compare with his subjective phenomena. It is explained that although the pitch in the recording may be different from that of his tinnitus, we are interested in knowing whether the tone quality, combinations, or effect in any way resemble his subjective sensations. Many patients will respond to the tinnitus identification record by picking out two or three components and giving dominance to certain of these components. All psychological tests carry the burden of interpretive, emotional, and other variables. This tinnitus comparison or identification test is a subjective test and falls heir to these inadequacies, but so does the threshold audiogram, and the test for recruitment.

**Management of Tinnitus**

**Specific otologic therapy.** It is important at the present time to re-evaluate critically many of the therapeutic techniques previously suggested to avoid therapeutic nihilism as well as mythical tinnitus cures. The organic otologic disease focus in such a case must be approached with the idea of therapy directed specifically to eradication of the tinnitus. In most instances, such therapeutic techniques will also improve the hearing. There are situations however, when only a slight hearing improvement induced by a particular therapy may be accompanied by a major diminution of tinnitus intensity. It should be the tinnitus that receives the stress of our therapeutic attack rather than other considerations. For example, the annoying pulsating visceral tinnitus of a tympanic glomus jugulare will usually disappear following surgical removal, yet the hearing may be poorer.

*Palliative Measures.* Simple reassurance as to the reality of the tinnitus accompanied by encouragement and good prognosis will go far in helping alleviate the anxieties of the patient with decompensated tinnitus.

*Acoustic Sedation.* Acoustic sedation is very helpful in many cases of tinnitus, especially in regard to the difficulty in sleep, which is a great problem with many patients. The reason for greater difficulty at that time is, of course due to the removal of ambient masking noise in the quiet of the evening which allows greater cerebral irritability by the ever-present auditory paresthesia. The use of a bedside or pillow radio or phonograph speaker is very helpful in providing an artificial source of ambient noise to mask out the subjective tinnitus.

*Drug Sedation.* Drug sedation is an important palliative measure, not only for daytime use but especially for bedtime tinnitus irritability. In this light it is valuable to rotate the simple barbiturates, bromides, and other substitutes. No one drug should be used for any long period. It is helpful psychologically to disguise the vehicles and to alternate the medications so that habituation and recognition by the patient are decreased.

*Surface Psychotherapy.* In most instances where the decompensated tinnitus is due to high intensity acoustically with little or no psychosomatic component, no further measures are necessary. In instances where the de compensated tinnitus is accompanied by major psychologic stresses and strains, a certain degree of surface psychotherapy by the otologist is helpful. Such surface psychotherapy should include a thorough explanation as to the real nature of tinnitus with assurance that it is neither an hallucination nor an illusion. Any expressed phobias should be carefully denied. An optimistic prognosis regarding duration and severity is not only justifiable but very helpful psychologically. A brief inquiry into personal problems may uncover the existence of major psychologic problems. In some instances, deep psychologic therapy at the hands of a psychiatrist is indicated.

*Major Psychotherapy.* Deep psychotherapy in psychiatric hands is indicated in every case of organized, symbolic, verbal or musical tune tinnitus. It is also indicated where surface psychotherapy, as described above, has not solved the decompensated tinnitus problem. Where deep psychotherapy is necessary, adequate otologic supportive therapy should not be denied the patient while he is under psychiatric management.

## BIBLIOGRAPHY

BLAKE, C. J., 1892. Operation for removal of the stapes. Boston *Med. Surg. J.,* 127, 551–552.

BORDLEY, J. E., and HARDY, W. G. 1949. A study in objective audiometry with the use of a psychogalvanic response. *Ann. Otol., etc., St. Louis,* 58, 751–760.

FLETCHER, H. 1953. Speech and hearing in communication (2nd ed.). New York: Van Nostrand.

GOODHILL, V. 1939. Syphilis of the ear: a histopathologic study. *Ann. Otol., etc., St. Louis,* 48, 676.

—— 1950a. The management of tinnitus. *Laryngoscope,* 60, 442–450.

—— 1950b. Nuclear deafness and the nerve deaf child: the importance of the rh factor. *Trans. Amer. Acad. Ophthal. Otolaryng.,* July-August. 671–687.

—— 1950c. The nerve-deaf child: significance of rh, maternal rubella and other etiologic factors. *Ann. Otol., etc., St. Louis,* 59, 1123.

—— 1952a. The use of cortisone in otosclerosis. *Trans. Amer. Acad. Ophthal. Otolaryng.,* July-August. 635–646.

—— 1952b. A tinnitus identification test. *Ann. Otol., etc., St. Louis,* 61, 778.

—— 1952c. Management of tinnitus: 1952 instruction section, course No. 430. *Amer. Acad. Ophthal. Otolaryng.* Pamphlets.

—— 1955c. Surgical audiometry in stapedolysis (stapes mobilization). *A.M.A. Arch. Otolaryng.,* 62, 504–508.

—— 1956a. Present status of stapedolysis (stapes mobilization). *Laryngoscope,* 66, No. 4, 333–381.

—— 1956b. Instruments for transtympanic surgery, including transincudal stapedolysis (stapes mobilization). *Trans. Amer. Acad. Ophthol. Otolaryng.,* July–Aug.

——, REHMAN, I., and BROCKMAN, S. 1954. Objective skin resistance audiometry. *Ann. Otol., etc., St. Louis,* 63, 22.

GOODHILL, V., and HOLCOMB, A. 1955. Cochlear potentials in the evaluation of bone conduction. *Ann. Otol., etc., St. Louis,* 64, No. 4, 1213–1233.

—— 1955a. Trans-incudal stapedolysis for stapes mobilization in otosclerotic deafness (under audiometric control). *Laryngoscope,* 65, No. 8, 693–710.

———— 1955*b*.　Surgical audiometry in stapedolysis (stapes mobilization). *Arch Otolaryng. Chicago*, 62, 504–508.

GUILD, S. 1944. Histologic otosclerosis. *Ann. Otol., etc., St. Louis*, 53, 246–266

HOLMGREN, G. 1923. Some experiences in surgery of otosclerosis. *Acta oto laryngologica*, 5:460.

JACK, F. L. 1891–1892. Remarkable improvement in hearing by removal o stapes. *Trans., Amer. Otolog. Soc.*, 5, 284.

KESSEL, J. 1876. Über das ausschneiden des trommelfelles und mobilisieren de steigbügels. *Archiv für ohrenheilkunde.*, 11, 199.

LEMPERT, J. 1938. Improvement in hearing in cases of otosclerosis: a new on stage surgical technique. *Arch. Otol.*, 28, 42–97.

———— 1950. Modern temporal bone surgery: history of its evolution. *Laryngo scope*, 60, 740–778.

MIOT, C. 1890. De la mobilisation de l'etrier. *Revue de laryngologie, d'otologi et de rhinologie.*, 10, 49–83–113–145 & 200.

ROSEN, S. 1955. Mobilization of the stapes for otosclerotic deafness. *A.M.A Arch. Otolaryng., Chicago*, 61, 2–197–206.

SCHUKNECHT, H. F. 1955. Presbycusis. *Laryngoscope*, 65, 402–419.

SIEBENMANN, F. 1900. Traitement chirurgical de la sclérose otique. *Trans., Int Con. Med.* 170. *Ann. Otol., etc.*, 26, 467.

SOURDILLE, M. 1929. Nouvelles techniques chirurgicals pour le traitment de surdites de conduction ou otosclérosis: presentation de la soc. d'otologie de hospitaux de Paris 16 December 1929. Académie de medicine, Paris.

# CHAPTER 10

# CLINICAL AND EDUCATIONAL PROCEDURES FOR THE DEAF

## • S. Richard Silverman, Ph.D.

THE EVOLUTION OF Western man's attitudes toward the deaf is perhaps most significantly reflected by his creation of arrangements and systems for their education. The history of our culture is marked by man's slow, faltering, and at times haphazard, frustrating, and irrational struggle toward enlightenment; and the history of the education of the deaf is no exception to this general rule (Silverman, 1947a).

The notion that deafness and muteness depend upon a common abnormality and that the deaf were poor if not impossible educational risks persisted through medieval times. The Justinian Code (sixth century) classified the deaf and dumb as mentally incompetent, and the Rabbis of the Talmud classified the deaf with fools and children (second century B.C.). Cardano of Padua in the sixteenth century asserted that the deaf could be taught to comprehend written symbols or combinations of symbols by associating these with the object, or picture of the object, they were intended to represent. Dalgarno, in 1680, suggested the possibility of preschool education, and de L'Épée of France and Heinicke of Germany argued the merits of the language of signs and speech for the intellectual development of the deaf. Edward Miner Gallaudet brought the French (language of signs) system to the United States, and Alexander Graham Bell applied a science of speech to teaching the deaf. Itard in France, and later Urbantschitsch of Vienna and his student Goldstein of the United States, suggested the values and techniques in training every residuum of hearing. Universality of educational opportunity for deaf children of school age has now become a reality in our country. The deaf have, by and large, become economically and socially productive men and women. This is an absorbing story that has been set down in many contexts by many writers and need not be elaborated here (Best, 1943; Farrar, 1923; Hodgson, 1953; Silverman, 1947a). Rather we shall take up the story in terms of present-day concerns—definition, magnitude of the problem, and the bases of educational procedures—that are likely to determine and to shape our approach to deaf children in the future.

## DEFINITIONS

A great deal of unnecessary confusion among the laity and well-intentioned professional workers alike has surrounded the precise classification of hard-of-hearing and deaf children and unfortunately has frequently obfuscated discussions of their problems. The confusion seems to grow out of the differences in frameworks of reference to which classification and nomenclature are related. For example, some workers classify the child who develops speech and language prior to onset of deafness as "hard of hearing" even though he may not be able to hear pure tones or speech at any intensity. This child, it is argued, unlike the congenitally profoundly deaf child who has not acquired speech naturally, behaves as a hard-of-hearing child in that his speech is relatively natural or "normal" and, therefore, he should be classified as "hard of hearing." It is obvious that a not-too-precise educational standard has guided the labeling if not the definition of the child. If, however, we consider the same child from a purely physiological standpoint, it is grossly misleading to term him "hard of hearing" when for all practical purposes he hears nothing at all.

The situation is complicated further by the use of terms that suggest not only physiological communication and educational factors but also gradations of hearing loss and time of onset. To this category belong such terms as *deaf and dumb, mute, deaf-mute, semi-deaf, semi-mute, deafened, partially deaf,* and others. These terms are of relatively little value from either the physiological, communicative, or educational points of view, and it would be well to eliminate them from general usage (Silverman, 1947b).

For purposes of our chapter we need to define the deaf child in terms of his educational and psychological potential. For some, the significant dimension related to the definition would be the child's ability to talk. In England, for example, under the School Health Regulations children are described as (1) deaf, and (2) partially deaf. The former are those who have no "naturally" acquired speech when they are admitted to school, the latter are those who have begun to talk naturally (however imperfectly) before being admitted to school. According to this scheme children with defective hearing are classified in three grades:

Grade   I. Children who are found to have defects of hearing (which in most cases are amenable to medical treatment) but who do not need hearing aids or special educational treatment.

Grade  II. Children who have some naturally acquired ability to talk but need special educational treatment, on either a part-time or full time basis. Many of these children need hearing aids.

Grade III. Deaf children who are without naturally acquired speech when admitted to school. Many of these children are not totally deaf and can be helped by hearing aids, in learning to talk and to speak distinctly (Ewing and Ewing, 1954).

For others, the important dimension is the hearing loss expressed by the child's ability to respond to various environmental sounds, speech, and pur tones. Itard, in the early nineteenth century, classified children according to their responses—to bells, drums, and flutes, and Urbantschitsch some years later used a harmonica with a six-octave range ($E^{-1}$—$e^4$) and an intensity regulator for the same purpose. Both of these workers also used speech stimuli, and Urbantschitsch's classification is fairly representative of the categories that emerge from these approaches—(1) total deafness, (2) tone-hearing, (3) vowel-hearing, (4) word-hearing, and (5) sentence-hearing (Wedenberg, 1951). Huizing's classification (1953a) relates to the loss as expressed by pure tone audiometry. He suggests the following categories:

*Grade    I.* 0–30 db = slight loss.
*Grade   II.* 30–60 db = moderate loss (practical speech span).
*Grade  III.* 60–90 db = severe loss.
*Grade  IV.* More than 90 db = deaf (no speech-understanding ability).

We quote Huizing's rationale:

The principles underlying this scheme have a logical base. An impairment of less than 30 db means only a remote loss of the whispering world and of the warning element of weak ambient sounds. Under certain circumstances this may be of biological importance. As long as the threshold loss for the middle frequencies (500–2000 cps) does not pass the 30 db level, *grownups* encounter no trouble in daily life (Grade I). At the 35 to 40 db level, however, discommunication troubles arise in auditoria, group conversation, etc.

It is very important to realize that in the case of a *young child* the critical borderline of handicap should be put at a lower level, say at 25 db. This is explained by a lack of communication experience and language skill. . . . For this reason the 30 db level appears to be a useful average as the general borderline of a Grade I handicap. The 60 db level is a more or less critical borderline for the natural development of speech in very young acoustically handicapped children. This is explained by the fact that in life situations the most important part of the speech span is covered by range II. . . .

Finally the 90 db line fences off that part of the audibility area in which, notwithstanding the severe loss, speech understanding in most cases is still possible provided that a modern hearing aid is used.

In most cases with more than 90 db loss there is no speech understanding left, unless it is mainly based on speech reading. Recognition of individual speech sounds has become impossible, although the perception of rhythm, melody and occasionally of some vowels may still provide important clues for understanding.

It is of incidental interest here that Silverman and his co-workers (1948), in relating loss of hearing for speech to the judgment of fenestrated patients as to how they got along in auditory communication, found significant cutting points at losses of 30 db and 60 db. It is not out of order to suggest that comparisons of European and American pure-tone audiometric data should be made with caution, since Dadson and King (1952) found discrepancies in the reference zero to which the respective audiometers are calibrated.

O'Connor (1954) suggests that

The deaf . . . may be described as those who are unable to hear spoken language either with or without amplification, if their hearing loss is profound, or who hear spoken language only imperfectly with amplification if they have some useful residual hearing and are only moderately deaf rather than profoundly deaf. They are the children whose hearing impairment is greater than 60 db.

For the National Health Survey of 1935 and 1936, Beasley (1940) classified hearing loss according to the extent to which the individual with impaired hearing performed everyday listening tasks. His classification was based on the following five groups:

*1. Partial deafness stage 1:* The individual has difficulty in understanding speech in church, at the theatre or in group conversation, but can hear speech at close range without any artificial assistance.

*2. Partial deafness, stage 2:* The individual has difficulty hearing direct conversation at close range, but can hear satisfactorily over the telephone or can hear loudly spoken speech.

*3. Partial deafness, stage 3:* The individual has difficulty hearing over the telephone at ordinary intensities, but can hear amplified speech by means of hearing aids, trumpets or other means of amplification.

*4. Total deafness for speech:* The individual cannot hear speech under any circumstances, but acquired the hearing defect after learning to speak language by ordinary means.

*5. Deafmute:* The individual was born deaf or acquired severe deafness sufficiently early in life to prevent him from learning speech through the usual means.

Of course, the time of onset of deafness affects the psychological and educational developmental patterns and should be borne in mind in labeling and classifying.

The important points along the "time-of-onset" dimension for the profoundly deaf are the age from three to five years and the time when adulthood has been reached. The war-deafened may be placed in the latter category (Levine, 1953). Children who are deaf before the age of three are not likely to retain normal patterns of speech and language. Obviously, from age three to five years on, the later a child has lost his hearing the more apt he is to retain "natural" patterns of communication by speech.

In 1937 the Committee on Nomenclature of the Conference of Executives of American Schools for the Deaf appeared to have been mindful of the dimensions of ability to speak, ability to hear (in the use of the word *functional*), and time-of-onset in proposing the following classification and definitions:

1. THE DEAF: Those in whom the sense of hearing is nonfunctional for the ordinary purposes of life. This general group is made up of two distinct classes based entirely on the time of the loss of hearing.
   a. *The congenitally deaf:* Those who were born deaf.
   b. *The adventitiously deaf:* Those who were born with normal hearing but in whom the sense of hearing becomes nonfunctional later through illness or accident.
2. THE HARD OF HEARING: Those in whom the sense of hearing, although defective, is functional with or without a hearing aid.

Hardy (1952) objects vigorously to the restricting influence of the definitions and classifications of impaired hearing contained in the proposals of the Conference of Executives. He maintains that increasing fundamental clinical, and therapeutic audiological knowledge precludes "static categorization." For example, study of the thresholds of tolerance for speech and pure tones has suggested that there is a potentially useful portion of the auditory area even beyond the range of classical audiometry (Silverman, 1947c). Consequently, some individuals who have heretofore been termed *totally deaf* as a result of audiometric tests may be reached by auditory stimulation through properly designed amplification devices.

Barker and his associates (1953) suggest that perhaps it will be more fruitful to classify the person with physical disability on some psychological scale of behavior that may be more descriptive as to how he lives with his disability.

We are aware that delimiting definitions are hazardous and we recognize that each child's potential must be assessed individually by the best methods available to us so that we avoid being restricted by the tyranny of classification. Nevertheless, we need some orientation to the kind of child we are writing about and we suggest, therefore, that in this chapter we are concerned with the child who, when we first encounter him, has not developed the expressive and receptive skills of communication prior to the onset of deafness. He cannot initiate language through speech nor can he understand the speech of others as is done by a normally hearing child at an equivalent level of maturation. This may include the child who has acquired some of these skills of communication prior to the onset of deafness but who is at a level of competence in language that requires special technique to develop it. For convenience, we shall refer to him as the deaf child.

## MAGNITUDE OF THE PROBLEM

If we examine the results of mass testing surveys among school children (Watson and Tolan, 1949) we find a range of about 2 to 21 per cent reported as having defective hearing. This great variability in reports of hearing impairment is undoubtedly due to differences in definition of hearing impairment, in techniques, apparatus, and conditions of testing, and in socioeconomic status and location of communities in which the surveys were carried out. Our best estimate from available data (Silverman, 1947b) is that 5 per cent of school-age children have a hearing impairment of some kind, and that one to two out of every ten in this group require special educational attention. The others are likely to respond to medical care or their hearing loss is not apt to reach the handicapping stage (Hardy, 1952). How the bulk of these children are handled we shall discuss in the following chapter.

As we have described them, how many deaf children are there in the United States? It is difficult to state precisely because the enrollment in our schools for the deaf is likely to include children who are hard of hearing or aphasic and is not likely to include all the children of preschool age and deaf children who are in schools for the hearing or in other kinds of schools. Our guiding figure is their reported enrollment of 22,100 children in all schools for the deaf (Doctor, 1954)—a formidable number, even if the figure is not quite accurate.

## THE GOALS OF EDUCATION OF THE DEAF

How we go about educating deaf children is obviously related to the goals we have set for them, and these goals are in turn determined by what we consider to be the over-all potential of the deaf—educational, psychological and social. Or, otherwise said, some of the sharp differences of opinion concerning the most desirable arrangements and methods for the education of deaf children really have their roots in fundamental differences about the long-range outlook for them.

The overwhelming amount of literature on the subject (a bibliography would probably exceed two thousand titles) ranging from school papers and convention resolutions to lengthy sections of books (Best, 1943; Ewing and Ewing 1947a; Hodgson, 1953; McClure, 1953) reveals an intense polemicism resting in the main on a nonexperimental empirical foundation. Of course, there are many shades of opinion, but stated views and observed practices suggest what we may term three "schools of thought." We are aware that we may be indulging in caricature and that "it all depends on the individual child," but we believe that a sorting out of views is desirable if we are to understand the rationale for particular views on the education of deaf children.

One group appears to stress the limitations, especially social, of deafness. It points up such issues as the exclusion of the deaf from certain types of desirable employment, the effect on the deaf of insurance practices and legislation, the implication of what amounts to minority status in certain educational and social contexts, the impact of isolation from other deaf people, the difficult if not impossible task for some of learning speech and lip-reading, and the misunderstandings of the general public concerning the abilities and aspirations of the deaf (McClure, 1949). This group would "suit the method [of communication] to the child," and its view is best summarized by the following statements (Hardy, 1952):

> The aim of the education of the deaf child should be to make him a well integrated, happy deaf individual, and not a pale imitation of a hearing person. Let us aim to produce happy well-adjusted deaf *individuals*, each different from the other, each with his own personality. If a child cannot learn to read lips well or cannot speak well, far better develop other modes of expression and communication, writing and gesturing, than make him feel ashamed and frustrated because he cannot acquire the very difficult art of speech and lip reading. Our aim must be a well-balanced, happy *deaf* person and not an imitation of a hearing one.

A second point of view emphasizes the great possibilities of the deaf, as yet untapped, particularly for education and participation in a world of hearing people (Fiedler, 1952). This group is likely to stress the importance of early education (Ewing and Ewing, 1947a), the great potential of auditory training (Fry and Whetnall, 1954; Huizing, 1953b), and is apt to emphasize the objective of "normalization," ". . . deviating only insignificantly from persons with normal hearing" (Wedenberg, 1951). In essence, there is "one world" in which the deaf person must function and that is a world of hearing and speaking people. There is no separate world for the deaf.

A third school of thought points to the record of economic, academic, and social achievement of deaf persons *among the deaf and the hearing* as strong, tangible justification for its belief that forward-looking, proper, and early fundamental training enables the deaf child to realize his potentialities (Hirsch, 1951). Yet it is apparent, at least in our present state of knowledge, that there are situations in which the deaf may always be marginal and our approach to them should be influenced accordingly. Realism impels us to spare parents and the child himself the psychological distress that stems from failure of the child to achieve what was set up as an attainable goal of "normalcy."

In the exhaustive critical treatment of the experimental work on somato-psychological significance of impaired hearing, Barker, Wright, Myerson, and Gonick (1953) indicate that the findings are inconsistent and those that are well established give little insight into how impaired hearing affects behavior. They suggest that concepts found to be useful for the study of the effects of other physical impairment be the basis for the studies of impaired hearing. Myklebust (1953), too, stresses the need for the study of the nature of deafness itself and its effect on the behavior of the total organism and not merely as a cause of inability to communicate verbally.

At any rate, until more facts are available to fill the open spaces now occupied by opinion, a rational attitude seems to point to a recognition that deafness imposes certain limitations that must be accepted, while at the same time proper education in its broadest sense strives to couple the deaf person to the world about him in a psychologically satisfying way. We now turn to consideration of what we judge to be a "proper education." It is both convenient and logical to organize our discussion around the following topics:

1. Organization and Administration of the Education of the Deaf in the United States.
2. The Rise of the Preschool Movement.
3. The Skills of Communication.
   a. Speech
   b. Auditory Training
   c. Lip-Reading
   d. Language
4. Extra-School Agencies and Resources.

Because there is universal agreement among educators of the deaf that every deaf child shall be given an opportunity to communicate by speech, our attention shall be directed solely to this approach which is called oralism. As implied in our consideration of the three schools of thought, some educators may advocate supplementing, or, if indicated, supplanting oral instruction with other forms of communication. One of these is the manual alphabet which is a method of forming the letters from A to Z by certain fixed positions of the fingers of one hand. This is a form of "writing" in the air. The language of signs is another form of communication. This is a system of conventional gestures of the hands and arms that by and large are suggestive of the shape, form, or thought which they represent. The combined method, which attempts to make available speech communication, the manual alphabet, and the language of signs, depends upon the aptitude of the child and the context of the communication. For example, the language of signs and the manual alphabet are frequently employed in public assemblies. The combined method is usually employed in public residential schools (Gallaudet College, 1951).

## THE EDUCATION OF THE DEAF

Perhaps the most significant fact about the education of the deaf in the United States is that it is universally available to all deaf children of school age. Of course, the quality of education may vary, but it is important that no child need be denied an opportunity for it. Where are these opportunities available?

Of 22,100 children enrolled in schools for the deaf in the academic year 1953–54 (Doctor, 1954), 14,157 attended public residential schools for the deaf. These schools, open to qualified children without charge, are either directly or indirectly supported by state tax funds. Most of the public residential schools are supported by legislative appropriation and hence come under the control of state authorities. The educational services of the remaining schools are purchased by the states on a per diem or per capita basis and are controlled by their own boards. Examples of the first group are the Indiana and Illinois Schools for the Deaf; in the second group we find such schools as the Lexington (New York) and the Clarke (Massachusetts) Schools for the Deaf.

Other tax-supported institutions for the deaf are public day schools and classes. A day school is usually large enough to be a separate entity; for example, Horace Mann School, Roxbury, Mass. Day classes are usually groups within a larger school unit and there may be as few as one in a school and as many as ten; for example, La Crosse, Wis. In 1953–54, 1954 children were being educated in public day schools and 4046 were in public day classes. The remaining children, 1943, were being educated in denominational or private schools, such as Lutheran School (Detroit) and Central Institute for the Deaf (St. Louis). The latter schools may be either day and/or residential. The number of children in each class ranges generally from five to ten. Some deaf children have been absorbed into classes for the hearing. Deaf individuals attend high schools and colleges for the hearing. Most public residential schools provide education at the secondary level and higher education exclusively for the deaf is available at Gallaudet College, Washington, D. C.

The difference of opinion about the merits of residential and day schools for the deaf range from the view that residential schools are superior because of homogeneity of grouping, constant guidance by "experts" (Silverman and Lane, 1947), and the feeling of security that comes from associating with other deaf children at all times (McClure, 1953) to the view that day schools are more desirable because of opportunities for use of speech through association with hearing people and of "normal" home experiences. There is little convincing evidence to guide us in the approach to this problem. Templin (1950) found that children in a residential school for the deaf were no more restricted in reasoning ability than children with equal amounts of hearing loss who attended a day school. Burchard and Myklebust (1942) found that children in residence four years or more were more retarded in social maturity than those who had been in the school a shorter time.

Until we have more evidence to support one or another point of view, we are obligated to study each child's situation thoroughly in order to determine what educational placement is likely to be most fruitful for him. This points up the crucial need for early diagnosis and sophisticated consideration of the child's potential for developing the skills of communication which in turn may effect his psychological and social growth. In addition to information about a child's hearing, among the significant aspects to be considered are age of onset, etiology, physical development, behavioral development, social maturity, home environment and parental insight (Hardy, Pauls, and Bordley, 1951).

## The Rise of the Preschool Movement

The encouraging progress in the assessment of hearing of young children has contributed to the increasing awareness of the value of preschool programs for deaf children. It is well known that the period from birth to the age of six is particularly critical for the learning and over-all development of children—hearing or deaf. Since the young deaf child is denied many of the normal experiences that further satisfactory socialization, it appears to be all the more essential that he be given guided opportunities for optimum development as early in life as possible. This means not just a sensible program for developing skills of communication which in a great measure contribute to socialization, but a regime that provides opportunities for removal of the barrier which in a sense isolates the deaf child from the world about him—the world of his home, his parents, his sisters and brothers, and other children. Formal and informal intercommunications (by whatever means) tend to attenuate the feeling of apartness of the child and hence should make him feel wanted and significant.

The child is thus motivated to communicate and it is the task of the parent and the teacher to demonstrate the usefulness of speech as a tool of com-

munication. What is of great importance is "that these situations do no
happen often enough by themselves; they must be anticipated and contrivec
frequently and deliberately" by all those who are in close contact with hin
(Ewing and Ewing, 1947a).

Although it is not generally mandatory for tax supported schools to provide preschool classes for deaf children, we note that in practice the need i
beginning to be recognized. In the academic year 1953–54, of 22,100 children enrolled in public residential schools for the deaf in the United States
593 were under the age of six; and of 6000 children in public day schools
and classes 729 were of preschool age. Incidentally, of the 1943 children ix
denominational and private schools, 577 were under the age of six. The pro
portions reflect the initiative of private groups in promoting programs fo
preschool deaf children. It is of more than passing interest to those who nee
to be convinced of the value of early training that Lane's (1942) long-rang
study showed greater post-elementary educational achievement for childre
who entered school before the age of five than for those who entered at th
regular school age.

It is not inappropriate in discussing the young deaf child to call attentio
to the mounting swell of activity to inform and guide parents of deaf children
Although here and there an effort may be misguided, the proliferation of par
ent institutes and clinics, correspondence courses, reading lists and literar
output (Ewing and Ewing, 1947b; Illinois, 1949; Lassman, 1951; Montague
1953; Myklebust, 1950) is one of the most constructive and forward-lookin
developments in the education of the deaf. One parent put it succinctly
". . . the tough thing about deafness is likely to be social isolation, socia
adjustment. There is no one in the world, and there never can be anyone, a
important in determining any child's social adjustment as that child's ow
parents and his own family at home. For that reason parents are important
(French, 1946).

Most of these commendable efforts in orientation and guidance have bee
directed at parents of preschool-age children. This is understandable, sinc
the initial shock of the discovery of deafness must be intelligently cushione
and crucial and immediate decisions must be made about the child's future
Even though we are here discussing preschool age children, it is pertinent t
emphasize that the placement of a child in a satisfactory educational situa
tion in no way decreases the need for guidance of parents. This was force
fully driven home to the writer in a survey made of the parents of preser
and former pupils at Central Institute for the Deaf. Parents of teen-agers an
young adults wanted an opportunity to share information and experience
about such problems as choices of occupation, marriage with the deaf c
hearing, the genetics of deafness, and choice of companions for the deaf. I
short, social adjustment is just as much a problem for the deaf youth as it
for the preschool child, and it is essential that parent institutes and clinics t
fostered about these problems too.

## he Skills of Communication

That the development of the skills of speech, of understanding of speech lip-reading and "hearing") and of language are interrelated is obvious. For onvenience of our discussion, however, and without slighting the interrela- on, we shall consider the following topics: speech, auditory training, lip- eading, and language.

**Speech.** Studies of the speech of deaf children have by and large dealt /ith differences between the speech of of the deaf and of normal hearing ubjects. By a technique of kymographic recordings, Hudgins (1934) found ie following abnormalities in the speech of the deaf: (*a*) slow and labored peech usually accompanied by high chest pressure with the expenditure of xcessive amounts of breath; (*b*) prolonged vowels with consequent distor- on; (*c*) abnormalities of rhythm; (*d*) excessive nasality of both vowels and onsonants; and (*e*) malfunction of consonants with the consequent addition f superfluous syllables between abutting pairs. Rawlings' (1935, 1936) re- ilts were similar to those of Hudgins. He found that normal speakers use pproximately the same amount of breath while speaking in a conversational ne as they use in quiet breathing over a similar period, while the deaf use great deal more breath while speaking. Voelker (1935) found that 80 per ent of deaf children had less average pitch changes than normal speakers. he maximum phonation duration for deaf children was more than four mes that of normal speakers and they took much longer to say a sentence.

Carr's (1953) study of the spontaneous speech sounds of five-year-old eaf-born children suggests that deaf children should not be taught vowel nd consonant sounds in the manner and order popular with many teachers f the deaf (Joiner, 1946; Yale, 1938). Neither do her data support "wholly ie notion that deaf school children can master vowel and consonant sounds the order in which hearing infants master these sounds." Carr's data agree ith those of Sykes (1940) that show a predominance of front consonants the spontaneous vocalizations of young deaf children. Kampik (1930) in iterviewing parents found that deaf children babble as hearing children do nd that their speech organs are as well developed as those of the hearing.

We gain a substantial insight into the speech of the deaf from the investi- ation of Hudgins and Numbers (1942), who departed from the usual ap- roach of comparing the speech of the deaf and of the hearing and studied ie relation between errors of articulation and rhythm and intelligibility of e speech of deaf school children. They used a technique of recording and ibsequent analysis by a group of auditors of ten sentences spoken by deaf hildren. They found two general types of errors: errors of articulation, in- olving both consonants and vowels, and errors of rhythm.

Consonant errors were classified into seven general types as follows: (*a*) iilure to distinguish between voice and breath consonants; (*b*) consonant ibstitutions; (*c*) excessive nasality; (*d*) malarticulation of compound consonants; (*e*) malarticulation of abutting consonants; (*f*) nonfunctioning o arresting consonants; and (*g*) nonfunctioning of releasing consonants.

The vowel errors were (*a*) vowel substitution; (*b*) malarticulation of diph thongs; (*c*) diphthongization of vowels; (*d*) neutralization of vowels; anc (*e*) nasalization of vowels. The rhythm of the speech samples were eithe correct, abnormal, or nonrhythmic.

In general, our experimental and empirical evidence indicates that the deaf child lacking an adequate auditory monitor is likely to develop, at leas by the way he has been taught till now, a breathy, nasalized vocal quality abnormal temporal patterns, and some surprisingly consistent errors o articulation. This judgment does not imply that deaf children cannot be taught to speak intelligibly—many do. It merely stimulates us to conside the areas that are the bases for developing speech in deaf children which we may study profitably to improve that speech. Silverman (1954) has delineatee these areas.

*Fundamental Attitude.* As we have indicated previously, all educators o the deaf endorse the proposition that all deaf children shall have an oppor tunity to learn to speak. But the implementation of this notion in everyda practice reveals fundamental differences in attitude.

For some, speech is a subject to be taught like a foreign language to those who can "benefit" from it. Practice and atmosphere are not aimed at vitaliz ing speech for the child. Rather, speech is viewed as an eminently desirabl but not essential skill to cultivate. For others, a corollary to the propositio of universality of opportunity to learn speech is inescapable; and that i that speech is a basic means of communication and hence is a vital mecha nism of adjustment to the communicating world about us. Therefore, w must so set the stage for the child *everywhere*—in the home, on the play ground, in the school room—from the moment we learn he is deaf, tha speech eventually becomes meaningful, significant, and purposeful for hir at all times. Parents, counselors, teachers, and all who are responsible fo the child's development need to share this attitude. Only practice stemmin from this attitude will realize the deaf child's maximum potential for com munication by speech. Actually, the Ewings (1954) suggest that the absenc of this kind of "living speech environment" may account for some of the so called oral failures in schools for the deaf.

*The Multisensory Approach.* Obviously the teacher must use optimall the sensory channels available for teaching speech to a deaf child. Of signif cance are the visual, the auditory, the tactile, and the kinesthetic, as well a the popular approaches associated with them.

When we consider the use to which we put the visual system in teachin speech we tend primarily to think of lip-reading as the child learns to watc with purpose the movements of the lips (and the expressions of the face) c those about him and to imitate, however imperfectly, these movements i attempts to express himself. This really is the initial technique with dea infants. In addition to lip-reading, well-known uses of vision include system of orthography, color codes (New, 1942) that differentiate the manner of production of phonetic elements, models and diagrams that show position and movement of the mechanisms of speech, acoustic translators of various sorts that display speech patterns visually and can carry information to the eye about time, frequency, and intensity. The latter range from pitch indicators (Ewing and Ewing, 1954; Sterne, 1939) to the elaborate and complex visible-speech apparatus designed and developed at the Bell Telephone Laboratories (Potter, Green, and Kopp, 1947).

We know that the literature even of the nineteenth century (Urbantschitsch, 1897) mentions the desirability of using the auditory system to aid in teaching speech to the deaf. But today we are better able to exploit this possibility because of the development of modern wearable, and of group, hearing aids designed to deliver speech to the auditory area useful to the child. We are aware that for the kind of child whom we are here discussing the auditory area is greatly restricted, but even limited perception of stress patterns can be helpful in achieving better rhythmic and voice quality and understanding of the talker.

The tactile or vibratory sense is most commonly used by stimulating the child's fingertips or hands in contact with his own or the teacher's face or head during speech or during phonation (Alcorn, K., 1938; Alcorn, S. K., 1941). Some techniques use sounding boards, including pianos, and diaphragms which are caused to vibrate by speech and music (St. Michiels-Gestel, 1940). Wedenberg (1951) suggests that Barczi (1934), even though he spoke words into the ear, selected them for their tactile value. Becking (1953) has demonstrated surprisingly good differential sensitivity to sound of the thoracic region of severely deaf children, although the sensitivity curves of human skin to mechanical vibration are not quite in agreement (Sherrick, 1953). Sherrick's is one of many promising investigations in vibrotactile sensitivity being carried on in the Department of Psychology at the University of Virginia. Wiener (1950) has suggested that the transfer to the sense of touch of the principle used in the visible-speech machine is possible. It was felt that the visible-speech instrument gave a measure of the amount of information which it was necessary to transmit for the intelligibility of speech. Rather than vision, the sense of touch was to be used. It is too early to assess the results of this approach.

The kinesthetic sense is used in "getting the feel" of certain articulatory and vocal movements and in tongue and lip exercises. Some teachers employ rhythmic gross-muscle movements to reinforce kinesthetically utterances consisting of connected speech and of suitable nonsense syllables.

Among the sources of variation in commonly used techniques to teach speech to the deaf are the differences of opinion concerning the relative emphasis to be placed on specific sensory pathways. The controversy ranges from the concept of mutual reinforcement by deliberately using the senses together—a co-ordinated sensory input—to the notion that speech will be better learned if stimulation by one sense is purposely excluded in order to achieve optimum performance by another sense. Hudgins (1953a) has shown that however small a fragment of hearing a child may have, it may be trained to supplement vision in visual-auditory presentation. In other words, the eye and the ear together perceive speech better than either one alone and hence the bisensory approach is likely to produce better speech. Sumby and Pollack (1954) showed how, among people untrained in lip-reading, visual perception was important for individuals listening in high-level noise. The desirability of reinforcing vision is indirectly suggested by the results of Myklebust and Brutten (1953) who found that the deaf child has more difficulty interpreting visual experience than does the hearing child. Incidentally this finding questions a commonly held view that the deaf have relatively superior visual perception because they must depend primarily on vision to make contact with the world and after all practice makes perfect. Huizing (1953b) argues that at least in the early stages lip-reading should be excluded from auditory training because it (lip-reading) is likely to divert the child from optimum use of his hearing. And S. K. Alcorn (1941) suggested shutting the eyes of the child during development of sensitivity to vibrations.

In developing techniques, it is desirable for the teacher to analyze the speech skill she is trying to cultivate and to select the combination of sensory channels best suited to stimulate the child. For example, the perception of the phonetic element *p* is best accomplished through vision reinforced by feeling, and vowel differentiation is greatly aided by a combination of auditory-visual and tactile stimulation. Watson (1951) has adequately epitomized what appears to be the forward-looking view that the sum of reinforced multisensory stimulation is greater than any of its parts. It is, in fact, "the nearest approach to the normal that can be made by the deaf child."

*Systems of Orthography.* Students of speech are aware of what amounts to irrationality of the choice and use of our symbols to stand for discrete units of speech. The shape and size of the letters of our alphabet bear no logical or consistent relation to the sounds they are intended to represent. Furthermore, most of our symbols represent more than one sound and most of our sounds are represented by more than one symbol. This situation has stimulated teachers of the deaf, among others, to devise or to adopt a system of orthography that would carry more information about speech units than the unrelated letters of the alphabet.

The Bells (1894) created their system of visible speech wherein four fundamental consonant curves related to the articulators—the back of the tongue, the top of the tongue, the point of the tongue, and the lips; and appropriate modification of the basic vowel symbol indicated the production of the vowels. For example, for the consonants ɑ = k, Ω = sh, and ʊ = t, ɒ = p.

The Northampton charts (Yale, 1938), popular with many teachers of the deaf, are arranged to give more phonetic significance to letters of the alphabet through their voice, breath, and nasal columns, and through their similarity-of-production rows for consonants and suitable categorizing columns and rows for vowels. The multiplicity of symbols representing the same ound is handled by a system of appropriately arranged secondary spellings under the primary symbol which presumably occurs most frequently in English usage. Thus *a–e* is the primary symbol for the diphthong in *cake,* the dash representing a consonant. A secondary spelling under *a–e* is *ay* as in *ay.*

The diacritical system used in our dictionaries is based on the concept of familiarity with the pronunciation of frequently used key words. Where one letter may represent more than one sound a differentiating symbol is used; thus *e* as in *be* is *ē,* and *e* as in *bed* is *ĕ.* Phoneticians and linguists generally use the International Phonetic Alphabet which has a single agreed-upon symbol for each sound and supplements the existing alphabet to fill out needed representation. Zaliouk (1954) has devised a "visual-tactile system of phonetic symbolization" which he suggests for teaching speech to the deaf. This utilizes two categories of symbols, static and dynamic. The static symbols represent the different organs—hard palate, tongue, teeth and lips—participating in the formation of the adequate articulatory positions. The dynamic symbols for finger and hand indicate movement.

There have been other attempts too numerous to mention that have sought through shorthand or other means to convey phonetic information through a logical and consistent system of symbolization. The search for these systems underlines the need it expresses. An ideal system of orthography would (*a*) convey information on how to articulate, (*b*) use symbols of the language, (*c*) be within the grasp of children, (*d*) be free of ambiguities. It is obvious that these criteria are in conflict and some compromises need to be made. For example, if we are looking for symbols that convey information on how to articulate we would probably choose the system of Bell or Zaliouk. The Northampton charts, with secondary spellings included, would probably be representative of the most frequently occurring symbols and symbol combinations in the English language, and hence would be likely to contribute to pronunciation. On the other hand, because there are so many secondary spellings and exceptions, the learned symbols may be confusing out of chart contexts. The diacritical markings are obviously useful, but everyday English symbolization does not carry the differentiating symbols. This is in essence one of the drawbacks of the International Phonetic Alphabet. Some teachers prefer to start children with the Northampton charts and then to teach the diacritical marks when children reach the appropriate academic level. These comments are by no means exhaustive but they may be useful as a guide in the choice of a system of phonetic symbolization.

*Units of Speech.* The various approaches to teaching articulation to the deaf may properly be placed on a continuum ranging from an elemental, analytical method to a patterned or "natural" approach. The former would emphasize the development of individual elements out of speech contexts and the latter would begin with words and phrases "as is natural for hearing children to do." The elementalists argue that in the absence of an appropriate auditory monitor, the kinesthesia of each phonetic element must be fixed before precise articulation can be achieved, lest fluency be attained at the expense of good articulation. The "naturalists" contend that we must take advantage of the spontaneous articulations, temporal patterns, and voice qualities of young children. These are not generally isolated elements and precision can be achieved within the framework of the natural spontaneous vocal output without sacrificing fluency.

The emphasis in present-day practice lies somewhere between the extremes of this continuum on the syllable as the basic unit. Stetson (1951) has shown that the syllable is the simplest possible utterance in a monosyllabic breath group. Individual "sounds" cannot be discussed without involving their function in a syllable. Stetson maintained that "when teachers and demonstrators give what they think are 'separate sounds' they are actually uttering syllables; the vowels and on occasion the liquids and nasals constitute separate syllables, as in 'oh, a, rr......, ll ......;' long drawn out fricatives, sss . . . etc. become vowel substitutes, the other consonants are given with a brief vowel as in 'buh puh' . . ." Of course, individual sounds may be corrected but they should not be considered complete until they are articulated properly in the kinds of syllables in which they are likely to occur. Furthermore, speech rhythm which contributes to intelligibility is primarily a matter of grouping, accentuating, and phrasing syllables (Hudgins and Numbers, F. C., 1942; Numbers, M., 1942). The use of the babbled syllable (Avondino, 1924) and the building of connected rhythmic speech from syllabic units feature popular approaches in the development of speech (Haycock, 1942).

It is not out of order here to mention our apparent failure to capitalize in later speech development on the spontaneous utterances of the very young child. Irwin (1947) has studied carefully the development of sounds in young hearing children and he has shown that by the tenth month practically all of the different sounds have appeared. Yet it is curious that even though a child may have produced *l* and *r* during his infantile babbling, he frequently cannot at the age of two or three produce these sounds correctly in English words (Jakobson, 1941). Apparently he finds it difficult to use the phonetic elements of his babbling as the phonemes of his language. This relearning comes about by perceptive development, both auditory and kinesthetic, and in the case of the deaf child by whatever sensory potential is available and in a relatively flexible and adaptive sequence.

*Evaluation of Speech.* Silverman (1943) has stressed the necessity for frequent critical evaluation of the speech *intelligibility* of deaf children, both as a guide to modifying existing approaches and, in the light of the controversy over how the deaf shall be taught, as a dispassionate assessment of the value of the oral method. Attempts to accomplish this may fall into two related categories, the first dealing with the periodic evaluation during the school career of the deaf child, in which he is exposed to formal training in speech, and the second carrying out long-range procedure designed to discover how effectively speech functions in post-school life.

Evaluative techniques used periodically to measure progress in speech ntelligibility have not yet attained the degree of objectivity and validity chieved by measuring instruments in the subject-matter and skill fields. Among the more popular techniques is the procedure in which a child reads selection and auditors indicate the extent to which the selection has been understood. Or carefully selected word samples (Hudgins, 1953) are read nd scored by the auditors. Although this evaluation technique may yield limited but fairly reasonable appraisal of the child's speech mechanics, it loes not simulate the pattern of usual oral intercourse which takes place vithout benefit of printed or written visual crutch. What is being evaluated s a form of *oral reading* and not speech in terms of broad social objectives. The translation of the child's *own* thoughts into intelligible speech is an ability neglected by this type of evaluation.

The use of memorized material without the aid of a visual crutch is subject to similar criticism, since the thoughts expressed usually do not originate n the child, and if they do, the process of memorization furnishes the child n advantage which does not operate in a normal speech situation. The interview approach to evaluation, in which the child is stimulated to talk freely, may approximate true appraisal of speech if it is conducted skillfully but, very often in this situation, anticipation of answers to questions may operate to the child's advantage and the technique fails to appraise the child's ability to take the initiative in speech. The use of speech recordings as a periodic evaluative technique has considerable value. However, the limitations of read or memorized selections or the question-and-answer type of sample should be kept in mind. Of course, it would be fruitful to capture for study the casual conversation of children.

The outcomes of speech-teaching which are most important in the long un are those that reveal the extent to which the child's training in speech unctions adequately when he has left school. Unfortunately, we are without satisfactory evidence in this area and the information that comes to us is frequently biased and invariably anecdotal. Here is a task to which zealous oralists may profitably apply their energies.

Our discussion of teaching speech to the deaf suggests the following guides to practice:

1. An environment must be created or maintained for the child in which speech is experienced as a vitally significant and successful means of communication. Oralism is as much an atmosphere and an attitude as it is a "method" of teaching.

2. Spontaneity of speech should be encouraged, but at the appropriate stage in a child's development formal instruction is necessary. Good speech in deaf children is not generated spontaneously. The Ewings (1954) say "The plain truth is that a deaf child cannot ever achieve the highest standard of intelligible speech that is possible in his case without such help [formal instruction individually or in small groups]."

3. The proper combination of the visual, auditory, tactile, and kinestheti pathways should be exploited rationally and vigorously.

4. The syllable is a suitable unit for the development of articulation an of desirable temporal patterns in speech. Through its use, adequate cc ordination of parts of the speech mechanism is more likely to be achievec

5. A functional system of orthography is essential.

6. Judicious correction of poor articulation, including individual pho netic elements, and of undesirable rhythm and voice quality is necessary i reinforcement of poor speech by acceptance is to be avoided. The teache in a sense, is the monitor of the child's speech and she needs to let hin know how he can improve it.

7. Periodic and long-range evaluation of the social effectiveness of th speech of the deaf, even though it may not meet rigid scientific requirements is useful for diagnosis and for educational planning.

**Auditory training.** The systematic use of residual hearing potential t improve communication of persons with impaired hearing has come to b labeled *auditory training.* We have seen previously how, as early as the be ginning of the nineteenth century, it was recognized that "very deaf" chil dren may have hearing which if stimulated or "trained" could serve a usefu communication purpose. The evolution of this movement has been discussec elsewhere (De Weerd, 1951; Goldstein, 1939; Silverman, 1949; Weden berg, 1951), but it is interesting to observe that awareness of the possibilit of auditory training was spotty and spasmodic during the nineteenth century perhaps because of wide use of the manual methods of instruction. The grea advance in electro-acoustic instrumentation of the past three decades, how ever, both for testing of hearing and for amplifying sound, brought about a revival of interest from many fields—otology, physics, engineering, psy chology, education—in auditory (sometimes in the past referred to a "acoustic" or "auricular") training that has been sustained and substantial

In discussing hearing "potential," particularly for profoundly deaf chil dren, we need to keep in mind the area available for hearing which we refe to as the auditory area. Silverman (1947c) has likened the auditory area t a building with the foundation represented by the threshold of sensitivity, th in-between stories corresponding to levels of equal loudness, and the roo represented by limits of tolerance. In attempting to determine the maximun desirable acoustic output of hearing aids, he "mapped out" the upper in tensity limits of human hearing. If it could be demonstrated that the limit of tolerance were higher than previously supposed, instruments could b designed with a higher level of maximum undistorted acoustic output anc thereby the auditory range of usefulness could be improved materially.

In Fig. 1 (Davis, 1947) with its accompanying explanation we see th auditory map for the normal hearing bounded at its upper portion by th three successive thresholds of tolerance as described by Silverman. In Fig. 2 (Davis, 1947) we see the auditory area severely reduced in size because a major portion of it is rendered useless by deafness. In the kind of childre

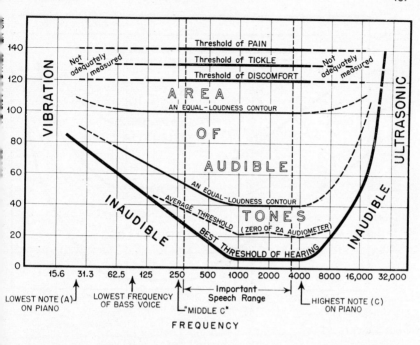

G. 1. The area of audible tones is bounded below and to the right and left by the threshold
 hearing. Below this curve tones are inaudible. The *average* threshold of hearing (zero hearing
ss on the 2A audiometer) lies considerably above the *best* threshold. To the left, at high
tensities, the auditory area is not clearly bounded as hearing merges into the sense of
bration. Above, the area is bounded practically by the successive thresholds of discomfort,
:kle, and pain. These thresholds have been carefully studied only over the middle range of
equencies, and the broken portions of the curves are quite uncertain. Above the threshold of
ain sounds are still audible and very loud, but auditory fatigue (and/or injury) becomes
ore and more rapid. The scale of sound pressures refers to pressures measured in the ear under
e receiver of an audiometer or hearing aid. (The points on the *average* threshold curve at 4096
d 8192 cycles per second represent measurements just under the receiver, while the
est thresholds were measured at the eardrum. The difference is important at high frequencies
d accounts for the lack of parallelism of the two curves at and above 4096 cycles per second.)
(After Davis, 1947.)

e are dealing with in this chapter, the area available for hearing is much
:ss than in Fig. 2. Therefore, our task is to "package" sound into the area
etween the elevated threshold of sensitivity (also greatly restricted in fre-
uency) and the threshold of discomfort. The sound must be intense enough
› be perceived in some form and not so intense that the child "can't take it."
he surprisingly high level-of-tolerance threshold reached experimentally
1ggests that in terms of the concept of the auditory area the "hearing" po-
:ntial is substantial, and it is likely that very few children are "totally" deaf.
1struments directed toward taking advantage of these possibilities have
een designed and are generally available commercially. In order to achieve
1e maximum operating range without exceeding desirable limits, they use
1e principle of compression amplification which is equivalent to an in-
antaneous automatic volume control (Silverman and Harrison, 1951).

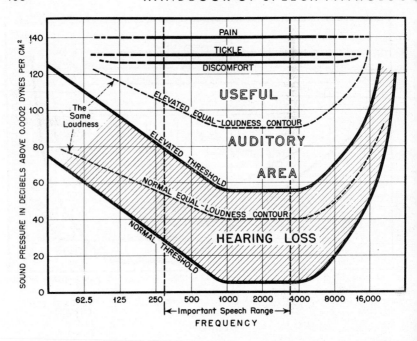

**FIG. 2.** Reduced auditory area in pure conductive hearing loss. This diagram represents hearing loss of 50 decibels at all frequencies, a so-called "flat" loss, produced by a purely conductive lesion. The case is theoretical, as such a severe conductive hearing loss is rarely perfectly flat and there is usually some high-tone nerve deafness associated with it. The equal-loudness contours are raised without distortion. The threshold of discomfort is almost up to the threshold of tickle. Nothing sounds very loud. The high equal-loudness contours have been elevated above the thresholds of tickle and pain. (After Davis, 1947.)

We must remind ourselves that in this chapter we are concerned with deaf children as we described them at the outset. They may be in the Grade IV of Huizing (1953a), the "deaf mute" group of Beasley (1940), or the "third group" of Hudgins (1954) with losses above 80 or 90 db. In other words, these are the children whose auditory area is about as restricted as it can be (sometimes as little as 10 db in the frequencies below 1000 cps with still some residuum of sensitivity. Through this limited sensitivity, however, the central nervous system may get sufficient information and contribute to the attainment of the objectives listed below.

The objectives of auditory training that are potentially attainable for this group are:

1. *Improvement in speech perception.* These children are not likely to achieve any appreciable level of auditory discrimination for speech, at least to the point where they can understand connected language through hearing alone. However, they can be led to appreciation of temporal patterns of speech and to improved control of the intensity and in some instances of the pitch of the voice. Refined appreciation of phrasing and stress patterns may be expected to improve the child's ability to attain the "rhythmic grouping"

which Hudgins and Numbers (1942) consider contributes greatly to the intelligibility of the speech of the deaf. Speech perception is improved through auditory training (Ewing and Ewing, 1938; Hudgins, 1953a; Johnson, 1939), particularly when it is combined with lip-reading. Failure to note improvement in communication by speech after a regime of auditory training may be attributed to the fact that the training was not begun early enough, actually in the first year of life (Wedenberg, 1951; Whetnall, 1952).

2. *Improvement in language skills.* Although there is no definitive experimental evidence to indicate that auditory training improves language skills, it seems likely that information carried by stressing and phrasing, not too discernible by lip-reading, adds to the meaning and significance of connected language. Vocabulary, particularly with auditory associations, may be enriched. For example, if a child reads that "the baby *cried,*" the word *cried,* which has auditory connotations, has limited meaning for him even though he is able to draw a line between it and the word *baby* in his workbook and he has seen a picture of a baby crying. On the other hand, a recording of the cry of a baby played over an amplifying system, though not perceived precisely, should enrich the meaning of the word *cry.*

3. *Improvement in psychological coupling to the hearing world.* Again, convincing experimental evidence is lacking. Nevertheless, consider the deaf child at a ball game. A thrilling play is made on the diamond that evokes a spontaneous outburst of yelling from the crowd. The child sees the hands clap and wave, the spectators rise from their seats, the mouths open, but he has not caught the emotional impact of the moment because its basic richness lies in yelling of the crowd and the accompanying noises—an auditory appeal. If the child could perceive just the presence of these noises, however distorted, through a hearing aid he would be a richer sharer in the group experience (Silverman, 1949). Perhaps "hearing" on this primitive level, as Ramsdell (1947) has pointed out, can relieve the feeling of isolation from the outside world that may characterize deaf people. Not to be overlooked are the esthetic appreciations which may result from auditory exposure to the rhythm of music. Many deaf children who have been trained to appreciate rhythmic cadences seem to enjoy dancing and eurythmics.

Although it is likely that the future will reveal additional and greater values resulting from auditory training, our statements of objectives-within-reach suggest that we must be cautious of extravagant claims adduced to the use of hearing aids by deaf children, particularly the notion that if equipped with a hearing aid even from infancy they do not need special education.

With these objectives in mind, we turn now to a consideration of the basis for practices in auditory training for the deaf child. It is important to realize that the child must form the *habit* of listening. Even the very young child under two should be talked and sung to close up to his ear and he should be encouraged to look at and to listen to sound-producing objects, be it the rattling of a paper bag or the noise of the wind-up toy. Actually, this is the first stage. As the child matures, he needs to develop an awareness for sound and a realization that it can have meaning. Therefore, it is essential that the child be surrounded by sounds that are intense enough to be "sensed." Then as Carhart (1947) has suggested, the other stages in auditory training are (a) the development of gross discriminations, (b) the development of broad discriminations among simple speech patterns, (c) the development of finer discrimination for speech.

Gross discriminations can be developed by using objects that produce unique and loud sounds. The child first associates the object with the sound and then is called upon to indicate which object, activated out of his sight, produced the sound. Whistles, drums, horns, bells, cymbals, and chimes are typical of the sound-makers found to be useful with this technique. The same techniques may be applied to identifying dissimilar musical sounds played either live on a piano or produced from recordings. Furthermore, discrimination may arise from association with common sound-generating activities and experience, such as clapping, crying, coughing, and running water. Sounds increasingly alike are used to refine the child's skills of discrimination.

The development of broad discrimination among simple patterns is merely a special application of the techniques used to develop gross discriminations. Dissimilar phonetic elements are contrasted, the child gives them back, and eventually he is exposed to words and phrases with varying rhythms. Here the child is likely to develop an appreciation for the regime of auditory training because it is related to speech expression and reception.

It is not likely that the deaf child can develop finer discriminations for speech like f as in fin and th as in thin. Of course, these should be tried, but in all stages of auditory training the teacher must be aware that the child's performance is eventually limited by his restricted auditory area and she should not spend what may be discouraging periods for both her and her pupil in trying to attain the impossible. This is implied in what are representative expositions of details of technique (Ewing and Ewing, 1954; Goldstein, 1939; Lexington School, Streng, et al., 1955).

*Hearing Aids and Auditory Training.* Electronic hearing aids for use with deaf children may be one of many varieties of three basic types—group, desk, or wearable. A group hearing aid consists of one or more microphones, amplifiers, and as many as ten pairs of over-the-ear earphones. Frequently a turntable is included for playing recorded speech, music, and sound effects. The advantage of this type of instrument appears to be in its greater power output and in a more desirable frequency response than the wearable aid and the possibility of minimizing acoustic feedback by keeping the microphone at a reasonable distance from the earphone. The improvements in wearable hearing aids, however, are increasingly reducing the areas of difference. Engineering details of the basic design and arrangement of group hearing aids have been described, among others, by Bangs and Shapley (1953), by Hudgins (1953b), by Silverman and Harrison (1951), and by

Wedenberg (1951). The latter has followed the principle of inserting appropriate filters "to compensate the lack of balance between the high and low portions of the speech frequency spectrum which accompanies auditory impairment. Thus the formant areas of higher frequencies valuable . . . to perceptibility may be 'raised' to a level at which they are audible along with the lower speech spectrum areas." This principle may be useful for children from whom we can expect to achieve refined auditory discrimination. Whether this type of frequency response or that suggested by Davis (*et al.,* 1947) and the Medical Research Council of Great Britain (1947) applies to hearing aids for deaf children remains to be investigated. Perhaps the energy should be concentrated in the auditory area which has marked limitations in the frequency range.

Desk-model hearing aids consist of microphone, amplifier, and usually a single pair of earphones, although it is possible to have multiple outlets. They are frequently recommended for individual instruction and have about the same advantages as group hearing aids over wearable instruments.

Wearable hearing aids are the familiar small instruments with microphone, amplifier, and power supply in one case—sometimes as small as a compact—and a small earphone (or, very infrequently, a bone-conduction unit behind the ear) coupled to a plastic eartip inserted in the external auditory canal. The major advantage for the child is that he can have it with him at all times and benefit continuously from stimulation. Frequently, children are first taught to appreciate sound over group instruments and then use the wearable instrument outside the classroom.

There are a number of problems concerning features of group hearing aids for deaf children about which there is little experimental information. The desirability of compression amplification is generally recognized but how restricted the dynamic intensity range of the compressed signal should be is another matter. For the deaf child who cannot make fine discriminations, the information contained in intensity changes in speech is important.

We also need more information about the value of binaural hearing aids for deaf children. We are not here referring to pseudo-binaural hearing aids that use one microphone, one amplifier, and two earphones, which according to Hirsh (1950) are no better than a monaural system even for localization of sound. Hirsh has suggested that a true binaural hearing aid would be possible if both ears are aided by systems that are fed from microphones that are mounted on the two ears. The advantage for a deaf child, in addition to his not too primary need for localization of sound sources, is yet to be determined.

Other features of group hearing aids that are proving useful in practice are insert-type earphones to increase comfort and to reduce acoustic feedback, ceiling-mounted microphones to increase freedom of action for the teacher, acoustically treated rooms to reduce reverberation and distortion, visual aids to reflect intensity or pitch changes, and outlet boxes at blackboards.

There is a great difference of opinion, again without much supporting evidence, as to when a child is "ready" to wear a hearing aid. One point of view holds that the early years are the years in which the child learns the meaning of sounds, particularly speech, and hence he should wear a hearing aid at all times from the moment it is discovered that he is deaf (Whetnall, 1952). On the other hand, some workers believe that the child must first be trained to some degree of awareness and discrimination of sound, since little value from the instrument will discourage its use (Carhart, 1947). Furthermore, some young children may fear the loud sound of an instrument and may be conditioned against it (Ewing and Ewing, 1954). The evidence from the relations of hearing loss to noise exposure (American Standards Association, 1954) suggest the possibility of damage to an ear exposed to the level of sound pressures generated by a hearing aid. Of course, some would "trade" the training in hearing for some damage. But it is difficult to determine the exact amount of hearing loss in infants. The cause of lack of response to sound may be other than hearing impairment, and it would be risky to damage an intact end organ.

Despite the unsolved problems that are still with us, experience indicates that there is no longer any question about the usefulness of the auditory system in the education of deaf children. Out of this experience grow the following guides for practice in auditory training:

1. There is an approachable and potentially useful portion of the auditory area beyond the range of usual audiometry. Consequently, many children who have been termed "totally deaf" as a result of audiometric tests may be reached by auditory stimulation through properly designed apparatus. Formal training is essential.

2. Auditory training tends to be more effective through mutual reinforcement when combined with the use of other sensory systems. There are, of course, times when hearing alone is used in order to assess a child's progress. Audiograms are not always indicative of a child's potential for appreciating speech.

3. The techniques should be geared to a child's auditory potential. This requires frequent assessment of his hearing.

4. Auditory training, with or without a hearing aid, should be begun as soon as it is determined that a child is deaf.

5. Formal techniques are directed at creating an acceptance for hearing aids through differential auditory experiences that are meaningful, through the development of gross discrimination of various environmental sounds and, within the limits of the child's hearing, through the development of discrimination for speech.

6. Informally, wherever practical, the child should have the benefit of amplified sound in all of his classroom work (either by group or wearable hearing aid), at home and at play.

7. Children should be taught as early as possible the management and care of instruments.

**Lip-reading.** Lip-reading, sometimes called speech-reading because it involves observing more than the lips, is the process through which an individual, regardless of the state of his hearing, understands speech by carefully watching the speaker (Silverman, 1948). It was not until the middle of the seventeenth century that John Bulwer, an English physician, in his *Philocopus* and the *Deafe and Dumbe Man's Friend* suggested the possibility of lip-reading as a satisfactory way for the deaf to understand spoken language. However, it may be that the rise of manual methods of instruction in the latter part of the eighteenth century and in the early part of the nineteenth century retarded the development of lip-reading despite efforts of German educators like Heinicke to popularize it. The latter half of the nineteenth century saw an increasing acceptance of oralism and with it an enthusiastic interest in lip-reading.

This writer (1948) has crystallized the latter-day evolution of lip-reading.

Since speech reading (or lip reading) appeared to have value for deaf children, it was inevitable that it should be taught to the deaf child and to the adult whose hearing was so impaired that communication by auditory means was impossible or severely limited. Teachers in schools for the deaf began to instruct adults and in 1902 Martha Bruhn established in Boston a school of speech reading for adults based on the system of Julius Müller-Walle, formerly a teacher in the school for the deaf in Hamburg, Germany. Miss Bruhn emphasized the importance of differentiating the movements of speech through syllable drills as they appeared to the speech reader. Immediately after Edward B. Nitchie founded his school of speech reading in which he stressed the importance of psychological factors in speech reading, primarily the ability to synthesize meaning from contextual clues. Emil Froeschels in Vienna also stressed the need for ability to get meaning of speech movements which were either hidden or ambiguous, teaching first only those with the help of a special phonetical alphabet. In 1917 the Kinzie sisters, Cora, Elsie, and Rose, founded a school in which they attempted to combine the best features of the Müller-Walle and Nitchie systems and they also introduced the idea of speech reading material graded to various levels of difficulty. Later Jacob Reighard of the University of Michigan translated the principles of Brauckmann's Jena method into English and advocated their adoption in America. The Jena method seeks to associate movements of speech with the process of speech reading. . . .

In recent years the emphasis has been on associating lip-reading instruction with hearing (Pauls, 1947; Ewing and Ewing, 1944), with kinesthesia, and with motion pictures that provide opportunities for learning and practice (Mason, 1946; Morkovin and Moore, 1949). Lip-reading has come to be accepted as an essential tool of communication for deaf and hard-of-hearing children and adults.

Children with normal hearing learn oral language primarily over the auditory system reinforced by other sensory experience. Frequent repetition leads to a functional hearing and spoken language that later incorporates the association with the symbols that stand for language—the reading process. The deaf child is denied the possibility of the primary auditory language association and is forced primarily to make visual language associations. The extent to which he is able to do this may depend upon a number of factors some of which are exceedingly complex and difficult to analyze. Significant among these are (*a*) factors concerning the speaker—distance, light, position, the character of the talker's speech which may be influenced by precision and rate of articulation, sectionalisms, and facial expressiveness, and, of course, the familiarity of the lip-reader with the speaker; (*b*) factors concerning the language material—the level of vocabulary and language structure; and (*c*) factors concerning the lip reader—his vision, his ability to synthesize from contextual clues, his intelligence, his general information, his ability to recognize discrete units of speech, his ability to associate his own "feel" for speech with the speech he sees on the lips, and finally the fundamental structure of his personality which may determine his attitude toward lip-reading.

Lip-reading is further complicated by the ambiguities that result from hidden movements, such as *h* and *k,* from homophenous words (words that look alike on the lips, *smell* and *spell*) and from the difficulty of appreciating patterns of stress, intonation, and phrasing.

Numerous attempts have been made to assess the role of these factors in the lip-reading process with a view to diagnosis of difficulties, to evaluation of progress and of methods of instruction, and to prediction of performance. With deaf children in advanced grades in schools for the deaf, Pintner (1929) found no correlation between intelligence and lip-reading. Heider and Heider (1940*a*) also worked with deaf children and found no correlation between lip-reading of nonsense syllables and general lip-reading ability, but they found significant correlations between lip-reading ability and ability to follow a rhythm in dancing and ability to recognize vowels. Utley (1946) and later Reid (1947) reported that the lip-reading ability of deaf and hard-of-hearing children could not be predicted from reading level, school achievement, chronological age, age of onset of deafness, grade placement, or length of training. Incidentally, the Utley test has been criticized by both G. M. Heider (1947) and by Di Carlo and Kataja (1951) on the grounds that there are many nonfunctional items and that the test may be sufficiently difficult to demoralize subjects. G. M. Heider felt it has greater possibilities for adults who are superior lip-readers than for deaf children. With the hard of hearing, attempts have been made to relate personality (Nitchie, 1917) and skill in synthesis (Kitson, 1915) to ability in lip-reading but the efforts to achieve the objectives of testing are limited by the adequacy of the tests themselves.

The test constructors are faced with formidable variables that are unique to the population to be tested. Among these are the degree and kind of hearing loss, the time of onset of impaired hearing, the language ability of the population, the standardization of test material, particularly of its presentation, and the difficulty of establishing norms for a hetergeneous population. And the validation appears to rely on teacher ratings which introduces a new set of problems.

Instruction in lip-reading for deaf children is usually not a thing apart. In the beginning, even before the child enters school, he is encouraged to watch the face of the talker. The deaf child is not as aware as the hearing child that he can get information (in its broadest sense) from the utterances of the speech mechanism. When formal instruction is begun the child is taught to associate movements of the lips with objects, feelings, and actions. The objective here is not merely the enlargement of lip-reading vocabulary but nurture of the idea that watching the face of the talker is useful. Finally, lip-reading pervades every act of speech perception of the child and it becomes an increasingly useful tool of communication as it is practiced in purposeful situations.

The frailty of our formal tools for assessment of lip-reading ability need not deter us from suggesting the following guides to practice in developing this valuable skill in deaf children.

1. As we said previously in our guide for teaching speech, an atmosphere of oral communication must be created and maintained. Lip-reading must be shown to serve a purpose.

2. Even if the child is not expected to understand every word of a spoken message, he should be talked to and he should be encouraged to take advantage of situational clues.

3. Lip-reading should be reinforced by other sensory clues whenever practical.

**Language.** In our discussion of the skills of communication to this point we have, in a sense, considered the development of the skills of talking and "listening"—speech, auditory training and lip-reading. We now turn to the message itself, the stuff of oral communication—language. Just as what Miller (1951) calls the "ear-to-voice link" is essential for talking and listening, it is the basis of a child's attachment of meaning—in speaking, in writing, in listening, in reading—to words and the combination of words. And, therefore, the absence of the ear can be catastrophic for the "natural" and complex development of association of language with experience.

It is the task of the teacher, nevertheless, to develop language in deaf children despite deprivation of their full use of the sensory channel considered essential for its growth. In the performance of this task she needs to be aware of the unique problems created by absent or severely distorted auditory verbal reinforcement of experience. Among the major problems are vocabulary, multiple meanings, verbalization of abstractions, and complexity of structure.

*a. Vocabulary.* It is difficult to determine when a child really "knows" a word. Is it in his spoken, written, reading, or listening vocabulary? This accounts for differences in the estimates of the functional vocabulary of children. At any rate, it is interesting that one representative study shows that hearing children "know" 272 words at the age of two, 1540 at four, and 2562 at six (Smith, 1926). Compare this with zero words that the deaf child is likely to know when he enters school, even at the age of three and more frequently at six.

*b. Multiple Meanings.* Single words in our language may have many meanings that are eventually clarified for hearing children by predominantly auditory usage denied the deaf child. Simmons (1945) found an average of almost four meanings per recurring word in twelve commonly used arithmetic textbooks. For example, the word *over* could mean *above* (the number "over" 5 is the quotient); *across* ("over" the Arctic Ocean); *again* (do your work "over"); *at an end* (the show is "over"); *more than* ("over" half the children); *besides* (left "over"); *during* ("over" a period of two years; *present* (turn meeting "over to"); *on the other side* (turn card "over"); *by means of* ("over" the radio).

*c. Verbalization of Abstractions.* Of course, hearing children and, for that matter, adults may experience difficulty in attaching words to abstract concepts, but the deaf child is in particular need of formal and informal but nonetheless deliberate instruction in the meaning of such relatively simple abstractions as *hope* and *want.*

*d. Complexity of Structure.* Smith has shown that by age five the spoken sentence has reached five words for the average child and about ten words for the superior child. This increase in length is inevitably accompanied by the usage of complex syntactical relations that clarify and enrich meaning. These involve such grammatical concepts as pronouns, connectives, tense, person, word order, and relations among clauses and among phrases of various sorts. If the hearing child reaches these levels of complexity at age five, we are again struck by the extent of the language gap between the deaf and the hearing. Heider and Heider (1940b), after their thorough comparison of sentence structure in the written compositions of deaf and hearing children, commented that the "whole picture indicates a simpler style [for the deaf] involving relatively rigid unrelated language units which follow each other with little overlapping structure or meaning."

In general, the deaf appear to be comparatively deficient in the flexible manipulation of our language to make optimum use of it as a tool of communication. This may be attributed to their educational retardation (although retardation may also be the cause) which has been variously estimated as ranging from two to five years (Pintner, 1918; Reamer, 1921; Schick, 1935); it may be due to the methods of teaching language (Fusfeld, 1954); or, in addition to these, to the idea that "the difference between the deaf and the hearing cannot be fully expressed in quantitative terms as the degree of retardation and that they represent differences not merely of skill in the use of language forms but in the whole thought structure" (Heider and Heider, 1940b).

*Methods of Instruction in Language.* Methods of instruction in language for the deaf can be conveniently divided into two major approaches—the natural method, sometimes known as the synthetic, informal, or mother method, and the grammatical method, sometimes referred to as the logical, systematic, formal, analytical, or artificial method (Nelson, 1949).

Historically, the grammatical method preceded the natural method (Far-

ar, 1923). It was based on the notion that after memorization of classifica-
ions of words and their conjugations and declensions, they could be used
is building blocks for connected language. This approach evolved into a
multiplicity of "systems" that were primarily created to provide for deaf
children a systematic set of visible symbols to guide them in the use of
language. These systems have been thoroughly reviewed by Nelson (1949).
We shall illustrate briefly the more popular ones.

1. *The Barry Five Slate System.* The assumption underlying this system,
developed by Katherine E. Barry (1899) at the Colorado School for the
Deaf, is that ability to analyze the relations among parts of sentences is
necessary to the "clear thinking" essential to an understanding of language.
Five slates or columns are visible on the walls of the schoolroom. The subject of a sentence goes into the first slate, the verb into the second, the object of the verb into the third, the preposition into the fourth and the object
of the preposition into the fifth. Children then learn the rationale of the
verbalization of their actions according to the visual aid afforded by the
slates. This system, it is believed, tends to stultify idiomatic expression and
actually may result in ungrammatical, stilted language.

2. *Wing's Symbols.* This system, devised in 1883 by George Wing of the
Minnesota School for the Deaf, is based on a set of symbols, mostly numbers
and letters, representing the functions of different parts of speech in a sentence. These symbols are placed over the word, phrase, or clause in order
to demonstrate the form, function, and position of the parts of a sentence,
rather than just to illustrate parts of speech. For example, *1* stands for the
noun, *2* for a possessive, and *0* for the object. Advocates of the system believe that it is of great value as a corrective tool throughout the child's career
and that it encourages correct grammatical usage (Minnesota School for the
Deaf, 1936).

3. *The Fitzgerald Key.* This system, first published in 1926, was developed by Edith Fitzgerald (1937), a congenitally deaf person, when she
was head teacher at the Virginia School. Miss Fitzgerald advocated developing "natural" language but felt that this could be aided by developing the
child's power of reasoning, judgment, and discrimination about language.
This is accomplished by a set of key words and symbols related to language
that was developed as it was needed by the children. There are six symbols,
one each for verbs, infinitive, present participles, connectives, pronouns,
and adjectives. For example, the symbol for a verb is ⹀. Among the advantages of the method, pointed out by Buell (1931), are its comprehensive-
ness, its flexibility, and the possibilities for self-correction.

The basic feature of the grammatical systems is the emphasis on getting
the child to *analyze* functional relations among discrete units of language
and, by repetition and visual aids, to impart to him an understanding of
language principles—groups of words whose arrangement affect the meaning of a sentence. Numerous guides for the sequential presentation of lan-

guage principles are available (Buell, 1954; Central Institute for the Deaf, 1950; Croker, Jones, and Pratt, 1939; Fitzgerald, 1937).

One of the early advocates of the natural method was D. Greenberger, who headed what is now the Lexington School for the Deaf in New York City. He felt that language was best learned by supplying it to children in the situations in which they had need for it. Practice was geared to actual and natural situations. A leading advocate of this approach is Miss Mildred Groht (1933), who suggests that prior to the time a language principle is to be introduced formally it should be used in natural situations through lip-reading and writing. It is then drilled on in various ways that are interesting and purposeful for the child. In essence, the teacher creates situations in which multiplicity of contact with language principles is stimulated. The method is claimed to be more consistent with the laws of learning of language by hearing children.

Until we gain more insight into how the deaf child conceptualizes, the teacher of language will need to use all the knowledge and ingenuity at her command to combine the best features of a grammatical method with the obvious excellent possibilities of the natural method. She will use such commonly accepted techniques as general conversation, composition, news items, trips, action work, topical essays, experience stories, letters, and descriptions of places, events, and persons, and their potential in developing language will be governed only by the extent to which she uses her own ingenuity, flexibility, and her knowledge of how children grow and develop. Perhaps she may find some help in the following guides to practice:

1. Language teaching should be related to significant and meaningful experiences of children.

2. Language should constantly be made to serve a purpose for the child.

3. All sensory channels should be used to teach language.

4. Teachers need to be alert to ideas that are developing in children so that they may furnish the language to express them.

5. Children need many varied contacts with the same language in order to make it theirs.

6. Many children need formal, systematic aids to acquisition of language. Many shun language when they feel insecure in its use.

7. Schools and homes should create an atmosphere where language is used and where books are read regularly.

In general, curricula, textbooks, and other teaching materials of schools for the deaf tend to follow those used in schools for the hearing, with appropriate adaptations for difficulties of verbal communication. There are also the usual provisions for instruction in art, physical education, and vocational subjects. Special textbooks for the deaf in reading and in content subjects have practically disappeared from the educational scene. The problem of the mentally deficient who are deaf or hard of hearing is difficult to solve. Its present management is far from satisfactory, according to Mac Pherson (1952).

## Extra-School Agencies and Resources

Elsewhere (1947*a*) the writer has said, "Society now understands that the deaf cannot only be educated but can also, with proper guidance and assistance, become economically and socially productive men and women." Their accomplishments in industry, in the arts, in certain professions, and in community activities attest to this (Gallaudet College, 1951*b*; Hirsch, 1951; Silent Worker, 1954). Responsible for the significant level of performance attained by the deaf, in addition to the schools themselves, are a number of agencies directly concerned with promoting opportunities for them. Among the more prominent agencies are the Convention of American Instructors of the Deaf and the Conference of Executives of American Schools for the Deaf, publishers of the *American Annals of the Deaf,* with headquarters at Gallaudet College, Washington, D. C.; the National Association for the Deaf, publishers of the *Silent World,* devoted to activities of the deaf, with editorial offices at 2495 Shattuck Avenue, Berkeley 4, Calif.; The National Fraternal Society of the Deaf, which operates an insurance company for deaf and arranges social activities, with headquarters at 433 Oak Park Avenue, Oak Park, Ill.; the Alexander Graham Bell Association for the Deaf, founded by Alexander Graham Bell and dedicated to the oral method of instruction. The Bell Association maintains an extensive library on the deaf, operates the Volta Bureau at 1537 Thirty-fifth Street N.W., Washington, D. C., which is a clearing house for information about the deaf, particularly for parents, and publishes the *Volta Review.*

The Office of Vocational Rehabilitation of the Department of Health, Education, and Welfare (formerly the Federal Security Agency) works closely with schools for the deaf and with various professional groups in broadening and upgrading opportunities for employment (Federal Security Agency, 1948, 1950). This writer cannot improve on a previous contribution of his as an appropriate conclusion to this chapter (1947*a*).

Although man has traveled a long tortuous road from the pre-Christian era in evolving an enlightened understanding of the social problems of deafness, a large portion of society still looks upon the deaf and hard of hearing as queer, dependent, and, sometimes, ridiculous. We are all familiar with the cheap humor of which they are often the target. Since their handicap is not as visible as that of the blind and the crippled, the deaf often find themselves in embarrassing and humiliating situations because others do not understand their special problems.

The answer of the deaf to such misunderstanding is to continue their social and economic achievements as self-respecting and productive individuals. Our social action for the deaf, therefore, should not aim for special privileges for them, but should constantly strive to provide opportunity without discrimination for the deaf to help themselves.

The achievements of the deaf in the United States since the founding of the first school for the deaf in Hartford in 1817 have been good, but the record can be improved. This is the conjoint task of the teacher, the parent, the scientist, the clinician, the social planner and, of course, the deaf person himself.

## BIBLIOGRAPHY

ALCORN, K. 1938. Speech developed through vibration. *Volta Rev.*, 40, 633–638

ALCORN, S. K. 1941. Development of speech by the tadoma method. *In* Report of the proceedings of the thirty-second meeting of the Convention of American Instructors of the Deaf. Washington: Government Printing Office Pp. 241–243.

American Standards Association. 1954. The relation of hearing loss to noise exposure. Report of Exploratory Subcommittee Z24–X–2 of the American Standards Association Z24 Committee on Acoustics, Vibration and Mechanical Shock. New York: Amer. Standards Assn.

AVONDINO, J. 1924. The babbling method: a system of syllable drills for natural development of speech. Washington: The Volta Bur.

BANGS, T. E., and SHAPLEY, J. L. 1953. Group auditory training unit for preschool children. *J. Speech Hearing Disorders,* 18, 366–372.

BARCZI, G. 1934. Bericht über die verhandlung des VI Kongresses der internationalen Gesellschaft für Logopädie und Phoniatrie, 153–160 *cited by* Wedenberg, E. 1951. Auditory training of deaf and hard-of-hearing children Stockholm: *Acta Otolaryngologica,* Supplementum 94, 1–129.

BARKER, R. G., WRIGHT, B. A., MYERSON, L., and GONICK, M. R. 1953. Adjustment to physical handicap and illness: a survey of the social psychology of physique and disability. Bull. 55. New York: Soc. Sci. Res. Council.

BARRY, K. E. 1899. The five slate system: a system of objective language teaching. Philadelphia: Sherman.

BEASLEY, W. C. 1940. The general problem of deafness in the population *Laryngoscope,* 50, 856–905.

BECKING, A. G. T. 1953. Perception of airborne sound in the thorax of deaf children. *In* Proceedings of the international course in paedo-audiology Groningen: Verenigde Drukkerijen Hoitsema N.V. Pp. 88–97.

BELL, A. M. 1894. Sounds and their relations. Washington: Volta Bur.

BEST, H. 1943. Deafness and the deaf in the United States. New York: Macmillan.

BUELL, E. M. 1931. A comparison of the Barry five slates system and the Fitzgerald key. *Volta Rev.,* 33, 5–19.

——— 1954. Outline of language for deaf children. Washington: Volta Bur

BURCHARD, E. M. L., and MYKLEBUST, H. R. 1942. A comparison of congenital and adventitious deafness with respect to its effect on intelligence, personality and social maturity. *Amer. Ann. Deaf* (Part 2), 87, 241–250.

CARHART, R. 1947. Auditory training. *In* Davis, H., Hearing and deafness. New York: Rinehart Books. Pp. 276–299.

CARR, J. 1953. An investigation of the spontaneous speech sounds of five-year old deaf-born children. *J. Speech Hearing Disorders,* 18, 22–29.

Central Institute for the Deaf. 1950. Language outline. *Amer. Ann. Deaf,* 95 353–378.

CROKER, G. W., JONES, M. K., and PRATT, M. E. 1939. Language stories and drills. Brattleboro: Vermont Pub.

DADSON, R. S., and KING, J. H. 1952. A determination of the normal threshold of hearing and its relation to the standardization of audiometers. *J. Laryngology Otology,* 66, 366–378.

DAVIS, H. 1947. Physics and psychology of hearing. *In* Davis, H., Hearing and deafness. New York: Rinehart Books. Pp. 23–49.

———, STEVENS, S. S., NICHOLS, R. H., HUDGINS, C. V. MARQUIS, R. J., PETERSON, G. E., and ROSS, D. A. 1947. Hearing Aids: an experimental study of design objectives. Cambridge: Harvard Univ. Press.

DE WEERD, M. J. 1951. The development of principles underlying auditory training. Unpublished Master's Thesis. Washington (St. Louis) Univ.

DI CARLO, L. M., and KATAJA, R. 1951. An analysis of the Utley lip reading test. *J. Speech Hearing Disorders,* 16, 226–240.

DOCTOR, P. V., editor. 1954. *Amer. Ann. Deaf,* 99, 2–219.

EWING, I. R. 1944. Lip reading and hearing aids. Manchester: Manchester (Eng.) Univ. Press.

―――― and EWING, A. W. G. 1938. The handicap of deafness. New York: Longmans.

―――― 1947a. Opportunity and the deaf child. London: Univ. London Press.

―――― 1947b. If your child is deaf. London: Deaf Children's Soc.

―――― 1954. Speech and the deaf child. Washington: Volta Bur.

FARRAR, A. 1923. Arnold on the education of the deaf (2nd ed.). Derby: Francis Carter.

Federal Security Agency: Office of Vocational Rehabilitation. 1948. Co-operative relations between public residential schools for the deaf and state rehabilitation agencies. Rehabilitation service series Number 68. Washington: Federal Security Agency: Office of Vocational Rehab.

―――― 1950. Rehabilitation of the deaf and hard of hearing. Washington: Federal Security Agency: Office of Vocational Rehab.

FIEDLER, M. F. 1952. Deaf children in a hearing world. New York: Ronald Press.

FITZGERALD, E. 1937. Straight language for the deaf: a system of instruction for deaf children (2nd ed.). Austin, Texas: Steck Co.

FRENCH, J. R. P. 1946. What can parents do? *Volta Rev.,* 48, 720–726.

FRY, D. B., and WHETNALL, E. 1954. The auditory approach in the training of deaf children. *Lancet,* March, 583–587.

FUSFELD, I. S. 1954. A cross-section evaluation of the academic program of schools for the deaf. Washington: Gallaudet College.

Gallaudet College. 1951a. The deaf child. Washington: Gallaudet College.

―――― 1951b. Diversification of employment for deaf college graduates. Washington: Gallaudet College.

GOLDSTEIN, M. A. 1939. The acoustic method for the training of the deaf and hard of hearing child. St. Louis: Laryngoscope Press.

GROHT, M. A. 1933. Language as taught in the Lexington school. *Amer. Ann. Deaf,* 78, 280–281.

HARDY, W. G. 1952. Children with impaired hearing. Children's Bureau publication number 326. Washington: Government Printing Office.

――――, PAULS, M. D., and BORDLEY, J. E. 1951. Modern concepts of rehabilitation of young children with severe hearing impairment. *Acta Otolaryngologica,* 40, 80–86.

HAYCOCK, G. S. 1942. The teaching of speech. Washington: Volta Bur.

HEIDER, G. M. 1947. The Utley lip reading test. *Volta Rev.,* 49, 457, 458, 488–489.

HEIDER, F. K., and HEIDER, G. M. 1940a. An experimental investigation of lip-reading. *In Psychol. Monogr.,* number 232, Studies in the psychology of the deaf., Columbus, Ohio: *Amer. Psychol. Assn.,* 104–123.

―――― 1940b. A comparison of sentence structure of deaf and hearing children. *In Psychol. Monogr.,* number 232, Studies in the psychology of the deaf, Columbus, Ohio: Amer. Psychol. Assn., Pp. 42–103.

HIRSH, I. J. 1950. Binaural hearing aids: a review of some experiments. *J. Speech Hearing Disorders,* 15, 114–123.

HIRSCH, J. G. 1951. Post-school adjustment of the deaf. Unpublished Master's Thesis. Washington (St. Louis) Univ.

HODGSON, K. W. 1953. The deaf and their problems. New York: Philosophica Library.

HUDGINS, C. V. 1934. A comparative study of the speech coordinations of dea and normal subjects. *J. genet. Psychol.*, 44, 1–48.

────── 1953a. The response of profoundly deaf children to auditory training *J. Speech Hearing Disorders*, 18, 273–288.

────── 1953b. Modern hearing aid equipment in schools for the deaf. *Volt Rev.*, 55, 185–186.

────── 1954. Auditory training: its possibilities and limitations. *Volta Rev.* 56, 339–349.

────── and NUMBERS, F. C. 1942. An investigation of the intelligibility of th speech of the deaf. *Genet. Psychol. Monogr.*, 25, 289–392.

HUIZING, H. 1953a. Assessment and evaluation of hearing anomalies in youn children. *In* Proceedings of the international course in paedo-audiology Groningen: Verenigde Drukkerijen Hoitsema N.V. Pp. 88–97.

────── 1953b. Paedo-audiology, its present status and future development. *I* Proceedings of the international course in paedo-audiology. Groningen Verenigde Drukkerijen Hoitsema N.V. Pp. 88–97.

Illinois Annual School for Mothers of Deaf Children. 1949. If you have a dea child. Urbana: Univ. Ill. Press.

IRWIN, O. C. 1947. Infant speech: consonantal sounds according to place o articulation. *J. Speech Hearing Disorders*, 12, 397–401.

JAKOBSON, R. 1941. Kindersprache, aphasie und allgemeine lautergesetze. Upp sala: Almquist & Wiksell. *Cited by* Miller, G. A. 1951. Language and com munication. New York: McGraw-Hill.

JOHNSON, E. H. 1939. Testing results of acoustic training. *Amer. Ann. Deaf*, 84 223–233.

JOINER, E. 1946. Graded lessons in speech. Danville: Kentucky School for th Deaf.

KAMPIK, A. 1930. Experimentelle untersuchungen über die praktische lei stungsfähigkeit der vibrationsempfindungen, Archives ges. Psychologie., 76 56–67. *Cited by* Sykes, J. L. 1940. A study of the spontaneous vocalization of young deaf children. *In Psychol. Monogr.* Number 232, 104–123.

LANE, H. S. 1942. Influence of nursery school education on school achievement *Volta Rev.*, 44, 677–680.

────── and SILVERMAN, S. R. 1947. Deaf children. *In* Davis, H., Hearing an deafness. New York: Rinehart. Pp. 367–391.

LASSMAN, G. 1951. Language for the preschool deaf child. New York: Grune & Stratton.

LEVINE, E. S. 1953. The deaf. *In* Garrett, J. F. Psychological aspects of physi cal disability. Rehabilitation service series number 210. Washington: Gov ernment Printing Office. Pp. 125–146.

Lexington School for the Deaf. The utilization of residual hearing. New York Lexington School for the Deaf (mimeographed).

McCLURE, W. J. 1949. Misleading information concerning the deaf. *Amer. Ann Deaf*, 94, 339–344.

────── 1953. The humane approach to the deaf. *In* Tennessee Observer. Knox ville: Tenn. School for the Deaf.

MACPHERSON, J. R. 1952. The status of the deaf and/or hard of hearing mentall deficient in the United States. *Amer. Ann. Deaf*, 97, 375–386, 448–469

MASON, M. K. 1946. Personal experience in teaching lip reading through motio pictures. *Volta Rev.*, 48, 661–663.

Medical Research Council. 1947. Hearing aids and audiometers. Special repor series number 261. London: His Majesty's Stationery Office.

MILLER, G. A. 1951. Language and communication. New York: McGraw-Hill.

Minnesota School for the Deaf. 1936. An exposition of the Wing's symbols in their relation to the teaching of language as used by the Minnesota School for the Deaf. Fairbault: Minn. School for the Deaf.

MONTAGUE, H. 1953. Parents of deaf children. *Amer. Ann. Deaf*, 98, 358–361.

MORKOVIN, B., and MOORE, L. 1949. Life situation speech reading through cooperation of the senses. Los Angeles: Univ. South. Calif.

MYKLEBUST, H. R. 1950. Your deaf child: a guide for parents. Springfield, Ill.: C. C. Thomas.

——— 1953. Towards a new understanding of the deaf child. *Amer. Ann. Deaf*, 98, 345–357.

——— and BRUTTEN, M. 1953. A study of the visual perception of deaf children. Stockholm: *Acta Otolaryngologica,* supplementum 105, 1–126.

NELSON, M. S. 1949. The evolutionary process of methods of teaching language to the deaf with a survey of the methods now employed. *Amer. Ann. Deaf*, 94, 230–294, 354–396, 491–499.

NEW, M. C. 1942. Color in speech teaching. *Volta Rev.,* 44, 133–138, 199–203.

NITCHIE, E. B. 1917. Tests for determining skill in lip reading. *Volta Rev.,* 19, 222–223.

NUMBERS, M. E. 1942. The place of elements teaching in speech. *Volta Rev.,* 44, 261–265.

O'CONNOR, C. D. 1954. Children with impaired hearing. *Health news,* New York State Depart. Health., 31, 4–16.

PAULS, M. D. 1947. Speech reading. *In* Davis, H., Hearing and deafness. New York: Rinehart. Pp. 257–275.

PINTNER, R. 1918. Measurement of language ability and language processes of deaf children. *Volta Rev.,* 20, 757–764.

——— 1929. Speech and speech reading tests for the deaf. *J. appl. Psychol.,* 13, 220–225.

POTTER, R. K., KOPP, G., and GREEN, H. 1947. Visible speech. New York: Van Nostrand.

RAMSDELL, D. A. 1947. The psychology of the hard of hearing and deafened adult. *In* Davis, H., Hearing and deafness. New York: Rinehart. Pp. 392–418.

RAWLINGS, C. G. 1935. A comparative study of the movements of the breathing muscles in speech and in quiet breathing of deaf and normal subjects. *Amer. Ann. Deaf,* 80, 147–156.

——— 1936. A comparative study of the breathing muscles in speech and in quiet breathing of deaf and normal subjects. *Amer. Ann. Deaf,* 81, 136–150.

REAMER, J. C. 1921. Mental and educational measurement of the deaf. *Psychol. Rev. Monogr.,* 29, number 3.

REID, G, 1947. A preliminary investigation in the testing of lip reading achievement. *J. Speech Disorders,* 12, 88–82.

Report of committee of inquiry into problems relating to children with defective hearing. 1938. London: Board of Education. Pp. 2–4 and 48–9. *Cited by* Ewing, I. R. and Ewing, A. W. G. 1954. Speech and the deaf child. Washington: Volta Bur.

St. Michiels-gestel Institute. 1949. Perception des vibrations comme bas de l'enseignement de la musique sensorielle et de l'enseignement chorégraphique. The Netherlands: À l'Institut des Sourds-muets de St. Michiels-gestel.

SCHICK, H. F. 1935. A five-year testing program to measure the educational achievement of the deaf child. Transactions of the eighteenth annual meeting of the society of progressive oral advocates. St. Louis: Laryngoscope Press.

SHERRICK, C. E. 1953. Variables affecting sensitivity of the human skin to me chanical vibration. *J. exp. Psychol.*, 45, 273–282.

Silent World. 1954. The status of the deaf in America yesterday, today, tomor row. Special Issue, Oct. 2495 Shattuck Ave., Berkeley 4, Calif.

SILVERMAN, S. R. 1943. The speech program of Central Institute for the Deaf *Volta Rev.*, 45, 12–15, 56.

———— 1947a. From Aristotle to Bell. *In* Davis, H., Hearing and deafness. New York: Rinehart. Pp. 341–351.

———— 1947b. Hard of hearing children. *In* Davis, H., Hearing and deafness New York: Rinehart. Pp. 352–366.

———— 1947c. Tolerance for pure tones in speech in normal and defective hear ing. *Ann. Otol., etc.*, St. Louis, 56, 658–678.

———— 1948. Educational therapy for the hard of hearing: speech reading. *In* Froeschels, E., Twentieth century speech and voice correction. New York Philosophical Library. Pp. 142–151.

———— 1949. The implications for schools for the deaf of recent research on hearing aids. *Amer. Ann. Deaf*, 94, 325–339.

———— 1954. Teaching speech to the deaf—the issues. *Volta Rev.*, 56, 385–389 417.

———— and HARRISON, C. E. 1951. The National Research Council group hear ing aid project. *Amer. Ann. Deaf*, 96, 420–431.

SILVERMAN, S. R., and LANE, H. S. 1947. Deaf children. *In* Davis, H., Hearing and deafness. New York: Rinehart.

SILVERMAN, S. R., THURLOW, W. R., WALSH, T. E., and DAVIS, H. 1948. Im provement in the social adequacy of hearing following the fenestration operation. *Laryngoscope*, 58, 607–631.

SIMMONS, A. A. 1945. Multiple meanings of words in arithmetic textbooks Unpublished Master's Thesis. Washington (St. Louis) Univ.

SMITH, M. E. 1926. An investigation of the development of the sentence and th extent of vocabulary of young children. Univ. Iowa Studies in Child Wel fare, 3, no. 5.

STERNE, T. A. 1939. The construction of a thyratron inflection indicator, it behavior with certain vowels, and its use in instructing deaf children. Un published Master's Thesis. Washington (St. Louis) Univ.

STETSON, R. H. 1951. Motor phonetics. Amsterdam: North-Holland Pub. Cc

STRENG, A., FITCH, W. J., HEDGECOCK, L. D. PHILLIPS, J. W., and CARRELL, J. A 1955. Hearing therapy for children. New York: Grune and Stratton.

SUMBY, W. H., and POLLACK, I. 1954. Visual contribution to speech intelligibilit in noise. *J. acoust. Soc. Amer.*, 26, 212–215.

SYKES, J. L. 1940. A study of the spontaneous vocalizations of young deaf chi dren. *Psychol. Monogr.*, No. 232, 104–123.

TEMPLIN, M. C. 1950. The development of reasoning in children with norma and defective hearing. Minneapolis: Univ. Minn. Press.

URBANTSCHITSCH, V. 1897. Des exercises acoustiques dans la surdi-mutité c dans la surdité acquise. (Translated by Egger, L.) Paris: A. Maloine.

UTLEY, J. 1946. A test of lip reading ability. *J. Speech Disorders*, 11, 109–11(

VOELKER, C. H. 1935. A preliminary strobophotoscopic study of the speech c the deaf. *Amer. Ann. Deaf*, 80, 243–259.

WATSON, L. A., and TOLAN, T. 1949. Hearing tests and hearing instrument Baltimore: Williams & Wilkins.

WATSON, T. J. 1951. Auditory training and the development of speech an language in children with defective hearing. *Acta Otolaryngologica*, 4( 95–103.

WEDENBERG, E. 1951. Auditory training of deaf and hard of hearing children. Stockholm: *Acta Otolaryngologica,* supplementum 94, 1–129.

WHETNALL, E. 1952. Deafness in children. *In* Diseases of the ear, nose and throat. London: Butterworth & Co., Ltd. Pp. 328–360.

WIENER, N. 1950. The human use of human beings. Boston: Houghton Mifflin.

YALE, C. A. 1938. Formation and development of elementary English sounds. Northampton, Mass.: Metcalf.

ZALIOUK, A. 1954. A visual-tactile system of phonetical symbolization. *J. Speech Hearing Disorders,* 19, 190–207.

# CHAPTER II

# CLINICAL AND EDUCATIONAL PROCEDURES FOR THE HARD OF HEARING

● *S. Richard Silverman, Ph.D.*

IN THIS CHAPTER we shall deal with children and adults with impaired hearing who have the ability or the potential for communicating by speech over the auditory system. We have seen in the previous chapter that precise classification is difficult and that the line of demarcation between what we have called the deaf and the hard of hearing is not entirely clear. Nor should it be, since individuals may differ greatly in the extent to which they are able to make use, for purposes of communication, of their residuum of hearing. Obviously, in addition to the amount of hearing loss itself, this may be influenced, among other things, by the age of onset and type of hearing loss, by intelligence, by training (particularly age at which it was begun), by acoustic environment, and by parental attitude and understanding of the significance of hearing impairment.

If we are guided by the dimension of hearing loss we are concerned with the person who falls in the category of *Grades I, II,* and the better hearing group of *Grade III* of Huizing (1953a), in the less than 60 db hearing-loss group of O'Connor (1954), and the three stages of "partial deafness" of Beasley (1940). (See the preceding chapter.)

Within the broad group of the hard of hearing there are, of course, gradations of social efficiency for communication by speech. These range from the mild loss of less than 30 db where there is little handicap, except perhaps for faint speech or for hearing at a distance, to the loss of about 60 db which, if it is congenital or of early onset, may require painstaking instruction in learning to hear, perhaps with a hearing aid, and in the understanding and use of language. The situation is complicated by the fact that hearing loss is not merely a loss of sensitivity that may be overcome by amplification, but may be a loss of ability to discriminate certain sounds that cannot be so overcome. This is true when there is marked reduction of sensitivity in the high frequencies. Furthermore, there are gradations in the quality and intelligibility of speech of the hard-of-hearing children that are related to hear

426

ing loss. These may range from inability of the lay observer to notice any deviation to inability to understand the speech.

There is not too much evidence about the relation of gradation of "adjustment" to hearing loss. Brunschwig (1936) and McCormick (1941) found correlations that indicated poorer adjustment as the amount of hearing loss increased. Springer (1938*a*, 1938*b*) found small and unreliable correlations between percentage of hearing loss and behavior ratings and neurotic score. Kirk (1938) found no significant difference in behavior-rating schedules between a group of children with an average hearing loss of 50 decibels and a group with an average loss of 72 decibels. Nor did Streng and Kirk (1938) find any significant difference in social competence between deaf and hard-of-hearing children. It is obvious that we are not now able to describe the individuals with whom we are concerned in this chapter on any scale of adjustment related to hearing loss.

On the other hand, hard-of-hearing and normal hearing persons have been compared on the basis of personality characteristics. Madden (1931), using a teacher-rating scale, found no difference in the two groups in attentiveness, obedience, and social attitude, but the hard-of-hearing group rated lower in aggressiveness and tended to be more shy. Habbe (1936) studied 48 adolescent hard-of-hearing and hearing boys with a variety of measures of personality including an analysis of autobiography and interviews of selected subjects. He found no significant differences among the groups, except that the hard of hearing tended to be more submissive and introverted. Pintner (1940) found the hard of hearing almost as well adjusted as the hearing child and he and his associates compared the groups for ascendance-submission, extroversion-introversion, and emotional stability. He found no great difference in ascendance-submission or in extroversion-introversion. There was a significant difference in emotional stability in favor of the hearing.

In studying hard-of-hearing adults, Welles (1932) and Pintner (1933) found the hard of hearing to be less stable emotionally, more introverted, less dominant, and equal in self-sufficiency. In their investigations, which included comparisons of urban and rural hard-of-hearing adults, they found no relation between neurotic tendency and age of loss of hearing, years of deafness, and hours of lip-reading instruction. Pintner stressed the value of educational measures because of the finding that those untrained in lip-reading had higher neurotic scores and the isolated group with less opportunity for training had more undesirable traits.

Ramsdell (1947) has described three psychological levels of hearing: (*a*) the primitive level at which we are aware that there is sound around us—the noises of the everyday world; (*b*) the signal or warning level at which we make use of certain types of auditory information—the ring of the telephone and the whistle of the traffic policemen; (*c*) the symbolic level at which we understand language. Ramsdell attributes the "depression" of the deaf to absence of hearing on the primitive level because it creates a sense of apartness from the world. Inability to hear at the warning level may cause a feeling of insecurity. Hearing at the symbolic level enables us to communicate experiences, to clarify and to organize our thoughts to achieve high-order knowledge, and in the growing child "to formalize and to bind those social prohibitions and permissions which make up the moral code."

Barker and his associates (1953) question the theoretical formulations of Ramsdell. They maintain that one would expect the totally deafened to be more frequently depressed than the hard of hearing, but this is contrary to some evidence; and Myerson (1948) found that in mild experimental conductive deafness the chief complaints related to difficulty in communication. Barker *et al.* mention the work of Dembo, Ladieu, and Wright (1948) who suggest that the loss of anything of value, a loved one, social status, or a physical function causes depression and suffering. Loss of hearing may be treated by the same psychological procedures and not as something, at least psychologically, that is in itself unique. We still do not have sufficient information to draw a composite picture of the structure of personality of the hard-of-hearing child or adult.

When we consider the subjects of this chapter from the point of view of intelligence we find, if nonlanguage tests are used (Pintner and Lev, 1939), that there is no real difference between the normal and hard-of-hearing child at the elementary school level. Waldman, Wade, and Aretz (1930) found, however, that for every five grade repetitions of good hearers there were nine grade repetitions of poor hearers. The lower grades seemed to be affected more than the higher grades, probably because of more oral instruction in the lower grades and greater dependence upon textbooks in the upper grades. Pintner, Eisenson, and Stanton (1941) also suggested some educational retardation of hard-of-hearing children.

It is of interest to us that educational retardation may be reduced by instruction in lip-reading (Caplin, 1937) and by the use of a good hearing aid (Gates and Kushner, 1946). Lane (1953) has suggested that "the loss in school achievement is extremely important in the attitude of the hard-of-hearing child toward school, toward his [normal] hearing companions, and toward the continuation of education beyond the legal age requirement. The future of the hard-of-hearing adult who had a hearing loss as a child is affected by the level and quality of his education."

For the purposes of this chapter, it is most convenient for us to describe the hard of hearing in terms of the extent to which their ability to understand speech and their ability to progress in school is affected by hearing loss. We shall assume that these hearing losses occurred prior to the development of speech and language. Of course, if speech and language have already been acquired, the deficiencies in these areas are absent or reduced depending on the age of onset of hearing impairment.

Our subjects are those who have a hearing loss (average at 500, 1000, 2000 cycles per second) of:

1. Less than 30 decibels: May have difficulty in hearing faint or distant speech, is likely to "get along" in school and have normal speech.
2. 30–45 decibels: Understands conversational speech at a distance of 3 to 5 feet without too much difficulty. May have some articulatory defects and have difficulty in school if talker's voice is faint or if face is not visible.
3. 45–60 decibels: Conversational speech needs to be loud to be understood and there is considerable difficulty in group and classroom discussion. Language, especially vocabulary, may begin to be limited and deviations of articulation and voice are noted.
4. 60–80 decibels: May hear voice about one foot from the ear, may identify environmental noises and may distinguish vowels but have difficulty with consonants. Voice may show signs of deviation, but speech and language need to be taught.
5. 80 plus decibels: May hear some loud sounds. Speech and language need to be developed through training.

In a study of adults who had had the fenestration operation (which indicated a predominance of conductive deafness) and who were asked to rate the social efficiency of their hearing, Silverman *et al.* (1948) found that social difficulty began at a loss of 30 decibels for speech, that threshold of "social adequacy" was a 45 decibel loss and that the limit of compensation by the human voice was at a level of 60 decibel loss for speech (without a hearing aid). Groups 4 and 5 above are, by and large, the subjects of the preceding chapter.

In an earlier chapter we discussed the prevalence of hearing impairment in the school population. For the entire population, the National Health Survey (Beasley, 1940) found that one in 78 males (the statistics are slightly less for females) has some impairment of hearing. The number of hard-of-hearing persons becomes less as the severity of the impairment increases, ranging from one in 152 for mild impairment to one in 2326 for individuals totally deaf for speech. And as age increases, the number of individuals in proportion to the population of the particular age bracket increases. The range is from one in 2041 under 5 years of age, through one in 34 in the 55–64 age group, to one in 6 in the 76-and-over group. It is likely that as screening techniques improve both in public schools and in industry we shall have more accurate information about the magnitude of the problem of impaired hearing.

## EDUCATIONAL PROCEDURES

The educational needs of the hard-of-hearing child are different from those of the deaf child discussed in the preceding chapter because he has the potential for learning speech, speech perception, and language by more natural means, primarily over the auditory system. Furthermore, with proper recognition of his difficulties and with proper auxiliary aid, his needs are apt to be met in a special class for the hard of hearing within a public school system or in the regular classroom itself. Where he is placed will depend on his hearing loss and the availability of special help. The aim should be to educate him wherever practical with normal-hearing children.

The particular needs are as follows:

1. Less than 30 decibel loss—lip-reading and favorable seating.
2. 30–45 decibel loss—lip-reading, hearing aid (if suitable) and auditory training, speech correction and conversation, favorable seating.
3. 45–60 decibel loss—lip-reading, hearing aid and auditory training, training in speech, special language work, favorable seating or special class.
4. 60–80 decibel loss—needs the kind of educational procedures for the deaf child described in the preceding chapter, with special emphasis on speech, auditory training, and language; with the possibilty that the child may enter regular classes.
5. 80-plus decibel loss—special class or school as described in the preceding chapter. Some of these children eventually enter high schools for the hearing.

Special help in developing the skills of communication may be available through a special class, an itinerant teacher, a speech-and-hearing clinic of a university or hospital or in a society for the hard of hearing. Pattee and Downs (1954) have published a list of centers that serve hearing-handicapped children and adults.

### Auditory Training

As we have seen in the preceding chapter, auditory training, primarily through amplified sound, is aimed at improving speech, speech perception (when combined with lip-reading), and at improved psychological well-being. For hard-of-hearing children, the potential for auditory training is greater than for deaf children. We may look for development not only of gross discriminations but greater development of discrimination of speech patterns and speech sounds. Actually, lip-reading is likely to be the supplementary (to hearing) means of communication for most hard-of-hearing children. Training should be pointed at more extensive discrimination of the kind suggested in the preceding chapter. Most of the techniques for both children and adults reflect the possibility of attaining discriminations sufficient to permit understanding of speech through the ear for all but the severely handicapped (Brentano, 1946; Browd, 1951; Goldstein, 1939; Kelly, 1953; Ronnei, 1951; Utley, 1951; Wedenberg, 1954; Whitehurst, 1947).

In general, hearing aids are useful to hard-of-hearing children and adult who have a loss of 30 decibels or more in the speech range and whose hearing loss is such that amplification will not distort speech to the point where the instrument not only does not help but may impair speech perception. Care must be taken not to force hearing aids on children or adults. As long as our culture stigmatizes hearing loss, people will hesitate to display evidence of it. This situation may be aggravated by the tendency of purveyors of instruments to base advertising on ingenious methods of concealing the hearing aid when it is worn on the person. This may be necessary to get people into the shop, but it may also heighten the feeling of stigma and keep the prospective client away. In a study of factors influencing the decision of children to wear hearing aids, Gates and Kushner (1940) found that fear of losing social status and concern over personal appearance caused some children to reject hearing aids. On the other hand, they found that hearing-aid users showed consistent improvement in school achievement and in participation in group activities.

Quantitative information available to us about the effect of auditory training for the hard of hearing is fragmentary. We have seen in the preceding chapter that Hudgins (1953) has shown the value of a bisensory approach for the deaf and Wedenberg (1954) reports encouraging results with selected children, the results varying with the amount of hearing loss. Morley (1948) and Kelly (1954) claimed some improvement in children for speech perception and social adjustment, and Silverman (1944) reported substantial gains by adults from auditory training in understanding of words and sentences. Siegenthaler and Gunn (1952) questioned some of the results and found in general that previous "acoustic rehabilitation" does not insure more threshold help with a hearing aid. These investigations suffer from the lack of adequate and valid measuring devices and criteria for gain from auditory training.

It is clear that we need more scientifically derived information about the factors that are associated with successful use and acceptance of a hearing aid.

## Lip-Reading

In the preceding chapter we discussed the evolution of lip-reading, its pedagogical basis, and the factors influencing its performance. For the hard-of-hearing child and adult, lip-reading instruction may be more flexible and varied because it is not subject to the restriction of limitations in language. As we have said previously, it is the supporting skill for hearing. The skillful teacher of lip-reading learns to create situations that stimulate taking advantage of contextual clues and to use material that appeals to the interests of her pupils. Many suggestions of this sort are contained in the recommendations of Bunger (1942), the Kinzies (1931), Nitchie (1950), Pauls (1947), Stowell *et al.* (1928), and Whildin and Scally (1939).

## Speech Development, Correction, and Conservation

We have already discussed the underlying considerations in the development of speech in the severely deaf. Our major speech problem with the hard of hearing is the correction and the conservation of speech. The hard-of-hearing person does not hear speech and speech patterns clearly and therefore has a poor model for imitation. This is particularly applicable to the person with a high-frequency loss. For example, French and Steinberg (1947), using low-pass filtering, found that when only the frequencies below 1000 were passed, 88 per cent of nonsense syllables were heard correctly; but when only the frequencies below 1000 cps were passed, the score fell to 27 per cent. Furthermore, defective hearing prevents adequate monitoring of articulation and phonation.

Characteristic errors of articulation involve the mutilation or omission of sibilants such as *s* and *sh* and of word endings. Deviations in voice that may tax listener effort are the soft voice (with relatively good articulation)—characteristic of conductive deafness; the poorly modulated voice (with incorrect articulations)—characteristic of perceptive deafness; and various combinations of these, depending, of course, upon the time of onset of hearing impairment and the kind and amount of corrective training. Many hard-of-hearing persons may have no detectable disorders of articulation or voice because of mildness or recency of onset of hearing impairment. Speech may deteriorate, however, with increase in the amount or the length of time of the deafness. It is, therefore, desirable, in order to prevent deterioration, that clinical and educational procedures for such individuals include work in speech conservation.

The procedures in speech correction and conservation for the hard of hearing should not differ too radically from the measures suggested in other parts of this handbook dealing with disorders of voice and articulation, except that consideration must be given to the difficulties of auditory perception (see Chapters 23, 24, 25 and 26). The techniques should include learning to listen to good models of speech over hearing aids, creating moto-kinesthetic awareness by feeling vibrations connected with the production of speech, and the encouragement of good speech by the people who live and work with the hard-of-hearing person (Carhart, 1947; Stone, 1954).

## EXTRA-SCHOOL AGENCIES AND RESOURCES

For the hard of hearing as well as for the deaf (see the preceding chapter), there are numerous organizations that are concerned with the interests of the hard of hearing. The American Hearing Society, 1800 H St., Washington 6. D. C., is composed of chapters in many cities of the United States and publishes a monthly *Hearing News*. The Society's purpose is "to serve as an information center on problems of defective hearing, to improve the educational, economic and social conditions among both adults and children whose hearing is impaired; and to stimulate scientific efforts in the prevention of deafness and the conservation of hearing."

Among professional groups is the Committee on Conservation of Hearing of the American Academy of Ophthalmology and Otolaryngology (100 First Avenue Building, Rochester, Minn.), composed of otolaryngologists, which is interested in state-wide programs of hearing conservation and, more recently, in the increasing problem of industrial noise, its prevention, and its medico-legal aspects. The American Speech and Hearing Association (the Secretary-Treasurer is located at Wayne University, Detroit) is composed primarily of speech and hearing therapists and investigators working in our universities, schools, and hospitals. The Association publishes a quarterly *The Journal of Speech and Hearing Disorders*. The Office of Vocational Rehabilitation of the Federal Security Administration has the same services for he hard of hearing as it does for the deaf, and out of programs for military personnel and veterans have grown useful suggestions for service (Bergman, 1950; Canfield and Morrissett, 1947; Stone, 1954).

The management of the hard of hearing requires:

1. Public information about hearing impairment and acoustic hygiene (Hardy, 1952; Silverman, 1950).
2. Case-finding through appropriate screening programs in clinics for babies, in schools, and in pre-employment physical examinations.
3. Complete diagnosis of hearing impairment.
4. Appropriate medical and surgical treatment.
5. Thorough assessment of hearing after all indicated medical and surgical procedures have been completed, with particular attention to educational and rehabilitative needs.
6. Special educational and rehabilitative measures that include auditory training, lip-reading, speech correction and conservation, vocational planning, and psychological guidance.

It is appropriate to conclude this chapter by venturing the judgment that recent intensification of interest and activity in problems of hearing impairment, as shown by advances in otological surgery, by improvement in electroacoustic instrumentation, by government and private support of clinical and research programs, by increased interest of workers in peripheral fields, and by increasing community awareness presages a brighter future for the hard-of-hearing child and adult.

## BIBLIOGRAPHY

ARKER, R. G., WRIGHT, B. A., MYERSON, L., and GONICK, M. R. 1953. Adjustment to physical handicap and illness: a survey of the social psychology of physique and disability. Bull. 55, New York: Soc. Sci. Res. Council.

EASLEY, W. C. 1940. The general problem of deafness in the population. *Laryngoscope,* 50, 856–905.

ERGMAN, M. 1950. The audiology clinic: a manual for planning a clinic for the rehabilitation of the acoustically handicapped. Stockholm: *Actaotolarynglogica,* supplementum, 89, 1–107.

RENTANO, L. 1946. Ways to better hearing. New York: F. Watts.

ROWD, V. L. 1951. The new way to better hearing: through hearing re-education. New York: Crown Pub.

RUNSCHWIG, L. 1936. A study of some personality aspects of deaf children. New York: Columbia Univ.

UNGER, A. M. 1942. Speech reading—Jena method. Danville, Ill.: Interstate Press.

ANFIELD, N., and MORRISSETT, L. E. 1947. Military aural rehabilitation. *In* Davis, H., Hearing and deafness. New York: Rinehart. Pp. 318–337.

APLIN, D. 1937. A special report of retardation of school children with impaired hearing in the New York City schools. *Amer. Ann. Deaf,* 82, 234–243.

EMBO, T., LADIEU, G., and WRIGHT, B. A. 1948. Adjustment to misfortune, Final Report to Army Medical Research and Development Board. Office of Surgeon-General, War Department. (Typescript.)

RENCH, N. R., and STEINBERG, J. C. 1947. Factors governing the intelligibility of speech sounds. *J. acoust. Soc. Amer.,* 19, 90–119.

GATES, A. I., and KUSHNER, R. E. 1946. Learning to use hearing aids. New York: Columbia Univ.

GOLDSTEIN, M. A. 1939. The acoustic method for the training of the deaf and hard of hearing child. St. Louis: Laryngoscope Press.

HABBE, S. 1936. Personality adjustments of adolescent boys with impaired hearing. New York: Columbia Univ.

HARDY, W. G. 1952. Children with impaired hearing. Children's bureau publication number 326. Washington: Government Printing Office.

HUIZING, H. 1953. Assessment and evaluation of hearing anomalies in young children. In Proceedings of the international course in paedo-audiology. Groningen: Verenigde Drukkerijen Hoitsema N. V. Pp. 88–97.

KELLY, J. C. 1953. Clinicians handbook for auditory training. Dubuque: W. C. Brown.

———— 1954. A summer residential program in hearing education. J. Speech Hearing Disorders, 19, 17–27.

KINZIE, C. E., and KINZIE, R. 1931. Lip reading for the deafened adult. Philadelphia: John C. Winston.

KIRK, S. A. 1938. Behavior problem tendencies in deaf and hard of hearing children in America. Amer. Ann. Deaf, 83, 131–137.

LANE, H. S. 1953. The deaf. In Garrett, J. F. Psychological aspects of physical disability. Rehabilitation service series number 210. Washington: Government Printing Office.

McCORMICK, H. W. 1941. Report of the subcommittee on acoustically handicapped children. New York: New York City Board Educ.

MADDEN, R. 1931. The school status of the hard of hearing child. New York: Columbia Univ.

MOSLEY, D. 1948. An experimental program for hard of hearing children. J. Speech Hearing Disorders, 13, 337–345.

MYERSON, L. 1948. Experimental injury: an approach to the dynamics of physical disability. J. soc. Issues, 4, 68–71.

NITCHIE, E. 1950. New lessons in lip reading. Philadelphia: Lippincott.

O'CONNOR, C. D. 1954. Children with impaired hearing. Health News. New York: State Department Health, 31, 4–16.

PATTEE, H. L., and DOWNS, M. P. 1954. A survey of hearing centers in the United States. Arch. Otolaryng., Chicago, 59, 413–430.

PINTNER, R. 1933. Emotional stability of the hard of hearing. J. genet. Psychol. 43, 293–311.

———— 1940. An adjustment test with normal and hard of hearing children. genet. Psychol., 56, 367–381.

————, EISENSON, J., and STANTON, M. B. 1941. The psychology of the physically handicapped. New York: Crofts.

PINTNER, R., and LEV, J. 1939. The intelligence of the hard of hearing school child. J. genet. Psychol. 55, 31–48.

RAMSDELL, D. A. 1947. The psychology of the hard of hearing and deafened adult. In Davis, H., Hearing and deafness. New York: Rinehart. P. 392–418.

RONNEI, E. 1951. Learning to look and listen. New York: Columbia Univ.

SIEGENTHALER, B. M., and GUNN, G. H. 1952. Factors associated with help obtained from individual hearing aids. J. Speech Hearing Disorders, 17, 338–347.

SILVERMAN, S. R. 1944. Training for optimum use of hearing aids. Laryngoscope 54, 29–36.

———— 1950. The hard of hearing child: how the classroom teacher can recognize and help him. J. nat. Educ. Assn., 39, 136–7.

————, THURLOW, W. R., WALSH, T. E., and DAVIS, H. 1948. Improvement in the social adequacy of hearing following the fenestration operation. *Laryngoscope*, 58, 607–631.

SPRINGER, N. N. 1938a. A comparative study of behavior traits of deaf and hearing children of New York City. *Amer. Ann. Deaf*, 83, 255–273.

————1938b. A comparative study of psychoneurotic responses of deaf and hearing children. *J. educ. Psychol.*, 29, 459–466.

STONE, R. H. 1954. Special considerations regarding the disability in the vocational rehabilitation of veterans who have hearing, speech or language impairments. Information bulletin, Department of Veterans Benefits. Washington: Veterans Administration.

TOWELL, A., SAMUELSON, E. E., and LEHMAN, A. 1928. Lip reading for the deafened child. New York: Macmillan.

TRENG, A., and KIRK, S. A. 1938. The social competence of deaf and hard of hearing children in a public day school. *Amer. Ann. Deaf*, 83, 244–254.

UTLEY, J. 1951. What's its name. Urbana: Univ. Ill. Press.

WALDMAN, J. L., WADE, F. A., and ARETZ, C. W. 1930. Hearing and the school child. Washington: Volta Bur.

WEDENBERG, E. 1954. Auditory training of severely hard of hearing school children. *Acta Otolaryngologica*, supplementum 110, 7–82.

WELLES, H. H. 1932 .The measurement of certain aspects of personality among hard of hearing adults. New York: Columbia Univ.

WHILDIN, O. A., and SCALLY, M. A. 1939. Speech reading for the hard of hearing child. Westminster, Md.: John William Eckenrode.

WHITEHURST, M. W. 1947. Train your hearing. Washington: Volta Bur.

# CHAPTER 12

# APHASIA IN ADULTS—
# CLASSIFICATION AND
# EXAMINATION PROCEDURES

• *Jon Eisenson, Ph.D.*

## NATURE OF APHASIC DISTURBANCES

APHASIC INVOLVEMENTS CAN be understood only if we begin with the basi
appreciation that aphasia constitutes a complexity of disturbances whic
may happen to a person. The aphasic individual had habits, attitudes, an
abilities, as well as capacities not yet translated into abilities, and a person
ality, before he became aphasic. If the individual is an adult, he had learne
to respond to illness, to incapacities, to frustration, and to the myriad c
influences that man is exposed to long before he became aphasic. How he
likely to respond to the immediate effects of aphasic involvements will de
pend to a large extent on the kind of person he was before he became aphasi
Aphasic involvements are likely to bring about modifications in the patient
premorbid personality. They are not likely to produce a new personalit
unrelated in any way to the individual's premorbid state and manner of be
having. A well-adjusted individual who becomes aphasic probably has
better chance of ultimate adjustment than a neurotic individual who becom
aphasic. The latter is likely to become a neurotic-aphasic with a reduce
chance of recovery from either his neuroticism or his aphasic disturbance

Aphasic disturbances, purely for convenience, may be divided into thre
major categories:

1. Symbolic (linguistic) and related disturbances
2. Intellectual change
3. Personality modification

In the given individual, these changes are interrelated. Each one necessari
affects the others. The result of these interactions, and their influence on t
individual in terms of his premorbid make-up, permit us to understand t
aphasic individual.

## PRELIMINARY CONSIDERATIONS

### anguage and Symbol Behavior

In order to understand the nature of the linguistic disturbances of aphasic atients, as well as to understand why under some conditions some language s available to almost all aphasic patients, we need to review briefly the ature of symbol behavior and of language as such behavior.

**Language is a system of symbols.** Symbols are arbitrary arrangements of udible or visible and sometimes of tactile signs which derive their meaning rrough a process of association. These symbols are usually produced ac- ording to conventionalized patterns of grammar, sentence structure, vocal ones, and manner of articulation. When the speech is written, spelling is ubstituted for articulation. The conventions of written language are gen- rally more rigid and, by the literate person, tend to be more strictly observed ran are the conventions of spoken language.

**Words and concepts.** *Concepts are generalizations* about experiences. A iven concept is a generalization about one experience, or about a series or roup of similar experiences. Words, whether spoken or written, are con- entionalized symbols of concepts. Concepts, for normal persons, are subject ) continued modification according to their continued experiences. These xperiences may be direct or vicarious. Modification may take place as a sult of teaching, which frequently constitutes a form of vicarious experi- nce.

A single word form may stand for one or more concepts, which may or ray not be related. Homonyms, such as *reign* and *rain, read* and *reed,* are xamples of audible word forms which have different and unrelated mean- gs. Other single word forms, such as *board* and *race,* have both related and nrelated meanings. The word *water* is an example of one of many English ords that have several meanings and concepts which, for the most part, are lated to the most common or core meaning of the word. Other such English ords are *run, head,* and *chief.*

**Nonintellectual use of word forms.** Most intelligent and normal human eings learn to use language symbols with sufficient proficiency to elicit ecific responses or to express specific ideas according to the needs of vary- g situations. Most human beings also learn to use language symbols with- ut regard to specific ideas or without intention of eliciting specific responses. Vords spoken under the influence of strong emotion, of anger, fear, and of ate, as well as words of a more tender emotion, are *nonspecific* and *non- mbolic.* The same word form, then, may have both abstract and specific ymbolic) meaning as well as nonabstract and nonsymbolic meaning. Some nglish words of Anglo-Saxon origin are rarely used except in nondenota- ve, nonsymbolic ways. It is possible, however, to utter any word, or any oup of words, in a manner which makes them devoid of intellectual sig- ficance. This point is being emphasized because an aphasic person is one *r whom intellectual and abstract meanings are disturbed.* An aphasic

person is one who suffers impairment of meanings more than he suffers los
of words.

Nonintellectual speech is not confined to emotional utterance. Othe
forms of nonintellectual speech are *automatic, serial-content,* and *socia.
gesture speech.*

*Automatic speech* consists of linguistic material which has been so ofte
repeated *in a given order* that the content has been memorized. Familia
verses, prayers, and songs are examples of speech content which initiall
may or may not have had intellectual significance but which became autc
matic and nonintellectual through repetition. Words of a song are usuall
automatic only when the melody as well as the words are produced. If th
melody is intentionally inhibited, it will generally be found that voluntar
effort is necessary to recall the words of the song.

*Serial content* consists of a series of words which have been learned an
memorized in a given order. The alphabet, numerical sequences, and aritl
metic tables are examples of serial-content speech. Automatic speech ma
become modified and require voluntary control when it becomes necessar
to begin at other than the habitual starting point.

*Social-gesture speech* is another form of linguistic content in which i
dividual words and their specific symbolic significance are relatively u
important. In the use of such verbal social gestures as "How are you?" an
"Pleased to meet you," we pay little attention to the specific symbolic c
denotative meanings of the words. At best, these words have "area mear
ings." Social-gesture words are appropriate in rather broad ways to the situe
tions in which they are used. In general, several possible choices may b
equally appropriate to the same situation. For example, when two acquain
ances meet it is not of great importance whether one greets the other wi
"Hello"; "How are you?"; or "How do you do?" It is usually equally u
important whether the response to the greeting is "Fine, thank you"; c
"How are you?"

Emotional utterance, automatic-content, serial-content, and social-gestu
speech are examples of linguistic word forms and word usage which rema
relatively intact for many aphasic patients. These are nonpropositional form
of speech.

**Propositional speech.** When linguistic symbols are used to communica
a specific idea or to elicit a specific response, we are dealing with *propo:
tional speech.* The unit of linguistic content with which the individual pr
duces specific symbol situations is termed the proposition. In a propositio
as the term was originally used by Hughlings Jackson (1893 and 1932), n
only the words but the manner in which the words are related and refer
one another within the unit become important. A proposition, Jackson er
phasized, implies an internal and external relationship. The words are r
lated to one another and to the situation in which they are used.

The aphasic individual's chief difficulty is in evaluating and in evoki
propositional units. From the point of view of productive speech, the apha:

person is not without words. He is rather one who cannot readily evoke the appropriate linguistic symbol or group of symbols for a given situation.

In the pages which immediately follow, we will discuss the forms of linguistic disturbance most frequent in aphasic patients.

## Linguistic Disturbances

From the linguistic point of view, aphasia constitutes an impairment in the individual's previously established ability to deal with symbols. Because all language requires the use of symbols, linguistic functions are disturbed. Aphasia, therefore, is a disturbance in symbolic formulation and expression (Head, 1926). The aphasic patient experiences difficulty in some degree in evaluating and in expressing meanings through the use of symbols.

Aphasic linguistic disturbances have been classified in numerous ways according to major type and specific form of defect. Very detailed classifications may be found in Nielsen (1946). Other, less detailed classifications may be found in Goldstein (1948), Wepman (1951), and Granich (1947). The classifications which will be followed in this chapter are modifications of a four-category classification of Weisenburg and McBride (1935). They used the following classifications for linguistic disturbances:

*Predominantly Receptive.* The greatest amount of disturbance is in the individual's ability to comprehend spoken or written symbols.
*Predominantly Expressive.* The greatest amount of disturbance is in the individual's ability to express ideas in speech or in writing.
*Amnesic.* The patient's chief difficulty is in the evocation of appropriate words as names for objects, conditions, relationships, qualities, and so on. Amnesic disturbances are in effect a subtype of expressive disturbance.
*Expressive-Receptive.* Both receptive and expressive language functions are extremely disturbed. In early stages of aphasic involvements, this is likely to be true of a great many patients. Only a comparatively few patients continue to manifest equally severe disturbances of both reception and expression. Usually, receptive functions improve spontaneously to a greater degree than do expressive functions.

The classifications about to be presented constitute an effort, on the part of the present author, to add clinically significant subtypes to the basic classifications of Weisenburg and McBride. From the point of view of the clinician, the classifications are intended to suggest where the major emphasis in the aphasic's language rehabilitation should be made.

**Evaluative.** The individual's area of greatest disturbance is in his evaluation of language symbols which come to him through a given sensory avenue, usually the ear or eye, or through a combination of sensory avenues. The category *evaluative* comprises what Weisenburg and McBride include under their heading of *receptive* and which some other authorities have included under the general heading of *sensory disturbances*.

Evaluative disturbances include the following subtypes:

*Auditory Aphasia.* This refers specifically to disturbances in the comprehension of audible speech which normally is received and evaluated through hearing. Perhaps more often than we might suspect, auditory aphasic disturbances become apparent only as the quantity or complexity of speech i increased. Occasionally, it will become readily apparent only when the pa tient is fatigued. Sometimes a patient's difficulty in auditory comprehension is manifest only when there is a fairly rapid change in the nature or conten of the what he hears.

*Alexia.* This is a disturbance in the comprehension of written symbols Alexic difficulties are difficulties in *silent reading.* These difficulties, as is th case with auditory aphasia, sometimes become obvious only as the patien is required to read comparatively difficult material or long, unbroken pages Occasionally, the difficulty is apparent chiefly in the evaluation of "smal words"—articles, prepositions, conjunctions, and others which are use semantically as connectives or to indicate relationships of words (ideas within a sentence. Sometimes it will be found that the rate of reading is im paired. A once proficient reader may read accurately but laboriously, an with a feeling of insecurity about his ability. Alexic disturbances may b tested by presenting a patient with written material varying in length an complexity which he is directed to read silently. When he is finished readin the patient is then required to answer questions or to carry out direction based on the reading.

**Productive (expressive).** This class of disturbances reveal the aphasic in dividual's disabilities in the production and expression of ideas through th use of spoken or written symbols. For the deaf person who previously em ployed manual sign language before becoming aphasic, the production visible (sign) symbols would be disturbed. Productive disturbances refer disabilities in the evocation of the symbol rather than to the motor aspect the productive act. The latter aspect will be considered separately as relate difficulties under the headings of apraxia and dysarthria.

There are several subcategories of productive disturbances which becom evident in the spoken and written efforts of the aphasic patient. As a gener rule, most aphasic patients manifest a greater amount of disability in one more of the productive disturbances and less difficulty in others. It is rare find an aphasic patient with an isolated difficulty for one type of producti disturbance. Rather frequently, we will find that involvements in speakin and writing parallel one another. The degree of defect, however, may greater in one than in the other.

*Anomia or Nominal Aphasia.* This is probably the outstanding and m frequent subtype of productive disturbance. Anomia refers to the patien difficulty to evoke an appropriate word regardless of the grammatical part cech of that word. The defect is most likely to be evident in the effort voke nouns (nominal words) because nouns constitute the bulk of m ocabularies. As the patient recovers, anomia is most likely to be the re dual disturbance. Most patients, unless they also have considerable evalu tive difficulty, are readily able to recognize and repeat words which th cannot easily evoke. A patient with anomic difficulty, consciously or

onsciously, may learn to substitute a synonym or a phrase with approxi-
ate meaning for the elusive word, or he may engage in circumlocution, or
se a gesture as a word substitute. This technique is not the special property
f the aphasic patient. Normal speakers use it when, under some temporary
ressure, they cannot readily find the most appropriate word to express an
lea.

Anomia or nominal aphasia may be tested by directing a patient to
ame objects or pictures, by having him supply words to complete sentences,
y requiring the patient to supply a synonym for a word or a phrase, or by
king the patient to summarize in his own words content he has heard or
ad.

The following is a sample of conversation which illustrates naming diffi-
lty. The patient, a 28-year-old infantry officer, suffered a penetrating
ound of the left cerebral hemisphere.

Examiner: What is that? (Examiner points to a tree outside of the window.)
Patient: It's, it's something that grows.
Examiner: What do you call it?
Patient: It's a thing—one of those things—it grows in Brooklyn.
Examiner: Is it a tree?
Patient: Yes, a tee, a tree.
Examiner: Did you read "A Tree Grows in Brooklyn?"
Patient: Yes, I did, before I got it, before I got hit.
Examiner: Can you say tree now?
Patient: A tree.

*Agraphia.* Writing disturbances may be manifest in all writing, or in the
riting of nominal words, as in anomia, or in faulty grammar, or by the omis-
on of articles, prepositions, conjunctions and other words which serve as
nnectives or to indicate relationships of parts of a sentence. These errors
ay appear in writing to dictation, in spontaneous writing, and even in
rect copying.

The following letter is an example of the spontaneous writing of a 49-year-
d male veteran. His aphasia was associated with cerebral thrombosis. The
ter was written six months after the onset of his disturbance. Errors of
nctuation, grammar, and sentence structure are evident.

June 12, 1949

ar ———

Soldier back is U.S., miles home farm 90,100 mi,. Do you live near ocean, 20
. A place you can swim.

Your

The following is an example of dictated material and writing of an aphasic
tient. The patient was a 48-year-old army sergeant who suffered a left
ontal-parietal brain injury as a result of a skull fracture. The dictated
aterial was:

Dear ——,

I am a patient at —— Hospital. I was injured in Korea. When I am we
enough to return to duty, may I have my old job back.

Thank you.

The patient wrote:

Dear A. J.

I am a patent. At —— navy hoptile.at. I want hurt korea when I hurtmeit t
duat. May I hurt made open down. Beause.
Thand you.

*Spelling.* Disturbances in written spelling may be considered a form o
agraphia. Written spelling difficulties may parallel those of oral spelling. A
a rule, oral spelling difficulties are more severe than those of written spelling
A likely reason for this is that when a patient writes, he may do so slowl
so as to avoid errors, or he may correct them as he proceeds. The mos
usual types of errors are letter reversals and omissions. In English writing
many patients write phonetically rather than conventionally. The followin
are typical examples of spelling errors of single dictated words. (The dictate
material is in parentheses.)

> (feeling)—filing
> (cabinet)—kamit
> (campaign)—campane
> (occur)—acor

*Acalculia (Arithmetic Disturbances).* These disturbances may be preser
on a twofold basis: (1) because of actual difficulty on the part of the patien
in dealing with arithmetic processes, or (2) because of related difficulty i
the oral or written production of the symbols involved in calculation. If th
latter is the case, the difficulty is really one of word-finding (anomia) rathe
than of acalculia.

Frequently we will find that an aphasic patient may do well in simpl
arithmetic computation, especially if he is permitted to write his response
This apparently well-retained ability can probably be explained by the aut
maticity with which most of us do simple arithmetic. The arithmetic table
have become automatic for most adults, so that most of our computatio
are carried on without the need for quantitative conceptualization or reaso
ing. Despite this general finding, it is not too rare to come across an aphas
who cannot perform simple arithmetic operations accurately but who ca
do fairly well in numerical problem-solving situations.

*Paraphasia.* In our discussion of anomia, agraphia, and spelling, note w
made of tendencies for substitutions of words, grammatical errors, lett
transpositions, and omissions which occur in the oral and written efforts
the aphasic. Taken as a group, these errors are referred to as *paraphasi*
Paraphasic errors continue, to some degree, to characterize the speech
many patients who have made a fairly good linguistic recovery. In som
"former" patients who seem to be free from these errors, one might note
slowness of rate in speech. This modified rate may be the way the individu

has learned to guard against his tendency to commit paraphasic errors. The prevalence of such faults should not surprise us. The slips of the tongue and occasional linguistic transgressions of nonaphasic persons bear evidence that the tendency toward paraphasia is a strong one. Persons without brain injury commit these errors when under emotional stress, or when fatigued, or when the "wish is father to the thought" but the thought is one which is not altogether situationally appropriate. The aphasic person's tendencies to paraphasia can be explained both by normal dynamics and psychodynamics as well as by reason of cortical damage.

Not infrequently, an aphasic's paraphasic errors may be attributed to the patient's basic evaluative (receptive) difficulties. An aphasic individual who is not secure in his understanding of what he hears or sees may well reflect some of his evaluative deficiencies in his own speech efforts.

*Dysprosody.* As the term is here used, *dysprosody* refers to disturbances of melody pattern which may influence speech. In a more extreme form, dysprosody may be used for all melody disturbances, in music as well as in speech. It is rare, however, for a patient with aphasia to lose his ability to reproduce a simple musical melody in some form. If he cannot sing, he may still be able to hum the melody or tune. The melody or intonation pattern of speech is more subtle than in music. In some languages, as in Chinese dialects, it affects meanings to a marked degree. In English, disturbances of melody are likely to be significant semantically only as they interfere with the patient's ability to suggest subtleties. To a larger extent, however, much of speech may be affected. The patient with dysprosody—and many manifest this as a residual of their aphasic disturbances—talks without the color normally provided by vocal inflections. A patient may speak English as if he were accustomed to some accent other than English. Actually, however, he is speaking *without accent*. For an excellent discussion of this little-appreciated form of aphasic disturbance, the author suggests an article by Monrad-Krohn (1947).

## Related Subsymbolic Disturbances

The aphasic disturbances which we have just considered were all on a high symbolic linguistic level of evaluation or production. They were disturbances of symbol association. Frequently, aphasic patients, especially in the early stages of their involvement, have related subsymbolic disturbances which impair their perception or expression of symbols. On the receptive side, these disturbances are collectively known as *agnosias*. On the productive side, they are *apraxias* and *dysarthrias*. The full appreciation of aphasic involvements requires an understanding of these related disturbances.

**Recognition (agnosias).** The ability to evaluate objects, representations of objects, or symbols is based on a primary ability of an individual first to recognize what he is expected to evaluate. Recognition, in and of itself, implies only the ability to perceive configurations of objects, representations (pictures), or symbols. *Agnosias* are disturbances in ability to recognize configurations through the various sensory avenues *when the disturbances are not present because of specific sensory loss.*

*Visual Agnosia.* This is disturbance of recognition of situations through the visual sense. The individual may sense that he is seeing something, but may not be able to recognize what he sees. Visual agnosias may be specific for objects, representations, geometric forms, colors, letters, words, or other special configurations. It is unlikely, however, that an individual will have an agnosia for pictures and not for objects; for letters, and not for words or for single words and not for words in context.

The importance of determining whether an individual has visual agnosia before deciding whether he has alexia is evident. If letters, or groups of letters, cannot be recognized they cannot be evaluated as symbols. It is essential, therefore, that a patient's ability to recognize configurations must be determined before a decision is made as to possible alexia.

*Auditory Agnosia.* This term refers to disturbances in the recognition of sounds or combinations of sounds without regard to the individual's ability to evaluate them. The disturbance may be for nonsymbolic (linguistic) sounds such as mechanical or animal noises; for human, nonlinguistic sound (coughing, sneezing, hand-clapping); or for sounds which are associated with spoken symbols (phonetic units, words, or groups of words). A patient who hears sounds which he cannot recognize will not be able to evaluate the auditory sensations. An individual with *auditory verbal agnosia* is not able to understand what he hears.

We may test for auditory agnosias by having a patient imitate sounds, or in some other way, as by pointing, indicate the source or origin of a sound. Verbal agnosias may be tested by repetitions of words or, on a higher level, by eliciting an appropriate motor response to a word or a group of words. A person who can point to the parts of his body when they are named reveals that he both recognizes and understands the words he hears.

A special form of auditory agnosia is *amusia*. Auditory musical agnosia (amusia) refers to a disturbance in a previously existing ability to recognize music. It is not to be confused with so-called tone deafness, or with a lack of singing ability which is fairly common among nonaphasic persons. If amusia is actually found to exist in a patient, the disturbance may impair the person's ability to respond appropriately to inflectional and intonational changes in speech. On the whole, however, amusia is not one of the more important disturbances related to aphasia.

*Tactile Agnosia (Astereognosis).* This disturbance is in the ability of an individual to recognize objects through the sense of touch. For the blind person, however, who has been trained in braille reading, tactile agnosia will impair reading ability.

We may test for tactile agnosias by presenting distinctive objects in the person's hand without permitting him to see them or to hear them if they make a characteristic noise. The patient may then be directed to name, match, or in some other way identify the objects.

**Production (apraxias and dysarthrias).** *Apraxias.* Apraxias are motor disturbances which are manifest in a patient's disability in the use of tools in purposeful and intended ways. The tools may be external to the human organism, such as hammers, knives, forks, pens, brushes, and so on. The tools may also be parts of the body such as the hands, arms, feet, the lips or other organs of articulation. When the tool is the hand, the apraxic disturbance directly impairs writing ability. When the tools are parts of the articulatory mechanism, the motor aspect of speech is directly affected.

Apraxias, it becomes evident, may be nonverbal or verbal. *Nonverbal* apraxies may disturb not only writing but the use of pantomime and gesture. They may also be manifest in a disturbance in oral nonlinguistic activity, such as in whistling or other forms of nonsymbolic sound production.

*Verbal or oral apraxias* are reflected in the purely motor aspect of speech. If a patient has severe verbal apraxia, he may be completely inarticulate even though the inner symbolic formulation may be completely or relatively intact. Less severe oral apraxia may be manifest in errors of articulation. Apraxic defects of articulation constitute one form of dysarthria.

*Dysarthrias.* The patient with productive (expressive) language disturbance frequently has associated dysarthric disturbance. *Dysarthrias* are defects of articulation on a neurological basis. The neurological lesion may be central or peripheral. For the aphasic, the associated lesion is most likely to be central. The brain damage responsible for the aphasic involvements may also be responsible for the dysarthric disturbances.

Dysarthric errors are manifest in distortions and omissions of the sounds of speech. Individual consonants, vowels, diphthongs, or blends of these sounds may be affected. Although dysarthric errors are not errors of symbolic function, an aphasic patient is likely to have increased difficulty in the dysarthric (motor) aspect of his speech as he experiences difficulty in the symbolic (aphasic) aspect of speech. It may also be noted that speech which readily available to the patient, such as emotionally-laden content, automatic content, and serial speech, is less likely to reflect dysarthric disturbance.

Aphasia, then, is an impairment in symbolic formulation and expression. It is primarily a disturbance in the ability of the patient to deal with symbolic (linguistic) situations. Nonpropositional speech may be relatively intact. Aphasic disturbances may be classified into those which are predominantly evaluative (receptive) and those which are predominantly productive (expressive).

Related subsymbolic disturbances of reception are agnosias. Related subsymbolic disturbances of production are apraxias and dysarthrias.

## EXAMINATION PROCEDURES

The approach to testing of aphasic patients, and specific procedures consistent with the approach, depend upon the examiner's philosophy of the

over-all nature and implications of aphasic disturbances. If the individual'
philosophy is one which looks upon the aphasic as a person who, because c
brain damage, has undergone permanent intellectual changes and ha
evolved a "new" personality, then the testing should seek to evaluate th
changes so that a therapeutic program consistent with the changes can b
undertaken. For example, for the clinician who accepts the point of view c
Kurt Goldstein (1948, Ch. IV) that the various dysfunctions of aphasia ar
the manifestations of a single disorder—the loss of ability to grasp the es
sential nature of a process—the approach should be one for determining th
extent of the basic disorder. Testing then would employ psychological tech
niques such as are used by Strauss and Lehtinen (1947) or by Goldstein an
Scheerer (1941) in their test for abstract and concrete behavior.

For the clinician who looks upon the intellectual and personality change
as temporary for most aphasics, and as manifestations of an underlying dis
order of language function, the examination approach would emphasize th
testing of language abilities. Psychological tests would be used, if they ar
used at all, as supplements useful only to estimate the over-all abilities of th
patient *at the time the tests are administered*. This is the point of view of th
author of this chapter. It is supported by his own observations (1947), b
test and retest scores, as well as by the findings of research workers an
clinicians such as Wepman (1951, pp. 70–72), who found that the intell
gence scores of a group of aphasics after training approximated their pre
traumatic (preaphasic) scores much more closely than they did their earl
posttraumatic scores. In addition, Wepman (1951, p. 24) again substantiate
the present author's observations that loss of abstract ability, even whe
measured by the Goldstein-Scheerer Tests, is subject to improvement wit
training. Wepman found that twenty of seventy-one aphasics had difficult
on the Goldstein-Scheerer Tests at the start of a training period. "When th
same subjects were tested at the end of training, only nine of the twenty sti
showed loss of abstracting ability."

### Examination Inventories

The examinations to be described are in current use in the United State
For the most part, with the exception of the Chesher Examination, they ar
used by speech clinicians, speech pathologists, and clinical psychologists, a
well as by neurologists and other physicians.

**Chesher's Technique for Clinical Examination in Aphasia (1937).** Th
examination is based on the Henry Head (1926) Serial Tests. Head publishe
a battery of tests which was designed specifically and directly to stud
aphasic language disturbances. This was a marked departure from the the
current practice of using psychological instruments and techniques to evalu
ate aphasic dysfunctions. Chesher's examination employs six common ob
jects: a pencil, button, scissors, comb, key, and hammer. The followin
functions area tested: naming, repetition, ability to execute oral command

oral reading, silent reading, writing, writing to dictation, copying, and oral spelling.

**The Wells-Ruesch Examination (1945).** Chesher's examination technique has been modified and somewhat elaborated by Wells and Ruesch (1945). Their examination requires the use of six common objects, six cards on which the names of the objects are printed, a match box, and a writing pad. The Wells-Ruesch examination tests for the following abilities:

1. Naming objects seen
2. Repeating the spoken word
3. Comprehension of the spoken word
4. Reading aloud
5. Comprehension of the written word
6. Writing (names of objects presented)
7. Writing from dictation
8. Copying the written word
9. Spelling the spoken word
10. Use of objects
11. Complicated actions
12. Tactile recognition of objects

Neither the Chesher nor the Wells-Ruesch examinations include grading of material. Because of this limitation, the examinations are recommended for use only as screening devices.

**Halstead-Wepman Aphasia Screening Test (1949).** This screening test provides material which the clinician uses to elicit linguistic responses from the patient. The responses enable the clinician to analyze the patient's language disturbances and to classify them into major types. A booklet describing the administration of the examination, and forms for entering the patients responses, are available. No objective score is derived from the test. According to Wepman (1951, p. 132) ". . . its only function is to give the therapist a rapid overview of the problem rather than a measurable quantity score."

**Eisenson's Examining for Aphasia.** This inventory was designed to provide the clinician with a guided approach for evaluating aphasic language disturbances and for disturbances related to language (symbol) functions. The various test items, some of which are taken directly or adapted from standardized educational achievement tests, are intended to reveal both the assets and liabilities of the patient at the time of testing. Much of the material is graded, so that level of ability within a given area of language function can be estimated. Test items are arranged to permit examination for evaluative (receptive) functions, subsymbolic and symbolic, and for productive (expressive) functions. The major types and subcategories of disturbance follow the classifications presented earlier in this chapter.

*Examining for Aphasia* includes a manual of directions and an entry form. The manual describes administrative procedures and scoring. It includes illustrative material used in the examination. The test form provides space for the patient to enter written responses and for the clinician to enter the patient's responses, as well as to make notes relative to the patient's re marks and behavior during the examination. A check sheet permits the clinician to make a profile of the patient's tested abilities.

The author has found the inventory useful as an initial examination fo estimating the areas and approximate levels of linguistic abilities as well a a retest instrument for measuring patient improvement. The entire inventory takes from about 30 to 90 minutes to administer, depending upon the sever ity of involvement and the rate at which the patient is able to work. The ex amination need not be given at a single session if the patient demonstrate fatigue or frustration. If it is desired to use the inventory for rapid screening then single items of each subtest may be administered.

### Additional Tests for Estimating Level of Ability

Unless the aphasic's linguistic disturbances are severe, it is not feasibl to determine the ceiling of the patient's abilities in the course of administer ing an aphasia inventory examination. The clinician who wishes to make thorough evaluations within an area of symbol function may use additiona "educational echievement" tests. For functions commonly considered part of the "three R's," standardized test batteries such as the Metropolita Achievement Tests, the New Stanford Achievement Tests, and the Progres sive Achievement Tests may be used. The last-named test battery is organ ized to permit diagnosois of type of difficulty as well as to determine leve of achievement. All of these test batteries, as well as others which are avail able, provide for graded series of test items, with norms for expected achieve ment for the various school grades.

It is recommended, if achievement batteries are used, that they be ac ministered as power tests with time limitations ignored by the examiner. H may, however, wish to make note as to the amount of time required by th patient to complete whatever was undertaken. That would enable the clin cian to compare improvement in rate even though the same number of item may be correctly completed in the retest. Achievement-test items, inc dentally, provide rated material which may be used for practice and drill i training.

### BIBLIOGRAPHY

CHESHER, E. C. 1937. Technique for clinical examination in aphasia. *Bu Neurol. Inst.* New York, 6, 134–144.
EISENSON, J. 1947. Aphasics: observations and tentative conclusions. *J. Speec Hearing Disorders,* 12, 290–292.
——— 1954. Examining for aphasia (rev.). New York: Psychological Corpor tion.
GOLDSTEIN, K. 1948. Language and language disturbances. New York: Gru and Stratton.
——— and SCHEERER, M. 1941. Abstract and concrete behavior. *Psych Monogr.,* 51, 9.

GRANICH, L. 1947. Aphasia: a guide to retraining. New York: Grune and Stratton.

HALSTEAD, W. C., and WEPMAN, J. 1949. The Halstead-Wepman aphasia screening test. *J. Speech Hearing Disorders,* 14, 9–15.

HEAD, H. 1926. Aphasia and kindred disorders of speech. New York: Macmillan. Part 2, Ch. 1.

JACKSON, H. 1893. Words and other symbols in mentation. *Med. press circular,* 56, 205–208.

——— 1932. On the nature of the duality of the brain. *In* Taylor, J., editor, Selected writings of Hughlings Jackson. London: Hodder & Stoughton. Vol. 2.

Metropolitan Achievement Tests. Yonkers: World Book Co.

MONRAD-KROHN, G. H. 1947. Dysprosody or disordered melody of language. *Brain,* 70, 405–415.

New Stanford Achievement Tests. Yonkers: World Book Co.

NIELSEN, J. M. 1946. Aphasia, apraxia, and agnosia (2nd ed.). New York: Paul Hoeber.

STRAUSS, A. A., and LEHTINEN, L. E. 1947. Psychopathology and education of the brain-injured child. New York: Grune and Stratton.

TIEGS, E. W., and CLARK, W. W. Progressive achievement tests. Los Angeles: S. Calif. Sch. Book Depository.

WEISENBURG, T., and McBRIDE, K. 1935. Aphasia. New York: Commonwealth Fund.

WELLS, F. L., and RUESCH, J. 1945. Mental examiners handbook (2nd ed.). New York: Psychological Corporation. 48–50.

WEPMAN, J. M. 1951. Recovery from aphasia. New York: Ronald Press.

# CHAPTER 13

# CORRELATES OF APHASIA IN ADULTS

• *Jon Eisenson, Ph.D.*

## NEUROLOGICAL CORRELATES

### Etiology

APHASIA IS ETIOLOGICALLY associated with damage to cerebral tissue. This does not mean that all persons with brain damage suffer from aphasia. It does mean that persons suffering from aphasic language disturbances are presumed to have brain damage.

The possible causes of cerebral damage with which aphasic disturbances are associated are many and varied. They include direct trauma by externally applied force, tumors, cerebral vascular lesions (embolisms, thromboses, aneurysms, hemorrhages), infectious diseases affecting brain tissue and degenerative diseases invading the brain. Of the factors just enumerated the vascular disturbances, embolisms, hemorrhages, and thromboses are the most frequent etiological associates during times of peace. Brain traumas resulting from head injuries, and brain penetrations from high-velocity missiles, are increased factors during war, both for the civilian and military population.

We may assume unanimity among workers in the field—neurosurgeons, neurologists, psychologists, and speech pathologists—only on the issue that aphasic patients all have brain damage. Beyond this, unanimity is not to be anticipated. Differences are to be expected as to the significance of the site, the cerebral dominance of the patient, and the extent and the type of lesion. Problems relative to the physical health of the individual and his personality prior to the onset of the disturbance are felt by some workers to be important factors related to the etiology and persistence of aphasic disturbances. Some of the areas of controvery, and their implications for therapy, will be considered in this chapter.

### Localization of Language Function

The literature on the subject of localization of brain function, and the effects of brain lesion on such localization, is long, frequently contradictory and except perhaps from the viewpoint of the individual interpreting his own findings, is likely to be inconclusive. Among contemporary investigators, the points of view continue to be diverse and extreme. One extreme point of view contends that specific lesions of the cortex are almost invariably associated with specific language dysfunctions. Henschen and Nielsen are among those who believe in strict localizations. At the other extreme are those who believe that the human brain cortex has very little localization relative to language function. They hold that language is a function of the brain as a whole, and that the effects of a specific lesion can be understood only insofar as the specific lesion modifies this general function. Foremost among the 'nonlocalizationists" is Kurt Goldstein. In between these extremes are some who are more moderate and take the general stand that language function may be localized in many areas, but in certain areas more than in others. Among the moderates we might include Hughlings Jackson, Henry Head, and Weisenburg and McBride.

The space limitations of this text do not permit the inclusion of a survey of the vast literature of localization theory as related to language function. The interested reader may find excellent surveys in Volume I of Henry Head's monumental work (1926) and in the first chapter of Weisenburg and McBride (1935). The attempt of this writer will be to present contemporary points of view and the implications of some of the older as well as the more recent investigations relative to therapy with aphasic patients.

## Early Localizationists

*Broca.* Present-day localization theory relative to aphasic disturbances had its origin in the presentation by Paul Broca of two papers in Paris in 1861.[1] At first Broca postulated that a lesion in the second or third frontal convolution was associated with aphasia of the motor (expressive) type. Later, Broca fixed the third convolution as the site of the lesion associated with expressive (spoken) disturbances of language function. This is the area which is included in Brodmann area 44.[2]

Other names prominent among the early localizationsts and "diagram-makers" are Bastian and Wernicke. Bastian (1880) went beyond Broca, and localized areas for auditory and visual functions. Wernicke (1874) located and described an auditory center in the temporal convolution.

## Contemporary Localizationists

*Nielsen.* The name of Dr. J. M. Nielsen is foremost among contemporary exponents of localization theory. He is, however, not as rigid and pedantic localizationist as is Henschen. Nielsen (1941, p. 227), for example, ad-

[1] An English translation of the original Broca article by J. Kann appeared in the *Speech Hearing Disorders,* 15, 1950, pp. 16–20.
[2] Brodmann divided and "diagrammed" the human cerebral cortex into areas according to cellular distribution. These have come to be known as Brodmann's cyto-rchitectonic areas.

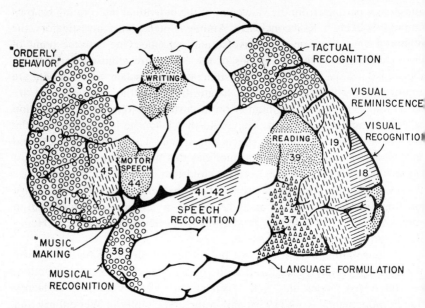

FIG. 1. Composite diagram of the supposed "association" areas of the human cerebral cortex. Many neurologists believe that the cortex functions in some such way as indicated; some do not. The scheme is worth while mainly to provide hypotheses for further research and to help in thinking about the role of the cortex in learning and memory. (From Morgan, C. T., and Stellar, E. 1950. Physiological psychology (2nd ed.). New York: McGraw-Hill, p. 514.)

mits that "Anatomy and physiology are still incompletely co-ordinated so far as the cerebral cortex is concerned." Though aware that ". . . logic would seem to stipulate that each area of a certain structure must have a function differing from that of other areas with different structures . . . ," Nielsen (1941, p. 229) observes that certain areas of the brain (e.g.—area 19 of Brodmann) ". . . [are] certainly divided physiologically." Nielsen (1941, Ch. 10) suggests several explanations for the apparent inconsistencies in localization theory. These include: (1) the possibility that ". . . even though the distribution of the cortical cells is the same throughout an anatomic area, the organization of the cells may be different in various portions of the same area"; (2) neurons establish different connections with use in order to subserve different purposes in the more minute and precise sense; and (3) an area can serve one purpose as a result of one method of training and another purpose as a result of different training.

Despite these reservations, Nielsen accepts localization theory in a comparatively strict sense both in his textbook (1941) and in his more specialized book on disturbances related to aphasia (1947). He lists and describes specific cortical areas and specific dysfunctions which are etiologically associated with lesions in these areas.

*Henschen.* Henschen, whose text on clinical pathology is referred to by Nielsen (1941, p. 306) as "a priceless classic," allowed for no leeway in his structural viewpoint. On the basis of 60 of his own cases and 1500 taken from the literature, Henschen (1926) worked out what he considered to be unfailing one-to-one relationships between defective cortical area and linguistic disturbance. He also specified centers for arithmetic and music.

*Morgan and Stellar.* An interesting composite diagram of the supposed "association" areas of the human cerebral cortex, and what appears to this writer to be a fair and objective attitude toward localization theory, is included in Morgan and Stellar (1950). It is presented here in place of a more conventional summary.

In the concluding paragraph of their section on the cortical areas, Morgan and Stellar (1950) say:

It is hard to tell how much truth there is in these ideas of localization of functions in different areas of the cortex. We can be sure that they are not entirely correct. Yet we cannot wholly reject them. For the time being, whether we accept them or not, we probably should consider them as hypotheses to keep in mind in interpreting further clinical studies and planning research programs in animals.

## Opposition to Strict Localization (the Moderates)

*Hughlings Jackson.* Opposition to the concept of strict localization of language function in specific cortical areas was not absent during the time of Broca and his followers and is vigorously present today. Hughlings Jackson, a chronological contemporary of Broca, was an early and outspoken oppositionist. Jackson emphasized the viewpoint that a knowledge of pathological conditions which disturb and impair language function does not per se provide information as to how the function is normally controlled in the healthy individual. Further, Jackson insisted that aphasic disturbances could not be understood without a knowledge of the patient who suffered the disturbances. He stressed the importance of observing the live aphasic patient rather than studying the autopsy findings of those who did not survive.

Jackson (1915 and 1931) did not deny that Broca's area was frequently damaged in patients who suffered from aphasic disturbances, especially when motor speech involvements were manifest. He refused, however, to localize language function in Broca's area alone, and stressed the notion that language was a psychological rather than physiological function. For language, as for other intellectual functions, the brain operates as a functional unit.

The concept that a destructive lesion can never be responsible for positive symptoms, and the much-quoted principle that "to locate the damage which destroys speech and to locate speech are two different things," were stressed by Jackson. Destruction, Jackson held, produces negative symptoms. Positive symptoms associated with destructions of cortical tissue are to be attributed to the effects of the released activity of the lower centers.

Among other contemporaries of Broca who opposed strict localization were Pierre Marie in France, Arnold Pick in Czechoslovakia, and W. R. Gowers in England. All three agreed with Jackson that while localized lesions could not be held responsible for language and speech disturbances, lesions in certain cortical areas can more readily disturb speech than do lesions in other areas.

*Henry Head.* The English neurologist Henry Head (1926) continued along the clinical, psychological paths of Hughlings Jackson. Head pointed out that the capacity to use language in any form is the result of physiological activities of certain parts of the brain cortex. All forms of language usage develop from the ". . . simple acts of speaking and comprehension of spoken words." Aphasia is defined as ". . . a disorder of symbolic formulation and expression." Symbolic formulation and expression is characterized as a mode of behavior in which some verbal or nonverbal symbol plays a part between the initiation and the execution of the act. Destruction of brain tissue is likely to result in an interference of normal fulfilment of some specific forms of behavior. The reaction which follows is an expression of the organism as a whole to the new situation.

Although Head emphasized the function of the brain as a whole, he observed that, in the event of pathology, certain types of aphasic language dysfunction can probably be associated with lesions in rather broadly outlined areas of the brain. For example, impairments in the capacity to understand the deeper significance of words and the wider meaning of a sentence as a whole (semantic aphasia) seems to be associated with lesions of the supramarginal gyrus. Similarily, Head postulated other likely areas of lesion associated with such subtypes of aphasia as the verbal, syntactical, and nominal. Head emphasized that aphasic disturbances are not discrete and noted that for the aphasic person there is a generalized defect in intellectual expression which requires symbolic formulation. The degree of defect is likely to be directly related to the propositional level of the expression.

*Weisenburg and McBride.* As a result of their clinical and psychological study of aphasic patients, Weisenburg and McBride arrived at a comparatively moderate stand on the issue of localization of function. They accepted relatively fixed localization for such motor and sensory functions as motion vision, hearing, and smell. In regard to intellectual functions such as language usage, however, they said (1935, p. 467):

. . . it is impossible to localize language. In the majority of individuals language permeates the thought processes to such an extent that the one cannot be separated from the other; and for the present at least it is impossible to give an adequate explanation of intelligence, much less to localize it. That it is the result of the activity of the entire brain, however, there is no doubt.

Weisenburg and McBride do not deny that lesions in certain parts of the brain are more likely to be associated with aphasic disturbances than are lesions elsewhere. Although they avoid specific localization, they observe that (1935, p. 468):

. . . in about 95 per cent of the cases the lesion must be in the dominant hemisphere; and that it must implicate the anterior and to a less extent the posterior part of the brain within certain limits, including the lower portion of the pre central convolution and probably the adjoining part of the frontal lobe, the lower portion of the parietal lobe, the upper part of the temporal lobe, and the anterior part of the occipital.

Weisenburg and McBride divided their patients into four clinical types on the basis of predominant linguistic disturbances. For patients whose greatest difficulty is in expression, they found the lesion to be in the anterior or motor part of the brain; for patients with predominantly receptive (comprehension) difficulty, they found the posterior part of the brain more involved than in the expressive group, and a likelihood that the anterior part of the brain was also involved, but less severely than for the expressive patients. Patients with almost equal amounts of expressive and receptive difficulties were found to have more extensive and more permanent involvements of both anterior and posterior parts of the brain. Amnesic patients—those whose difficulty was in recall of names with relatively good ability to recognize the names not able to be recalled—were found to have no definitely localizable lesions.

### Recent Research

Opponents to strict localization theory can find support for their views in some recent research findings. Although the persons engaged in the research were not always primarily interested in language function per se, some of their observations have direct bearing on the problem.

Mettler and his associates—a team of workers which included neurosurgeons, psychiatrists, neurophysiologists, and psychologists—carried on a study of a group of patients who were subjected to bilateral topectomies or "standard lobotomies." Although they were not primarily concerned with the problem of aphasia, two of their cases had surgery which included bilateral removal of Broca's area. In regard to these cases, Mettler says (1949, pp. 433–434): "Our two cases . . . of bilateral removal of Broca's area militate against the views (a) that destruction of the left Broca's area in right-handed individuals necessarily results in anarthria or motor aphasia: and (b) that the opposite Broca's area takes over function. Mettler (p. 195) notes that one of the patients who had been mute several months prior to having Broca's area removed bilaterally ". . . began to speak about one month after operation and spoke clearly and distinctly." Of the other patient, described as being extremely verbal, who had Brodmann's area 44 (Broca's area) removed bilaterally, Mettler (pp. 194–195) observes that she began to speak immediately after recovery from anesthesia and that "no traces of aphasic disturbance could be detected."

Penfield and Rassmussen (1950), working with epileptic patients, observed that as a consequence of electrical stimulation of areas of the brain cortex, either arrest of speech (difficulty in speaking applied to all words alike) or vocalization may be produced. Two of these areas are the (bilateral) Rolandic and superior frontal areas. In addition: "Outside these Rolandic and superior frontal vocalization areas, interference with speech was pro-

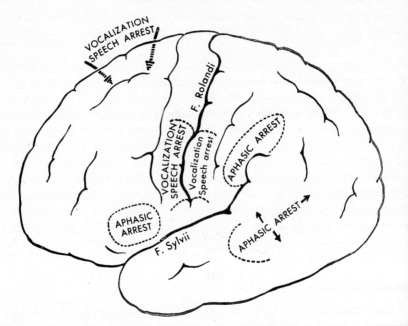

FIG. 2. Summary of areas in which stimulation may interfere with speech or produce vocalization in the dominant hemisphere. Speech interference produced by stimulation of the superior intermediate frontal area within the longitudinal fissure has in certain cases produced evidence of aphasia rather than simple arrest, an observation that calls for further study. (From Penfield, W. and Rasmussen, T. 1950. The cerebral cortex of man. New York: Macmillan, p. 107.)

duced by stimulation in three cortical areas of the dominant hemisphere —frontal, parietal, and temporal."

It should be pointed out that Penfield and Rasmussen were observing epileptic patients, so that the implications of their findings may not pertain to normal patients who suffer permanent brain lesions. Nevertheless, the possibility that the effects of a brain lesion on aphasic disturbances may vary with the individual patient is one that suggests itself (Fig. 2).

Blatt (1950) studied a group of seventeen male veterans in a Veterans Administration Hospital. All of the patients had unilateral lesions such as tumors, healed abscesses, and cortical cicatrices which were localized on the basis of surgical findings, pneumoencephalography, and angiography. (Patients classified as suffering from recent cranio-cerebral trauma or from pathology of the cerebral blood vessels were eliminated from the Blatt study.) None of the subjects was mentally defective, psychotic, or otherwise suffering from disease. Blatt considered 48 aphasic signs as a basis for possible correlation with localized lesion. Using the Eisenson test, *Examining for Aphasia*, Blatt found that 26 signs predicted for the cortical areas were confirmed while 22 of the expected signs were not confirmed. He concluded that: ". . . the predicative value of using psychological tests alone in localizing the exact site of a brain lesion is questionable."

## Extreme Opposition to Localization

*Kurt Goldstein.* There is probably no present-day neurologist or psychologist who is more vigorous in his opposition to localization theory than is Goldstein (1948). Among his stated objections are the following (1948, p. 47):

The so-called classic theory of localization is based mainly on the material gained from postmortems. It should be observed that the objections against the theory stem first from a more careful consideration of the *pathologic-anatomic* data. There are so-called negative cases: on the one hand, absence of symptoms in a lesion affecting an area which was considered characteristic of this locality; on the other hand, appearance of symptoms wthout the presence of a correspondingly localized lesion.

Goldstein, however, does more than present a negative attitude toward localization. He discusses in his writings some of the positive factors which make strict localization theory difficult for him to entertain (1948, p. 48):

It is very difficult, indeed, to evaluate the degree of damage; it is not only dependent on the direct destruction of the nerve cells but also on the condition of the glia, blood vessels, etc. Further, we have no idea of the relationship between a definite anatomic condition and a specific performance. *We are far from being able to decide whether the preserved tissue is still functioning sufficiently to allow for a certain performance or not.*

On the question of the inconsistency of symptoms as related to local brain injury, Goldstein holds (1948, p. 48):

Whether certain symptoms will appear or not on account of a local injury certainly depends on many factors other than locality: i.e., on the nature of the disease process, on the damage of all or only some structures of the cortex, on the condition of the rest of the brain, on individual differences in co-operation of both hemispheres, . . . on the state of circulation in general, on the functional reactions of the organism to the defect . . . on the psycho-physical constitution of the personality, etc.

A very important point relative to the effects of a lesion is made by Goldstein. He points out that "A lesion of a special locality in different cases may vary very much regarding the degree to which the substratum in general is affected, and particularly its different striata. Such a selective character of the process may be of paramount significance for the development of symptoms (1948, pp. 47–48).

Goldstein's interpretation of localization is best understood in terms of Gestalt psychology which emphasizes the function of the organism as a whole and the effects of a specific performance only as it is related to the organism functioning as a whole. With this in mind, it becomes possible to appreciate Goldstein's concept of cortical localization: ". . . *each performance is due to the function of the total organism in which the brain plays a particular role.* In each performance, the whole cortex is in activity, but the excitation in the cortex is not the same throughout (1948, p. 50).

From the above, it would appear that Goldstein does not completely reject cortical localization. Actually, he redefines localization in terms which are consistent with his own thinking. For Goldstein, localization is acceptable only in so far as an individual performance is considered. The role of a given cortical area is significant according to the particular influence it exerts on the excitation of the cortex as a whole, and so as to the total dynamic process which occurs as a result of the functioning of the entire nervous system.

With this concept of localization, Goldstein is able to accept and define symptom complexes as being related to definite areas. Indeed, for practical purposes, Goldstein and Weisenburg and McBride are in agreement. Goldstein accepts the likelihood that a motor (expressive) language disturbance will usually be correctly localized in the expanded Broca's region of the left hemisphere and that sensory (receptive) disturbances will usually be correctly located in the temporal lobes.

## Summary of Thinking Opposed to Strict Localization Theory

Present-day opposition to strict localization theory relative to language function and its breakdown come from many sources and for diverse reasons. Some of these include:

1. Observations that patients with similar lesions do not always suffer from the same defect.
2. Observations that the same defects may be associated with lesions in different parts of the brain.
3. Failure of clinicians to recognize and appreciate the existence of symptoms other than the ones with which a specific lesion is allegedly associated.
4. Failure of clinical findings—including those of autopsies—consistently to substantiate the pathological predictions of localizationists.
5. Failure of the localizationists to appreciate the varying effects of brain pathology associated with physical and psychological premorbid factors in the individual.
6. Failure of research workers to find consistent deviations through the use of psychological instruments among patients presumed to have the same cortical involvements.
7. Failure, in general, to differentiate through the use of psychological instruments among patients with presumptive damage to specific and different areas of the brain.[3]

The point of view of the author relative to localization is one which accepts the thesis of Hughlings Jackson, Henry Head, and others, that normally language reception, formulation, and expression are *functions of the brain as a whole.* Under normal conditions, broadly outlined areas of the brain exercise more or less specialized influences relative to language reception, the selection and formulation of symbols, and the expression of these symbols in the various ways and for the various purposes for which linguistic symbols may be used.

Under conditions of pathology involving the cerebral cortex, language

[3] Recent literature on the subject is reviewed by Klebanoff, Singer, and Wilensky (1954), and Milner (1954).

function may be disrupted. Where language is disrupted, for clearly right-handed persons, the lesion may regularly be expected to be in the left cerebral hemisphere. Beyond this, no consistent correlation can be found between site of lesion and type of language dysfunction (Eisenson, 1947). In general, however, the broad regional localizations of Weisenburg and McBride seem to be acceptable.

## Implications for Therapy

*Strict Localization.* Neurologists who, like Nielsen, are strict localizationists and who are interested in therapy, assume logically that during the course of therapy the minor (nondominant) area of the brain takes over the function of the injured dominant area. In Nielsen's writings (1941, pp. 276–277) we find such statements as: "It is evident that the minor area of Broca is more difficult to train than is the minor area of Wernicke." And, perhaps more significantly, he says: "All of our hope in retraining aphasics depends on the functional capacity of the minor cerebral hemisphere."

Consistent with this point of view is the concept that learning consists in the formation of engrams in different parts of the cerebral cortex. These engrams—or brain tracings—are destroyed as a result of brain pathology. With retraining, engrams are formed in the corresponding areas of the noninjured hemisphere. As engrams are formed on the minor side, function is restored.

*Nonlocalizationists.* In contrast with this point of view relative to therapy, the nonlocalizationists hold that training influences and affects the activity of the entire noninjured or remaining healthy cortical tissue. Wepman (1951, p. 18), who accepts this point of view, presents the following as his working principle:

> *Aphasic language disorders are considered as affecting all the language modalities and cannot be limited to specific language skills. The recovery process must include a program leading to reintegration of the activity of the cortex and not to specific skills . . . recovery follows reintegration of the remaining cortical tissue into a functioning whole.*

## Cerebral Dominance and Laterality

**The development of cerebral dominance.** By the time an individual has become an adult, cerebral dominance is normally established. Such dominance tends to be the same for most or all of the individual's sensory and motor functions. Mixed dominance, however, is by no means unique. Many persons may, for example, be right-handed and left-eyed. Some have been found to be left-footed, left-handed, and right-eyed. It is not unusual to find preference for the use of the left ear in right-handed persons. In short, though there is a general tendency toward unilaterality of function, mixed laterality is not unusual.

*Degree of Dominance.* Dominance need not be an all-or-none affair. Not only is there evidence of mixed dominance, but there are obviously differences in degree of dominance. Persons who are referred to as *ambidextrous* have more nearly equal capacity for both hands than do clearly right-handed or left-handed persons. Most left-handed persons, however, can use their right hands with greater dexterity than right-handed persons can use their left hands.

*The Establishment of Dominance.* How dominance is established is still a moot question. Dominance is either congenital or acquired. If it is congenital, we may still look upon the development of dominance as something the individual is predisposed to, but which may be altered by environmental influences. If cerebral dominance is thought to be acquired, then its acquisition must be attributed entirely to environmental influences. The relative "normality" of right-handedness, and right laterality in general in the Western world would then have to be ascribed to the influences in Western culture which tend to make persons right-sided. This is essentially the point of view of Blau (1946, p. 181), who holds that "Dextrality is a cultural and not an organic heritage." Persons become left-brain dominant because they yield to the influences in their culture which encourage greater use of the right side than of the left in the handling of tools and instruments. The infant has no lateral preferences. Preferences appear only after the infant has engaged in certain activities and has learned certain skills.

Preferred laterality begins to appear at about 9 months and is not definitely established until about 1½ to 2 years. This is the age when the first peak of postnatal neurological maturation takes place. However, preferred laterality is not completely formed at this point, but continues to develop until childhood and even later. The incidence of dextrality in children increases with age as they are exposed to more and more educational and cultural influences (Blau, 1946, p. 182).

**Left-laterality (sinistrality).** Right laterality, either because of inheritance, predisposition, or training, is the expected normal development. Left-sidedness, then, needs to be explained as a deviation from the expected norm. Possible explanations include the following: (1) atypical formation of the left cerebral hemisphere prevents the development of right laterality; (2) a physical defect of an organ or organs on the right side compels use of the corresponding organ or organs on the left; (3) imitation of another person who is left-sided; (4) emotional negativism expressing itself in the child in the use of the left hand;[4] (5) and finally there is the possibility that in identical twins, the left "mirror-image" member has a cerebrum which predisposes the twin to left-sidedness.[5]

One may believe that left cerebral dominance is usually predetermined on a genetic basis or that a person is born without cerebral dominance but with a brain ready for training so that the establishment of dominance is deter-

---

[4] Blau (1946, p. 183) holds that "This is probably the most common type of sinistrality—the product of an emotional contrariness in early childhood."

[5] The possibility of negativism expressing itself in one member of identical twins cannot be altogether overlooked.

mined by, instead of a determinant of, function. Regardless of the point of view, the fact remains that by the time most children begin to talk, right laterality is the rule, and left cerebral dominance is generally assumed.

A review of the literature indicates that there is little disagreement as to the role of the left cerebral hemisphere in right-handed persons and its significance for language function. The left cerebral hemisphere is accepted as the "dominant" hemisphere. By "dominant" most persons interested in the subject mean the cerebral hemisphere in which special areas for speech elaboration are located.

Most observers agree that though left-sided brain injury is not always followed by the production of aphasic symptoms in right-handed persons, when such symptoms do appear, injury to the left brain hemisphere is present.

*The findings for left-handed persons* are by no means as consistent or clear. For example, Penfield and Rasmussen (1950, p. 96) observed that ". . . among left-handed people speech may have its representation in either the right or the left hemisphere."

An implication along the same line for left-handed persons is made by Grinker and Bucy (1951) who hold that "Aphasia and related conditions result from lesions of the left cerebral hemisphere in true right-handed individuals and of the right hemisphere in some left-handed persons."

In a recent study, Humphrey and Zangwill (1952) selected ten World War II cases of unilateral brain lesion in "naturally left-handed patients of good intelligence" for special study. All of the patients had suffered penetrating brain wounds. Five of the patients had lesions of the left and five of the right cerebral hemisphere. Humphrey and Zangwill found that aphasia was present in all cases of left-hemisphere lesion and in four of the five cases of right lesion. The left-hemisphere cases had more severe aphasic involvements than did the righ-hemisphere cases. Defects of calculation, however, were more prominent among the right-hemisphere lesion patients.

Wepman (1951, p. 81), after reviewing the recent literature and his own data relative to the role of the so-called dominant hemisphere, offers the following tentative conclusion: "It is suggested . . . that only the left cerebral hemisphere in all people is concerned with language on the symbolic level . . . in other words, that speech and language may be the function of the left hemisphere of the cortex only."

Wepman is careful to distinguish between aphasic disturbances (language disturbances on the symbolic level) and dysarthric (articulatory) disturbances. The latter may occur with damage to the right hemisphere. Occasionally, aphasic-like disturbances do follow right cortical lesion, but these are likely to be of a temporary nature.

The author's observations of his own patients coincide, essentially, with those of Wepman for all cases where the cortical lesion was of traumatic origin. For patients with nontraumatic lesions of the cortex, the picture does not seem to be as clear. But even for these patients, if we assume the preferred hand to be an index of dominance, relatively few left-handed persons with right-sided brain lesions appear to be truly aphasic. On the other hand, at least two patients who believed themselves to be left-handed and who used their left hands for writing did become aphasic following cerebral thrombosis with right hemiplegia. This observation is in general agreement with that of Weisenburg and McBride to the effect that: "The dominance indicated by handedness is a criterion of the crucial hemisphere for speech in about 95 per cent of cases." (1935, p. 452).

**The role of the nondominant hemisphere in right-handed persons.** One of the striking behavior characteristics of aphasic patients is the comparatively well-retained capacity to evoke affectively laden speech content. Hughlings Jackson, more than three-quarters of a century ago, held that emotional expressions are the function of the nondominant (right) side of the brain. Similarly, we may assume that other "lower language functions," such as serial speech, singing, and the reproduction of thoroughly memorized language content are controlled by the nondominant hemisphere and so are usually more available to the aphasic patient than propositional speech. Although this concept of the role of the nondominant hemisphere was met with considerable opposition when first announced by Jackson, it is now rather generally accepted as the explanation for the observation that expressive aphasic patients are "not wordless but speechless."

Weisenburg and McBride believe that the nondominant hemisphere has functions other than that of the control of affective speech. They compared 22 cases of patients with right-sided cerebral lesions without aphasia with a group of matched normals and found that the brain-injured patients ". . . showed distinct mental deterioration, which is not at all like that found in aphasia . . ." and concluded that ". . . the nondominant hemisphere is apparently concerned with normal language function; but to a limited degree" (1935, p. 453).

Goldstein is inclined to accept the point of view that the nondominant hemisphere plays a role which makes it differ in degree rather than in kind from that of the dominant hemisphere. Goldstein (1948, p. 53) holds that directly after birth and during the first years both cerebral hemispheres act together in all functions: ". . . the whole brain cortex represents a unitary apparatus in which functional differentiation between the two hemispheres does not exist." The development of dominance of one hemisphere takes place while higher mental functions are being developed. After one hemisphere has gained dominance, all new performances are related to the dominant hemisphere so that, as Goldstein (1948, p. 54) puts it, ". . . the difference between the two hemispheres becomes increasingly more outspoken." It should be emphasized, however, that the "minor" hemisphere does not ever totally give up its functions to the "major" hemisphere, so that differences are always quantitative rather than qualitative and vary according to different performances.

**The nondominant hemisphere and restoration of function.** The role of the nondominant hemisphere in the event of restoration of function—spontaneous or occurring during a therapeutic program—cannot be definitely determined. It is generally assumed, however, that the minor (nondominant) hemisphere assumes or takes control of functions from the damaged major (dominant) hemisphere. Workers as diverse in their points of view as Nielsen (1947, p. 155) and Goldstein (1948, p. 53) are on common ground in their belief that "The minor cerebral hemisphere assumes the function of the major in language with great facility in some instances, with difficulty in others, and not at all in some persons." We do not know what the factors are which permit virtually complete assumption of functions in some instances, and virtually no assumption in others. In those comparatively rare cases where an entire cerebral hemisphere is destroyed and where some degree of function is restored, it is apparent that restoration of function is a result of the activity of the remaining cortical tissue. It is possible also that persons with "incomplete" dominance may have more facility in the taking over of function by the minor hemisphere than would be the case with individuals having strong or complete one-sided dominance.[6] Another possibility is that dominance need not be unilateral for all cerebral functions, and so what is assumed to be a taking over of function is actually only a resumption of function after the generalized effects of trauma have worn off or have been significantly reduced (Eisenson, 1947).

## PSYCHOLOGICAL CORRELATES

Earlier in this chapter it was pointed out that not all persons who incur damage to the dominant cerebral hemisphere become aphasic. Further, it has been observed by this author (Eisenson, 1947) and others, that the known extent of brain damage is of little use in predicting how much disturbance an individual will suffer, or what bearing the extent of damage will have on the progress and improvement of the aphasic. It would be helpful to know what factors, other than brain damage to the dominant hemisphere, are associated with the likelihood that a person will become aphasic. Is there a pre-aphasic personality? Does level or type of intelligence make a difference? Is education a contributing factor? Does imagery type affect the outcome? These are questions for which there are no definitive answers. To get such answers, a controlled experimental situation would have to be set up with a population exposed to environmental risks likely to result in head injury and brain damage. Pretesting for personality traits and types and for the other factors suggested would have to be done. Then, after the inevitable brain damage, correlations could be made which should reveal to us whether positive, negative, or no relationships exist between any psychological factors

---

[6] This is the point of view of the Russian psychologist, Alexandria Luria, cited in Wepman (1951, p. 12).

and aphasic disturbances following brain damage. As far as this writer knows, there have been no such controlled experimental studies. Some workers in the field have, however, exercised clinical judgments. These, for what they may be worth, will now be considered.

## Personality

Goldstein (1948, p. 48), it was pointed out earlier, argued that whether certain symptoms will appear or not following a brain injury depends upon a number of factors, one of which is the "psycho-physical constitution of the personality." Unfortunately, Goldstein does not elaborate on the premorbid personality or behavioral characteristics of the aphasic. The author believes that such traits as rigidity and tendencies toward concretism are premorbid characteristics of many, but not of all, persons who become aphasic. This conjecture is made as a result of conversations he has had with parents, wives, and other relatives of young aphasic persons who suffered penetrating wounds in combat and became aphasic, and with relatives of older aphasics who suffered vascular brain insults. The so-called "organic personality" is not a result of brain damage per se. It is, rather, the effect of brain damage on a person with premorbid tendencies to behave as he comes to behave. It is likely that prior to the onset of the effects of brain damage, the same tendencies were present. The individual, having some awareness of these tendencies, or at least of his being different from other persons in his environment, exercised special effort to make acceptable adjustments. The effect of the brain damage on the individual is probably to reduce his capacity to make the necessary adjustments, or to reduce the drive to overcome latent undesirable behavioral inclinations.

Rigidity and concretism, though frequently associated with withdrawal behavior, may also be discovered in aggressive and openly hostile persons. The general effect of brain damage, this writer believes, is to make more readily apparent all undesirable behavioral traits. Thus, tendencies become exaggerated and the latent becomes the actual. Essentially, then, the so-called "organic personality" is what he might have been in any event. Wepman (1951, p. 88), recognizing this in his aphasic patients, observes:

> It also seems more and more apparent that the patient's reported on did not develop a so-called "organic personality," but rather seemed to possess and to project the same basic personalities they had in their premorbid condition. The major sign of change was not in their personality type but in the manner in which it was projected.

## Imagery

About seventy years ago Charcot observed that persons with essentially the same neurological defects nevertheless frequently behaved differently. To account for these divergencies in behavior, Charcot theorized that there were different kinds of individuals according to predominant imagery. The predominant imagery of the individual determines the nature of his inner speech. Thus, for some persons, inner speech consists of motor images, for others of visual images, and for still others, inner speech consists mostly of auditory images.

A person who has incurred brain damage in his auditory center would be likely to suffer from considerably more impairment if he were auditorally minded than if he were visually or motor-minded. In contrast, a visual-minded person would suffer more from brain damage to the visual center than he would if the damage were in the motor or auditory center. Charcot apparently assumed imagery type to be innate. We need not make such an assumption. It is conceivable that a person can become a given imagery type as a result of training. The immediate effect of brain damage, if it is in a so-called center which is positively related to the individual's imagery type—innate or developed as a result of training by a teacher, parent, or other environmental influence—is to disturb inner speech and produce aphasic manifestations. When there is no positive relation between sensory area of damage and imagery type, aphasic impairment may be much less severe.

## Intelligence

During World War II, the writer obtained the impression from studying pre-injury records of army personnel, that there was a disproportionate number of persons with high intelligence among the aphasics. He gathered data at two Army General Hospitals which were neurosurgical centers. Army General Classification Scores[7] of 69 aphasic patients were distributed as follows: Grade I—5; II—25; III—25; IV—13; V—1.

From these figures it may be noted that 55 of the patients were average or better in intelligence and only 14 were in the below-average group. Perhaps of greater significance is the observation that 30 of the patients were above-average and, of this number, five were in the superior grade. This compares with 13 in the dull-normal group and only one in the definitely below-average group.

At the present time, based on his experience with civilian patients, the writer's early impression has been strengthened. It is his belief that persons of above-average intelligence are more likely to suffer from aphasic disturbances following brain damage than are persons of below-average intelligence. It is possible, of course, that the factor of intelligence is related to many others in regard to the effects of brain damage. Language ability is in itself known to be positively related to intelligence. Awareness of disturbance to language ability may create anxieties on the part of the more intelligent which less intelligent persons may not experience. The anxiety may perhaps be an important factor in the failure of the patient to make a rapid and

---

[7] The lower the grade the higher the score. These grades roughly approximate intelligence groupings as follows: I = superior intelligence; II = above average intelligence; III = average intelligence; IV = dull normal intelligence; V = below average intelligence.

spontaneous recovery. In any event, whether the influence is direct or in-direct, from the point of view of possible aphasic involvement associated with brain damage, above-average intelligence may be included among the premorbid factors associated with aphasic disturbance for persons with cortical pathology.[8]

## Educational Achievement

Of a group of 64 aphasic patients with traumatic brain damage hospital-ized at an Army General Hospital during World War II, 30 were found to have completed 12 years or more of formal education. The distribution of the group as a whole was as follows:

| Years of Education | Aphasic Patients |
|---|---|
| 16 or more (college graduate) | 3 |
| 13 to 15 | 4 |
| 12 (high school graduate) | 23 |
| 9 to 11 | 18 |
| 8 (elementary school graduate) | 9 |
| 6 to 7 | 6 |
| Less than 6 | 1 |
| Total | 64 |

In Wepman's group of 68 aphasics studied at another Army General Hos-pital, 51 had either completed high school or were within the high school range at the time of their completion or interruption of their formal educa-tion (Wepman, 1951).

Since the end of World War II, the writer has seen a large number of aphasics whose pathologies were nontraumatic in origin. His initial impres-sion was reinforced to the effect that aphasics—at least those who do not recover spontaneously—come from the better educated part of the popula-tion. This, of course, is not too surprising because, in general, years of edu-cation and level of intelligence are positively related.

## BIBLIOGRAPHY

BASTIAN, H. 1861. The brain as an organ of the mind. London: Paul, Trench, and Trubner. New York: Appleton, 1896.

BLATT, B. 1950. The problem of language localization into specific brain areas. Unpublished Ph.D. Dissertation. New York Univ.

BLAU, A. 1946. The master hand. New York: Amer. Orthropsychiat. Ass.

BROCA, P. 1861. Remarques sur le siège de la faculté du language articulé, suives, d'une observation d'aphemie. Bull. Soc. Anat. de Paris. Ser. 2, 36, 330–357; and Nouvelles observations d'aphemie produite par une lesion de la moitié posterieure les deuxieme et troisieme circonvolutions frontales. Ibid, 398–407.

EISENSON, J. 1947. Aphasics: observations and tentative conclusions. J. Speech Disorders, 12, 290–292.

[8] It may be of interest to note that a high level of intelligence is not necessarily a poor prognostic factor in terms of expected improvement. Wepman, for example states that a ". . . more successful resolution of the language problem can be expected when I.Q. level at the pre-injury state is found to be high" (Wepman, op. cit., p. 79).

GOLDSTEIN, K. 1948. Language and language disturbances. New York: Grune and Stratton.

GRINKER, R. R., and BUCY, P. C. 1951. Neurology (4th ed.). Springfield, Ill.: C. C. Thomas. P. 410.

HEAD, H. 1926. Aphasia and kindred disorders of speech (2 vols.). New York: Macmillan.

HENSCHEN, S. E. 1926. On the function of the right hemisphere of the brain in relation to the left in speech, music, and calculation. *Brain,* 49, 110–123.

HUMPHREY, M. E., and ZANGWILL, O. I. 1952. Dysphasia in left-handed patients with unilateral brain lesions. *J. Neurol. Neurosurg. Psychiat.,* 15, 184.

JACKSON, H. 1915. Selected writings of J. Hughlings Jackson, H. Head, editor. *Brain,* 38, 1–90.

———— 1931. Selected writings of John Hughlings Jackson, J. Taylor, editor. London: Hodder & Stoughton.

KLEBANOFF, S. G., SINGER, J. L., and WILENSKY, H. 1954. Psychological consequences of brain lesions and ablations. *Psychol. Bull.,* 51, 1–42.

METTLER, F. A., ed. 1949. Selective partial ablation of the frontal cortex. New York: Paul Hoeber.

MILNER, B. 1954. Intellectual function of the temporal lobe. *Psychol. Bull.,* 51, 42–64.

MORGAN, C. T., and STELLAR, E. 1950. Physiological psychology (2nd ed.). New York: McGraw-Hill, p. 516.

NIELSEN, J. M. 1941. A textbook of clinical neurology. New York: Paul Hoeber.

———— 1947. Agnosia, apraxia, aphasia (2nd ed.). New York: Paul Hoeber.

PENFIELD, W., and RASMUSSEN, T. 1950. The cerebral cortex of man. New York: Macmillan, p. 107.

WEISENBURG, T., and MCBRIDE, K. E. 1935. Aphasia. New York: Commonwealth Fund.

WEPMAN, J. 1951. Recovery from aphasia. New York: Ronald Press.

WERNICKE, C. 1874. Der aphasische Symptomencomplex. Breslau.

# CHAPTER 14

# THERAPEUTIC PROBLEMS AND APPROACHES WITH APHASIC ADULTS

● *Jon Eisenson, Ph.D.*

## MOTIVATION

### Need for Motivation

The need for an aphasic patient to improve his linguistic ability is usually so strong that motivation for improvement may ordinarily be expected to come from the patient. This is generally so in the period immediately following awareness of the existence of impairment. Unless values become established that make linguistic improvement less worth while than the maintenance of these values, motivation for language rehabilitation may be assumed. Occasionally a patient may learn that it is possible to impose tyranny without words where tyranny with words could not previously be imposed. Such a patient may, for a short or an indefinite time, resist the reacquisitions of language habits and will require external motivation to modify his attitude toward relearning. One of the advantages of early training is that the patient does not have an opportunity for realizing that there may be values in not using language, so that self-motivation rather than external motivation can function.

As a rule, the problem of motivation, if it occurs at all, is one which begins to take place when the aphasic reaches his first plateau in learning. Then, having relearned some language, and having improved to some extent in communicative, expressive, and comprehension ability, he may require urging to make the necessary effort for further progress. If effort has been great, and progress small, the discouraged patient may prefer not to try but to resort instead to wishful thinking that spontaneous improvement will occur. It is also possible that the patient may accept himself with all his limitations and feel little need for further improvement. This attitude may in fact be nurtured by members of his family, or by his friends, who may over-estimate gains, or who may begin to understand his nonlinguistic behavior or to anticipate his wants and so reduce the need for conventional language usage.

## Degree and Direction of Motivation

Perhaps the most significant problem in regard to motivation is the problem of how much and to what degree. Should the highly educated patient be encouraged to believe that in a short time he may expect to be as linguistically proficient as once he was? Should the engineer, the mathematician, the lawyer, the teacher, or the physician be encouraged to believe that he will again have control of all he once knew and be able to return to his profession? No categorical answer can or should be given to these questions. At the present time we do not know how close to a former level of proficiency in dealing with symbols a given patient can approximate. To promise too much may lead to disappointment and frustration. To promise too little may result in reduction of effort. The approach used by the author is to set up a series of short-term objectives which the patient can recognize, and to raise the sights and the objectives as the individual patient's rate and amount of improvement warrants. To the patient's insistent question, "Will I be able to talk and read and write as well as I once could?", the safest and most honest answer is "We'll see as we go along."

The goals and achievement objectives should be correlated with the overall training program planned for the patient. Questions about the patient's possible vocational training or retraining must be considered and answered. His sensory and motor limitations, if they are likely to be permanent, must necessarily be considered. His past interests, his hobbies, his avocations, must all be evaluated. If a patient, because of permanent motor or sensory disability, cannot possibly resume an occupation, even should complete linguistic recovery be possible, the new vocation, if any, should determine in large part the ultimate objective of the rehabilitative program, and so the degree and direction of motivation.

## Level of Aspiration

It is understandable that most aphasic patients wish to become restored to a previous level of ability in the shortest possible time. Unfortunately, few if any normal persons ever know what level of ability they have. Normal persons may either underestimate or overestimate ability levels. So also may the aphasic patient. It is likely, however, that the aphasic may not appreciate how long it took him to achieve whatever premorbid level he thinks he had attained, and so he may become impatient to be restored to that level. A danger also exists that more often than not the patient will overestimate previously developed abilities and set himself too high an aspiration level for rehabilitation. In language performance this tendency may be expressed in the wish to speak in long sentences and in polysyllabic terminology when short, simple sentences could do as well.

The author has worked with several patients who failed to evoke a common word because they were hunting for more elusive, less frequently used synonyms. Such patients should be encouraged to accept the common words as their immediate objectives, and to postpone gaining control over less frequently used words for a later time. One patient with this tendency was trained by the author to evoke the common (more frequently used) word for a list of synonymous terms. The less frequently used synonym was presented by the author, and the common term by the patient for a list which included the following:

> Lofty . . . . . . . . . . .  high
> Depressed . . . . . . .  sad
> Powerful . . . . . . . .  strong
> Obese  . . . . . . . . . .  fat

In each instance, the patient knew the common word but preferred not to evoke it. Yet he could not readily utter the less frequently used synonym. The author learned what the patient was trying to do, and what he was inhibiting, when the patient finally succeeded in uttering or in writing the elusive word.

The relationship between motivation and level of aspiration is apparent. The role of the therapist in helping the patient modify or reduce, *as an immediate objective,* a very high level of aspiration should be equally apparent.

## Low Aspiration Level

Not infrequently a patient will become apparently satisfied with a relatively low level of achievement. There may be several possible reasons for this tendency. The patient may be one who in his premorbid state never tried particularly hard for any high level of achievement and was easily satisfied with what he could readily do. On the other hand, the patient may be one who reduced his level of aspiration to avoid frustration and repeated experiences of failure. His acceptance of a low-level achievement as an aphasic constitutes a continuation of a pre-injury attitude and conduct pattern. A third possibility is that the aphasic patient has re-evaluated his present assets and liabilities and has reached a decision as to how much language he needs to get along. In arriving at his evaluation, he has included the privileges and exemptions of the physically disabled. His aspiration level is a reflection both of what he expects of himself and what he expects others to do for and about him. Such a patient will require motivation to continue to make new evaluations in terms of amount of improvement. He must have his assets and his potentialities brought to his attention so that his low aspiration level does not become a persistent liability. The clinician should, however, be able to recognize that the acceptance of a low aspiration level may in effect constitute a patient's mechanism for avoiding future failure and frustration. With this awareness, he may be able to help the aphasic patient to accept occasional failure in learning experience as a normal aspect of living as well as of the process of rehabilitation and training.

## CONCRETISM

Earlier it was indicated that the aphasic patient's tendency toward concretism was not found by this author to be as prevalent as other workers in the field have found it to be. Where it exists, it may be an expression of an attitude rather than an inherent aspect of the aphasic's involvement. There is little question, however, that occasionally an aphasic patient does manifest concretism and indicates a preference to deal with situations that touch upon his immediate, personal experiences rather than to assume a more difficult abstract attitude. For the therapist, the tendency toward concretism should constitute an additional challenge. Except with very old patients, concretism as an attitude and a mode of behavior can probably be modified to the patient's advantage in the rehabilitation process.

The author has been successful in modifying aphasic patient's tendencies towards concretism by creating an awareness of such tendencies when they become apparent. If the patient can understand speech, a frank discussion of the implications of concretism—its limitations in relearning and in dealing with the world at large—should be of help.

The therapist should also be aware that concretism as a tendency may be developed by faulty training techniques. If, for example, a therapist working to build up an aphasic's vocabulary has the patient learn to identify and name objects such as a black pencil, a crayon pencil, and an automatic pencil, and fails to emphasize that despite the differences, all the objects are *kinds of pencils,* serve a common function, and are to be called *pencils,* an opportunity to abstract and generalize has been lost. Instead, a patient's tendency to be specific and concrete may be reinforced. In teaching names for objects, situations, or relationships, the therapist should emphasize the generic aspects of the names wherever and whenever the opportunity permits. Thus, a lesson on paper should include different kinds of paper, one on apples should include apples of different size, shape, and color, and so on. All this need not be accomplished in a single teaching session or in a given day. The therapist may confine the teaching to two or three members of a generic family, one during one learning period, and then begin a second period with a statement such as the following: "Yesterday you identified and named an apple when I showed you a red apple (presenting picture or actual apple). Today we have a green apple. It is shaped like the red one, and is about the same size, but it is green. Some apples are red, some are green and others are yellow. In fact, apples may have several different colors or shades."

In re-establishing a patient's naming ability, the therapist should go out of his way to provide manifold stimulation for the name category. This means that the therapist's "bag of tricks" must be large, and the individual items must be changed quite frequently so that the associations the patient makes will not be limited to a single item under a general category. Specifically, not one comb but several combs of various sizes, shapes, and colors should be included to establish not only the *name* comb but the *concept* comb as well. So with other objects such as forks, books, brushes, and so on. The generic term should be taught as well as the specific term. It is the therapist's task to direct the patient's attention to why, *despite some differences, essential similarities make things belong to the same category and call for their having the same family name.*

Although the discussion above dealt with object-naming, the principle is intended for naming in general. Relationships, representations, and situations in general which have either common or proper names can be similarly presented so that specific as well as generic names are learned at the earliest possible time. If this is done it is likely that a patient's tendency, if it exists, to be concrete-minded will be discouraged. Moreover, the therapist himself will avoid training the patient in a manner which might help to establish a concrete attitude that otherwise would not exist.

## PERSEVERATION

Earlier it was indicated that the perseverating tendency was probably the most frequently found characteristic of persons with organic brain involvement. Perseveration was defined as the tendency for an act of behavior to persist or remount into consciousness spontaneously after it has once occurred. We can understand the significance of the perseverating tendency and will be better able to deal with it therapeutically if we have some insight into the dynamics of perseverations.

In general, perseveration may be thought of as a disturbance of volition. Perseveration becomes manifest when the usually potent tendencies for a given performance task are somehow blocked, diverted in some way by an inhibiting event or idea, or completely overcome by an interfering (previously performed or entertained) act or idea. Landis and Bolles (1950) explain the perseverating tendency as follows:

> The perseverating individual attempts to respond (there is a tendency toward a genuine decision); he attempts to carry out the required act (there is a tendency to voluntary action); but the act does not succeed because the favoring circumstances for goal achievement (or of insufficient motivation) are lacking. Hence, the previously executed activity is maintained in a repetitive, secondary fashion. The continuing behavior is carried on automatically in the form which is most readibly available, but without the formation of a new determining tendency.

Normal persons tend to perseverate when they are fatigued; they also tend to perseverate under conditions which demand more rapid and more frequent change than they can achieve. Epileptic persons increase their frequency of perseveration after seizures. Perseveration, in general, may be the human mechanism's way of reacting to situations which demand adaptations and call for responses which the individual is not capable, momentarily or chronically, of making. If the failure to make the adaptation is momentary, the repetition of a previous act which requires little or no conscious effort

ffords the individual opportunity to select or to organize a new response
vhich he hopes is appropriate. If, for organic or psychogenic reasons, the
nability to make ready adaptations is chronic, the repetition of a response
lls a void which would exist if no response were made. The individual,
ware that some response is expected, repeats an old response to avoid the
mbarrassment of failing to make any response. In general, perseveration
aay be regarded as a manifestation of inadequacy on the part of the per-
ormer. When the aphasic patient perseverates, he is in effect saying, "I am
ot able to do what is expected, so I am doing something I have previously
one which was appropriate. I hope it is better than doing nothing." Beyond
nis, however, he is saying something which is of greater significance to the
nerapist. He is signaling that the therapist's demands, at the given moment
n the given situation, are excessive. It becomes the problem of the therapist
o discover why the demands are excessive, and to modify them in keeping
vith the aphasic's present abilities.

The first recommended step for the therapist is to present a situation to
ne patient for which the perseverated act is appropriate. If, for example,
 patient has named one of series of objects correctly and then, because of
nability to name a new object, repeats the name of a previous one, that one
nould again be presented. The response then becomes appropriate. Then
ne therapist should review the series up to the point where perseveration
ad occurred. At this point the therapist should himself offer the name and
sk for the patient to repeat it. If blocking or perseveration reoccurs, the
erapist should again call for a previously successful naming performance
nd put aside for a later time the learning of the new object. It is then usually
ise for the therapist to change the situation and the type of task required
 that the patient's inadequacy will not be recalled and so interfere with
w learning or relearning. In reply to my question, "What is the significance
 perseveration in a learning situation?" a recovered aphasic told me, "It
eans that the therapist is not aware of what is going on with the patient.
ood therapy avoids the need for perseveration. When it occurs, the thera-
st has failed to do a good job."

Although perseveration cannot always be avoided, awareness on the part
 the therapist that his patient is showing signs of fatigue, irritability, or dis-
terest will go a long way to reducing its incidence. Moderation of pace,
 a change of activity, frequently will be all that is needed to eliminate
rseveration when it becomes evident, or to prevent the need for it to be-
me evident.

## THE CATASTROPHIC RESPONSE

The *catastrophic response* may be characterized as a "psychobiological
eakdown" involving the organism as a whole in a situation where a suc-
ssful performance does not seem possible. Vascular changes, irritability,
asiveness, or aggressiveness may precede or accompany the catastrophic

response. An extreme catastrophic response may take the form of a loss of consciousness. The dynamics of the catastrophic response are comparable to those of perseverating behavior. The patient is revealing inadequacy and a wish to avoid the need to make a response. If a way out is not available and escape from the situation, psychological or physical, is not permitted, the catastrophic response may occur. Frequently, it will be preceded by perseverating behavior. Some patients resort to catastrophic behavior more immediately and more frequently than do others. It is the author's belief that these patients are ones who, prior to brain insult, were likely to resort to psychosomatic symptoms such as headache or fatigue to avoid difficult or demanding situations.

The significance of the catastrophic response for the therapist is essentially the same as that of perseveration. If it occurs during the course of therapy the catastrophic response signifies that the therapist's demands, at the given moment, have exceeded the patient's ability in producing an appropriate response. Reduced demand or change of activity is indicated. It is best, of course, to avoid an extreme catastrophic response if this can be done. Alertness to signs of irritability, such as apparent disinterest, sweating, or excessive eye-blinking, should serve as cues to the therapist that the patient is finding the situation, or the changing situations, too difficult for his adaptive abilities. A brief recess in which a cigarette may be smoked, or a piece of candy eaten, or casual conversation undertaken, may be all that is needed to avoid pushing the patient into a catastrophic manifestation. Once the catastrophic response has been resorted to, a sensitive patient may need considerable time as an ego-saving measure. If he is not sensitive, there is danger that the patient will become consciously aware of a device he may use in the future to avoid difficult situations. In a large measure, the manifestation of the catastrophic response, as well as of perseveration, reveals failure on the part of the therapist to recognize the needs and abilities of his patient as well as inadequacy on the part of the patient to meet the needs of his situation.

## PSYCHOTHERAPY

### The Place of Psychotherapy

There is probably less question as to the aphasic patient's need for psychotherapy than there is as to whether and how this need can be met. It is fairly obvious that any individual whose thinking and communicative ability has been disturbed and who has awareness of these disturbances must reorient and readjust himself to the modifications which they impose. Any person deprived of a means of being economically self-supporting, or who is able to continue only with the help of others to whom he recognizes an obligation, can benefit from psychotherapy to assist him in making the necessary adjustments. If, in addition, an individual is suffering from varying and changing degrees of sensory and/or motor disability, there can be little doubt that psychotherapy, if it can be made available, is indicated. This includes most, if not all, aphasic patients. There is, however, considerable doubt that psychotherapy can be made available to most aphasics. It is the author's belief that, in many instances, more harm than good is accomplished through any *direct attempt* at psychotherapy. The basic reason for this attitude is the appreciation that, despite the aphasic's need, language—the instrument for direct psychotherapy—is impaired. Without assurance that the patient is able to understand, to reveal the amount of his understanding or misunderstanding, direct psychotherapy is precarious. Certainly, direct psychotherapy should not be undertaken unless the aphasic patient has sufficient language ability to expess himself and to understand what is being explained to him as well as the need for the explanation.

The therapist who undertakes to work directly and individually with an aphasic must not only be qualified in psychotherapy but must have specific experience with aphasic patients. He must be constantly aware that he cannot assume that the patient completely understands on even an intellectual level what he is trying to have him understand. The usual test of understanding—an appropriate verbalization—is not to be expected of the aphasic.

Beyond this precaution, there is another which should be observed. The aphasic patient should probably not be given direct psychotherapy if his problems, were he not an aphasic, would otherwise not come to the attention of a psychotherapist. An aphasic patient is entitled to a certain number of problems because he is a human being. As such, he, in common with other human beings, should be permitted to work his problems through himself. It is only when his problems are too severe, or too numerous, that psychotherapy should be considered.

An essential aspect of therapy for the aphasic, which can usually be worked out indirectly and without the direct intervention of an especially-trained psychotherapist, is the patient's necessary acceptance of himself as himself, disabilities included, on a temporary basis. The patient should be encouraged to postpone a "final assessment" and to make re-evaluations of his changing self as language, sensory, and motor improvements take place. The aphasic must be given time to adjust to his disabilities and limitations, and to the attitudes of his family, relatives, friends, and other members of his environment.

## Dependency Relationships

Because of the aphasic's communicative, expressive, and frequent physical disabilities, there is a strong likelihood that he will quickly become dependent on the first person who understands him and apparently accepts him as he is. Frequently, such a person will be the language therapist. For the welfare of the aphasic patient, and to some degree for the therapist, it is important that dependency be avoided. There is grave danger that the aphasic who finds acceptance and understanding in the therapist will become satisfied with that relationship and so avoid others which may be less satisfactory.

Having made one adjustment and worked out one relationship, he will nc undertake the risks of other adjustments and relationships. Even in regard t language which is recovered, the aphasic patient may limit his linguisti attempts to situations in which the therapist is involved. Doing so, he reduce the likelihood for disapproval, often more imagined than real, for communi cative failure. Unfortunately, this limitation also restricts practice in expres sion and communication, with resultant undesirable effects for ultimate socia adjustment as well as language improvement.

From the point of view of the therapist, a dependency relationship is als undesirable. The tendency for a therapist to become subjectively and pei sonally involved in working with a handicapped individual is understandabl Frequently, such a relationship satisfies a need which the therapist may ur consciously have—a need to be needed. It is, however, difficult for effectiv therapy to be carried on when a patient's failure becomes one which th therapist shares. When the patient's moods, frustrations, successes, or de feats are felt by the therapist, he cannot do justice to the individual patier whose experience he is sharing subjectly. Nor, under the circumstances, ca he work effectively with other patients with whom he has a different relatior ship.

The therapist must maintain objective interest and avoid subjective ir volvement. One way of doing this, if the rehabilitative program permits, to have a team of therapists working with several aphasic patients individe ally, as well as in a group. If the therapist is in private practice, and does nc have a group of aphasic patients, he must maintain objectivity though work ing individually. If he finds this too difficult, in fairness to the patient as we as himself, the patient should be referred to another therapist for treatmer

## GROUP THERAPY

The question of whether aphasic patients should have the benefits of grou therapy is one which cannot be decided solely on the basis of the values c of the shortcomings of group work per se. As a practical matter, few clin cians who do private work, and relatively few clinics, except those in larg urban areas, are likely to have a sufficient number of aphasics in treatment any one time to make the group approach possible. One might, of cours follow the practice of Backus (1947) and have aphasics included in a grou with nonaphasic speech patients. Although this practice might be feasib in large clinics, in private practice strong resistance might be anticipate from nonaphasic speech patients.

### Values of Group Therapy

Where feasible, group therapy for aphasics is recommended for the fc lowing assumed values:

1. Group training provides an *opportunity for socialization*. The aphasi because of his communicative handicap, cannot socialize with normal pe

sons as an equal. As a member of a group of similarly handicapped persons, socialization becomes more possible. In setting up a group, it is essential that a relaxed attitude prevail. Blackman (1950) set up a group situation for aphasics and was able to report that the individual aphasic lost his feelings of isolation and apparently enjoyed the friendly competitiveness and social acceptance of the others. Activities that may successfully be included to increase socialization and group belongingness include: singing of both well-known and current popular songs; practicing "social-gesture" speech such as acknowledgements of greetings, introducing a new member to a group, and leave-taking from a group. These activities provide situations for the practice of linguistic units which most aphasic patients can evoke with relative facility.

In these group activities, the patient must be encouraged to do as well as he can. If he cannot sing with words, but can hum or whistle a tune, then the humming or whistling should be approved. One way of establishing group approval for nonlinguistic expression is to begin by setting up a music situation in which, initially, some individuals are asked to hum, some whistle, and some sing the words of the song. In response to a greeting, if the patient finds it difficult to respond with a "Fine, thank you" to a "How are you?" or "How do you do?" then a gesture or a simple "O.K." plus a gesture should be encouraged.

When the group has "jelled" and the members have built up an *esprit de corps,* then more ambitious projects such as skits, charades, and quiz programs may be included. With an advanced group, discussions of current problems may be introduced. Such discussions may be preceded by a reading of highlights of the day's news or a period of listening to a radio news broadcast. It is important to bear in mind that in the early stages of group work, participation and not accuracy of information is the objective. As the individuals of the group find participation becoming easier, other aspiration levels and objectives may be set.

2. Group training provides an opportunity for *motivation from peers* rather than from the superior clinician. It is easier for an aphasic to try to evoke a response, or read a phrase if another patient has tried, failed at first, and succeeded after a second or third attempt. The motivation of "You can do it, Joe. You saw me try and finally get it" coming from one aphasic is more readily acceptable to another than when it comes from a therapist who has no linguistic impairment.

3. The group approach provides a situation in which awareness of certain aphasic *speech "habits,"* such as telegraphic and agrammatical language structure, become apparent. The aphasic who uses telegraphic speech, who omits prepositions and conjunctions, will appreciate the difficulty of understanding such language when he hears it from others. Such appreciation should provide motivation for improvement. The verbalized "I don't know what you mean when you talk like that," or the implied failure of comprehension which one aphasic can read from the faces of others who are listen-

ing and trying to understand him, should stimulate an attempt at a more conventional language pattern so that "I-fish-Sunday" may be changed to "I'm going fishing next Sunday."

4. Group training provides an aphasic patient with an opportunity to observe the techniques of other aphasics for evoking speech and for getting speakers to make themselves understood. The individual patient also has in the group a ready-made and sympathetic audience for the testing of his own techniques for oral expression. The techniques which prove to be successful can then be used outside of the group. The unsuccessful techniques can be delayed for outside use until further testing indicates whether it is inappropriate for the given patient and should be put aside for another technique. In brief, the group provides an opportunity for vicarious as well as active learning. The aphasic can learn by observation without direct ego-involvement and risk of failure.

5. Still another advantage of group training is that it provides the aphasic with an opportunity in a learning situation to respond to more than one manner of speech and language usage. The clinician has habits of speaking which are peculiar to him. The aphasic whose learning is associated with the person becomes accustomed to the manner of this person. When others are introduced, learning is not limited to one speaker, and adjustments to others are not as difficult to make as they may become without group training.

6. The last of the advantages of the group approach to be considered is the opportunity it provides for *ventilation of feelings and an airing of grievances*. Aphasic patients, in common with most handicapped persons, develop feelings of hostility and aggression. Some of these are undoubtedly realistically justified; others are not. The expression of these feelings as well as their evaluation can be accomplished in a group situation. The knowledge and assurance that an aphasic patient gains when he learns that others feel or have felt like him, and have to a large extent gotten over their feelings, is of invaluable help. This constitutes psychotherapy without imposition. With it, the aphasic is likely to feel less isolated, and in time, less hostile to the nonaphasics with whom he must live.

## Shortcomings of Group Therapy

The group approach is not without some possible disadvantages as compared with individual training. For the most part, the disadvantages to be considered can all be overcome with skilled handling on the part of the clinician directing the group, or in individual training which should supplement group work.

1. *Withdrawn patients* may find it difficult to attempt expression as members of a group. They may inhibit even the small amount of speech available to them rather than risk faulty expression before a group. Instead of attempting speech, as they may be encouraged to do in individual treatment, withdrawn patients may develop techniques of avoiding response, or may

"hide behind" talkative members and limit their own production to simple gestures of agreement or disagreement.

2. *Group pressure* may provoke some patients into talking about personal problems before they are entirely ready for such revelations. Patients not adequately able to define their problems may find their explanations misunderstood or improperly evaluated. The impact of such a reaction may set the patients back considerably in their rate of progress. Although an alert group therapist tries to avoid this situation, avoidance is not always possible.

3. *The rate of a group* is usually slower than the best member can manage and somewhat faster than the weakest member can progress. Patients who have made considerable improvement may be irked by having to slow down. Patients who are slow learners may find the pace uncomfortable, become confused, and cease trying to maintain the group's pace.

Despite these possible shortcomings, the author's experience with patients working in groups has been generally favorable. It should be emphasized, however, that group training is recommended to supplement and not to replace individual training. If proper precautions are exercised, and no aphasic patient is introduced into a group until he has shown some readiness for it, the advantages of group training will by far outweigh any possible disadvantages.

## LEARNING TECHNIQUES

The basic principles which govern the language learning of normal persons, adults as well as children, hold for aphasics. Associations are strengthened if they are rewarded. If information and insight can be added to or become an integral characteristic of the reward, learning progresses more smoothly and reliably than with noninformative, noninsightful rewards. Other things being equal, frequency of occurrence of an association helps to strengthen it. Learning situations which have an objective, meaningful, and significant objective for the patient, help to motivate and direct the relearning.

There are some essential similarities between an aphasic's relearning and the learning of a new (foreign) language by an adult without brain injury. There are, however, a few important differences which must be understood if a rehabilitative program with an aphasic adult is to be successful.

### Differences Between Aphasic's Relearning and Normal Adult Language-Learning

1. The normal adult who learns a new—for him a foreign—language does so with unimpaired cortical association areas and with an intact neuromotor mechanism. For the aphasic, the association areas are, by definition, injured; and the neuromotor mechanism may also be impaired.

2. The normal adult who learns a new language is not disturbed by rem-

nants of what he once knew. He is aware that he is starting with a "clea slate." The aphasic in "relearning" is often hindered as well as helped b what he once knew. Established habits may interfere with the new teachin (learning) techniques.

3. The normal adult in a new learning enterprise cannot hope that pat terns and associations will come to him spontaneously. He knows that h must apply himself to establish patterns and associations. For the aphasic some associations do come back spontaneously, and it is understandable tha he will hope that spontaneous recovery will continue. This hope may, an frequently does, interfere with voluntary efforts at relearning.

### Reinforcement Through Reward

The adult aphasic is susceptible to reward, but the rewards must not be to obviously made. The lollipop or the gumdrop following an appropriate as sociation may do very well for a child. For the adult, a more mature rewar may consist in the information that he is "right." This information may com in the form of a verbal response, a gesture of approval, or the continuation c a conversation which incorporates the appropriate word in the therapist' response. After a series of correct responses, a general type of reward migh be given in the form of a drink, a smoke, or some other pleasant break i the session. A break, however, should not be made if the patient is doin well and obviously enjoying his successes. It is better made when the patien shows first signs of fatigue, tension, or anxiety.

### Intensification of Stimulation

Intensification of stimulation can be achieved through an actual increas in the size or loudness of the material presented, or through repetition of th material, or through both. If visual material is used, the print size, at lea at the outset, should be relatively large. Type at least twice the size of th type of this book is recommended. If the material is audible, volume ma be increased simply through talking more loudly than for ordinary conver sation. Care should be exercised, however, that increased volume does n *suggest yelling.* If a patient seems embarrassed by the increased volume c the clinician's voice, an amplifying unit may be used. In early stages, e pecially for patients with auditory aphasia, increased volume may help t break down the "barrier of auditory resistance." Some patients prefer t have the audible material personalized by listening with earphones. Th technique serves as an ego-saving device. No outsider becomes aware tha loud sounds are being poured into the patient's ears when head-set earphon are used.

Repetition of stimulation is most successful when it is not too obviou The child may learn to read by being exposed to a sentence such as "Ti saw the rabbit go hop, hop, hop." The adult prefers to have his "hops" bett distributed. More subtle distribution is recommended for all forms of prese tation. If, for example, a "new" word is to be added to the patient's function

anguage inventory, the word should be incorporated in the therapist's responses several times during the course of a session rather than be successively repeated.

## Negative Practice

The conscious and deliberate use of an inappropriate word or phrase—
he technique of *negative practice*—has for some time been recognized as
an excellent technique for eliminating unintentional errors. This technique
is described in some detail by Van Riper (1954) as a method of correcting
articulatory defects. For the aphasic, a modification of the technique of
negative practice along the following lines is suggested.

If a patient evokes a wrong response in answer to a question such as:
"What do you use for cutting meat?" and says *spoon* instead of *knife,* the
therapist should explain that "We use a spoon for eating soup. We use a
*knife* for cutting meat." This should be followed by presenting the patient
with an opportunity to use the word *spoon* as an *appropriate response,* and
then by a second opportunity to use the word *knife* correctly. If the word
*knife* still cannot be readily evoked, further opportunity for the appropriate
use of *spoon,* or whatever other word tends to be evoked, should be offered
the aphasic. Through this approach, even though the word *knife* is not forthcoming, the patient has been enabled to learn correct associations for the
word *spoon,* and an appropriate association has been formed.

For the correction of dysarthric errors, the conventional approach to the
use of negative practice is recommended. Attention is directed to the error
which the patient is making. The patient is then directed to repeat his error
as closely as he can with awareness of how the sound or sound combination
being produced. The correct sound or combination is then presented for
imitation and for contrast with the defective articulation.

Negative practice for dysarthric errors provides practice in recognition of
sounds, in the controlled production of sounds, and practice in the habitual
formation of the desired sound combinations.

## Determining the Original Approach

Learning for the aphasic will frequently be facilitated if the therapist can
determine how the content or process was originally learned, and in what
way the learning was symbolized or recorded. For example, if a patient
learned manuscript writing before cursive writing, it may help considerably
if the manuscript approach is used with the patient who has writing difficulty. If the patient learned to tell time by adding the minutes to the hour
6:40 (six-forty), 7:10 (seven-ten), and so on), he should be taught time-
telling that way rather than to say twenty minutes to seven, or ten minutes
after seven. In writing numbers for division, some patients used the arrange-
ment X $\overline{)\text{XX}}$ for both "short" and long division; others used X $\overline{)\text{X}}$ for "short"
division and XX $\overline{)\text{XXX}}$ for long division; still others used X $\overline{)\text{XX}}$ for all
division. Information about the habit of the patient can frequently be ob-

tained from members of the family. If this information is not available, the age of the patient and his place of education may provide clues as to the likely approach to school learning. Most young patients probably learned to subtract by the additive process so that $-2$ will be worked as "Two and what make six? Two and four make six." Older patients may have been taught to subtract by the "take-away" process—"Six minus two is four." If the patient has used the phrase "take-away" instead of "minus," then the therapist should use that term with him.

Essentially, it should be remembered, most aphasic learning is actually reawakening or re-establishing of associations. This can usually best be accomplished by determining how the old associations were formed in the first place rather than by imposing the therapist's own way of making associations on the patient.

### Raising the Level of Response

Earlier it was pointed out that there is a considerable amount of speech which remains relatively intact for most aphasic patients. These forms include emotionally laden speech content, automatic and serial speech, and social-gesture speech. Use can be made of these "low level of intellect" linguistic contents for "higher level" speech purposes.

A patient who cannot readily evoke the name of a number can be trained to *count* serially until that number comes up in the sequence, and then to stop at it. Later, he can be taught to say the sequence quickly and silently and then to utter aloud only the numeral which is appropriate. In this way patients can learn to give their telephone numbers, their home addresses, the date, and other functionally useful number-phrases. Similarly, patients can be taught to evoke a particular day of the week, or month of the year.

Automatic content such as prayers, familiar verse, songs, can be used to evoke significant words and phrase. *Good* and *morning* can be evoked separately through the relatively automatic gesture phrase, "Good morning." A physician, Dr. Rose (1948), who suffered a stroke and associated aphasic involvement described his own retraining through his recollection and memorization of familiar lines of poetry, psalms, and other material which, according to him, "At one time I could almost say it in my sleep." In his account of his recovery, Dr. Rose explained that he also memorized or near memorized considerable amounts of "new poetry." He recommends "Read often aloud and you will come close to memorizing. . . ."

Where bodily action is customarily or frequently associated with given locutions, as is often the case with gesture phrases, the patient should be encouraged to engage in such action as an aid in the evocation of the desired words. Terms of greeting, as well as the single word responses *Yes* and *No* can frequently be evoked more readily when associated with bodily action than when attempted alone. This technique, and its wider application in the use of skits and other pantomimic activity, is described by Backus (1947).

Emotionally laden speech can also be "elevated" and used to evoke significant intellectual-level language. One of the author's military patients was speechless until a ward mate provoked him to say "Get the hell out of here!" Later, he was reminded of this evocation and could use the individual words by recalling the words of his emotional outburst. From time to time he was reminded of other useful phrases at his command which he became able to use in nonemotional, propositional situations.

## Handedness Change

For many aphasic patients the need for changing handedness, generally, from the right to the left hand, is an essential and inevitable procedure. If the paralysis of the preferred hand is severe, a shift in handedness must be accomplished if the patient is to relearn writing. For the patient with residual weakness, the desirability for effecting the change has not yet been experimentally proven. The desirability of handedness change is consistent with the theoretic concept that improvement in aphasia is associated with the assumption of control of language function by the originally nondominant cerebral hemisphere.

The idea of handedness change is frequently resisted by patients who still have some amount of control of the preferred hand. It is probable that the patient's wish to be as much like his former self as possible is responsible for this resistance. Change of handedness is recommended by the author based upon his observations that, in most instances, improvement has been accelerated not only in the motor aspect of writing but in the accuracy of spelling and written word usage as well. To overcome resistance, the author has suggested to his patients that they try writing with the nonpreferred hand for a period of a month. If, at the end of the period, the patient wished to resume writing with the original hand, no objection would be made. Almost all patients who agreed to the month's trial period continued, as a matter of choice, to write with the alternate hand. Some were pleased that they had become ambidextrous. Several patients admitted that they began to feel more secure about what they were writing, that "things clicked right inside their heads" shortly after they attained some degree of skill with the nonpreferred hand.

The accomplishment of a shift in handedness seldom takes more than three or four weeks—providing that resistance to the change has been overcome. Gardner's (1945) manual for left-handed writing has been found most useful for establishing the new writing technique.

## When to Begin Training?

The author's answer to the question above is "Just as soon as the patient is able to take notice of what is going on about him." It is not so long, however, since this writer, in common with other speech clinicians during World War II, met with objections to training such as the following: (1) eventually, aphasics recover spontaneously if they are to recover at all; and (2) in any event, training should be delayed at least until after the first six months of the patient's involvement because that is the period of greatest spontaneous improvement.

The observations of the present writer, and of several of his colleagues with whom he conferred during World War II, urged him to insist on an early initiation of a training program. At the Army General Hospital where the author was in charge of language rehabilitation, training was initiated at bedside, even if the patient was seen for no more than five minutes a day during the first week of the re-educational program. Today, the therapist or clinician who recommends early training can find support in a study by Butfield and Zangwill (1946) on a group of British aphasic patients. They compared a group of 36 aphasics who began their training before the end of the first post-traumatic year with a second group of 32 patients who began their training after the end of the first post-traumatic year. Their results at the end of the training period, as measured by total progress in educational achievement, *speech per se not included,* was in favor of the group that began early training. This finding is consistent with the present writer's more subjective observations of factors related to recovery in aphasic patients (Eisenson, 1949).

Even if there were no objective findings to support the recommendation for beginning re-education early, the following argument could be made. A delay in training permits aphasic patients to resort to and develop nonlinguistic methods of communication, or to reconcile themselves to being cut off from communication with their environment. For some patients, secondary gains from noncommunication might be established. Patients may expect that their needs and wishes will be anticipated, and so reduce their attempts at making their wants known. Once this attitude is assumed, its modification may be difficult.

Another approach to the problem is the need to appreciate that, except for physical therapy and re-education, aphasic patients have little that they can do. The psychological support afforded the patient by the therapist, the awareness that the patient is having something taking place in which he is an *active participant,* all undoubtedly help to accelerate improvement. Even if we should admit that the only real value of training is psychotherapeutic and arises out of a relationship between the patient and the therapist, early re-education is recommended. Wepman (1951, pp. 98–99) argues for early training with reasons which include the following: a failure to begin training may result either in the rejection of the patient, or in the patient becoming infantalized; patients who do not receive training may tend to become reconciled to their limitations and to withdraw from social intercourse; and later, they may resist attempts at assistance and evidence irritability or yield readily to catastrophic behavior reaction patterns if frustrated.

### How to Begin Training

Training of a patient should begin with an evaluation of his assets and limitations. These should include a knowledge of what the patient can do, as well as what he cannot do, at the time the evaluation is being made. This knowledge should go beyond estimating the patient's present linguistic and general "educational performance" level. The complete picture should include an assaying of the patient's complete health history, his premorbid manner of reacting to illness, to frustration, and to the need to exert intellectual effort. This information will determine, to a large measure, how the patient is likely to respond to his present limitations.

An evaluation of linguistic ability can be made through the use of aphasia inventories and educational achievement tests. These will be discussed later. An estimate of premorbid tendencies should come through an interview with responsible members of the family. An evaluation of present behavioral tendencies should come from direct observation. When these areas of information are obtained, the therapist will know what the patient is presently able to do, as well as what kind of a patient he has for re-education. The therapist will then be ready for the next question: Where and how do I begin specific linguistic re-education?

Probably the best broad answer to the question is: Begin in an area in which the patient can be stimulated. More particularly, the area will depend upon the individual patient's immediate needs as well as his ultimate objectives and the strength of inner motivation in arriving at the objectives. If these are not known to the therapist, and occasionally they may not even be known to the patient, a trial-and-error, or better, a "trial-until-success," period is indicated. A failure to elicit a favorable response may merely mean that the area of stimulation, for the time being, is not an appropriate one. Another should then be tried.

Frequently, the obvious needs of the patient may serve as a guide. If the patient is still in the hospital, words such as *nurse, water, comb,* or better, terms which include such words, might well become an immediate starting point. The patient who can call attention to his needs, and who can thereby save himself embarrassment, has been helped to rediscover how functional language can be. The patient who can acknowledge a greeting, who can thereby indicate that he is still a vital human being, will command some respect and will ward off injury to his ego. Language which will help to achieve this end is a good area in which to begin to stimulate a patient.

The patient's less immediate objectives will depend upon a number of factors. Among these are the type and amount of sensory and motor involvement, the degree to which these involvements are likely to be permanent, the effect of these upon his re-employability, and the linguistic needs of the patient in the light of his vocational goal. If this goal is too remote as a basis for stimulation, then the patient's avocations and hobbies should be considered. A reservation, however, must be made in regard to this area. If the patient's physical disabilities are such that the avocations may forever need to be put aside, stimulation in this area should be avoided. Failure to do so may merely remind the patient of what was and can no longer be, and frustration rather than successful stimulation may be the result.

Some specific examples of what can be done may be of help. One patient with right hemiplegia who had been a golf enthusiast was stimulated to start language training after he was provided with a set of left-handed golf clubs, and received instruction in their use. He then was willing to learn to read a manual on how to play golf, to learn to spell and say such words as *hole, tee, fairway, par, birdie,* and to read numbers which approximated "average duffer" golf scores. Another patient wanted most to learn to read his young wife's letters and to be able to say in his own words "How much I love her." A middle-aged woman patient wanted to be taught "how to talk back" to her nurse.

### The Pathway for Stimulation

In general, the best pathway for stimulation will be the sensory and motor avenues which are intact or relatively unimpaired. Which these will be will depend, of course, upon the individual patient and can usually be determined after an adequate physical and linguistic examination. The information provided by the neurologist as to sensory and motor abilities and disabilities is essential. Questions of hearing loss as well as auditory aphasia apraxic involvements, and so on, must also be answered. With such information, the therapist can usually decide whether the sensory avenue should be through vision, hearing, or possibly through the tactual pathway. He should also be able to decide whether the primary motor expression or output should be through speaking, writing, or through the use of symbol gestures. A selected "complete circuit" may, for an individual patient, be aural for reception and graphic for production; for another it might well be visual for reception and oral for production.

Unless the patient, for reasons which cannot always be determined, rejects the avenues selected on the basis of physical examination, the "circuit pathways" should be developed until the patient is able to achieve a fair degree of facility in revealing his moods, attitudes, and thoughts. If the patient rejects or resists the use of these avenues, then the therapist must accept those which the patient himself prefers. In any event, it should be made clear that other receptive and productive avenues are not to be ignored. As soon as possible, practice through other avenues should be provided so that multiple associations may be made.

It should not be taken for granted that every aphasic patient is readily available for re-education. Some patients require a considerable amount of stimulation in order to become available for therapy. Along this line, Wepman (1953) characterizes appropriate stimulation as "What is done externally to the patient which produces some heightening of his efforts. This includes ... every possible form of persuasion."

## SPECIFIC TECHNIQUES

It is not possible, and probably not desirable, to present numerous specific techniques for the rehabilitation of aphasic patients. The best techniques are those which are designed for the individual patient. The therapist will find some useful advice and information in texts and articles on the subject of remedial education. He should not, however, assume that teaching a person to *read again* presents the same problems as teaching a poor reader, or a slow-to-get-started-reader, how to read in the first place.

At all times, the therapist must bear in mind that his patient is going to relearn considerably more than he can possibly be directly taught. The basic job of the therapist is to get the patient going, to help him to realize that he can relearn. Once the patient appreciates this, neither he nor the therapist will be surprised at the large amount of spontaneous linguistic recovery which takes place.

The literature on aphasia therapy has grown large during the past quarter-century. Much of what has been published might well be evaluated as descriptive of successful approaches with individual patients rather than as positive suggestions on treating specific patients. In the writer's Army Rehabilitation Clinic during World War II he had several therapists working under his supervision, each using different approaches with their patients for the "teaching" of the same content. One, a former English teacher, was an efficient drillmaster who was successful with drills for "reading, writing, and arithmetic." Another, who had a clinical psychological background, was successful with conversational therapy and limited drill. Each therapist used techniques according to the inclinations and directions of his training and personality. The only principle that governed all therapy was that *under no circumstances was the personality of the patient to be violated.*

To these words of precaution, one more will be added. The techniques and approaches which are about to be discussed are to be regarded as *suggestions rather than prescriptions.*

### Therapeutic Techniques for Evaluative (Receptive) Disturbances

**Agnosias.** Visual agnosias, as we indicated earlier, must be determined if the patient manifests any reading disability or, more generally, a disability in responding appropriately to visual configurations. An agnosia for visual form may explain a patient's inability to read. If this form of agnosia is discovered, retraining techniques along the following lines may be tried:

The patient may be given two types of "blocks" (e.g., squares and triangles) to arrange in groups or piles. If he is successful, he should be given the names of these blocks. A third type, circles, should then be introduced and the patient is directed to proceed with the new groupings. Appropriate naming should follow correct performances. The patient should be encouraged to repeat the names after the therapist if he cannot spontaneously utter the appropriate name for each of his selections. Discrimination practice for the geometric forms should continue until the most usual ones (star, square, circle, cross, triangle) are learned and can be selected from a random assortment of forms when each is named by the therapist.

Sometimes the mere handling of the forms by the patient is not sufficient to bring about discrimination. Some therapists have found that directed tracing of a form, either with finger pantomime or with a pencil or crayon, while the form is on a piece of paper, is of help. Wepman (1951, p. 186) suggests that the patient be directed to trace each form or to copy it in a paper or blackboard presentation. This technique is recommended by the present writer as a regular procedure because it permits the patient to compare a two-dimensional representation with one which is three dimensional.

Occasionally, a patient will fail because the size of the configuration is too small. In keeping with the principle of intensification of stimulation, it is recommended that larger configurations be tried. When recognition is established with the larger ones, then the therapist should introduce smaller configurations until ones approximating those most commonly found are used.

If the patient demonstrates an agnosia for flat representations of forms, and can recognize three-dimensional forms, he should be given practice in associating one with the other. Such practice might consist of his placing three-dimensional configurations on sheets which have two-dimensional ones. That is, he is directed to place a rectangular block on a rectangle, a triangular block on a triangle, and so on. When he succeeds in doing this, the process should be reversed, and the patient is asked to place a cut-out of a two-dimensional figure on the actual object. A final step should be the appropriate and ready selection of the flat figure named by the therapist.

Visual agnosia becomes a significant problem for aphasics if it involves *letter recognition*. In not all cases, however, are the two necessarily related. This writer has examined many patients who could recognize and read aloud whole words but who could apparently not recognize individual letters of the words. It is possible that these patients learned to read by the word or sentence recognition method. For them, individual letters do not have the same significance as for persons who have learned to read by building up words from synthesizing letters and sounds. Because of this, the attitude of the patient may be such that he finds no reason for concerning himself with letter recognition. In effect, such persons manifest a disinclination rather than a disability in a recognition function.

For patients with actual *visual letter agnosia,* remedial procedures along the following lines may be tried. An alphabet book, or a series of alphabet cards, with pictures or pictures and words for each letter may be arranged. Children's alphabet books are not recommended because the representations are on a level which might cause ego insult. It is usually no great problem to get colored illustrations from magazine advertisements. Each picture should be edited so that the representation to be associated with the object is most readily evident. If possible, a single object representation should be used. So, a single picture of a book and the word *book* should be associated with the letter *B*. If it is possible to find common object-pictures the form of which suggests the letter, as, for example, a telegraph pole for the letter *T*, such pictures are especially worth while. The patient may be directed to copy these letters. If he cannot copy, then he should be asked to trace them, and later to copy them when tracing is easily accomplished. Again, the principle of intensification of stimulation may be used, with the ultimate objective of decreasing the intensity (size) of the letter to usual book-size print. The final step, of course, is for the patient to learn to write letters from dictation.

Some patients who were not readily able to learn to recognize words by the approach just described were helped through body pantomime. For example, a large letter *T* was attached to the corner of a large mirror before which the patient and therapist stood. The therapist stretched his arms out at shoulder height, said "*T*" and asked the patient to imitate the action he saw in the mirror. Later, the patient was able to respond with pantomime to the picture of the letter *T*. Finally, the patient learned to recognize the letter without resorting to pantomime.

These techniques, it is again emphasized, are suggestions. The therapist, using his own resources, should be able to invent suitable ones for his individual patients. Discussions of other successful techniques for dealing with the problem may be found in such texts as those of Goldstein (1932), Granich (1947), Wepman (1951), and Longerich and Bordeaux (1954).

**Reading disturbances (alexia).** Although some of the techniques of remedial reading for children may be applied to aphasic adults, there are several fundamental differences between the reading disturbance of the aphasic and the reading disability of the child. First, as Backus (1947, p. 461) points out, the aphasic was once able to read. (If he was not, if the aphasic was illiterate, then the reading disability should not be considered part of the aphasic's problem per se. This writer does not recommend that the therapist undertake to teach an illiterate aphasic how to read.) The aphasic's linguistic disabilities are likely to be more numerous, and his abilities less even and consistent, than the child's. For the aphasic, productive as well as evaluative disturbances are likely to be present, and to interfere directly and indirectly with reading function.

With these precautions in mind, the underlying approach to remedial reading may be considered. Dolch (1939) lists five steps in a remedial-reading program. These steps, somewhat modified for aphasic patients, may be stated as follows:

1. Begin remedial work at the patient's present level of ability.
2. Build up a sight vocabulary and work for speed recognition.
3. Teach self-help sounding, providing the patient has no marked oral paraphasia or dysarthria. (If he does, this step should be omitted, because these disturbances will impair rather than improve reading comprehension.)
4. Develop comprehension.
5. Secure interesting reading material at the individual's present level.

Each of the Dolch principles include special problems for the aphasic. Some of the problems are implied in the rewording of the Dolch principles.

*To begin at the patient's level of ability* requires an evaluation of that ability. The usual standardized tests for reading achievement may be used for this purpose, with the recommended modification that the time allowance for testing be ignored.[1]

Eisenson's *Examining for Aphasia* (1954) includes a series of reading items which are usually sufficient for preliminary purposes for moderately alexic disturbances and are sufficient for evaluating the reading level of severe alexic patients.

The *building up of a readily functional sight vocabulary* should be determined in part by the patient's needs and interests as an adult and in part by the provision of words selected from lists incorporating words and phrases most frequently found in the patient's language. Several such lists have been prepared for American-English-speaking persons. Buckingham and Dolch (1936) published a combined word list which indicates the sources and overlapping of eleven word-count studies. A relatively short list of 220 words was compiled by Dolch (1939, p. 154). This list, according to Dolch, makes up from 50 to 75 per cent of all ordinary reading matter. A second Dolch list of *One Thousand Words* was published in 1950. Another widely used list, on which many primers are based, is one by Gates (1935). The Gates list includes 1811 words which were selected as highly suitable for the primary grades. In his *Improvement of Basic Reading Abilities,* Durrell (1940, pp. 345–354) includes a special primary-grade-level list of words which were compiled for older children. This list according to Durrell (p. 345) "contains 90 per cent of the words ordinarily used in the written compositions of children in the intermediate grades. . . ." In the same book, Durrell includes a somewhat lengthy *Intermediate Vocabulary List* (pp. 360–388).

Techniques for the building up of sight vocabularies are described by the cited authors in their texts. A good discussion, but by no means the only good one, on the subject of building up word recognition may be found in the Gates (1950, Ch. 9, 3rd ed.) *Improvement of Reading.*

It is well to remember that published lists can only suggest words the aphasic should know. In the final analysis, aphasics should be helped to recognize and read the words *they* need to know according to their situations and their objectives.

The present writer prepared a list of words and phrases based upon the first 1000 most frequently used words in English as determined by Thorndike and Lorge (1944). The words and phrases were printed in large type, with more than the usual amount of space between lines. A card with a slot

---

[1] The recommendation that time allowances be ignored holds for all educational testing of aphasic patients. Testing should be stopped when it becomes obvious that the patient cannot continue with any degree of success as the items increase in difficulty. Note should be made as to the amount of time the patient needed to complete the number of items attempted before successive failures occurred.

was given to each alexic patient. This permitted the patient to see, concentrate, and respond to a single word or phrase at a time.

The use of a card with an "exposure slot" was found helpful for many aphasic patients in the early stages of reading re-education. Many patients become overwhelmed when confronted with large amounts of material. They were found to respond better when a small amount was presented at one time. The card served the purpose of helping patients to believe that they were making progress, a little at a time, and reducing the size of the task. For some patients, pointing to each word as the word was read was found to serve the same purpose. Ultimately, of course, the patient should be encouraged to try to do without this kind of an aid. It is well to remember that, for the aphasic, security and accuracy of comprehension are more important than speed of reading. As training progresses, speed of reading may be improved through the use of flash cards, or by having phrases or short sentences exposed for brief periods on a screen.

Many patients enjoy building up their own stock of reading cards. These may be prepared by the patient with illustrations cut from magazines. A sentence relating to the picture, with the most significant word or words underlined may be typed under, over, or to one side of the picture. A key word or phrase may be typed or written in one corner. If the patient is able to write, his own writing may appear under the printed material. The patient, in adding to his card list, may go over them by himself, or review them with a relative, friend, or another patient. Periodically, the stock may be separated into cards always read easily and correctly, ones usually read easily and accurately, and others "not yet" read easily and accurately. Through this device both the patient and the therapist can estimate improvement in single-sentence reading based on material selected by the patient.

Vocabulary-building cards such as the Dolch Sight Vocabulary Cards and Sight Phrase Cards can be used to considerable advantage. Although these sets of cards were prepared primarily for teaching children to read, their small size and general appearance make them suitable for adult use.

*The development of comprehension* cannot be taken for granted merely because a patient learns to read words and sequences of words aloud. It is essential—even more so than for children who do not read well—that comprehension be constantly checked. This may be done by having the patient indicate *in some form most readily available to him* that he understands what he has read. The patient may retell the content in his own words, complete sentences with key words, or even use gestures to reveal his comprehension. As the patient improves, he may enjoy taking self-administered reading tests, such as are provided in many primers and in texts for teaching language to foreign-born persons. Considerable use can also be made of reading paragraphs and test materials of standardized reading scales.

*Securing reading material* at the present level of the aphasic is frequently a real problem. If the patient's alexia is severe, something comparable to a primer is needed. Primers, however, are infantile both in content and in format. The author undertook to "translate" a primer story for use with his patients. He found the task of using a simple vocabulary and casting the words and ideas into an adult form a much more difficult one than he anticipated. The results, however, were rewarding. In his "translation" he used black-line drawings and photographs to replace the multicolored pictures of the primer. The story including illustrations was then bound in hard covers. The aphasics did not suspect that they were reading a paraphrased primer story, and seemed pleased that they had a "book" especially prepared for them.

Probably the best type of initial reading material is that which is especially prepared for the individual patient. As patients improve, edited (rewritten) news reports are useful. They have the advantage of being timely, and so are usually of immediate interest.[2]

**Auditory disturbances.** It is fortunate that most aphasic patients spontaneously recover considerable auditory comprehension in the early stages of their aphasic involvement. It is probably also true that patients and clinicians both tend to overestimate the amount of recovery which seems to have taken place. Much of what we say to patients in conversation, regardless of specific content, can frequently be answered by a single word, or a nod of the head. A patient who just has the merest hunch of what is said to him can frequently determine by observing the speaker's face whether a "Yes" or "No" is expected. Often the patient catches the rudiments of what is said, but if no specific response is expected of him he does not have any check or test of how much he really understood. Some patients stop listening, or become "functionally deaf," when they cannot readily understand what they hear. By doing this they avoid the challenge, the effort, and the possible frustration, of trying to comprehend. One of the author's patients, a highly social person, almost always took the initiative in conversational situations. He spoke with relevantly fluent circumlocutions and seldom permitted other persons in a conversational group to say much in response to him. By con-

---

[2] The author has found general acceptance by aphasics of specially prepared newspapers such as *Young America* (Eton Publishing Co., Silver Springs, Md.) and the special *Reading Skill Builder Series* (Reader's Digest Educational Service, Pleasantville, N. Y.). Among other books prepared for special groups of readers which the author recommends as useful for aphasic patients are the following:

The *Everyreader Library Series* (Webster Publishing Co., St. Louis, Mo.) includes classics and biographies adapted by remedial reading experts for use with slow readers. A basic vocabulary and simple sentence structure are employed. Titles include *Ivanhoe*, *A Tale of Two Cities, The Gold Bug, Cases of Sherlock Holmes*, and *Simon Bolivar*.

The *Oxford English Course* (Oxford University Press, New York) consists of a graduated course intended for persons for whom English is a second language. The vocabulary for each course is based upon a selected list of essential words. The entire series includes language books for presenting basic vocabularies and teaching grammar. *Language*, Book One, Part One, introduces the alphabet arranged for reading and writing. The supplementary readers include simplified versions of classics which employ limited (basic) vocabularies. Titles which employ vocabularies of from 1500 to 2000 words include *The Merchant of Venice, The Tempest, Pilgrim's Progress, Tales from the Arabian Nights,* and *The Purloined Letter*.

trolling the conversation, the patient seemed to understand conversational speech. When this patient's device of taking the initiative was evaluated for him, he accepted the evaluation and began to listen as well as to speak. By doing so, the first principle of training for a patient with auditory disturbances became established: *patients must learn to listen if they are to learn to understand what they hear.*

Earlier, in our discussion of therapeutic problems and approaches, the technique of intensification of stimulation was considered. The auditory aphasic needs intensification. He also needs constant encouragement and reassurance that in time comprehension will come and two-way communication will be re-established.

For the auditory aphasic, television observation is strongly recommended, especially for dramatic plays. The frequent close-ups permitting the patient to concentrate on the facial movements of speech, which may be associated with the total background situation, constitutes excellent therapy as well as educational recreation. Newscasts, whether on television or radio, are also highly recommended. If possible, a discussion between patients and clinician should follow listening to news broadcasts. Such discussion, which should be held informally, will serve as a reinforcement of understanding. If a given newscast involves a matter about which there may be differences of opinion, then the patients may be encouraged to give their reactions or opinions about what was said.

For more formal teaching situations, Schuell (1953) offers a number of suggestions for determining whether a patient understands what he hears. Schuell emphasizes that the only way to be certain whether an aphasic patient understands what he hears is to ask him to respond in some way. The nature and particular type of response which the patient should be encouraged to make will depend both upon the patient's productive abilities and the specific situation. Among the type of responses which may be elicited, Schuell suggests the following:

1. Identifying objects in a picture. This may be used in going over illustrations in magazines, books, or specially arranged cards.
2. Following directions.
3. Answering questions, formally or informally, in conversation with the therapist.
4. Completing sentences intentionally left incomplete by the therapist.
5. Answering specific questions presented by the therapist.
6. Identifying, by pointing, underlining, or naming specific words or sentences for a given context.
7. Paraphrasing in the patient's own words, or in words he recalls, what the patient heard.
8. Writing answers, especially if the patient can write more readily than he can use oral speech.
9. Presenting oral opposites of single words, phrases, or sentences: for example, high—low; come here—go away; it is early—it is late.

To this list, which is merely suggestive, the therapist can add his own devices to insure the second basic principle of training for auditory disturbances: *the patient must understand what he hears.* Severe auditory aphasics, who may have auditory agnosia as well as auditory aphasia, need training which begins with establishing associations between objects and sounds. The sound of a bell ringing may become established by having a patient hold a bell in his hand and imitate the therapist's action in ringing the bell. The noise of a hammer may similarly become associated with the object hammer and with the action of banging a hammer on a nail, or a block of wood. So, also, noises of other mechanical objects may be established.

Animal noises may become identified by association between the animal, or a representation (picture), and the conventional sound the animal is assumed to make. Most children have learned to make such identifications and associations, so that this form of training usually recalls what the patient once learned. Nonverbal human sounds can also be re-established. *Coughing* and *sneezing* in the manner most cultured human beings eventually permit themselves are conventionalized and characteristic nonverbal sounds.

Recognition of articulate sounds, for the rare patient with auditory agnosia, must also be established. The author taught one of his patients to recognize, and later to imitate, articulate sounds through the following approach. He and the patient sat before a large mirror. The author produced several of the more easily recognizable vowel sounds, such as [u] (oo) and [i] (ee) and had the patient imitate the oral movement. When the imitation was successful, and the sound was produced by the patient, snapshots were taken of the patient's face. The pictures were later presented to the patient so that he could, when alone, practice imitating himself. This approach, while comparatively expensive, was effective. It is not, however, likely to be a necessary one for many patients.

### Therapeutic Techniques for Productive (Expressive) Disturbances

At the outset, it is well that productive disturbances as well as evaluative ones are seldom found as pure or isolated disabilities in the adult. Not infrequently, the patient's concern with one aspect of his disturbance may make him oblivious to other aspects. Without thorough examination, areas of productive defect may not become apparent to either the clinician or to the patient. This statement is not intended to imply that the clinician or therapist has an obligation to "reveal all" to the patient just as soon as "the all" is discovered. It is intended to imply that the ultimate objective should be improvement, to whatever degree seems possible, in all areas of disturbance.

**Nonverbal apraxias.** The space limitations of this text do not permit any detailed discussion of this form of subsymbolic productive disturbance. It is obviously important, as indicated earlier, to determine whether a particular productive disturbance is one related to the symbol per se, or to the motor act per se. In the case of writing disturbance, it is essential to know whether the patient's basic difficulty is in knowing how to use a tool external to the body —a pen or pencil—intentionally and meaningfully, or to use the arm-hand-finger tools intentionally or meaningfully. For the most part, the speech therapist is not likely to be concerned with the patient's use of tools which are not part of the body. Such training is likely to be provided by other members of the therapeutic team. It may, however, become necessary to teach the patient how to handle writing equipment such as pencils, pens, chalk, the blackboard, and so forth.

Probably the best initial approach to the handling of writing tools is to have the patient imitate the therapist's act as a whole in a relatively simple movement. The first tool should be large, easy to grasp, and one that offers little resistance. Soft chalk and a large blackboard, soft black crayons and a large sheet of paper mounted on a blackboard, are good instruments for a start. If the patient cannot directly imitate the writing of a simple word outline such as *cat,* then the therapist may try placing the writing instrument in the patient's hand and moving the hand for the execution of the word outline. From soft chalk or crayon, the patient should progress to using a large, oversize pencil. If the patient finds it difficult to grasp a pencil, its width and tenability can be enhanced by tying multiple-strand string around the bottom of the pencil. If the notion of grasping itself needs to be established, the use of a half-filled bean bag or a sponge rubber ball is recommended. Other suggestions for this type of training may be found in some of the texts already referred to on aphasia therapy. The problem of the teaching of writing as an aphasic difficulty will be considered later.

**Oral apraxia**. Earlier, in the discussion of auditory agnosia, one approach which may be used for the patient with oral apraxia was presented. This approach consisted of imitation by the patient of simple articulatory movements made by the therapist. Imitation may be direct, with the patient observing the therapist, or may be mirror imitation, with the patient observing the therapist and himself in a large mirror. The use of photographs to enable the patient to imitate himself was also suggested.

From single sounds such as [i] (ee), [u] (oo), and [ɑ] (ah), which, fortunately, have some word value in English, the patient should be helped to consonant-vowel combinations. To begin with, the readily visible consonants should be taught. The sound [p] is a good one because of its distinctive lip movement and breath characteristics. It can be combined with each of the vowels mentioned above to constitute three word forms. The patient then is not only making sounds, but to a degree may be making sense. It is not recommended that the sound [m] follow the teaching of [p]. The partial similarity in lip activity may confuse some patients. It is recommended instead that a sound differently produced, such as [t] or [n] be taught next. Fortunately, [t] plus each of the three vowels adds at least two more word forms for most American speakers, and three word forms for American speakers who use Standard Eastern or British (London) dialect.

The concept of voiced and unvoiced sounds should be established after sound as such is appreciated. If the patient does not spontaneously vocalize sounds, the patient's hand may be placed at the therapist's larynx while the therapist produces voiced sounds. The author has found that frequently all that is necessary for the patient to produce vocalized sound is to place his (the patient's hand) on his own larynx in imitation of the therapist. In this way, differences between cognate sounds are usually readily established.

The next step is to establish not readily visible speech sounds such as [s], [z], [r], [k], and [g]. These again may be taught in isolation and in combination with vowels in addition to the first three which have been suggested. Wherever possible, chosen combinations should be ones which are word forms rather than nonsense syllables. Word forms may be used, or recognized, in speech. For a patient with disturbances so severe as to include oral apraxia, the ability to use a few words may be a great morale booster.

It is a fairly common observation (Wepman, 1951, p. 218) that it is rarely necessary to teach a patient all sounds, or many combinations of sounds. Once the idea of articulatory activity is established, most apraxic patients progress by themselves in making additional sounds, and in going from sounds to attempts at words.

**Writing (agraphia).** We shall begin with the assumption that the patient has no external tool apraxia, or has overcome this form of disability and now must be trained to learn to form letters and to write words and sentences. The suggestion has already been made that, unless the patient shows resistance, a change of handedness is recommended. If the patient has a hemiplegia or a severe paresis which involves his preferred hand, a change of handedness is essential. The use of Gardner's manual for this purpose has already been indicated. Visual disturbances, especially those involving visual field, must also be considered. It is essential that the patient be able to see as well as feel the materials he is to use. If the material is to be copied, it should be placed so that it can be seen. If this can be accomplished, almost all aphasic patients can succeed in copying. Retraining might well begin with copying material on a blackboard. Next steps might include copying with a soft crayon on a large sheet of newsprint, copying with a pencil, and copying with a pen. Many patients are able to proceed directly from blackboard to pencil and paper. It is again emphasized that the therapist must assume the responsibility for the good working condition of the equipment. Mechanical difficulties should not be permitted to aggravate the patient's efforts at improvement.

If a patient cannot copy readily by looking at material above his writing space, he may be helped by placing letters underneath thin, transluscent paper, through which the letters underneath may be seen. The letters should be clear and simple in outline. If possible, they should be enlargements of the kind of writing the patient himself habitually used. Almost always, some specimen of the patient's own writing may be obtained from a member of his family.

Occasionally, a patient, for reasons not always apparent, has persistent difficulties with one or more letters. It frequently helps to personalize these letters. One patient learned to write the letter *I* by standing straight and tall, with his hands close to his sides, so that he looked like an *I*. Another, who was fond of smoking a pipe, associated the letter *P* with the picture of a pipe placed so that it suggested the letter *P*. The resourceful clinician may arrive at his own devices which meet the needs and interests, as well as the disabilities, of his particular patient. For further suggestive techniques, the clinician is referred to texts by Granich (1947) and Goldstein (1932), and to an article by Smith (1948).

Copying should be followed by writing from memory after visual presentation. The time period of stimulation-presentation should be reduced progressively to a brief period, sufficient only for the patient to read what is presented. Following this, the patient should be encouraged to write from dictation, beginning with single words and proceeding, as early as possible, to short phrases and short sentences. Eventually, short paragraphs should be used for dictation material.

In his attempts at writing, the patient should never be required to struggle for the letter or word he cannot evoke from memory. The elusive word should be made available to him so that he can copy what he cannot recall.

*Spelling disability,* in the sense that the appropriate sequence of letters cannot be recalled for a given word, is not an apraxic disturbance as the term *apraxia* has been used in this chapter. It is a higher level symbolic disturbance, and therefor is classified as agraphia. Many patients with writing disturbance have this form of difficulty. Some have both apraxic and spelling involvements. A few will have little difficulty with spelling as such once they overcome their apraxic disability.

For the patient with both forms of writing disturbance, practice in copying and writing from dictation has incidentally provided practice in spelling. Continued practice may be given in flash-card presentations, and in spontaneous writing with word lists available for copying when necessary. If it is determined, as is sometimes the case, that the patient's oral spelling is more accurate than his written efforts, then the oral approach should be emphasized. Similarly, if the patient seems to learn better through the auditory than through the visual avenue, the words should be spelled aloud for the patient, and he should practice writing while he spells aloud.

In teaching spelling, the selection of words to spell should primarily be determined by what the patient will need to write. The essential objective for spelling instruction, for aphasic adults as for children, is to equip them to write what they need and want to write. The needs of the mason and a lawyer are likely to be more divergent for the building of a writing vocabulary than for a speaking or reading vocabulary. This, however, should not overlook the possibility that some masons have avocations which include the need to write and spell to a greater degree than some lawyers.

Spelling lists serve as a guide to ultimate objectives. The lists previously suggested for basic reading vocabularies may obviously be used for spelling as well. These lists should be supplemented by special ones that are related to the patient's interests, and should include vocational and avocational vocabularies if the patient is likely to return to them.

It will frequently be found that many patients' spelling difficulties are similar to those usual with children. Devices such as enlarging the letters of the troublesome parts of the word, or writing the letter in colored ink or crayon, may be of help. Other suggested techniques have been given by Fernald (1943) and Gates and Russell (1937). The patient should be encouraged to keep his own list of troublesome words, written in a fashion best suited to help him to learn the correct spelling of the words. In this regard, it is hoped, that the patient will pride himself on an ever decreasing rather than increasing list size.

**Paraphasia.** Paraphasic errors—the errors of omission, substitution, or transposition of sounds or words—frequently constitute a final therapeutic problem for both the patient and the therapist. These, together with word-finding (anomic) difficulties, may persist as residuals of aphasic involvement. In some instances, there is little to do but to become resigned and adjusted to their continued presence, especially under conditions where intellectual vigilance is reduced.

Some patients evolve oral and written speech which is characteristically agrammatical. Their speech suggests the economical form of a message prepared as a telegraph or a cablegram. So-called "unessential" words—the connectives, prepositions, and conjunctions—are often omitted. A sentence such as "Let us go for a walk" may be reduced to "Go walk" or simply to "Walk." According to Goldstein (1932), many patients lose their attitude toward grammar and need to be reoriented to grammatical practices. This reorientation is not always possible, especially with a patient who has accepted his disabilities and the immunities associated with them. For such a patient, his new point of view seems to be "I am a patient, and I have many disabilities. It is up to others to make adjustments to me and to exert effort to figure out what I mean."

For patients who are motivated to make themselves understood, it is of some help to record their oral speech and to play it back. Then the patient may be asked to indicate what words he omitted that another speaker is likely to use to convey the same meaning. The patient is then encouraged to fill in the omitted words. The author has found that it may also be of help to reduce his own speech to telegraphic style when speaking to the patient, so that the patient can appreciate that such speech is difficult to understand. Where possible, this exercise should be given to a group of patients who may correct one another. Written speech may be corrected by having the therapist indicate the places within a sentence where words were omitted. The patient is then encouraged to fill in the omitted words. If he cannot do this, the words should be inserted for him, and the patient is then directed to rewrite the sentence with all words in conventional order.

Errors of sound reversal may be treated in a similar way. For some patients, the technique of negative practice may be used with success to create awareness of error. Fortunately, for most aphasics, severe paraphasic errors tend to disappear as improvement in general takes place. If paraphasic errors are relatively infrequent, it may not always be worth while to correct them. It is well to remember that even normal nonaphasic persons sometimes commit paraphasia. We call them slips of the tongue. Their psychodynamics, from which aphasics are not free, cannot justifiably be discussed here.

**Word-finding difficulty (anomia).** Both logically and psychologically, the aphasic patient's language needs are greatest for oral speech, and training should, wherever possible, begin here. Unless he is an extremely withdrawn person, a patient can learn to get along without all other forms of productive language except oral speech. Word-finding difficulty is both the most common characteristic of the aphasic's disturbances and the most persistent even after considerable over-all improvement has taken place. It is the form of difficulty most likely to return under conditions of tension, excitement, or fatigue. For many, and perhaps for most aphasics, it is to some degree a permanent residual problem. Sometimes, the substitute word may not readily suggest, in sound or meaning, the desired word. Some patients prefer to say something, in the remote hope that they may guess right, or because of an attitude that saying something—anything—is better than saying nothing. Most patients are able to recognize their errors and try to correct them. If, as indicated earlier, the word evoked in error is one which may be functionally useful, an attempt might be made to establish that word. If this is not the case, the therapist should patiently return to trying to establish the originally selected word.

In establishing a name of an object, the function of the object should be demonstrated, and the object should be named. The patient may then be asked to repeat the name after the therapist. If he can write, he should be asked to write and say the name, alone if possible, otherwise with or after the therapist. Finally, the patient should be given an opportunity at some later time in the therapeutic session to evoke the name by himself.

Once the naming process gets under way for descriptive action, as well as for nominal terms, progress may be accelerated and considerable spontaneous improvement may be expected. Improvement as a result of direct training may also be more rapid. Most patients, however, will continue to find that a few words are ever elusive, and will not be theirs for ready evocation. Some patients will learn to speak slowly, as if they are always hunting for words. Others will become adept in using synonymous terms and phrases. Still others will indulge in lengthy circumlocutions to suggest the meanings of the precise words which will not readily roll off their tongues.

As soon as possible, it is recommended that the patient incorporate the words which have become established, or which are being established, into conventional oral sentence form. All too frequently patients become satisfied with naming as a sentence function. This device, though economical of effort, does not help the individual concerned, or others, to think of him as a recovered person rather than as a patient.

Training to overcome anomia takes place informally whenever a patient is spoken to about things around him, or about himself, or other persons known to him. It would probably be more effective if the talking were about objective things, with simple names, which are familiar to and needed by the patient. If possible, the same object, and the same names, should be used by all persons who have contact with the patient. To insure this, the names can be printed on cards and placed next to the objects, or pinned on the objects. The patient, if he is able to read, may then associate the written word with the object, and he will hear the same name for it spoken by several persons. Through repetition, the oral name word may become established. Most anomic patients, unless they have auditory difficulty, can readily recognize an appropriate name when they hear it. They are usually able to imitate the word name. Their chief difficulty is in the spontaneous evocation of the appropriate word.

Formal training, and if possible informal training, should be limited at first to a few word names of immediate functional value to the patient. If he is a bed patient, such names as *pillow, water,* and *towel* may be good starting words. At first appropriate naming may be slow. A patient may evoke a word somewhat similar in sound, as *owl* for *towel,* or related in meaning, as *wash* or *dry* for *towel.*

It is assumed that the reader will review the general principles of therapy and apply these to the training of the patient with anomia. For useful word lists, the reader is referred to the discussions on reading and spelling.

**Arithmetic difficulty (acalculia).** Arithmetic disturbances may arise because of linguistic aspects per se, or because of the special processes involved in calculation and problem-solving.

Fortunately, much of arithmetic effort is entirely automatic by the time the individual becomes an adult. Because of this, many aphasics can arrive at correct results without being able to name the numerals or tell what they did to arrive at their results. Speed of calculation can be enhanced by making the patient aware of automatic arithmetic series, and by showing him how he can make use of them. After relative automaticity is established, the patient may be shown the rationale of the various arithmetic tables. For example, the patient may be shown that the series 2, 4, 6, 8 . . . is arrived at by adding the amount 2 to each previous amount.

The need for reteaching arithmetic in a manner as close to the one in which the particular process was originally learned has already been discussed under General Principles of Training. Additional suggested approaches to calculation difficulties may be found in texts which deal with the teaching or the remedial teaching of arithmetic. The books by Hildreth (1947) and Fernald (1943) should be of help.

As with other symbolic functions, the amount and kind of calculation to be taught should be determined by the individual patient's immediate needs and later objectives. If the patient is ambulatory, counting sums for payment of purchases and making change should probably have priority.

The linguistic aspect of calculation, that is, the naming per se, is one which should be approached through the techniques for vocabulary building and anomia. Here, patient interests may also be put to good use. One patient who was a stamp collector relearned number-naming by going over his stamp collection. Another, a baseball fan, was strongly motivated to read the box scores and talk about the club standings in the major baseball leagues. The specific approaches to naming may be as varied as the interests of the patient and the resources of the therapist will direct.

**Dysarthria.** Dysarthric (articulatory) difficulties other than those on an oral apraxic basis, may be a concomitant aphasic disturbance. These difficulties may be present because of peripheral nerve involvements of the face, lips, tongue, and the palate, or because of central (cortical) involvement. If the involvements are peripheral, the patient is likely to distort or slur sounds, or to speak slowly and laboriously because his articulatory mechanism has become cumbersome. Improvement is likely to take place spontaneously as innervation improves. If there is residual paresis, the patient, through a basic phonetic approach, may be taught compensations for some of the speech sounds which continue to be difficult to produce. Articulatory drill may be of some help, as will any drill which improves the tonus and control of the articulatory muscles. "Tongue twisters" are not recommended by this author because they require a degree of facility beyond the ordinary needs of the patient.

If the dysarthria is of central origin, it may be of help in *later stages of training* to make the patient aware of his errors and to use a phonetic approach in training. The writer agrees with Wepman (1951, p. 241) that a patient should be encouraged to feel free to express himself. Early self-consciousness inhibits communicative effort and impairs expression. Fortunately, the problem of dysarthria becomes a reduced one as the patient improves. Niceties of articulation should be an objective only if the patient himself chooses it. Unless the patient or the therapist is a perfectionist, this is not likely to be chosen as one of the more important goals of therapy.

## BIBLIOGRAPHY

BACKUS, O. 1947. The rehabilitation of persons with aphasia. *In* West, R., Kennedy, L., and Carr, A. The rehabilitation of speech. New York: Harper. Ch. 25.

BLACKMAN, N. 1950. Group psychotherapy with aphasics. *J. nerv. ment. Dis.*, 111, 154–163.

BUCKINGHAM, B. R., and DOLCH, E. W. 1936. A combined word list. Boston: Ginn.

BUTFIELD, E., and ZANGWILL, O. L. 1946. Re-education in aphasia; A review of 70 cases. *J. Neurol. Neurosur. Psychiat.*, IX, New Series, 75–79.

DOLCH, E. W. 1939. A manual for remedial reading. Champaign, Ill.: Garrard Press.

———— 1949. Basic sight vocabulary cards. Champaign, Ill.: Garrard Press.

———— 1948. Sight phrase cards. Champaign, Ill.: Garrard Press.

——— 1950. Teaching primary reading. (2nd ed.). Champaign, Ill.: Garrard Press.

DURRELL, D. D. 1940. Improvement of basic reading abilities. Yonkers: World Book Co.

EISENSON, J. (1954). Examining for aphasia (rev. ed.). New York: Psychological Corporation.

——— 1949. Prognostic factors related to language rehabilitation in aphasic patients. *J. Speech Hearing Disorders*, 14, 262–264.

FERNALD, G. M. 1943. Remedial techniques in basic school subjects. New York: McGraw-Hill.

GARDNER, W. 1945. Left-handed writing. Danville, Ill.: Interstate Press.

GATES, A. I. 1935. A reading vocabulary for the primary grades. New York: Bureau of Publications, Teachers College, Columbia Univ.

——— and RUSSELL, D. H. 1937. Diagnostic and remedial spelling manual. New York: Bureau of Publications, Teachers College, Columbia Univ.

——— 1950. The improvement of reading (3rd ed.). New York: Macmillan.

GOLDSTEIN, K. 1932. After effects of brain injuries in war. New York: Grune and Stratton.

GRANICH, L. 1947. Aphasia: a guide to retraining. New York: Grune and Stratton.

HARRIS, A. H. 1940. How to increase reading ability. New York: Longmans, Green.

HILDRETH, G. 1947. Learning the three R's (2nd ed.). Minneapolis: Educational Test Bureau, Educ. Publ.

LANDIS, C., and BOLLES, M. M. 1950. Textbook of abnormal psychology (rev. ed.). New York: Macmillan. P. 507.

LONGERICH, M. C., and BORDEAUX, J. 1954. Aphasia therapeutics. New York: Macmillan. P. 109.

ROSE, R. H. 1948. A physician's account of his own aphasia. *J. Speech Hearing Disorders*, 13, 294–305.

SCHUELL, H. 1953. Auditory impairment in aphasia: significance and retraining techniques. *J. Speech Hearing Disorders*, 18, 14–21.

SMITH, M. 1948. Teaching an aphasic how to write again. *J. clin. Psychol.*, 4, 419–423.

THORNDIKE, E. L., and LORGE, I. 1944. Teachers word book of 30,000 words. New York: Bureau of Publications, Teachers College, Columbia Univ.

VAN RIPER, C. 1947. Speech correction (3rd ed.). New York: Prentice-Hall. pp. 258–261.

WEPMAN, J. M. 1951. Recovery from aphasia. New York: Ronald Press.

——— 1953. A conceptual model for the process involved in recovery from aphasia. *J. Speech Hearing Disorders*, 18, 4–13.

## CHAPTER 15

# APHASIA IN CHILDREN—
# LANGUAGE DEVELOPMENT
# AND LANGUAGE PATHOLOGY

### ● Helmer R. Myklebust, Ed.D.

THE USE OF LANGUAGE is one of the basically distinguishing characteristics of man. Man's behavior is predominantly symbolic in nature. Thus, the process of language acquisition and language functioning become fundamental problems in the scientific appraisal of human behavior. The importance of the symbol has been stressed by Cassirer (1944) when he states:

> Yet in the human world we find a new characteristic which appears to be the distinctive mark of human life. The functional circle of man is not only quantitatively enlarged; it has also undergone a qualitative change. Man has, as it were, discovered a new method of adapting himself to his environment. Between the receptor system and the effector system, which are to be found in all animal species, we find in man a third link which we may describe as the *symbolic system*. This new acquisition transforms the whole of human life. As compared with other animals man lives not merely in a broader reality; he lives, so to speak, in a new *dimension* of reality. There is an unmistakable difference between organic reactions and human responses. In the first case a direct and immediate answer is given to an outward stimulus; in the second case the answer is delayed. It is interrupted and retarded by a slow and complicated process of thought.

Symbolic behavior is not limited to language symbols. Music, art, and religion entail symbols which are not specifically language symbols. Therefore, man's symbolic behavior is not limited to language, but language is his most predominant type of symbolization and is the main basis of his ability to communicate. This discussion is limited essentially to that aspect of man's symbolic behavior which can be described as being attributed to the use of language.

#### THE NATURE OF LANGUAGE AND SYMBOLIC BEHAVIOR

Language is an organized set of symbols which may be either auditory or visual. It is the task of every infant to acquire the particular set of symbols which are characteristic of his culture. The auditory symbol is basic to the total language process. Genetically, it is the first language symbol which is acquired. Furthermore, it is the auditory or spoken symbol which is predominant in any cultural group. Man's symbolic behavior is determined predominantly by this auditory symbol.

It is language which makes symbolic behavior possible. Symbolic behavior is that behavior which occurs on the basis of a sign or symbol instead of the actual object, idea, or feeling. After the symbol has been acquired, an individual can relate to another individual on the basis of this symbol and this in turn makes the presence of the actual object, idea, or feeling unnecessary. When this occurs, abstract behavior has been achieved and such behavior occurs only under the circumstances of symbolization. Langer (1942) has emphasized the difference between the language of people and the language of lower animals. She emphasizes that lower animals have a language of "signification"; that is, they can signify the presence of certain phenomena, such as food, anger, and danger, but they cannot symbolize such phenomena. In this respect man differs greatly from the lower animals. The most primitive of people have a highly developed language and behave in a highly symbolic manner. Nevertheless, it seems possible that abstract behavior is rather directly related to the subtlety of the language system which any specific group of human beings uses. Likewise, in language pathology, when the symbolic process has been disturbed, man is reduced in his abstract functioning; this varies greatly with the type of language pathology encountered. Before considering the complex problem of disturbed language functioning in children, it is necessary to explore the basic problem of how the normal child acquires language.

## LANGUAGE DEVELOPMENT IN CHILDREN

The process of language acquisition in children has been studied mainly in terms of normative data. For example, the age at which a child first speaks a single word and then speaks in sentences has been well established (McCarthy, 1946). Such information is only indirectly suggestive of the process of language acquisition itself. Furthermore, the study of language has been primarily in terms of expressive language. Other aspects, such as inner and receptive language, only recently have been considered scientifically. Similarly, the study of language acquisition traditionally has considered mainly organic factors and has tacitly assumed psychological factors. It is now apparent that this is an oversimplification of the process of language acquisition. Language acquisition and language pathology are interrelated theoretically, and inclusive consideration entails concern for organic and psychological aspects simultaneously. However, the infant first lives through a nonsymbolic period. An excellent discussion of this period and its importance is given by Sullivan (1953).

Functionally, language can be divided into three types: inner, receptive, and expressive (Myklebust, 1954). Genetically, inner language is acquired first, receptive language is acquired next, and expressive is acquired last.

*Inner language* can be described as the use of language symbols for purposes of inner life or thought; that is, it might be described as that language which the individual uses for autistic purposes or for "talking to himself." As the individual matures (on the average after six years of age), this inner language might be either auditory or visual; one might think in "heard words" or "seen words." *Receptive language* might be considered as that language which an individual uses to understand others. This, too, might consist of either spoken or written symbols after a certain degree of maturation has occurred. Genetically, the ability to understand the spoken word precedes that of being able to understand the written word by approximately five years. *Expressive language* can be viewed as that language which the individual uses to make himself understood to others. Again, such symbols may be either spoken or written. In general, the functional classifications of language can be viewed simply in these terms: inner language is that language which the individual uses autistically, receptive language is the language which he uses for the purpose of comprehending others, and expressive language is that language which he uses in making himself understood to others.

As indicated previously, although expressive language has been studied more extensively than either inner or receptive language, it seems that the expressive use of language can occur only after both inner and receptive language have been partially established. This is emphasized by the genetics of language development, which indicate that inner language must have been established before receptive language can become functional and expressive language occurs only if inner and receptive language have become useful within certain minimal levels of adequacy. During approximately the first eight months of life, the infant receives sensations and through gradual integration he develops basic and fundamental inner language. At the age of approximately eight or nine months he has acquired sufficient inner language so that he begins to comprehend some of the spoken language which he hears. He then begins to use receptive language, which is the second step in the genetics of language development. After he has received or comprehended the spoken word for approximately another four months, he begins to use expressive language. It is a well-established finding that children on the average use their first word at approximately 12 to 13 months of age. It is apparent that much of the language process in terms of language acquisition has preceded this specific occurrence of being able to use a word expressively.

## Language Pathology and Language Development

This functional classification of language has certain advantages in terms of the problems encountered in language pathology. The traditional classification of language disorders has been expressive aphasia, receptive aphasia, and central (global) aphasia (Goldstein, 1948). Therefore, if an individual had a disturbance characterized by interference with the use of language for purposes of thinking or communicating with himself—that is, a disturbance of inner language—it was referred to as *central aphasia*. If the symbolic disturbance caused impairment of the ability to interpret the symbols as spoken by others—that is, a disturbance of receptive language—it was referred to as *receptive aphasia*. Similarly, if the symbolic disturbance interfered primarily with the ability to express language, it was referred to as *expressive aphasia*.

If a symbolic disturbance occurs in the young child during the time that he is acquiring language, then certain reciprocal relationships between inner, receptive, and expressive language might be inferred. For example, if the child's capacity to integrate sensations is impaired and thereby his inner language is retarded, it might be expected that both his receptive and expressive language will be delayed reciprocally. Furthermore, if the child's receptive language has been impaired, it might be expected to delay the development of inner and expressive language. Normal development of inner language assumes integrity of the reception of sensations and of integrative capacities. Therefore, impairment of receptive function would impede development of inner language. Likewise, until inner language is acquired within certain limits, expressive language apparently cannot occur. This reciprocal relationship between inner, receptive, and expressive language seems to be a fundamental concept relative to language acquisition and language pathology as revealed by normal language development and by aphasia in young children.

Normal language development assumes integrity of the organism in several respects. Perhaps one of the limitations of some of the points of view of language acquisition is that it has been assumed that if the organism has normal sensory functioning and normal integrity of the central nervous system, language would be acquired automatically. Experience, especially with language pathology in children, is not in agreement with this theoretical frame of reference. Rather, the organism must have adequate integrity both organically and psychologically if language is to be acquired in a normal manner. Normal language development can be impeded by peripheral nervous system damage, such as deafness or blindness; by central nervous system damage, resulting in aphasia or mental deficiency; or by psychological disturbances which interfere with the processes of integration. Basic psychological disturbances such as childhood schizophrenia, infantile autism, and severe anxieties might impair normal integrative processes and thereby impede inner language (Mykelbust, 1954). Likewise, psychological disturbances might cause psychic deafness and interfere with normal receptive language development. Such disturbances would be expected to interfere reciprocally with expressive language, but psychological disturbances might impede expressive language directly, such as in the child with psychogenic mutism. Psychological processes which seem to be directly related to language acquisition are identification, internalization, and imitation (Mowrer, 1950). Various authors have emphasized the importance of these processes in language development (McCarthy, 1954). Sullivan (1953) provides discussion

/hich reveals the importance of anxiety in early infancy relative to the de-
elopment of language. In view of these various evidences, it seems that
ormal language development occurs only when the organism has adequate
ntegrity of the peripheral and central nervous systems, and when psycho-
ogical integrity is present at the required level.

## THE PROBLEM OF APHASIA IN CHILDREN

There is agreement that the term *aphasia* should be limited to language dis-
rders which derive from organic impairments. Language disturbances
aused by deafness, blindness, or by various psychological disorders should
ot be referred to as aphasias. There is good agreement in that aphasia is
aditionally and typically viewed as a language disorder which results from
amage to the brain. Conditions such as dysarthria are not included under
phasia because such conditions, although neurological in nature, are not
ue symbolic disorders. The term *aphasia* is further defined as meaning that
n impairment in the use of language symbols has been incurred. In children
is highly desirable to distinguish between the aphasias and the dyslexias.
phasia becomes apparent in the child long before the problem of dyslexia.
he characteristic age for encountering the problem of aphasia in children
between two and four years, while dyslexias do not become apparent until
me time after six years of age. Although the term *aphasia* is sometimes
sed with adults to mean a disturbance of either auditory or visual symbolic
nctioning, this use of the term does not serve the purpose of classification
children in a desired manner. Thus, in the area of language pathology in
oung children it seems necessary to differentiate between aphasia and dys-
xia. *The term aphasia as used here includes all degrees of disturbance of
e of the verbal symbol.* Recognition is made of the fact that the term
ysphasia is becoming more widely used and perhaps is the term which will
 used extensively in the future because it emphasizes that, while a symbolic
sorder is present, a complete loss of symbolic functioning has not occurred.

### lationship Between Aphasia in Children and Adults

There has been rather wide confusion relative to the area of aphasia in
ildren. Much of this confusion is due to semantic difficulties. For example,
me adhere to a literal definition of the term *aphasia,* which is "the loss of
eech." This literal definition of the word *aphasia* perhaps is inaccurate
d inappropriate as far as any language or symbolic disorder is concerned,
hether it be in children or adults, because as indicated in the discussion
der language and symbolic behavior, aphasia is not a speech disorder as
ch. Rather, it is an impairment or inability to relate a language symbol to
perience. There are aphasics, both children and adults, who have no speech
pairment but who have marked disorders in ability to function symboli-
lly from the point of view of language usage (Wepman, 1951). This has
en recognized over a period of approximately 125 years and the term

*aphasia* now has taken on the meaning of symbolic disturbance; or mor
broadly, a problem in language functioning. A certain confusion persist
because some authorities continue to think of aphasia as a "loss of speech
and imply that, if an individual has not acquired speech, he has no speec
that he can lose and thus cannot be correctly or appropriately referred t
as an aphasic. This problem of terminology has been present in various othe
areas, such as in the area of deafness. In such areas clarifying terms usuall
have been used with the basic term for classification and confusion has bee
greatly reduced. For example, we speak of "congenital deafness" to diffei
entiate it from deafness which has been sustained after birth. Likewise, i
aphasia the causal concept, that is, a symbolic disorder due to neurologic;
involvements, should not be confused with the time concept of when such
difficulty was sustained (Mykelbust, 1954). The term *congenital* appropr
ately used is simply a time-of-onset concept. Therefore, congenital aphasi
simply means that neurological involvements which have caused the verb;
language disorder have been present from the time of birth. Most aphasia i
children seems to be congenital from the point of view of timing or age c
onset. This is discussed further in connection with etiology.

It has not been necessary traditionally, as other areas of pathological b
havior in the human being have been studied and classified, to use differe
classifications for the same problem in children and adults. This is illustrate
by the use of the terms *congenital deafness* and *childhood schizophrenia,* an
by use of the terms *exogenous* and *endogenous* to distinguish between cla
sifications based on causal concepts and those based on time of onset. Fu
thermore, the similarities of the problem of aphasia in many children ar
adults are sufficiently great to make diverse classification on the basis of a§
of onset unnecessary and unwarranted. It is true that the language disord
present in the young child can be fully ascertained and appraised only aft
a certain degree of maturation has occurred, but this is true also of vario
other areas of the study of pathological behavior in human beings, such ;
in the area of deafness. Rather then the age of onset being the predomina
factor relative to classification, it is necessary for us to consider the bas
problem and then classify on the basis of the fundamental nature of the di
order. Inasmuch as the aphasic child's problem is a language disorder
should be so classified; thus the classification of aphasia which has been w
developed for adults seems to be the logical and appropriate one to be us
for the same disorder in the child, despite the fact that he must be of a certa
maturational level before such a classification can be made.

## NONSYMBOLIC LANGUAGE DISORDERS

Language pathology in children is not limited to aphasias and other typ
of symbolic disturbances. It is helpful to contrast the symbolic and nonsy
bolic language disorders when considering the problem of aphasia in you
children.

## The Deaf

Nonsymbolic language disorders are of various types. For example, children who are congenitally deaf have a marked disturbance of language development and functioning. Their language difficulties derive from their being unable to hear the auditory verbal symbols with which they are surrounded. Because they do not acquire oral language at any level, that is, inner, receptive, or expressive, they also present marked limitations in the area of read and written language. This further illustrates the importance of oral or spoken language relative to the genetic aspects of language development. Deaf children are not typically deprived in visual capacities. Because they are limited in the acquisition of spoken language, they are likewise and reciprocally impeded in the acquisition of read and written language. The deaf child illustrates the importance of the acquisition of spoken language relative to inner, receptive, and expressive language functioning. Apparently the basic language system in any human being is essentially auditory and oral in nature, and when this basic type of language is impeded relative to development from early life, then all other language functioning is reciprocally affected. It should be emphasized that the congenitally deaf child's language disorder is not a true symbolic impairment and therefore should not be classified as an aphasia. Comparative studies of deaf and aphasic children continue to be highly revealing relative to various aspects of language development and of language pathology in general (Mykelbust, 1954). Furthermore, studies of the type of symbol system which the congenitally deaf child does acquire can be considered as being important in the understanding of all language and symbolization in children or adults (Mykelbust and Brutten, 1953). The differential diagnosis between congenital deafness and congenital aphasia also is an important facet of the total problem of language disorders in children; it has implications for appropriate methodologies and training programs to be instituted. This aspect of the problem is discussed in the following chapter.

One of the challenging problems presented by the congenitally deaf child from the point of view of language behavior is that he does organize his world and he does become an integrated symbolic organism with greater ease and greater facility than the child with a basic problem of congenital aphasia. The deaf child seems to be able to organize his world and his experiences visually and to develop an inner language, despite the fact that his language is devoid of verbal symbols and is essentially visual and tactual in nature. Further understanding of the congenitally deaf child's language can be expected to be useful and revealing regarding all types of language pathology in young children.

## The Blind

Another form of nonsymbolic language disturbance is that which is found in the congenitally blind child. From the point of view of language pathology only, the blind child's language impairment is perhaps less basically disturbing than that of the deaf child. The blind child does acquire verbal language but is lacking primarily in being able to acquire normally the read and written symbol system. It is significant that clinical experience suggests that congenitally blind children typically are delayed in the acquisition of verbal language as compared to normal children. This emphasizes the supplementary functioning of audition and vision in acquiring oral language, although usually we think of hearing alone as being responsible for the acquisition of spoken language. As with the deaf child, studies of the symbolic functioning in the blind can be expected to reveal significant information relative to language acquisition and language behavior in general. Congenitally blind children, too, do organize their world and integrate their experiences and they do behave in a symbolic manner, despite the fact that their symbolization lacks visual symbols. Such studies are useful in ascertaining the nature of sensory processes as they relate to language development and language functioning. The scientific observer who is confronted with young children presenting problems of language pathology is continually impressed by the excellent symbolic behavior encountered in both the deaf and the blind as contrasted with the young aphasic child. This emphasizes the need of a diagnosis of aphasia in early life; because in terms of the debilitating effects on the organism when it is unable to function symbolically, such diagnosis is most important. Even children who are both deaf and blind seem to be able to acquire an inner language through their residual sensory capacities and do achieve a level and type of symbolic behavior. The deaf-blind child, moreover, presents a challenging problem and opportunity relative to the study of language development and language disorders in young children.

## Auditory Perception

A nonsymbolic language disturbance might derive from impairment of perceptual functioning. The perceptual capacities which are most directly related to language development and behavior are auditory and visual perception. Auditory perceptual capacities are fundamental to acquisition of spoken language. Visual perceptual disturbances commonly are associated with auditory perceptual disturbances, but are less directly influential on oral language acquisition (Strauss and Lehtinen, 1947). They might be directly influential in the acquisition of reading and writing. On the basis of experience and studies of young children with auditory perceptual disturbances, it seems that the infant normally must gradually develop auditory perceptual capacities. At birth the infant cannot select sounds from his environment which are immediately pertinent to his needs and circumstance. Rather, the auditory world impinges upon him in a conglomerate, unselected and unstructured manner. As he begins to associate meaning to his auditory world, he gradually learns to select those sounds which are most useful to his immediate needs and adjustment. For example, as he matures he is able to select the sound of his mother's voice and the sounds associated with feed ng on the basis of their immediate suitability and usefulness relative to his maintaining a firm and wholesome homeostatic relationship with his environment. To the extent that such behavior develops, the child is structuring his auditory world appropriately for his own well-being. Before he can acquire inner, receptive, or expressive language it is necessary for him to select speech sounds from the total conglomerate world of sound in order that he can listen to such speech sounds and integrate them meaningfully. A disturbance in auditory perception precludes this achievement in the typical or normal manner. Such an incapacity apparently can be due to either organic or emotional disturbances. Auditory perceptual disorders are common in the brain-injured child. Such disorders are not true symbolic disorders and therefore should not be considered the equivalent of aphasia (Myklebust, 1954). Presumably if auditory perceptual disturbances are of sufficient severity, they might cause a true symbolic incapacity because the organism is incapable of psychologically organizing its sensations sufficiently to make symbolic behavior possible. It seems that perceptual disturbance usually should be considered as being distinct from true symbolic disorders. Methods and procedures for training of children with perceptual problems are discussed in the following chapter.

## Auditory Agnosia

Agnosia is a nonsymbolic language incapacity. Agnosia, like perception, usually is prefaced by a term indicating the area of sensory functioning. The sensory areas which are most important in agnosias as they relate to language are the same as those encountered in perceptual disturbances; that is, hearing and vision. Hence auditory and visual agnosia are the types which are significant in connection with language disorders. As in the discussion of perception, only the auditory will be considered.

Auditory agnosia must be differentiated from the aphasias. The primary contrasting aspect of an agnosia as compared to an aphasia is that the agnosia is not specifically or essentially only a symbolic disturbance. The aphasic child has a basic impairment of his ability to use spoken sounds. He is not disturbed or incapable of using his auditory sensations in other respects; that is, the aphasic finds all sounds in his environment useful and meaningful with the exception of the spoken word. In contrast, the auditory gnosic not only cannot use these spoken sounds in his environment but he cannot attribute meaning to any sounds in his auditory world. For example, he cannot associate meaning to the sound of an airplane, the ringing of a telephone or the closing of a door. Presumably agnosia occurs only on an organic basis and is due to a generalized damage to the auditory cortex (Gardner, 1948). Severe auditory perceptual disturbances and auditory agnosia are highly similar in symptomatology but comparatively the condition of agnosia seems to be considerably more severe. It seems that an auditory agnosia does not occur unless an aphasia also is present. Auditory agnosia is primarily related to receptive language disorders.

## Apraxia

Another nonsymbolic language disorder which is frequently considered in relation to the aphasias is apraxia. Its importance in young children seems to be relatively less than that of perceptual disturbances, but an apraxia usually must be considered comparatively with an expressive language disorder such as expressive aphasia or agraphia. An apraxia of the speech motor system is highly similar to an expressive aphasia. An apraxia is not limited to the motor aspects of language; rather, it is a generalized inability to use the particular motor system for any purpose. Perhaps the classic description as given by Head (1926) that the apraxic "cannot do what he wants to and the aphasic cannot say what he wants to" is a useful means of clarifying the concepts of apraxia and aphasia.

## Dysarthria

Frequently it is necessary to make a comparison between apraxia and dysarthria. As indicated above the motor incapacity of the apraxic is more generalized than that which is found in the dysarthric. Both conditions are due to neurological involvement but dysarthria is limited to a paralytic involvement of the tongue, whereas apraxia is considered a more generalized but nonparalytic impairment of a motor function (DeJong, 1950).

## Psychological Disorders

Emotional disturbance, like organic involvements, might cause language deficiencies of the nonsymbolic type. Perhaps the most widely recognized conditions in this respect are childhood schizophrenia and infantile autism (Kanner, 1948). As stated previously, severe anxieties and other types of behavior problems might be influential in causing a delay in language acquisition or in the normal use of language which has been acquired. This type of language pathology, while highly relevant to the study of language development in children and to the problem of differential diagnosis, will not be considered in detail in this discussion. The problem of differential diagnosis is further discussed in the following chapter.

## Mental Deficiency

Various studies have revealed a significant relationship between mental capacity and language acquisition and development (Karlin and Strazzula, 1952). Thus, any broad consideration of language pathology in young children must include the concept of mental development and mental deficiency. The study of language behavior in the mentally deficient presents intriguing possibilities in terms of further determining the relationship between intelligence, abstract behavior, and language functioning. This consideration beyond the scope of this discussion except as it relates further to the problem of differential diagnosis which is discussed in the following chapter.

## SYMBOLIC DISORDERS IN ADDITION TO APHASIA

In young children it seems desirable to distinguish between the symbolic disorders in spoken language as contrasted with those in written or read language. The classification of aphasia in young children usually does not include symbolic disorders in reading or writing. But as a frame of reference, it is essential to include all symbolic disorders of language; hence the problems of alexia and agraphia must be included in the area of symbolic language disorders in children (Orton, 1937). The term *alexia* is used only when a true symbolic disorder of reading is present. Likewise, the term *agraphia* is used only when a true symbolic disorder of writing is present. Problems of peripheral vision and visual perceptual disturbance should be differentiated from alexia. Similarly, motor disorders should be differentiated from the true inability to associate the symbol with the appropriate motor function such as is found in agraphia.

## BIBLIOGRAPHY

CASSIRER, E. 1944. An essay on man. New Haven: Yale Univ. Press.

DE JONG, R. N. 1950. The neurologic examination. New York: Paul Hoeber.

GARDNER, E. 1948. Fundamentals of neurology. Philadelphia: Saunders.

GOLDSTEIN, K. 1948. Language and language disturbances. New York: Grune and Stratton.

HEAD, H. 1926. Aphasia and kindred disorders of speech. Cambridge: Cambridge Univ. Press.

KANNER, L. 1948. Child psychiatry. Springfield, Ill.: C. C. Thomas.

KARLIN, I. W., and STRAZZULA, M. 1952. Speech and language problems of mentally deficient children. *J. Speech Hearing Disorders,* 7, 286.

LANGER, S. K. 1942. Philosophy in a new key. New York: Penguin Books.

MCCARTHY, D. 1946. Language development in children. *In* Carmichael, L., Manual of child psychology. New York: Harper.

———— 1954. Language disorders and parent-child relationships. *J. Speech Hearing Disorders,* 19, 514.

MOWRER, O. H. 1950. Learning theory and personality dynamics. New York: Ronald Press.

MYKLEBUST, H. R. 1954. Auditory disorders in children. New York: Grune and Stratton.

MYKLEBUST, H. R., and BRUTTEN, M. 1953. A study of the visual perception of deaf children. Stockholm: *Acta-Otolaryngologica,* Supplementum 105.

ORTON, S. T. 1937. Reading, writing and speech problems in children. New York: Norton.

STRAUSS, A., and LEHTINEN, L. 1947. Psychopathology and education of the brain-injured child. New York: Grune and Stratton.

SULLIVAN, H. S. 1953. The interpersonal theory of psychiatry. New York: Norton.

WEPMAN, J. 1951. Recovery from aphasia. New York: Ronald Press.

# CHAPTER 16

# APHASIA IN CHILDREN— DIAGNOSIS AND TRAINING

● *Helmer R. Myklebust, Ed.D.*

APHASIA DOES NOT PRESENT a syndrome which is dichotomous as compared to other types of language pathology in early life. The primary complaint by parents of aphasic children usually includes the question of why the child is not beginning to speak. Frequently these parents have observed that the child presents other types of problems such as inattention, hyperactivity, restlessness, and inconsistency. But such parental observations overlap with those which are found in children with deafness, emotional disturbance, and to some extent in the mentally deficient. While it is apparent that the primary concern of the parent of an aphasic child is his lack of normal acquisition of speech, parents of deaf children and of certain types of emotionally disturbed children, likewise, give this as their basic concern. Therefore, the nature of the diagnostic problem relative to aphasia in young children is to differentially determine which of the total group of young children who are not acquiring speech normally have aphasia and which do not. More specifically, the diagnostic task becomes one of ascertaining whether a symbolic involvement is present or whether the problem consists of a type of language pathology without symbolic disorder. This diagnostic problem is complex and presents a challenge to various professional groups. Usually the diagnosis entails the professional efforts of several specialists. Perhaps those who are most commonly involved in the diagnosis of aphasia in young children are the neurologist, the clinical psychologist, the child psychiatrist, the pediatrician, the otolaryngologist, the audiologist, and the speech pathologist. This discussion does not presume to include a consideration of the importance of the work of all of these specialists. Rather, the problem of diagnosis as discussed here is intended primarily for the audiologist and the speech pathologist. It is assumed that these workers would find it necessary to rely on the assistance and opinions of various other diagnosticians.

## DIFFERENTIAL DIAGNOSIS

Perhaps the most limiting aspect of the diagnostic approach to aphasia in young children in the past is that it has been essentially unitary. The child has been viewed basically as a speech problem and a diagnosis of delayed speech has been considered sufficiently comprehensive. The emphasis contemporarily is on a multiphasic approach. The child is not viewed as presenting a problem only in the area of communication; he is considered as an organism which necessarily manifests alterations in its behavior and development in various ways. The diagnostic problem is viewed as being inclusive and presenting the possibility of ascertaining corroborative data from the child's total incapacities. Usually a diagnosis of aphasia is made only when such corroborative evidence is found. Characteristically, a diagnosis of aphasia in young children consists of a three-step procedure. These three steps are: taking a differential history, making clinical observations of behavior and administering suitable and appropriate objective tests (Mykelbust, 1954). The history, clinical observations, and testing usually include six different areas of functioning or capacity. Each of these areas is considered briefly below.

## Hearing

Aphasic children frequently are presumed to have peripheral deafness. Although it is possible for the aphasic child to have a peripheral hearing loss, typically he should not be thought of as having a hearing loss. His auditory incapacities usually derive from causes other than reduced acuity, such as a disturbance of auditory perception. Inasmuch as most hearing tests assume integrity of auditory perception, the aphasic child frequently cannot respond normally to such tests. This is especially true if the auditory tests are of the normal type and require intact listening capacities and behavior. In daily life the aphasic child frequently is inconsistent in his auditory functioning. Parents often report that at times he seems quite deaf but at other times he hears even faint sounds. This is consistent with expectation when auditory perceptual problems are present. In certain situations, the auditory world is much more readily structured than in other situations. Usually the aphasic child responds in a way so as to reveal normal auditory acuity when the situation is one in which he is capable of structuring his auditory environment. Many of these children respond consistently only to one or two sounds. For example, one such child responded normally only to the sounds made in connection with opening a cookie jar; he had been able to learn to select this sound from the auditory environment and responded to it from a considerable distance even though it was faint.

Ingenuity and caution relative to the ascertainment of auditory acuity in children presumed to be aphasic is of critical importance. In general, the more formal the hearing test, the more it is dependent on a high degree of structuring and listening behavior and the more inappropriate it is for the ascertainment of deafness in these children. This is not only because of their frequently marked inadequacies in listening and in auditory perception but also because of their disinhibition and inattention. Considerable discussion of the problem of determining auditory capacities in young children is available (Barr, 1955; Myklebust, 1954).

## Motor Capacities

Motor and neurological capacities are related. The specifically neurological considerations relative to aphasia will not be included in this discussion. Excellent presentations of neurological aspects as viewed diagnostically and therapeutically are available in standard references (DeJong, 1950; Goldstein, 1948). Wide interest persists in the area of motor functioning and in the area of dominance and laterality. This interest is highly desirable and significant as far as the problem of diagnosis of aphasia in young children is concerned. Most of these children show definite and distinct motor signs in the history, in the clinical observations, and on motor tests. Presumably the central nervous system involvement is not limited to language capacity, but characteristically includes other functions. This is logical in view of the generalized organismic disturbance typically found in aphasic children. A disturbance of motor co-ordination can be considered as characteristic of the aphasic child. This motor disturbance can be described as mildly diffuse in-co-ordination, inferior grasp, and awkwardness rather than as obvious disabledness or cerebral palsy. Genetic aspects of motor development also are disturbed. This has been revealed by a comparative study of normal, deaf, emotionally disturbed, aphasic, and mentally deficient children. The aphasic child is delayed both in the age of sitting and walking as compared to the normal (Myklebust, 1954).

In the differential diagnosis of aphasia in young children, possible motor involvements should be explored through the differential history, through clinical observations, and through tests of motor capacity. Several useful motor tests are available (Cassell, 1950; Gesell, 1940; Heath, 1942). Tests which require the organism to function as a total unit have been found to be the most revealing diagnostically. Motor appraisal of a specific area, such as of the speech mechanism, is unlikely to reveal the presence of motor incapacities satisfactorily. Rather, tests of grasp, balance, kicking, throwing and locomotor co-ordination are most likely to reveal motor disturbances of the type commonly associated with aphasia in the young child.

Determination of dominance and laterality is a significant aspect of the motor evaluation. Disturbances of laterality are encountered frequently in the aphasic child (Orton, 1937). He might be predominantly right-handed but predominantly left-legged. Such mixed laterality is a typical motor sign in these children. Presumably the neurological involvement has precluded normal development of sidedness, and the organism is compensating by developing normal dominance for one limb but dominance for the other limb has been transferred to the other side. Such natural compensation by the organism seems the most successful possible, because attempts to shift such dominance often are unsuccessful.

The area of general motor functioning and its relationship to aphasia an other types of language pathology seem well established. Many specific aspects of this relationship remain to be clarified. This is a challenging problem for the speech pathologist and other specialists involved in the problem of language development and language behavior as it relates to the young child.

## Social Maturity

Considerable work has been achieved relative to the significance of social maturity as an aspect of growth and development in the human being. Social maturity as viewed and defined by Doll (1947) includes the extent to which the individual has achieved independence of behavior, that is, the extent to which he has learned to care for himself and is able to assist with the care of others. The appraisal of social maturity consists largely of determining the extent to which the individual remains dependent on his parents or on society. Perhaps one of the most significant results of any handicap is that it increases the need for dependence on others. Sometimes this is the basis of the emotional adjustment problems encountered by handicapped people. It is apparent that the aphasic child faces a significant problem in this connection. One of the basic avenues through which an individual acquires social maturity is that of communication. However, the aphasic child's limitations in regard to social competence are not limited to inabilities specifically in this area. It has been suggested previously that the brain-injured organism is diffusely affected. Hence problems related to social maturity might derive from disinhibition, motor disturbances, perceptual disturbances, and from other difficulties. Diagnostically and therapeutically, ascertainment of the child's level of independent behavior is practical and beneficial in various respects.

The most satisfactory method for ascertaining social maturity in aphasic children is through the use of the Vineland Social Maturity Scale (Doll, 1947). Comparative studies of aphasic, deaf, emotionally disturbed, and mentally deficient children have revealed that on the average the young aphasic child makes approximately three-fourths of normal progress in development of independence during the preschool years. This increased dependence is greater than that found in deaf children and equal to that found in certain emotionally disturbed children. It is significantly above the level of independence achieved by comparable mentally deficient children. This manifests the significance of determining the level of social competence diagnostically and therapeutically. Determination of social maturity can be expected to be useful in differentiating aphasic children from those who are deaf and from those who are mentally deficient. Such determination reveals the basic nature of the problem of aphasia relative to the development of independence—ability to care for one's self and to assume one's role in society. It provides a conceptual frame of reference for the handicap of aphasia and the needs of the individual relative to therapy.

Comparable to other scientific procedures, training and experience in the administration and interpretation of the Social Maturity Scale is essential for its maximum usefulness by the clinician or the research worker.

## Mental Capacity

Various authorities have studied the effect of a brain injury on mental functioning and capacity (Doll, 1951; Strauss and Lehtinen, 1947). The area of clinical psychology is making progress in objectifying the disorders in psychological functioning which are commonly associated with brain damage. One of the fundamental problems in this connection is that of distinguishing between basic mental retardation due to diffuse involvement of the brain and more specific disorders such as perceptual disturbances. The more conceptualization is affected, the more the child is similar to the mentally deficient. On the other hand, the extent to which basic perceptual involvements can be ascertained and alleviated by training, to this extent the child's mental functioning will approximate the normal. However, there is a reciprocal relationship between perceptual and conceptual development. If perceptual development is disturbed fundamentally, conceptual development seems to be reciprocally retarded. Therefore, the differential diagnosis of an aphasic child frequently becomes a problem of ascertaining whether true perceptual disturbances are present with reciprocal retardation in abstract behavior and development, or whether generalized involvement of the central nervous system has caused a basic mental retardation. Characteristically, the young aphasic child presents a problem of perceptual disturbance without marked generalized retardation. Viewed psychologically the most common effect of brain injury in a child or in an adult is the way in which it impedes normal integrative functioning. The aphasic child can be described as having mental capacity and receiving sensations but as being unable to integrate these phenomena and to develop a logicalness of experience. This is revealed in the aphasic child's lack of normal ability to focus his attention, to behave selectively, by his disinhibition, and by his perseveration. (This behavioral syndrome is discussed below under training.) These attributes of the brain-injured child cause a difficult problem in the use of objective tests. The assumptions made when administering a psychological test usually do not apply when they are used with the brain-injured aphasic child. The use of such tests for this purpose requires considerable training and experience if validity and reliability are to be inferred.

The findings from tests of mental functioning should be corroborated by evidence secured from the appraisal of other areas of the child's behavior such as motor capacity, social maturity, and hearing. A diagnosis of aphasia can be made with considerably more assurance when data from various areas of behavior reveal consistent results in terms of the syndrome of the aphasic child. A number of tests of mental capacity and mental functioning have been adapted for use with aphasic children (Myklebust, 1954). However, a great deal of research effort will be necessary before such a battery of tests will become highly definitive relative to differential diagnosis in young chil dren. One of the fundamental requirements of such tests is that they must be essentially free of language usage in both administration and response.

## Emotional Aspects

The differential diagnosis of aphasia in young children includes the problem of distinguishing between those who are inferior in language for reasons of emotional disturbance and those who have an aphasia. Perhaps the most frequent differentiations that must be made are those between aphasia, childhood schizophrenia, and infantile autism. Inasmuch as these children typically are unable to use language either receptively or expressively, most standard techniques for the appraisal of emotional factors cannot be used. The behavioral symptomatological approach is necessary when making such a differential diagnosis. This approach assumes that the organism behaves primarily on the basis of its major deprivation (Myklebust, 1954). If the problem is peripheral deafness, the organism will behave on the basis of sensory deprivation because alteration on the basis of this deprivation is necessary if it is to maintain adequate relationships to its environment and survive. If the basic disorder is emotional in nature, the organism will behave on the basis of psychological deprivation and will function bizarrely and disintegratively with a characteristic symptom complex.

The aphasic child behaves primarily on the basis of brain injury and his inabilities symbolically. The rationale for this approach and a discussion of behavioral symptomatology accordingly has been presented elsewhere (Myklebust, 1954). It is apparent that a differential diagnosis of emotional factors versus brain injury requires careful study by various specialists usually including child psychiatry, clinical psychology, and pediatric neurology. A highly definitive differential history is essential, just as it is with other aspects of this diagnostic problem.

## Language Capacity

One of the most fundamental responsibilities faced by the speech pathologist in connection with the differential diagnosis of aphasia in young children is the appraisal of the child's total capacities in communication. Perhaps one of the limitations of the work of the speech pathologist has been his specific concern with the production of speech. After evaluating the speech production and classifying the child on the basis of delay or retardation of speech, he has concluded that a differential diagnosis has been made. It is evident that a child might have a delay in his speech acquisition and production for at least four primary reasons: deafness, emotional disturbance, mental retardation, and aphasia. Therefore, to refer to the child's condition as a delay in speech usage is unsatisfactory relative to differential diagnosis and planning for therapy. Usually it is essential to ascertain the reason for the lack of or delay in speech behavior. It seems reasonable to assume that a certain number of the children who are now commonly referred to as being delayed in speech are actually aphasic children.

All young children who present a problem of limitation in oral communication should have the benefit of an examination of language development and language functioning. Such an examination can be described as an analysis of his symbolic behavior, but primarily as it relates to language. However, total symbolic functioning is appraised in such an evaluation. The use of gesture, facial expression, crying, laughing, or whining might be highly indicative of the symbolic capacities and should be included in the history, clinical observations, and examination.

In evaluating the child's language behavior it is helpful to proceed on the basis of the functions of language as discussed in the previous chapter. This means that the examination should include a specific appraisal of the child's inner, receptive, and expressive language. Characteristically, appraisal of language-functioning has been limited largely to expressive abilities. One of the ways in which to proceed with securing information relative to the child's language abilities is to engage him in a spontaneous activity. The activity should be deliberately planned and presented, because it is essential to consider the child's total capacities of attention, inhibition, and integration. The activity must not exceed his level of functioning in these respects in order to assure definitive information in regard to his symbolic functioning. The most suitable type of activity for evaluation of language is one which provides an opportunity to make associations between objects. For example, if the child is given toys, including kitchen utensils, bathroom, living room, and bedroom furniture, it is possible to observe his organization and structuring of these objects. Commonly he is presented also with doll figures representing both children and adults. If he proceeds by associating the objects appropriately and relating them to his daily experience, certain inferences can be drawn relative to his inner language capacities. The objects which are used in such language-testing can range from the highly concrete to the very abstract. This permits an opportunity for noting considerable difference in functioning from child to child. Similar procedures have been used with adults and have been described by authorities in the study of the brain-injured (Goldstein, 1948).

Receptive and expressive language can be evaluated simultaneously as inner language behavior is being observed. This is done by asking the child to "show me the bed" and "show me the chair." This is the naming level of receptive language ability. It ascertains the extent to which the child has been able to establish names of objects as a beginning of the development of receptive language. The examiner then can increase the complexity of the language and the abstractness of the situation by giving instructions, such as "show me what we sit on," "show me what mommy cooks on," or "show me what keeps us warm," "show me what makes a noise," and many other increasingly difficult language situations.

Expressive language can be appraised by having the child become interestedly engaged in the activity and then casually but in a highly structured manner ask, "What is that?" This provides an opportunity to ascertain whether the child has expressive oral language at the level of naming the common objects in his environment. Engaging the child in an activity is a significant aspect of the total appraisal because it presents a real situation and one in which he is motivated to use the language of which he is capable. As he continues to be engaged in the activity, it is possible to present an increasingly complex language situation. After the naming level has progressed, it is common to ask him, "What are you doing?" This can be varied in many ways so that if he is attempting to place a doll figure in the bed he can be asked, "What is the baby doing?" and many variations accordingly.

To specifically appraise the child's language in this manner is a critical aspect of the diagnosis of aphasia. It is characteristic for the aphasic child to function below the level of the deaf child as far as engaging himself projectively and imaginatively in a play situation. Furthermore, characteristically the aphasic child is inattentive and distracted in the total situation. Many other qualitative indications are apparent to the trained clinicians who use such a procedure for the evaluation of symbolic behavior. The information which is secured from the language evaluation, like the information secured from the other areas of examination, requires corroboration. If the child is reduced in his language-functioning as revealed by the appraisal of language ability and if he shows evidences of motor disturbance on the motor appraisal, as well as in other areas, a diagnosis of aphasia can be made with substantially greater assurance and conviction. However, a diagnosis of aphasia should not be made unless the language evaluation reveals reduced or disturbed symbolic functioning in language. This means that the language evaluation is a critical aspect of whether the child should be classified as having an aphasia. Unless symbolic disturbance is revealed, such a classification should not be made. Training and experience in the appraisal of language disorders is necessary in order for such an evaluation procedure to be highly meaningful and valid.

## ETIOLOGY OF APHASIA IN CHILDREN

Although the problem of etiology of aphasia in children has not been studied extensively, it is evident that there are a number of causations. These causations can be classified on the basis of time of onset or on the basis of the nature of the defect itself. The time concept frequently is useful; onset can be classified on the basis of prenatal causes, damage at the time of delivery, and postnatal traumas. Most aphasic children seem to sustain their damage either prenatally or at the time of delivery.

Another consideration in the etiology of aphasia in young children is the nature of the central nervous system involvement. This usually is referred to as (1) agenesis or (2) damage due to trauma. The concept of agenesis implies that the organism deviated from the time of conception and therefore it is basically a maldevelopment phenomenon. In trauma or damage the concept assumes normal development until the time at which some insult occurred and resulted in the central nervous system disorder. This approach to the study of etiology is highly significant, because it seems that there is a relationship between the specific etiology and the nature of the language disorder most likely to be present. This is revealed by children with expressive aphasia because they are organismically considerably less affected as compared with children with receptive aphasia. This advantage of the expressive aphasic is challenging relative to the implications concerning language development and symbolic behavior. Most frequently he has good, if not intact, inner and receptive language. Hence he has two of the fundamental types of language and is confronted with a much less debilitating psychological situation than the receptive aphasic child. There are other challenging aspects to this comparison. The expressive aphasic child frequently does not have a history of disease or trauma. Etiologically considered, he is found by inferential determination to be an agenetically involved child, whereas the receptive aphasics more often are found to have a history and other evidence of actual trauma of the disease or damage type. Thus, neurologically, too, the expressive aphasic child perhaps has an advantage in that his involvement conceivably does not cause as diffuse a disturbance in central nervous system integration. This remains to be further ascertained by research in pediatric neurology and in other areas.

There are many other reasons for viewing the etiological aspects of aphasia in children as an important area for study and for increasing knowledge about this complex disorder. Perhaps the most commonly found causative factors in the histories of these children are anoxia, Rh incompatibility, rubella, cerebral hemorrhage due to birth injury, and encephalopathic diseases such as meningitis and encephalitis. Anoxia can be considered as a contributing cause in various ways, including anoxia at the time of delivery and anoxia due to complicating factors during early life. Studies of this condition are increasingly helpful in the determination of the specific etiology and its effects from the point of view of a resultant aphasia (Council for International Organizations of Medical Sciences, 1953). Such studies of children who have sustained anoxic effects from Rh incompatibility are contributing to greater understanding of brain injury and aphasia in early life. In general it seems that factors such as anoxia, rubella, and Rh incompatibility are more likely to cause aphasia with mild diffuse involvements of the total organism than are such factors as cerebral hemorrhage due to forceps injury at the time of delivery.

## EDUCATION AND THERAPY

Perhaps the most fundamental problem confronted by the aphasic child is his reduced capacity for normal integration. He sees, hears, and feels; but he cannot integrate this sensory information into an experience pattern which is logical and reliable for purposes of understanding his environment. While this disturbance of the process of integration typifies aphasic children, it characterizes the receptive aphasic to a considerably greater extent than it does the expressive aphasic.

In view of this disturbing incapacity to relate to the environment in an integrated manner, it is essential that the training program assist the child in structuring and organizing his internal world. Such an educational and therapeutic program usually is divided into the nonlanguage and language aspects. The aphasic child's environmental field needs to be planned and structured carefully in order to simplify the task of integration and organization of his subjective experience. There are various procedures and techniques which can be used accordingly.

## Nonlanguage Aspects

**Age for beginning training.** A basic concern relative to education and therapy for young aphasic children is the age at which training should begin. Aphasic children vary considerably in their readiness for therapy, but their needs can be considered sufficiently similar so that a statement can be made regarding the most suitable ages for beginning the training program. In this connection it is important to distinguish between speech and language therapy. By two years of age many children are seen for appraisal in regard to their retarded speech development. If the evaluation at this age is conclusive concerning the presence of brain injury with aphasia, nonlanguage-training can be started immediately. It is not uncommon for the nonlanguage-training to begin before the specific language-training. The language-training usually is started by three years of age; and if management and handling of nonlanguage aspects has been successful in the home, language-training can be inaugurated earlier. However, many children are not appraised and classified as aphasic until after three or four years of age. Such children usually are started on the nonlanguage and language aspects of the therapy program simultaneously. One of the most significant beginning steps in the therapy program for an aphasic child is to give specific assistance to the parents in understanding the child's problem and to outline with them the type of management which is most beneficial in the home. Usually this is done during the first contact with the child and his parents irrespective of his age.

**Group or individual therapy.** Another question which must be considered in planning therapy is whether the child's needs can be served best by group or individual training. Usually expressive aphasics can be classified into small groups immediately. Three to six expressive aphasic children have been worked with successfully in a group. Such children have ranged in age from three and a half to five years. Because of their greater capacity to integrate and to tolerate stimulation, these children can be expected to respond well to group training. Furthermore, experience and research suggest that the interaction and identification which is achieved by having these children together in small groups is desirable from the point of view of language-training.

Receptive aphasic children often are so disintegrated, especially at the preschool age, that they must have individual therapy. If this therapy is successful and if gradual generalized improvement is occurring, they can be classified into groups of two, three, four, or five children when they have reached the age of four or five years. By six years of age many of these children have been classified in regular public-school classes; usually after entering the regular public school they still are in need of assistance by the speech therapist.

**The training room.** The training room should be small and free from distracting influences. The size of the room is significant because the proximity of the therapist to the child is an important aspect of the training situation. Many young aphasic children can cope with the demands being made of them more successfully when they are permitted to remain close to the therapist. The therapist's immediate presence helps them to structure and to give sustained attention to the training tasks which have been placed in the foreground of their attention. The ingenious therapist soon becomes aware of the distance which she can permit successfully between herself and the child. An objective of the training program is to assist the child in gaining control of himself and in attending to the foreground activity although the therapist is not immediately present. Many aphasic children require the therapist to be side by side with them in the beginning of their training. Gradually the distance between the therapist and the child can be extended to two feet, four feet, six feet, and then within more normal proximities.

Another significant aspect of the training room is that it should be free from distractions. It should not have the usual decorations such as pictures, toys, and other training materials immediately apprehendable to the child. Preferably the room should be painted or papered in a solid color. Coloring should be subdued but pleasant. All materials should be concealed in drawers or cabinets so that the only materials present at the time of training are those which the therapist is using and to which the child is expected to give his attention. Such a structured environment is highly desirable from the point of view of assisting the child to organize his experiences and to relate satisfactorily to his environment. As soon as the child becomes familiar with this environment, he unconsciously prefers it because he becomes aware that his world is more logical and satisfactory when he is not being overstimulated. The room should be quiet but not necessarily soundproofed. Excessive traffic or other sounds in the background tend to be distracting and disturbing. Pilot studies suggest that a highly soundproofed room creates other problems and does not provide the ideal opportunity for the child to improve his perceptual functioning and to reduce his distractions. The use of controlled sounds projected into the room through electronic equipment provides an opportunity for exploration of the child's auditory perceptual behavior and furnishes a uniform background which assists the child in reducing his auditory distractibility. Floor-carpeting is highly desirable because it assists the children in standing and walking and it reduces undesirable noises produced from movement of chairs and from other activities in the room.

**Distraction, disinhibition, and perseveration.** As indicated throughout this discussion, a basic problem confronted by the aphasic child is his inability to control his behavior and to integrate his experiences. Several workers have referred to this problem in terms of distraction, disinhibition, and perseveration (Strauss and Lehtinen, 1947). Aphasic children tend to be characterized by one of these difficulties. For example, the behavior of a specific child might be characterized by distractibility, whereas the behavior of another child might be characterized primarily by disinhibition. This disintegrated behavior frequently becomes the first problem which must be dealt with when considering the nonlanguage aspects. Many children have such severe difficulties of this type that unless they can be assisted with them, it is unwise, if not impossible, to proceed with the specific language-training.

Clinically, it is helpful to analyze carefully the nature of these disabilities. Distraction means that the child engages in forced responsiveness to stimuli from without. He cannot control his behavior to the extent that he can receive visual or auditory sensations without reacting to them immediately and without plan or objective. As a result, he runs and grabs objects in a fleeting, random manner. Disinhibition by contrast is characterized by an inability to control distractions from within. This is most apparent when the child is expected to wait for an occurrence in a normal manner. For example, if the child has been told that at a certain time he is to go with his mother to the store (assuming that the child has comprehended this situation and is aware of this anticipated occurrence, and assuming that he has even a small amount of verbal language), he is likely to say continuously, "Go, go, go, go." The mother will state "not now, after awhile," but the child is unable to inhibit this internal distraction and continuously makes demands that they go immediately. This inability to inhibit can become so severe that the child is completely disintegrated. All explanations might be of no benefit because his disinhibition has become so marked that he can do nothing but behave in a seriously disintegrated manner. It is of critical importance that the therapist be aware of this problem of disinhibition and plan her therapy program accordingly; also, that she assist the parents with the control of this highly disturbing circumstance which occurs so frequently in the homes of aphasic children. In general, the child with this problem of disinhibition should not be expected to be able to engage in normal "waiting-behavior." Usually, when therapy is beginning he would not be told that at some time in the future something is to occur. Rather, he is not informed of the occurrence until it is imminent.

Perseveration, which is frequently observed simultaneously with distraction and disinhibition, seems to be an attempt on the part of the organism to maintain equilibrium with its environment. After an activity is begun, that activity serves the purpose of making a relationship to the environment;

hence it can be relinquished only with urging and appropriate assistance. From this point of view, perseveration is a method which the child has of preventing fearful disintegration; the activity is continued because it prevents disintegration, but it has no immediate goal or objective such as is characteristic of the normal child's behavior. Perseveration takes a great many forms. Some children will engage in "running behavior" until exhaustion causes them to disintegrate further. Such disintegration can be noticed frequently through the child's beginning to "laugh" or "giggle" in a compulsive, defensive manner and not in the usual manner of enjoyment of the situation.

Distraction, disinhibition, and perseveration frequently can be dealt with successfully by the principle of *firmness with acceptance and without anger*. This entails knowing the level of the tolerance that the child can sustain and stimulation only within the limits of his capacity to integrate. If he is engaged in marked distraction, disinhibition, or perseveration a firm and deliberate procedure is indicated. This might mean removing the child from the immediate situation, using mild restraint by having him close to the therapist, using simple and pleasant vocalizations, and assisting him to relinquish the behavior which has caused his disintegration. Awareness of the total situation under such circumstances is essential.

### Language-Training

Although nonlanguage aspects often are emphasized in the beginning of the training program, usually nonlanguage and language therapy proceed simultaneously. In the discussion of the examination of language capacity it was suggested that inner, receptive, and expressive language should be considered separately. This is true also in connection with language-training. Some children require emphasis on inner language before receptive or expressive language are stressed. If the child has developed sufficient inner language, the program would begin by emphasizing the receptive aspects of language acquisition. Expressive aphasic children usually have well-established inner and receptive language and thereby are essentially in need of training in expressive language. It is apparent that each child's language training program should be based on his specific readiness in terms of the function of language which it has been possible for him to acquire.

### Materials

The selection of materials for language training of aphasic children becomes a most significant aspect of the success of the therapy program. Experience suggests that toy objects which are realistic and highly symbolic of the child's daily life experiences are the most suitable for such training. Pictures and drawings are more abstract and do not provide the child with an opportunity for tactile experience. As the child progresses and becomes more integrated and more perceptually mature, the use of pictures is more suitable.

## Training for Inner Language

Inner language training consists of assisting the child to structure his experiences so that they become meaningful and so that he can relate more effectively to his environment. Usually this is done through play activities which are appropriate to his total behavioral circumstances. In some children, these activities must be highly rudimentary and simple. The child is presented with meaningful toys representing his daily experiences. Such toys include toy furniture which is the most meaningful to him, such as furniture for the kitchen, bathroom, and bedroom. Human figures which represent members of his specific family also are included. The therapist then assists the child in using these toys to "act out" the routines of his daily experiences. As this therapy proceeds, the child gains ability to engage in imaginative or "pretend" behavior. Until he reaches the level of being able to engage in such behavior, inner language seems to be at such a low level that training on receptive or expressive aspects is not readily successful or beneficial.

## Receptive Language-Training

Most aphasic children are in considerable need of assistance with receptive-language development. As stated previously, receptive language follows inner language genetically. This requires emphasis because traditionally language-training has consisted primarily of expressive language. It is noteworthy that experience in training young aphasic children reveals that expressive language often does not require emphasis if receptive language is given appropriate consideration and if it develops satisfactorily. This again reveals the reciprocal relationships between the various types of language-functioning.

The principle described under inner language is used also for training of both receptive and expressive language. After the child can engage himself meaningfully with toy objects, and reveals imaginative and "pretend" play behavior, he is given the names of the objects with which he is engaging himself. Words such as *mommy, daddy, chair, table, shoe,* and *baby* are given first. Although emphasis is given to the recognition of the names of the objects, no demands are made on expressive language. Usually receptive language must have reached the level of being able to recognize the names of a number of objects in his daily environment before the child is ready for the use of expressive language. If expressive-language demands are made simultaneously with emphasis on receptive language, the total process and progress are confused and delayed. After the child has acquired some facility in recognizing the names of objects, he can be asked to "show me the baby," "show me the chair," and "show me the car." The therapist should be highly sensitive and insightful regarding what the child is doing in his play activity and refer only to the objects he is using, inasmuch as this procedure capitalizes on the greatest possible motivation for language development. As the child achieves success in recognizing the names of objects, and as he identifies the objects by name, the next step is introduced. This consists of the therapist using more complex receptive language. As she observes his play she participates with him and leads his activities by such verbal direction as "put the mommy on the chair," "the baby wants to go to sleep," and so on. These directions should be immediately appropriate to the child's activities so that they are not confusing but are related directly to his play activity.

Because of the distractibility and disinhibition of the receptive aphasic child, the therapist must simultaneously be aware of his need for structuring and his inability to tolerate normal stimulation. The activities in which the child is asked to engage must be appropriate for his total perceptual and conceptual capacities. Furthermore, the factor of proximity between the therapist and the child is often critical.

A number of children with receptive aphasia require training in listening. These children usually have marked inabilities in auditory perceptual capacities. Because they cannot integrate the auditory world, they cannot select those sounds which are useful at any specific moment and attend normally to these sounds; they become inattentive to all sound. They are deficient in their ability to listen. Training in listening usually does not begin with words or verbal comprehension. Instead, sounds which are concrete and which lend themselves well to motivation are used in the initial stages. If the child's attention can be directed to the ringing of a bell (toys which produce sounds or realistic sounds from daily life can be used for this purpose), the therapist and the child each should have a similar bell. The therapist rings her bell in full view of the child and attempts to get the child to ring his bell simultaneously. Some training usually is needed to get the child to start and stop his ringing in imitation of the therapist's. The next step is for the therapist to ring the bell and the child to ring his only after the therapist has ceased. This is done in full view of both the child and the therapist initially. After the child can begin and stop his ringing of the bell by "taking turns" with the therapist, the therapist puts the bell behind her back and again rings it. The child is to imitate by taking his turn, just as when both bells were in full view. As he succeeds in this activity, the therapist hides so that both she and the bell are out of the view of the child. Now she rings the bell and the child is to ring his bell in turn; the child is to go and find the therapist after he has *listened* and heard the bell. Such activities have been found beneficial in getting children to attend to the world of sound and to associate the world of sound meaningfully with experience. The therapist gradually introduces demands for listening to the spoken word.

### Expressive Language-Training

Receptive aphasic children usually do not require major emphasis on expressive language. As they acquire inner and receptive language, their expressive language develops reciprocally. This means that expressive language-training is emphasized primarily with children who have a specific expressive involvement. Perhaps the greatest limitation of the therapeutic work done traditionally with expressive aphasic children is the undue demand to imitate what the therapist says. In contrast to this emphasis, it has been found beneficial to allow the child to use whatever vocal expression he can. These children frequently have vocal utterances which have meaning to them. These utterances should be comprehended by the therapist as soon as possible in order to establish a basic communication process between herself and the child. In this way the child's utterances become symbolic and are language in the true sense of being useful for purposes of communication. The sooner, and the more often, the child can use utterances which serve the purpose of communication, the greater his motivation for acquiring the verbal language which is characteristic of his culture. Furthermore, it seems that as soon as these utterances become symbolic and are useful for communication the child's total progress is improved reciprocally; it is possible for him to make greater progress in his general psychological development. In the beginning the therapist might even imitate the child's utterances, in order to establish the process of communication, but gradually she uses words for the objects and activities in which she and the child are engaged.

Another significant factor in expressive language-training is that emphasis on correction of the attempts to imitate words defeats the purpose of development of expressive verbal language. Even though articulation is highly deficient, corrections are not made until verbal language has become rather fluent, or at least useful for the child's purposes of making himself understood by others.

The principle of language-training suggested under inner and receptive language can be used in the training of expressive language. As the child is engaging himself in activities in a meaningful play situation, the therapist begins by having him attempt the names of the objects with which he is playing and, as stated previously, she accepts whatever vocal utterances he uses for any specific object. As he can make himself understood and acquires the names of objects, the therapist gradually introduces the next step which is simply asking the child to make a statement about what he is doing. The therapist does this first in a concrete and then gradually in a more abstract manner. For example, if the child places the mother figure on the bed the therapist might ask, "What is mommy doing?" The child now can respond in a one-word sentence such as, "Sleeping." There are many such demands which the therapist can introduce and gradually extend the child's use of expressive language. These requests include, among others, "What are you doing?" and "Where did you and daddy go yesterday?" Just as in the training of receptive language, these requests should be appropriate to the child's activity and tolerance in order to be most useful from the point of view of language development.

## PROGNOSIS AND INCIDENCE

Although much knowledge remains to be established regarding the diagnosis and training of aphasic children, it is apparent that the prognosis for many of these children is substantially better than has been assumed. Many aphasic children who have received language-training have entered regular public school classes and have made a successful adjustment. Often these children have continued to receive some assistance from the speech therapist in the school system. It should not be inferred, however, that children with aphasia and other symbolic disorders have been adequately provided for in the public school systems. Further consideration must be given to the special needs of children with symbolic disorders after they enter school. This presupposes the training of therapists to work with children who have symbolic difficulties.

Unfortunately, the number of aphasic children in any given population has not been well established. It seems that the incidence of aphasia and related symbolic disorders is substantially greater than has been assumed traditionally. There is some possibility that there are as many children with handicaps of this type as there are children with handicaps such as hearing impairment. This estimate does not limit the problem of symbolic disorders to aphasia but includes symbolic disorders in reading, writing, and arithmetic. One of our greatest needs is to develop further diagnostic procedures which can be used in surveying school populations and thus ascertain the incidence of symbolic disorders in children. Further study of the aphasic child can be expected to increase our knowledge relative to the nature of language pathology and of symbolic behavior in the human being.

## BIBLIOGRAPHY

BARR, B. 1955. Pure tone audiometry for pre-school children. Stockholm: *Acta Oto-laryngologica*, Supplementum 121.

CASSELL, R. H. 1950. The Vineland adaptation of the Ozeretsky tests. Vineland: *Train. Sch. Monogr.*, Suppl. No. 1.

Council for International Organizations of Medical Sciences. 1953. Anoxia of the new-born infant. Springfield, Ill.: C. C. Thomas.

DE JONG, R. W. 1950. The neurologic examination. New York: Paul Hoeber.

DOLL, E. A. 1951. Neurophrenia. *Amer. J. Psychiat.*, 108, 50.

——— 1947. Vineland social maturity scale. Minneapolis: Educ. Test Bur.

GESELL, A., HAVERSON, H. M., THOMPSON, N., ILG, F. L., CASTNER, B. M., AMES, L. B., and AMATRUDA, C. S. 1940. The first five years of life. New York: Harper.

GOLDSTEIN, K. 1948. Language and language disturbances. New York: Grune and Stratton.

HEATH, S. R. 1942. Railwalking performance as related to mental age and etiological type among the mentally retarded. *Amer. J. Psychol.*, 55, 240.

MYKLEBUST, H. R. 1954. Auditory disorders in children. New York: Grune and Stratton.

ORTON, S. T. 1937. Reading, writing and speech problems in children. New York: Norton.

STRAUSS, A., and LEHTINEN, L. 1947. Psychopathology and education of the brain-injured child. New York: Grune and Stratton.

# CHAPTER 17

# SPEECH PROBLEMS OF THE MENTALLY RETARDED

● *Jack Matthews, Ph.D.*

## INTRODUCTION

**Terminology**

IN CITING STUDIES FROM the field of mental retardation, we do not find a consistent terminology employed. The same term may be used by two different investigators to describe two different degrees of mental retardation. The same degree of retardation may be designated by different writers by different terms. Wallin (1949) has suggested terminology that is widely but by no means uniformly employed. He lists the following terms to represent the range from high degree of retardation to average or normal intelligence: idiot, imbecile, moron, borderline, backward or dull, retarded, average.

Among many workers in the field of mental retardation, the term *idiot* has become widely accepted to designate individuals whose retardation as measured on intelligence tests places them in the I.Q. range below 25. Individuals in the I.Q. range roughly 25–50 are frequently referred to as imbeciles. The term *moron* is often applied to the I.Q. range approximately 50–70.

We will use mental retardation as a generally inclusive term, following the usage suggested by the Nomenclature Committee of the American Association on Mental Deficiency (Sloan, 1954).

Mental Retardation refers to that group of conditions which is characterized by: 1. slow rate of maturation; 2. reduced learning capacity; 3. inadequate social adjustment present singly or in combination, and associated with below average intellectual functioning, and is present from birth or early age.

Mental Retardation is an inclusive term incorporating all that has been meant in the past by such similar terms as mental deficiency, feeblemindedness, etc.

We also follow the thinking of the Nomenclature Committee in accepting the premise that in mental retardation we are dealing with a symptom complex which may result not alone from defects of the central nervous system but from defects "in the psychological and sociological spheres" (Sloan, 1954).

531

While the latter conditions [defects in the psychological and sociological spheres] are recognized as causative mechanisms in their own light, they may also, and frequently do, play significant roles in influencing the degree and nature of the mental retardation resulting from cerebral defects. The implication of this premise also involves the conception of mental retardation as a dynamic rather than static condition, amenable in many cases to treatment through therapeutic procedures even though the basic cerebral defect is irreversible.

The term *speech therapist, speech correctionist,* and *speech pathologist* will be used interchangeably. *Speech disorder* will be used as a general term to indicate disorders of speech or language. The term *communication disorder* will be employed as a general term to include speech, language, or hearing disabilities.

### The Role of the Speech Pathologist

Aside from the family doctor, the speech pathologist is often the first professional person to evaluate the mentally retarded child. Frequently a child may first be recognized as mentally retarded when his inability to express himself becomes obvious. The speech pathologist may not treat the speech problem per se but may initiate the series of referrals to physician, psychologist, social worker, educator, and so on, which results in parents coming to understand that they have a mentally retarded child. The chief contribution of the speech pathologist can often be an intelligent sympathetic interpretation of the diagnosis of mental retardation. Such an interpretation may help parents to take their focus off the speech problem and to place it on other problems which must be recognized and dealt with in mental retardation. Some of these other problems often need attention before consideration can or should be given to the speech problem.

The role of the speech pathologist in the area of mental deficiency is certainly not limited to that of diagnostician, interpreter, and referring agent. We feel there is also a very important role for speech therapy in the field of mental retardation. The decision as to whether or not a given speech therapist wishes to work in the field of mental retardation will of course have to be made by each speech therapist. It is the feeling of this writer that although speech pathology as a profession may not have actively discouraged speech therapy for the mentally retarded, certainly there has been little encouragement given by the profession to devote attention to communication disorders associated with mental retardation.

As long as speech correctionists deal with the problems of language and speech retardation, they will almost of necessity be confronted with problems of mental retardation. In our own clinical experience, mental retardation has been one of the most frequently encountered factors associated with language and speech retardation. With the increased attention currently being given to mental retardation will come more and more pressures on the profession of speech pathology to devote greater attention to speech problems associated with mental retardation. This will require that speech pathologists not only increase their knowledge of the speech of the mentally retarded but of the field of mental retardation itself.

## LANGUAGE AND SPEECH RETARDATION

The dependence of language on intelligence can be illustrated by observing the frequent absence of language and speech in the severely mentally retarded. Absence of these functions has actually been employed as a basis of classification of the mentally retarded. Binet and Simon (1914) have employed this principle in defining the idiot.

An idiot is any child who never learns to communicate with his kind by speech —that is to say, one who can neither express his thought verbally nor understand the verbally expressed thought of others, this inability being due solely to defective intelligence, and not to any disturbance of hearing, not to any affection of the organs of phonation.

Tredgold (1947) has observed that in idiocy, "Speech is usually absent, although a few do learn to articulate such simple monosyllables as man, cat, eat, etc., but none of them can form sentences."

Few statistical studies have been made to determine the relationship between intelligence and speech retardation. We have little accurate information concerning the average age at which individuals with varying degrees of mental retardation begin to babble, use words meaningfully, combine words into phrases and sentences, and so forth.

In her examination of the speech status of 32 idiots (I.Q.'s below 20 and chronological ages from 7 years 9 months to 38 years), Kennedy (1930) found 22 were altogether mute, nine could produce only jabbering, and only one produced recognizable words. In this one instance, however, the words were used in nonmeaningful and irrelevant contexts. Kennedy reported that some idiots gave evidence of understanding simple commands.

**TABLE I. Language Development of Idiots (Town)**

| Language Character-istics of Idiots | % Present in 17 Low-Grade Idiots | % Present in 8 Middle-Grade Idiots | % Present in 25 High-Grade Idiots |
|---|---|---|---|
| Understand gestures | 2 | 2 | 23 |
| Imitate gestures | 0 | 1 | 20 |
| Make voluntary gestures | 4 | 2 | 22 |
| Understand a few words | 1 | 3 | 14 |
| Speak a word or two | 0 | 1 | 10 |

Town (1913), studying 50 idiots, divided his sample into low-, high-, and middle-grade intelligence levels. His data (Table 1) suggest that among idiots, the degree to which language develops is directly dependent on intelligence. At all levels, more children used voluntary gestures than imitated them. Town observed that where voluntary gestures develop before ability to imitate gestures develops, the voluntary gestures seem to be limited to prehension or a direct need for expression of repulsion. Many of the high-grade idiots who could say nothing except perhaps "mama," "yes," and "no," understood the names of many familiar objects.

Lapage (1911) noted that high-grade defectives acquired speech at 20 months compared with 41 months for low-grade defectives. In this study neither "high-grade" nor "low-grade" defectives is defined.

In an investigation of 1000 boys and girls whose I.Q.'s ranged from 10 to 159, Abt, Adler, and Bartelme (1929) correlated age of speech onset (time child first associated a word with an object) with intelligence (Stanford-Binet). The correlation between age of speech onset and intelligence was —.41 for boys and —.39 for girls.

Mead (1913) studied 92 feeble-minded children (not defined in terms of I.Q.) and reported that the "typical" feeble-minded child uses a word meaningfully at 34.44 months and that this behavior may have its onset at 12 months or up to 156 months.

Karlin and Strazzulla (1952) investigated age of babbling, word use, and sentence use in three groups of mentally retarded. Their data are summarized in Table 2. Karlin and Strazzulla's data on the use of the first word by children in the I.Q. range 51–70 are in substantial agreement with the earlier work of Mead (1913).

TABLE 2. Age of Speech Acquisition (Karlin and Strazzulla)

| Activity | I.Q. 15–20 | I.Q. 26–30 | I.Q. 51–70 |
|---|---|---|---|
| Babbling | 25 months | 20.4 months | 20.8 months |
| Word use | 54.3 months | 43.2 months | 34.5 months |
| Sentence use | 153 months | 93 months | 89.4 months |

Meader (1940) compared the age of speech onset of a mentally retarded group with the group of gifted children studied by Terman (1925). In Terman's genius group the incidence of delayed speech was one per cent. In Meader's group with I.Q.'s of less than 66, the incidence of delayed speech was 44 per cent. In the group with I.Q.'s of 67 and higher the incidence was 25 per cent.

Wallin (1949) examined 272 "subnormal" children and found that this group used single words at an average age of one year and 8 months. Sentences were used at 2 years 6 months. "Mentally defective" children (164 in number) used single words at 2 years and sentences at 3. Morons used words at 1.6 years and sentences at 2 years and 3 months. Imbeciles used single words at 2 years and 3 months and sentences at 3 years and 7 months.

Ingram (1935) and Gesell and Amatruda (1937) present some general tables outlining the progress that a mentally retarded child can be expected to make. Although these tables contain items concerned with the onset of speech, no information is given about the sample from which these norms were derived.

TABLE 3. Summary of Studies on Use of First Word by Mentally Retarded

| Investigator | Type Population | Time of Use of First Word | |
|---|---|---|---|
| Karlin & Strazzulla (1952) | I.Q.'s from 15–20 | 54 | months |
| Karlin & Strazzulla (1952) | I.Q.'s from 26–30 | 43.2 | months |
| Lapage (1911) | Low-grade defectives | 41 | months |
| Karlin & Strazzulla (1952) | I.Q.'s from 51–70 | 34.5 | months |
| Mead (1913) | Nondefined retarded population | 34.44 | months |
| Wallin (1949) | Morons | 18 | months |

Table 3 summarizes the findings of studies of the time of use of the first word in groups of mentally retarded.

The studies concerned with time of speech acquisition in mentally retarded children do not provide us with normative data we can accept with confidence. Various indices of speech acquisition have been employed by different investigators. Definitions of intellectual levels of subjects are not always presented nor are they comparable from study to study. The sampling procedures and statistical treatment are subject to question. In spite of these limitations, the studies do point out clearly that on the average the mentally retarded child acquires language and speech considerably later than the child of normal intelligence.

## INCIDENCE OF SPEECH PROBLEMS

Not only is speech frequently delayed in the mentally retarded but when it does emerge it is often defective. The incidence of speech problems among mentally retarded has been reported in a number of studies and the incidence figures vary widely. Variations in the incidence figures are probably due to differences in criteria of what constitutes a speech defect and to differences in the composition of the mentally retarded groups studied.

Sir Cyril Burt (1937) studied the speech of children in typical schools in London and Birmingham. In the group with I.Q.'s 70–85, he found 9 per cent of the children with mild speech defects and 5 per cent with severe speech defects. In the group with I.Q.'s 50–70 there were 13 per cent with mild speech defects and 11 per cent with severe defects. Burt estimated that at least 25 per cent of retarded children are speech defectives.

American incidence statistics are considerably higher than those of Burt. However, most of the American studies have been carried out in institutionalized populations and have included the speech of children too retarded to have ever entered regular schools. Such a population would never have been part of that on which Burt's figures are based.

Lewald (1932) investigated 533 patients in an institution and found that 56 per cent of all the patients had speech defects. Sirkin and Lyons (1941) examined 2522 institutionalized mentally retarded. They reported that 50 per cent had speech defects and 17 per cent had no speech at all. Schlanger

(1953c) found that 68 per cent of 74 children in a private school for retarded children had speech defects. Kennedy (1930) studied speech defects in an institution population and found that 71.87 per cent of 27 imbeciles had dyslalic speech. Of 249 morons 42.57 per cent had speech disorders ranging from slight to severe in nature. All of 32 idiots studied lacked language beyond jabbering, crying, and utterance of isolated words.

Sachs (1951) examined 210 morons and imbeciles who were inmates at the Lynchburg State Colony in Virginia and found that 57 per cent had speech defects. Eighteen per cent of the borderline group were defective in speech, whereas 44 per cent of the moron group and 79 per cent of the imbecile group had defective speech. Sirkin and Lyons (1941) found 31 per cent of their institutionalized mentally retarded with I.Q.'s over 69 had speech defects. In the moron group 47 per cent had speech defects and in the imbecile group 74 per cent had speech defects.

**TABLE 4. Summary of Studies on Incidence of Speech Defects Among Mentally Retarded**

| Investigator | Type Population | Incidence of Speech Defects (per cent) |
|---|---|---|
| Sirkin and Lyons (1941) | 2,522 institutionalized defectives | 67 |
| Lewald (1932) | 500 institutionalized defectives | 56 |
| Sachs (1951) | 210 institutionalized imbeciles, morons, and borderliners | 68 |
| Schlanger (1953) | 74 private school retardates | 57 |
| Burt (1937) | Mentally backward school children (I.Q.'s 70–85) | } 9 mild } 5 severe |
| Sirkin and Lyons (1941) | Institutionalized defectives (I.Q.'s over 69) | 31 |
| Sachs (1951) | Institutionalized borderliners | 18 |
| Burt (1937) | Severely retarded school children (I.Q.'s 50–70) | } 13 mild } 11 severe |
| Kennedy (1930) | Institutionalized imbeciles | 71.87 |
| Sachs (1951) | Institutionalized imbeciles | 79 |
| Sirkin and Lyons (1941) | Institutionalized imbeciles | 74 |
| Kennedy (1930) | Institutionalized morons | 42.57 |
| Sachs (1951) | Institutionalized morons | 44 |
| Sirkin and Lyons (1941) | Institutionalized morons | 47 |
| Sirkin and Lyons (1941) | Institutionalized idiots | 100 |

An examination of Table 4 indicates that incidence figures vary from 5 per cent to 79 per cent. Such variations are attributable in part to differences among investigators' definitions of speech defects and to differences in the various populations studied. Although the incidence figures reported in Table 4 vary greatly, the data permit us to conclude that the incidence of speech defects in populations of mentally retarded is high—considerably higher than in the general population.

## TYPES OF SPEECH PROBLEMS

We have established that the mentally retarded are slower than the normal in acquiring speech. We have also shown that when speech is acquired, it i

ite likely to be defective in the mentally retarded. We can now ask if the
eech defects found among mentally retarded are essentially different in
nd from those found in nonretarded populations. Irwin (1942) is one of the
w investigators who feels that the mentally retarded child is not only de-
yed and defective in speech but that his entire course of development of
unds is different from that exhibited by normal children. Irwin studied
n children having I.Q.'s (as measured by the Kuhlman and the Binet) rang-
g from 7 to 48. He made transcriptions of their speech sounds twice with
interval of a year between times of testing. He found these children used
ck vowels more infrequently than front vowels. In this respect their speech
sembled that of infants more than that of adults. Since the chronological
es of the children ranged from two to five years, one would expect to find
ck vowels in greater use. The retarded children showed concentration in
e labial, postdental, and glottal sounds; whereas infants show the greatest
ling up among the glottals and adults among the postdental sounds. The
tio of vowels to consonants in the speech sounds of this retarded group
is 1:1; whereas the adult ratio is 1:2. The ratio for newborns is 3:2. Ir-
n's study of infants is the only one of its kind and suggests that in the
entally retarded the course of development of sounds is different from that
und in normal children. However, most investigators of the speech of older
entally retarded children find that speech defects in the mentally retarded
e similar in kind to those found in a nonmentally retarded population of
eech defectives.

Karlin and Strazzulla (1952) listed consonant defects in order of occur-
nce in a population of retarded. The most frequently occurring defective
nsonant was [s] followed by [z], [l], [r], [tʃ], [dʒ], [ð], [ʃ], and [θ]. This is
nilar to the order of occurrence of articulation errors that would be found
a nonretarded population. Karlin and Strazzulla's findings are similar to
ose reported by Kennedy (1930), Lapage (1911), Lewald (1932), and
chs (1951).

The most systematic study of the kinds of substitutions, omissions, and
ditions in the speech of mentally retarded was made by Bangs (1942). He
ected a homogeneous group of primary aments from an institution and
ve them articulation tests by using 65 picture cards as stimuli. Bangs's
ta in general indicate that the speech of primary aments tends to corre-
ond very closely to that of normal children insofar as sounds avoided and
unds most frequently substituted are concerned. Bangs concluded that the
eech of the primary ament shows the same retardation as all of his other
ictions. Bangs noted that the aments differed from normal children in the
eat number of omissions made in the final position. Normal children gen-
lly do not leave off their final consonants as frequently as the aments do.
ngs suggested that the omissions may be due to the inability of the ament
concentrate on one act until full completion. He further noted that al-
ough in general there were no significant differences between the sort of
ors made by normal and ament children, sometimes the retarded children

made minor substitutions which were very bizarre and not of the sort eve
found among normal children.

In special syndromes of mental retardation such as mongolism, cretinisn
or microcephaly no special speech pattern or particular type of speech ha
been reported in any systematic investigation. There is, however, a certai
amount of opinion expressed in the literature concerning speech problem
"typical" of certain syndromes. West, Kennedy, and Carr (1946) note tha
mongols have very hoarse voices and that they are frequently afflicted wit
nerve deafness. Their voices are supposed to be loud and inflectionles
Mongols are supposed to have difficulty in the articulation of [k], [g], [ŋ] an
the back vowels. No data are presented to support any of these contention
Benda (1949) states that mongoloid children often have very deep voices an
that these are so typical of the syndrome that often a diagnosis of mongolis
can be made on the basis of hearing the child speak. The voice is raucou
low in pitch, and sounds masculine and mature. Again no data are presente
to support these conclusions.

In one of the few objective studies of the speech of mongoloids, Gott
leben (1955) reported the incidence of stuttering in a group of 36 mongoloic
to be 33 per cent. In a control group of nonmongoloid mentally retarded tl
incidence of stuttering was only 14 per cent. The high incidence of stutterir
in mongolism found by Gottsleben is consistent with observations made t
Travis (1931), Gens (1951c), and Schlanger (1953). Although there is son
evidence to suggest that the incidence of stuttering in mongoloids is high
than that in the nonmongoloid mentally retarded population, there is r
evidence to suggest that mongolism could be recognized on the basis of tl
speech symptoms alone.

Gens (1950) studied the speech of a group of 1252 epileptics. He four
that 73.6 per cent had defective speech. He did not find any typical epilept
pattern of speech, but instead found the same disorders that are found in
nonepileptic population.

Although one may find in the literature references which attempt to d
scribe the "typical" speech of certain syndromes in mental retardation, the
are no systematic studies to bear out such a contention. There is clear-c
evidence to indicate that the incidence of speech disorders among mental
retarded is considerably higher than in a nonretarded population. There i
however, no evidence to suggest that the speech defects of the mentally r
tarded differ in kind from those of a nonretarded speech-defective popul
tion.

## RELATIONSHIP TO OTHER FACTORS

### Intelligence

In studies which have related I.Q. and onset of speech, or I.Q. and spee
proficiency, low correlations have been reported. Abt, Adler, and Bartelr
(1929) studied 1000 children excluding those with I.Q.'s below 70 and tho
who did not begin to talk until after five years. The correlation between a

of onset of speech and Binet I.Q. was —.41, indicating that the earlier the onset of speech is, the more intelligent is the child. Bangs (1942) found that when chronological age was held constant there was a correlation of .39 between speech proficiency and mental age. In a study of twelve birth-injured children with defective speech, Doll (1932) reported a correlation of .02 between I.Q. and severity of the speech defect. Schlanger (1953c) found a correlation of .37 between mental age and articulation proficiency. Although all of the correlations just cited are low, they do point to a relationship between intelligence and degree of speech involvement.

## Handedness

The role of handedness in speech disorders has not been adequately determined. It is interesting to note that there is a higher incidence of left-handedness in mentally deficient populations than in normal groups. Karlin and Strazzulla (1952) reported 16 per cent of the mentally retarded children they studied were left-handed as compared to 3 per cent in a normal population. The percentage of established handedness increased with I.Q. level. Lewald (1932) found approximately 20 per cent of 466 mentally retarded either left-handed or without hand dominance. Hawk (1950) in a study of 53 cases of dull normal children found that next to the speech handicap the most frequently occurring difficulty was with establishing handedness and poor use of the right hand. Burt (1937) reported that 7.4 per cent of the mentally deficient children in Birmingham and 12.3 per cent of those in London were left-handed. Left-handedness and lack of hand dominance is found much more frequently in populations of mental defectives than in the normal population.

## Hearing Loss

A high incidence of hearing loss is found in populations of mentally retarded. Tredgold (1947) has stated:

Defects of hearing are fairly common in the aments and include complete deafness, tonal deafness, and word deafness. Some of these conditions may be due to developmental anomalies or disease of the peripheral organ, but others are of central origin. Even where no actual deafness is present the acuity and range of auditory perception are usually below normal.

Burt (1937) reported that slight hearing defects were present in 4 per cent of the normal school children in London. In backward children, hearing defects were present in 6 per cent and these defects were severe in nature. Twelve per cent of the backward children had slight hearing defects. Burt also records the fact that boys who are backward seemed to have more hearing defects than girls who are in a similar I.Q. group.

Abernathy (1938) administered pure-tone audiometer tests to children with I.Q.'s ranging from 20 to 69 and with chronological ages ranging from to 20. Children with ear pathologies or who were deaf or extremely hard of hearing were excluded from the study. He computed the median thresholds (in sensation units) for 373 subjects for eight frequencies. His resul are summarized below.

| Frequency | 64 | 128 | 256 | 512 | 1024 | 2048 | 4096 | 819 |
|-----------|----|-----|-----|-----|------|------|------|-----|
| Sensation Unit Loss | 10 | 15 | 15 | 20 | 10 | 10 | 15 | 1 |

Birch and Matthews (1951) found that over half of a mentally defectiv population of 247 persons from 10 to 39 years of age had hearing losses. C this group with hearing losses, 32.7 per cent had severe enough losses to **handicapped in some activity. Depending upon which frequency was beir used for comparison, the incidence of hearing loss was two and one-half **18 times greater than that found in a normal population. Schlanger (1953₄ in a study of 70 mentally retarded children reported data on hearing loss substantial agreement with Birch and Matthews.

MacPherson (1952) sent questionnaires to various institutions for mer tally retarded and inquired about the status of deaf patients committed fc mental retardation. He found that 22 schools considered 50 per cent of the patients to be either deaf or very hard of hearing. Fourteen schools est mated that about 50 per cent of their patients had at least moderate hearir losses.

Johnston and Farrell (1954) studied 270 mentally retarded with ment ages from prekindergarten to fifth-grade levels of functioning. The mea chronological age of his population was 12 years 9 months. He found th₂ 24 per cent of the children had hearing losses greater than 20 db. This pe centage, according to the author, is five times the percentage of hearing lo found in an audiometer survey made in the public schools in Massachusett

Foale and Paterson (1954) measured the hearing loss of 100 juveni patients at Lennox Castle Institution for Mental Defectives in Scotland. Th mean I.Q. of the patients was 66. Of the boys tested 67 per cent had goc hearing in both ears and approximately 13 per cent were handicapped t their hearing impairment. Although the incidence of hearing impairment Lennox Castle was lower than that reported by Birch and Matthews (195 at Polk, the incidence of hearing loss in the retarded children at Lennc Castle is considerably higher than that found in normal populations surveye in Scotland.

Table 5 summarizes studies of hearing loss in mentally retarded childre

TABLE 5. Summary of Studies of Hearing Loss in Mentally Retarded Populations

| Investigator | Per Cent with Hearing Loss |
|--------------|----------------------------|
| Burt (1937) | 6 per cent severe, 12 per cent slight |
| Abernathy (1938) | Median thresholds 10–20 sensation un below normal |
| Birch and Matthews (1951) | 50 per cent some loss, 32 per cent severe lc |
| Macpherson (1952) | 50 per cent severe loss |
| Schlanger (1953c) | 30 per cent |
| Foale and Paterson (1954) | 33 per cent some loss, 13 per cent severe lc |
| Johnston and Farrell (1954) | 24 per cent loss greater than 20 db |

Although there is not complete agreement among all the investigators as
) the incidence of hearing loss in mentally retarded cases, there is a clear-cut
ndication that the incidence of hearing loss among mentally retarded is con-
iderably greater than that in a nonretarded population.

## DIFFERENTIAL DIAGNOSIS

In view of the high incidence of speech and hearing problems among
mentally retarded children, it is not surprising that communication disorders
re often thought to result from mental deficiency. The well-trained speech
nd hearing therapist should recognize that there may be many explanations
f delayed or defective speech which have no relation to intellectual re-
ardation. Brain injury, glandular dysfunction, emotional disturbances, and
earing loss all may cause retardation in the development of language or
esult in poor articulation. Becky's (1942) study of 50 children with delayed
peech revealed a number of constitutional, environmental, and psychologi-
al factors other than mental retardation.

Kanner (1948) believes there are groups of individuals who may be called
pseudo-feeble-minded," since their over-all abilities may not be retarded.
Ie includes in this group individuals with delayed speech but well-developed
onverbal abilities. Matthews and Birch (1949) have pointed out some of
ae problems encountered in evaluating the intelligence of speech and hear-
ng handicapped.

The responses required in many tests are verbal. Children with speech defects
ften are very self-conscious about speaking. They will sometimes feign ignor-
nce rather than make a speech attempt that will lead to their embarrassment.
Often the responses of a child with defective speech cannot be understood by the
xaminer. This difficulty is especially noticeable in testing individuals with severe
rticulatory problems or with delayed speech; both conditions often found in
everely involved cerebral palsy cases.

These problems can be overcome in part by making use of tests requiring non-
erbal performance. Many such tests, however, depend almost exclusively on
erbal directions for administration. For the child with a hearing loss such direc-
ons have an obvious weakness. In certain cases, e.g., in delayed speech, speech
aay be a relatively unimportant entity. A child may be habitually inattentive
) the speech of others. In certain instances there may actually be a negative re-
ction to speech. Under any of these circumstances the use of verbal instructions
aay place the speech and hearing clinic case at a disadvantage; he may not get
om the directions of the test an adequate knowledge of what is expected of him.

In administering intelligence tests to hearing handicapped, psychologists
ave attempted to replace verbal instructions with pantomime. When the
ester is able to use pantomime freely—and many psychologists find it hard
) do so—it is difficult to standardize. Matthews and Birch (1949) suggested
ome of the requirements of an adequate intelligence test for use with in-
ividuals with speech and hearing problems.

Such a tool while meeting the usual requirements of objectivity, reliability,
nd validity should also conform to additional specifications. It should not re-
uire verbal responses. The instructions should not involve speech or complicated

pantomime on the part of the test administrator. The test should be relativel free from time limits and scoring based on speed. The test should impose a little penalty as possible on the handicapped child when he lacks experience which are commonplace to normal youngsters.

Hardy (1948) feels that the child with hearing loss in certain frequencie who presents a picture of inconsistent responses to speech along with delaye speech or defective articulation may be superficially diagnosed as feeble minded. Jellinek (1941) has described phenomena resembling aphasia, ag nosia, and apraxia in mentally retarded children and adults. Myklebus (1954) describes a number of clinical-observational techniques which ma be employed in the differential diagnosis of hearing loss, aphasia, menta retardation, and emotional disturbance. Nance (1946) devised a scale i which an attempt is made to differentiate aphasia and mental retardation The directions are given in pantomime and the scale includes items fron well-known standardized intelligence tests. Strauss and Lehtinen (1947) hav developed tests which attempt to differentiate brain damage from menta deficiency.

Most of the differential diagnosis techniques referred to are based on ricl clinical experience. There is little validation information about any of th procedures. The speech pathologist should remember that in mental retarda tion we are dealing with a symptom complex which may result not alon from defects of the central nervous system but from defects "in the psycho logical and social spheres" (Sloan, 1954). Defects "in the psychological an social spheres" can themselves be causative mechanisms and can also influ ence the nature and degree of mental retardation caused by cerebral defects This implies that mental retardation is "amenable in many cases to treatmen through therapeutic procedures even though the basic cerebral defect is ir reversible" (Sloan, 1954). The speech therapist must be alert to the roles o aphasia, hearing loss, and emotional disturbance in influencing both th nature and degree of mental retardation. Mental retardation is no vaccina tion against emotional maladjustment, brain damage, or hearing loss. Th speech pathologist must be equally careful that the role of mental retarda tion as an etiological factor be considered in all cases of language and speec retardation even though the primary problem may appear to be aphasia hearing loss, or emotional disturbance. It is all too easy to forget that th child we have labeled psychotic or aphasic may also be mentally retarded. I the realm of mental retardation, it is extremely important for the speec pathologist to recognize the role of the pediatrician, audiologist, psycholc gist, neurologist, psychiatrist, and other specialists in making a differenti; diagnosis.

## THERAPY

### Prevailing Attitudes

For some years good educational practice has called for the exclusion o the mentally retarded child from the regular classroom. This has not mear

otal exclusion from formal education, however. Instead special classes have
een established for the mentally retarded. These classes have been set up to
1eet his special needs. Techniques have been developed for teaching the
1entally retarded. Education in 1955 is no longer asking, "Can we provide
1n education for the retarded child?" Instead, the questions are concerned
vith finding the best techniques for training and educating.

In many speech clinics, little provision is made for the mentally retarded
hild with a speech problem. In some clinics, no cases with an I.Q. of less
1an 70 are admitted. West, Kennedy, and Carr (1946) state, "the true mon-
ol is particularly unresponsive of speech rehabilitation and it is practically
seless to attempt such training." In the introduction to Stinchfield and
ʻoung (1938), Immel gives a similar opinion. "Mental subnormality is still
fact and when a child fails to learn to talk because of real mental deficiency
ope is still an illusion and must remain so under the limitations of our pres-
nt knowledge." Backus (1943) has pointed out that a low I.Q. is not neces-
arily "a death warrant" for a child and that the child's handicap may be
·ssened by improving his articulation. At the same time, she implies that
vorking with a severely retarded child who has an I.Q. below 70 is likely to
e a waste of time. This point of view has been quite widely accepted by
pecialists in speech pathology. Its acceptance by specialists in mental re-
1rdation is not as widespread. There is little research data to guide us in the
cceptance or rejection of the advisability of attempting speech therapy with
1e severely retarded—those whose I.Q.'s fall below the almost mystical
,Q. of 70.

### valuation of Therapy

There have been relatively few attempts to evaluate speech therapy with
1entally retarded children. Sirkin and Lyons (1941) selected 169 institu-
onalized patients for a three-and-one-half-year therapy program. The mean
·ngth of treatment was five months with two or three sessions weekly. Pa-
ents were selected on the basis of intelligence, co-operation, and likelihood
f receiving parole. Nineteen borderline, 104 moron, and 4 imbecile patients
·ere in the therapy group. Seventy patients achieved satisfactory speech
:vels and 17 cases were still under treatment and progressing well at the
me of the writing. These 87 cases comprised 52 per cent of the therapy
roup. Seventy-three cases, or 48 per cent of the group, had to be dropped
·om the program because they had insufficient intelligence or were too un-
o-operative to make any progress. At the end of three and one half years,
4 of the cases had retained the improvement. Thirty out of the 44 cases
ad retained this improvement from one to three years or more. Ten of the
ases had retrogressed, and 14 cases could not be contacted by the authors.
ʻwo cases had died. The I.Q.'s of those who had retained the correction
anged from 43 upward, but only eight of this group had I.Q.'s below 50. In
10se who had retrogressed, I.Q.'s ranged from 48 to 67, but only five had
,Q.'s above 53. In percentage terms, 52 per cent of the total group bene-

fited from the therapy; 79 per cent of the borderline group, 59 per cent of th moron group, and 26 per cent of the imbecile group had profited by the experience. Because no control group was used, it is difficult to determin how much of the improvement may have been due to factors other tha speech therapy.

Schlanger (1953b) carried out speech therapy with 62 mentally retarde children in special classes in Madison, Wis. The mean chronological age the group was 11 years 11 months, and the mean mental age was 7 years an 2 months. The I.Q. range extended from 39 to 77. Significant improveme was noted in articulation, mean sentence length, and percentage of comple sentences used. No significant improvement was noted in number of word spoken per minute or in sound discrimination. The speech therapy progra included many activities structured to encourage spontaneous conversatic and listening. Schlanger felt that desirable changes in attitude, responsiv ness, self-confidence, and so on, were brought about not entirely because c speech therapy but as a result of establishment of group unity and the ir fluence of the therapist. Because Schlanger employed no control group, it difficult to separate the improvement which came as a result of Schlanger program from the improvement which may have come from maturation c other factors in the total school program.

Schneider and Vallon (1955) at the end of one year of a speech therap program carried out at the Westchester School for Retarded Children cor cluded: "On the basis of our experiences, there is definitely a place fc speech therapy in the educational or training programs for the moderatel and the severely retarded child." The Schneider and Vallon (1955) progra involved a very small number of cases and did not utilize a control grou

The conclusions of Schneider and Vallon (1955), Schlanger (1953b and Sirkin and Lyons (1941) certainly do not rest on as firm an experiment and statistical basis as one might desire. However, they indicate that speec therapy with mentally retarded can produce beneficial results. These cor clusions are closer to the author's clinical experiences than are the mor pessimistic views cited earlier.

## Approaches to Therapy

The speech therapist must learn to accept and to strive for language an speech appropriate to mental age rather than chronological age. Prognos for the severely retarded is not favorable. We can turn to no studies whic have compared the effectiveness of various types of speech therapy in worl ing with the mentally retarded. Our therapy guides for the present will com largely from the techniques employed by teachers of the mentally retarde To these techniques might well be added the speech-improvement prc cedures which speech correction has developed for use in kindergarten an elementary grades. Speech therapists will have to plan activities suited to th mental age of the child and which will be appropriate to his short attentio span. Rote memory drills will probably have little value. Group activiti can no doubt be profitably employed. Principles of mental hygiene will be applicable. The speech-correction and speech-stimulation program which is integrated with the entire educational and training program of the retarded child will probably be more successful than a speech-correction program lacking such integration. All of the general suggestions just set forth are the author's clinical judgments which will require considerable testing prior to their acceptance as guides in carrying on speech therapy with the mentally retarded. A sampling of some other clinical judgments may be suggestive of additional procedures.

Twitmyer and Nathanson (1932) stress the importance of integrating speech-training with other aspects of training the mentally retarded.

The employment of technical speech training alone yields scanty results. On the other hand in those cases of amentia where the general condition improves through education, environmental control, and the like, the employment of specific speech training incidental to the general training is indicated and is usually followed by improvement in speech and increased ability to enjoy communication with fellow human beings.

Schlanger (1953d) has offered the following suggestions for developing speech in institutionalized mental defectives.

1. The speech situation should always be a pleasant one whether the child is learning his first word, or learning to correct a faulty sound.

2. The child should be stimulated verbally a great deal with short sentences and simple sounds.

3. When the child has no language he should be encouraged to babble and his babblings should be repeated so that the child develops an awareness, interest, and need for speech.

4. The child should be encouraged to name persons and objects in his environment.

5. Any effort that he makes toward communication should be encouraged even if his meaning is not clear or if he does not express himself well.

6. Once the child attempts a word it should be repeated and used by the attending adult even if the production is faulty.

7. A multisensory approach should be utilized in teaching language. The child should hear the word, feel the resonance of the nose, lips, or larynx, and should receive help through jaw manipulation, and so on.

8. Time should be set aside for listening by the patient and for listening to the patient who needs an audience to practice on.

9. Doing and talking about what has been done is more meaningful to the child than rote drill. Group participation and social activities should be planned for speech.

10. The child can learn to imitate noises of animals, trains, airplanes, etc., as part of learning to be aware of sound.

11. The child can learn conventional greetings and social phrases.

12. He can learn speech by participating in life-like situations, by participating in creative drama situations built around familiar relationships, and by being encouraged to talk out and work through his personal problems.

13. Smaller children can be stimulated to speak with View Master slides, stories, and naming of activities such as clapping, stamping, jumping, and so on.

Kirk and Johnson (1951) try to improve the child's language facility by discussion of situations within the child's range of experience. The weather, the home, and personal activities including the walks the child has taken, the pictures he has seen, and the stories he has heard are all topics of discussion and part of a vocabulary- and concept-increasing program.

West, Kennedy, and Carr (1946) stress the importance of simplifying directions for the mentally retarded child. They feel that motivation and praise of the child may be factors determining the success or failure of the program. The therapist is warned that improvement if it comes at all will come very slowly. Wallin (1924) has stressed the importance of developing a speech-therapy program in which the mentally retarded child is accepted with all his limitations for what he is. His personal problems and needs must be attended to instead of routinely giving him practice in speech improvement.

An examination of the various suggestions for speech therapy for the mentally retarded indicates that many of the recommended procedures might be difficult to carry out in the traditional one-or-two-sessions-per-week kind of individual speech therapy offered in many speech clinics. Much of the suggested speech-correction program may not be carried out by the speech therapist but by parents, teachers, and others who spend considerable time with the retarded child. Perhaps the pessimism about the success of speech therapy with the mentally retarded is based to a large extent on the failure to apply to the retarded therapy procedures suited to their needs and capacities.

### Justification of Therapy

If we grant that speech-correction procedures can be successful with the mentally retarded, we still must make a value judgment as to the worthwhileness of such activities. There is now, and will continue to be, a shortage of speech therapists to work with children with normal intelligence. Should we add to the shortage by diverting speech therapists to work with the mentally retarded? In making a decision it would be well to remember that in high grade defectives adequate speech may make the difference between self sufficiency and dependency—between a lifetime in an institution at tax payers' expense and vocational adjustment in society. Blanton and Blanton (1924) raised the question as to the amount of time the speech therapist is justified in spending on the mentally retarded. Their answer, given over quarter of a century ago, seems to this writer equally valid today.

This [the amount of time the speech teacher is justified in devoting to the mentally retarded] must be decided on the merits of each individual case and of the learning ability and temperament of the child. While with the present scarcity of trained teachers in the speech field it would hardly be wise that the abnormal should be cared for and the normal child not; still, the speech defect may be the one added handicap that makes of the high-grade deficient a pauper or a criminal.

To the research-oriented speech therapist, the field of mental retardation offers an excellent laboratory. The institutional setting in which many retarded children grow up provides unusual opportunities for experimentally manipulating environmental factors. In classrooms for the retarded child there is freedom from pressure to "stick to the curriculum." Such freedom makes possible types of experimentation which might be considered too disruptive of established routine in the normal class.

We have learned that the normal child can benefit from many of the techniques which were originally developed many years ago for teaching the exceptional child. It is equally possible that research in the area of speech development and correction in the mentally retarded will make valuable contributions to our knowledge of normal speech development and to the field of speech pathology in general.

## SUMMARY

Our survey of current research and clinical judgments has shown that in the population of mentally retarded there is a high incidence of speech and hearing disorders. Even though the speech pathologist might wish to avoid contact with the field of mental retardation, it is unlikely he will be able to do so. The speech pathologist often performs the first evaluation which leads parents to recognize that what appears to be a speech problem is actually a more basic problem of mental retardation. Many speech therapists provide no time for the retarded child. Such an exclusion of the retarded child from speech therapy grows out of pessimism on the part of many speech pathologists concerning the feasibility of speech correction for the mentally retarded. There is no research evidence to show the inability of the mentally retarded to profit from speech therapy. The literature does contain a few studies showing the effectiveness of speech therapy with mentally retarded and a number of suggestions for modifying traditional speech-therapy techniques to meet the needs of the mentally retarded. For the speech therapist who is careful in diagnosis, adapts techniques to the capacity of cases, and sets realistic goals, there can be challenges and successes in working with the mentally retarded. For the profession of speech pathology we feel an obligation to explore further the field of communication disorders in the mentally retarded.

## BIBLIOGRAPHY

ABEL, T., and KINDER, E. 1942. The subnormal adolescent girl. New York: Columbia Univ. Press.

ABERNATHY, E. R. 1938. The auditory acuity of feeble-minded children. Unpublished Ph.D. Dissertation. Ohio State Univ.

ABT, I. A., ADLER, H. M., and BARTELME, P. 1929. The relationship between the onset of speech and intelligence. *J. Amer. Med. Assn.*, 93, 1351–1355.

ANDERSON, V. A. 1953. Improving the child's speech. New York: Oxford Univ. Press.

BACKUS, O. L. 1943. Speech in education. New York: Longmans, Green.

BAKER, H. J. 1945. Introduction to exceptional children. New York: Macmillan.

BANGS, J. L. 1942. A clinical analysis of the articulatory defects of the feebleminded. *J. Speech Disorders*, 7, 343–356.

BARR, M. W. 1904. Mental defectives. Philadelphia: Blakiston.

BECKY, R. E. 1942. A study of certain factors related to retardation of speech. *J. Speech Disorders*, 7, 223–249.

BENDA, C. E. 1949. Mongolism and cretinism. New York: Grune and Stratton.

——— 1952. Developmental disorders of mentation and cerebral palsies. New York: Grune and Stratton.

BENNET, A. 1932. A comparative study of subnormal children in the elementary school grades. *Teach. Coll. Contr. Educ.*, No. 510. New York: Teachers College, Columbia Univ.

BERRY, M. F., and EISENSON, J. 1942. The defective in speech. New York: Appleton-Century-Crofts.

——— 1956. Speech disorders. New York: Appleton-Century-Crofts.

BERRY, R., and GORDON, R. G. 1931. The mental defective. New York: McGraw-Hill.

BEST, H. 1943. Deafness and the deaf in the United States. New York: Macmillan.

BIBEY, M. 1951. A rationale of speech therapy for mentally deficient children. *Train. Sch. Bull.*, 48, 236–39.

BIJOU, S. W., and WERNER, H. 1945. Language analysis in brain injured and non-brain injured mentally deficient children. *J. genet. Psychol.*, 66, 239–254.

BINET, A., and SIMON, T. 1914. Mentally defective children. London: Edward Arnold.

BIRCH, J. W., and MATTHEWS, J. 1951. The hearing of mental defectives: it measurement and characteristics. *Amer. J. ment. Defic.*, 55, 384–393.

BLANTON, M. G., and BLANTON, S. 1924. Speech training for children. New York: Century.

BRODBECK, M. E. 1941. Remedial speech in a special school curriculum. *Amer J. ment. Defic.*, 45, 598–601.

BUCK, P. S. 1950. The child who never grew. New York: John Day.

BURT, C. 1937. The backward child. New York: Appleton-Century.

CABANAS, R. 1954. Some findings in speech and voice therapy among mentall deficient children. *Folia Phoniatrica*, 6, 34–37.

CARRELL, J. A., and BANGS, J. L. 1951. Disorders of speech comprehension associated with idiopathic language retardation. *Nerv. Child*, 9, 64–76.

DESCOEUDRES, A. 1928. The education of mentally defective children. Chicago Heath.

DOLL, E. A. 1940. The nature of mental deficiency. *Psychol. Rev.*, 47, 730–780

——— 1941. The essential of an inclusive concept of mental deficiency. *Amer J. ment. Def.*, 46, 215–217.

———, PHELPS, W. M., and MELCHER, R. T. 1932. Mental deficiencies du to birth injuries. New York: Macmillan.

DORCUS, R. M., and SHAFFER, G. W. 1945. Textbook of abnormal psychology Baltimore: Williams & Wilkins.

EISENSON, J. 1940. The psychology of speech. New York: Crofts.

FOALE, M., and PATERSON, J. W. 1954. The hearing of mental defectives. *Amer J. ment. Defic.*, 59, 254–258.

GARRISON, K. C. 1950. The psychology of exceptional children. New York: Ronald Press.

GENS, G. W. 1949. Let's be realistic about aphasics. *Train. Sch. Bull.,* 46, 49–57.

———— 1950. Correlation of neurological findings, psychological analyses, and speech disorders among institutionalized epileptics. *Train. Sch. Bull.,* 47, 3–18.

———— 1951. The speech pathologist looks at the mentally deficient child. *Train. Sch. Bull.,* 48, 19–20.

———— 1952. Congenital aphasia: a case report. *J. Speech Hearing Disorders,* 17, 32–38.

GESELL, A. 1926. The mental growth of the preschool child. New York: Macmillan.

———— and AMATRUDA, C. 1937. Developmental diagnosis and supervision. *In* Brennemann's practice of pediatrics. Hagerstown, Md.: W. F. Prior.

GIANNINI, M. J., SNYDER, E., SMITH, H. M., and SLOBODY, L. B. 1954. Home training program for retarded children. *Pediatrics,* 13, 278–282.

GODDARD, HENRY H. 1914. Feeblemindedness; its causes and consequences. New York: Macmillan.

GOLDENBERG, S. 1950. An exploratory study of some aspects of idiopathic language retardation. *J. Speech Hearing Disorders,* 15, 221–233.

GOLDSTEIN, M. 1939. The acoustic method for the training of the deaf and hard of hearing child. St. Louis: The Laryngoscope Press.

GOTTSLEBEN, R. H. 1955. The incidence of stuttering in a group of mongoloids. *Train. Sch. Bull.,* 62, 209–217.

HARDY, W. G. 1948. The relations between impaired hearing and pseudo-feeblemindedness. *Nerv. Child,* 7, 432–445.

HAWK, S. S. 1950. Speech therapy for the physically handicapped. Palo Alto: Stanford Univ. Press.

HOLLINGWORTH, L. S. 1921. The psychology of subnormal children. New York: Macmillan.

INGRAM, C. 1935. Education of the slow learning child. New York: Ronald Press.

IRWIN, O. C. 1942. The developmental status of speech sounds of ten feebleminded children. *Child Developm.,* 13, 29–39.

———— and SPIKER, C. C. 1949. The relationship between the IQ and indices of infant speech sound development. *J. Speech Hearing Disorders,* 14, 335–43.

JELLINEK, A. 1941. Phenomena resembling aphasia, agnosia, and apraxia in mentally defective children and adults. *J. Speech Disorders,* 6, 51–62.

JOHNSON, W., BROWN, S., CURTIS, J., EDNEY, C., and KEASTER, J. 1948. Speech handicapped school children. New York: Harper.

JOHNSTON, P. W., and FARRELL, M. J. 1954. Auditory impairments among resident school children at the Walter E. Fernald State School. *Amer. J. ment. Defic.,* 58, 640–643.

KANNER, L. 1948. A miniature textbook of feeblemindedness. New York: Child Care Publications.

KARLIN, I. W., and STRAZZULLA, M. 1952. Speech and language problems of mentally deficient children. *J. Speech Hearing Disorders,* 17, 286–294.

KASTEIN, S. 1951. The different groups of disturbances of understanding language in children. *Nerv. Child,* 9, 31–42.

KENNEDY, L. 1930. Studies in the speech of the feebleminded. Unpublished Ph.D. dissertation. University of Wisconsin.

KIRK, S. A., and JOHNSON, G. O. 1951. Educating the retarded child. Boston: Houghton Mifflin.

LAPAGE, C. P. 1911. Feeblemindedness in children of school age. Manchester: Univ. Press.

LEHERFELD, D. T., and NERTZ, N. 1955. A home training program in language and speech for mentally retarded children. *Amer. J. ment. Defic.*, 49, 413–416.

LEWALD, J. 1932. Speech defects as found in a group of five hundred mental defectives. *Proc. Amer. Assn. Study Feeblemindedness*, 37, 291–301.

McCARTHY, D. 1954. Language development in children. *In* Carmichael, L., Manual of child psychology. New York: Wiley. Pp. 492–631.

MACPHERSON, J. R. 1952. The status of the deaf and/or hard of hearing mentally deficient in the United States. *Amer. Ann. Deaf*, 97, 375–386.

MAKNEN, G. H. 1898. Training of speech as a factor in mental development. *Bull. Amer. Acad. Med.*, 3, 501–505.

MARTINSON, B., and STRAUSS, K. A. 1940. Education and treatment of an imbecile boy of the exogenous type. *Amer. J. ment. Defic.*, 45, 274–280.

MATTHEWS, J., and BIRCH, J. W. 1949. The Leiter International Performance Scale—A suggested instrument for psychological testing of speech and hearing clinic cases. *J. Speech Hearing Disorders*, 14, 318–321.

MEAD, C. D. 1913. The age of walking and talking in relation to general intelligence. *Pedagogical Seminary*, 20, 461–484.

MEADER, M. H. 1940. The effect of disturbances in the developmental processes upon emergent specificity of function. *J. Speech Disorders*, 5, 211–220.

MYKLEBUST, H. R. 1954. Auditory disorders in children. New York: Grune and Stratton.

NANCE, L. S. 1946. Differential diagnosis of aphasia in children. *J. Speech Disorders*, 11, 219–223.

NEHAM, S. 1951. Psychotherapy in relation to mental deficiency. *Amer. J. ment. Defic.*, 55, 557–572.

RIDENOUR, N. 1943. Mentally retarded preschool children; suggestions to doctors and nurses in well-child clinics. *Amer. J. ment. Defic.*, 48, 72–78.

SAAIJENGA, H. 1954. Do's and dont's for speech correctionist. *Except. Child.*, 20, 322–324.

SACHS, M. H. 1951. A survey and evaluation of the existing inter-relationships between speech and mental deficiency. Unpublished Master's Thesis. University of Virginia.

SARASON, S. B. 1953. Psychological problems in mental deficiency (2nd ed.). New York: Harper.

SCHLANGER, B. B. 1953a. Speech measurements of institutionalized mentally handicapped children. *Amer. J. ment. Defic.*, 58, 114–122.

——— 1953b. Speech therapy with mentally retarded children in special classes. *Train. Sch. Bull.*, 50, 179–186.

——— 1953c. Speech examination of a group of institutionalized mentally handicapped children. *J. Speech Hearing Disorders*, 18, 339–350.

——— 1953d. Suggested practices for developing speech in speech handicapped children in institutions. Unpublished manuscript.

SCHNEIDER, B., and VALLON, J. 1955. The results of a speech therapy program for mentally retarded children. *Amer. J. ment. Defic.*, 49, 416–424.

SHUTTLEWORTH, G. E. 1900. Mentally deficient children. London: H. K. Lewis.

SIRKIN, J., and LYONS, W. F. 1941. A study of speech defects in mental deficiency. *Amer. J. ment. Defic.*, 46, 74–80.

SLOAN, W. 1954. Progress report on special committee on nomenclature of the *Amer. Assn. ment. Defic.*, 59, 345–351.

SMITH, M. E. 1935. A study of some factors influencing the development of the sentence in the preschool child. *J. genet. Psychol.*, 46, 182–212.

STINCHFIELD, S. M., and YOUNG, E. H. 1938. Children with delayed or defective speech. Palo Alto: Stanford Univ. Press.

STRAUSS, A. A., and LEHTINEN, L. E. 1947. Psychopathology and education of the brain injured child. New York: Grune and Stratton.

TERMAN, L. M. 1925. Mental and physical traits of a thousand gifted children. Genetic studies of genius, I. Palo Alto: Stanford Univ. Press.

TOWN, C. H. 1913. Language development in 285 idiots and imbeciles. *Psychol. Clinic,* 6, 229–235.

TRAVIS, L. E. 1931. Speech pathology. New York: Appleton.

TREDGOLD, A. F. 1947. A textbook of mental deficiency. Baltimore: Williams & Wilkins.

TWITMYER, E. B., and NATHANSON, S. Y. 1932. Correction of defective speech. Philadelphia: Blakiston.

VAN RIPER, C. 1947. Speech correction principles and methods. New York: Prentice-Hall.

WALLIN, J. E. W. 1916. A census of speech defectives among 89,157 public school pupils—a preliminary report. *Sch. and Soc.,* 3, 213–216.

———— 1921. Problems of subnormality. New York: World Book.

———— 1924. The education of handicapped children. Boston: Houghton Mifflin.

———— 1949. Children with mental and physical handicaps. New York: Prentice-Hall.

WEISS, D. A. 1951. Speech in retarded children. *Nerv. Child,* 9, 21–30.

WEST, R., KENNEDY, L., and CARR, A. 1947. The rehabilitation of speech (rev. ed.). New York: Harper.

# CHAPTER 18

# AN APPROACH TO SPEECH THERAPY FOR THE CEREBRAL-PALSIED INDIVIDUAL

● *William H. Perkins, Ph.D., and Victor P. Garwood, Ph.D.*

THE CEREBRAL-PALSIED PERSON is above all else a human being. He is a unique human being with an injured neuromuscular control system, and the ramifications of this injury may be imperceptible or they may be extensive. They are usually most evident in his comparative lack of motor control. But a neuromuscular disorder does not relegate the victim to another species. Although he most certainly has problems peculiar to his disorder, the majority of his needs are common to us all. His is the problem of finding suitable means within his capacity for meeting these needs. Speech therapy for the cerebral-palsied should begin with a clear recognition that the patient is a person, an individual with a personality, who strives and feels like all other persons. He is a person who must, despite a largely hostile and at the same time pitying society, almost bend over backward to fit himself in somewhere in our culture. Even with nation-wide campaigns to educate the public about the disability, person-to-person relationships remain difficult, to say the least.

The obviousness of the muscular disability is an enticing lure for the speech therapist. The patient's inability to manipulate his speech structure normally seems so evident a cause for the disordered speech, particularly to the beginning clinician, that the therapy may easily become focused on the muscular defect itself rather than on the person with the defect. Setting sub goals to be achieved in the course of rehabilitation has an excellent rationale and the more objectively success can be demonstrated, the greater the mutual satisfaction for both patient and clinician. Little wonder, then, that objectively measurable muscle exercises and speech drills frequently dominate the therapeutic proceedings. That this is so may be attested by a preponderance of literature on the subject (National Society for Crippled Children and Adults, Inc., 1953). Important as is this aspect of rehabilitation, it can become just busy-work if the gratification of demonstrable achievement prove too appealing. How many times per minute the tongue can be elevated or how long a vowel can be sustained become such dominant issues that th patient may almost be delegated the role of an automaton to be manipulated. This process in turn reduces the therapist to the role of one who reminds, a checker, an onlooker. The clinician is safe, his job is clear-cut: eliminate the *defect* but avoid the *person;* his problems are discouraging and threatening.

On the other hand, the therapist who can maintain his perspective, who can exercise constant vigil over his clinical endeavors and evaluate each procedure against the total needs of his patient, demonstrates his excellence. This attitude presupposes a discriminative recognition of the patient's difficulties, a recognition which allows an ordering of the rehabilitative events in the sequence of their importance.

Such an attitude is difficult enough to achieve wtih the physically "normal"; it is especially elusive with the physically handicapped. However, the objective when physical barriers to normalcy are present is to prevent, minimize, or delimit their distorting effects on growth and development whenever possible. Here the proverbial ounce of prevention has inestimable value over the pound of cure. But so often preventive measures are not undertaken in time to obviate maldevelopment. When to start, granted, is a moot point. There seems to be a growing concern in the field of special education that the preschool age is far advanced—in some cases, too far—along the growth curve. Information on maturation levels is at best sketchy and incomplete. More thoughtful exploration should be pursued at the prespeech period, more specifically the 18-month to 3-year level. This level is being seriously examined, for example, by researchers in the field of the acoustically handicapped (Whetnall, 1952), and is thoughtfully discussed by Lehtinen (1955) in the area of the brain-injured child. However, late as it might be, the therapist must make the most of an unfortunate situation and adjust his objectives accordingly. He should endeavor to prevent further faulty development and undo, insofar as they are reversible, those behavior patterns that have gone awry. In other words, he should help the physically handicapped person to achieve his maximum potential within realistic limits.

## PREVENTIVE TREATMENT

The urgency for early treatment of the cerebral-palsied child cannot be overestimated (Sharpe, 1952). Crippling disabilities will compound themselves if left untended. Even motor involvements that in the beginning were mild can ramify so extensively that they may threaten the patient's life. Muscles will grow according to the genetic blueprint, provided they are stimulated and respond to a normal work load. Their growth and strength is dependent on proper exercise. Consider, then, the plight of the cerebral-palsied youngster whose parents are, perhaps, too keenly aware of his disability. The child may have difficulty maneuvering a bolus of food with his tongue and trouble maintaining head balance when most children his age can sit erect unaided. Parental concern is natural, but too often it takes the form of unbridled assistance. By inference, the mother's feeling would seem to be, "as my child is not normal, he needs more help. His difficulty with chewing and swallowing is self-evident, so I must do as much for him as I can and guard against overtaxing him." Accordingly, soft foods are literally poured into him to the exclusion of all other kinds. In some cases, what the mother cannot do for her child's food ingestion, she arranges to have gravity do for him. Thus, even an expenditure of energy for swallowing, probably an essential progenitor of speaking, is minimized. The assistance, of course, does not stop with feeding. The child may be sheltered in his every activity. If he cannot keep up with other children in their play, then he can stay in his room and study the four walls. If he cannot stand up, then he can sit; and if he cannot sit up, then he can lie in one spot for hours on end, deadening his curiosity with the view of things long since grown familiar. This "compressed" environment undoubtedly encourages a passivity and phantasy life at periods during the developmental continuum which normally calls for action and not introspection. His social world becomes egocentric, a world of "I" and not "we."

The consequences of such oversolicitous treatment are not difficult to discern. Obviously, the speech musculature will have very little opportunity to develop and strengthen; so, too, the arms and legs will atrophy with disuse. We knew one girl for whom these consequences were tragic. She had a relatively mild spastic condition as a small child, but it was sufficient to arouse excessive maternal concern. She was overly sheltered and was rarely provided an opportunity to play. The less she exercised, the weaker she became, so the less she was able to exercise which, of course, furthered her debilitation. What little speech she had was virtually unintelligible. By the time she was 10 she was bedridden and had developed a severe spinal scoliosis. Three years later the spinal condition became so acute that it contributed to a continual state of nausea. A generally lowered resistance led to a cold which developed into lobar pneumonia and quickly resulted in her death.

Unfortunately, the effects of overprotection are not solely physical in nature. The psychic development may never progress much beyond the early symbiotic relation with the mother. An increasing accumulation of clinical and research evidence points to the relative immutability of early learning (Hebb, 1949; Munn, 1946; Lewin, 1935; Beach and Jaynes, 1954). This is merely confirmation of the homely expression, "as the twig bends, so grows the tree." New learning occurs in relation to what a person anticipates (Woodworth, 1938; McGeoch, 1942; Ruesch and Bateson, 1951). For example, if two blind men were to feel the trunk of an elephant, and if one man were certain from his past experience that it was an elephant's trunk, whereas the other was equally convinced it was the body of a large snake, they would undoubtedly have vastly different tales to tell of this incident. Similarly, the cerebral-palsied child is influenced in his learning by what he anticipates. If his every need is met as soon as it arises, even after he has developed sufficiently to do things for himself, then he will have little, if any, opportunity to learn methods of dealing with the normal stresses of life. In his later years he will be forced to establish dependency relationships to maintain his previously encouraged passivity, for he will have no other frame of reference by which he can learn from new experiences.

Habits of independence must be acquired progressively (Hebb, 1949; Allport, 1955). Each successful step on the road to independence has to be assimilated before the next one can be anticipated and performed. One of the cruelest travesties on rehabilitative efforts occurs when the sheltered cerebral-palsied patient reaches adulthood. Not only are the job opportunities for self-support relatively limited, but so often the physically handicapped person has had practically no emotional preparation for the constant buffetings of independent existence. No longer protected and cared for, he may be overwhelmed with a sense of helplessness (Barker *et al.,* 1953).

There is a point here specific to speech. Many speech disorders develop and are maintained by dependency needs. Even though no organic cause may exist, the defect frequently will not yield to treatment until the underlying need is met. With the cerebral-palsied, this problem is intensified, because a physical basis for the disorder greatly complicates the task of correcting it. The motivation needed to overcome the obstacles must be unlimited, yet during the formative years many a physically handicapped person learns little about self-service and much about being served.

There is no doubt that a healthy baby will explore his environment until he feels thoroughly familiar with it. At first a thumb, a toe, a rattle, or his gurgling may preoccupy him. After an exhaustive investigation of the little world of his crib, he will lose interest in it and turn his attention to bigger worlds. Normally, his is a constantly expanding curiosity with comparatively few regressive excursions. The cerebral-palsied child's curiosity, though, may be thwarted by two forces. First, he may be ennervated by his physical injury. Hence, he will devote little attention to exploring his environment, and vocal play from which speech would evolve will be minimal. Second, if his parents feel an undue urge to intercede for him, they may inadvertently circumscribe his environment and stop short any curiosity he may have energy enough to exhibit. If he is confined to bed or even to his house, social interaction from which language development gains impetus is limited.

Concurrent with the normal expansion of curiosity is the increasing complexity of the socially prescribed ritual for satisfying one's demands. As an infant, no controls are usually imposed on biological needs. The infant eats, sleeps, and eliminates as soon as the urge is upon him. But as he grows older, he discovers that he can only meet his wants in certain ways, in certain places, at certain times. No longer is the desire tantamount to its fulfillment. What he wishes to do today must frequently be postponed until tomorrow. How to manage this delay and still obtain satisfaction obviously requires more than a few gestures. If the child wants what he wants badly enough, and if he must conform to a social formula for getting it, he will feel a strong need for a communication system that will permit the expression of his desires.

But the cerebral-palsied child may not experience this communicative need keenly. If he is carefully watched lest any desire go untended, he is not being indoctrinated into the socially acceptable methods of drive reduction, most of which involve waiting. The immediacy with which his demands are met forestalls frustration he might have over the inadequacy of communicating by gesture. Why should he trouble to learn a name for an object if he can point to what he wants and get it? Then, too, if his living is circumscribed by overindulgent parents, he may spend a major portion of each day in a wordless world, so his perceptions of objects and events and their relationships will develop without associations with the spoken word. Thus, he may accomplish the babbling and echolalic activities that prepare him for the next stage of speech development (Piaget, 1948); but if his perceptual organization has not been accomplished in a speech-rich milieu, and if he is vegetating without need for an abstract communication system, then he is not ready to progress beyond the autistic stage of sound production (Mowrer, 1952). Attempts to teach such a child to talk by direct attack are clearly destined for minimal success.

The clinical precept we have connoted throughout this discussion is to treat the cerebral-palsied child as normally as his probable capacities will permit. What is once done cannot be completely undone. If preventive therapy could be instituted as soon as a neuromuscular disorder becomes apparent, there would be much less demand for corrective measures and far fewer seriously disabled persons. The task of preventive therapy falls squarely on the parents. They do not have to be taught speech-correction methods to do their job effectively. They may, however, need counseling to permit them to function wisely (Bice, 1955). To have a physically handicapped child can be, and generally is, a severely traumatizing experience. The parents will perhaps feel grief, pity, remorse, and particularly guilt. They may try to appease themselves by lavishing attention on their injured child, or they may wish him out of the way. In any event, if they do have troubled feelings they will have difficulty relating to him normally. Thus parents will be hard-pressed to evaluate his capabilities accurately. Such an evaluation is particularly important with the cerebral-palsied child. To push him beyond his capacity is a disservice, but to hold him back, especially during the first years of life, for fear of exceeding his capacity is perhaps an even greater disservice. Counseling that provides parents with an opportunity to recognize their feelings *accurately* and that provides them with information about what they can do to help has immeasurable value. If parents can be made aware of the tremendous importance to speech development of exercising their child's oral musculature by encouraging vigorous chewing, sucking, and swallowing; of stimulating his curiosity; of helping him to establish healthy social relations with children outside of the home as well as with themselves; and if they will foster his sense of independence and responsibility, then they can frequently do more in his early years to set his speech right than can be expected of the finest clinical regimen during the remainder of his life.

## CORRECTIVE SPEECH THERAPY

The writers were impressed, while reviewing the literature on techniques of speech therapy for the cerebral-palsied, with the paucity of information on the feelings of the therapist. What are the mainsprings which channel speech clinicians into this area? Working with brain-damaged children, although richly rewarding, is a slow, tortuous process. It requires a rigorous self-discipline on the part of the therapist. Patient-oriented goals with the cerebral-palsied may extend temporally over periods of months or years rather than days or weeks.

Who does this work? Originally it was the job of the institutional nurse trained in specialized techniques for working with the orthopedically handicapped child. The work is now done by physiotherapists, occupational therapists, classroom teachers, "special" teachers, and trained speech and hearing therapists. Why do these people work with the cerebral-palsied child? Is there some deep-seated need which appeals for expression, which can only be satisfied in working with the crippled? Are these therapists different dynamically from the therapist working with physically normal children?

We feel that these are important questions which must be answered if we are to further the significance of our profession. If we could get some answers, we could selectively encourage students to go into this highly publicized area of speech therapy. Our problem is not one of random recruitment but one of careful selection. Excellence of academic performance may not be the most thoughtful criterion. Perhaps doggedness and single-mindedness might be more adequate measures. In a sense, selecting and training therapists to work with the physically handicapped is a pre-eminent challenge in our profession.

We make no attempt in this brief chapter to detail clinical techniques for implementing the treatment principles.[1] Rather, we are concerned with delineating an approach to therapy that gives broad perspective to the speech clinician's task. We sense a growing tendency toward specialization among speech pathologists, a tendency which implies that the problems peculiar to the various speech disorders are so divergent as to have little in common. This notion may lead some therapists to the unhealthy belief that the cerebral-palsied are a breed unto themselves, to be treated as being essentially different. The neuromuscular differences obviously are unique. They exist; they must be recognized; they must be dealt with. But they should not obscure the clinician's awareness of how similar in most other respects the cerebral-palsied person's troubles are to those of other brain-injured patients in particular and of the speech-defective population in general.

[1] The National Society for Crippled Children and Adults, Inc., issues periodical bulletins apprising the profession of new contributions to the rehabilitation process.

Knowledge of brain function is scanty, especially regarding its role in complex processes and organizations. We know slightly more about response, receptive and perceptual processes. At an operational level, we are hard put to separate the processes of growth and development from the process of habilitation. Thus, for lack of scientific verification we must at present speak of highly developed therapies validated mainly by clinical evidence.

Speech disorders of the cerebral-palsied population can be more effectively minimized by preventive than by corrective measures, but the majority of these patients are not seen for therapy until correction is mandatory. The speech pathologist's province in the total rehabilitative effort then is to assist the development of more desirable speech habits and speech musculature adjustments. He should be prepared, though, to encounter problems requiring his attention other than those directly associated with sound production and muscle activity, paramount as these may be. He can anticipate singular personality, perceptual, emotional, motivational, and hearing (see Chapters 9, 10, and 11) difficulties which may be partially attributable to the brain injury and partially to unfortunate developmental circumstances in the cerebral-palsied person's growing-years.

### Sensorimotor Treatment

The development of neuromuscular training for the cerebral-palsied has taken some surprising turns during these last several decades. Modern explorations in neurosurgery and neurophysiology have changed our concept of the developmental interrelationship between the central nervous system and the body periphery. Much of the earlier muscle training for cerebral palsy consisted of treating the neuromotor system as an entity, a one-way discharge system, stimulus to response. We have no quarrel with the methodology employed in that motor-speech training; it worked despite the theoretical framework.

The emergence of the "moto-kinesthetic method" (Stinchfield and Young, 1938) revolutionized thinking about motor-speech training for the cerebral-palsied, if for no other reason than for its implication that motor disabilities were only part of a larger sensorimotor disturbance. Viewing this concept in the broad perspective of cybernetics, Wiener has stated (1948, p. 15):

The central nervous system no longer appears as a self-contained organ, receiving inputs from the senses and discharging into the muscles. On the contrary, some of its most characteristic activities are explicable only as circular processes, emerging from the nervous system into the muscles, and re-entering the nervous system through the sense organs, whether they be proprioceptors or organs of the special senses.

Among the training procedures that implement this multiple-sense modality approach are audio-visual-kinesthetic speech-therapy methods described by such writers as Westlake (1951a), Huber (1951), Rutherford (1950), Harrington (1950), Cass (1951), Gratke (1947), and Di Carlo

(1955). Another technique based on the principle of sensorimotor inter-action is one developed by the Bobaths (1948, 1950, 1952, 1954). They have said (1953, p. 102):

> Our technique is a mixture of proprioceptive stimulation of righting reflexes and equilibrium reactions, while at the same time we inhibit undesired tonic reflex activity at whatever stage of movement it may interfere.

Their technique apparently calls for close co-operation of the speech thera-pist with the physiotherapist. For example, with patients who exhibit a pre-dominant flexion pattern, the physiotherapist sets the stage with a "reflex inhibiting posture" such as the prone position, arms fully extended forward and neck extended, a posture contrary to the usual supine position for such patients, and then the speech therapist takes over the training (Marland, 1953). The Kabat (1947) resistive measures have been utilized by Lefevre (1952) for speech-training. She resists movements of the jaw, lips, tongue, and of respiration to call forth strong contractions of the affected muscle or muscle group. She suggests that the patient's response to this technique might be a useful screening prognostication for later training. Rood's (1954) physi-cal-therapy methods which can be adapted to the speech clinicians' needs provide a final example of the sensorimotor approach. She regards the sensory system as the mediator through which the motor system responds reflexively. By applying selected sensory stimuli according to basic develop-mental gradiency, the proper motor act will occur. By applying cold, for example, to a restricted surface area above the diaphragm and in some cases over the sternocleido-mastoid and scaleni fibers, better breathing response patterns have been secured. By lightly stroking the cutaneous surfaces con-taining sensory endings related to fine muscle movement, such as areas on the fingers, tongue, lips, velum, or pharynx, Rood believes that these muscles can be stimulated into action. Moreover, she indicates that the stroking effects better circulation which is basic to muscle and nerve reaction.

One of the most potent forces affecting methodology in speech therapy for the cerebral-palsied case was Gesell's (1941) developmental theory. He pointed up the differential maturation of sensorimotor modalities and their effect on personality development. The implication for speech-training was evident; there is a progression of physiological and psychological events following a relatively prescribed space-time order that normally culminate in the acquisition of speech. Therefore, delay in attaining speech connotes a disruption in the normal progression of these events. To put it plainly, the speechless child is not *ready* to speak; he has not yet mastered the prerequi-sites. Froeschels and Jellinek (1941) and Palmer (1947), recognizing the physiological prerequisites, have described the need for utilizing the early prespeech movements of sucking, chewing, and swallowing as precursors to speech. Westlake (1951b) too has been cognizant of the great significance of differential development. He has presented a systematic program for acquiring speech that emphasizes the necessity for psychosocial and physiological readiness to talk before formal speech-training is attempted as a major undertaking. A significant feature of this system is the development on a vegetative or involuntary level of the movements desired for speech production. Then, as awareness of these movements is heightened, the patient assumes voluntary control of them. Clearly, to achieve the necessary readiness for speech, a concentrated co-ordinated effort by parents, physicians, psychologists, physical therapists, occupational therapists, as well as by speech therapists, will be needed.

A fascinating subject for speech therapists that we have purposely avoided is the differential handling of the cerebral-palsied. Much has been said about differences among the subtypes, particularly among spasticity, athetosis, and ataxia. There is an abundance of literature available on this subject, and the interested student should consult the periodical bibliographies of the National Society for Crippled Children and Adults, Inc., for exhaustive references. In our opinion, the larger issue of sensorimotor training for the cerebral-palsied has been too often obscured by preoccupation with the subtype, which in turn may be so obscure as to defy accurate classification in the first place.

### Nonmotor Problems

Brain injury involving the motor system creates the commanding muscular disability in cerebral palsy. However, Wechsler (1947) notes that the pathology in postmortem specimens shows widespread manifestation of damage in addition to the tissue of the motor area. Indeed, Pohl (1910) describes "mental confusion," "poor direction sense," and "inattention" as proof of sensorimotor complications. But the effects of damage to the brain, even when restricted to the motor areas, may spread far beyond the motor dysfunctions. The nervous system is an almost unbelievably interrelated complex of neural circuitry. An anatomically isolated cerebral insult has far-reaching neurophysiological reverberations (Cruickshank, 1955; McCullough, 1944; Lashley, 1942; Strauss and Lehtinen, 1947). Accordingly, a therapist should anticipate more than muscular barriers to speech improvement in the cerebral-palsied.

The tendency toward increased emotional lability, psychomotor disinhibition, and distractibility are consequences that have a direct bearing on muscle treatment. As the new brain developed phylogenetically and ontogenetically, it progressively softened and inhibited excessive emotional reactions and hyperactivity of the old brain while providing more discriminative control of behavior. When cerebral damage impairs the new brain's dominion, unchecked emotional outbursts are readily provoked, attention wanders distressingly, and excitement is easily stimulated (Strauss and Lehtinen, 1947).

None of these conditions is conducive to the acquisition of new speech patterns. If the therapist is attempting to train the tongue, for example, in a new movement, the greater the precision of that movement, the better will be the patient's opportunity to observe it and preserve it accurately. The observation is complicated, though, by the neuromuscular proclivity to gross random action and the voluntary efforts to prevent the randomness which instead heighten it. The observational difficulties are further complicated by the weakened emotional control and the hyperexcitability which serve to exaggerate the neuromuscular disorder. As if these were not sufficient barriers to learning, the cerebral-palsied person may have insult heaped on injury. Not only will he have difficulty achieving precise movements that allow for accurate observation, he will probably also have perceptual disturbances that would make effective observation difficult under the most ideal circumstances. He may attend to insignificant details and fail to perceive essential cues to improved speech. He may, too, be unable to concentrate long enough on the proper cues to perceive them adequately even if he manages to isolate them (Goldstein, 1936). Thus, the cerebral-palsied patient attempting to learn a new tongue movement may not only have difficulty making his tongue move as he wishes, he may also have trouble attending well enough to that movement which he is trying to learn to be able to learn it.

Emotional and perceptual consequences of brain injury pose barriers to more than just muscle-training. Interpersonal relations may be strained by decreased frustration tolerance. Situations that would be mildly frustrating to the normal person can provoke vehement responses from the brain-injured. Disrupted connections between the *telencephalon* and *diencephalon* in these patients free the old brain to overreact to environmental stresses. Most people, for instance, are irritated by unavoidably broken appointments or unkept promises, but they can temper and control their frustration by maintaining a certain perspective. They evaluate their disappointment realistically and modify their reactions accordingly. On the other hand, the brain-injured will tend to have more difficulty behaving rationally under the same circumstances. With weakened emotional control, they may be unable to prevent a violent outburst even if they recognize it as being ill-advised. Too, their powers of abstraction, foresight, and concept formation may also be impaired (Strauss and Werner, 1943). Hence, their perspective is apt to be limited; they may be unable to tolerate frustration today for a bigger gain tomorrow. Today is here and now, it is real. Tomorrow is only a vague abstraction, it is frequently too difficult for the brain-damaged to grasp and appreciate.

Many of the nonmotor characteristics of the cerebral-palsied seem closely akin to those commonly attributed to neurotics. Certainly the physically handicapped are often exposed throughout life to conditions which create emotional maladjustment (Cruickshank, 1948). They are made to feel unwanted either by overprotection or by outright rejection; their physical limitations render them relatively helpless, and their body concepts may well be distorted (Bender and Silver, 1948). The physically normal person disabled by psychic conflict may not function any better during his mental illness than will the brain-injured. However, most physically normal neurotics have the capacity to achieve perspective and exert control over their troubled feelings as they are exposed and resolved either in psychotherapy or in the normal course of living. Brain-injured persons are limited in this capacity, although there is evidence that the limitation is not absolute (Wepman, 1951). Accordingly, the resolution of psychic trauma in these patients should be undertaken with great caution, if it is undertaken at all. Exposure of feared antisocial feelings may arouse such intolerable frustration that the brain-injured person will be incapable of restraining himself from social aggressions.

On the other hand, we know of one successful attempt to treat the emotional disorders of a group of cerebral-palsied children in an all-day play-therapy situation. This was a unique psychotherapeutic arrangement, though, in which the mothers as well as the clinicians actually participated in the play-therapy treatment. The children were allowed to release their feelings without any limitations, and they were continued in this completely unrestricted situation long enough for their emotional needs to be largely resolved. One remarkable result was that some of the children in the group with severe muscular involvements showed great gains in controlling their random movements without any specific muscle-training!

Whether or not the success achieved would have been possible in a more orthodox psychotherapeutic setting is questionable. Under typical play-therapy circumstances, these children would have been seen a few times a week for limited periods. They would have been allowed the free expression of feelings with minimal restrictions, but they would have been required to discriminate as to what could be done and when it could be done and to govern themselves accordingly. Such control in a comparable situation is a major problem for any normal child with emotional troubles. He is frustrated when allowed to vent his feelings and then finds that he must not transgress the therapeutic limits, low as they may be. He is frustrated still more when he discovers that he cannot release his emotions at home or at school in the same manner permitted him in therapy. And he would be frustrated even further if therapy were terminated *after* his control of the dangerous feared feelings had been weakened but *before* a satisfactory resolution for these feelings has been worked out. In effect, any child in a typical play-therapy situation is told, "We are going to start something that you are not going to want to stop, but you must stop when we tell you, whether you like it or not." The normal child will be hard-pressed to obey these instructions. The brain-injured child may find the restrictions intolerable.

With cerebral-palsied adults we have seen remarkable improvement in oral-motor activity accompany improved interpersonal relations. One young man with ataxia worked for months attempting to correct a grotesque facial expression accompanying speech. Very little improvement occurred until he became interested in a young lady. The changes were then rapid and startling. The facial grimace was soon eradicated, the slurred speech became readily intelligible, and his stumbling gait gave way to a somewhat purposeful stride. In fact, he even learned to dance! With another case, a woman who had extensive athetoid involvements, speech therapy was eventually combined with psychotherapy to effect improvement. Extensive efforts to increase her oral-motor control were rewarded with little success. Her personal troubles proved so pressing, however, that the majority of each hour was finally devoted to working on her emotional problems. Some time later the clinician was amazed to find upon returning to oral-motor exercises that her tongue was no longer immobile. Whereas earlier she had been unable to achieve any noticeable tongue elevation, she now found that she could touch it to the alveolar ridge. These encouraging results are supported by Cowen's (1955) report on the use of limited psychotherapy methods with cerebral-palsied cases.

The obvious point we are making is that emotional problems left untended will frequently interfere with progress in treating the cerebral-palsied individual. Psychic conflicts cause great anguish and distress for the person who is physically sound. For the brain-injured person these tensions are even more intolerable, since they aggravate his other disabilities. They make him more distractible, more irritable, more irrational in his behavior, more prone to failure. Obviously, the need for their reduction is great. Unfortunately, brain injury tends to leave the victim an unlikely candidate for psychotherapy, but this is not universally true. The critical question is not whether the person has suffered brain damage, but rather whether the brain damage has impaired his self-control and resistance to frustration. Stated in Freudian terms, the issue is whether or not the patient has sufficient ego-strength to *tolerate* therapy.

Another closely related consequence of cerebral palsy that complicates treatment is the devastating effect of failure. Again, the difference from the normal is more quantitative than qualitative. Failure for anyone is discouraging, but if the brain-injured person attempts and fails a task beyond his ability he may experience what Goldstein (1939) calls a "catastrophic reaction." In addition to the somatic disturbance he becomes enraged, anxious, and depressed. Instead of seeking adequate, rational, satisfying solutions to a problem, he becomes disorganized and almost desperately attempts any response regardless of how inappropriate it may be. The after-effect of a catastrophic reaction leaves the patient physically exhausted, discouraged, and unable to cope with difficulties he could normally meet easily.

Unhappily, cerebral-palsied individuals tend to be predisposed to failure by their neuromuscular condition. Furthermore, cerebral palsy may alter the patient's perceptual experience. Instead of grasping the relation of parts to the whole normally, he may misperceive the whole and focus on some detail that the normal person would disregard. Moreover, the figure-ground relations he does perceive may be unstable, so that he experiences constant fluctuations in his thinking and a disturbing inability to concentrate (Strauss and Kephart, 1955). He may be quite distressed by any form of disorder, so he may strive to hold things constant by being compulsively neat, exact, and meticulous. These perceptual disturbances are not readily understood by most of those whom the cerebral-palsied will encounter in their daily living, yet these are the people who may frequently judge the performance of the brain-injured. Friction is almost unavoidable and failures are predestined when the patient in a normal environment demands extreme orderliness, finds himself unable to concentrate on a task, and attends to insignificant details because of his lack of foresight and perspective and limited ability to perceive essentials.

## CONCLUSIONS

The problems facing the cerebral-palsied person are immense, and we have made no attempt to minimize them. The patient will frequently experience difficulty in every phase of learning. His *need* to learn will be minimized if he has been overprotected. His perceptual deviations will disturb his *discrimination* of what it is he is trying to learn. His neuromuscular disabilities will interfere with *practicing* accurately the movements to be learned. And his reduced need to learn in the first place will weaken any *rewards* for learning. We have presented the issues bluntly, not with an intent to discourage, but rather with a desire to acquaint the speech clinician with difficulties he can anticipate which so vitally affect therapy. The ostrich approach to rehabilitation, that of ignoring problems with the hope that they will somehow go away, merely serves to distort the treatment. Obviously, the person's needs cannot be met until they are recognized. To search for them with the preconceived certainty that the bulk of the troubles can be explained in terms of muscle disorder, or in terms of perceptual disturbance, or in terms of emotional upset is to gather more and more evidence about less and less of the bigger issues in the patient's life.

The cerebral-palsied persons who have not developed adequate speech are faced with an acute multifaceted predicament. As we have already indicated, a certain amount of environmental complexity and frustration is necessary to foster speech development in the normal child. With cerebral-palsied people their need to talk must be considerably greater, since they must overcome serious perceptual and muscle-control handicaps to master the most elementary speech skills. Yet for this need to be effective, the patient must be able to tolerate much tension for prolonged periods while acquiring communication skills that will reduce his frustration. His troubles would be sufficiently grievous if they stopped here, but his already overloaded pain tolerance may be taxed further by "catastrophic reactions" to failures, of which he will probably have more than a normal share; by hyper-irritability in interpersonal relations; by emotional conflicts which he may have to tolerate if their relief through psychotherapy proves unfeasible; and, if he has lived long enough in a sheltered environment, by consternation at finding his mode of living disrupted by demands that he meet his own needs. The approach to speech therapy for the cerebral-palsied patient is dictated by these obstacles with which he struggles. Above all else, he must feel a need for improved speech. Collateral rewards such as a piece of candy or a gold star after each successful performance have value, but their worth is dubious if they are expected to provide the patient with sufficient desire to submit to the rigors essential to speech acquisition. But even an overwhelming need is not enough. Undirected, such urgency can generate more frustration than it relieves. Each skill to be learned should be isolated cleanly to reduce figure-ground confusion. Clinical situations should be arranged to provide success without prolonged concentration. Free-play activities, for instance, are not conducive to clear perceptions because they foster rapid shifts of attention, and the cues to be brought into focus blend into the background, blurring sensory impressions. Once the task is accurately perceived, its execution should be undertaken with calm determination. Any disturbing influence during therapy should be eliminated if possible whether it be emotional upset, physical discomfort, excessive enthusiasm, or too complex a performance such as speaking while writing or while walking or even while standing. Finally, it is critical that the patient succeed in his efforts. His disabilities may predispose him to failure but the effects of failure can devastate him. Thus, each task should be calculated to provide him with some measure of success.

We have posed a dilemma. First, we indicated the necessity for submitting the cerebral-palsied child to as normal a socialization process as he can tolerate. To do this he must be frustrated. Then, we discussed the reduced frustration tolerance of the brain-injured which would seem to make normal socialization almost impossible. This dilemma cannot be resolved easily. If there is a key, it is to effect a lifelong delicate balance between protection and stress. The patient's first two or three years should be carefully sheltered, but then a continuous series of stresses should commence that never exceed his power to handle yet constantly approximate his limits of pain tolerance. This procedure should, ideally, be followed with any child. It is more critical, though, with the brain-injured ones, for if they fall behind by being protected too long or pushed too hard, they have relatively little reserve capacity for meeting increased strain. Just as an athlete would not wait until the day of a contest to start conditioning nor would he overtax himself at any time during training, so, too, the cerebral-palsied person must have his frustration tolerance carefully nurtured. His needs are not uncommon, but to satisfy them he must contend with extraordinary obstacles. The earlier in his life his problems are met squarely, the greater will be his chances in society for a normal existence.

Until recently, the environment has imposed severe restrictions on the cerebral-palsied population. Only those who could appear as nearly normal had much hope of employment or social acceptance. The more severely involved cases were truly in "the farthest corner." Today the prospects are better, but there are still limitations. Although an increasing segment of the population is achieving a more rational attitude toward the problem, this does not yet, and probably never will, assure automatic approval for cerebral-palsied people regardless of their disability. Socially desirable traits, such as good grooming, a pleasant voice, attentive listening, thoughtfulness, good humor, and flexibility will continue to be criteria for acceptability. Unfortunately, the muscular and emotional disorders of the cerebral-palsied child or adult are not conducive to these qualities. As for employment possibilities, the frequent impression that only certain jobs are available is misleading. Several studies (Glick, 1953; Brinn and Smith, 1951) have shown a wide range of occupations from the professional to the unskilled in which the cerebral-palsied members of society have been successful. Selective placement and personal-adjustment counseling provide the key to success on the job. Selective placement emphasizes the best matching of the individual's abilities with the specific requirements of the task. This method is in contrast to that of listing occupations available for each type of disabled worker, a method that ignores the great variation of individual handicaps within a diagnostic category. Personal-adjustment counseling before commencing the job has been shown to be critical to stable employment. Such counseling is a time-consuming procedure, so this is one reason why the placement facilities for the cerebral-palsied are limited (Garrett, 1955). However, opportunities are increasing. The future for those handicapped individuals who wish to help themselves is brighter. The challenge of rehabilitation is becoming more attractive.

Our final conclusion has been connoted throughout this chapter. Much of what we have written has been from clinical supposition, not from experimental certainty. The cerebral-palsied persons particularly need the advantage of the most beneficial treatment from birth if they are to conquer their handicaps. But what is the most beneficial treatment? Among the various techniques now used to improve the speech of the cerebral-palsied case, which are the best? Are there better principles and methods of therapy that we have hardly tried? Even in the area of greatest endeavor, muscle-training, basic questions remain unresolved. Tentative knowledge of maturation levels and neural patterns have led to some hypotheses about the acquisition of skills, but these theories still need further testing. For instance, to what extent is the development of an oral-motor skill a function of organismic maturation as opposed to being a function of learning? Presumably, a skill cannot be learned if the organism has not matured sufficiently but, conversely, the question remains whether the skill can be acquired if the person *passively* awaits the necessary level of development. Research (Cruze, 1935) indicates that the acquisition of many skills in lower animals is not dependent upon prior training, but with man's oral-motor activities this conclusion is dubious. For the cerebral-palsied patient the question is critical. Treatment of the speech musculature is predicated on the belief that function will improve with exercise. Still, we do not know how much exercise to use and when it should begin for maximal improvement. For that matter, we do not know enough about muscle activity and learning to be certain that the training which supposedly accounts for muscle-strengthening also accounts for muscle fatigue. These are questions in an area that has received extensive attention in cerebral-palsy rehabilitation. We know even less about problems of personality development and intellectual impairment, especially as they relate to the acquisition of speech. At an operational level, we cannot say with great assurance what activities specifically the parents of an infant suspected of cerebral palsy should encourage. Answers to these problems do not lie just in the realm of speech therapy, they must come from all of the professions concerned: from neurology to physical therapy, from occupational therapy to psychology. The pattern of interaction among these specialties should carefully follow lines of mutual understanding of part functions as they relate to the total problem.

## BIBLIOGRAPHY

ALLPORT, F. H. 1955. Theories of perception and the concept of structure. New York: Wiley.

BARKER, R. G., ROGER, G., WRIGHT, B. A., MEYERSON, L., and GONICK, M. R. 1953. Adjustment to physical handicap and illness: a survey of the social psychology of physique and disability. New York: Social Science Research Council.

BEACH, F. A., and JAYNES, J. 1954. The effects of early experience upon the behavior of animals. *Psychol. Bull.*, 51, 239–263.

BENDER, L., and SILVER, A. 1948. Body image problems in the brain damaged child. *J. soc. Issues.*, 4, 84–89.

BICE, H. V. 1955. Parent education and counseling. *In* Cruickshank, W. M., and Raus, G. M. Cerebral palsy: its individual and community problems. Syracuse: Syracuse Univ. Press. Pp. 411–428.

BOBATH, B. 1948. The importance of the reduction of muscle tone and the control of mass reflex action in the treatment of spasticity. *Occup. Therapy Rehabilitation.*, 27, 371–383.

—— 1953. Control of postures and movements in the treatment of cerebral palsy. *Physiotherapy*, 39, 99–104.

—— 1954. A study of abnormal posture reflex activity in patients with lesions of the central nervous system. I, II, III, IV. *Physiotherapy.*, 40, 259–267; 295–300; 326–334; 368–373.

—— and BOBATH, K. 1952. A treatment of cerebral palsy. *Brit. J. phys. Med.*, 15, 1–11.

BOBATH, K., and BOBATH, B. 1950. Spastic paralysis. *Brit. J. phys. Med.*, 13, 121–127.

BRINN, C., and SMITH, E. E. 1951. Opportunities limited. San Francisco: Calif. Soc. Crippled Children.

CASS, M. T. 1951. Speech habilitation in cerebral palsy. New York: Columbia Univ. Press.

COWEN, E. L. 1955. Psychotherapy and play techniques with the exceptional child and youth. *In* Cruickshank, W. M., Psychology of exceptional children and youth. New York: Prentice-Hall. Pp. 520–575.

CRUICKSHANK, W. M. 1948. The impact of physical disability on social adjustment. *J. soc. Issues.*, 4, 81–82.

—— 1955. Psychological considerations with crippled children. *In* Cruickshank, W. M., Psychology of exceptional children and youth. New York: Prentice-Hall. Pp. 284–344.

CRUZE, W. W. 1935. Maturation and learning in chicks. *J. comp. Psychol.*, 19, 371–409.

DI CARLO, L. M., and AMSTER, W. W. 1955. Hearing and speech problems among cerebral palsied children. *In* Cruickshank, W. M., and Raus, G. M., Cerebral palsy: its individual and community problems. Syracuse: Syracuse Univ. Press. Pp. 166–255.

FROESCHELS, E., and JELLINEK, A. 1941. Practice of voice and speech therapy. Boston: Expression.

GARRETT, J. A. 1955. Realistic vocational guidance and placement. *In* Cruickshank, W. M., and Raus, G. M., Cerebral palsy: its individual and community problems. Syracuse: Syracuse Univ. Press. Pp. 429–461.

GESELL, A., and AMATRUDA, C. 1941. Developmental diagnosis. New York: Hoeber.

GLICK, S. J. 1953. Vocational, educational, and recreational needs of the cerebral palsied adult. New York: United Cerebral Palsy.

GOLDSTEIN, K. 1936. The modification of behavior consequent to cerebral lesions. *Psychiat. Quart.*, 10, 586–610.

———— 1939. The organism. New York: American Book.

GRATKE, J. M. 1947. Help them help themselves. Dallas: Texas Soc. Crippled Children.

HARRINGTON, R. 1950. The speech rehabilitation of the cerebral palsied. Chicago: Nat. Soc. Crippled Children Adults.

HEBB, D. O. 1949. The organization of behavior: a neuropsychological theory. New York: Wiley.

HUBER, M. 1951. Speech rehabilitation of the cerebral palsied. *West. Speech.*, 15, 13–16.

KABAT, H. 1947. Studies on neuromuscular function, XI: New principles of neuromuscular reeducation. *Permanente Foundation Bull.*, 5, 111–123.

LASHLEY, K. S. 1942. An examination of the "continuity theory" as applied to discrimination learning. *J. genet. Psychol.*, 26, 241–265.

LEFEVRE, M. C. 1952. A rationale for resistive therapy in speech training for the cerebral palsied. *J. except. Child.*, 19, 61–64.

LEHTINEN, L. E. 1955. Preliminary conclusions affecting education of brain-injured children. *In* Strauss, A. A., and Kephart, N. C., Psychopathology and education of the brain-injured child. New York: Grune and Stratton. Vol. 2. Pp. 165–191.

LEWIN, K. 1935. A dynamic theory of personality. New York: McGraw-Hill.

MCCULLOUGH, W. S. 1944. The functional organization of the cerebral cortex. *Physiol. Rev.*, 24, 390–407.

MCGEOCH, J. A. 1942. The psychology of human learning. New York: Longmans, Green.

MARLAND, P. M. 1953. Speech therapy for the cerebral palsied based on reflex inhibitions. *In* Van Riper, C., Speech therapy: a book of readings. New York: Prentice-Hall. Pp. 235–238.

MOWRER, O. H. 1952. Speech development in the young child: 1. The autism theory of speech development and some clinical applications. *J. Speech Hearing Disorders*, 17, 263–268.

MUNN, N. L. 1946. Learning in children. *In* Carmichael, L., Manual of child psychology. New York: Wiley. Pp. 370–441.

National Society for Crippled Children and Adults, Inc., The. 1953. A selective bibliography on cerebral palsy. 11 S. LaSalle St., Chicago 3, Ill.

PALMER, M. 1947. Studies in clinical techniques. II, normalization of chewing sucking and swallowing reflexes in cerebral palsy: a home program. *J Speech Disorders*, 12, 415–418.

PIAGET, J. 1948. The language and thought of the child. London: Routledge & Kegan Paul.

POHL, J. F. 1950. Cerebral palsy. St. Paul: Bruce.

ROOD, M. 1954. Neurophysiological reactions as a basis for physical therapy. *Phys. Therapy Rev.*, 34, 444–449.

RUESCH, J., and BATESON, G. 1951. Communication: the social matrix of society. New York: Norton.

RUTHERFORD, B. R. 1950. Give them a chance to talk. Minneapolis: Burgess.

SHARPE, W. 1952. Brain surgeon. New York: Viking.

STINCHFIELD, S. M., and YOUNG, E. H. 1938. Children with delayed or defective speech. Palo Alto.: Stanford Univ. Press.

STRAUSS, A. A., and KEPHART, N. C. 1955. Psychopathology and education of the brain-injured child. New York: Grune and Stratton. Vol. 2.

STRAUSS, A. A., and LEHTINEN, L. E. 1947. Psychopathology and education of the brain-injured child. New York: Grune and Stratton. Vol. 1.

STRAUSS, A. A. and WERNER, H. 1943. Impairment in thought processes of brain-injured children. *Amer. J. ment. Defic.*, 47, 291–295.

WECHSLER, I. S. 1947. A textbook of clinical neurology. Philadelphia: Saunders.

WEPMAN, J. M. 1951. Recovery from aphasia. New York: Ronald.

WESTLAKE, H. 1951a. Muscle training for cerebral palsied speech cases. *J. Speech Hearing Disorders*, 16, 103–109.

——— 1951b. A system for developing speech with cerebral palsied children. Chicago: Nat. Soc. Crippled Children Adults.

WHETNALL, E. 1952. Deafness in children. *In* Scott-Brown, W. G., Diseases of the ear, nose, and throat. London: Butterworth. Vol. 2. Pp. 328–360.

WIENER, N. 1948. Cybernetics. New York: Wiley.

WOODWORTH, R. S. 1938. Experimental psychology. New York: Holt.

# CHAPTER 19

# PATHOMORPHOLOGY OF CLEFT PALATE AND CLEFT LIP

● *Herbert Koepp-Baker, Ph.D.*

CONGENITAL CLEFT LIP and cleft palate produce the most profound of speech disturbances. The disconfiguration of so many speech structures is reflected in serious alterations of the processes of articulation and resonation. Indirectly, it also modifies unfavorably the functions of phonation and respiration. Its adverse effects upon audition, together with the deformities of the face which so often accompany this oro-naso-pharyngeal teratism, impose further penalties and limits upon speech behavior. Being present before birth and in varying degrees during the period in which speech is learned, this condition is a deterrent to the acquisition of speech-production skills.

Circumstances dictate that the relationship between the speech clinician and the child with the cleft palate seldom begins until the child is learning to talk, and often much later. Rarely, therefore, does the speech clinician have an opportunity to see the child before reconstructive surgery is done or prosthetic service is provided. The many effects of this aberrancy of structure upon the speech processes can be appreciated only when the original condition is understood.

Cleft lip and cleft palate are deformities of tissue disposition, specifically of disjunction and inadequacy (occasionally overdevelopment) of the tissue of the lip, nose, jaw, hard palate, velum, pharynx, and cranial base. The varieties of cleft lip and palate may be grouped into four general categories based upon embryological, anatomical, and physiological considerations: (1) those involving the lip alone; (2) those involving the lip, palate, and velum; (3) those in which the palate and velum only are affected; and (4) those in which the palate is congenitally insufficient.

## Clefts of the Lip

Nonunions limited to the lip may appear in varying degrees, ranging from minimal defects of the vermeil portion of the lip to complete extension into the nasal vestibule. When one side of the lip alone is involved, it is described as unilateral; when both are involved, bilateral. Bilateral clefts of the lip may be asymmetrical, since one side may be cleft to a greater extent than the other. When the cleft of the lip is complete on one side only, the

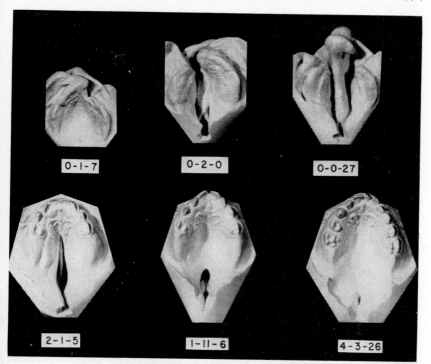

FIG. 1. Representative examples of the common clefts of the lip, alveolar process, hard palate, and velum. The age of the patient appears beneath each figure and is stated in years, months, and days. These are illustrations of casts made from impressions of the mouth before surgery.

is commonly marked displacement of the nasal alar cartilage on that side and of the tip of the nose. In bilateral clefts that are complete, the median portion of the lip, containing the philtrum, is isolated and remains attached to the premaxillary bone and columella. This isolated portion of bone and lip protrudes forward in the facial profile and both nasal alae are depressed and rotated laterally. The columella is usually deficient.

The alveolar defects which accompany divisions of the lip may range from small grooves or dimples, which can be detected only by palpation and which tend to fill in as the jaw grows, to total unilateral or bilateral clefts of the bony process. The extent to which the tissue of the lip shows disjunction is an index of considerable reliability of the probable extent of involvement of the alveolar process at the same site. On the other hand, it is not possible to predict accurately the degree of palatal involvement from the extent of the cleft or clefts of the lip.

The effect upon the pattern of dental eruption of the alveolar defects accompanying cleft lip is not clear. The form of the dental arch and the arrangement of the anterior teeth are often disturbed. A number of clinical observers have emphasized the intimate embryonic relationship between the lip and the anterior portion of the alveolar arch (Pruzansky, 1953; Fogh-Anderson, 1942). Sicher (1949) has offered an embryological explana-

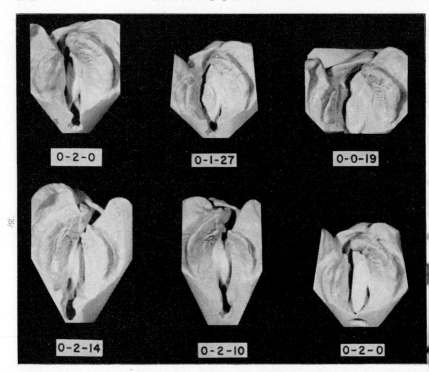

FIG. 2. Varieties of unilateral complete clefts. Though they are all of one "type," they show great differences; and these differences are often more important than the general classification.

tion for these observations. He has pointed out that the entire palate does not develop from the primitive palatine anlage. Rather, the maxillary alveolar processes arise from the mesoderm in the depths of a sulcus which separates the lip and the palate, while the tegmen oris gives rise only to the soft palate and the central part of the hard palate.

### Clefts of the Lip and Palates

Both unilateral and bilateral clefts of the lip may be associated with complete or incomplete clefts of the palate and velum. The palatine processes of the maxillae form the floor of the nose as well as the roof of the mouth. Hence, a division of the lip, jaw, hard palate, and velum obliterates the dividing wall between the nasal and oral cavities on the side of the cleft. There is much individual variation in the adequacy of tissue and the degree of separation and tilt of the palatal processes of the maxillae, and hence in the width of palatal clefts. In unilateral clefts of the palate and velum, the vomer bone and nasal septum are attached to the palatal process on the side opposite the cleft, maintaining on that side the normal separation between the nasal and oral chambers. The palatal process on the side of the cleft is often tilted medially and upward. There may be deviation of the vomer and sep

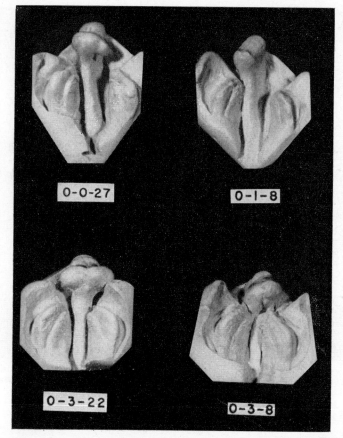

FIG. 3. Varieties of bilateral complete clefts. The individual differences are impressive.

tum along the line of their attachment to the palatal process on the noncleft side.

Bilateral clefts of the lip and palates may also be complete or incomplete, symetrical or asymetrical. In bilateral complete clefts of the lip and palates, both nasal chambers are in direct communication with the oral cavity. The rudimentary vomer and nasal septum form a midline structure which is attached firmly to the base of the skull, but somewhat movable at its anterior end where it supports the premaxilla and columella. The premaxilla may, in bilateral clefts of the palates, be large or small, extended or rotated on its supporting septovomer stalk. Its growth having been unrestrained, the premaxillary bone with the portion of the lip which covers it is usually protrusive and greatly alters the facial profile.

## Clefts of the Palates

In this class neither the lip nor the alveolar process is involved. The nonunion may be limited to the velum alone, or may involve both the velum and

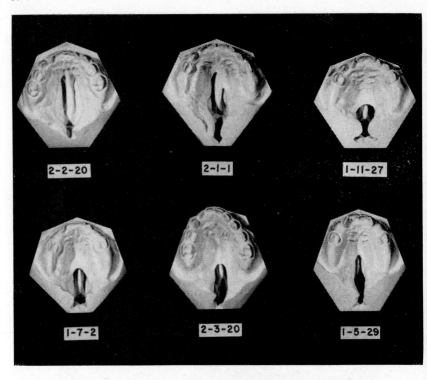

FIG. 4. Varieties of incomplete clefts of the palates in which neither the alveolar process nor the lip is involved. The variation in size and shape of the clefts is noteworthy.

the hard palate. Most embryologists are agreed that the fusion of the parts forming the hard and soft palates proceeds anterio-posteriorward. This is supported by the clinical observation that clefts involving the palates appear in varying extent: a division of part or all of the horizontal palatine processes beginning at the anterior palatine foramen; all or part of the velum; and a bifidated uvula. An underdevelopment of the horizontal bony palatine processes is also not an unusual finding in clefts which involve the velum and/or uvula only. As is the case in unilateral and bilateral clefts of the lip and palates, the extent of the cleft on either or both sides will determine the degree to which the nasal chambers are exposed. As in lip-and-palate clefts, the vomer will be in the midline or be fused to one or the other of the palatal maxillary processes, but is often of a different shape and size. These palatal clefts may be V-shaped or pyriform. They may be narrow or wide, with more or less obliteration or displacement of the palatal processes. In clefts of the hard palate and velum the maxillary dental arch may also be wider than normal, this being advertized by the mandibular arch lying in complete lingual relation to the upper arch. A number of authorities have also commented on the high incidence of mandibular micrognathia associated with clefts of the palates.

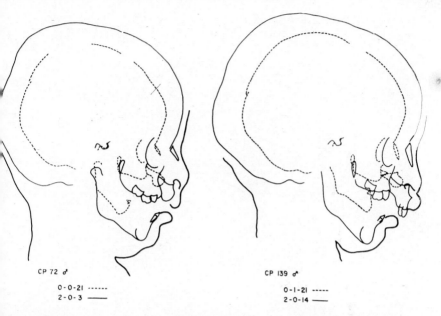

CP 72 ♂

0 - 0 - 21 ------
2 - 0 - 3 ——

CP 139 ♂

0 - 1 - 21 -----
2 - 0 - 14 ——

FIG. 5. Differences in the pattern of growth of two children with a cleft of the same "type" and each treated in a similar fashion. These are tracings of the roentgenocephalograms made of each child at two different times, as indicated below the illustrations. The differences in growth patterns are reflected in the internal structures and in the profile.

## Congenital Insufficiency of the Palates

Speech pathologists and surgeons have observed that in patients in whom the uvula is divided or the soft palate is cleft in varying degrees up to the palatovelar aponeurosis, a concomitant submucous cleft of the hard palate also exists. The degree of cleft in the bones of the palate may range from a simple absence of the posterior palatal spine to a marked inadequacy of the horizontal process of the palatal bones. The mucous membrane over the bony defect is usually intact, though often attenuated. Dorrance (1933) was of the opinion that these forms are accompanied by an underdevelopment of the velum as well, and that this created a significant reduction of the total anterio-posterior palatal axis. However, since Dorrance made these observations in surgical anatomy, our understanding of variations in the structure of the pharynx and its supporting and contiguous structures has also been extended. Kirkham (1931), Wardill (1928), and Psaume (1950) studying skeletal material and McCarthy (1925), Schüller (1929), Ricketts (1952), and Subtelny (1953) employing radiographic techniques have made it evident that there are very important anatomic variations of the cranial base, the pterygoid plates, the hamular processes and the cervical structure of persons with cleft palate. The pharynges of cleft-palate patients tend to be wider and deeper. In such pharynges the velum, whether of normal or less-than-normal length, is at a functional disadvantage.

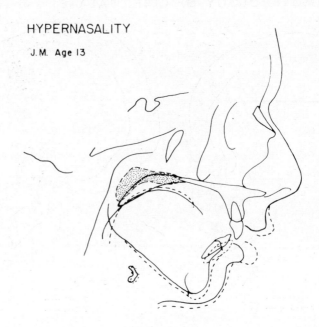

HYPERNASALITY

J.M. Age 13

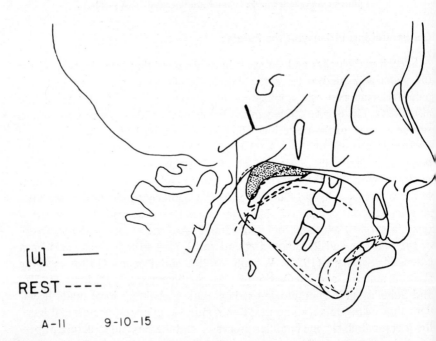

[u] ——

REST - - - -

A-11      9-10-15

FIG. 6. Top, tracing of the roentgenocephalogram of a child with palatal insufficiency. The solid line indicated the structures at rest, the broken line and stippled area show the structures during phonation of a high back vowel. Bottom, a tracing of the roentgenocephalogram of a normal subject provided for comparison.

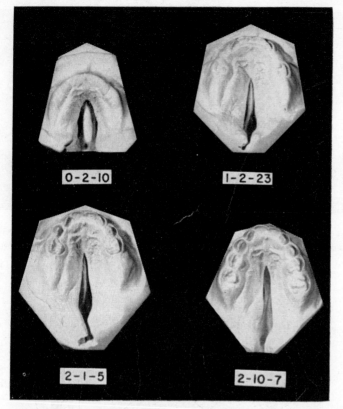

FIG. 7. A series of casts of the same child beginning at the age of 2 months to age 2 years, 10 months. No treatment of any kind was instituted. Note the dramatic decrease in the width of the cleft. Some, but not all, show such changes. Some grow wider.

## The Myopathology and Myodynamics of Cleft Lip and Cleft Palate

Since speech production is the result of complex myosynergies, it will be useful to extend our examination of cleft palate and cleft lip beyond the osteal and connective framework of the face and mouth. Two features of the problem are noteworthy: (1) the effect of structural aberrancy upon muscular growth, and (2) the maldevelopment of the muscular behavior subserving the speech process.

### Effect of Nonunions upon Muscle Growth and Function

It is evident that the vectors of growth are modified extensively by the absence of union of strategic parts of the cranio-facial skeleton. The critical relationship between (1) muscle growth and function and (2) growth of the skeleton is well established. The circumstance in which a lip is divided unilaterally or bilaterally illustrates this dramatically. The mass of the lip is principally muscle. When it does not unite at the appropriate embryological time, the usual directive, facilitative, and inhibitive forces of growth are disturbed. There is, as a result, certain disposition, underdevelopment, and over-

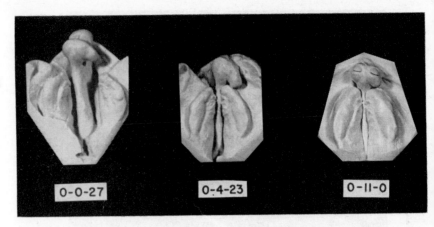

0-0-27    0-4-23    0-11-0

FIG. 8. The effect of primary lip closure upon the size of a bilateral cleft is illustrated here. First one side was closed, then the other. Oral orthopedics will later improve the arch form.

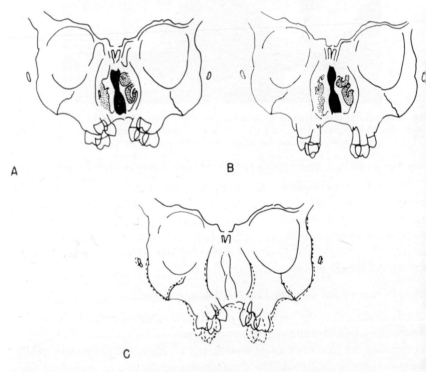

A          B

C

FIG. 9. The effect of oral orthopedics (orthodontia) in a case of bilateral complete cleft. The severe contraction of the maxillary arch has been greatly improved. That this improvement is not confined to the arch alone but is shared by many other contiguous structures of the head is evidenced by the tracing of the x-ray laminagram of the patient before and after treatment. A, these structures before oral orthopedics was begun; B, after it was completed. The extent and locations of these changes are shown by superimposition of one tracing upon another in C.

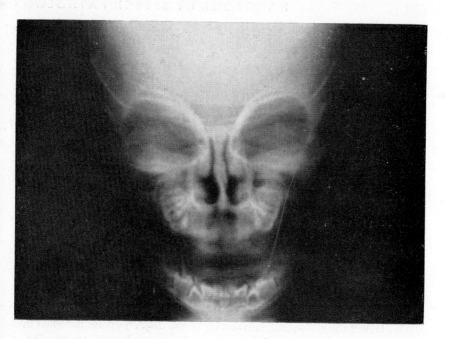

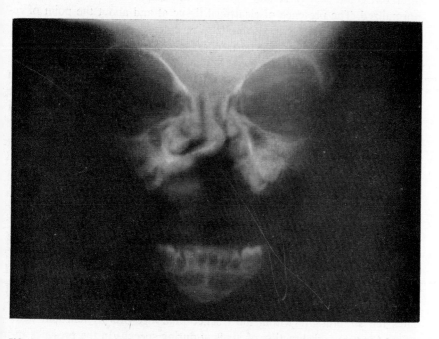

FIG. 10. Top, a frontal laminagraphic section of a normal subject. Bottom, a patient with uni-lateral cleft reflecting the profound alteration of the interior structures of the nose in some cleft-palate individuals.

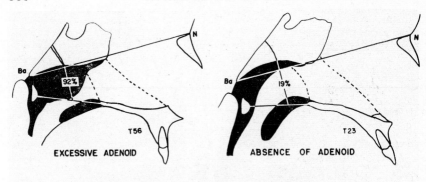

AVERAGE TISSUE OCCUPIES 56% OF NASOPHARYNX

FIG. 11. The role played by lymphoid (adenoid) tissue in nasopharyngeal valving. The speech of subject on the left was hyponasal. That of the subject on the right was hypernasal.

development of the structure itself and of contiguous structures (the nose, dental arch, and dentition). It is well established that the primitive alimentary movements are present *in utero*. That these functional movements emerge gradually is probable. That they involve both the lip and the mouth is also likely. Hence the embryonic movements of the divided lip are modified both because of the division and because of the gradual variant alteration of growth of the parts. Even though the lip will be reunited surgically sometime after birth, the structural and kinetic relationships cannot be completely normalized. The presence of cicatricial tissue at and about the point of re-union will, to some degree, also inhibit movement.

Intraorally, the major myosystems of speech are the tongue and velo-pharyngeal complex. The muscular systems which elevate, depress, extend, and retract the mandible are also very important. It has been observed that the division of the jaw and palates permits early maladaptation of the tongue to its oral environment. The implications of this maladaptation are important both in terms of growth of lingual tissue and its behavioral patterns. If the palates remain open during the early years of life and are uncorrected sur-gically or prosthetically, growth patterns of the tongue will be further altered and it is reasonable to assume that the lingual behavior will assume aberrant forms. Even if the palate is closed surgically or prosthetically in early life, lingual form and behavior will still have been, to some degree, prede-termined.

In deglutition the velopharyngeal mechanism functions to occlude the nasopharyngeal isthmus. In the normal individual, this closure is vigorous. In speech production, though less energetic, it regulates the dimensions of the nasopharyngeal isthmus from complete closure to full patency for coupling and uncoupling the oro-pharyngo-nasal resonators. It also regu-lates the air pressure within the tracheo-pharyngo-oral system and deter-mines the rate and direction of air flow during speech. In the presence of a divided palate and/or velum, extensive compensatory movements of the pharyngeal wall and tongue tend to develop. This general compensation

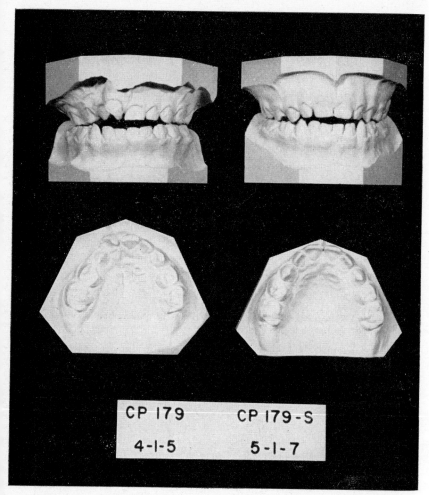

FIG. 12. Orthodontic correction of a child in the stage of deciduous dentition and with a surgically treated unilateral cleft. The occlusion before and after is shown in the picture at the top. A palatal view of the maxillary arch is depicted below. Note the correction of the typical cross-bite.

causes the total oropharyngeal muscular synergies of speech to be to some extent perverted. As has been pointed out, it is clear from radiographic studies that in persons with cleft palate, important variations in the cranial base, the pterygoid plates, the hamular processes, and cervical structure are also present. The effect of these skeletal variations in regions contiguous to the velum has great significance in any analysis of the myodynamics of cleft palate speech. Though cleft palate affects the form and adequacy of the velum, any full assessment of the defect must be made in terms which take into account the concomitant variations in those structures functionally related to it.

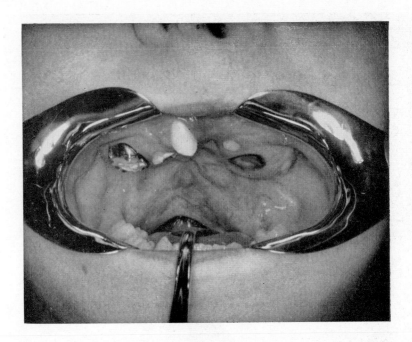

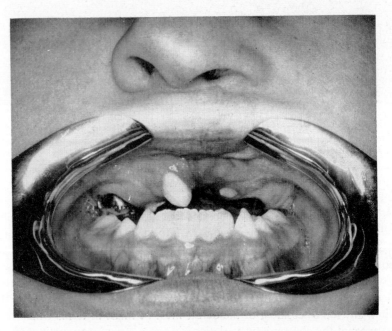

FIG. 13. This child shows profound loss of dental tissue, severe contraction of the maxillary arch, generalized scarring of the palate, and a foreshortened and immobile velum. Top, palatal view. Bottom, in occlusion.

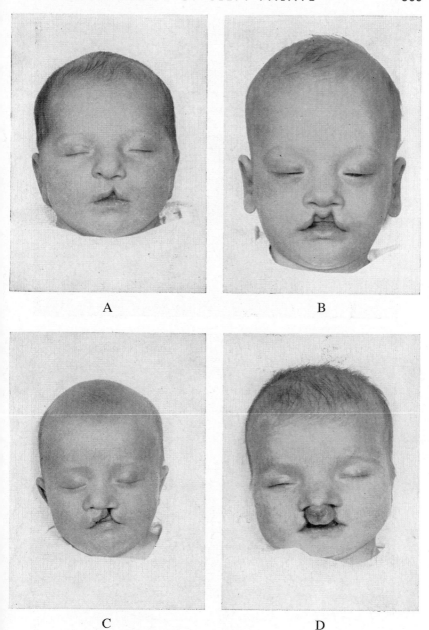

A        B

C        D

FIG. 14. A, unilateral incomplete cleft of the lip; B, bilateral incomplete cleft of the lip; C, unilateral complete cleft of the lip; D, bilateral complete cleft of the lip.

## The Patterns of Dental Growth in Cleft Lip and Cleft Palate

The effects of divided lips-and-palates upon dental development are manifest both in the shape and location of individual teeth, in their relationship

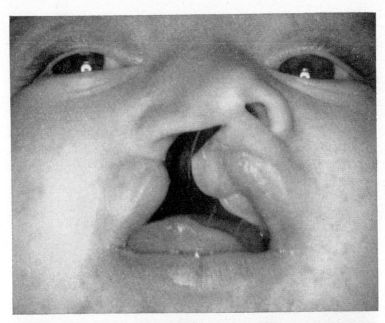

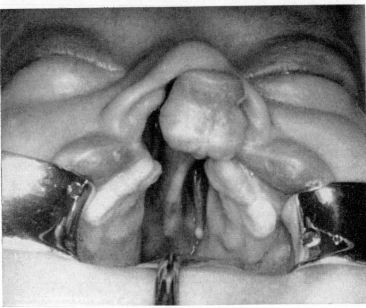

FIG. 15. Top, unilateral complete cleft of the lip, alveolar process, palate, and velum; bottom, bilateral complete cleft.

to each other in the upper dental arch, and in the relationship of the two dental arches. Deformity and absence of both deciduous and permanent teeth in or near the line of cleft are not unusual. After surgical closure of the lip, the occlusion in both deciduous and permanent arches is often in cross-bite relation on the side of the cleft. In bilateral lip-palate clefts the premaxillary support of the two central incisors may be insecure, the whole segment being somewhat movable. Though the surgically restored lip will tend to retropose the premaxillary segment into a reasonably satisfactory anterior occlusive position, it may at times also distort its position.

## Otologic and Audiologic Considerations in Cleft Palate

The muscles of the epipharynx are largely responsible for the air pressure regulation in the middle ear. The interference with velopharyngeal action imposed by cleft palate and by palatal insufficiency has long been suspect as a factor in the high incidence of middle-ear disease in children and adults with cleft palate. Since the external and internal deformities of the nose characteristic of cleft lip-and-palate interfere with ventilation and drainage, these congenital deformities seem to add further hazards to pharyngeal and otological health. The hearing loss that frequently attends middle-ear disease plays an important role in the speech and in the general behavior patterns of cleft-palate persons.

In this connection, the role of lymphoid tissue in the individual with cleft palate should also receive consideration. Whether Waldeyer's ring develops atypically in cleft-palate patients is not known with certainty. However, speech pathologists have been impressed by the severe effects of adenoidectomies upon speech in certain cases. Our understanding of the critical part which the pharyngeal tonsil (adenoid) plays in the velopharyngeal closure makes it evident that the removal of the central portion of this lymphoid mass in individuals having potential short vela and marked variation in the architecture of the base of the cranium and cervical regions may have serious speech consequences. When indicated as treatment of ear disease in children in whom palatal deformity or variations in the cranial base are suspected, otorhinolaryngologists now often recommend a partial extirpation of the lymphoid mass, limiting it to the region around the eustachian meatuses.

In summarizing the major effects of pathomorphology the following frame is helpful: (1) the adequacy or inadequacy of parts; (2) the distortion of parts; (3) the spacial relationship of parts; (4) the relationship of the palate to contiguous structures; and (5) the dimension of time. Any estimate or prediction regarding function of the speech structures must take into account the information in these areas.

## MEDICAL, DENTAL, AND SURGICAL TREATMENT OF CLEFT-PALATE CHILDREN

### Implications of Reconstructive Surgery

The technical details of surgical procedure lie outside the concern of the speech clinician. However, a full understanding of the principles guiding surgical manipulation of the tissues of the speech organs is essential to his

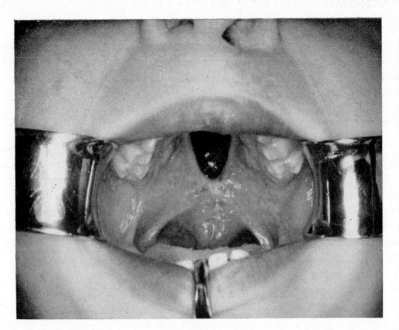

FIG. 16. A velum that has been closed and the residual opening in the hard palate later covered with a palatal prosthesis. The speech result was good. Sometimes the palate is closed surgically. These methods, however, can be employed only in carefully selected cases.

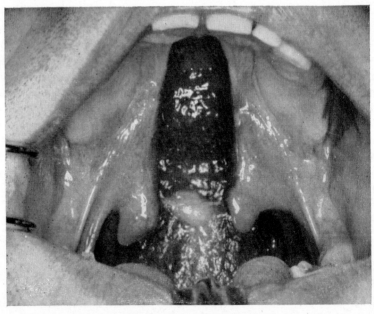

FIG. 17. Cleft of the hard palate and velum in an adult and not amenable to surgical closure. Fitted successfully with a speech-aid.

sessment of cleft lip and palate and their effect upon speech development
nd production. Specific surgical procedures, and the events of recovery
ay affect speech behavior favorably or unfavorably. However, conditions
ithin the patient are often more determinative than the choice or execution
the surgery. From the standpoint of reconstructive surgery the disunity of
e lip or palates per se may be of secondary significance. The lack of union
tiates important inhibitors and facilitators of the growth process *in utero*.
he result is dislocation, overdevelopment, and underdevelopment of parts.
hese variations of tissue location and proportion create much more critical
oblems for surgical reconstruction than the mere disunity of parts.

Lip surgery is usually performed during the first six months of the child's
e, the exact time being dictated by both pediatric and surgical considera-
ns. Initially the restoration of the lip is primarily concerned with mus-
lar realignment, and secondarily with cosmetic improvement. It aims to en-
urage proper growth and the correct development of the function of the lip
d of the contiguous structures in the mouth. The resulting lip may be
ght, overlong or overshort for reasons that may be quite beyond the control
surgical insight or skill. At some later time, secondary plastic operations
ay be done to bring the parts into improved relationship and toward a more
rmal appearance. Even though the surgery is limited to the lip, the effect
lip closure upon the divided alveolar process in complete clefts is pro-
und. It tends to mold the dental arch and to narrow the alveolar and palatal
eft. Not uncommonly, the unopposed forces of the restored lip musculature
vercorrect" the arch form, bringing the segments of the jaw and palate
to a temporary unsatisfactory relationship. If surgery on the palate is post-
ned, oral orthopedics (orthodontia) may be used to relocate the alveolar
d palatal segments when the deciduous teeth have erupted. It must be
inted out, too, that surgical correction of the lip often involves manipula-
n of the tissues of the nose—alae, septum, vomer, and columella. It may
necessary to use surgery in several stages to achieve a reasonably satis-
ctory result in both the internal and external regions of the nose.

The surgical closure of the hard palate and velum involves a number of
portant principles. The choice of procedure should be conditioned by the
dividual characteristics of the patient. The speech clinician may be asked
treat children who have had operations in which the bony substructure of
e palate has been moved and fixated. In recent years this type of procedure
s been less used. Much present-day surgery involves the movement of the
ucoperiosteum and mucous membrane of the palate in such a way as to
hieve a coaptation of the margins of the cleft. In some surgical hands these
sues are elevated and then moved mesially. In those children who have
adequate soft tissue, such mesial displacement may produce a reduction
the length of the anterio-posterior palatal axis. In other instances, the
vation and repositioning of soft tissue may be attended by such extensive
atrization that the height of the palatal vault is reduced or the movement
the velum is inhibited. Even under the most favorable anatomic circum-

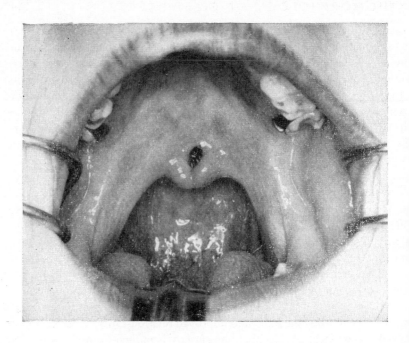

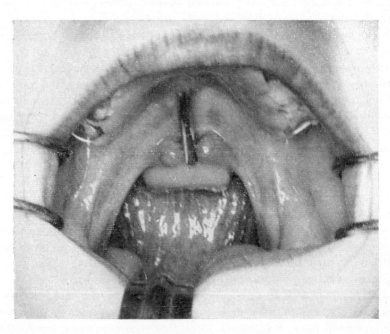

FIG. 18. Top, postsurgical condition frequently encountered by the speech clinician in which the resulting velum is too short and too tight to function in a pharynx of large dimension. Botton, fitted with a speech-aid.

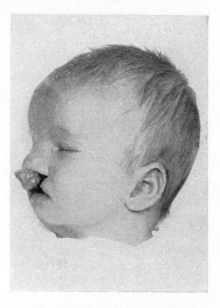

FIG. 19. The protrusive premaxillary segment in bilateral complete cleft.

ances, the palatal vault is lowered by the necessary conjunction of the soft
ssue to close the cleft.

Frequently the cleft in the velum is closed at the same time the hard palate
closed. This often produces a velum too short to participate efficiently in
elopharyngeal valving for speech. Some surgeons close the velum before
losing the hard palate, believing that the muscular effect of this procedure
ontrols or reduces the spontaneous widening of the posterior portion of the
ental arch in the region of the maxillary tuberosities and produces longer
nd more functional vela. Still other maxillofacial surgeons elevate and retro-
ose the soft tissue of the hard palate as a part of the closing procedure, or
fterward, with the aim of placing the palatovelar aponeurosis and velum
a more favorable position for velar action.

It is reasonable to assume that in cleft palate the muscles which produce
ction of the velum may also be underdeveloped and possess other atypical
eatures. For many reasons, therefore, the reunion of the edges of the cleft
the divided velum may not accomplish a restoration of satisfactory myo-
ynamic and myokinetic relationships. It is for these reasons that, in the
xperience of the speech clinician, palates which are closed and present
easonably good anatomic appearance postsurgically, may not necessarily
unction satisfactorily in speech. It must be emphasized, also, that the func-
onal integrity of the velopharyngeal valve is not exclusively determined by
ne length or mobility of the soft palate, but rather by the nature and position
f the surrounding structures of the base of the skull and the pharynx as well.
Modern x-ray procedures now make it possible to assess these local and more
emote structures and guide the surgeon in his choice of procedure.

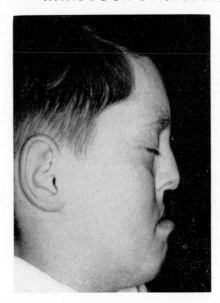

FIG. 20. The profile of a patient in whom the premaxillary segment was poorly managed in t initial surgical closure. It was probably excised! Great improvement in this profile and occlusion can be brought about by dental prosthesis.

Longitudinal growth studies of the heads of cleft-palate children tend confirm the opinion that surgical closure of the palate and velum is not a ways a wise procedure if the goal of improved speech is to be attaine Fortunately, there exist other rehabilitative procedures which promi speech improvement in these children. In the view of the speech clinicia there are many children in whom no surgery of the palate or velum shou ever be performed. His experience impresses him with the discouraging fa that many children appear to be helped but little and often are permanent prevented from having good speech. He recognizes that when palates of i adequate tissues substance have been closed, the velopharyngeal mechanis is left in a state of great functional disadvantage. Later prosthetic treatme of these children is also often made much more difficult.

## The Rationale of Prosthetic Treatment of Cleft Palate

It is apparent that only by surgery can a divided lip be returned to reaso able function and appearance. In the case of cleft palates, however, anoth approach is possible. It is often feasible to design, construct, and fit pro thetic devices which encourage and assist the child to develop acceptab speech. Basically, a cleft-palate speech-aid is a device which, when wo in the mouth, makes it possible for the speech organs, even though deforme to meet the physiological and acoustic requirements for speech productic For illustration, a prosthetic speech-aid for a cleft of the hard and soft pala will be described. Three principal ends must be accomplished by a speech-ai t must be possible to wear it comfortably in the mouth. This means that it must have some support and attachment in the mouth to remain in proper functional position. It is, therefore, anchored to the teeth but is removable for care and hygiene. Secondly, it must obturate the cleft in the palatal vault. This is accomplished by the inclusion of an artificial palatal covering. Third, it must provide assistance to the muscles of the nasopharyngeal valve so that the pneumatic and acoustic traffic in the throat, nose, and mouth may be directed and controlled. For this purpose a pharyngeal section is added to the palatal portion. It should be observed that a speech-aid does not attempt to mirror the natural anatomic structures or their natural functional relationship. It is, essentially, a mechanical device to assist the speech organs in a compensatory way. In the case of a divided velum only, the instrument is so designed as to assist in nasopharyngeal closure, but it does not need, of course, to provide obturation for the palatal vault since this is intact.

Speech-aids may be constructed for and worn by children as soon as a sufficient number of deciduous teeth have erupted. Orthodontic bands are usually affixed to teeth. Into these bands are incorporated mechanical devices for retaining the tooth-embracing bent-wire clasps of the speech-aid. This same mechanical arrangement is usually employed during the period of mixed dentition. In children whose permanent teeth have erupted, it is usual for the retention clasps to be made of cast metal and so constructed as to be self-retaining without dental bands. The palatal portion and the pharyngeal section are constructed of one of the plastic dental materials. Since these devices must fit perfectly and be carefully adapted to the tissues for function and comfort, it is necessary to make impressions of the mouth of the patient in much the same way as an impression is made for the design and construction of upper and lower dentures. The retention clasps and the palatal and pharyngeal sections are constructed upon the working models made from these impressions. As the mouth structures of the child grow, the speech-aid must be modified. An important modification must be made in the size and shape of the pharyngeal portion of the aid since, with speech stimulation, the muscles of the pharynx develop and hyponasality may appear in speech unless at intervals it is adjusted in size. These adjustments must be guided by observations of the individual's growth patterns.

### Oral Orthopedics in Cleft Palate

The inclusion of orthopedic treatment of the mouth (orthodontia) in the program of care for the cleft-palate child is, from the view of the speech clinician, not a desirable luxury but an imperative. Since modern orthodontia contemplates much more than merely achieving proper alignment of the teeth, but also aims at guiding the development of the bones and muscles of the whole head, it has, as a clinical science, much to contribute to the restitution of the speech function in the person with cleft palate. It has been traditional for orthodontia to be postponed until a child is about twelve years old and the permanent dentition is in place. It may appear unusual,

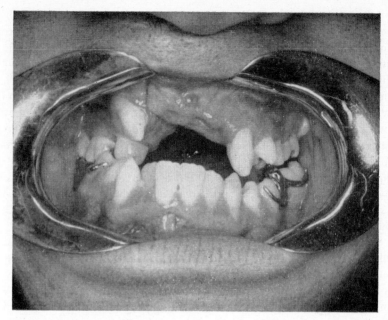

A

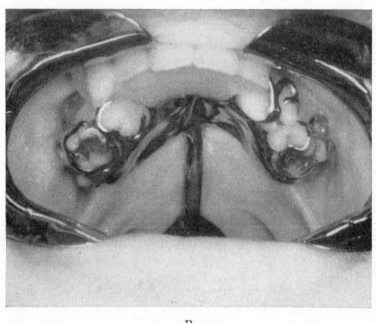

B

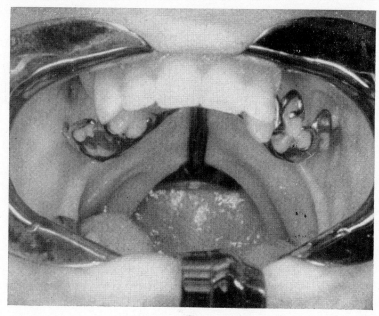

C

IG. 21. Prosthetic treatment of a post-surgical patient in whom poor speech persisted. A, without the speech-aid. B, shows the cast metal clasps embracing the supporting teeth, the palatal section which also carries anterior teeth and plumps the lip, and the carrier bar supporting the pharyngeal section is shown in position in C.

herefore, to stress the importance of early oral orthopedics in cleft-palate children. It should be begun in the stages of deciduous dentition, or at least luring mixed dentition. Though technical details of orthodontics do not concern us, it is helpful to the speech clinician to know that the structures of the mouth, face, and head generally may, by the use of early orthodontia, be rought into greatly improved positions for function and appearance. It is now not unusual to incorporate orthodontic devices into speech-aids so that a child may have early speech help while undergoing oral orthopedic correction. In some cases oral orthopedics must precede prosthesis in the sequence of treatment. In others it is important for it to be spaced between primary and secondary surgical procedures on the lip and palates. The serious deformities and constrictions of the upper dental arch and palate, which otherwise impose severe limits on the articulatory processes, may be reduced through properly timed orthodontic treatment of appropriate type. Important, too, are the very favorable effects upon the nasal structures and spaces achieved by early oral orthopedic treatment. It should not be neglected in older children, however, even though it was not begun at the more favorable early age. The marked cosmetic improvements that can be made in the cleft-palate child's facial appearance, with its valuable socioemotional effects, is another justification for its inclusion in the treatment program. Close cooperation of the surgeon, the oral orthopedist, the prosthetist, and the speech

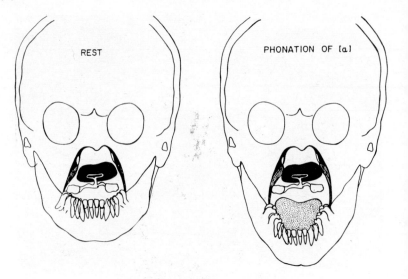

**FIG. 22.** Tracing of a frontal laminagram of patient wearing a speech-aid, showing the par
played by the lateral pharyngeal walls in phonation.

clinician in planning the stages of treatment produce much more desirable
outcomes than when each specialist proceeds alone.

### Otorhinolaryngologic Care in Cleft Palate

The great structural and functional intimacy of the mouth and nose ha
already been stressed. Many ear, nose, and throat specialists feel that there is
a higher incidence of upper-respiratory disease in cleft-palate children than
in noncleft-palate children. In the care of the cleft-palate child, the neglec
of continuous otorhinolaryngologic surveillance and treatment may have
serious consequences for speech habilitation. Modern and enlightened medi
cal treatment for diseases of the head spaces can often control and reduce
the exaggerated penalties of these conditions in cleft-palate individuals. The
prompt treatment of pharyngeal and otologic diseases can control their
destructive effects upon the processes of audition. The implications of con
trolling threats to hearing are obvious to the speech clinician. It is equall
important for him to warn the surgeon that injudicious and careless remova
of tonsils and adenoids may, through damage to the palatoglossal and palato
pharyngeal muscles, vitiate the good results of the maxillofacial surgery
Surgical procedures must also include strict considerations for the structure
and spaces of the nose.

### General Dental Care

It is known that cleft-palate children are more prone to dental caries an
to diseases of the investing tissues of the teeth. Many factors present in th
mouth having cleft palate may contribute to this vulnerability to oral dis

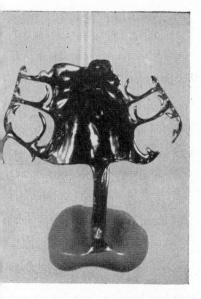
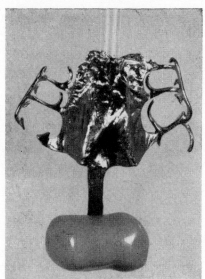
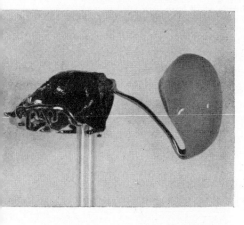
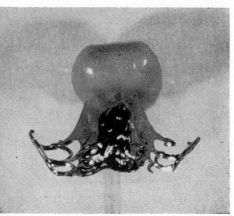

FIG. 23. Speech-aid for an adolescent. Top left, the lingual aspect; top right, the nasal aspect; middle left, the lateral aspect; bottom left, the labial aspect. The component parts are clear: the cast-metal dental clasping system, the palatal portion, the pharyngeal section and its carrier

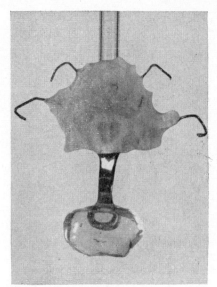 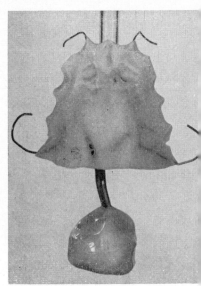

FIG. 24. Two children's ad interim speech-aids. These have bent-wire clasps that are retained by lugs soldered on orthodontic bands which have been fitted to the deciduous teeth.

ease. The general unfavorable state of oral hygiene and the imperfect arrangement and occlusion of the teeth are thought to be causative factors in the dental and oral problems of cleft-palate children. It is also not uncommon to find these children suffering from rampant caries. Since the presence of teeth figures importantly in the growth of the jaws and of the whole head and face, it is necessary to apply the best measures of dental treatment and restoration in these cases so that the loss of dental tissue may be minimized. Especially critical is the treatment and restoration of deciduous teeth, even though it is generally assumed by parents that restorative treatment should be reserved for the permanent dentition. The presence of sound or carefully restored teeth predetermines whether a speech-aid can be fitted properly and effectively worn.[1]

[1] For bibliographic reference, *see* Bibliography at end of Chapter 20.

The illustrations appearing in this chapter were provided by the *Cleft Palate Center and Training Program* of the Professional Colleges and the Division of Services for Crippled Children of the University of Illinois, Chicago.

# SPEECH PROBLEMS OF THE PERSON WITH CLEFT PALATE AND CLEFT LIP

*Herbert Koepp-Baker, Ph.D.*

FOR CONVENIENCE of discussion, the important characteristic features of the uncorrected speech of the person with cleft palate will be described as disturbances of intelligibility and alterations of voice quality. From a functional standpoint, such a division of the speech syndrome labeled "cleft-palate speech" is, of course, artificial, since the speech act cannot be fractionated. The process of phonation, resonation, and articulation are so intimately interassociated that a disturbance in one is reflected to some degree in the others. The close physiologic unity of these speech processes becomes apparent in this speech disorder.

## The Articulatory Defects of Cleft-Palate Speech

Practically all of the articulatory movements in these speakers are subject to defect to a greater or lesser degree. With the exception of the nasal sounds, a large number of consonantal release-and-arrest movements of syllables are modified by the congenital organic variation. The plosive sounds are commonly absent, weak, or distorted. If the palates are open and no obturation by a speech-aid is present, it is impossible to achieve the necessary air pressure within the oral cavity for the implosive phase of consonant production. If intactitude of the palatal vault has been produced by surgical repair but the velum remains short and immobile, the functional inadequacy of the velopharyngeal sphincter still makes it impossible to impound air within the mouth. The usual substitution for plosives is a nonphonetic laryngeal or pharyngeal stop. The relative ease of producing an occlusion at a lower level in the airway and at a point ahead of the usual and normal point of articulatory contact for the plosive encourages this type of substitution. There is considerable variation from speaker to speaker in the omission or substitution in plosive production. The resulting speech lacks the sharp definition produced by normal syllable boundaries. In some speakers, sufficient reduction of the nasopharyngeal port can, in deliberate and careful speech, be

597

achieved by compensatory pharyngeal movement so that weak or transient
oral occlusives can be produced. In syllable production at normal or mo
rapid rates, the plosives drop out or glottal or deep pharyngeal stops a
substituted.

When the consonant-movement does occur in the mouth, phonokinesi
graphic and palatographic records of cleft-palate speakers show extensiv
variation as to locus of oral occlusive contact and the temporal features o
organ movement. The total consonant co-ordination appears to be modifie
There is also some modification of voicing and unvoicing of consonan
with a tendency toward partial voicing.

The fricatives, in cleft-palate speech, are either absent or suffer distortic
because of the substitution of characteristic pharyngeal fricatives or the in
proper posture-movement sequences. The loss of air pressure by leakag
into the nasopharynx and nose during the production of fricatives is ve
apparent in cleft-palate speech at normal and rapid rates. In some speaker
the compensatory pharyngeal and posterior lingual adjustments reduce a
leakage sufficiently so that weak fricatives are heard in some positions. Hov
ever, their acoustic qualities are usually changed. The voiceless fricatives a
frequently voiced with stress or effort of production.

Many clinical observers feel that the lingual synergies for both plosiv
and fricatives reflect characteristic malhabits. These have been describe
as (1) a reduced activity of the anterior tongue and tongue tip and (.
atypical postures of the dorsum of the tongue. Some studies suggest th
the tongue is habitually retroposed and lowered. Subtelny (1956) has pr
duced evidence that a dependable frame of reference is highly important
making accurate measures and judgments of tongue positions in cleft-pala
speakers. There is little doubt, however, that the mode or manner of tong
use in cleft-palate speakers is basically variant and affects practically a
articulations. This generalized disturbance also affects the articulation o
vowels, the vowel-to-consonant and consonant-to-vowel transitions. N
should the effects of mandibular adjustments in consonant production l
neglected. Clinically, the reduced intra-oral space and the concomitant r
duction and irregularity of lingual movement appear to be related. In chron
cleft-palate speech, the degree of mandibular depression during consona
production is reduced. Whether this is due to a continuing malposition of t
tongue for compensatory reasons which restrict the mandibular moveme
is not known. There are sound phonetic reasons why this relationship m<
exist. There are, however, other organic factors which may also affect ma
dibular habits. As has been pointed out earlier, the cleft-palate speaker fr
quently has gross alterations of upper dental arch form, dental occlusio
and form and height of palatal vault. These variations in the areas of occl
sive contact available to the tongue, particularly anteriorly, impose limi
tions upon tongue movement. Great individual differences make generaliz
tions of the effect of these maxillary factors difficult or impossible. Size
tongue and individual characteristics of lingual dynamics also play a role

determining how, in a given speaker, the maxillary deformities will affect the range and character of tongue movement and posture.

In the early years of the life of many cleft-palate speakers, after surgery and before oral orthopedic correction, it is not unusual for the mandibular dental arch to lie outside the maxillary arch. This may operate to modify the characteristic lingual and mandibular rest-position as well, and hence affect the position from which lingual movement sequences start and to which they return. That this may encourage lower or more retroposed tongue positions has been suggested by some clinicians.

The function of repaired lips in cleft-palate speakers is probably not normal. The degree of disturbance is determined by the extent of the original labial deformity, the inadequacy or superfluity of tissue, and the final results of surgical reconstruction. The repaired lip is often less flexible and its range of movement reduced. Since lip movement in the articulation of bilabial sounds is, in the normal person, relatively gross, the effect of lip deformity is probably less critical than is supposed. Dental irregularity in the anterior region of the upper dental arch, common to cleft-palate persons, may be a disturbing factor in articulation of the labiodentals.

Because of the generalized malarticulation of both plosives and fricatives, it is to be expected that affricate production is also modified. If the implosive component of the affricate is omitted, the entire affricate will be omitted or executed with an extensive acoustic change. The semivowel and glide articulations are thought to show less phonetic change in cleft-palate speakers than those of the fricative and plosive groups.

The principal deterrent to an understanding of the variations of consonant production in cleft-palate speakers is the difficulty of obtaining adequate *dynamic* records of these movements in the release and arrest of the breath pulse. The full implication of disturbance of movement cannot be perceived by typical palatograms which record only the occlusive-contact phase of consonant production. Cinefluoroscopic records are of some help, but the present definition and clarity of screen-image, together with reliable measurement techniques, are not yet adequate for exact description. This technique, and especially that of sagittal x-ray have, however, added considerably to our understanding of vowel articulation in these speakers.

## Disturbances of Vowel and Consonant Resonation

The disturbance of vowel quality in cleft-palate speech is one of its most conspicuous features. The quality is usually described as "hypernasal." The phenomenon of nasality in speech is a highly complex acoustic matter. Our understanding of the relationship between organ position, physiologic function, and the acoustic pattern of vowels is by no means clear. It appears tenable that the basic physiologic mechanisms are determinants of vowel quality. In recent years much attention has been directed to the velopharyngeal valve and its role in speech production. There is some radiological evidence that for the production of consonants requiring steep intraoral pressure gradients,

the valve must be closed or nearly closed. The degree of occlusion of th·
pharyngonasal airway appears to be dependent upon the kind of consonan·
the function of the consonant, the rate of speech, and the syllabic stress.

In the production of vowels or vowel-like sounds, the patency of the nas·
pharyngeal airway also appears to be variable. The degree of closure for
sound of any class is related to the total synergic adjustments of the palat·
pharyngeal, palatoglossal, salpingopharyngeal complex, the muscles of th·
superior constrictor, and the lingual and mandilubar adjustment. It is gen·
erally assumed that the "normal" vowel quality is the product of the com·
bined effects of the pharyngeal, oral, and nasal resonators upon the laryngea
tone. In the presence of complete or partial stenosis of the nasal airways, th·
vowel quality becomes "hyponasal." From this and experimental studies ·
has been inferred that, in the normal speaker, the epipharynx and nasa
cavities contribute characteristic components to the acoustic spectrum of th·
vowel. The adjustment of the velopharyngeal valve that is necessary for th·
proper oro-nasal acoustic balance is one of great physiological nicety. I·
must provide appropriate regulation of pneumatic traffic and, at the sam·
time, be sensitively responsive to the vocalic needs through coupling an·
uncoupling the oral and nasal resonators. In cleft-palate speakers the exter·
and character of the original oral and pharyngeal deformity must be take·
into full account, if the disturbance of resonation is to be understood. Th·
character and the effects of reconstructive surgery or of prosthetic inter·
vention are also important conditioners of the kind of resonator relationship·
that will be available to the speaker during the period of speech-learning·

Three types of postsurgical conditions of the palate and velum are usua·
The first is a closed palate and closed velum in which the disturbance of th·
architecture of the palatal vault and arch form is slight; the vault is of nor·
mal or near-normal height; and the velum is united, of adequate length, an·
of satisfactory mobility. In these patients the internal nasal anatomy ·
also usually relatively normal. The faucial pillars are in normal position an·
their mobility unaltered. The second type is that in which extensive change·
in the arch form and palatal vault dimensions are present. These also prese·
a partially closed or closed velum, but the tissue in the velar region is und·
tension, attenuated, and the velum inadequate in length. The pillars are als·
abnormal in position and changed in form. The nose is often deflected an·
the columella shortened. The third class of postsurgical states is that ·
which the lip and alveolar process have been closed, with much or little res·
dual deformity in the dental arch, but the palatal vault and velum are ope·
It is obvious that each of these classes produces different effects upon th·
mechanism of resonation. It is of interest to note, however, that in the fir·
type described the voice may still be strongly hypernasal even though th·
structures of the mouth and throat appear relatively normal.

Though a variety of secondary surgical procedures have been devised an·
advocated for providing more mobile and adequate vela, their speech valu·
is often questionable. Their sequelae of extensive cicatrization sometim·

actually produces velar shortening and immobility. Lengthening or retro-posing the velum also appears to leave unaffected the residual inadequacies in the total musculature of the pharynx. The malarticulations have often been so thoroughly habituated that little change in the hypernasality of the patient can be detected following this type of surgery. In some cases, attempts are made to ameliorate the hypernasality by pharyngeoplasty or by the intro-duction of a prosthetic speech-aid. The conditions for optimum success of prosthesis in this type of patient are rarely present. In recent years, oral prosthetists have devised a variety of aids to assist these speakers in con-trolling hypernasality. The margin of success is far less than ideal.

The second class (that in which the serious alterations of arch form, dental occlusion, and vault dimension together with a partially closed or closed velum exist) is more amenable to prosthetic treatment for control of hypernasality. In these cases the pharyngeal portion of the speech-aid may be placed in a more functional position in the nasopharynx because of the velar cleft. Better adaptation of the speech appliance to the functional musculature of the pharynx makes possible an improved or adequate naso-pharyngeal valve for pneumatic and resonation control. The speech-aid may include additional features for the improvement of dental occlusion, better maxillomandibular and lip relationships and facial contour.

When, as in the third postsurgical class, the palates are open and clinical judgment dictates no further surgical intervention, a prosthetic speech-aid is the only means by which the patient may be prepared for effective speech re-education. In this instance the prosthetic speech-aid is so designed as to provide satisfactory obturation of the cleft of the hard palate, as well as pro-viding prosthetic assistance for nasopharyngeal valving. An increasing num-ber of speech clinicians and speech-oriented surgeons feel that in many cleft-palate children, little or no surgery should be performed beyond that of closing the lip and restoring continuity of the alveolar arch. This, then, should be followed by prosthetic help. Speech improvement, by this com-bined surgical and prosthetic procedure, is obtained more quickly and more effectively.

It is essential to point out that prosthetic assistance should not be delayed. Satisfactory speech-aids can be designed for and worn comfortably and use-fully by young children who are in the stage of deciduous dentition. It is also often practical to use a speech aid as an *ad interim* assistance in patients for whom further palatal surgery is projected but, for good reasons, is post-poned. There is at present no common agreement among maxillofacial sur-geons as to how much surgery should be performed on patients with clefts of the palates, nor at what age it should be done. Therefore, there are good clinical speech reasons for employing prostheses in young children. This makes it possible to intervene early with speech-training and decelerate or prevent the establishment of the profound speech malhabits which attend cleft palate.

Longitudinal radiologic cephalometry provides an excellent basis for more secure diagnosis and encourages a more specific and adaptive surgical and/or prosthetic treatment. Moreover, it increases greatly the accuracy of prediction of the outcome of treatment. It underscores the clinical significance of individual anatomic differences and reveals how unsafe any routine surgical or prosthetic treatment which aims merely to "correct cleft palate" may be. It may be observed that cephalometric growth-and-development research assures us that cleft-palate children are more often distinguished by their anatomic and physiologic differences from each other than by their similarities. It is these individual variations of skeletal and soft-tissue growth which are clinically more significant than the general fact that they are born with a nonunion of the palate and lip.

## THE SPEECH HABILITATION OF CHILDREN WITH CLEFT PALATE AND CLEFT LIP

This discussion of cleft palate and cleft lip will not include a review of the principles and technologies of speech therapy. These are very competently and completely discussed in other sections of this book. It is appropriate however, to examine with considerable care and detail the special implications of this congenital deformity for speech therapy. The special problems it poses for speech examination, speech diagnosis, treatment-planning and conduct, psychosocial guidance, and educational and vocational direction are often discouraging because of their complexity, uniqueness and resistance.

### The Speech Examination

The clinical examination made by the speech therapist includes a systematic study of the patient's speech organs at rest and, insofar as possible in function.

The mouth and its contiguous structures are, for the cleft-palate child highly charged with components of fear, anxiety, and embarrassment. Previous medical, surgical, and dental treatment of these regions have often been very painful, and examination of his speech structures requires adequate and sensitive preparation. Sudden or rough manipulation of his mouth will be threatening and will defeat the purposes of a satisfactory physical examination. Preparatory contact with young cleft-palate children through friendly, indirect play situations will build up the young patient's confidence. The structures of the facial mask may, in a young child, be examined without in any way making physical contact with him. The shape and contour of the external nasal structures will be apparent. The extent and character of tissue displacement should be noted. The external disfiguration will, in many patients, be related intimately to internal nasal deformity. When the light adequate and when the head of the patient is slightly tilted backward, the nasal vestibules may be inspected. The speech clinician will not be experienced in the use of a nasal dilator or speculum, but this is not necessary.

Any marked stenosis or atresia caused by displaced or deformed alae, columella, septum, or anterior nasal floor will be manifest without dilation.

In recording the observations, the correct and specific anatomic designation should be used. If the observations can be even grossly quantified it will be useful. The amount of cicatricial tissue present in the lip, its location and distribution, should be described. The general mobility of the upper lip should be assessed. The nose and lip must be studied from both cosmetic and functional standpoints. The labial rima and the mucodermal border will provide the most important observational landmarks. When the child has sufficient confidence in the examiner, the dental structures and the interior of the oral cavity may be examined. One of the most important observations is that of dental occlusion. The child should assume a natural bite relationship for this inspection. It is usual for a child to protrude his lower jaw when asked to "bite his teeth together." Sometimes the mandible may be gently guided in its upward path to proper position. If the child is asked to place the tip of his tongue as far back on his palate as possible and to press it firmly while he comes into a bite position, his usual maxillomandibular relationship is more likely to be achieved. A wooden tongue-blade will be useful in retracting the buccal surfaces for examining the relationship in the molar area.

The speech clinician is not expected to make as experienced and detailed examination of the jaw and dental relationship as would the oral orthopedist, but he should be sufficiently acquainted with normal external tooth structure, interdental and jaw relationships to make reasonable judgments of irregularity. The most obvious deviations will be on the side of the line of cleft in unilateral cases, and on both sides in bilateral. Cross-bite on either or both sides is not uncommon. In addition, in bilateral cleft palate the premaxillary segment which carries the two central incisors may show marked deviation of position. Individual teeth at the line of cleft and on the cleft side should be included in the general inspection. General health of the dental and investing tissue should be noted, even though carious areas on the teeth need not be counted or detailed, since this is done expertly by a dentist when he examines the mouth, explores the teeth, and charts the carious regions. It is, however, highly important that the speech clinician determine the general extent of dental disease, for the health of the teeth and the need for restorative treatment is a critical determinant in a child's speech recovery, especially if he is to be fitted with a speech-aid.

A simple way to make a preliminary inspection of a child's palates is to ask him to look up at a point on the ceiling and to open his mouth as he does so. The child's mouth will not need to be touched at this stage. This head posture places the palates in direct view. A flashlight is a convenient source of light. An orderly sequence for examining the palates is to observe first the general upper dental arch form as a palatal boundary. Degrees of contraction of the arch and any asymmetricality should be estimated. The height and shape of the palatal vault should be studied next. The amount and distribution of cicatricial tissue and the degree of depression of the

zenith of the vault are important points for observation. As inspection pr(
ceeds posteriorward, the point of muscular flexion will suggest how far for
ward the anterior border of the velum is placed. Extensive scarring in th
region may obscure this point. Asking the patient to phonate the vowel [(
while the tongue is lightly depressed will usually cause sufficient elevatio
of the velum for this observation. Care should be exercised with regard t
the degree of depression of the mandible and depression of the tongue wit
the depressor. The movements of the velum in surgically operated cleft-pala(
children are apt to be limited at best. If the mouth is opened too widely an
the tongue depressed too much or too forcibly it will produce marked tensio
in the faucial pillars and restrict the upward and backward movement of th
velum.

The patient can be examined best if he is placed high enough so one o(
tains a fairly direct line of vision of his posterior oral cavity. If he is not s
seated and is asked to tip his head back, his cervical structures are retr(
flexed and serious distortion of the pharynx is produced. He should be seate
with head erect. The muscles of the tongue, the velum, the lateral walls (
the oropharynx, and the posterior pharyngeal wall are so intimately relate
mechanically that any marked displacement of one changes the postures ar
range of movement of the others. Peroral inspection of the form and fun(
tions of the velopharyngeal valve is limited to its oral aspect and informatic
provided by this view is limited. Hence, it is important that the cervical su|
ports and the cranial base be so positioned as to cause the least possib
distortion of the pharyngeal tube and its contiguous structures. If necessar
stimulation of the tongue to elicit the gagging reflex will also elicit maxim
elevation and depression of the velum. It is difficult to see this fleeting mov
ment unless the patient's head is stabilized with one hand and the tong(
depressor firmly held. The examination of the posterior of the oral cav(
should be extended to include the position, form, and movement of t|
palatoglossal and palatopharyngeal muscles. In certain surgical procedur
the anterior faucial pillars are united with each other superiorly or with t|
free posterior borders of the divided velum, in order to reduce the later
dimensions of the oropharyngeal and nasopharyngeal isthmi. Of particul
interest is the amplitude of mesial movement of the anterior pillars.

The inspection of the extent and character of occlusive movement of t|
total nasopharyngeal valve is a difficult one to make, and especially diffic(
is any objective estimate of the completeness of closure during speech. Abo
all that may be accomplished in this direction is to examine the valve |
reflected light during phonation of a low mid or back vowel. The best instr
ment for this visualization is a nasopharyngeal mirror of generous diamet(
The tongue is controlled but not depressed with a metal tongue depress(
and the mouth slightly more open than in the rest-position. The illuminati(
must be directed upon the mirror's face. If the examiner is skilled in the u
of the Garcia head mirror it is even better. The nasopharyngeal port c
be viewed if the mirror is held at the appropriate angle. Care must be tak

o reduce the possibility of the patient's gagging. Even under the best conditions with the most skillful instrumental manipulation and posture and
co-operation of the patient, the view obtained is not always adequate or
meaningful. If the nasopharyngeal port is wide during phonation of a low
vowel, the vowel [i] should be tried. The elevation of the front of the tongue
must be controlled, however. X-ray records of velopharyngeal closure of
normal subjects suggest that the maximum closure on the vowel series is for
[i] and [u]. Sometimes this part of the examination is more dramatic and impressive than useful. It is, with experience, possible to educe in a general
way the extent of velopharyngeal closure from direct observation of the
velum, pillars, and posterior throat wall during deglutition (with the tongue
controlled) and during phonation. In many ways, the most significant picture
is that of the general lateral dimensions of the oropharyngeal isthmus and
the distance between the posterior margin of the velum and the posterior
pharyngeal wall in rest. This description of examinative procedure has been
limited to the cleft that has been closed by surgery.

When the palate and velum are open, the view into the inferior regions
of the nasal space is available. This examination should include an estimate
of cleft width and shape, as well as a description of the inferior turbinates
and should reflect an impression of the location, shape, and size of the vomer
bone. In these cases careful study of the extent and path of movement of the
divided velar remnants is necessary. The adjustment of these velar tags,
together with that of the palatoglossal and palatopharyngeal muscles and
the posterior pharyngeal wall are important in visualizing the adaptation
to a speech-aid. This judgment will also be useful in estimating the length
of the final palatal axis and ultimate velar size and shape following classical
surgical closure.

## Audiometric Assessment

Periodic study of the hearing status of cleft-palate children is an important part of the regimen of care. The middle-ear infection so common in
these children begins early and even with the best otological care frequently
reduces auditory acuity in amounts that interfere with speech-learning and
the auditory training procedures. Otologic disease must not be neglected.
Since the advent of antibiotic drugs, conscientious medical care makes it
possible to reduce greatly the threat to hearing by otologic infections.

Auditory training must be an integral part of the speech-training program.
The reduction of hypernasality and the modification of the malarticulatory
patterns of cleft-palate children requires the most sensitive auditory self-
monitoring of speech that can be attained. Though the auditory training
procedures employed with these children do not differ importantly from
those used with other articulatory and voice patients, its inclusion is very
urgent.

## THE GENERAL PROBLEMS OF SPEECH HABILITATION OF
## CLEFT-PALATE CHILDREN

It has been suggested earlier in this section that the feature of hyper nasality in the cleft-palate person is a product of the total mode or manner of speech production. It is most economic of clinical time, therefore, to change those malhabits which will result in the greatest and earliest change in the total speech act. It is now generally agreed by speech clinicians that the initial attack should be made upon the defects of articulation. A revision of malarticulatory habits will at the same time affect favorably the improper resonation and result in the largest and most immediate change in the intelligibility of speech and quality of voice. This is encouraging to both the patient and the clinician. Cleft-palate speech has been generally regarded as a very resistant type of speech disorder. This has been due in a measure to the fact that the clinician has concerned himself initially, and often exclusively, with the phonatory features of the disability. It is doubtful, too, whether nonphonetic exercises for the improvement of vowel quality are clinically justified. Experience demonstrates that a revision of the articulatory defects in these patients produces an impressive and gratifying change in their speech. Much of the hypernasality disappears as the oral movement and postures of syllable production are normalized.

The dictum that "speaking is learned by speaking" applies especially in this disorder. The malarticulation can best be revised by training with fractions of speech no smaller than the physiologic syllable and prompt inclusion of the phrase appears to produce the earliest and most lasting change. Many clinicians combine the anterior plosives with low vowels and proceed gradually to the fricatives with low and mid vowels. Syllables with a high-vowel core are apt to be the most resistant. The general habit of speaking with the mandible and tongue elevated and retracted encourages a resonation pattern that is strongly hypernasal. The use of syllables with low vowels in early training discourages this tendency. It makes it possible for the patient to hear early his *own* production of those vowels which are relatively free from hypernasality and refines his auditory speech-sound discrimination that is so imperative in this disturbance. It is essential, too, to observe that in the young cleft-palate child, the preparation for speech-training by a speech-readiness program on the part of the parent and the clinician will hasten the effects of later and more intensive speech education.

Psychosocial counseling forms an important part of the clinical speech program. This assistance must be directed at an improvement of parent-child relationships and the social hygiene of the family unit. To the extent to which the parents' sophistication permits, they should be used in the training program. The parents must be helped to understand the child's problems, the details and nature of his medical, dental, surgical, and speech care. They must also be helped to understand that changes will be slow and that they must be spaced appropriately in the child's whole developmental schedule.

# BIBLIOGRAPHY

DORRANCE, G. M. 1933. The operative story of cleft palate. Philadelphia and London: Saunders.

FOGH-ANDERSON, P. 1942. Inheritance of harelip and cleft palate. Copenhagen: Nyt Nordisk Forlag—Arnold Busck.

KIRKHAM, H. L. 1931. *Quoted* by Peyton, W. T., The dimensions and growth of the palate in the normal infant and in the infant with gross maldevelopment of the upper lip and palate. *Arch. Surg.,* 22, 704–737.

McCARTHY, M. F. 1925. Preliminary report of studies on the nasopharynx. *Ann. Otol., Rhinol., Laryngol.,* 34, 801–813.

PRUZANSKY, S. 1953. Description, classification, and analysis of unoperated clefts of the lip anl palate. *Amer. J. Orthodontics.,* Vol. 39, No. 8, 590–611.

SAUME, J. 1950. Contribution a l'Étude du Squelette du Bec de Lièvre et de la Division Palatine Non-Opérés. Thése Doctorat en Médecine, Paris.

RICKETTS, R. M. 1952. The significance of variation in the cranial base and soft structures. Newsletter, Amer. Assoc. Cleft palate rehabilitation, 3, 5–6.

SCHÜLLER, A. 1929. X-ray examination of deformities of the nasopharynx. *Ann. Otol., Rhinol., Laryngol.,* 38, 108–129.

SICHER, H. 1949. The development of the face and oral cavity. *In* Orban, B., Oral histology and embryology (2nd ed.). St. Louis: Mosby.

SUBTELNY, J. 1956. Unpublished Doctoral Thesis. Northwestern Univ.

SUBTELNY, J. D. 1953. Width of the nasopharynx and related anatomical structures in normal and unoperated cleft palate children. Master's Thesis. Univ. Ill.

WARDILL, W. 1928. Cleft palate. *Brit. J. Surg.,* 16, 127–148.

CHAPTER 21

# SPEECH DEFECTS ASSOCIATED WITH DENTAL ABNORMALITIES AND MALOCCLUSIONS

• H. Harlan Bloomer, Ph.D.

## INTRODUCTION

THE SUCCESSFUL diagnosis and treatment of defective speech rests ultimate
upon an understanding of the relationships existing between structure an
function in the human organism. It is thus that a discussion of speech a
normalities logically includes reference to the teeth and their occlusal pa
terns. The teeth, however, exist in the body only in relation to other tissu
of the oral cavity and the face—the jaws, the alveolar arches, the palate, th
lips, and tongue—all of which with the teeth provide a complex of orofaci
structures. It is through the relative positional changes of these hard an
soft tissues as they inflect the outgoing air stream and the vocal tone th
speech emerges in normal or abnormal patterns. Except for the fact th
cleft lip and palate are excluded from this chapter, a more accurate chapt
heading would be "speech defects associated with orofacial abnormalities

The term *orofacial abnormalities* implies reference to the hard and rel
tively immobile framework of the mouth and face, and the soft muscul
tendinous tissues which are highly motile and which by their pressures an
tensions are partially responsible for molding the osseous structures to whic
they attach. The term includes "dental abnormalities" and "malocclusions
which are not synonymous but refer respectively to defects of tooth d
velopment and defects of tooth relationship. Dental abnormalities incluc
such deviations in development as the number, shape, texture, and positic
of the teeth (Watson and Lowrey, 1954, p. 272). Malocclusions are defin
as any deviations from the "normal" relation of the teeth to each other in t
same dental arch and to the teeth of the opposing arch (Anderson, 1948,
18).

The discussion which follows pertains to the function of orofacial stru
tures in normal and abnormal speech, the classification and etiology of or
facial abnormalities, and the significance of these abnormalities to the wo
of the speech clinician. Although the authors of most textbooks of spee

pathology include reference to dental malocclusions as etiological factors in defective speech, most of them are careful to indicate that the relationship is seldom a simple and clear-cut one. Reports of the clinical observations correlating certain aspects of defective speech and abnormalities of dentition and occlusion (Fymbo, 1936; van Thal, 1936; Wolf, 1937; Herman, 1943; Frowein and Moser, 1944; Kessler, 1953) are somewhat contradictory. In general they support the concept that whereas structural abnormalities are found more frequently among those individuals whose speech is defective, the abnormalities may influence speech patterns adversely but generally do not serve as primary causes of the speech defects.

Normal speech can be achieved only when certain appropriate movements of the orofacial structures occur. Abnormal orofacial structures which move maladaptively produce defective speech. It is, of course, also possible to have normal structures which move maladaptively to produce defective speech, or conversely, to have abnormal structures which function adaptively and thus produce good speech. In short:

    Normal structure + normal movements = normal speech
    Abnormal structures + maladaptive movements = defective speech
    Normal structures + maladaptive movements = defective speech
    Abnormal structures + adaptive movements = normal (compensated) speech

Speech defects which arise in connection with orofacial abnormalities are mainly those in which the articulation of the vowels and consonants is disturbed by functional maladaptations of the various structures of the mouth during speech. The effects upon speech may be both direct and indirect: *direct,* through the mechanical difficulties which they impose upon a person attempting to achieve the proper positioning and movement of the articulators of speech; and *indirect,* through the influence which the deformities may have upon the physical and mental health of the individual. An instance of direct interference is found in a person whose teeth are protruded in such a way that the lips cannot meet for normal production of bilabial consonants. An example of indirect influence is to be seen in a person whose reaction to an orofacial deformity is such that he has developed certain personality traits which interfere with his speech even though the deformity of itself may not cause any true mechanical obstacle to tongue or lip movement.

From this viewpoint, any osseous, muscular, dental, or soft-tissue deformity which impairs the movement or appearance of the organs of articulation may contribute to defective speech. A discussion which includes all of these factors, however, would be too extensive for full presentation here. In this chapter we shall confine our discussion mainly to the osseous, dental, and muscular tissues which may be directly involved in the act of speech or in shaping the course of development of the facial bones and teeth in the maturing individual.

Considered diagnostically, the relationship between speech and orofacial structures is a complex one. Any decision as to the etiological significance of orofacial abnormalities in accounting for the defective speech of an individual must, therefore, be made with great care and due regard to the total dynamics of speech. The speech clinician must consider the multiple causalities of speech characteristics (normal or abnormal), the effects of physical growth, the timing of environmental and physio-anatomical forces as they inflect the emerging patterns of speech, and the ways in which behavior in turn modifies the directions of growth. He must consider not merely the effects of orofacial structures upon speech but also the possible effects of speech habits upon the developing dental arches and dental occlusion. The clinician will need to weigh the effects of personality upon orofacial growth and speech, and the effects of these functions upon the personality of the individual. He will look for the clues which dental development and occlusal relationship can give to the history of the patient—as a record of his earlier nutrition, his disease history, his oral habits, his heredity, his stages of physical growth and maturation, and even as to the kind of home environment which can be deduced from indications of oral hygiene and parental concern for his dental health.

It is a wise man who can know enough to correlate all this information in a meaningful way. Nevertheless, such a correlation must be the goal of the well-trained speech clinician. It is to this end that in the following pages of this chapter we shall discuss:

1. Orofacial structures in the production of normal speech
2. Classifications of dental malocclusion and dental anomalies
3. The development of the teeth and other orofacial structures
4. Orofacial abnormalities and their effects on speech
5. The role of the speech clinician in relation to members of other professions concerned with the care of persons with orofacial abnormalities

## OROFACIAL STRUCTURES AND THE ARTICULATION OF SPEECH

The teeth and their supporting structures are directly involved in the production of those consonants for which accurate pneumatic control is required to create fricative and plosive characteristics. The teeth and dental arches play a significant role with the tongue and lips in occluding, constricting, or opening the passageways through which the air must pass during speech. They probably play some part also in the accurate formation of the vowels and diphthongs of speech, but this role is a less critical one (Spannenberg, 1937) and hence not so likely to contribute to defective vowel formation as to the defective enunciation of consonants. The effect of palate shape upon voice quality has also been suggested (Greene, 1937; Juste, 1948), but experimental evidence in support of these suppositions is lacking thus far. Dental diseases are reported by Tarneaud (1946) to cause voice disorders through paralysis of the vocal cords.

### The Musculo-skeletal Valves of Speech

The production of consonant sounds is achieved in part by a series of variable musculo-skeletal valves which modify the breath stream as it is ex-

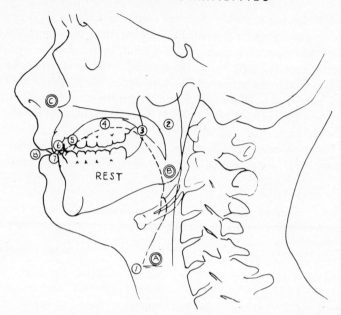

**FIG. 1.** Tracing of lateral head x-ray study. Numbers show the areas at which occlusions or constrictions normally occur in the production of speech sounds. Letters indicate location of maladaptive valving.

haled for speech. These valves are functionally created by (1) the glottis, (2) the palatopharyngeal mechanism, (3) the tongue and soft palate, (4) the tongue and palate, (5) the tongue and alveolar ridge, (6) the tongue and teeth, (7) the lips and teeth, and (8) the lips in relation to each other (Fig. 1). In functioning, the valves close, constrict, or open the channels through which the respiratory air must pass, and by these modifications determine to a large extent the physical conditions of pressure change and air vibration which initiate the acoustic patterns of the consonants. As substitutes for the normal valving of orofacial structures, compensatory valves are sometimes developed—adaptively or maladaptively. Certain of these are indicated by (A), (B), and (C) enclosed in the double circles in Fig. 1. A relatively common maladaptation is the use of the back of the tongue (B) for the production of the consonants *k* or *g* by making occlusive contact with the posterior pharyngeal wall, or by pinching the nares (C) to produce an accessory valve in persons who cannot effectively close the palatopharyngeal valve. (A) represents false vocal-cord constriction as in dysphonia plica ventricularis.

Although consonants are formed by a complex series of movements which continuously modify the speech sounds, these articulatory movements may be described as "articulatory positions" and the consonants may be classified so as to call attention to certain important conditions for their production. Table 1 presents a classification of consonant phonemes according to: (1) the presence or absence of voicing; (2) the anatomical structures by which the valve is created; and (3) the degree of valve closure required to produce the phoneme. Reference to such a chart can help us to see how abnormalities of structure and maladaptive movements may interfere with the normal production of consonant phonemes and thus result in dyslalia. Such charts are by no means new, but have been used in many forms to illustrate the conditions of consonant production. N. W. Kingsley in his *Treatise On Oral Deformities,* published in 1880, presents an incomplete chart of this type. West, Kennedy, and Carr (1947, pp. 104–105) describe in some detail the circumstances which distinguish the various consonants. Other systems of classification, based on acoustic differences, are frequently used, but are not as appropriate to a discussion of orofacial defects as the one suggested in Table 1.

**TABLE 1. Physiological Classification of Consonant Sounds**

| STRUCTURAL COMPONENTS OF THE ARTICULATORY VALVE | CLOSED VALVE | | CONSTRICTED VALVE | | |
|---|---|---|---|---|---|
| | *Voiceless (Surd)* | *Voiced (Sonant)* | *Voiceless (Surd)* | *Voiced (Sonant)* | *Voiced Nasals* |
| Bi-labial ............... | [p] | [b] | [ʍ] | [w] | [m] |
| Labio-dental ............ | | | [f] | [v] | |
| Linguo-dental ........... | | | [θ] | [ð] | |
| Linguo-alveolar ......... | [t] | [d] | [s] | [z] [l] | [n] |
| Linguo-palatal .......... | [tʃ] | [dʒ] | [ʃ] | [ʒ] [r] [j] | |
| Linguo-velar ............ | [k] | [g] | | | [ŋ] |
| Glottal ................ | | | [h] | | |

The construction of Table 1 suggests that the locus of the articulatory valve is the most significant factor in consonant production. In actuality the placing of the valve is important only insofar as it makes possible characteristic phonemic patterns which are recognized by the listener as correct. Thus, although the phoneme [s] is ordinarily produced with the tongue grooved and in contact with the alveolar ridge of the maxilla as far forward as the incisors (see Figs. 3 and 4), it is possible to produce an acoustically acceptable [s] in other ways. One of the variant forms most commonly used is to bring the tonguetip in contact with the lingual surface of the lower incisors and the grooved blade into contact with the maxillary alveolar ridge (Kanter and West, 1941; Froeschels, 1933). No published data have been found to indicate the prevalence of these two methods of producing the [s] phoneme. The author has made a number of spot observations of normal speakers selected at random and has found the two methods about equally distributed. It is quite possible, of course, that every speaker uses each method to some extent depending on the sound which immediately precedes or follows the [s] sound.[1] Individual preference may also be related to general tongue posture and dental occlusion, but this has not yet been determined objectively.

It is not intended that this chapter shall contain a complete discussion of

[1] Other modifications of compensatory articulatory adjustments are described in the section of this chapter dealing with orofacial abnormalities and defective speech.

the characteristics of the various phonemes or the requirements for their production. It is pertinent to the problem of orofacial anomalies and speech defects, however, to pursue somewhat further the positional relationships which characterize oral structures during consonant articulation. Much information can be derived from direct observation of articulatory movements, or by the use of such a simple device as the "hearing tube" as suggested by Froeschels (1933). Two of the most important objective means for study of articulatory positions and oral structures are provided by palatography and x-ray. With an improvement of techniques, electro-myography (Moyers, 1949) may also provide a useful research method in experimental phonetics.

Palatography is a method employed by phoneticians to study the areas of linguo-dental and linguo-palatal contacts made during the articulation of discrete consonant or semivowel sounds or of consonants in combination with a vowel or diphthong. The process requires the construction of a thin plate (pseudo-palate), made from a dental base-plate material (shellac, ash metal, or acrylic compound) or other relatively stable material which can be shaped to form an exact replica of the contours of the hard palate from the gingival borders of the palate to the posterior border of the hard palate. A dental cast of the informant's palate and teeth is used as a mold for the pseudo-palate. The lingual surface of the false palate is dusted with powder and placed in the mouth of the informant, who then produces the sound which is required for study. The moist surface of the tongue removes the powder from the palatal area contacted, thus defining the linguo-alveolar or linguo-palatal pattern which is required to produce the sound. The procedures used in palatography are described by Roussellot (1910), Moses (1939), Kantner and West (1941), and others.

In the production of consonant and vowel combinations, or consonant clusters, the position of the tongue in relation to the teeth and palate is determined in part according to the other sound which precedes or follows the consonant under study (Muyskens, 1925; Moses, 1936).

Palatograms ordinarily show two-dimensional patterns, thus ignoring the depth dimension by which steepness of slope, the height of the palatal vault, and details of palate shape are revealed. This limitation of palatography can be overcome by the use of a palatopograph (Bloomer, 1943), an instrument which surveys the palate by means of a stylus which can be set at various depths. The stylus is mounted on a surface gauge which is connected to a scriber so that the perimeters of various parallel planes of the palate may be drawn.

The palatograms of Fig. 2 present such a topographical record of the informant's palate. The contour lines are 5 millimeters apart in vertical dimension. The height of the palatal vault, the angle of slope, and the area of the successive planes are to be interpreted in the same manner as a contour map of the earth's surface. Starting with the gingival border of the palate as a zero line, this palate is slightly over 15 millimeters high.

The relationship between palatal contour and linguo-alveolar contacts for

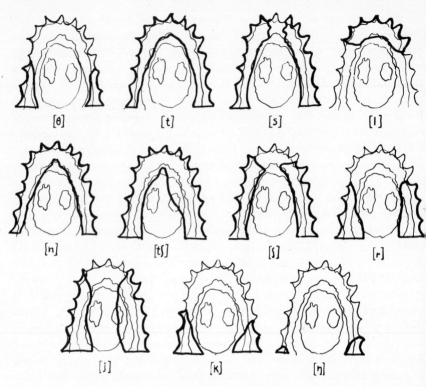

FIG. 2. Palatograms shown in relation to palatal contours (palatopograms). Contour lines are 5 millimeters apart. The areas of linguo-alveolar or linguo-palatal contact are circumscribed by the heavy lines.

speech has not yet been worked out. The study of Crane and Ramstrum (1943) has indicated that three basic classifications of normal palate shapes can be identified according to their *configuration* (trapezoid, tapering, or ovoid) and the *ratio of antero-posterior slope* (in the mid-sagittal plane) *to the medial slope* (coronal plane when measured at the mesio-lingual groove of the upper first permanent molar). Fig. 3, taken from the reference cited, indicates the three basic configurations described.

Further appreciation of the interrelationship of oral structures in speech

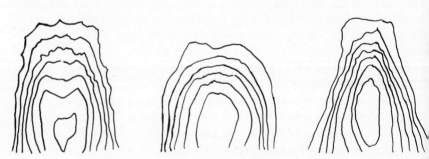

FIG. 3. Basic types of palatal shapes: trapezoid, ovoid, triagonal.

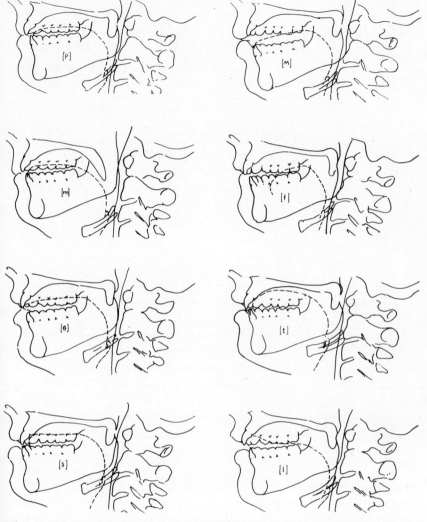

**FIG. 4.** Tracings based on x-ray films of a subject during a distinctive moment in the production of certain consonants. Exposure time .4 sec. The subject also produced the palatograms shown in Fig. 2.

can be obtained from lateral x-ray films of the head during the "contact" phase of consonant articulation. Tracings outlining structures directly involved in articulation of the consonants and semivowels [p], [ʍ], [m], |f|, [θ], [t], [s], |l|, [n], [tʃ], [ʃ], [r], [j], [k], [ŋ] and [h] are shown in Figs. 4 and 5. The informant for the x-rays also made the palatograms shown in Fig. 2.

Interesting woodcuts intended to depict similar information are to be found in Kingsley (1880). Barclay and Nelson (1922) presented one of the early reports on x-ray in the analysis of speech sounds. Russell (1934) described some x-ray studies of consonant sounds. The most detailed study

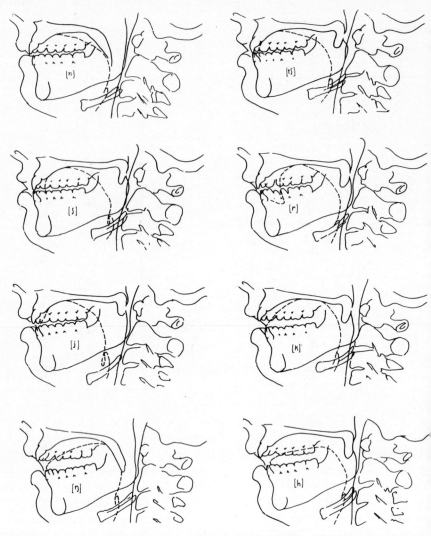

**FIG. 5.** Further tracings based on x-ray films of a subject during a distinctive moment in the production of certain consonants.

to date, although mainly concerned with vowel sounds, is that reported by Holbrook (1937) and assembled and arranged by Francis Carmody after the author's death.

It must be presumed that the character of the linguo-alveolar and linguo-palatal contacts during speech will be determined at least in part by the occlusal relationships of the maxillary and mandibular dentures and the configuration of the hard palate.

The data and study methods suggested above are adequate for the description of consonant production as it relates to average normal structures of the mouth and face. The phonetic values of an individual speaker must be studied with reference to his own peculiar physio-anatomical structures. The basis for distinguishing and describing these individual characteristics of orofacial form are discussed in the section which follows.

## OROFACIAL ABNORMALITIES

A majority of the orofacial abnormalities which may be associated with defective speech are of developmental origin—that is, they come about because of some condition effective during prenatal or postnatal growth of the individual. Trauma and disease play their part, but usually during the period of growth and development, so that the effective processes become complexly and almost inextricably interwoven.

It is important that the speech clinician have some understanding of the etiology of certain of these abnormalities and an awareness that structural anomalies which appear to be similar may come from quite different origins —a fact which may be of great importance in the diagnosis of the speech disorder and in establishing a prognosis for treatment. He should be aware of the dynamic interplay of forces which takes place between the function of speech and the structures of the body which to some extent govern that function. The clinician should know that it is possible for the informed diagnostician to read in the teeth and their supporting structures an indelible record of certain aspects of the life history of the individual. Through a knowledge of the causes of orofacial deformity, the speech clinician may play some part in the prevention of these deformities if he recognizes the early signs of pathological development. He should realize that the etiological forces which produce structural maldevelopments may also forecast functional maldevelopments in speech. The disease or nutritional deprivation which brings about bone deformities may affect speech through damage to the neuromuscular system which regulates the speed and accuracy of muscle movements. A genetic approach is much needed by specialists in our field, not only for the diagnostic and therapeutic orientation it makes possible, but because it can help the speech clinician to understand the problems and treatment limitations of the dentist or surgeon who may also be involved.

The brief summary of orofacial development which is presented in this section is admittedly fragmentary. Since the description and classification of the relationship of the dental arches provides one of the best means of classifying orofacial defects pertaining to speech, our discussion of orofacial development will refer especially to the teeth and their immediately supporting structures. The true nature of their development and their effect on the growth of other structures, however, must be seen against a background of the growth of the entire facial skeleton.

Man's face is his most distinguishing morphological characteristic. Above all other human anatomical units, the face represents the phylogenetic end-product of evolutionary development. It is the physical expression of the properties and qualities which differentiate man from other forms of animal life. Moreover, the

growth of the face is extremely sensitive to disturbances of the mental and physi
cal coordination which determines the extent to which each individual progresses
along the road to his potential growth, development and attainment. For these
reasons the face cannot be studied without consideration of the body, and the
body can be better understood by knowledge of the face. (Noyes, Schour, and
Noyes, 1948, p. 35)

The development of the normal structures of the face and mouth occupies
a period of approximately twenty years in the life of a human being, begin
ning late in the first month of intra-uterine life and ending sometime between
the eighteenth and twenty-fifth year of adult life. By the third week in utero
the fetus develops two primitive structures (the frontal process and the man
dibular arch) from which the maxillary and mandibular processes grow
joining with the frontonasal process to become the differentiated tissues of
the face and mouth. The cranial skeleton develops first as a framework of
connective tissue followed by the formation of cartilage and, during the
second month of intra-uterine life, by the formation of bone. While the bony
and muscular parts are developing, a concomitant development of the
sense organs of the oral and nasal cavities is taking place. (For a more complete description of these processes, reference should be made to such standard works as Arey, 1954, or Patten, 1953. An excellent summary of the
growth of the cranio-facial skeleton is provided by Hemrend and Moyers,
1953.)

The various parts of the head at birth are not merely small versions of the
parts of an adult skull but differ in proportional size and potential rate of
growth. The face at birth is oftentimes less than one-eighth the size of the
cranium, whereas the adult face is one-third to one-half the size of the adult
cranium. Hemrend and Moyers (1953) note that the cranium has completed
90 per cent of its growth by four years of age, and maximum growth by 10
to 12 years; the nasomaxillary complex is about 90 per cent complete by
the age of 12 and nearly complete by 18 years; whereas the mandible may
continue to grow until 25 years of age. It is important to remember these
facts when discussing abnormalities of facial growth and the factors which
cause them, since the time at which the cause is an effective agent determines
in large part the structure which is affected. Easlich and Moyers (Watson
and Lowrey, 1954, pp. 254–255) note that:

The cranial base is the most stable area of the skull during growth. Because the
cranial vault and the nasomaxillary complex are attached to the cranial base, it
growth is a determining or limiting factor in the growth of the rest of the skull
The cranial base increases in width by sutural growth in the sphenoid region and
in height by apposition. Its length is increased by sutural apposition in the spheno
occipital and spheno-ethmoidal sutures. The spheno-occipital synchondrosis contributes to growth in an anteroposterior direction until some time after puberty
Different investigators suggest that this stops between the ages of twelve and
twenty. The spheno-ethmoidal synchondrosis contributes to growth in length for
a longer time and at a faster rate than the spheno-occipital suture.
The nasomaxillary complex at birth is farther from its adult dimensions than
is the cranium. Height and length are less developed than width because they are

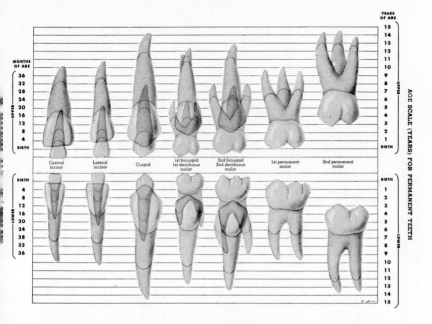

FIG. 6. Chronology of tooth development. (By I. Schour and H. G. Poncher. Based upon their original unpublished studies, also data of Logan and Kronfeld.) The position of the crown of the tooth on the chart indicates the age at which formation and calcification of the tooth begins. The horizontal lines indicate the approximate time of formation of that part of the tooth adjacent to each line. The dotted line on the root indicates the age of the child when the tooth erupts, as well as the size of the tooth at that age. Formation continues from the time of eruption to the age shown for the complete formation of the root. For example, the chart shows that the deciduous mandibular canine begins its formation at six months in utero, erupts about the 20th month of life, is fully formed at the 30th month; and that the permanent canine starts forming about the sixth month (before the deciduous tooth erupts), erupts at 11 years, and is fully formed between the 14th and 15th year. The deciduous teeth all start forming in utero. It normally takes about three years after eruption for the roots of permanent teeth to complete their formation. The sequence of eruption (relative position of dotted lines on the roots) is much more important for normal occlusion than the exact chronologic time. Thus the canine, for example, is guided by the adjacent teeth into its correct position. The chart makes it possible to determine the approximate age period at which a particular defect in tooth formation occurred, and was recorded in the growing tooth. (From Salzmann, J. A. 1950. Principles of orthodontics. Philadelphia: Lippincott. Fig. 122, pp. 242–243.)

largely dependent on alveolar growth which is yet to come. The body of the maxilla will also be increased in height and length by sutural growth. At birth the orbits have attained more of their adult size than any other portion of the face. The uppermost boundaries of the nasal cavities have also attained most of their adult size.

From this it is clear that all parts of the orofacial region are not equally susceptible to maladaptive forces. The various structures differ not only in the timing of their development and rates of maturation but also in the nature of the process by which growth occurs. Thus we will find that the cranial base may be little affected by local influences such as the existence or condition of the teeth or the forces of muscular contraction, whereas certain aspects of

**TABLE 2. Chronology of the Human Dentition**

| | Tooth | Hard Tissue Formation Begins | Amount of Enamel Formed at Birth | Enamel Completed | Eruption | Root Completed |
|---|---|---|---|---|---|---|
| **Deciduous dentition** | | | | | | |
| Maxillary | Central incisor | 4 mo. in utero | Five-sixths | 1½ mo. | 7½ mo. | 1½ yr. |
| | Lateral incisor | 4½ mo. in utero | Two-thirds | 2½ mo. | 9 mo. | 2 yr. |
| | Cuspid | 5 mo. in utero | One-third | 9 mo. | 18 mo. | 3¼ yr. |
| | First molar | 5 mo. in utero | Cusps united | 6 mo. | 14 mo. | 2½ yr. |
| | Second molar | 6 mo. in utero | Cusp tips still isolated | 11 mo. | 24 mo. | 3 yr. |
| Mandibular | Central incisor | 4½ mo. in utero | Three-fifths | 2½ mo. | 6 mo. | 1½ yr. |
| | Lateral incisor | 4½ mo. in utero | Three-fifths | 3 mo. | 7 mo. | 1½ yr. |
| | Cuspid | 5 mo. in utero | One-third | 9 mo. | 16 mo. | 3¼ yr. |
| | First molar | 5 mo. in utero | Cusps united | 5½ mo. | 12 mo. | 2¼ yr. |
| | Second molar | 6 mo. in utero | Cusp tips still isolated | 10 mo. | 20 mo. | 3 yr. |
| **Permanent dentition** | | | | | | |
| Maxillary | Central incisor | 3 – 4 mo. | ——— | 4 – 5 yr. | 7– 8 yr. | 10 yr. |
| | Lateral incisor | 10 –12 mo. | ——— | 4 – 5 yr. | 8– 9 yr. | 11 yr. |
| | Cuspid | 4 – 5 mo. | ——— | 6 – 7 yr. | 11–12 yr. | 13–15 yr. |
| | First bicuspid | 1½– 1¾ year. | ——— | 5 – 6 yr. | 10–11 yr. | 12–13 yr. |
| | Second bicuspid | 2 – 2¼ yr. | ——— | 6 – 7 yr. | 10–12 yr. | 12–14 yr. |
| | First molar | At birth | Sometimes a trace | 2½– 3 yr. | 6– 7 yr. | 9–10 yr. |
| | Second molar | 2½– 3 year | ——— | 7 – 8 yr. | 12–13 yr. | 14–16 yr. |
| | Third molar | 7 – 9 yr. | ——— | 12 –16 yr. | 17–21 yr. | 18–25 yr. |
| Mandibular | Central incisor | 3 – 4 mo. | ——— | 4 – 5 yr. | 6– 7 yr. | 9 yr. |
| | Lateral incisor | 3 – 4 mo. | ——— | 4 – 5 yr. | 7– 8 yr. | 10 yr. |
| | Cuspid | 4 – 5 mo. | ——— | 6 – 7 yr. | 9–10 yr. | 12–14 yr. |
| | First bicuspid | 1¾– 2 yr. | ——— | 5 – 6 yr. | 10–12 yr. | 12–13 yr. |
| | Second bicuspid | 2¼– 2½ yr. | ——— | 6 – 7 yr. | 11–12 yr. | 13–14 yr. |
| | First molar | At birth | Sometimes a trace | 2½– 3 yr. | 6– 7 yr. | 9–10 yr. |
| | Second molar | 2½– 3 yr. | ——— | 7 – 8 yr. | 11–13 yr. | 14–15 yr. |
| | Third molar | 8 –10 yr. | ——— | 12 –16 yr. | 17–21 yr. | 18–25 yr. |

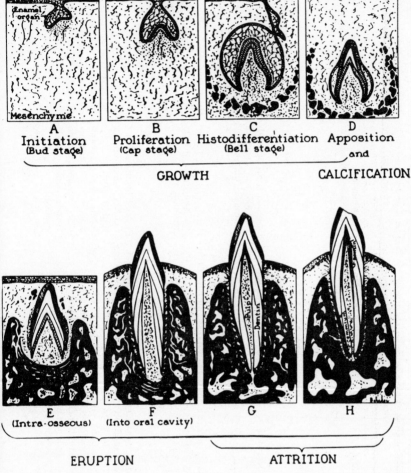

FIG. 7. Diagrammatic representation of life cycle of a tooth. During the period of growth, the following stages are shown diagrammatically: A, the initiation of development of the enamel organ or tooth bud; B, the stage of proliferation, or the cap stage; C, further histologic differentiation, or the bell stage; D, stage of apposition and calcification. The dark area surrounding the tooth shows the progress of calcification of the alveolar bone; E, intra-osseous eruption, the crown of the tooth is approaching the overlying mucosa; F, the tooth has erupted into the oral cavity and there has been a further growth of the alveolar bone; G, shows the fully formed tooth with the beginning of attrition during function; H, shows a further stage of attrition of the crown of the tooth. Courtesy, I. Schour and M. Massler. (From Salzmann, J. A. 1950. Principles of orthodontics. Philadelphia: Lippincott. Fig. 101, p. 213).

total mandibular growth are directly affected by muscular function, the eruption of the teeth, and the growth of the condylar region of the mandible (Walpole-Day, 1951).

The teeth begin their first visible evidences of growth at about the fourth month *in utero*. From this beginning, dental development continues successively through the formation, eruption, and exfoliation of the primary teeth, and the formation and eruption of the permanent teeth, ending in adult life

**TABLE 3. Developmental Physiology of the Tooth (Schour and Massler)**

| Phases in Development | Physiologic Characteristics | Sensitivity to Experimental Interferences | Methods of Measuring | Aberrations in Development | Experimental Conditions Showing Specific Disturbances |
|---|---|---|---|---|---|
| Growth (a) Initiation and proliferation | Cell multiplication | Low | Number of mitotic figures | Disturbances of all subsequent phases of growth | Colchicine and lead poisoning (deficient proliferative growth) Hypovitaminosis A (uninhibited proliferation of enamel epithelium and invasion into pulp) |
| (b) Histodifferentiation | Cell differentiation and assumption of definitive form plan (e.g., outlining form of tooth) | Increased | Cytologic changes and positioning of cells | Irregular form of tooth and atypical structure of matrix formation | Hypovitaminosis A (atypical dentin formation and form of pulp) |
| (c) Apposition | Secretion and deposition of matrix by formative cells | Most sensitive phase in growth | Vital staining (alizarin, sodium fluoride, trypan blue, etc.) | Hypoplasia (deficient amount of matrix formation) | Hypovitaminosis A (markedly disturbed gradient of growth; enamel hypoplasia and vascular inclusions in dentin) |
| Calcification | Precipitation of calcium salts in protein matrix, following apposition in close incremental succession Enamel and dentin, unlike bone, not subject to calcium withdrawal | Most sensitive phase in development: sensitive to even normal variations in body metabolism; constitutional status reflects of individual (neonatal adjustment, weaning, infancy, etc.) | (a) X-ray densiometer (b) Histologic staining reaction (c) Degree of fusion of calcospherites (d) Vital staining | Enamel immature and acid resistant, chalky and fragile Dentin showing nonfusion of calcospherites (interglobular and fragile dentin), wide predentin Cementum and bone with wide osteoid and precementum borders | Hypovitaminosis D (wide predentin and interglobular dentin) Parathyroidectomy (interglobular dentin) Fluorosis (chalky-white opacity of enamel) |

| | | | | | |
|---|---|---|---|---|---|
| Eruption | Extrusion of the formed and calcified tooth into the oral cavity by a force acting at its basal end. Opposition by incisal or occlusal stresses so that the eruption potential is not fully expressed | Very easily affected by local conditions; less readily affected by systemic factors | Marking of tooth by notching; x-rays | Deficient eruption, submersion. Excessive eruption, supra-occlusion (supra-occlusion). Perverted eruption, malposition of tooth | Local: Traumatic occlusion causing decreased rate of eruption; removal or fracture of antagonists allowing for increased rate of eruption. Systemic: Hypophysectomy, thyroidectomy; decreased rate and final cessation of eruption |
| Attrition | Result of functional wear, compensated by continuous eruption of tooth and growth of periodontal tissues | | Marking of tooth by notching | Deficient attrition, elongation (supra-occlusion). Excessive attrition, abnormal wearing of crown | Local: Deficient wear due to removal of antagonist; abnormal wear due to excessive muscular function. Systemic: Deficient calcification of enamel (fluorosis) resulting in abnormal attrition |

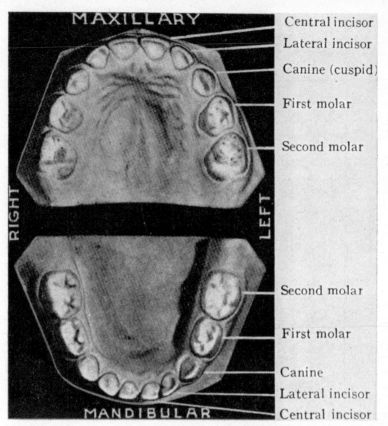

FIG. 8. Designation and arrangement of deciduous teeth. (From Wheeler, R. C. 1940. Textbook of dental anatomy and physiology. Philadelphia: Saunders. P. 2.)

with the completion of the roots of the third molars. The chart of tooth development by Logan and Kronfeld (1933) (after Anderson, 1948, p. 70) is presented in Table 2. Similar data are presented in pictorial form in the excellent chart by Schour and Poncher, Fig. 6 (from Salzmann, 1950, p. 242).

The teeth go through various stages of development from the initial formation of the crown to the eventual completion of the root. Even then the life history of the teeth is not complete, for they continue to meet and be affected by the hazards of the life of the individual, the wear from contact with other teeth, and often by decay. Schour and Massler (1940) distinguish and picture the stages in the life of the tooth in the drawings reproduced in Fig. 7.

The significance of such information for the student of speech lies in the record of growth which is traced indelibly in tooth structure as it is affected by developmental epochs through which each individual passes. Massler and Schour (1946) note that these events are reflected "accurately and permanently within the structure of the dental tissues forming and calcifying at that particular time . . . To the pedodontist, the pediatrician, and others dealing with children, the quality of the dental tissues should serve as a valuable index of the prenatal care of the mother and of the feeding of the child during infancy and childhood." The period of development and the aberrations of development are shown in Table 3, adapted from Schour and Massler (after Salzmann, 1950, p. 222).

In undergoing eruption the tooth moves from its developmental crypt and emerges into the oral cavity in occlusion with its antogonist. Although there are approximate ages at which certain teeth erupt (Fig. 6), there is considerable variation in these times of eruption in different individuals and it is oftentimes difficult to ascertain the cause or to determine the significance of premature or delayed eruption. Easlick and Moyers (Watson and Lowery, 1954) state that probably the moment of eruption is not so very important, but that the order and site of eruption, especially of the permanent teeth, are very important to the development of normal occlusion.

The normal sequences of eruption of the permanent teeth occur in subsequent relationship to the exfoliation of the deciduous teeth, a fortunate process of timing whereby adequate space for the permanent teeth is maintained in the alveolar bone. If the sequence of events is broken either by premature loss of the baby teeth or the eruption of the permanent teeth out of normal order, the positional relationship of these teeth may be disturbed and result in malocclusion. The normal and hence the optimal order of eruption is shown in Table 4 (Watson and Lowery, 1954, p. 260).

**TABLE 4. Normal Sequences of Eruption of Permanent Teeth\***

| Mandible | Maxilla |
|---|---|
| 1. First molar | 2. First molar |
| 3. Central incisor | 5. Central incisor |
| 4. Lateral incisor | 6. Lateral incisor |
| 7. Cuspid | 8. First bicuspid |
| 9. First bicuspid | 10. Second bicuspid |
| 11. Second bicuspid | 12. Cuspid |
| 13. Second molar | 14. Second molar |

\* The numbers indicate the usual sequence of eruption (From Watson and Lowery, 1954, p. 260).

The deciduous teeth are 20 in number, arranged in each dental arch so that the mandibular teeth normally fit within the circumference of the maxillary teeth when the jaws are closed (Fig. 8).

There are 32 permanent teeth in the normal maxillary and mandibular dentures. Their arrangement and the standard system of numbering are indicated in Fig. 9, from Wheeler (1940, p. 7). Indicated also are the terms *distal, medial, labial, buccal,* and *lingual,* which are frequently used in describing the positional relationship of the teeth to each other and to other structures of the oral cavity.

### Dental Occlusion

The term *dental occlusion* has been specifically defined in many different ways. In a general sense it refers to the natural closure and fitting together

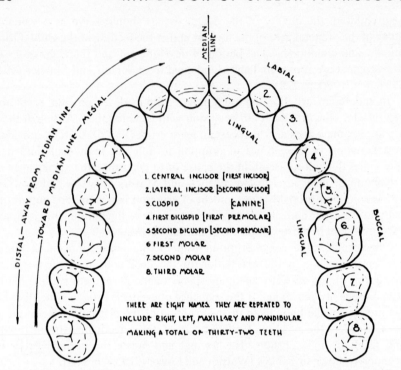

FIG. 9. Permanent teeth of an adult dental arch, showing arrangement and terms of orientation. (From Wheeler, R. C. 1940. Textbook of dental anatomy and physiology. Philadelphia: Saunders. Fig. 7, p. 7.)

of the upper and lower teeth (Wheeler, 1940). The term also implies certain concepts pertaining to (1) the alignment of the teeth in the upper and lower arches, (2) the relationship of these arches to each other, (3) the axial inclination of the individual teeth, and (4) the biting height of the teeth when the jaws are in contact relationships (Salzmann, 1950).

"Normal occlusion" in the adult mouth assumes that the dental arches are

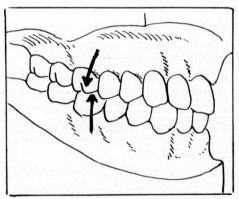

FIG. 10. Maxillary and mandibular teeth in normal occlusal relationship with reference to the first permanent molars.

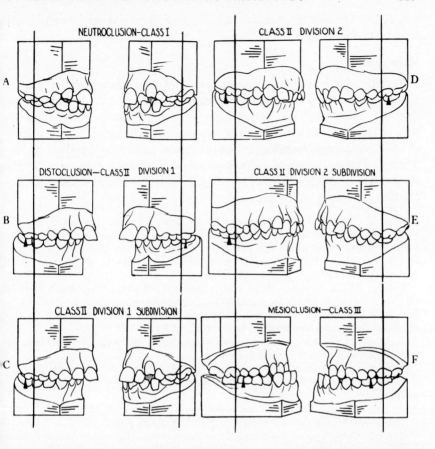

FIG. 11. Clasification of malocclusion according to Angle. A, neutroclusion, Class I; B, distoclusion, Class II, division 1; C, Class II division 1 subdivision; D, Class II division 2; E, Class II division 2 subdivision; F, Class III. (From Salzmann, J. A. 1950. Principles of orthodontics. Philadelphia: Lippincott. P. 475.)

arranged in concentric parabolic curves in which the outline of the maxillary arch is slightly larger than the mandibular arch (Wheeler, 1940). As a feature of this relationship between the two jaws, the mesiobuccal cusp of the maxillary permanent first molar occludes in the buccal groove of the mandibular permanent first molar (Fig. 10). This is an important characteristic and forms the basis for various classifications of malocclusion which will be discussed later.

The teeth of the maxillary arch normally overhang the teeth in the mandibular arch labially and buccally—a condition described as *overjet* of the maxillary teeth. The incisal ridges of the maxillary anterior teeth also extend below the incisal ridges of the mandibular anterior teeth when the teeth are placed in natural occlusion, a characteristic known as *overbite*. The amount of overbite is considered to be normal when the maxillary incisors overlap the mandibular incisors one-third of the mandibular incisor crowns (Anderson, 1949). The lack of, or excess of, either overbite or overjet are considered forms of malocclusion.

## Malocclusion

The classifications of malocclusion in current use are nearly all based upon a system originally worked out by Edward H. Angle (1907). In general, the system assumes a certain "normal" antero-posterior (mesio-distal) relationship of the jaws to each other. The key point of orientation is the position of the maxillary and mandibular first permanent molars, as described above. The following discussion of malocclusions is an adaptation of Moyer's (1955) restatement of Angle's original classes. The classical forms of these malocclusions are shown in Fig. 11.

*Class I* (Neutrocclusion)—those malocclusions wherein there is a normal antero-posterior relationship between the maxilla and mandible. The mesio-buccal cusp of the maxillary first permanent molar articulates in the buccal groove of the mandibular first permanent molar (Fig. 10). Anterior malocclusions of various types are present (Fig. 11, A).

*Class II* (Distocclusion)—those malocclusions in which the mandible is "distal" (in posterior relationship) to the maxilla. The mesial groove of the mandibular first permanent molar articulates posteriorly to the mesio-buccal cusp of the maxillary first permanent molar (Fig. 11, B, C, D, E).

1. Division 1—distocclusion cases in which the maxillary incisors are typically in extreme labioversion (protrusion).

2. Distocclusion cases in which the maxillary central incisors tend to be in linguoversion (retruded) while the maxillary lateral incisors are tipped labially and mesially.

3. Subdivisions—the distocclusion occurs on one side only of the dental arch.

*Class III* (Mesiocclusion)—those malocclusions in which there is "mesial" (anterior) relationship of the mandible to the maxilla. The extreme form is seen with the prognathous jaw. The mesial groove of the mandibular first permanent molar articulates anteriorly to the mesiobuccal cusp of the maxillary first permanent molar, the lower incisors protruding (Fig. 11, E).

In addition to the relative positions of the dental arches it is useful to the dentist and speech clinician alike to have means of indicating the positions of individual teeth in relation to each other and in relation to their position within the dental arch. Lischer (1912) has proposed the following terms (modified by Salzmann, 1950) which have won general acceptance in the field of dentistry.

*a.* Linguoversion—toward the tongue
*b.* Labioversion (or buccoversion)—toward the lip or cheek
*c.* Mesioversion—mesial to the normal position
*d.* Distoversion—distal to the normal position
*e.* Infraversion—not reaching the line of occlusion (thus, higher in the maxilla and lower in the mandible than the line of occlusion)
*f.* Supraversion—extending beyond the line of occlusion (thus, lower in the maxilla or higher in the mandible, than the line of occlusion)
*g.* Torsiversion—rotated on its long axis
*h.* Axiversion—wrong axial inclination
*i.* Transversion—wrong sequential order of position in the arch

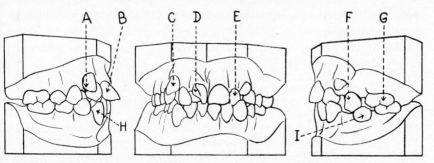

FIG. 12. Lischer's method of designating malposition of individual teeth. A, lateral incisor in transversion; B, central incisor in labioversion; C, canine in axiversion; D, central incisor in torsiversion; E. lateral incisor in linguoversion; F, first premolar in supraversion; G, first molar in mesioversion; H, mandibular canine in infraversion; I, first premolar in distoversion. (From Salzmann, J. A. 1950. Principles of orthodontics. Philadelphia: Lippincott. p. 486.)

These malpositions of individual teeth are illustrated in Fig. 12.

The Angle classification system tends to concentrate attention merely upon the relative position of the dental arches with respect to each other and to ignore such factors as discrepancies in the vertical or lateral planes and the general relationship of the teeth to the facial skeleton (Moyers, 1955).

The Simon system of classification takes these factors into account by utilizing cephalometric measures derived from landmarks of the cranium. This system uses three planes established with reference to cranial landmarks—the Orbital, the Mid-sagittal and the Frankfurt planes, from which antero-posterior, medio-lateral, and vertical relationships may be ascertained and described (see Fig. 13 and Salzmann, 1950, p. 486, Fig. 272). A denture which is placed too far forward with respect to the orbital plane is said to be in *protraction;* a denture in abnormally posterior placement is in *retraction.* If a denture is nearer to the midline (mid-sagittal plane) than normal, it is said to be in *contraction;* when expanded abnormally, it is said to be in *distraction.* A denture which is abnormally high (nearer than normal to the Frankfurt plane) is said to be in *attraction;* one abnormally low with respect to that plane is in *abstraction.*

Moyers (1955) indicates that only three of these terms are in current usage—protraction, retraction and contraction. The main advantage of the system is that it relates the dentures to the facial skeleton and thus makes possible a more accurate diagnosis of the basic dento-facial problems. From the standpoint of the speech clinician, the system's employment of antero-posterior, medio-lateral and vertical relationships is useful, especially in describing the position of the dental arches in relation to tongue positions and movements during speech.

## ETIOLOGY OF MALOCCLUSION AND DENTAL ABNORMALITIES

Abnormalities of orofacial tissues which affect speech may be of traumatic, pathological, or developmental origin acting prenatally or postnatally.

Moyers (1955) cites an equation attributed to Dockrell (1951) to illustrate the dynamic character of these forces of origin: Cause + Time + Tissue → Result. His further discussion of the origins of dento-facial abnormalities is reproduced in part below:

> Since investigators cannot isolate and identify all of the original causes, they may be studied best by grouping them as follows: (1) heredity, (2) developmental causes of unknown origin, (3) trauma, (4) physical agents, (5) habits, (6) diseases, and (7) malnutrition. It will be seen that there is a certain overlapping among these groups. The duration of the operation of these causes and the age at which they are seen, are both functions of time, and thus may be grouped together under this heading. The primary tissues principally involved are: (1) the bones of the facial skeleton, (2) the teeth, (3) the neuro-muscular system, and (4) the soft parts, excepting muscle. Rarely one tissue alone is involved; usually other tissues become affected, and one tissue may be termed primarily involved, and the others considered as being secondarily concerned. The result of the action of the factors is malocclusion, malfunction or osseous dysplasia; more probably a combination of all three. . . . If the primary tissues concerned involve the teeth, malocclusion is the result. If they impede the normal working of the neuro-muscular system, the result is malfunction. If they alter the growth plan of the bones, an osseous dysplasia is the result. Most clinical problems are a combination of these three aberrations.

In short, constitutional factors, trauma, or malnutrition may operate as causes; their relationship to time may be continuous or intermittent; the tissues affected may be dental, osseous, neuro-muscular, or soft tissues; the result may be malocclusions, osseous dysplasias (abnormalities of bone development), or malfunction of muscles.

1. *Osseous defects* occur when one or more of the bones of the face develop in a perverted, delayed, advanced, or other asynchronous pattern of growth. Although each bone has a growth potential which is genetically determined, this potential may be altered by disease or by environmental forces such as mechanical interferences and habits of use, with the result that the growth of the lower jaw (mandible) or the upper jaw (maxilla and the naso-maxillary complex) may be so distorted that severe deformities of the dental arches and tooth relationships occur. Hypertrophy of the mandible due to hyperpituitarism may bring about a Class III malocclusion (mandibular protraction), or underdevelopment of the mandible may result in a Class II malocclusion (mandibular retraction).

Treatment and prognosis depend upon accurate diagnosis in such cases. Alveolar bone can be shaped and altered by tooth movement or by the forces of muscular contraction; basal bone is generally unaffected by such forces. Distortions of dental-arch relationships may result from aberrant growth of either basal or alveolar bone, but only the latter can be altered effectively by orthodontic treatment or by the use of corrective muscular training.

2. *Muscular dysfunctions* which persist throughout critical periods of oro-facial growth can distort the direction of facial development so that the width of the maxillary dental arch, the inclination of the teeth, or the habitual positioning of the mandible may result in permanent deformities. In this

connection, it should be remembered that the musculature of the face is well defined before ossification of the face and cranium get under way, so that the growing muscles exert a molding influence upon bone development. Muscle groups which may affect orofacial formation include: (1) the muscles of mastication, (2) the muscles of facial expression, and (3) the muscles of the tongue. These muscles, acting in response to their motor innervators (Cranial nerves V, VII, and XII respectively) and sensory fibers of pain, temperature, and proprioception, develop habits of muscular contraction. These habits, in turn, exert forces of pressure or contraction which, acting postnatally, determine to some extent the directions of bone growth. A state of physiological balance between the forces of these three muscle groups encourages normal growth and shaping of the bones (Cooper, 1930). Distorted growth will occur if the forces are asynchronous or otherwise unequal. Zappler (1949) states that deformities of the dental arches and malocclusion come about because of abnormal muscular contraction in cerebral palsy.

Swinehart (1950) notes that although orthodontists agree that the tongue in habitually abnormal movement can cause a variety of malocclusions, little concerted study has been made to determine whether the tongue is an important factor in forming the arches originally. He speculates that an instance of congenital aglossia reported by Eskew and Shepard (1949) supports a contention that normal tongue function is necessary to normal arch development.

Detrimental neuromuscular habits which cause pressures on the developing oral structures and hence affect facial form and the development of malocclusions include: abnormal patterns of mandibular closure, abnormal habits of swallowing, incompetent lip postures, tongue- or lip-biting, the biting of hard objects (such as nail-biting), and abnormal habits of pillowing the head during sleep (Stallard, 1930).

The effects of thumb- and finger-sucking upon occlusion have been much debated. There is much evidence to show a positive relationship, although Ruttle et al. (1953) state that their effects are mainly recorded on the anterior maxillary tooth placement. Mouth-breathing also is a factor producing malocclusion. With respect to this, Salzmann (1950, p. 424) observes:

Whether or not mouth-breathing is a primary cause of malocclusion is relatively unimportant. The fact remains that in the mouth-breather a muscle complex is present which tends to produce narrowing, or interference with, the lateral widening of the maxillary arch. When the lower lip in the mouth-breather falls lingual to the normally erupted maxillary incisors, protrusion of the maxillary incisors and narrowing of the lateral segments of the dental arches is encouraged.

In consideration of the influence of muscular function upon bone growth it follows logically that whereas speech may be affected by the growth of the face and jaws, the habits of speech can also play their part in inflecting growth, an observation that has been made by Froeschels (1933), Greene

(1937), Palmer (1948), and others. Henry (1937) suggested speech drills as a means of improving occlusion.

3. *Dental defects* involving malpositioning of individual teeth, gross variations in size and shape, abnormalities of number and sequence of eruption, constitute a third site of origin. These defects and the primary malpositioning of the teeth in relationship to each other (malocclusion) give rise to malfunction, which in turn can bring about alterations in bone development.

4. "*Soft parts*" (excluding muscle) probably also play a role although a less clearly marked one. A list of these tissues would include the periodontal membrane, the mucous membrane, skin, tendons, etc. Changes in these tissues due to infections, abnormal pressures, or other adverse conditions alter the normal physiology of the masticatory system and hence may contribute to aberrant patterns of growth.

The orofacial defects produced by abnormal growth of the facial bones, distortions of the direction of growth due to muscular forces or the effects of external pressures, and the various anomalies of tooth development may, to superficial study, appear to be quite similar in form. The differences in origin, however, determine to a large extent the degree to which alteration of the orofacial growth and proportion may be obtained by treatment. It also should determine the nature of the treatment undertaken, such as medical treatment to correct glandular dyscrasia, surgical treatment to alter the size and shape of bone or to improve the function of muscular tissues, orthodontic intervention to change tooth and alveolar arch relationships, or "habit-training" to allow muscular postures and patterns of movement to assist rather than impede normal development. Whatever the form of treatment, or whether the forces of maldevelopment seem to come from physical, psychological, or environmental sources, it is evident that the individual grows and behaves as a whole. It is thus that the development of speech and orofacial structures may be mutually inflected.

## OROFACIAL ABNORMALITIES AND THEIR EFFECTS ON SPEECH

A viewpoint has been expressed repeatedly in a variety of ways to indicate that abnormalities of orofacial structures cannot of themselves alone be considered as prime causes of defective articulation. As Van Riper puts it (1954 p. 192), ". . . the presence of some anatomical abnormality is of no importance in itself unless it stands in functional relation to defective speech sounds." The trick which the diagnostician must perform, of course, is to determine whether a "functional relationship" exists. West (1947) has advanced good arguments to show that a speaker is capable of many articulatory adjustments by which he can produce clear speech even though his orofacial structures are abnormal. Van Thal (1936, p. 256) concluded that "There is sufficient evidence available to prove that adaptability and skill in the use of the tongue compensate for many dental malformations." And yet the pure mechanics of articulatory adjustment is not the only thing involved for the way an individual feels about his abnormality (his acceptance, defensiveness, or discouragement) may partly determine whether he learns to use his speech mechanism effectively or poorly. The following observations in this section dealing with the relationship of orofacial abnormalities and speech defects are advanced with due regard for the intricate nature of the functional interdependencies which must be assumed to be present always in the act of speaking.

Defective consonant sounds are produced if the essential valves described in Table I are not properly created because of abnormal oral structures or maladaptive patterns of articulatory movement. The nature of the articulatory defects thus caused is usually one of distortion rather than complete omission or substitution, although almost any form of defective articulation can conceivably occur in some way related to the structural or functional abnormalities. Deformities important to the etiology of disorders of articulation may include the *soft tissues* (lips, tongue, or palatopharyngeal regions), *bony structures* (the jaws, the hard palate, the temperomandibular joints), *dentition* (malocclusions and certain dental deformities), and *dental appliances* (orthodontic or prosthetic). We have noted earlier that the effect of such structures on speech must always be evaluated in terms of the interrelated positional changes which occur during consonant production.

The speech sounds most likely to be affected by abnormalities of these orofacial structures are:

1. Fricatives [s], [z], [ʃ], [ʒ], [f], [v], [θ] and [ð]
2. Affricates [tʃ] and [dʒ]
3. Plosives [p], [b], [t], [d], [k], [g]

In addition to these consonants, the semivowels and nasals [l], [r], [j], m], [n], [ŋ] occasionally may be distorted because of deformities or the maladaptive function of defective structures.

## Astomia

In rare instances children may be born without a mouth opening (astomia, or atresia of the mouth). Such deformities result from a failure of the developmental processes which should normally occur before the end of the first nine or ten weeks of fetal growth. The case reported below (from records of the University of Michigan Hospital) illustrates this type of deformity and indicates the nature of speech defect associated with it.

L. W. was born with an atresia of the mouth, characterized by micrognathia, a continuous wall of mucous membrane, and congenital bilateral fusion of the mandible and maxilla and the lateral pterygoid plates. An anterior aperture was created shortly after birth by extraction of a left central incisor so that the infant could be fed. Several subsequent attempts were made surgically to give the patient a functional jaw, but after each operation heavy scarring prevented sustained mobilization of the lower jaw. Although it appears that the temperomandibular joint is potentially functional, the mandible is underdeveloped, and the range of mandibular movement at six years of age is scarcely one-fourth of an inch.

Speech evaluations on three occasions between two and six years of age showed delay in the initiation of speech and subsequent articulatory defects after functional speech developed. At six years her anterior teeth are in open-bite relationship, lingual movements are poorly controlled in both speech and deglutition, and the speech is markedly defective in articulation. She has had no speech-training and the parents have evidently made comparatively little effort to provide speech stimulation or to encourage function and growth of the oral structures.

### Lip Deformities and Malfunctions

Among the lip deformities (exclusive of cleft lip or repaired cleft lip) which may contribute to articulatory defects are (1) labial underdevelopment, (2) labial deficiency due to trauma, (3) restricted mobility of the lip due to scar tissue or a short labial frenum, (4) inadequate motility due to muscular weakness, (5) marked asymmetry of muscular contraction, (6) tumors or mucoid cysts of the lip, and (7) excessive fullness or thickness of the lips. Even though the lips may lack intrinsic deformity, they may be functionally inadequate because of the mechanical interference of protruding teeth or an excessively protracted or retracted mandible or maxilla.

Closure of the lips provides a pneumatic valve for the articulation of the bilabial consonants [p], [b], [m]. Labial constriction has an important acoustic function in the articulation of [w] and [ʍ], the rounded vowels [ɔ], [o], [ʊ], [u], and the diphthongs [au] and [ɔi]. Although these sounds can be imitated approximately by linguo-dental and linguo-palatal movements, the acoustic effect is never quite the same as that produced with normal lips. An effect of lip function on voice quality is described by Froeschels (1940), who notes excessive tension of the lips as responsible for one of the "hyperfunctions" of voice. It should be noted also that abnormal lip postures and malfunction may be significant in the diagnosis of abnormal habits of swallowing (see below).

The correction of labial malfunction may be accomplished by surgical alteration, the use of dental prosthesis, or by exercises for strengthening the lips. Congenital shortness of the upper lip may require surgical modification by a lengthening procedure (Ford, 1944). The appearance and function achieved thus may improve speech directly. It also has cosmetic (and hence psychological) values for improvement of speech and also assists in the correction of mouth-breathing. The restoration of a functional balance between the lips, tongue, and cheeks is important also, since an imbalance of the muscular pressures exerted by these three organs is one of the causes of dental malocclusion.

In cases of maxillary deficiency, the upper lip may be so far retruded in its relationship to the lower lip that normal bilabial function is difficult. If enough lip tissue is available and flexible, it is sometimes possible to "plump" the upper lip by the use of an anterior maxillary dental prosthesis to provide structural support for the lip, bringing it into normal or nearly normal anatomic position with respect to the lower lip.

Certain forms of lip dysfunction contributing to dental malocclusion may be improved by the use of exercises designed to strengthen the lips and to develop proper habits of use. Johnson (1940) advises a series of exercises developed by Lloyd Lourie, and the use of phonetic drills involving the sound [p] as suggested by Lightoller.[1] These exercises are supposed to restore functional muscle balance for lip-opening and closure, and to assist in the development or maintainance of normal occlusion. They are especially adapted to overcome the hyperfunction of the mentalis muscle believed to be responsible in some cases of protrusion of the maxillary incisors (see myofunctional therapy below).

In those instances in which correction of the labial deformity is not possible, adaptations for speech can be made by substituting the upper lip for the lower, as in producing the phonemes [f] and [v]. The lower lip may be brought into compression against the upper teeth for labial plosives. The tongue may be used to approximate the labial sounds if no lip is present. A patient whose upper lip had been surgically removed (Bloomer, 1953) was able to speak with moderate intelligibility even though the upper lip, the anterior two-thirds of the maxilla and all of the teeth were missing. Palmer (1948) describes the case of a nine-year-old boy whose face was paralyzed by bulbar polio. He was successfully trained to substitute tongue tip for labial movements. Substitutions of this sort are basic in ventriloquism.

## Maxillary Protraction (Distocclusion)

The discussion of speech defects associated with maxillary protraction includes all of those dental malocclusions in which the mandibular teeth are posterior (distal) to their normal position with respect to the maxillary teeth. This condition may be present in maxillary protraction, mandibular retraction, protrusion of the maxillary incisors, or retrusion of the mandibular incisors. Thus the anomalies affecting speech may include the various forms of Angle Class II malocclusion, those Angle Class I malocclusions in which the maxillary teeth are in marked labioversion to the mandibular anteriors, the condition of micrognathia, and certain defects of the temporomandibular joints.

The influence of maxillary protraction (or mandibular retraction) upon speech should always be considered in relation to the adequacy of tongue and lip function. A mild labioversion of the maxillary incisors may impede the correct formation of the bilabial plosive consonants if the upper lip is short or lacking in mobility, whereas a speaker with normal lip function may, under similar or even extreme conditions of labioversion of the maxillary incisors, make correct bilabial approximations for these sounds.

In general, excessive protraction tends to (1) increase the difficulty in producing normally articulated bilabial sounds (Greene, 1937), (2) make it more difficult for the speaker to form acoustically acceptable sibilants (Wolfe,

[1] See L. R. Johnson (1940) for details of exercises and drills developed by Lourie and Lightoller.

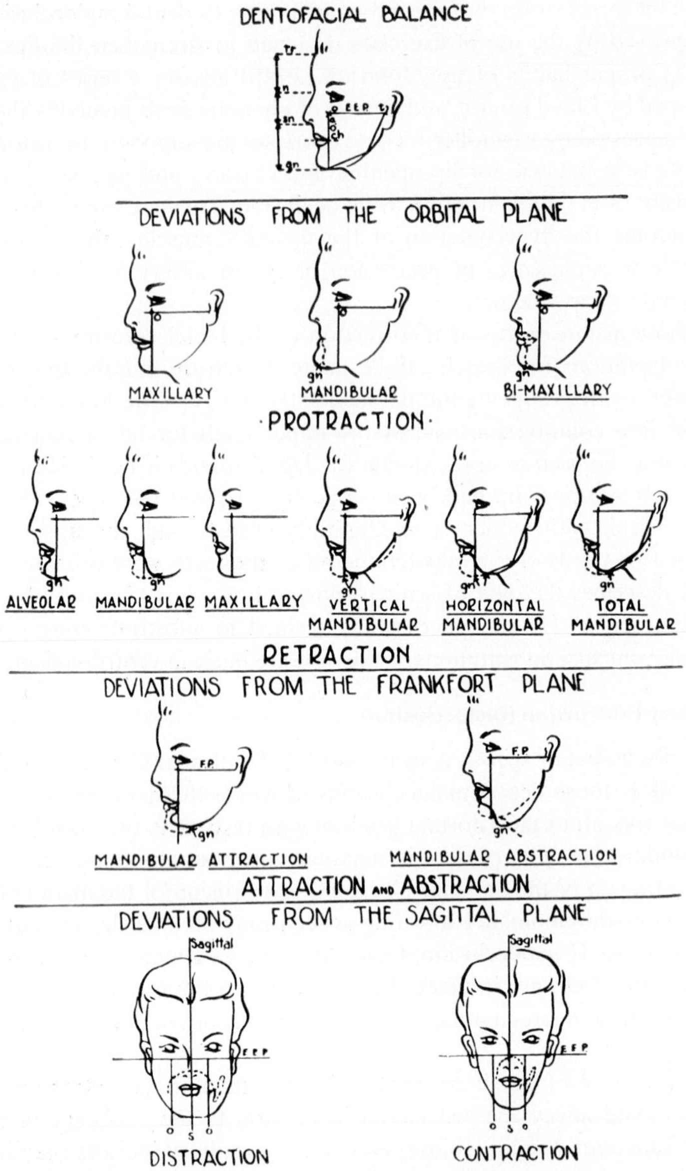

FIG. 13. Designations of dentofacial deviations from the three planes of space according to Simon, reading from above downward as follows: Dentofacial balance showing the following landmarks—TR, trichion; N, nasion; SN, subnasion; GN, gnathion; CH, cheilion; OP, orbital plane; O, orbitale, E.E.P., eye-ear plane; T, tragion. Deviations from the orbital plane—protraction indicates protrusion; retraction indicates retrusion. Deviations from the Frankfort plane— attraction indicates a shortening of the vertical dimension; abstraction indicates a lengthening of the vertical dimension from the eye-ear plane. Deviations from the sagittal plane—distraction indicates an increase in the horizontal dimension from the sagittal plane; contraction indicates a decrease in the horizontal dimension from the sagittal plane. (From Salzmann, J. A. 1957. Principles of orthodontics. Philadelphia: Lippincott. Fig. 272.)

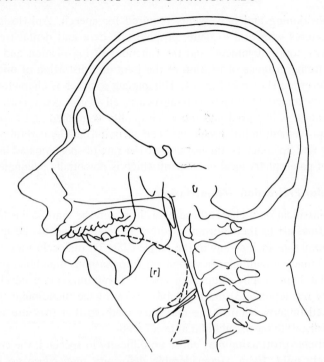

FIG. 14. Subject with ankylosis of the temperomandibular joints, with subsequent micrognathia and mandibular retraction.

(937), and (3) modify the quality of the sibilants in characteristic ways. The acoustic effect on the sibilants has to do presumably with the difficulty which the speaker finds in directing the air current in relation to the teeth. West (1949) and others have emphasized the need to have a narrow air blade directed against the cutting edge of a tooth for the production of an [s] sound. It can be shown, however, that the cutting edge of the teeth, although it undoubtedly contributes to sibilance, is not essential to it. It has been noted clinically that patients who have a severely protracted maxilla or who may even have lost all anterior teeth, may use the upper or lower lips to create the requisite air turbulence for satisfactory sibilant consonants (Wolfe, 1937).

A man whose mandibular deformity was similar to that shown in Fig. 14, except that the temperomandibular joint was not ankylosed, was able to produce good [s] and [z] consonants when the lip and tongue movements were properly co-ordinated during speech. When the lower lip was pulled away from the [f] position which it characteristically assumed during the production of sibilants, the [s] and [z] were no longer clear.

Malfunction of the temporomandibular joint is often associated with micrognathia. Fixation (ankylosis) of the joint prevents normal motion which should be a combination of hinge and gliding movement occurring at the articulation of the mandibular and temporal bones. This form of articulation permits extensive movements of the mandible for chewing and facilitates the tongue-positioning and movements required for speech. Ankylosis of the joint interferes with oral hygiene, prophylactic care and dental treatment, jaw growth, tooth alignment, and the functions of mastication and speech.

An extreme instance of fixation of the joint and distortion of micromandibular form are shown in Fig. 14. This patient's speech is characterized by articulatory maladaptations involving nearly all of the consonants. Vowel differentiation is impaired and the voice quality is muffled and hypernasal. Some improvement in his speech has been accomplished by careful attention to tongue and lip contacts, the use of a slower rate of speaking and increased control of palatopharyngeal movement which is potentially adequate.

### Mandibular Protraction (Mesiocclusion)

This classification includes those cases in which the mandibular teeth are anterior (mesial) to their normal position in relationship to the maxillary teeth. It may thus include any of the Angle Class III malocclusions, whether due to (1) macromandibular development (prognathous mandible, progenia, mandibular hypertrophy, Hapsburg jaw), (2) micromaxillary development (maxillary retraction), (3) marked labioversion of the mandibular teeth, or (4) marked linguoversion of the maxillary teeth so that they are in retroposition (distal) to the mandibular anterior teeth.

Mandibular protraction may cause no difficulty in speech if the condition is relatively mild. Even a considerable deformity may cause no obvious articulatory defect if the lips and tongue can adapt to the structural handicap. Frequently, however, individuals who have this type of malocclusion have a tongue posture which is habitually low and somewhat flaccid so that a constriction of the linguo-alveolar valve necessary for sibilants is not effectively produced. A further complication is often found in the relative distraction (abnormal expansion) of the mandibular arch (conversely, the relative contraction of the maxillary arch), so that the tongue is habitually brought into contact with the occusal edges of the maxillary teeth instead of being brought into proper contact with the alveolar arch and the linguodental surfaces. In such individuals the [f] and [v] consonants may be formed habitually by bringing the upper lip into contact with the incisal edges of the lower teeth or by approximating the two lips. The condition of mandibular protraction is oftentimes complicated by open-bite, and the speech symptoms are accentuated by missing teeth or malpositioned teeth which hamper adaptive articulatory movements.

In severe malocclusions of this general type, correction of the speech usually requires improvement or correction of the osseous or occlusal deformity. Depending on the nature and etiology of the abnormality, treatment may require osteotomy (bone surgery) such as that described by Dingman (1944), orthodontic treatment, the use of an anterior maxillary dental prosthesis, or a combination of procedures. In some cases the structurally rehabilitated patient is able to achieve clear speech without special instruction; others may require speech-training. In these instances the therapist will need to study carefully the posture of the body of the tongue, working with the patient to develop habits of mandibular position and linguo-palatal contacts which are specifically adapted to his structures.

## Open-bite (infraclusion), Overbite (supraclusion), Collapsed Bite, and Cross-bite

The references to open-bite in connection with speech defects usually designate or assume an anterior open-bite relationship involving the incisors of both dental arches. There is also the possibility of a lateral open-bite which may impede linguo-alveolar contact on the affected side (Greene, 1937). If the anterior open-bite is extreme, it may interfere somewhat with bilabial and labiodental sounds (Gardner, 1949).

The most noticeable defect of speech associated with open-bite is likely to be distortion of the sibilants [s], [z], [ʃ], [ʒ], and possibly the [tʃ] and [dʒ]. There is a tendency for the speaker to produce these consonants interdentally. Even if the tongue does not protrude interdentally, however, the sound may lack sibilance.

An adaptive constriction adequate to produce sibilance can be achieved, however, by placing the lower lip in relation to the air blade created by grooving of the tongue so that the requisite air turbulence is developed. Some attention may profitably be directed also to the general posture of the tongue within the mouth cavity to make sure that it occupies the best adaptive position for articulatory contact with the dental arches.

Open-bite can occur in all types of malocclusion, and is often attributed to habitual interposition of the tongue, lips, fingers, thumb, or other objects between the teeth frequently enough, and with sufficient pressure, that the teeth are prevented from developing normal occlusion with the teeth of the opposing dental arch. Congenital growth factors may also be responsible. Abnormal swallowing may initiate and perpetuate the open-bite (Salzmann, 1950).

Many forms of open-bite are responsive to treatment by orthodontic means, and the patient should be referred for orthodontic examination and advice as soon as the condition is recognized to exist. Inasmuch as sucking habits often are of etiological significance in such cases, proper planning in the early stages of development may prevent a disfigurement which would be difficult to treat in adult life.

Extreme forms of cross-bite may interfere with linguo-alveolar contact (Palmer, 1948) and thus be a factor in the etiology of lateral lisping. Supralusion (overbite) is not generally considered to contribute significantly to defective articulation of speech, although Kessler (1953) suggests that speech may be adversely affected by inadequate lingual space in closed-bite relationships. The effect of "collapsed bite" in the deciduous dentition is noted by Forde (1951) as responsible for preventing the full eruption of the posterior permanent teeth. The collapsed bite is said to force the tongue to a position of retraction deep into the throat, thus contributing to tonsilar and adenoidal complications.

## Anomalies of Individual Teeth and Groups of Teeth

The condition, size, or texture of individual teeth probably has relatively little direct influence on speech. The presence or absence of teeth and the position which they occupy in the dental arches may, however, directly or indirectly affect the quality of a speaker's enunciation.

Lischer's system of designating the malpositions of individual teeth has already been described in a preceding section of this chapter (Fig. 11). Other useful terms, similar in function, include *ectopic eruption* (eruption out of normal position), *supernumerary teeth, diastema* (abnormal spacing of the teeth), *missing teeth* (whether due to extraction or failure to erupt), *anodontia* (congenital absence of teeth), and *oligodontia* (the presence of only a few teeth).

Teeth in ectopic eruption or in malposition (especially in linguoversion) due to forces creating malocclusion may make clear articulation difficult because of their interference with linguo-alveolar, linguo-dental, or bilabial contact.

It is very doubtful if the absence of individual teeth in adult life can be considered to be a significant cause of articulatory disorders. Wolfe (1937) indicates that missing teeth or widely spaced teeth are secondary factors not closely related to the occurrence of lisping. Excessively wide spacing of the central incisors (diastema) may affect the quality of the sibilants somewhat but cannot be considered a primary cause of sibilant defects.

Anodontia or oligodontia may be found rarely in the child with a delayed speech or a dyslalia, although it is dubious whether the absence of teeth alone can be the basic cause of the disorder. It is more likely that predisposing factors of a congenital nature are responsible for the speech pattern. Nevertheless, artificial dentures may be beneficial to speech and are esthetically important. The problem of premature loss of deciduous or permanent teeth in children should not be ignored by the speech clinician, however, since these losses may contribute to eventual malocclusion of a serious nature. The child in adapting to premature dental loss may also develop habits of lingual movement which are retained even after the second teeth have erupted. This is not so likely to be true of the child whose speech is normal before loss of the teeth, and even the loss of the central incisor oftentimes produces no noticeable effect on the child's speech (Froeschels, 1941). The significance of premature loss of teeth is related to the general health of the individual, and if the pattern of loss results in facial disfigurement, the personality of the individual may be impaired.

A completely edentulous person may have some difficulty in making fricative sounds clearly, and the [f] and [v] may be particularly difficult to enunciate. Properly constructed artificial dentures will usually bring a return of correct articulation if they are made with due regard to the articulatory habits of the patient and the pattern of occlusion present in his own teeth before their loss.

## Asymmetry and Malformations of the Dental Arches

In discussing the relationship of the teeth to speech, Greene (1937) states that the ". . . existence or non-existence of the teeth is not so important for good speech as the shape and roof of the mouth. . . . Defects in enunciation can also be caused by the condition of the arches, especially the side arches. In 92 per cent of all cases of lateral lisp, the larger arch is on the lisping side." Herman (1943), in comparing the palatal configurations of lispers and normal subjects, found no significant differences between the palates of 26 lispers and 400 random selections used by Crane and Ramstrum (1943) in classifying palate shapes. Clinical observation of patients with deformities of the hard palate and alveolar arches subsequent to surgery for congenital cleft suggests, however, that there is a general tendency for the lingual groove to follow the direction of the palatal groove, and usually there is a distortion of sibilant sounds in the speech of such patients.

The matter of palate height in relation to articulatory defects is sometimes mentioned as an etiological factor in dyslalia. The author recalls a case in which a dentist was so impressed by the high narrow arch of a patient that he constructed a small prosthetic palate to fill in the vault of the patient's hard palate. The prosthesis was, of course, more hinderance than help, since there is relatively little relationship between palatal height and articulation unless for some reason the range of lingual movement is abnormally small. It is usually the restriction in arch width preventing or making difficult the lingual contacts around the alveolar borders of the maxillary teeth which impedes articulation. This is particularly true if the mandibular arch is of comparatively greater width, so that the tongue is able to contact only the occlusal surfaces of the maxillary teeth. If the arch is abnormally flat, the speaker can usually be taught to make the necessary lingual adaptations for clear speech.

Angle (1907, p. 413) describes a case in which ". . . the vault of the arch and bones of the nose . . . became involved until normal breathing became impossible, and as the space for the tongue was so greatly restricted, it was with much difficulty that the man could enunciate his words sufficiently to be understood." The relationship between maxillary contraction and mouth-breathing have long been noted, and thus the significance of the structural defect may be useful to the speech clinician in his study of the history of his patient. As described by Massler and Schour (1946), mouth-breathing leads to upper respiratory infection. The growing structures of the face are affected so that the face becomes markedly elongated and narrowed (adenoid facies), caused by dropping of the mandible into open position and by constriction of the upper arch and the palate. The nostrils are narrowed from disuse, and the facial expression becomes dull and drawn. The habit of mouth-breathing and enlargement of the pharyngeal tonsils both contribute to the typical facial configuration. Correction of the deformity requires removal of the nasopharyngeal obstruction, orthodontic treatment, and muscle exercises to strengthen the lips.

The significance of mouth-breathing to the speech clinician lies in the concomitant effects of the habit upon orofacial structures and their function. The lips become slack, the upper lip shortened and elevated over the maxillary incisors, the lower lip lies beneath and behind the upper incisors, and the upper teeth become spaced and protruding. There is hypertrophy of the gingival tissues. The tongue is suspended between the arches or lies on the floor of the mouth so that its molding action is lost to the upper jaw. The unopposed pressure of the cheek muscles gradually forces the maxillary arch to become narrowed and V-shaped, with a high palatal arch. The mandible is retruded and the mouth hangs open. The maxillary sinuses and the nasal cavity become narrowed as the upper arch is contracted. The turbinates become swollen and engorged. The nasal mucosa become atrophic from disuse and the alae nasi are red and pinched. The sense of smell is dulled, often accompanied by loss of taste sensation and decrease in appetite. Hyperplasia of the lymphoid tissues around the Eustachian tube may close it and contribute to hearing loss.

The speech of such individuals is more than likely to show a composite of symptoms in which the etiology is appropriately complex. The symptoms will probably include hyponasality (Gardner 1949) or perhaps a mixed (hyper-hypo-) nasality, and articulatory distortions which result from interference with the normal mechanics of articulation and also from a loss of the normal auditory monitoring of speech.

The shaping of the alveolar arch of the maxilla can be important in the articulation of linguo-alveolar sounds. The arch contours shown in Fig. 3 indicate clearly that there are marked differences in shape and angle of slope of the palate in adults. The speaker with a protracted maxilla or a retracted mandible (as in Fig. 14) will be aided in articulation of the consonants [s] and [z] if his maxillary alveolar arch rises gradually instead of abruptly behind the incisors.

### Lingual Deformities and Lingual Habits

The importance of the tongue to speech is clearly indicated in the very term *language,* which comes from *lingua,* the Latin word for tongue. Goldberg (1939) notes that language means tonguing, or wagging of the tongue, attributable to the observation of our remote ancestors who, by figure of speech, chose the tongue as the chief representative of all of the organs of speech. Froeschels (1933), Greene (1937), and others have stated, however, that the tongue is not essential to speech, and that congenital absence or adventitious loss of the tongue need not prevent a victim of such loss from learning to talk. Despite this claim, the tongue is extremely important; and it is due to the adept action of the tongue that most of the compensatory movements of speech are achieved by those patients whose oral deformities preclude the development of normal articulatory movements. The importance of the tongue in the development of normal occlusion has already been indicated (Swinehart, 1950). The general posture and habits of lingual movement have been shown by Wright *et al.* (1949) to determine the stability and comfort with which artificial dentures are worn.

Lingual deformities of various sorts include tongue-tie (ankyloglossia), macroglossia (enlarged tongue), long tongue, microglossia (undersized tongue), aglossia (absence of the tongue), tumors, malfunctions due to scarring, paralyses, bifid or trifid tongue due to developmental arrest (Arey, 1954, Brown, 1938), and various degrees of glossectomy (removal of the tongue). Any one of these abnormalities may affect speech, but the degree to which they may affect any individual case varies in accordance with factors other than the mere extent of lingual abnormality. Backus (1940) describes the case of a boy who lost the tongue-tip, but was able to learn to speak adequately. Frowine and Moser (1944) present an account of a boy whose tongue was severely scarred as a result of lye taken intraorally; his speech was satisfactory despite a limited range of tongue movement. Goldstein (1940) presents photographs of tongue movements and refers to a monograph by Twistleton in 1873 which reported several cases in which the tongue had been amputated or torn out, yet many of these unfortunate individuals recovered speech. Keaster (1940) cites evidence that the speech of tongueless people is less interfered with than is their chewing and swallowing. Kremen (1953) found that in cancer of the tongue requiring radical neck dissection, the speech was impaired in the early postoperative period but later improved so that the patients were able to converse.

Froeschels states (1933, p. 178) that he has many reports of persons whose tongue was removed surgically. Muscle contractions are said to appear postoperatively in the stumps of muscles that were left, and compensatory adjustments of the remaining oral structures are developed, enabling the person to speak. The lower lip can be pressed against the incisors to substitute for lingual sounds; [s] and [ʃ] can be made by blowing the air through the teeth or the protruded lips; [r] can be produced by quivering of the vocal cords or the uvula; [l], [j], [i], and [e] can be produced by raising the floor of the mouth to approach the palate; [k] and [g] can be formed by movements approximating the palatal arches.

The case of a twenty-two-year-old Chinese man with congenital aglossia is described by Eskew and Shepard (1949, p. 116). The man spoke but had a definite speech impediment. "In speaking, the buccinator muscles were very noticeable in their movement, as were the muscles of the floor of the mouth. Also in speaking there was a clearly audible intake of air, and a tendency for saliva to escape from the corners of the mouth." The floor of the mouth of this patient was smooth, but could be elevated in a tongue-like structure which could contact the incisal edges of the maxillary anterior teeth. The maxillary arch was constricted and triangular in form, and in malocclusal relationship with the maxillary arch. For the [k] sound he

established contact of the buccinators and the molars; [tʃ] was made similarly, with some difference in breath-stream control to differentiate it from
[k]. All of the vowels were made clearly except [e] and [i].

Tongue-tie is commonly diagnosed by the layman as a cause of speech
disorder, and physicians sometimes resort to "clipping" the tongue as a
remedy for a recognized disorder of articulation. The term *tongue-tie* refers
to abnormal shortness of the frenum of the tongue, a condition which limits
the range of movement of the tongue-tip. Greene (1945) indicates the comparative rarity of tongue-tie as a cause of speech defects. In more than 40,-
000 cases examined, not more than 10 or 12 cases of real tongue-tie were
recorded. McEnery and Gaines (1941) state that in observing a large number of infants and children they have never seen a tongue that had to be
clipped. Inasmuch as clipping can result in infection, with subsequent ulceration and scarring, hemorrhage, or extreme mobility leading to asphyxia
caused by swallowing of the tongue, they recommend that the operation, if
performed, be attempted with caution. In one thousand cases of speech disorders seen in the clinic in which they worked, only four had seriously
shortened frenums. In two cases of serious tongue-tie, one showed no defect
of articulation and the other overcame a slight [r] defect without surgery.

### Effects of Malocclusion on Hearing

The claim has been made in several publications that there is a relationship
between occlusion and hearing loss. Pryor (1933) in a description of the
dental problems of George Washington speculates that his considerable hearing loss in his latter years may have been due to an excessive closed bite
which allowed the mandibular condyles to encroach on the external auditory
meatus. Costen (1936, p. 1015), describes ear symptoms which include impaired hearing, tinnitus, a stuffy sensation in the ears, pain, and nystagmous.
He states:

> During the act of swallowing the tensor palatini muscle should be tensed, and
> effect a temporary opening of the tube. This function cannot occur during over-
> closure, and the result is a derangement of introtympanic pressure, and dizzi-
> ness . . . [This] brings about a catarrhal or adhesive deafness exactly as produced
> by inflammation or pressure from the nasopharynx. The catarrhal deafness
> improves more or less after repositioning the jaw.

Ronkin (1953) notes similar symptoms but ascribes their origin to the loss
of tone of the internal pterygoid muscles, which immediately causes a deviation from the norm of both the tensor palatini and the tensor tympani
muscles. Treatment consists in opening the bite, thus allowing the internal
pterygoid to resume its normal tone, with consequent effect on the associated muscle groups.

Harvey (1948) undertook an extensive and well-designed study of the
relationship of malocclusion and ear symptoms, with particular reference to
altitude changes and pain in the ears. Careful anatomical studies produced
no evidence that shortening of the tensor veli palatini could have any effect

on the ear, since both the tensor and levator insert into the maxilla, but not into the mandible. With respect to relaxation of the pterygoid muscles and pressure on the Eustachian tube, he found that the internal pterygoid and Eustachian tube are widely divergent in three planes, and concluded that it would be very difficult to see how these structures could possibly compress the tubes. In brief, he found no support whatever for the assertions made by earlier investigators of this topic.

### Artificial Dentures and Dental Appliances

Not much has been written, and apparently very little study has been made, of the effect of dental appliances on speech. Van Thal (1936) states that, "The wearing of an appliance appears to have little effect on speech once the wearer has got accustomed to it. Only in 13 cases (out of a total of 180 children studied) was articulation actually worse when wearing a plate or springs; and in five cases it was better . . . with the appliance than without it." Kimball and Muyskens (1937) report a case of speech improvement after prosthetic reconstruction, indicating that the placement of the bars of the supporting frame is important to the patient's speech adaptations. Palatograms illustrate how linguo-palatal contacts were improved by correct denture design.

The four main requirements for satisfactory artificial dentures are that they shall be pleasing in appearance, mechanically adequate for the mastication of food, noninjurious to oral tissues, and structurally and functionally adapted to normal speech habits (Pound, 1953). The latter requirement has probably received the least attention of all, although the jokes and imitation of people who wear artificial dentures have been a standard part of our national humor for a long time.

Tench (1927) suggests a number of mistakes in denture design which contribute to unsatisfactory speech of patients who have lost their natural dentures. The design and construction of artificial dentures should always be undertaken with reference to the functional relationship of tongue size and habits of movement to the position of the teeth and their supporting materials. An unusually broad tongue, or a tongue which is habitually retracted, may require a cross-bite arrangement of the molar teeth to provide enough lingual space so that the lingual denture is not unseated as the tongue returns to its normal rest position. If the incisors are not placed sufficiently far forward, [θ] may become [d]. The sibilants [s] and [z] may be impaired by abnormal thickness of the incisors, by incorrect antero-posterior positioning of the incisors, or by excessive width of the maxillary arch at the first bicuspids. Correction of the resulting speech defects, Tench indicates, can be achieved by adapting the dentures to the speech habits of the patient.

Slaughter (1945) advocates the construction of two ridges one millimeter thick, curving toward the midline of the palate from the lingual cusps of the first bicuspid and reaching back opposite the first molar. This is said to improve articulation by helping the patient direct the air stream during speech.

Landa (1935) states categorically that the rugae should be omitted from the palatal surface except in special instances, since they add thickness to the palatal surface of the denture and thus use valuable tongue room. Pound (1951) states that the positioning of the teeth, the preservation of adequate tongue room, the correct amount of clearance between the anterior teeth, and the reconstruction of the natural plane of occlusion are all considered to be important. Wepman (1937) indicates that the patient should be warned ahead of time that his speech may be different with the new appliances and that the patient and dentist should discuss the possible adjustments that must be made.

There is undoubtedly much that can be done to improve denture construction for speech and thus to improve the psychological comfort of the patient.

**Dental Anomalies and Personality**

One of the indirect ways in which dental and orofacial anomalies can affect speech is through their relation to personality. Personality, in turn, affects speech through the influence which anxiety, feelings of inferiority, and psychological resistance to the learning of new habits exert on the normal development and use of speech. Personality also is a factor in the development of the orofacial anomalies which affect speech.

Reference has already been made to the ways in which personal habits such as thumb-sucking, finger-sucking, nail-biting, and tongue-sucking contribute to malocclusion. Such habits are based in the personality structure and needs of the individual. Many parents and dentists feel that thumb-sucking is a habit which is to be eliminated as early as possible, without reference to its meaning to the child. This sometimes results in forcible correction of the habit or resort to methods which are more damaging to the personality of the child than the muscular habit is to the orofacial structures. Pearson (1948) reports a case of thumb-sucking in which severe restraints to thumb-sucking brought on stuttering which ceased after the father apologized to the child and permitted her to resume the thumb-sucking. Pearson states that thumb-sucking is a necessary means of gratification for young children, does not deform the mouth or face and, if stopped severely or suddenly, affects the personality adversely. Gesell and Ilg (1943) state that its harmfulness varies greatly with the type of child and associated behavior, but doubt if it has a permanent effect upon denture and occlusion if discontinued by the age of five or six years.

The effects of sucking habits on occlusal development are well documented by Gwynne-Evans (1951) and Rix (1953). The speech clinician who is aware of the complex origins of the habit may discover as much about the etiology of the child's speech defect through an interpretation of the sucking habits in relation to personality as can be learned through a consideration of the mechanical interference which the distorted occlusion imposes upon speech.

The effect of malocclusions upon personality was noted early in the development of medical science. Walker (1941) quotes Albucasis, who lived in the years 936 to 1013 A.D. and wrote in *De Chirugia,* "When a tooth is irregularly placed or projects above the level of the others, a deformity ensues which is particularly displeasing in women." Walker is of the opinion that an inferiority complex, and attitudes of superiority, timidity, selfishness, jealousy, or oversensitiveness all are to be found in people who have dental anomalies. Indications are strong (Glaser, 1946) that dental and surgical treatment cannot always be carried to a successful conclusion as long as the damaging forces of personality distortion persist in counteracting the beneficial effects of the surgical, prosthetic, or orthodontic treatment. Kimball and Muyskens (1937) found that the personality improved in an individual for whom speech was corrected in connection with construction of a dental prosthesis. Kempner (1943) states that carious or missing teeth, unsightly dentures, dental discoloration, malocclusions, or malpositioned teeth cause people to hide their mouths, or talk with their lips together. Gibbin (1939) reported a case of a girl, thirteen, whose morbid consciousness of a dentofacial deformity was supplanted by self-confidence, poise, and sociability after orthodontic treatment and myofunctional therapy. Speech was also greatly improved.

## RESPONSIBILITIES OF THE SPEECH PATHOLOGIST IN RELATION TO DENTAL TREATMENT

The speech pathologist has a number of important functions to perform in relation to the dental specialist and to the patient. These include:

1. Speech diagnosis and professional consultation with the dental specialist
2. Referral of speech patients suspected of having dental conditions which may currently interfere with speech, general health, or personality adjustment
3. Speech therapy and consultation in connection with patients undergoing orthodontic treatment, the construction of artificial dentures or other dental prosthetic devices, or surgical corrections or restorations

The average dental specialist is not a student of speech with enough detailed information about the various anomalies of speech to enable him to make an adequate diagnosis of the patient's speech problems. The speech pathologist should give a clear statement of his evaluation of the patient's speech problem, the probable etiological factors, and the importance of dental treatment in the eventual speech rehabilitation of the patient. A careful speech diagnosis can be helpful to the dentist in planning the time of corrective dental intervention and can help both the dentist and the patient to make a better prognosis of the final results of treatment.

The speech pathologist and speech therapist must be alert to the various conditions which may be present or which are incipient in the pattern of development which the individual seems to be following. Oftentimes the advice of the speech therapist will be a means of getting a child to the dentist for a preventive program which can result in the improvement of oral hygiene, the preservation of the permanent teeth, and the normal development of facial growth. The speech therapist can also be influential in letting parents know how important it is to preserve the deciduous teeth for the health and dental integrity of the growing child.

In referring the child or the adult patient to a dental or surgical specialist, it is important that the speech clinician be conservative in his estimate of the physical changes which can be accomplished. There is a tendency on the part of many individuals to "oversell" the patient on what can be accomplished by adjunct services, with the implication that if failure in the total rehabilitation program falls short of the desired objective, it is the fault of the adjunct service rather than the referring specialist.

The patient who is a candidate for orthodontic treatment frequently will need speech-corrective work at some stage of his treatment program if he is to receive full benefit from the dental correction. A decision must often be made as to whether or not speech-correction measures should await completion of the dental treatment, should be instituted and maintained concurrently with it, or begun prior to dental or surgical treatment. There is merit in any of these choices for certain patients, and the determination as to which shall be chosen should be made by the speech therapist in consultation with the dentist or surgeon.

As a matter of general policy, correction of those speech defects which cannot be directly attributed to the dental or structural anomaly may be undertaken without awaiting dental treatment, but due allowance should be made for the effects which dental appliances may have upon speech. In instances in which a definite relationship between structure and speech function can be established, it is sometimes appropriate to wait for a short time after completion of the dental work to see if the patient can successfully achieve self-correction of his speech.

In some cases it will be helpful to the program of dental treatment if the speech therapist can undertake to train the patient in habits of muscle movement for speech which will be in accord with the pressure patterns designed to promote or maintain the structural changes which the dental specialist is attempting to bring about. Johnson (1940) shows a number of cases in which overdevelopment of the mentalis muscle and underdevelopment of the upper lip may have been a factor in development of the malocclusion (protrusion of the maxillary incisors). For such cases he advises myofunctional therapy timed to accord with the progress of orthodontic treatment. Such therapy includes muscular exercises for development of the upper lip, and similar procedures involving the production of the phoneme [p] in syllable, word, and sentence drills.

One of the foremost advocates of myofunctional therapy was A. P. Rogers (Salzmann, 1950), who contributed significantly to the development of the viewpoint and methods used. Under this theory, muscular imbalance of the

orofacial muscles is considered to be one of the major causes of malocclu-
ion. It is thus a primary tenet of the theory that the re-establishment of
muscular balance is an essential adjunct to mechanical forces, proper nu-
rition, and general health as stimuli to normal growth. His procedures in-
lude attention to general facial and body posture and exercises for the
•terygoid, masseter-temporal, and tongue muscles in addition to those in-
·olving the mentalis and orbicularis oris muscles as described by Johnson
above.

In the construction of complete or partial dentures the speech therapist
may assist the dentist in determining the placement of cross-bars and some-
imes in the placement of the anterior teeth so that the [s] sounds will not
become either strident or occluded. A careful evaluation of the tongue-tip
movements and the labiodental contacts during speech will aid the dentist
n deciding whether or not the teeth are properly positioned to enable the
patients to speak properly.

## BIBLIOGRAPHY

ANDERSON, G. M. 1948. Practical orthodontics (7th ed.). St. Louis: Mosby.

ANGLE, E. H. 1907. Malocclusion of the teeth (7th ed.). Philadelphia: S. S.
White Dental Mfg. Co.

AREY, L. B. 1954. Developmental anatomy (6th ed.). Philadelphia: Saunders.

BACKUS, O. L. 1940. Speech rehabilitation following excision of the tip of the
tongue. *Amer. J. Dis. Child.*, 60, 368–370.

BARCLAY, A. E., and NELSON, W. 1922. The x-ray analysis of the sounds of
speech. *J. Radiology*, 3, 277–280.

BLOOMER, H. H. 1943. A palatopograph for contour mapping of the palate. *J.
Amer. Dent. Assn.*, 30, 1053–1057.

——— 1953. Observations on palatopharyngeal movements in speech and deglutition. *J. Speech Hearing Disorders*, 18, 230–246.

BROWN, G. V. I. 1938. The surgery of oral and facial diseases and malformations. Philadelphia: Lea and Febiger.

COOPER, H. K. 1930. Some thoughts concerning muscle exercises. *Int. J. Orthodontia Oral Surg. Radiography*, 16, 527–534.

COSTEN, J. B. 1936. Some features of the mandibular articulation as it pertains
to otolaryngology. *Int. J. Orthodontia Oral Surg.*, 22, 1011–1017.

CRANE, E., and RAMSTRUM, G. 1943. A classification of palates. Unpublished
Master's Thesis. Univ. Mich.

DINGMAN, R. O. 1944. Osteotomy for the correction of mandibular malrelation
of developmental origin. *J. Oral Surg.*, 2, 239–259.

DOCKRELL, R. B. 1951. A classification of post-normal occlusions. London:
Saward and Co.

ESKEW, H. A., and SHEPARD, E. E. 1949. Congenital aglossia. *Amer. J. Orthodontics*, 35, 116–119.

FORD, J. F. 1944. A plastic operation for lengthening the congenitally short upper
lip. *J. Oral Surg.*, 2, 260–265.

FORDE, T. H. 1951. Oral dynamics. *Dent. Digest*, Jan., Feb., Mar., April.

FROESCHELS, E. 1933. Speech therapy. Boston: Expression Co.

——— 1940. Laws in the appearance and development of voice hyperfunctions.
*J. Speech Disorders*, 5, 1–4.

———— and JELLINEK, A. 1941. Practice of voice and speech therapy. Bostoɪ
Expression Co.

FROWINE, V. K., and MOSER, H. 1944. Relationship of dentition to speech.
Amer. Dent. Assn., 31, 1081–1090.

FYMBO, L. H. 1936. The relation of malocclusion of the teeth to defects of speecʜ
Arch. Speech, June, 204–217.

GARDNER, ALVIN F. 1949. Dental, oral and general causes of speech patholog
Oral Surg., Oral Med., Oral Pathol., 2, 742–751.

GESELL, A., and ILG, F. 1943. Infant and child in the culture of today. Neᵛ
York: Harper.

GIBBIN, F. E. 1939. Macromaxillary and micromandibular development. Ame
J. Orthodontics Oral Surg., 25–7, 657–663.

GLASER, C. G. 1946. Psychotherapy in orthodontics. Amer. J. Orthodontiᴄ
Oral Surg., 32, 341–354.

GOLDBERG, I. 1939. The wonder of words. New York: Appleton-Century.

GOLDSTEIN, M. A. 1940. New concepts of the functions of the tongue. Laryʀ
goscope, 50, 164–188.

GREENE, J. S. 1937. Speech defects and related oral anomalies. J. Amer. Denɪ
Assn. Dent. Cosmos, 24, 1969–1974.

———— 1945. Anomalies of the speech mechanism and associated voice anɪ
speech disorders. N.Y. J. Med., 45, 605–608.

GWYNNE-EVANS, E. 1951. The organization of the oro-facial muscles in relatioɪ
to breathing and feeding. Brit. Dent. J., 91, 135–140.

HARVEY, W. 1948. Investigation and survey of malocclusion and ear symptoɱ
with particular reference to otitic barotrauma (pain in ears due to chang
in altitude). Brit. Dent. J., 85, 219–225.

HEMREND, B., and MOYERS, R. E. 1953. The growth of the carnio-facial skelᴇ
ton. Toronto: (privately printed).

HENRY, O. 1937. Phonetics in orthodontia. Int. J. Orthodontia Oral Surg., 2ɜ
456–461.

HERMAN, G. 1943. A study of palate shape and its characteristics in lispers. Uɾ
published Master's Thesis. Univ. Mich.

HOLBROOK, R. T. 1937. X-ray studies of speech articulations. Berkeley: Uniᵛ
Calif. Press.

JOHNSON, L. R. 1940. Problem of the mentalis muscle in the treatment of maloᴄ
clusion. J. Amer. Dent. Assn., 27, 1046–1054.

JUSTE, J. C. 1948. The masticatory face and the voice. Dent. Record, 6ɛ
309–310.

KANTER, C. E., and WEST, R. 1941. Phonetics. New York: Harper.

KEASTER, J. 1940. Studies in the anatomy and physiology of the tongue. Laryɴ
goscope, 50, 222–257.

KEMPNER, R. D. M., and CHOCK, K. T. 1943. Dentistry in neuropsychiatry, thᴇ
significance of oral sepsis and cosmetic effects. J. Amer. Dent. Assn., 3ᴄ
416–420.

KESSLER, H. E. 1953. Dentistry's part in speech production. Oral Hyg., 43, 108ᴄ

KIMBALL, H. D., and MUYSKENS, J. H. 1937. Speech reconstruction after proᴤ
thesis. J. Amer. Dent. Assn. Dent. Cosmos, 27, 1158–1168.

KINGSLEY, N. W. 1880. A treatise on oral deformities. New York: Appletoɴ

KREMEN, A. J. 1953. Cancer of the tongue. Minn. Med., 36, 828–830.

LANDA, J. H. 1953. The importance of phonetics in full denture prosthesis. Denɪ
Digest, 41, 154–160.

LISCHER, B. E. 1912. Orthodontics, principles and methods of. Philadelphiᴀ
Lea and Febiger.

LOGAN, W. H. G., and KRONFELD, R. 1933. Development of the human jaws anɪ surrounding structures from birth to the age of fifteen years. *Amer. Dent. Assn. J.*, 20, 379–427.

McENERY, E. T., and GAINES, F. P. 1941. Tongue-tie in infants and children. *J. Pediat.*, 18, 252–255.

MASSLER, M., and SCHOUR, I. 1946. Growth of the child and the calcification pattern of the teeth. *Amer. J. Orthodontics Oral Surg.*, 32, 495–517.

MOSES, E. 1936. Palatography, a critical study and analysis of sound-image contacts. Unpublished Doctoral Dissertation. Univ. Mich.

———— 1939. Palatography and speech improvement. *J. Speech Disorders*, 4, 103–114.

MOYERS, R. E. 1949. Temperomandibular muscle contraction patterns in Angle class II, division I malocclusions: an electromyographic analysis. *Amer. J. Orthodontics*, 35 (II), 837–857.

———— 1955. A handbook of orthodontics. Chicago: Year Book Pub.

MUYSKENS, J. H. 1925. The smallest aggregate of speech movement, the hypha, analyzed and defined. Unpublished Doctoral Dissertation. Univ. Mich.

NOYERS, F. B., SCHOUR, I., and NOYES, H. J. 1948. Oral histology and embryology. Philadelphia: Lea and Febiger.

ORBAN, B. 1944. Oral histology and embryology. St. Louis: Mosby.

PALMER, M. F. 1948. Orthodontics and the disorders of speech. *Amer. J. Orthodontics*, 34, 579–588.

PATTEN, B. M. 1953. Human embryology (2nd ed.). New York: Blakiston.

PEARSON, G. H. J. 1948. The psychology of finger-sucking, tongue-sucking, and other oral habits. *Amer. J. Orthodontics*, 34, 589–598.

POUND, E. 1953. Esthetics dentures and their phonetic values. *Dent. J. Australia*, 25, 150–158.

———— 1951. Esthetic dentures and their phonetic values. *J. Prosthetic Dentistry*, 1, 98–111.

PRYOR, W. J. 1933. The closed bite relation of the jaws of George Washington, with comments on his tooth troubles and general health. *J. Amer. Dent. Ass.*, 20, 567–579.

PULLEN, H. A. 1927. Abnormal habits in their relation to malocclusion and facial deformity. St. Louis: Mosby.

RIX, R. E. 1953. Some observations upon the environment of the incisors. *Dent. Record*, 73, 427–441.

RONKIN, S. H. 1953. Improvement of low-tone deafness and tinnitus by mandibular repositioning. *A. M. A. Arch. Otolaryngology*, 56, 669–673.

ROUSSELOT, L. P. J. 1910. Principes de phonétique expérimental nouveau ed. Paris. Paris: Libraire universitaire.

RUSSELL, G. O. 1934. First preliminary x-ray consonant study. *J. acoust. Soc. Amer.*, 5, 247–251.

RUTTLE, A. T., QUIGLEY, W., CROUCH, J. T., and EWAN, G. E. 1953. A serial study of the effects of finger-sucking. *J. Dent. Research*, 32, 739–748.

SALZMANN, J. A. 1950. Principles of orthodontics. Philadelphia: Lippincott.

SCHOUR, I., and MASSLER, M. 1940. Studies in tooth development; the growth pattern of human teeth (Part I). *J. Amer. Dent. Assn.*, 27, 1778–1793.

SLAUGHTER, M. D. 1945. Speech correction in full denture prosthesis. *Dent. Digest*, 51, 242–246.

SPANNENBERG, H. D. 1937. Effects of dental prosthetic appliances on voice quality. Chicago: Year Book Pub.

STALLARD, H. 1930. A consideration of extraoral pressures in the etiology of malocclusions. *Int. J. Orthodontia Oral Surg. Radiography*, 16, 475–526.

WINEHART, D. R. 1950. Importance of tongue in development of normal occlusion. *Amer. J. Orthodontics*, 36, 813–830.

TARNEAUD, J. 1946. La voix et les affections dentaires. *Le Progres Medical,* 17, 374–375.

TENCH, R. W. 1927. The influence of speech habits on the design of full artificial dentures. *J. Amer. Dent. Assn.,* 14, 644–647.

VAN RIPER, C. 1954. Speech correction, principles and methods (3rd ed.). New York: Prentice-Hall.

VAN THAL, J. 1936. The relationship between faults of dentition and defects of speech. Cambridge: Cambridge Univ. Press, 254–257.

WALKER, M. B. 1941. Psychologic effects of malocclusion of the teeth. *Amer. J. Orthodontia Oral Surg.,* 27, 599–604.

WALPOLE-DAY, A. J. 1951. The effect of the condyle on the growth of the mandible. London: Saward and Co.

WATSON, E. H., and LOWREY, G. H. 1954. Growth and development of children (2nd ed.). Chicago: Year Book Pub.

WEPMAN, J. M. 1937. Anatomic speech defects. *J. Amer. Dent. Assn. Dent. Cosmos,* 24, 1799–1804.

WEST, R., KENNEDY, L., and CARR, A. 1947. The rehabilitation of speech (rev. ed.). New York: Harper.

WHEELER, R. C. 1940. Textbook of dental anatomy and physiology. Philadelphia: Saunders.

WOLFE, I. J. 1937. Relationship of malocclusion to sigmatism. *Amer. J. Dis. Child.,* 54, 520–528.

WRIGHT, C. R., STRONG, L. H., KINGERY, R. H., MUYSKENS, J. H., WESTERMAN, K. N., and WILLIAMS, S. T. 1949. A study of the tongue and its relation to denture stability. *J. Amer. Dent. Assn.,* 39, 269–275.

ZAPPLER, S. 1949. Dentistry and the cerebral palsied child. *J. Dentistry Child.* 2nd quar.

# CHAPTER 22

# VOICE DISORDERS ASSOCIATED WITH ORGANIC ABNORMALITIES

## *Paul Moore, Ph.D.*

IN THE academic area known as the field of speech, communication by voice has been divided traditionally into five primary elements: (1) the phonetic and phonemic segments which comprise words and word groups; (2) the sequence of these words and word groups in the rhythmic pattern of the language; (3) the general vocal pitch level and the variations of pitch from moment to moment, often called the melody pattern; (4) the quality or timbre of the voice; and (5) its loudness related to place and circumstances. Speech correctionists routinely relate speech disorders to these five elements, and they consider speech to be defective when any one, or more, of them differs noticeably from that which is customary for the age and sex of the speaker in his particular language and environment. More particularly, when the deviation involves phonetics and phonemics the disorder is labeled "articulatory"; when the rhythmic pattern is interrupted by linguistically meaningless pauses, prolongations, or repetitions, the problem is known as stuttering; when the offending differences are composed of pitch, loudness, or quality deviations, they are classified as voice disorders.

Since the focus of attention in this chapter is on organic voice disorders, the discussion will center on those defects of pitch, loudness, and quality which are related to abnormalities in size, shape, tonicity, surface conditions, and muscular control of the phonating and resonating mechanisms. These differences result from such causes as heredity, disease, injury, abuse, and surgery.

The foregoing statement suggests three levels or types of phenomena which are present in voice defects and which are basic to the present discussion. The first is the symptom, the acoustic element—that which is heard and labeled as the voice defect. The second is the abnormal function of the mechanism which produces the acoustic deviation; and the third is the pathology, the basic condition of disease, injury, and so on, which is of primary concern in diagnosis and treatment. Each of these three levels is intertwined with the others, but for systematic presentation each requires separate consideration.

The problems which are heard as abnormal pitch, intensity, or quality ar
directly related to the mechanisms of the respiratory tract and to their as
sociated structures. When voice defects are present, it means that the voca
cords or the resonators are not functioning normally. This may result from
the way the individual learned to use these structures, that is, *functiona*
problems; or it may stem directly from growths, diseases, loss of tissue, sys
temic conditions, structural anomalies, or paralysis, which may be con
sidered as *organic* causes of voice defects.

It should be emphasized at the outset, however, that there is no shar
division between organic and functional voice problems. It is rather a con
tinuum, since malfunction often produces structural change and, conversely
vocally detrimental habits may develop in the presence of structural anoma
lies or disease, the alleviation of which sometimes allows the malfunction t
remain.

## PHONATORY THEORY

It is not the province of this section of the book to consider the variou
theories of voice production, but since different points of view do exist, an
since certain voice defects must be discussed in relation to theory, there ar
a few fundamental concepts which should be reviewed here briefly.

In normal vocalization, the breath meets the approximated vocal cord
and forces them apart, thereby allowing the air to escape until the elasticit
of the cords and the reduced lateral pressure in the glottis resulting from
the flow of air closes them. When the air pressure below the cords again
becomes great enough to overcome the cord resistance, they are forced open
and so the cycle of vibration is repeated. This alternating flowing and stop
ping, or slowing of the breath, creates pressure changes in the air of the
respiratory tract which are transmitted to the external atmosphere, an
hence to the ear of the listener. In the present discussion, it is relativel
unimportant as to whether the sound is generated entirely by the air pulse
and the cavity resonances, by the surfaces of the cords, or by a combination
of phenomena. As Fletcher (1953) points out, the phenomena can be de
scribed in several ways, with each serving the needs of the user. However
it is important for the student of voice disorders to understand the laryngea
physiology related to pitch, loudness, and quality if he expects to diagnose
and treat voice disorders successfully.

The pitch of the voice is directly related to the frequency of movement o
the vocal cords, and this factor is determined primarily by their mass and
stiffness, or elasticity, in relation to their length. The heavier and more mas
sive the cords, other factors constant, the slower they will vibrate and the
lower will be the pitch of the voice. Conversely, the greater the elasticity o
the cords, the quicker they will tend to return to their position of rest whe

disturbed by the breath stream; hence the faster the rate of movement and the higher the pitch. In two sets of vocal cords having the same cross section and the same tension, but of different length, the longer cord will vibrate more slowly. On the other hand, the lengthening—stretching—of a given set of vocal cords causes a decrease in cross-sectional area and an increase in elasticity. The latter two changes offset the increased length and the frequency increases. If one or both cords have their mass increased by a growth, swelling, or other causes, the frequency decreases and the pitch is lower. These relationships may be expressed by the equation:

$$\text{Frequency} = \tfrac{1}{2} \text{ Length of vibrator } \sqrt{\frac{\text{Tension}}{\text{Mass}}} \text{(Gray and Wise, 1947, p. 114)}$$

The loudness of the voice is produced by the pressure of the released pulsations. Additional pressure causes an increase in the amplitude of the movement of the air molecules, with a consequent increase in the excursion of the eardrum, and hence a louder sound. Greater pressure is acquired through a delicate balance between increased resistance at the vocal cords and greater air flow.

The quality of voice is determined both by vocal cord vibration and resonance. The phonatory aspect includes the manner of air release related to the vibratory pattern of the vocal cords.

If, for any reason, the breath flow is not completely interrupted or the air escapes in such a way as to create turbulences, noises are produced which are heard as breathiness or hoarseness. Other noise elements, particularly those heard in "wet hoarseness," probably result from transient disturbances on the surfaces of the vocal cords and within the substitute sound generators of surgically altered structures.

To reiterate, the movements of the vocal cords, caused by the breath pressure, determine the pitch, intensity, and some of the qualities of the voice, especially the varieties of hoarseness.

## DESCRIPTION OF VOICE DISORDERS

### Phonatory Voice Deviations

**Pitch.** There are three types of vocal-pitch deviations: (1) those which are consistently higher (in relation to the musical scale) than are customarily found among persons of the same age and sex in a particular cultural group; (2) those which are lower (in reference to the same circumstances); and (3) those which do not fit the meaning being expressed, including such deviations as bizarre melody patterns, monotone, and tremulousness.

**Loudness.** Disorders of loudness may be described similarly to those of pitch: (1) too loud in relation to the place and circumstances; (2) inadequate loudness related to the environmental needs; and (3) variations which are not appropriate to the meaning.

**Quality.** Quality deviations are the most common and the most comple
of the voice problems. There are two general types: (1) those associated wit
the sound generation at the vocal cords—phonatory; and (2) those related t
sound modification—the resonance problems. The phonatory defects, liste
as dysphonias, should be thought of on a continuous scale extending fror
aphonia (no phonation) through intermittent phonation, breathiness, dr
hoarseness, wet hoarseness, and rough hoarseness.

The aphonic voice is a whisper. In some aphonic patients the whispere
speech flows smoothly. The vocal cords do not interfere with the outgoin
breath and they do not vibrate. In others, however, the air flow is inter
rupted by momentary, spasmodic closure of the glottis, which causes th
speech to be halting and arhythmic. Occasionally, as the spasmodic closur
is released, there will be a moment of voiced sound. When this occurs fre
quently it produces one type of intermittent phonation. Another form o
intermittency may occur in direct relation to the force of the exhaled ai
stream. In this instance, the voice breaks suddenly from a whisper to pho
nated sound and back again at frequent intervals, often several times within
word. Almost always the phonated portions are of defective quality, eithe
breathy or hoarse.

The breathy voice is composed of relatively weak vocal cord sounds an
whisper sounds. Usually some pitch variation is present, and almost alway
the general intensity is diminished. The breathy voice is apt to suggest a lac
of physical vitality.

The acoustic characteristics of dry hoarseness are somewhat similar t
those which distinguish breathiness. The former is louder, and the breatl
sounds are more prominent. The speaker often shows signs of strain whil
speaking; the blood vessels and muscles of the neck may become prominen
Some persons who have a breathy voice under ordinary circumstances wil
have a dry hoarseness when they attempt to speak loudly. The problem i
common, and there are many who have a dry hoarseness at all times.

Wet hoarseness has been produced at times by most persons during a
attack of laryngitis. The acoustical structure of this voice quality is quit
complex. It derives its characteristic quality from three separately audibl
components: (1) a low-pitched sound from the cords; (2) a breath nois
similar to that heard in whispering; and (3) a sound which is closely relate
to the breath noise, and may be likened to the relatively constant static o
"frying" noises from a radio. These latter give the "wet" sound to the hoarse
ness and result from pressure changes in the breath stream, probably pro
duced by transient disturbances in the mucus on the cords, and on the othe
soft, moist surfaces which may contribute to sound generation. An extrem
example of the latter is often found in esophageal speech.

The term *rough hoarseness* indicates a severe phonatory defect which i
very complex acoustically, and which has a specific identifying characteristic
There are two vocal cord sounds present simultaneously: one at the expecte
pitch for the age and sex of the individual, the other at a very low pitch. Th

combination of pitches is usually accompanied by a wet hoarseness. The double pitch is present when the vocal cords vibrate at different frequencies. This condition may be caused by a unilateral vocal-cord paralysis, a change in the mass of one cord resulting from a growth or disease, or a surgical modification.

### Resonance Voice Problems

At this point it is appropriate to add a description of the resonance voice defects to distinguish them from the phonatory defects just considered. There are two which are associated closely with organic conditions and which, therefore, deserve mention here. These are excessive nasality and its physiological opposite, denasality.

**Nasality.** Nasality is a general symptom classification including all those voices which have an excessive nasal component. Acoustically, the nasal voice is composed of the customary sounds of speech with a simultaneous overlay of nasal sound. That is, the vowels are recognizable, yet they are distorted by the additional nasal element. The intensity of the audible portion of the nasal component determines the severity of the voice defect. This variation seems to be directly related physiologically to the size of the velopharyngeal opening and the degree of closure of the mouth cavity. It may be related acoustically, also, to the formants of the vowels in such a way as to emphasize the characteristic nasal frequency components with some vowels and to suppress the nasal component with others.

Nasal voices of organic origin vary considerably in quality and severity. Some are almost unintelligible, while others differ only a little from normal speech. The quality may be openly resonant, as found typically with cleft palate, paralysis of the velopharyngeal constrictors, congenitally short palate, or perforated palate; or the quality may be "twangy," such as that which anyone can produce by pinching the nostrils and "talking into the nose." Frequently the open nasality (rhinolalia aperta) is accompanied by superfluous noises caused by the uncontrolled rush of air through the air passages during the production of plosive and fricative consonants. The "twangy" voice referred to is caused by the combination of an anterior blockage in the nasal passages and an open velopharyngeal area. This allows the nose to serve as a resonator as far forward as the region of blockage, thereby emphasizing the nasal formants; and hence the characteristic quality. This voice (rhinolalia clausa anterior) is not accompanied by the extra air noises of the rhinolalia aperta.

**Denasality.** Denasality, another resonance problem, is acoustically quite different from excessive nasality; but because they are both associated with abnormalities of the nasal passages, they are usually discussed together. Denasality results from the reduction in, or absence of, the normally expected nasal component. It is most obvious in the production of the nasal consonants. The quality has been exhibited by most persons during a severe "head cold," when the nasal passages are blocked. When the voice defect is chronic, it means that there is a relatively constant obstruction in the naso-pharyn or posterior part of the nasal passages. A common term for this voice i *rhinolalia clausa posterior.*

Rhinolalia becomes complicated further in those instances where ther is a partial posterior obstruction associated with inadequate velopharyngea closure. This voice may be illustrated by the person with a head cold wh purposely tries to nasalize his speech. Those sounds which are normall nonnasal become somewhat nasal, and the nasal consonants are more or les denasal. Both qualities are audible in the same voice.

## THE PHYSIOLOGY OF ORGANIC VOICE DEFECTS

In the foregoing section, an attempt has been made to describe the acousti aspects of voice defects. These are the symptoms of abnormal behavior o function of the voicing mechanism. In the present section, the acousti phenomena will be linked with the organic deviations causing the atypica behavior. Somewhat later in this discussion, the underlying pathologies whic produce the organic changes will be introduced.

### Pitch Defects

**Chronically high pitch.** A consistently high-pitched voice in the late ado lescent and adult male is one of the most distressing of voice defects. Th resemblance to the female voice suggests a lack of masculinity. It is thi implication, with its psychosocial sequelae, which creates the seriousness c the disorder, since the voice proper does not interfere with communicatior nor would it be unpleasant if it were produced by a female.

Most "juvenile voices" are functional, but there are three organic origin which are found occasionally. The first of these is where the larynx fails t develop to the necessary size to produce a masculine pitch. In this instanc the cords are small, as in the female larynx, and therefore vibrate mor rapidly, producing a higher pitch than is normally expected. Sometime this small larynx accompanies a general structural retardation, or is part c a characteristic familial body size. The larynx may fail to develop, also, a a result of insufficient gonadal influence. This glandular lack is usuall demonstrated simultaneously in the retardation of other secondary sex cha acteristics.

The second organic cause of high-pitched voice is laryngeal web. Usuall this is a congenital condition, but may be cicatricial. Webs vary considerabl in size, and when large will interfere with breathing, thereby demandin early medical attention. Those which are small enough to go undetecte until the voice is observed as being different constitute the focus of attentio here. This is justified by the fact that the speech therapist is apt to be th first professional worker concerned with the problem.

A web is a shelf-like membranous development usually extending fro the anterior portion of the larynx and ordinarily attached to the vocal cord

ts effect is to shorten the vibrating portions of the cords, and hence to produce a faster oscillation and a resultant higher pitch. Sometimes hoarseness
s also present, accompanied by the audible evidence of strain, particularly
with the adult males who have attempted to force a lower pitch.

The third organic cause for a chronically high pitch is an abnormal approximation of the vocal cords. In this condition, a structural asymmetry
causes one vocal process of an arytenoid to slide under or over the other so
that the posterior segments of the vocal cords are pressed together, thereby
damping the movement in these areas and effectively limiting the vibrating
portions to the anterior sections. This increases the vibrating rate and raises
the pitch.

**Abnormally low pitch.** A masculine-type voice in a female is as distressing
to the one possessing it as the high-pitched voice in the male, and for the
same types of psychosocial reasons. An excessively low pitch in the male
may also constitute a voice defect, and it also frequently interferes with
communication. The persistent low pitch is generally caused by an organic
change in the larynx. The cords will vibrate slowly when they are weighted
by edema or growths, or when they are flaccid as the result of nerve damage.

Three possible pathological causes of low pitch have been observed in
the clinic with which the writer is associated: hormonal therapy, growths,
and nerve damage. A masculine type of voice developed rather suddenly in
two adult females following a period of male-hormone therapy, and the defect persisted after the cessation of the therapy. Mirror examination of the
larynx failed to show any significant changes. An assumption of psychogenic
involvement is not justified by the data. This leaves the possibility of either
internal changes in the vocal cords, modification of cartilagenous articulations, or edema along the under surfaces of the vocal cords. Any one, or a
combination of these, could produce the deviation. Continuing observation
and study should eventually provide an answer.

Weighting of the cords by tumors and other growths produces a low pitch
and hoarseness. Growths anywhere on the vocal cords tend to increase the
mass in two ways: (1) by direct addition of tissue; and (2) by edema and
inflammation caused by the growth. The additional mass slows the vibration rate, and thereby produces a lower pitch. Usually, a growth which is
extensive enough to cause a defectively low pitch will also produce a hoarseness, and the voice is apt to be classified under the latter heading.

Damage to the nerve supply of the larynx may cause a flaccid paralysis in
one or both cords, and, consequently, a low pitch. With both cords involved,
there may be an aphonia unless the arytenoids can be approximated. In the
latter instance, and also where only one cord is paralyzed, the elasticity of
the cords is reduced, thereby causing them to vibrate more slowly. The low
pitch of paralysis is often accompanied by hoarseness, which is usually more
prominent than the low pitch, and therefore represents the customary classification of the defect.

In the preceding description of pitch defects, a reference was made to tremulousness and similar pitch disorders. Most of these are functional rather than organic, and, therefore, are discussed in the appropriate chapter of this book. However, there is an occasional tremulous voice, or a voice without pitch changes, which is caused by deterioration or injury to the central nervous system. In these cases, the other physical symptoms are so pronounced that the voice is of relatively minor importance, and deserves no more than simple recognition here.

### Loudness Defects

Voices which are too loud or not loud enough are usually functional in origin. The most evident partial exception to the general statement is in those loudness differences which are associated with hearing loss. In this situation the symptom is corrected by improving the hearing rather than by attention to the voice.

Weak voices are often caused by paresis, or paralysis, in the larynx or in some of the muscles of respiration. When the cords cannot interrupt the flow of breath enough to allow subglottal pressure to develop, or when the muscles of exhalation are unable to provide sufficient air pressure in the trachea for vigorous activation of the cords, then a weak voice will result.

### Quality Defects

**Aphonia.** The absence of vocal sound indicates that the vocal cords are not vibrating. There are two general organic conditions under which this may occur: when the vocal cords cannot be approximated sufficiently to be set in motion by the air stream; and when the cords themselves are not capable of vibrating, even when approximated. The former condition may occur under three circumstances: (1) adductor paralysis; (2) ankylosis of the crico arytenoid joint or joints; or (3) the presence of an interarytenoid mass large enough to prevent approximation.

The second general condition exists, or tends to be present, under three circumstances also: (1) when one or both cords have been surgically removed; (2) when there is a growth on, or adjacent to, the cords in such a position as to prohibit their vibration; or (3) when they are too stiff with scar tissue, thickened tissue, or edema to oscillate in the air stream. These concepts may be restated for diagnostic application by saying that when there is an organic aphonia there is either a paralysis, a fixation of the crico arytenoid joints, a massive growth, the absence of one or both cords, a destructive disease, or a systemic condition producing extensive edema.

Occasionally there are persons who are intermittently aphonic. Their voices represent a wide range of vocal inadequacy. Some are aphonic most of the time, others are so only occasionally. The underlying conditions in these patients are similar to the chronic aphonics, but the paralysis, joint fixations, and so on, are less severe than in complete aphonia.

Breath pressure may also be an important factor in intermittent aphonia

Sometimes the cords may be vibrated by sharply increasing the flow of air in exhalation.

Some persons exhibit an intermittency in which the whispered and phonated sounds change from one to the other rapidly and repeatedly, often several times within a word. This condition frequently accompanies large vocal nodules or edematous cords. The phonated portions of this speech are always defective, and may be so prominent that the casual listener does not notice the intermittency.

The continuum of voice defects mentioned earlier is undoubtedly evident to the reader in this discussion of aphonia. Within this single term, there has been a range from complete voicelessness to almost unnoticeable intermittency associated with defective voice quality, usually of a breathy type. Therefore the transition to a discussion of breathy voice is only a progression along the scale of voice defects.

**Breathy voice.** The vocal cords vibrate in the production of a breathy voice, but they are unable to hold back the air stream long enough for much increase in infraglottal pressure. There is either a very short closed phase in the vibratory cycle or, as is more commonly present when breathiness results from organic disorders, the glottis cannot close completely. The air flows more or less continuously, thereby producing audible turbulence with a weak phonated component.

The organic conditions related to breathy voice are similar to those associated with aphonia, but there are some differences. The most prominent are: (1) the involvement of one cord rather than two; and (2) smaller growths, or more restricted areas of pathology. Each of the organic conditions deserves brief mention.

Adductor paralysis of one cord allows that cord to remain in an abducted position. The unaffected cord moves to the normal position of phonation; or it may have developed the capacity to cross beyond the midline and to approach the paralyzed cord. As a general rule, the closer the approximation, the stronger the voice (the less the breathiness).

A breathy voice may occur also with tensor paralysis which involves the cords proper and may be present even when the arytenoids move normally. In this condition the cords are bowed, thereby allowing wastage and turbulence of the air. A person with this type of voice exhibits considerable effort in speaking. "A little conversational use causes the patient to say his 'voice is tired,' or his 'throat is tired.' " (Jackson and Jackson, 1937, p. 299.)

A similar bowed appearance and voice defect as that observed with tensor paralysis may result, also, from myasthenia. The vocal difference between tensor paralysis and myasthenia is greater variability in the voices of patients with myasthenia. ". . . in paralysis the muscle is permanently out of function; whereas in myasthenia there is great irregularity, sometimes tension is fairly good, at other times it fails. Moreover, a regime of silence will temporarily restore activity in myasthenia laryngis; it will not do so in paralysis." (Jackson and Jackson, 1937, p. 301.)

The breathy voice produced when an arytenoid cartilage is paralyzed in an abducted position is duplicated when an arytenoid is fixed in a similar position by ankylosis of the crico-arytenoid joint. Jackson and Jackson hold the opinion that the condition is more common than is indicated in the literature, and that it is often misdiagnosed as recurrent paralysis (Jackson and Jackson, 1937, p. 102).

The common factor responsible for the breathiness in the conditions just discussed was the inability of the vocal cords to approximate properly. This lack of approximation permits air to rush through the larynx more or less continuously and to be made noisily turbulent by the irregular structures protruding into the air stream. There are other organic disorders which also affect the approximation of the arytenoid cartilages and which produce a breathy voice. These are the growths and other conditions which are on the medial surfaces of the arytenoids or in the posterior commissure. They include contact ulcer, thickened tissues, and benign and malignant tumors.

It should be noted that these conditions do not invariably cause breathiness. The amount of relaxation, the degree of approximation permitted by the obstruction, and the urgency of the vocal effort, as reflected in both the flow of air and the muscle tension in the larynx, will determine whether the voice is aphonic, breathy, or hoarse at any particular time.

Growths on the glottal edges of the vocal cords proper provide another mechanical interference which may cause a breathy voice. During the vibratory cycle of the cords, any protrusion on the cord edge will meet the opposite cord and prevent an adequate closure. Very little infra-glottal air pressure can be developed, and the constantly escaping air creates turbulence which is the source of the defective sound.

Both the size and degree of hardness of the growths are related to the voice quality. Generally, a large mass produces more breathiness. However, an equally faulty voice may be caused by a smaller growth which is hard and not compressible. As indicated previously, the quality will also vary in a given case with the amount of vocal effort; that is, a growth which causes a breathy voice in quiet conversation may produce hoarseness when the individual attempts to speak loudly.

The common growths on the cords which are responsible for breathiness and other voice deviations include nodules, hematoma, papilloma, polyps, keratosis, and, of course, malignant tumors. The speech correctionist does not diagnose such disorders, but he is obligated to understand their causes when they can be known, as well as their implications related to voice therapy.

When part of one vocal cord has been removed, three conditions remain which affect phonation: (1) the missing tissue, usually in the anterior section creates a concavity which the unaffected cord cannot close and through which air escapes, causing turbulence. The excision of the whole cord produces a larger opening, and, from the phonation standpoint, approaches the situation which is present in adductor paralysis or ankylosis of the cricoarytenoid joint, when the arytenoid is fixed in a lateral position. (2) Scar tissue forms at the site of the surgery, thereby presenting a relatively stiff shelf which has little or no vibration, but which may assist the mobile cord toward a vibratory closure through its passive position. At best, the function is inefficient, and there is considerable air wastage. (3) The removal of some or all of the thyro-arytenoid muscle tissue limits the adducting movement of the arytenoid cartilage, with the result that any portion of the cord remaining after surgery can be made only incidentally effective in the vibratory movement.

Edema may be associated with various conditions and diseases, which will be discussed later, but the important fact is that the swelling interferes mechanically with a normal vibratory pattern and may cause a breathy voice. The movements of vibration can change in several ways. The data are not conclusive at this time, but clinical observations suggest that edema, either inflammatory or noninflammatory, causes a stiffening of the cords. This is somewhat analogous, in effect, to the inflation of a balloon: the extent of inflation determines the degree of stiffness. The stiffness reduces the flexibility of the cords so that the undulating movements, which begin just anterior to the midpoint of the cords at the moment of the cord separation in the vibratory cycle and progress toward both ends, are reduced or eliminated. This allows much more air to be released suddenly in each cycle, with a consequent complex turbulence just above the cords.

Another factor which should be noted is that the constantly changing muscle tension in the cords is also related to the effects of the edema. That is, a relatively small amount of swelling might produce breathiness only at higher pitches, when the cords are stretched and the muscles of the cords are tensed. At this point, the swelling becomes effective by adding to the stiffness. On the other hand, at the lowest pitches, when the cords are shortened and relatively flexible, the edema may serve only to weight the cords; that is, to increase their mass, slow their rate of movement, and cause a lower pitch.

Discussions of breathy voice usually imply some association with the adequacy of breath supply. Adequacy may be expressed in two ways: the amount of air available; and the force with which it is expelled. Clinical evidence indicates that a reduced air supply, such as that resulting from the collapse or removal of one lung, is not, in itself, a cause of breathiness. The condition may result in shorter phrases and "shortness of breath," particularly under stress, but this is not a true breathiness. There are many persons with a low vital capacity who have normal voices. There is also substantial clinical evidence that reduced breath pressure alone is not a cause of breathiness. If low pressure produced the defect, a person with a normal voice would necessarily have a breathy voice whenever he uttered a tone of low intensity. It is obvious that trained singers can intone a clear nonbreathy voice which is scarcely audible. The critical element is the adjustment of the vocal cords in relation to the breath pressure.

In view of the foregoing observations, recognition should be made of the

fact that persons who are fatigued or ill, or who have a paralysis involving
the muscles of breathing, often have a breathy voice. Under most circum
stances, this is only part of the involvement. In these cases, the condition i
usually not limited to the muscles of respiration but includes also the muscle
of the larynx. The laryngeal component is responsible for the voice defect
but the combination of reduced breath pressure and weakened vibrator
control in the larynx tends to exaggerate the vocal defect which would have
resulted from the laryngeal weakness alone. The heightened effect comes
at least in part, from the person's lessened ability to compensate in som
measure for the reduced muscular control. That is, patients with only th
laryngeal involvement probably learn to regulate the breath stream for maxi
mum possible efficiency of voice production. Those with paralysis in th
breathing musculature only probably learn compensatory laryngeal adjust
ments.

**Dry hoarseness.** Each term which is used to label a voice problem en
compasses a variety of similar problems scattered along a section of th
continuum of voice defects. The differences between some of the voice de
fects may be so slight that their classification becomes somewhat arbitrary
Furthermore, as has been indicated previously, the voice of a person ma
vary from day to day in relation to his physical condition; or it may diffe
from moment to moment in accord with pitch and loudness changes. On
example of the similarity between types of voice defects may be noted i
breathiness and dry hoarseness. These qualities are somewhat alike, but i
dry hoarseness the voice is louder and has a relatively stronger phonate
element.

The physiology of dry hoarseness is similar to that of breathiness. Th
reader need only substitute the concept of dry hoarseness for breathiness i
the foregoing section of the physiology of breathiness, and add the minut
laryngeal differences which are necessary for the production of the louder
less breathy voice to obtain an understanding of the laryngeal behavior i
"dry hoarseness."

**Wet hoarseness.** Wet hoarseness is quite different from breathiness an
dry hoarseness. It occurs when something in the larynx creates noises which
are heard as part of, and in addition to, vocal-cord sounds. These noise
seem to arise from transient disturbances on the surfaces and edges of th
cords. To understand this type of voice, it is helpful to keep in mind th
processes of transient-wave generation and to relate them to the variou
organic conditions associated with wet hoarseness.

Transients are relatively brief disturbances which occur in structure
electrical circuits, resonators, and so on, as the result of a sudden change c
conditions (Beranek, 1949). Transient waves are created in a vibrating soun
source, as in a string, when it is touched, struck, or shortened suddenly
These transients can be created on the vocal cords, also, by any conditio
which would interfere momentarily with the normal cycle of vibration. Suc
interferences with vocal-cord movement can be grouped into four categorie

for this discussion: (1) excessive sticky mucus on the vocal cords; (2) relative flabbiness of one or both of the vocal cords; (3) additions to the mass of the cords; and (4) the destruction of all or part of a cord. Each of these deserves brief consideration as a basis for diagnosis and investigation.

When there is too much mucus on the cords, from any cause, there will be a wet hoarseness. The characteristic sounds of this voice defect seem to be produced by either of two factors, or their combination. First, excessive mucus tends to interfere with the normal undulating movements of the cords by weighting them unevenly, and by damping their excursion through causing them to adhere to each other. Accumulations of sticky mucus, particularly at the anterior and posterior commissures, appear to cling to the cords and to act as elastic bands or membranes between the cords. These probably slow the rate of vibration of the cords, thereby producing a lower pitch. It is probable, also, that mucous sounds are produced when the cords pull away from each other during the opening phase of the vibratory cycle. The elastic mucous particles stretch and break, producing many transient disturbances. It is possible that this action is somewhat similar to separating pieces of lightly adherent tape. The adhesive action would be more pronounced, of course, when larger areas of mucous membrane are brought into contact, a condition which is present, for example, when the person with a normal larynx purposely produces a wet hoarseness. The cords are squeezed together tightly so that their contacting portions are flattened against each other, and these surfaces are thereby enlarged during the closed phases of the vibration. This provides much more mucus to stretch and break as the cords separate in the opening phase of the cycle.

The second way in which mucus may contribute to wet hoarseness is through the vibration of mucus globules. These accumulations on the surfaces of the vocal cords become secondary vibrators which are agitated by the vocal cords, and thereby probably produce many transients. This phenomenon is commonly visible in high-speed motion pictures of the vocal cords.

Flaccidity of the vocal cords can exist with adductor paralysis, with the lateral fixation of an arytenoid cartilage, or with loose mucous membrane over the cords. The first two conditions have been related to breathiness and dry hoarseness, but it is obvious to the clinician that they also cause wet hoarseness. It appears that the affected cord may interfere with the unaffected cord, or the flaccid cord may be set into somewhat independent vibration. Either of these situations could create transient disturbances. It should be observed, too, that excessive mucus is usually present in these conditions, which contributes to the voice characteristic.

When there is difficulty in approximating the cords, as in these conditions, there is often a compensatory sphincter-like contraction of the superior parts of the larynx. The ventricular cords may be pressed together, and the epiglottis frequently meets the anterior surfaces of the arytenoids to create constrictions which have been seen to vibrate in the production of sound. These adjustments always produce wet hoarseness, probably because there are extensive areas of flabby, moist membranes which are pushed apart by the air stream, thereby creating the transient phenomena thought to be responsible for the voice defect.

Loose mucous membrane has been observed in high-speed motion pictures of the vocal cords. In this condition, the membrane seems to slide over the firmer underlying structures somewhat as the skin moves on the head of a bloodhound. This mucosa is sometimes free enough to swing over the glottal rim to meet the opposite member following the impact of the cords upon each other. The surface disturbances are irregular in shape, and probably create many high-frequency transient sound waves.

It was pointed out previously that a mass on a vocal cord may cause a pitch change, breathiness, or hoarseness by weighting it, by stiffening it, or by keeping the glottis from closing completely. A growth may rest on one or both cords in such a way that it is vibrated with the cord, thereby becoming a secondary sound source; or it may be jiggled if it rests more or less loosely on a cord. In the latter case, it interferes with the vibration of the cords and creates additional noise. Furthermore, a growth is usually accompanied by excess mucus which contributes to the generation of wet hoarseness, as described in a preceding paragraph.

Hypertrophic conditions in areas adjacent to the cords may also cause wet hoarseness. An example of this was observed in a patient who had an enlarged left ventricular fold which covered the left vocal cord and also rested on part of the right cord during phonation. The false cord in this instance interfered with the motion of the true cords and, in addition, was jostled into movements of its own. Flabby, moist surfaces contributed to the complex vibratory disturbances which were present.

The surgical removal of all or part of a vocal cord often causes wet hoarseness. The vocal sound is produced by a constriction in the superior part of the larynx sufficient to interrupt the breath stream. This may occur at the ventricular folds, or at the contact point between the posterior surface of the epiglottis and the anterior surfaces of the arytenoids. The membranes in these areas are supplied generously with mucus. The situation is similar to that described earlier under flaccidity of the cords when caused by unilateral adductor paralysis or the fixation of an arytenoid cartilage.

**Rough hoarseness.** The voice quality called "rough hoarseness" is similar to wet hoarseness, but it contains additional low-pitched sounds which give the "rough" characteristic. Those anomalies previously associated with wet hoarseness may also cause rough hoarseness if the growth, paralysis, and so on, creates a secondary sound source which vibrates at a low frequency.

It has been observed that when one vocal cord is flaccid it tends to flutter at a low frequency, while the other cord moves in a relatively normal manner. The flutter is most apt to occur when there is a vigorous breath stream.

Growths cause rough hoarseness in either of two ways: (1) by weighting one cord in relation to the other, thereby slowing the vibration rate of the heavier cord and causing a double tone; or (2) by the growth extending outward from the cord so that it rests on the opposite cord, or otherwise interferes with the vibratory pattern. The presence of a growth frequently produces excessive mucus which contributes to the general hoarseness. The result is a low-pitched component combined with the sounds of wet hoarseness.

## Resonance Defects

**Nasality.** Any condition which prevents the closure of the velopharyngeal area will produce excessive nasality. The organic causes for this voice defect may be grouped under two general headings: (1) the absence of sufficient structure to make the closure; and (2) the inability to manipulate the structure. The absence of tissue may be congenital, as with the cleft palate and short palate; or it may be the result of destructive disease, such as tumors or syphillis; or it may follow surgery, either on the palate or for the removal of adenoids. In the latter instance, the excessive nasality sometimes resulting from the removal of the adenoid growth indicates that this tissue occasionally contributes to the velopharyngeal closure, and that upon removal the other structures are unable to compensate.

The inability to manipulate the structures is associated primarily with paralyses. Unilateral or bilateral involvement of either velar or pharyngeal muscles will interefere with the proper closure. It should be noted that the opening into the nasopharynx need not be very large. This means that relatively little organic involvement may cause a marked nasalization of speech. It also means that vocal recovery may be slower than the functional recovery in cases of paralysis, surgical repair, etc. It is not unusual to observe adequate velopharyngeal control for swallowing and the production of isolated sounds, but at the same time to discover inadequate closure in the rapid movements required for speaking.

**Denasality.** This voice deviation is usually an organic problem, and results from obstruction in the posterior portion of the nasal passages or nasopharynx. The organic conditions are varied and include: (1) growths of many types; (2) hypertrophy associated with chronic nasal disease; (3) allergies which cause swelling of the nasal membranes; and (4) trauma, with its sequelae of deviated septum, nasal spurs, and congestion.

This voice deviation is most evident on the normally nasal sounds, but it gives the whole speech pattern a characteristic dullness, similar to that observed in persons having a "head cold."

Obstruction of the nasal passages produces other problems, also, which are potentially significant in evaluating the vocal re-education for the patient. The obstruction causes mouth-breathing, which results in drying of the pharyngeal and laryngeal mucosa and which might adversely affect phonation.

## Summary of Categories of Organic Voice Defects

The normal physiology of sound generation and resonation may be altered by diseases, growth, paralyses, malformations, loss of tissue, and so on. From the physio-acoustic standpoint, the importance of these anomalies in causing voice defects is in the way they modify the basic functional pattern of voice production. These modifications may be grouped into six categories: (1) those which destroy the customary resonances by blocking or compressing the upper parts of the respiratory channel, or by eliminating the capacity to control the size of the orifices which connect the sections of the resonators (growths, velopharyngeal paralysis, congenitally inadequate palate, cleft palate, and nasal diseases); (2) those which interefere with the movements of the arytenoids and the adduction of the cords (adductor paralysis, arthritis and ankylosis of the cricoarytenoid joints, interarytenoid growths, and hypertrophic tissue); (3) those which interfere mechanically with the vibrations of the cords (growths, edema, engorgement, scars, asymmetrical arytenoid approximation, and excessive mucus); (4) those which alter the contractile ability and tonicity of the cords (tensor paralysis, and myasthenia laryngis); (5) those which change the mucosal surface conditions of the cords causing extraneous noises (excessive sticky mucus, loose mucous membrane, dry mucosa, and scars); and (6) those in which essential tissue is absent (surgical removal, injury, destructive diseases).

## ETIOLOGIES OF THE ORGANIC CONDITIONS WHICH CAUSE VOICE DEFECTS

In the foregoing parts of this discussion, an attempt was made, first, to describe the sound characteristics—the audible symptoms—of the various voice defects which have an organic basis; and, second, to present the physiology of these problems, with particular attention to the organic deviations causing the vocal defects. The purpose of the present section is to present the underlying organic pathologies, in so far as that can be accomplished in this type of discussion. This is not done to suggest that the voice therapist should attempt any type of medical diagnosis, but rather to provide some insight into the basic causes for the voice defects. It is these, of course, which are the foci of therapy.

Jackson and Jackson (1942, pp. 47–48) list over sixty specific diseases associated with hoarseness in adults, and more than thirty-five in children. Some are chronic, others acute. The voice therapist must be concerned primarily with the chronic conditions, since they are associated with the voice problems requiring voice therapy. The etiology of chronic laryngeal disease is complex, but must be a part of the thinking of those who work with voice problems. Similarily, the chronic diseases of the nose and nasopharynx should be kept in mind, since they are direct causes of resonance faults and may also be indirect causes of phonatory defects.

The list of chronic laryngeal disease etiologies used by Jackson and Jackson (1942, p. 38) is the most detailed in the literature and forms a perspective for the present section:

| | |
|---|---|
| Age and sex | Lack of personal hygiene |
| Vocal abuse | Clothing |
| Tobacco | Climate |
| Alcohol | Environment |
| Dust | Allergy |
| War gases and other vapors | Trauma |
| Mouth-breathing | Instrumentation |
| Air-borne infections | Medication and medicaments |
| Vulnerability to infection | Cough |
| General diseases | Hammer and anvil |
| Impaired systemic elimination | Tumors |
| Dietary deficiency | Anomalies |
| Endocrine disturbances | |

It is obvious that there is considerable interrelation among the categories listed, and that some are more specific than others. This allows for combinations of factors and the simplification of the discussion. For the present purposes, the various problems are discussed under three general headings: (1) Modification of structures resulting from mechanical or chemical injury; (2) Diseases and growths; and (3) Hereditary factors.

## MODIFICATIONS OF STRUCTURES RESULTING FROM MECHANICAL OR CHEMICAL INJURY

### Injury

**Abuse of the voice.** According to Jackson and Jackson (1942, pp. 39–40):

Unquestionably the greatest of all causes of laryngeal disease [and hence phonatory problems—*author*] is the excessive use of one of its normal functions, phonation . . . The patient with chronic laryngeal disease is almost always a person who either talks constantly or uses his voice professionally, or often, both. There is little use asking the patient if he talks much. For some curious reason a patient who talks all the time he is awake will insist he talks little. It is not only the singer, the lecturer, and the huckster who suffer from occupational abuse of the larynx. Teachers are especially frequent sufferers and persons who talk in noisy places such as factories where machinery is running often develop chronic hoarseness . . . There is a great variation in the amount of abuse the larynx of different individuals will stand; but every larynx has its limit. To go beyond this limit means thickening of the cords, and a thickened cord means a hoarse voice. Not only is a thickened cord a poor vibrator but it throws great additional work upon the thyroarytenoidei. These muscles instead of growing stronger grow more and more feeble, less and less able to cope with the increased requirements. A vicious circle is established and this renders cure a long tedious process.

This weakness of the vocal muscles, primarily the thyroarytenoids, produces the condition known as *myasthenia laryngis*. It is very common, but often overlooked.

There are six classes of cases (of myasthenia laryngis) observed clinically; those due to (*a*) damage of the muscles by violent shouting, shrieking, screaming, cheering at football games and other brutal abuses of the larynx; (*b*) muscular fatigue from prolonged, excessive though not violent use; (*c*) excessive load imposed by a tumor, or an arthritic crico-arytenoid joint; (*d*) invasion by neighboring inflammatory conditions; (*e*) general systemic conditions; (*f*) association with chronic laryngitis caused by the abuse. (Jackson and Jackson, 1937, p. 313.)

Vocal abuse often leads, also, to other types of laryngeal disorder. Vigorous shouting and cheering may cause vascular engorgement, injury to the joints or musculature resulting in arthritis or myositis, or more often, hematoma. These subepithelial hematoma "do not always become absorbed; often they become organized into fibrous tumors that increase in size as the result of irritation and inflammation" (Jackson and Jackson, 1942, p. 378). They are often on the cord edges, where they cause either a dry or wet hoarseness according to associated conditions.

Prolonged vigorous use of the voice may also produce vocal nodules. These are fibromata "consisting of layers of stratified squamous epithelium." (Ballenger & Ballenger, 1954, p. 147.) Usually they are bilateral, and are always located approximately at the junction of the anterior and middle thirds of the cords.

Vocal nodules, usually associated with chronic hyperplastic laryngitis in singers and public speakers, are due as a rule to improper or overuse of the voice. The overtension of the muscles of the larynx causes attrition of the cords with the formation of the nodules. They are seen more frequently in women than in men. Children who habitually shout or scream while playing occasionally develop the nodules. (Ballenger and Ballenger, 1954, p. 174.)

Another disease which is caused chiefly by vocal abuse is contact ulcer. This entity is an ulceration which occurs on the medial surface of one or both arytenoids where they meet each other. It is related in the literature to a "throaty" method of phonation (Jackson and Jackson, 1942, p. 163; Peacher, 1948). The term *throaty* probably means that the person is using a habitual vocal pitch at the lowest part of his range and that there is audible evidence of muscular effort to keep it there. These patients, who are generally adult males, do not speak loudly, but they talk more or less continuously. They give the impression, and some have admitted this, that they use the low, effortful pitch in an attempt to sound more masculine.

Jackson and Jackson attribute the formation of the ulcer and its site on the arytenoid cartilage to the "trauma of the hammer and anvil." They suggest that the constant hammering of the arytenoids against each other is the chief mechanical cause of the ulceration.

The thin mucosa, which over the vocal processes amounts to little more than a thin layer of epithelium without any submucosal cushion, is constantly traumatized in a way which may be metaphorically described as being between the hammer and the anvil. The pinching may cause necrosis of the epithelium or may introduce infective agents under the epithelial barrier . . . Three additional perpetuating factors enter when the tip of the vocal process of the arytenoid cartilage becomes necrotic: (1) the roughened surface of the cartilage becomes potentially a greater traumatic agent; (2) necrotic cartilage is very slow in its repairative process; and (3) the surrounding ulcer cannot heal until after the necrotic cartilage is completely healed. (Jackson and Jackson, 1942, p. 164.)

The trail which starts with vocal abuse produces inflammation that soon leads to structural changes which, in turn, require compensatory adjustments that cause additional vocal misuse, and so on and on. It is an example of a very complex cause and effect spiral.

**Vocal abuse plus infection.** There are some phonatory problems which are related to misuse of the voice, as described in the preceding section, but in which infection is also present. This combination produces a chronic laryngitis:

. . . a chronic inflammation of the laryngeal mucosa . . . is an exceedingly common disease, standing, perhaps, next in frequency to chronic rhinitis. . . . Broadly considered, the cause of chronic laryngitis is *often-repeated infection, plus constant irritation.* . . . The irritation may be in part the product of infective foci above and below the larynx and these foci may be the source of the reinfection of the laryngeal mucosa. . . .
The most characteristic changes are noted on the vocal cords. Their edges are thickened and rounded, usually somewhat granular. Instead of the usual deceptive flat and band-like appearance there is a thickened rounded form. . . . Vessels may be seen on the upper surface but quite often the patchy redness of the thickened mucosa diminishes the visibility of individual vessels; the increased vascularity of all the capillaries, however, gives the eye well-trained on the normal the impression of chronic inflammation. (Jackson and Jackson, 1937, pp. 136–137.)

The wet hoarseness which is usually present in chronic laryngitis is a signal of potential structural changes of considerable extent and seriousness. As Jackson and Jackson (1937, p. 146) point out:

Chronic thickening of the larynx with permanent impairment of the voice is a common sequel. Chronic edema, hyperplasia, hypertrophy, fibroid tumors, and chronic polypoid corditis are very frequent if the etiologic factors are allowed to continue. The mucosa in chronic laryngitis is good soil for malignant growths. *Myasthenia laryngis* is a common and very intractable sequel.

In addition to the general chronic laryngitis, there are various types of localized laryngitis in which the inflammation is limited to a part or all of one or both cords. The condition is a chronic corditis. "The amenability of corditis to a regime of silence indicates that the irritation is a factor." (Jackson and Jackson, 1937, p. 140.)

The same authors point out that there may be general or localized thickening of the mucosa, in which case it ". . . is referred to as a *hypertrophic laryngitis.*" (Jackson and Jackson, 1937, p. 140.)

A similar condition is *hyperplastic laryngitis* in which there is abundant proliferation of connective tissue cells that do not go on to complete organization and contraction. All the layers of the mucosa and sometimes even deeper tissues are involved. (Jackson and Jackson, 1942, p. 152.)

Ballenger and Ballenger (1954, p. 173) point out that

". . . hyperplastic laryngitis frequently occurs in singers due to incorrect methods of voice training and singing, using the voice during or after a cold, or from repeated attacks of throat inflammation both infectious and allergic. . . . The usual location of the hyperplastic growths is on or under a portion of the vocal cords or in the interarytenoid space. . . . (This tissue) may interfere with the movements of the cords so that approximation is often incomplete. . . . The color of the hyperplastic tissues varies from a pale pink to a deep red. In some cases edema is present.

When there has been prolonged inflammation of the cords, chronic atrophy may develop. Ballenger and Ballenger (1954, p. 175) indicate that the condition

. . . is usually secondary to an atrophic process in the nose and pharynx. . . . Examination shows the mucous membrane to be pale and dry, with crusts on the cords, in the interarytenoid space, or upon the posterior wall of the larynx.
    The prognosis for improvement of the larynx is bad except in those cases in which the atrophic changes have progressed but little.

**Mechanical and chemical irritants.** Irritants produce inflammation which causes organic change. There are several types of substances which can influence the membranes of the respiratory tract, and which should be considered when dealing with voice problems. Some are carried in the air, others are applied to the mucosa directly or indirectly.

The airborne irritants include dusts and powdered substances of various kinds. Jackson and Jackson (1937, p. 52) indicate that continuous exposure to these substances

. . . can easily lead to chronic inflammatory changes in the mucosa, the submucosa and secondarily in the musculature. Dusts may be (a) mechanically irritating . . . (b) biochemically irritating . . . (c) allergic.

These same authors include tobacco smoke as an irritant and add

The effect of tobacco in producing chronic disease of the larynx is local not systemic. It is not the nicotine but the empyreumatic oil produced by the destructive distillation of the burning tobacco that causes the injury to the laryngeal mucosa. . . . (1937, p. 51.)

They say further on this subject:

Fumes, irritating vapors and war gassing are certainly factors in the causation of tumors. (1937, p. 316.) We have seen quite a number of cases of chronic laryngeal disease due to the exposure to smoke and chemical fumes in the case of firemen. In all these exposures, of course, the larynx suffers most in the case of mouth breathers. . . . (1937, pp. 52–53.)
    Even such a common factor as *dry indoor air* of winter in northern climates is a large etiologic factor in laryngeal disease . . . [and] it becomes desiccating,

almost cauterant, to the delicate laryngeal mucosa, especially of the mouth breather. (1937, p. 52.)

In addition to the airborne dusts, powders, and so forth, there are chemical irritants of potential importance to the voice therapist.

Silver nitrate locally applied is a common cause of hoarseness and the damage done by the prolonged applications of even dilute solutions will produce chronic inflammatory changes that may render the patient hoarse for life. (Jackson and Jackson, 1937, pp. 54–55.)

**Substances and conditions causing noninflammatory edema.** One of the causes of hoarseness, which has been mentioned several times in a variety of ways, is edema. Edema causes a change in the mass and sometimes the elasticity of the vocal cords. In the preceding discussion, most of the edematous conditions have been associated with inflammation. It is evident, however, that edema may occur also without inflammation, and be just as detrimental vocally.

Internal medicaments, such as iodides and acetylsalicylic acid, frequently produce edema (Ballenger and Ballenger, 1954, p. 166).

. . . of the internal medicaments potassium iodide is the commonest as a cause of hoarseness. Its selective effect on the larynx may go so far as to produce acute edema of the larynx or a chronic engorgement; . . . (Jackson and Jackson, 1937, pp. 54–55.)

Noninflammatory edema may be caused also by mechanical compression of the venous return flow (Jackson and Jackson, 1937, p. 83). This mechanical compression may be a growth pressing on a vein, or any condition which would reduce the flow of blood.

Various authors (Ballenger and Ballenger, 1937, p. 166; Boies, 1949, p. 284; Jackson and Jackson, 1942, p. 79) have indicated that noninflammatory edema may also be caused by glandular imbalance and allergy. The mechanisms of these relationships are extremely complex and are not completely understood, but a statement by Jones, Muckelston, and Hilger (Jones et al., 1953, pp. 1145–1169) simultaneously accounts for the frequent edematous conditions and organizes the multiple underlying causes:

Allergic reactions, states of autonomic dysfunction, and of endocrine imbalance, can produce identical clinical symptoms. . . . The common denominator . . . is abnormal extra vascular fluid. It creates the immediate problem in the end organ. The method of its formation in the precipitor states of allergy, autonomic dysfunction, and endocrine imbalance may vary but the end result in local symptoms is the same when excessive extra-vascular fluid is established in the end organ tissue. . . .
Autonomic balance is mediated through the basal nuclear aggregates of the brain stem. In this central switchboard the neurovascular, neuromuscular and neurosecretory activities of the vegetative nervous system are integrated. Reflexes from body surface receptors stimulated by heat, cold, light, barometric variations, etc., and impulses from higher psychomotor areas play through these centers upon the autonomic activity of peripheral organs. Unbalanced expression in peripheral organs results when integration is faulty. Faulty neurovascular im-

pulsion has its principal influence on the arteriolar bed. Here sphincteric spasm indistinguishable from the antigen-antibody conflict of the narrow allergy can result in similar damage to the capillary endothelium and capillary leak. The resulting transudate problem is indistinguishable from that of the narrow allergy....

Endocrine imbalance has a less well-defined mechanism of transudate. The thyroid, the gonadal and the adrenal cortical hormones all are important to the proper position of body fluids.

Jackson and Jackson (1937, p. 54) comment specifically on allergy by saying:

The reaction of the mucosa to foreign proteins and other substances is a factor in laryngeal disease. It is a very direct and important factor in such a condition as angioneurotic edema.

In the condition of endocrine imbalance, clinical observations and systematic research suggest a very close relationship between hypothyroidism and voice problems. Hypothyroidism produces edema. There is evidence that the amount of imbalance need not be great to cause hoarseness, and it is recognized that many borderline hypothyroid persons are not aware of their condition. It follows that some of the unsatisfactorily diagnosed cases of hoarseness may be caused by a hypothyroid condition (Luse, 1948).

**Engorgement.** The effect of vasodilation and engorgement on the function of the vocal cords is similar to that of edema. In both instances the mass and contractility are affected. According to Jackson and Jackson (1937, p. 51):

... alcohol is a potent cause of laryngeal disease ... Observation in thousands of patients justifies our opinion that it is the prolonged, peripheral, vasodilator effect of alcohol that is so injurious to the laryngeal mucosa. ... The mucosa of the larynx of the victim of alcohol ... was always engorged. It was evidently the chronic engorgement of the cords that was responsible for the hoarseness. ... It is the constant repetition of alcohol that results in the vasomotor condition resembling paralysis and the chronic engorgement.

**Destruction of laryngeal tissue.** The absence of laryngeal tissue, particularly when it involves the vocal cords, almost always causes a voice defect. There are three primary causes for the loss of such tissue: surgery, trauma, and disease.

Surgical procedures may affect the vocal cords, and hence the voice, in one of two ways: (1) directly through the removal of part or all of the larynx; or (2) indirectly through injury to the nerve supply. In the former, the absence of cord tissue precludes the normal vibratory closure and results in an abnormal voice. In the latter, except in abductor paralysis, there is an incomplete closure of the glottis and sometimes an atrophy of the involved cord tissue. This problem is discussed later, along with other neurological conditions.

The removal of structures is made necessary usually by some form of tumor. The location and the amount of material taken out varies, of course, from patient to patient. It should be noted, however, that the absence of even a small amount of the glottal border causes a marked hoarseness; and furthermore, that the voice may not be appreciably worse when one complete cord has been removed.

When the diseased condition extends beyond certain limits, the laryngeal surgeon usually performs a laryngectomy. The total absence of the larynx produces complete aphonia, and necessitates the development of a substitute type of phonation. This is not difficult for most patients to accomplish, and some suggested procedures are available in the section on therapy.

Another, but relatively uncommon, cause of tissue destruction in the larynx is trauma. Blows on the larynx which fracture the cartilages may result in the deterioration of the thyroid cartilage and the loss of tissue support. "Unless special precautions are taken to prevent it, any injury to the laryngeal cartilages usually results in cicatricial stenosis." (Jackson and Jackson, 1937, p. 95.)

There are some diseases which cause tissue destruction and which, when present in the larynx, can result in voice problems. The two which are referred to most commonly are tuberculosis and syphilis.

## Diseases and Growths

**Infections.** In the preceding discussion of the misuse of the voice, particular reference was made to the interrelationship between vocal abuse and certain infections. There are other infections which may cause organic voice defects without the association of vocal abuse. These infections are of four general kinds: (1) airborne; (2) contactual (kissing, silverware, cups, etc.); (3) focal; and (4) specific (tuberculosis, mycoses, syphilis, measles). The common routes of invasion are: (a) flotation (from some area on the mucosa of the larynx); (b) the air current; (c) the lymph channels; and (d) blood vessels (Jackson and Jackson, 1937, p. 53).

Infections influence the voice through the modifications which they produce in the vocal cords. The changes take many possible forms, including scars, tumors, thickening of the membranes, atrophy, fixation of the cricoarytenoid joint, and paralysis. The influences of these conditions on the action of the vocal cords have been discussed previously, and therefore need not be reviewed here. The reason for including this general reference to infections is to stress, for the voice therapist, that there are many kinds of damaging infections, and that their detrimental effects may last a long time.

**Paralyses.** In the preceding parts of this chapter, several references were made to the relationship between paralyses and voice problems. The importance of the various kinds of paralyses and their causes deserve special consideration.

The organic paralyses may be subdivided into: (1) congenital; (2) central (cortico or bulbar); (3) peripheral; and (4) myopathic. (Ballenger and Ballenger, 1954, p. 178.)

The first, or congenital, is rare. Regarding the second, the cortical or bulbar group, these authors say:

> It is generally agreed that a bilateral center for the larynx exists; therefore a unilateral lesion of the cortex would not produce a paralysis. . . .
>
> In paralysis of the vagus nerve due to a bulbar lesion the involvement of the other nerves readily establishes the diagnosis. (1954, p. 179.)

This is the type of complex condition found in those "post-polio" patients who present the characteristic combination of hypernasality and weak, breathy phonation.

Peripheral lesions causing a paralysis of the cords may be located anywhere along the course of the vagus down to and including the recurrent laryngeal. Among the lesions in this locality causing paralysis of the nerves are enlarged cervical lymph nodes, traumatisms, goiters (before and following operations), aneurysms, mediastinal tumors, tumors of the esophagus and the pharynx, pleurisy, scoliosis of the cervical vertebrae, tuberculosis of the apices of the lungs, and even paricarditis or mitral stenosis.

The most common cause of laryngeal paralysis is trauma incident to thyroidectomy. The entire trunk of the nerve may be involved or one of the extralaryngeal subdivisions. (Ballenger and Ballenger, 1954, pp. 179–180.)

Damage to the peripheral nerve supply to the larynx can result in several types of malfunction. If the superior laryngeal branch is damaged, the external tensor (crico-thyroid muscle) is paralyzed, and the sensory nerve to the interior of the larynx, which travels with the motor fibers, also ceases to function. In tensor paralysis, the cords are bowed allowing air waste, weakness, and huskiness.

A lesion of the recurrent laryngeal nerve may produce either an abductor or an adductor paralysis, or a complete paralysis. The form depends upon the branch of the nerve which has been damaged and the extent of the lesion (Morrison, 1952).

Myopathic.—This form of paralysis is characterized by some form of pathologic process in one or more of the intrinsic laryngeal muscles. It may be of the toxic origin such as typhoid fever or tetanus, or it may follow trichinosis, tuberculosis, local infections, and tumors of the vocal cords. (Ballenger and Ballenger, 1954, p. 181.)

The crucial question for the voice therapist concerns the probable outcome of a paralysis. Jackson and Jackson say, "A vocal cord that has remained motionless from interrupted innervation for a long time will never recover its motility." (1937, p. 287.) These same authors report that the maximum time of inactivity followed by recovery which they have observed was four months in adults and six months in children.

**Growths.** Growths in the larynx cause voice defects when they interfere with the normal adjustment and function of the cords. From the vocal standpoint, the type of growth is unimportant except where vocal nodules or contact ulcers are present. These signal the presence of vocal abuse, and have been previously discussed. Other growths which should be known to the voice therapist are cysts and tumors. The latter include benign growths such as papillomas, fibromas (polyps), granulomas, lipomas, hematomas, and malignancies (carcinomas). There are certain other subdivisions and less common neoplasms, but the ones mentioned constitute the more important ones numerically.

## Congenital Factors

An infant may be born with a laryngeal paralysis, a cyst, syphilis, papilloma, abnormally large structures, a laryngeal web, and so on. If any one of these is marked enough to receive medical attention, it may be remedied. On the other hand, those which go unnoticed, or are recognized as relatively insignificant anomalies, may become important later as causes for voice defects. Since these minor difficulties are apt to be observed only after some years, and since they may develop subsequent to the time of birth, it would be difficult or impossible to determine whether or not they were congenital in any particular case.

**Congenital web.** One of the exceptions to the preceding statement is the congenital web, which is not too uncommon.

The causes of congenital web are unknown, but are possibly atavistic.
The most frequent location for congenital web is the level of the glottis, usually in the anterior portion where it attaches the two cords together for more or less of their anterioposterior extent. (Jackson and Jackson, 1942, p. 60.)

The web is apt to cause a high-pitched voice, accompanied by effortful phonation. Therefore, wherever pitch problems are present, the possibility of a web should always be considered.

## Organic Causes for Resonance Voice Defects

The organic etiologies of the resonance voice defects might have been discussed along with the organic etiologies of laryngeal problems, since many of the causitive conditions are common to both. However, for simplicity of treatment, they have been considered separately.

**Excessive nasality.** It was pointed out earlier that there are two principal resonance defects associated with organic etiologies: too much nasal resonance, and insufficient nasal resonance. The former defect is caused by incomplete nasopharyngeal closure, and results from four possible organic causes: (1) congenital deformity; (2) paralysis; (3) destructive disease; and (4) surgery.

The congenital deformity takes two forms: cleft palate and short palate. In both conditions, the nasopharyngeal closure cannot be made, thereby allowing sound from the larynx to pass into the nasopharynx and nose.

Paralysis of one or both sides of the pharyngeal constrictor muscle groups, or of the velum, will prevent a velopharyngeal closure and will therefore provide a condition similar, in effect, to a cleft or short palate. Such diseases as poliomyelitis and measles can cause the lesions in the nerves to the muscles of the pharynx and velum.

The destructive diseases which have produced excessive nasality include malignant tumors on the hard or soft palates, and syphilis with a gumma extending through the hard palate. The voice quality is similar to that accompanying paralysis or cleft palate.

Surgical removal of adenoid tissue sometimes results in excessive nasality. When adenoid tissue in the nasopharynx has contributed to the velopharyngeal closure, thereby reducing the amount of velar movement necessary, and is then removed, excessive nasality will result until the habits are modified and the closure is again established. When the palate and the other velopharyngeal structures are not adequate to make a closure without the adenoid tissue, the voice will remain hypernasal.

**Denasality.** There are four conditions which commonly cause denasality: (1) growths; (2) hypertrophy resulting from chronic disease; (3) allergies; and (4) trauma. Growths may be of several types, such as adenoid tissue, polyps, papilloma, and nasal spurs. The diseases include chronic rhinitis and sinusitis. The allergies represent sensitivity to airborne irritants, which cause the membranes of the nose to be swollen. Traumatic occurrences, such as a broken nose, also produce swelling which may become chronic.

In all these conditions, the acoustic results are essentially the same. The exception exists when a growth or spur is located well forward in the nose, thereby allowing the posterior part of the nose to act as a resonator. In these instances, hypernasality rather than denasality, may be associated with a stoppage of air in the nasal passage.

### Summary of Pathologies of Voice Defects

The pathologies of the organic phonatory defects are extremely complex and often interrelated. The discussion just presented has arbitrarily grouped the various pathologies into the following six categories to simplify presentation:

1. Modification of structures resulting from misuse of the voice, including such conditions as thickened vocal cord tissue, myasthenia laryngis, vocal nodules, and contact ulcer. This section also touched on vocal abuse combined with infection in the production of such pathologies as chronic laryngitis and thickened cords, chronic corditis with hypertrophic and hyperplastic laryngitis, and chronic atrophic laryngitis.
2. Mechanical and chemical irritants as causes for laryngeal and consequent voice problems. The factors mentioned here included fumes, irritating vapors and gasses, dry air, dusts, allergens, and silver nitrate.
3. Substances and conditions causing noninflammatory edema, that is, internal medicaments, mechanical compression of venous blood flow, glandular imbalance, and allergy. The condition of engorgement and vasodilation related to alcohol was also included within this division.
4. Destruction of laryngeal tissue by surgery, trauma, or disease.
5. Diseases and growths, particularly infections not related to vocal abuse; paralyses of central, peripheral, and myopathic origin; cysts; and both benign and malignant tumors.
6. Congenital factors, in which most of the emphasis was placed on congenital web.

The organic causes for the more common resonance problems were discussed separately under two headings: those which cause excessive nasality; and those which produce insufficient nasal resonance. The former included such conditions as cleft palate, congenitally short palate, paralyses of the velopharyngeal constrictors, and surgery. The latter was related to growths, trauma, and allergies.

The successful management of organically caused voice defects requires an extensive understanding of the pathologies involved. It is imperative that the voice therapist be aware of, and informed about, the various anomalies of the respiratory tract. This does not imply any encroachment upon, nor functioning within, the field of medicine; it simply recognizes the fact that the laryngologist, the rhinologist, and the voice pathologist must work together, and must understand each other to do so effectively.

## MANAGEMENT OF ORGANIC VOICE DISORDERS

The management of organic voice disorders encompasses two distinct stages: diagnosis and therapy. The former has four well-defined steps which include: (1) analysis of the voice in terms of pitch, quality, and loudness; (2) investigation of the history of the voice problem; (3) examination of those structures potentially related to the voice defect—nose, mouth, pharynx, or larynx; and (4) evaluation of the nonspeech skills and abilities, including intelligence, emotional stability, motor skills, general health, systemic conditions, and hearing. Briefly and for practical purposes, these diagnostic steps might be reduced to: first, listen; second, question; third, look; and fourth, test. The data from these four steps determine the recommendations and the specific steps in therapy.

### Diagnosis

Diagnosis should be done systematically. However, it should be pointed out that the order of items in the suggested four-part diagnosis is not fixed. The situation and persons involved will determine the procedure. Furthermore, the experienced diagnostician knows that data for several parts of the diagnostic examination may be gathered simultaneously; that is, the history interview provides an excellent opportunity to hear the voice in conversational use. To gather information in an orderly manner then, and at the same time to maintain a flexibility of approach, makes it imperative that the examiner have a carefully prepared outline with which he is thoroughly familiar. In most situations this outline should be used as the data-collecting form, and should be standardized to fit the needs of each school system or clinic.

To systematize the immediate discussion of the diagnosis of organic voice defects, the previously suggested four steps of the diagnosis will be briefly elaborated in order, with each step containing items which could be used as the outline of an information form.

**Analysis of the voice.** Since the voice is the focus of interest, its analysis begins with the first words spoken at the initial interview, and continues throughout the time the patient or student is present. The examiner may wish to converse casually about some local event, or he may prefer to gather the identification data which usually occupy the first part of an information questionnaire. These identification data include name, address, telephone number, date of interview, birth date, school and grade, or occupation, parent or guardian, number of siblings and the patient's position in the series, the name of the informant (if different from the subject), the referral source, and the interviewer.

During this interview, the examiner should note the habitual pitch level and its normalcy in relation to contemporaries of the same age and sex. He should also observe the loudness and its suitability to the situation; and, at the same time, he should be aware of the quality of the voice. This type of voice evaluation is to be considered as a supplement to the more formal testing to be reviewed later.

By the time the identification data have been recorded, the examiner should have a fair estimate of the patient's ordinary vocal usage. The subject usually has some concept of his difficulty, and is willing to supply his own evaluation of his voice problem. It is important to know what he thinks is wrong with his voice, and why he wants to improve it. He should be asked to report the comments which have been made by teachers, friends, or employers. His report should also contain his reason for seeking help with his voice at this particular time. If the voice defect which the examiner has observed is not mentioned by the subject, leading questions should be asked to learn the true extent of his information and comprehension.

The next logical item under the analysis of the voice is the examiner's description and evaluation of the voice. This should contain comments on pitch, quality, intensity, rate, and other speech problems. Sometimes the interviewer will wish to complete the case history before carrying out the formal steps of the voice evaluation. Under these conditions, he would explore next the questions pertaining to the development and history of the voice problem. However, where the examiner uses the same office space for interviewing and voice evaluation, and where one person makes the analysis and takes the history, the vocal analysis can be carried out with some advantage at this point in the procedure. As an aid to the examiner in the analysis, the voice should be recorded on tape whenever possible for use in subsequent checking of initial impressions.

Voice-testing should concentrate on one vocal element at a time. With experience, of course, the examiner will be able to note quality differences while testing the pitch, and so on. However, even those who are thoroughly familiar with voice problems should establish a routine procedure which includes tests for pitch, loudness, and quality. Unintentional variations in procedure are apt to produce incomplete data and "improper diagnosis." Careful, systematic, routinized procedure is essential in diagnosis.

The tests of pitch should discover the total pitch range and the voluntary control of pitch. The subject should be asked to sing or hum a tone near the middle of his range (the examiner may need to supply a starting tone for imitation), and then to go by scale steps to the lowest note possible and to he highest, including falsetto. If an instrument (pitch pipe or piano) to determine the notes used is not available, the estimate of "adequate" or "inadequate" range will be necessary. At the same time, the control of pitch can be noted by observing the ease and accuracy with which the subject moves from one musical tone to the next. A "speaking" test should also be given in which the subject is asked to repeat a few questions with rising inflection, such as, "Oh?" or "Are you going home?" Some persons cannot voluntarily change from one scale note to another, yet they use normal inflectional patterns in speaking. The primary concern in diagnosis, of course, is whether or not the activity can be performed. It is secondary to discover how well it can be done.

If the voice is completely monotonous in both sung and spoken sounds and is also somewhat hoarse, the superior laryngeal nerve, or its central attachments, or the muscles supplied by it, are suspect. It must be remembered, however, that monotonous pitch can be habitual; and that it can be related to emotional problems. The latter are more apt to be evidenced in unusual melody patterns rather than in the absence of pitch change.

If the pitch is regularly very low combined with a rough hoarseness, some weighting of the cords is to be considered, as with edema or growths.

When the pitch remains high, particularly in the adult male, the most probable cause is functional, but it may also be a failure of laryngeal development or the presence of a laryngeal web. The delay in laryngeal development in the male is usually paralleled by inadequate hair growth on the face, obesity, and other signs which the physician can observe.

There are two factors in loudness which should be noted: (1) its suitability in the conversational situation, which has already been noted; and (2) the maximum loudness. The latter may be obtained by turning down the volume control on the recorder and asking the person to speak as loudly as he can. Many people are more willing to try to speak loudly "for a microphone" than for a person only a few feet away. If the patient is unable to produce a loud voice, it is either because the tension in one or both vocal cords is inadequate, because the breath pressure is insufficient, or because the individual is embarrassed. Questions about the patient's ability to call to someone at some distance or to cheer at a sporting event may help to differentiate the causes. If the quality becomes breathy or hoarse when a loud voice is attempted, an organic involvement is to be suspected.

Analyzing the quality of the voice means systematically listening for six qualities under different conditions of pitch and loudness. These qualities are: breathiness, dry hoarseness, wet hoarseness, rough hoarseness, excessive nasality, and denasality. Usually the interview conversation and the vocal use during the checks of pitch and loudness will provide adequate material for classifying the quality, but it may be desirable to use a standard test passage, such as those to be found in speech correction texts. In this instance, the patient should read and record the test paragraph in the habitual manner, then repeat it loudly. He should also produce sustained tones softly and loudly at several pitches. If the voice becomes increasingly breathy at higher pitches, it suggests a growth, such as a nodule, on the glottal border or perhaps inadequate arytenoid approximation. If the voice is hoarse at low pitches and becomes clearer at higher pitches, it creates suspicion of some inflammatory condition producing excess mucus, or of edema or growths.

Resonance problems may accompany the phonatory deviations just referred to. They are vocally important, sometimes are organically critical and always deserve careful evaluation.

The listening for nasal sound deviation is carried out very easily and simply. If the test passage selected previously for reading be one without nasal sounds, the presence of excessive nasal resonance will be markedly evident. Resonance of the aperta type immediately suggests an organic pathology in the velopharyngeal area. The presence of nasal twang indicates either a growth anteriorly in the nose or a functional problem.

If the opposite condition of denasality is present, there is almost certainly a partial or complete obstruction in the nasopharynx or posterior nasal passages.

The previous suggestion of recording the voice tests was to provide material for objective listening to the voice. It is advisable to rehear the voice from a recording to separate the voice from the person producing it. Sometimes the appearance of the patient influences the auditory judgment of the examiner. It is always advisable to listen to the recorded voice (from a good recorder) before making a final evaluation of the patient's voice.

The terminology of voice defects is notoriously inexact. There are several reasons for this, and they do not properly belong in this discussion. It is possible, however, to indicate the relative severity of each type of deviation noted, and it is advised that at least three modifiers be used, such as *mild, moderate,* and *severe.* These terms will be useful to the therapist as a device for noting progress, or the lack of it, in therapy.

**Investigation of the development and history of the voice problem.** The collection of the identification data at the beginning of the information form gives the interviewer some idea of the patient's background, family size, type of work, and so on. The description and evaluation of the voice by the patient and the examiner identify the problem and focus the attention of the patient upon it. Ordinarily, at this stage, questions about the voice difficulty will be answered readily and as completely as memory will allow.

To simplify the discussion of the development and history of the voice problem, a series of key questions have been presented, and are used to outline the steps in gathering pertinent information. These questions have been thoroughly tested in clinical situations. The student is advised to relate the previous discussions of organic pathology to the questionnaire items if the purpose and significance of the questions are not evident.

What were the circumstances under which the voice problem was first noticed? The informant frequently will give this information when he is describing his voice difficulty. However, it usually needs some elaboration through such questions as: Was the voice problem noticed suddenly, or have you been aware of it for some time? How long has it existed? Who first noticed it? Had you done any shouting, singing, extensive speaking, and so forth, before the problem was noticed? Had you been ill, in an accident, or had any surgery about this time?

It is extremely important to distinguish the problems of sudden onset from those of long or indefinite development. The former may indicate a condition which is a threat to life, and although all patients with phonatory problems should be examined by a laryngologist, the acute problems demand urgent referral.

What do you think caused the voice difficulty? If a specific statement has not been made previously to answer this question, the direct question should be asked. The answer may provide insight into the individual's concept of his problem.

Does it vary in severity? Has it become better or worse recently? Does it vary during the course of a day? Do seasons or daily weather changes seem to affect it? Does it vary with your feelings of happiness or discouragement? Does it vary significantly with the degree of fatigue? The longtime trend and the daily or short-term variations can suggest a variety of potential causes, such as developing growths, allergies, glandular imbalance, anemia, and disease.

Is your voice similar to that of anyone else in your family? It is often necessary to ask the patient if his voice is confused with that of anyone else on the telephone. Where the voice is similar to that of another member of the family, it usually indicates an imitation factor. However, in a large family, there is often vigorous vocal competition which may cause thickening of the vocal cord tissue, or nodules, or other vocal cord damage. It is not unusual to find several in a family who demonstrate this vocal similarity.

Are there any speech defects or other voice problems in your family? (Include aunts, uncles, and grandparents.) Sometimes the answer to this question reveals other speech problems and gives insight into family attitudes regarding speech deviations generally. Occasionally, also, when nasality is the voice defect, the patient may reveal cleft palate or other structural anomalies which have potential significance and which necessitate further questioning.

What remedial attempts have been made? Frequently, the answer to this question is given in the discussion of the first awareness of the problem. The information is important, and should include the names and addresses of physicians and teachers who have worked with the patient on his problem. It is also helpful to discover what therapy was administered, what its effects were, and why the work was stopped.

It may be desirable to get additional information from previous therapists, and it is always wise to learn all one can about previous therapeutic experiences. Successful voice therapy requires careful, serious work. There is no magic. It is helpful to be able to recognize the person who "shops around" looking for a ready-made "cure."

Do you have any information about your early vocal usage? As an infant, was there excessive crying, screaming, or yelling? Was there any abnormality in respiration, such as noisy breathing? Excessive vocal use in young children often produces vocal nodules, sometimes called screamer's nodes. Stridorous breathing may mean a laryngeal abnormality, with obvious potential relationship to the voice defect.

As a child, were you talkative and vocally noisy? Did you ever lose your voice? Was there anything unusual about the change of voice? When did it occur? Have you ever been a cheerleader? A singer? Did you ever work in a noisy place where it was necessary to speak loudly? It is obvious that these questions are intended to probe into areas of vocal misuse. Occasionally the answers to them are very revealing, and lead to more specific search.

The previous questions have concentrated on the origin and development of the voice problem itself. The following group of questions focus on the individual's general development and health history. These questions are particularly important in chronic voice cases of indefinite origin.

What diseases have you had, and at what ages? (Note particularly, measles, scarlet fever, diphtheria, poliomyelitis, mumps, ear trouble, or any other high fever diseases diagnosed or undiagnosed.) Special attention should be given to the so-called childhood diseases named, to their after-effects, and to their time relationship to the origin of the voice problem. Peripheral or central nerve damage may be associated with any of them.

What injuries have you had? The nature, extent, and date of injuries, particularly in the head and neck area, should be investigated thoroughly. If one of these is related in time to the start of the voice problem, a report should be obtained from the attending physician if possible.

What operations have you had? Usually, when an operation is related to a voice defect the patient is aware of the association. The voice therapist is interested in knowing the nature of the surgery, and whether the resultant voice defect is caused by tissue removal or nerve lesion and paralysis. A report from the surgeon is particularly advisable when the surgery is of recent date.

Do you have any allergies? What is your "blood count?" Do you know what your metabolic rate is? The conditions of allergy, anemia, or glandular imbalance should be suspected, particularly where a voice defect exists without a visible pathology. When a laryngologist refers a patient for speech therapy and reports no visible laryngeal pathology, a basal metabolism rating and a red cell determination are very desirable. The person with sufficient allergic reaction to produce a voice problem usually knows that he has an allergy, although he may never have associated the voice problem with it. The mechanism of the voice deviation in these conditions is edema.

When the voice therapist must carry out his diagnostic procedure without the immediate assistance of a physician, he must have some evidence of need before referring an individual to a medical doctor for metabolic tests or general physical evaluation. The following questions are not diagnostic, and no question is significant alone, but if there are a number of positive answers, the therapist can feel justified in suggesting a medical examination: (1) Have you ever had a basal metabolism test? What was your rating? (If the rate named is −15, or below, it could be significant in the voice defect.) (2) How long ago was this determined? Who suggested that you have it, and what was the circumstance? Did you take any medication? How long did you continue with it? (3) Is your pulse rate a little slower than the average? (4) Is your temperature usually a little lower than 98.6°? (5) Do you often feel tired without real cause? (6) Do you often have bodily aches and pains without specific cause? (7) Do you have an abnormal dryness in your nose and throat? (8) Do you have sinus infection? (9) Do you have dry skin and hair? (10) Do you perspire less than the average person? (11) Do you perspire more than the average person? (Either of these last two symptoms may be present with hypothyroid imbalance.) (12) Do you often feel chilly when others are comfortable or warm? (13) Do you have any eye trouble? (14) Do you have any ear trouble? (15) Do you have any dizziness? (16) Do you have any pain or sensation of pressure in the region of the larynx? (Luse, 1948).

Where there has been a previous history of thyroid imbalance, the physical condition is suspect as a cause of the voice problem, and the patient should be urged to report regularly to his physician if he is not already doing so. If a recent metabolic rating is not available, the voice therapist should be reluctant to accept a "functional" diagnosis, and should insist upon a reliable medical opinion.

Do you smoke? How much? How long have you been smoking? The amount of smoking and the length of time the subject has been smoking may have etiological importance. Heavy smoking associated with hoarseness, particularly if the hoarseness has developed recently, deserves careful and immediate laryngological attention.

Has swallowing ever been difficult? Has food often become lodged in the throat, causing coughing and discomfort? Have foods or liquids ever gone into the nasopharynx during swallowing? Has water ever escaped from the nose while drinking from a fountain? When either nasality or denasality has been noted in the patient's voice, these questions may be diagnostically revealing. If he answers affirmatively to one or more, it can be assumed that there is, or has been, a structural inadequacy or a paralysis.

Observation of the facial structures may be as diagnostically revealing as careful listening when considering nasal stoppage. Interference with the flow of air through the nose causes mouth-breathing, which, after a time, is usually accompanied by a shortened upper lip and a large, pendant lower lip.

Questions about difficulty of breathing through the nose and whether or not the stoppage occurs at certain seasons, in particular geographic locations, or such, will usually reveal the general nature of the problem.

By the time the examiner has progressed this far in the diagnostic procedure, he should have formed a rather detailed description of the voice defect and should also have acquired a substantial understanding of the patient, along with a concept of the origin and development of the voice problem. At this point in the procedure, there should be a careful study of the structure and function of the voice-producing mechanism. The tentative assumptions which have been made need to be confirmed or rejected.

**Examination of the vocal mechanism.** There is a tendency to think of the examination of the vocal mechanism as being identical with the examination of the larynx. The latter is very important, and persons specializing in voice therapy should become skillful examiners, although it should be remembered that the careful observer can learn a great deal without instruments and without attempting to see into the larynx. It should be noted, too, that in most school systems the examination of the larynx may be done only by a physician, which undoubtedly is a wise practice.

Observation requires a bright light which can be directed easily onto any desired area, and two chairs placed to allow the examiner to face the patient. The simplest light source is a flashlight, which is completely adequate for everything except examination with instruments. In the latter case, a concave mirror with a hole in the center is supported over one eye by a headband in such a position that light from a light bulb can be directed and focused onto a specific spot. The hole in the mirror allows shadow-free observation.

The examination should start with a scanning of the face and neck areas for scars or asymmetries. Usually this is done unobtrusively during the interview, but where such have been observed, further questioning at this time i indicated. These items may be clues to structural anomalies, injuries, o neural lesions which were not revealed previously.

The functioning and control of the facial muscles should also be checkec not because they are directly related to voice defects, but because a deviatio1 may indicate a neurological problem which also involves the velopharyngea area, or the larynx. This is accomplished by observing asymmetry when th patient is asked to pucker his lips and to smile, alternately.

A similar type of interest motivates the observation of the tongue. Th patient should be asked, first, to protrude the tongue beyond the lips. If i deviates definitely to the right or left, there may be a unilateral paralysis o1 the side toward which the turning occurs. Next, he should be asked to pas his tongue completely around his lips. Failure in any part of the movemen again suggests neurological involvement. The third test of tongue movemen is done by asking the patient to speak a word, such as *kitty* or *Tucker,* slowl at first, and then to accelerate to the highest rate possible. Persons with : co-ordination problem in the tongue will reveal it in a quick failure of th( diadochokinesis.

Light directed into the oropharynx will reveal the position of the sof palate, the contours of the faucial pillars, the presence of scars, and so forth Of greatest importance, however, is the observation of the movement of the velum and the related pharyngeal walls. A simple procedure is to ask the patient to open his mouth, to protrude his tongue, curl it down toward the chin, and to voice a prolonged "eh," as in *end.* The normally active soft palate will lift vigorously against the forward displacement of the tongue. A1 this time, it is easy to see any irregularities in palatal elevator and tensor action. A further test of the velopharyngeal closure is to ask the patient to produce a loud, prolonged "th" sound, as in *thin.* If he can accomplish this without nasal escape, the closure is potentially adequate.

The openness of the nasal passages can be determined if the examiner will press the nostrils closed, alternately, while the patient is humming a long "m" sound. Partial, or even complete, blockage of one side may not affect the voice noticeably, but it should be investigated further through proper referral unless the patient reports adequate medical care.

If a phonatory problem exists, the diagnosis cannot be considered complete until the larynx has been carefully observed. The examination of this structure with a mirror is relatively simple in principle. In practice, however, it is apt to be difficult, because most people have sensitive pharyngeal reflexes which interfere with the proper placement of the mirror in relation to the vocal cords and the light source. The examination technique can and should be learned by the voice pathologist, since it is a help to be able to observe laryngeal conditions and to follow the changes which occur in the course of therapy. It should be emphasized, however, that the diagnosing of laryngeal diseases and disorders is the province and responsibility of the

ryngologist. This implies at once that the laryngologist is a necessary and
xtremely important person in the management of voice defects.

It is obvious that a complete diagnosis of a phonatory problem cannot
e made until a laryngologist has examined the patient and reported his
ndings. This means that one of three procedures can be followed: (1) have
laryngologist as a regular member of the diagnosing team; (2) ask all per-
ons requesting assistance to be examined by a laryngologist before they
ome for the initial interview; and (3) refer all patients who have phonatory
roblems to a laryngologist after voices have been evaluated and other data
ollected. The last is the least desirable, since it delays the completion of the
iagnosis.

Where a close working arrangement can be made with laryngologists and
hey can be informed of the types of information which the voice therapist
eeds, it often helps to use a prepared form for acquiring data. Some pub-
ic-school speech correctionists have developed such forms, with the assist-
nce of the local laryngologists. These forms should be clear to everyone
using them, and it is important that they be brief.

Those speech pathologists who plan to concentrate on voice disorders, and
vho should learn, therefore, to examine the larynx skillfully, are advised
o follow three steps: (1) study the examination procedures set forth in at
east two books on laryngology; (2) arrange a light and mirrors for self-
examination; and (3) practice on some friends. It is emphasized that two
r more descriptions of laryngeal examination technique should be studied,
or the various authors follow somewhat different procedures.

The self-examination can be worked out in several simple steps, as fol-
ows: first, buy a #3 or #4 laryngeal mirror from a surgical supply house;
econd, fasten a flashlight, with a strong light, horizontally at the level of the
mouth when you are seated; third, attach a small mirror of the type found
n a woman's purse to the side of the flashlight, making it possible to see into
your own mouth when you are seated in the proper position and the flash-
ight is turned on; fourth, protrude your tongue, and hold it down toward
your chin, grasping it with a piece of sterile gauze; and, fifth, with the other
hand, place the laryngeal mirror back in the pharynx. By adjusting the
mirror properly, the interior of the larynx will come into view. The development of the technique is a substantial reward for the necessary patience and
practice.

When the time comes for practice on friends, the examination equipment
must be changed to conform with that described in the laryngology texts.
Practice in the manipulation of the head mirror and laryngeal mirror should
be accomplished before an examination is attempted, even on friends. The
examiner should approach even these practice examinations seriously and
with a sincerity of purpose. There is certainly no place for levity in such
situations.

**Evaluation of nonspeech skills and abilities.** The fourth step in the diagnostic procedure is the evaluation of certain nonspeech skills and abilities.

These include intellectual ability and emotional stability, motor skills, general health, systemic conditions, and hearing. If the patient's general level of skill and abilities are not included within the diagnostic evaluation, the stated causes of the voice defect may be inaccurate; and the plan for therapy is almost certain to be incomplete.

There is no implication here that organic voice disorders result from low intellectual ability or emotional instability. However, these factors influence learning ability, and they need to be evaluated as part of the plan of therapy. Furthermore, their intimate association with the psychogenic voice disorder causes them to be importantly present in the diagnostician's thinking.

Ideally, a clinical psychologist should be a part of the diagnostic team, but where this is not feasible, a qualified person should be available for referral. It is not necessary for all, or even a majority, of the voice cases to be examined by a psychologist. Usually the patient's reactions to the interview and the testing procedure, plus the school and employment records, provide sufficient evidence to determine the advisability of referral.

Occasionally, an individual who shows in-co-ordination of the face or tongue, peculiarities of gait, or random movements, will seek assistance for a voice defect. It may be obvious that there is a neurological disorder, but it may not be possible to determine immediately whether that problem has any influence on the voice. Observation and questioning will usually indicate whether the patient should be seen by a neurologist, a laryngologist, or a psychiatrist.

During the case history interview, it is usually possible to conclude whether or not further information on general health and the systemic conditions, such as glandular imbalance, is indicated. If it is, the referral should be made, with specific questions to the physician.

The hearing acuity of a person rarely contributes significantly to his voice defect. The exception is where it causes him to speak very loudly, and thereby produces vocal abuse. Such a hearing loss would be quite evident and would require immediate referral to an otologist or audiologist. A milder hearing loss should be known to the voice therapist if it exists, because it may make certain phases of the therapy more difficult. It follows that an audiometric evaluation should be a routine part of each voice diagnosis, and a qualified audiometrist should be a member of the diagnostic group.

The processes of listening, questioning, looking, and testing which have been described provide basic information about voice problems and the persons having them. The study of the relationship between these data, the elimination of nonapplicable items, and the final synthesis of the pertinent factors provide the diagnosis. Usually it can be set forth briefly in two parts: first, a classification, or descriptive statement, of the voice problem; and, second, the factors which seem to have caused it.

Such a diagnostic statement constitutes a hypothesis on which to base recommendations. These ordinarily take one of three directions. When voice therapy is indicated, the patient is either scheduled for remedial work with he diagnosing clinic, or he is referred to another voice therapist, if one happens to be more conveniently located. When voice therapy is not recommended, the decision is explained to the patient in terms most beneficial to his welfare and, when it will be helpful, he is referred to another type of service.

The preceding diagnostic routine has implied a need for a complete effect-to-cause investigation. This is not always necessary, however, since some surgical conditions are immediately evident and do not need a detailed diagnostic procedure. The primary example of this situation is the laryngectomized person. Ordinarily, the laryngeal surgeon's report is available, which, in combination with a few basic questions, will establish the advisability of vocal re-education.

In the case of the laryngectomee, the therapist needs to know something about him as a person, and about his presurgical and postsurgical history. The following questions have been found to be helpful in a clinical situation as items on a brief questionnaire:

When and where was the surgery performed? Who was the surgeon? Were there any complications? Before the operation, was there hoarseness or aphonia? When, and under what conditions? Was speech important to the patient's occupation? Did he sing? Did he smoke? How much? How long? Since the operation, what is the patient's attitude toward his condition? (Upset and disturbed; unconcerned acceptance; eager to develop speech.) Has there been any attempt to learn to speak? When? Where? What procedures were used? Were they successful? Have artificial devices been tried? What type? What is the reason for the present interest in voice therapy?

What is the laryngectomee's present level of speech ability as indicated by the following scale:

1. No sounds
2. Occasional sound, uncertain control
3. Single sounds and short words under voluntary control
4. Words and short phrases used in communication
5. Sentences used frequently, occasional sound failure
6. Fluent speech

## Therapy

The diagnostic procedures outlined above stressed the close affiliation of voice therapy with laryngology and other medical specialities. When an organic anomaly is present, the condition of the patient must be improved as much as circumstances will allow before active voice therapy starts. The following discussions are based on the assumption that all such treatment has been done, or is being done.

The therapeutic approach described here recognizes the individual nature of voice defects and the need for planning each remedial program specifically for the person and his voice problem. Certain principles of therapy, however, are applicable to many kinds of voice problems, which makes it possible to offer some generalizations about treatment.

690 HANDBOOK OF SPEECH PATHOLOG

There are two therapeutic approaches to organic voice problems: one i restorative; the other, compensatory. The one chosen for a particular re medial program will depend upon the extent to which the vocal structure can be restored to normal. That is, if the condition can be alleviated b vocal therapy alone, or if surgery and medicine can provide a normal struc ture, the vocal therapy attempts to re-establish normal vocal sound produc tion. On the other hand, if the mechanism and voice are permanently altered the voice therapy has three compensatory objectives: (1) to establish th greatest possible efficiency in the use of the remaining structures; (2) t develop physiological compensations; and (3) to help the patient accept hi "different" voice.

**Restorative therapy.** Restorative therapy applies to the following thre conditions: first, voice problems resulting from vocal abuse which has pro duced the intermediate mechanisms of thickened cord tissue, myastheni laryngis, vocal nodules, contact ulcer, or chronic laryngitis related to th combination of infection and vocal abuse; second, voice problems remain ing after any surgical correction which leaves the larynx normal, or nearl so; and, third, voice problems resulting from endocrine imbalance or anemia and persisting despite medical treatment.

The procedures in restorative therapy are both psychological and physio logical. Their combined aim is to establish a method of voice production i which the natural rejuvenating processes can occur, for normal structure tend to re-establish themselves when given the opportunity.

*Therapy for Problems Related to Vocal Abuse.* The psychological factor which are applicable in this type of problem include informing each patien as completely as his ability to understand will permit, that continued misus of the voice will create serious vocal problems in the future, that vocal re covery is a long process, that it will occur in relation to the completenes with which he follows the therapeutic program, and that he must learn t eliminate his vocal noisiness and to talk less. Throughout his therapy h should be encouraged to maintain the best vocal usage possible at all times in order to avoid the recurrence of the anomaly. Vocal improvement i these cases occurs slowly, and the therapist must be sensitive to those form of encouragement and motivation which apply to the individual patient an which can provide a favorable atmosphere for progress.

The physiological aspects of the therapy must be concrete and positive In many instances, a request should be made that the patient adopt com plete silence. This means that all communication must be by pencil an paper for a period of from two weeks to several months. If the patien claims he cannot avoid talking, he should be helped toward silence b placing strips of adhesive tape across his mouth for several hours at a tim over a period of a few days. This will help him to realize how much he talk ordinarily, and how necessary it is for him to learn to be quiet.

Jackson and Jackson (1942, p. 53) emphasize this type of therapy by say ing:

The first step in the treatment of almost all forms of benign disease of the arynx is rest of the larynx. If we do not stop the *vocal abuse* of the constant talker or the professional user he will utterly frustrate any remedial measures we may undertake. This is most important in the treatment of the inflammatory diseases such as contact ulcer but applies with almost equal force to pachydermia, keratosis, vocal nodules, chronic laryngitis, inflammatory tumor-like formations and even benign true neoplasms. Any such general instructions as "don't talk so much," or "rest your larynx" are worse than useless. A rigid *regime of silence*, the patient writing everything he has to say, for a few months is to be followed by a gradual resumption of very moderate use of the voice. During the silent period twenty-five to fifty words may be allowed to prevent atrophy but they must be spoken in a low tone in a quiet place and they must be counted. By low is meant low as to loudness, not pitch. . . . The patient must never talk in a noisy place, such as an automobile, subway car, omnibus, railroad train or even in a city street.

Silence alone, however, is not enough to produce the required change. Silence will not improve the *habits* of voice any more than absence from a piano will give the pianist a new pattern of finger movements. The period of silence provides the environment for vocal recovery, but the patient will use the only habits he knows, which are the abusive ones, when he resumes talking, unless he has been taught a new and nondamaging method of phonation.

The second specific step in the re-educative process is to train the patient to phonate in a relaxed, easy manner. This instruction can proceed during the period of communicative silence, and its importance should be vigorously emphasized. Training in relaxed phonation provides a bridge from the previous type of vocal abuse to the recommended way of phonating.

Relaxed voice production can be acquired through a combination of at least five types of training, which include: (1) learning general physical relaxation; (2) development of emotional control; (3) training in the recognition of adequate and inadequate voice production; (4) development of the awareness of tense and relaxed phonation; and (5) learning to produce voice without strain.

General physical relaxation will result from systematic training. Relaxation, as discussed here, encompasses two concepts. The first is that relaxation is a general reduction in muscular activity, causing the individual to be motionless and flaccid. The second is that relaxation is a dynamic balance, in which the opposing groups of muscles exert just enough reciprocating tension upon each other to accomplish the desired movement with perfect control. It is this concept which applies in efficient phonation. Training in general relaxation is desirable as an aid to the functional, dynamic relaxation. The patient can learn to relax the extremities and other voluntary muscle groups before he can manage the involuntary muscles, many of which are active in phonation. Dynamic relaxation as presented here is the basis for muscular co-ordination, and good co-ordination of the phonatory musculature is essential for good voice production.

Several methods and techniques have been advocated (Parry, 1947) for general and differential, or localized, relaxation, and each has claimed suc cess. The three ingredients which seem to be necessary for general relaxation are: (1) a comfortable position for the patient; (2) skill in the recognition and localization of muscle tension; and (3) the ability to release excessive tension either directly by voluntary attention to it, or indirectly by substitut ing another sensation, such as "heaviness" or "lightness." The amount of training required to achieve relaxation will vary widely with the attitude of the patient toward the process and toward his voice problem. Unless he is able to practice several hours a day and unless there is real motivation, re laxation will probably not be achieved. It hardly needs to be added that the voice therapist should be thoroughly familiar with the various relaxation techniques and should be able to apply them to himself.

The mere technique of general physical relaxation is relatively ineffective if the individual who is trying to relax is chronically worried or easily upset emotionally. It follows that learning to relax requires personal insight and control of emotional responses, as well as the physical ability to release muscular tension. This discussion cannot touch on the psychological and counseling techniques which are useful in this phase of relaxation, but it can stress the fact that the voice therapist should be thoroughly familiar with such procedures. It can point out, also, that the counselor, the psychol ogist, and the psychiatrist can aid in dealing with excessive muscular tension in vocal defects.

The principles of general relaxation which have been mentioned estab lish the environment for relaxed phonation. Next it is desirable to direct the patient's attention to the phonatory process proper, in order to help him gain control over it. As indicated earlier, the aspects of phonation to which he must attend before starting direct vocal training are the acoustic and the kinesthetic. The patient must learn to hear the characteristics of other voices as well as his own; and he must develop the ability to recognize the sensa tions of tension and relaxation which are present when he voluntarily pro duces various kinds of voice quality.

Learning to hear one's own voice, and particularly learning to recognize vocal faults in one's self and others, requires training in listening. The most direct approach to this learning is through the combination of a good teacher and a good recording machine. The teacher's role is to help the patient re cord many samples of his voice, and, as they listen to the recordings, to point out to him the good and poor characteristics of the various qualities. This often requires several lesson periods and may be facilitated by critically listening to samples of other voices.

After the patient has learned to hear vocal differences, he can be taught to associate various kinds of vocal sound with the kinesthetic sensations of their production. Specifically, he can learn to recognize hypertension both by hearing the sound and by the concurrent kinesthetic sensation. At this stage, the individual begins to gain a positive control of phonation, and he is ready to start direct vocal training.

Direct training in voice production is the last part of the re-educative program for a defective voice produced by a relatively normal larynx. The general aim of the program is to teach the patient to produce a pleasant and serviceable voice which will allow the larynx to function in a normal manner. This helps the natural healing and rejuvenating processes to occur, and prevents the recurrence of vocal abuse and its sequelae. The re-educative program is composed of five well-defined types of exercise and instruction. Each deserves a brief review:

1. From the moment phonation is resumed, both in and out of the lesson situation, the voice must be used quietly. The patient should realize that he must speak in this subdued way, without any exceptions, for a year or two. The therapist will need to remind the patient frequently, particularly at the beginning of corrective work, but it is a necessary part of the therapy.

2. Phonation should be started with a breathy quality. To establish this concept, one helpful exercise is to instruct the patient to produce a phonated sigh on a downward inflection. He is asked to inhale deeply, to let the air out as in a sigh, and, at the same time, to produce a vowel sound on a downward pitch glide. This exercise can be modified rather quickly to a gently phonated downward pitch glide which is breathy, but without the extreme air escape of the sigh.

As work progresses, another exercise which can be used is the quiet production of words and sentences containing initial aspirate sounds, such as *home, hurry, He hit Henry's hat, Hold hope high,* and so on. When the patient can manage these materials, he should be encouraged to read ordinary prose and poetry in a slightly breathy voice.

Breathiness, purposely produced, keeps the vocal cords from striking each other as vigorously as in other types of phonation, and the closed phase of the vibratory cycle is shortened, thereby reducing the time in which the cords are in contact. The relaxed, breathy voice production also reduces the pressure between the arytenoid cartilages, which is particularly advantageous with contact ulcers.

3. The patient must be instructed and helped to use a middle pitch range. Quiet, breathy phonation can be of maximum benefit only if the individual uses a pitch which averages at least four or five tones above the lowest note of his range. When the vocal pitch is held within one or two notes of the bottom of the range, there is excessive muscle tension evident in the larynx. This type of voice production is often associated with contact ulcer.

Exercises for learning to raise the average pitch level begin with listening to recorded pitch changes and comparing them with the patient's habitual pattern. The individual should listen to recordings of his own voice and that of his teacher, in which the two have alternately produced sounds with rising and falling inflections. Such vowels as "ah" and "oh" spoken as though asking questions and the speaking of actual questions are useful drill materials. A successful ear-training technique for pitch discernment is the "saying" of a sentence with the lips closed. This effectively eliminates the words but

leaves the tune of the sentence. Variations in meaning produce differen
melody patterns. The preceding exercise can be extended easily into phrase
and sentences, spoken with several melodies to express different meaning:
For example, "*I* am going down town.", "I *am* going down town.", "I ar
going *down* town." Eventually the patient can learn to read prose quietl
and with meaningful pitch changes, which is an excellent pitch exercise. Thi
must be delayed, however, until he can both hear and control the pitch c
his own voice. Many good exercises for varying the pitch and for using th
most advantageous average pitch can be found in voice and diction text:
The pitch exercises mentioned in this section have been included to stres
the need for attention to pitch when working for effortless phonation.

The point which should be emphasized is that variation in pitch at onc
eliminates monotony and raises the average level of a pitch that is too low
The attempt to change the average pitch level by direct instruction to "Rais
the pitch," or through chanting and singing exercises, is usually unsatis
factory. Ordinarily the patient is unable to comply with the first request, an
he is apt to feel silly trying to carry out the second. Furthermore, it is difficul
to make a transition from the sung tones to normal speech. On the othe
hand, an emphasis on meaningful expression of ideas through pitch variatio
accomplishes the change of pitch level in a normal way and generally im
proves the expressiveness of the speech.

4. The patient must be taught to use the breath efficiently. To learn t
hear one's own voice defects and to develop the ability to phonate easily a
a comfortable pitch are fundamental to vocal rehabilitation. However, th
ability to sustain single sounds and otherwise to use the breath stream effi
ciently must be learned and practiced if the habits of easy phonation are t
be made permanent.

There can be little doubt that many persons with harmful vocal habit
expend more effort on breathing than is necessary. Most patients have a
adequate vital capacity, but have poor vocal control. Some persons, particu
larly those who do sedentary work, develop breathing habits in which th
expansion and contraction of the thoracic and abdominal regions are asyn
chronous. That is, when they depress the rib cage they not only move ai
through the trachea and larynx, as they intended, but the intrathoracic pres
sure also forces the diaphragm downward, and hence distends the abdomina
wall. This breathing pattern seems to contribute to undesirable, compen
satory muscle tensions in the neck and larynx, particularly when additiona
vocal effort is necessary.

Usually it is possible to improve the efficiency of breath use withou
specific attention to the respiratory movements. This can be done mos
simply by improvement of posture, combined with the sustaining of tone
and the uttering of progressively longer sentences on one breath. The latte
of course, does not imply that the patient should say as many words a
possible on one breath in ordinary conversation. The prolongation is a dri
and should be so explained to him.

A breathy type of phonation was recommended earlier to avoid hypertension in the laryngeal musculature and to foster a subdued type of voice production. This voice quality, however, is not desirable if it can be improved. One of the simplest and best methods of reducing the breathiness without increasing harmful tensions is to sustain tones as suggested above. This is another aspect of efficiency in the use of the breath in vocalization.

5. Frequent, short practice sessions are necessary in restorative voice therapy. Overuse of the voice is always detrimental and must be avoided. Furthermore, the rest periods have a positive benefit, for they provide the opportunity for recovery if misuse happens to occur. The frequency of the practice sessions will be determined by many circumstances, but an ideal schedule, which has been found to be practical in many cases, is to practice the last few minutes of each hour. At first, three minutes of active practice are enough. If that is tolerated, the time can be increased one minute in each period. If the individual demonstrates improvement and no detrimental effects are apparent, additional minutes can be added until the period reaches ten minutes. At this point, an occasional practice session of thirty minutes should be tried. When this period can be handled with ease, more responsibility for the vocal usage should be given to the patient. Regular instructional sessions should be continued at weekly intervals for several months and, if the patient demonstrates sufficient progress, he should be started on a series of lessons in which the time interval between sessions is gradually increased. This gives the voice therapist an opportunity to guide the patient into a sound program of self-directed vocal hygiene which he can manage alone.

Restorative therapy for organic voice problems usually is a long re-educative process. As indicated in the preceding paragraphs, it requires the understanding and co-operation of the patient, a period of vocal rest, and specific re-educative procedures. These include relaxation and the use of quiet phonation, a breathy type of voice production, attention to the pitch level and the speech melody, the sustaining of tones and the production of progressively longer sentences for phonatory control and breathing efficiency, and the use of frequent, short practice periods. The specific exercises and their use must be determined by the therapist as he arranges the therapeutic program to fit the needs of the patient.

**Compensatory voice therapy.** At the beginning of the discussion of therapy, a differentiation was made between treatment for persons with essentially normal structures and those who have had structural modifications which are permanent and which preclude the likelihood of normal voice production. The pathologies which illustrate the latter situation include the surgical removal of all or part of the larynx, destructive diseases, ankylosis of the joints, and paralysis. The purpose of the voice therapy, where these structural changes exist, is to help the patient acquire as effective a voice as possible without developing harmful vocal habits or unpleasant associated behavior. This therapy, therefore, has been labeled "compensatory."

The discussion of compensatory therapy has been divided into two parts first, procedures for patients who have a larynx; and, second, procedure for the laryngectomized. Again it should be stressed that each person re quires careful planning of therapy to fit his particular case. However, there are some suggestions which can be generally applied in compensatory ther apy.

The voice program for a person who has a modified larynx ordinarily does not require a period of silence beyond that necessary for the proper healing of the surgically treated areas. When the patient is released by his physician for voice therapy, it may begin immediately with a systematic and careful sampling of what the patient can do vocally. The patient should be asked to attempt tones over his complete pitch range to discover whether or not certain parts of his range are less hoarse, louder, or produced with less effort than others. These pitch changes should be tried with many vowels and with variations in intensity. Frequently, particularly in cases having one cord re moved, there will be a significantly better quality with one vowel sound at a particular pitch.

There are several other investigations which should also be made. One is to ask the patient to cough in order to note the presence or absence of com plete laryngeal closure. He should be asked, also, to turn his head first toward one shoulder then the other, and to produce selected sounds and words. When the head is in the rotated position, the internal laryngeal structures are sometimes more nearly approximated and the voice is improved. A similar assistance may result from asking the patient to press lightly on the sides of the thyroid cartilage while attempting to phonate. The effect of this manipu lation is to improve approximation. Turning the head and pressing the thy roid cartilage are devices only, and do not represent any real advancement in vocal recovery. They are valuable in therapy in two ways: they sometime encourage the patient to greater effort; and they may be useful "crutches" in difficult communicating situations, such as with the telephone or in noisy places.

These investigative procedures are at once both diagnostic and therapeu tic. Ordinarily they are extended over a period of weeks, and often a favor able response does not come until after some considerable training and trial period. Discovering what the patient is capable of doing is the real beginning point in therapy. Exercises to help him improve and extend what he can do constitute the second step in therapy, and require all the imagination and ingenuity the clinician has. Adaptations of the types of vocal drills suggested in the discussion of restorative therapy are very useful.

This type of patient requires careful management and supervision to avoid excessive practice and vocal use. Short practice periods are imperative. Some of these people need a great deal of encouragement, since their progress is apt to be slow and therefore unrewarding. On the other hand, as long as the therapist believes some additional progress can be made, the patient should not be allowed to become satisfied with his results. The person who loses his desire for improvement has ended his advancement.

The second type of compensatory therapy applies to persons without a larynx. It is commonly known that any complex sound put into the upper respiratory tract can be formed into audible speech by the adjustments of the articulating and resonating mechanisms. It follows that a laryngectomized person can learn to speak again if he can introduce or create a sound in his pharynx or mouth. The focus of the therapy, then, is the production of the necessary sound.

There are three common substitute sound generating mechanisms used by laryngectomees. One is the reed type of artificial larynx in which the reed element is activated by the exhaled air which passes through a tube from the tracheostomy. The sound which is generated by the reed travels through another tube into the mouth, where it is articulated into speech. A second type of sound producer is the Electrolarynx, a battery operated buzzer which is placed against the neck in such a position that the vibrations activate the air in the pharynx, and the resulting sound is articulated in the customary manner. The third mechanism is a body structure which is trained to function as a pseudoglottis. This is a constriction capable of vibrating, and is usually located at the junction of the esophagus and pharynx. However, it may occur higher in the pharynx or in the mouth. The air is customarily taken into the esophagus and expelled as in eructation, and is, therefore, called "esophageal speech." The skillful esophageal speaker presents an entirely normal appearance, his speaking is fluent, he can often change the pitch of his voice, and, although there is always some hoarseness present, the quality of his voice is relatively normal. The laryngectomized usually prefer esophageal speech, not only because it is the most nearly normal procedure but because there are fewer esthetic problems and because the artificial devices occasionally fail to function or are not always within easy reach when needed. (Moore, 1955.)

It is desirable to begin speech therapy as soon as possible after it is known that a laryngectomy is necessary. In some situations, training may be started before surgery (McCall, 1943). However, the voice therapist ordinarily does not see the patient until after the operation. Usually vocal restoration occurs more quickly when therapy is started as soon after surgery as healing permits. However, many have learned esophageal speech after years of voicelessness or use of an artificial device. Therefore, both the patient and the therapist should expect success, providing there is proper motivation and adequate structure.

The first step in speech-retraining with a laryngectomee is to ask him if he can belch voluntarily. If he cannot, or if he is not sure, ask him to imitate either you or a good laryngectomized speaker who can be present at the lessons. The teacher should produce a sound and ask the patient to follow immediately with his own effort. It is helpful if the instructor demonstrates with a word, such as "yes" or "no," rather than an ordinary eructation. The formation of a word is esthetically more pleasant, and also indicates specifically what the patient is expected to do.

If the individual cannot imitate, ask him if he has produced a belch noise at any time since his laryngectomy. If he has, and almost everyone is able to, it indicates that he probably can learn esophageal speech. However, if he has not done so, the voice therapist should talk with the surgeon, if this is possible, to learn if there are any structural reasons why the patient cannot be expected to develop esophageal speech. If there are, it might be wise to consider the immediate acquisition of an artificial reed larynx, or an Electrolarynx. The need for these devices, however, is extremely rare.

When imitation does not produce sounds in three or four lessons, it is wise to add description and explanation in the teaching of esophageal speech. The first step is to inform the patient, if he does not already know, that his larynx was only a sound producer, and that the tongue, soft palate, lips, and so on, formed the sound into speech. He should be told that any other sound which can be put into the mouth can also be used for speech, and that the best sound is the natural one made by the escape of air from the esophagus—a kind of belch sound. Through descriptions and diagrams, he can be told about the structural changes which have occurred and why he needs to learn to take air into the esophagus. This instruction reduces the patient's reluctance to try and prepares him to follow the therapeutic program.

Another phase of the preparatory motivation is the presentation of a good esophageal speaker to the new patient. This is often the most important single step in therapy. It should be pointed out, however, that if a speaker is not available the therapist should not substitute recordings of other laryngectomized speakers. It is usually very difficult to obtain a faithful recording of esophageal speech, and, as a result, the recording may be more disturbing than helpful. Later, after the patient has some skill, he can appreciate a recording of a fluent speaker and will profit from hearing it.

There are several methods used to teach laryngectomized persons to take in the air for speech. The therapist should be familiar with all of them, since one approach may be successful with one patient and another one with a second.

Perhaps the most normal-appearing way of taking air is called the "inhalation" technique, and for this reason it should be tried first. In this approach, the therapist simply asks the patient to open his mouth, to relax the mouth and throat areas, and to inhale suddenly. Often the reduction of pressure within the thorax causes the air in the pharynx to be drawn into the esophagus. It will help if the patient places his finger over his tracheostomy momentarily at the start of inhalation so that the inhalation movement will inflate the esophagus. If he is successful, he should be encouraged to expel the air immediately with as much noise as possible. It should be emphasized that the momentary obstruction of the tracheostomy is a device for helping the patient in his first attempts at speaking. It should not, and need not, be continued.

Another temporary assisting device used with the "inhalation" technique is a forward and upward projection of the chin. This pulls the anterior structures of the neck forward, thereby helping to open the entrance to the esophagus. The head movement should be stopped after the patient learns to inhale the esophageal air, since it is not necessary for speaking and calls attention to itself as an abnormality.

If the patient is not successful with the "inhalation" technique, or if he generates air noise at the tracheostomy, he should be taught the "injection" technique of obtaining air. The critical element in this method is pressure on air held in the mouth and pharynx of such nature that the air is forced, or "injected," into the esophagus. When the velopharyngeal closure has been made and the mouth passage occluded at the lips, alveolar ridge, or velum, as in the formation of plosive sounds, there is a certain amount of air enclosed within the oral and pharyngeal areas. When pressure is exerted on this air, it will move if an opening is available. In this instance, the only place the air can possibly go is through the esophageal sphincter into the esophagus. The air in the esophagus is then expelled by an increase in intrathoracic pressure, as in respiration. The sound is made by vibratory interruptions to this air movement at one of several places in the pharynx or mouth.

The patient may be taught to "inject" the air in either of two ways. The first starts from the "b" position, the second from the "d" position. In either instance, the patient is asked to place his lips or tongue in the position for one of these sounds, and then to "squeeze" the air in the mouth. The tongue and cheeks compress the air and force it into the esophagus. The patient should be instructed to expel the air immediately in an attempt to produce sound.

A variation of this procedure has been described by Moolenaar-Bijl (1953), who believes that some of the articulatory movements of speech, particularly the plosives, produce pressure pulses which move into and out of the esophagus several times during the utterance of a phrase or sentence. This may account for the long sentences which some speakers can produce.

The first purposeful sound is usually a great encouragement to the patient. Often, however, he will be unable to repeat it immediately, since his excitement and desire to speak create excessive pharyngeal tensions which he cannot control. This may disturb him unless the therapist explains what has happened. This offers an excellent opportunity to point out the need for regular and frequent practice periods in a calm, quiet atmosphere. The ability to produce controlled sounds varies widely. A few patients produce words in the first lesson, but most require from several weeks to several months. Those who believe they cannot learn require a little longer.

The controlled production of sound is of greatest importance, but it is only part of the development of esophageal speech. In addition, the patient must learn to increase the number of words spoken on one "breath," and he must eliminate the individual eccentricities which sometimes develop.

The speech rehabilitation process usually advances rapidly after the patient knows how to produce esophageal sounds voluntarily. For a short time, while he is concentrating his attention on the control of sound, he should be allowed to produce single vowels, but it is advisable to substitute real words soon. Single-syllable words which begin with a vowel or voiced consonant (particularly "b" and "d") and end with an unvoiced sound are especially valuable—*oat, boat, at, bat, ate, eat, it, but, boot,* and so on. In these, the final sound is added after the phonation has ceased, and requires no more esophageal sound than the single vowel or the consonant-vowel combination. The patient, however, feels that he is actually speaking, and thus is motivated more than with the semantically meaningless saying of vowels.

Two and three syllables in words and phrases should be introduced as soon as there is a reasonably consistent production of monosyllabic words. Usually the patient is so anxious to talk he will indicate what he is able to do, and hence will determine his own progress. Talking in conversation is perhaps the best possible practice so long as the patient makes a consistent effort to speak well.

Environmental factors can also contribute to the success of the re-educative program. The therapist should explain to the patient that the ease of speaking will vary with fatigue, excitement, and the speaking situation. It will also be helpful to have conferences with members of his family to explain what is being done and the need for patience with the laryngectomee in his attempts to learn to speak again.

From the very beginning of therapy, the patient should be instructed regarding the esthetic aspects of his problem. He must be encouraged to keep the neck area and the tracheostomy tube clean. Men should keep their shirt collars closed, and should wear a tie when in the presence of others. This not only protects the patient by shielding the opening, it also keeps the exhaled air from striking persons standing in front of the patient. Women can be shown how to wear neckerchiefs, collars, and brooches on special neck bands to cover and protect the tracheal opening. Such esthetic care will help the patient to be more socially acceptable and will, in consequence, add to his opportunities for conversational practice.

**Therapy for resonance problems.** The resonance problems of organic origin which have been discussed in this chapter have included excessively nasal and denasal voices. The causes of the former include cleft palate, congenitally short palate, surgical procedures, and paralyses of the velar and pharyngeal muscles. The organic causes of the latter are stoppages of various kinds in the nasal passages or nasopharynx.

The voice defects associated with a cleft palate deserve every consideration, but since they are only part of the total problem they should be discussed in their proper perspective in an integrated therapy. For this reason, the reader is referred to the chapter of this book which deals with cleft palate.

The congenitally short palate is, first of all, a medical and surgical problem. After repair has been accomplished, the voice therapist can contribute by providing appropriate palatal and pharyngeal exercises, and by supervising their use. These are identical with those used in postsurgery speech-training for cleft palate. Therefore, to avoid needless duplication, the reader is referred again to the section on cleft palate.

Surgical procedures, primarily tonsillectomy and adenoidectomy, sometimes leave scar tissue in the faucial area which reduces the mobility of the velum. If the disability is extreme, additional surgery by an expert can reduce the scar tissue and improve the mobility. Following corrective surgery, velopharyngeal exercises of the type recommended for paralyses, in the paragraphs below, are helpful.

When the removal of adenoid tissue produces hypernasality, it means that this tissue was being used to form the velopharyngeal closure. If the velum and other structures are normal, the ordinary swallowing and articulatory movements will modify the habits, and normal action will be developed. Sometimes voice exercises to stimulate velar activity are indicated to accelerate the speech improvement. These exercises are the same as those suggested in the following section on paralysis.

Paralysis in the velopharyngeal area may be slight, or it may be extensive. Where it affects many muscles, the prognosis for speech is unfavorable. Ordinarily, however, therapy should be tried even in severe cases on the chance that there may be some beneficial development. The less extensive the involvement, of course, the greater the expected response.

Exercises can begin with the passive lifting of the velum with a tongue blade or the handle of a spoon. In addition, the eliciting of a gag reflex is also beneficial. When some constrictive motion or lift of the palate is present, the patient should be shown how to observe his own structures with a mirror so he can develop his voluntary control to the fullest extent. This can be facilitated by having the patient protrude the tongue and say such vowels as "ah," "uh," "eh." Thrusting the tongue out pulls actively against the palatal elevators and tensors, thereby stretching and stimulating them. It should be pointed out to the patient that one of the best exercises is swallowing, which he should practice regularly and frequently. Liquids should be taken with many small sips, and the swallowing act carried through as completely as possible each time.

The types of speech exercises which are applicable to paralysis include: (1) teaching as wide-mouth opening on all sounds as is both possible and consistent with sound production; (2) alternating open vowels with nasal sounds; (3) blowing exercises, in which the air is directed through the mouth as completely as possible and in which the blowing is frequently changed into "oo" and "oh" sounds without altering the positions of the articulators; (4) developing gentle plosives to reduce the apparent nasality and air noises; and (5) the development of the patient's ability to listen carefully to his own voice and speech in an effort to produce the most intelligible communication possible.

Organically caused denasality always represents an obstruction in the airway above the soft or hard palate. These obstructions are not amenable to voice therapy; they can be remedied only by surgery or medical treatment, depending upon the nature of the obstruction. The voice therapist is often the first person consulted professionally by the patient with denasality. Proper referral to a rhinologist or a rhino-laryngologist constitutes a service to the patient, and usually alleviates the voice problem.

## SUMMARY

This discussion of organic disorders of voice has been developed through six main divisions, which included: (1) introductory perspective; (2) phonatory theory; (3) descriptive definitions of organic voice defects; (4) physiology of organic voice defects; (5) etiologies of organic voice defects; and (6) management of organic voice disorders, which touched both diagnosis and therapy.

The presentation attempted to be practical, to relate practice to theory, and to stimulate a research interest in this extremely complex field. The author is aware that there is much yet to be learned before voice problems can be managed adequately. Careful observation, systematic study, and detailed reporting should eventually provide answers to most of the problems.

## BIBLIOGRAPHY

ARNOLD, G. E. 1955. Vocal rehabilitation of paralytic dysphonia. II. Acoustic analysis of vocal function. *Arch. Otolaryng.,* 62, #6, 593–601.

ASH, J. E., and SCHWARTZ, L. 1944. The laryngeal (vocal cord) node. *Transactions Amer. Acad. Ophthal. Otolaryng., Supplement* 48, 323–331.

BALLENGER, H. C., and BALLENGER, J. J. 1954. A manual of otology, rhinology, and laryngology (4th ed.). Philadelphia: Lea and Febiger.

BERANEK, L. L. 1949. Acoustic measurements. New York: Wiley.

BERRY, M., and EISENSON, J. 1956. Speech disorders. New York: Appleton-Century-Crofts. Chs. 9 & 10.

BOIES, L. R. 1954. Fundamentals of otolaryngology (2nd ed.). Philadelphia, London: Saunders.

BRODNITZ, F. S. 1953. Keep your voice healthy. New York: Harper.

BULLIS, R. O., and KISSELBURGH, A. 1955. Vocal technique for treatment of certain speech difficulties. *Ann. Otol., Rhinol., Laryng.,* 64, #2, 443–450.

CURRY, E. T. 1949a. Hoarseness and voice change in male adolescents. *J. Speech Hearing Disorders,* 14, 23–25.

—— 1949b. Voice breaks and pathologic larynx conditions. *J. Speech Hearing Disorders,* 14, 356–358.

CURRY, R. O. L. 1940. The mechanism of the human voice. New York, Toronto: Longmans, Green.

FLETCHER, H. 1954. Speech and hearing in communication. New York: Van Nostrand.

GOLDMAN, J. L., and SOLMON, U. J. 1942. Effect of androgen therapy on voice and vocal cords of adult women. *Ann. Otol., Rhinol., Laryng.,* 51, 961–968.

GRAY, G. W., and WISE, C. M. 1947. The bases of speech (rev. ed.) New York, London: Harper.

HARRINGTON, R. 1944. A study of the mechanism of velopharyngeal closure. *J. Speech Disorders,* 9, 325–345.

HOLINGER, P. H., and JOHNSTON, K. C. 1951. Benign tumors of the larynx. *Ann. Otol., Rhinol., Laryng.,* 60, 496–509.

JACKSON, C., and JACKSON, C. L. 1937. The larynx and its diseases. Philadelphia: Saunders.

———— 1942. Diseases and injuries of the larynx. New York: Macmillan.

JONES, I. H., MUCKLESTON, H. S., and HILGER, J. A. 1953. Nutrition and related problems. *Laryngoscope,* 63, #12. 1145–1169.

KALLEN, L. 1934. Vicarious vocal mechanisms. The anatomy, physiology and development of speech in laryngectomized persons. *Arch. Otolaryng.,* 20, 460–503.

KING, B. T., and GREGG, R. L. 1949. Anatomic reason for various behavior of paralyzed vocal cords. *Transactions Amer. Goiter Assoc.,* 386–390.

LEDERER, F. L. 1947. Diseases of the ear, nose and throat (5th ed.). Philadelphia: F. A. Davis.

LEVIN, N. M. 1952. Speech rehabilitation after total removal of the larynx. *J. A. M. A.,* 149, 1281–1286.

LUSE, E. M. 1948. A study of vocal structures and speech in relation to metabolic rate. Unpublished Dissertation. Northwestern Univ.

McCALL, J. W. 1943. Preoperative training for development of the esophageal voice in laryngectomized patients. *Ann. Otol., Rhinol., Laryng.,* 52, 364–376.

MILLER, G. A. 1951. Language and communication. New York, Toronto: McGraw-Hill.

MOOLENAAR-BIJL, A. 1953. The importance of certain consonants in esophageal voice after laryngectomy. *Ann. Otol., Rhinol., Laryng.,* 62, #4, 979–989.

MOORE, P. 1955. The treatment of voice defects following surgery. *Connecticut State Med. J.,* 19, #3, 180–184.

MORRISON, T. F. 1952. Recurrent laryngeal nerve paralysis. *Ann. Otol., Rhinol., Laryng.,* 61, 567–592.

MULLENDORE, J. M. 1955. Pre-operative consultations in organic voice disorders. *Virginia Med. Monthly,* 82, 141–143.

MYERSON, M. C. 1950. Smoker's larynx; a clinical pathological entity. *Ann. Otol., Rhinol., Laryng.,* 59, 541–546.

———— 1955. Observations and considerations on cigarette smoking. *Ann. Otol., Rhinol., Laryng.,* 64, 412–417.

PARRY, R. A. 1947. An experimental evaluation of training in suggestion relaxation and speech exercises. Unpublished Dissertation. Northwestern Univ.

PEACHER, G. 1947. Contact ulcer of the larynx. *J. Speech Disorders,* 12, 67–76 (part 1)., 12, 177–190 (part 2).

ROBE, E. Y., MOORE, P., ANDREWS, A. H., and HOLINGER, P. H. 1956. A study of the role of certain factors in the development of speech after laryngectomy: 1. Type of operation. 2. Site of pseudoglottis. 3. Co-ordination of speech with respiration. *Laryngoscope,* 66, #3, 173–186 (Part 1); 66, #4, 382–401 (Part 2); 66, #5, 481–499 (Part 3).

VAN RIPER, C. 1954. Speech correction (3rd ed.). New York: Prentice-Hall. Ch. 8.

WEST, R., KENNEDY, L., and CARR, A. 1947. The rehabilitation of speech (rev. ed.). New York: Harper. Chs. 6 & 7.

WHITE, F. W. 1946. Some causes of hoarseness in children. *Amer. Acad. Otol., Rhinol., Laryng.,* 55, 537–542.

WILLIAMSON, A. B. 1944. Diagnosis and treatment of eighty-four cases of nasality. *Quart. J. Speech,* 30, 471–479.

———— 1945. Diagnosis and treatment of seventy-two cases of hoarse voice. *Quart. J. Speech,* 31, 189–202.

# PART III

Speech and Voice Disorders
Unrelated to Organic
Abnormalities

# CHAPTER 23

# FUNCTIONAL DISORDERS OF ARTICULATION–SYMPTOMATOLOGY AND ETIOLOGY

• *Margaret Hall Powers, Ph.D.*

## GENERAL CONSIDERATIONS

ARTICULATION PROBLEMS have long been recognized as the most prevalent of all the disorders of speech. Because this is true and since only a small fraction of articulation cases are organically based, functional articulation problems constitute a highly significant group of disorders in the total field of speech pathology. They merit serious study and much greater scientific investigation than they have yet received, not only because they are so common but also because they are by no means so simply explained and treated as many people have assumed.

How can *functional articulation disorders* be defined? Let us examine the words of the term separately. *Articulation* can be defined as the production of speech sounds by the stopping or constricting of the vocalized or non-vocalized breath stream by movements of the lips, tongue, velum, or pharynx. *Disorders* of articulation are faulty placement, timing, direction, pressure, speed, or integration of these movements, resulting in absent or incorrect speech sounds. *Functional* is more difficult to define. The term originated in the field of medicine but has been widely adopted in speech pathology, where it has come to have a meaning practically synonymous with *nonorganic*. Some speech pathologists use it in such a way as to suggest the even narrower meaning of *nonstructural,* though most prefer to think of it as having physiological and neurological connotations as well as anatomical significance. Some of the writers in speech pathology have discussed the concept of *functional* in the following ways.

On the basis of determined or inferred organic pathology and the lack of such we classify disorders of articulation and phonation as organic and functional respectively. (Travis, 1931, p. 196.)

When no apparent organic or physiological cause can be discovered we assume the speech disorder to be functional and physiogenic. (Eisenson, 1938, p. 136.)

In other cases it [faulty articulation] may not be directly attributable to imperfect structures, but rather to a disturbance in the *function* of these structures and is then termed a non-organic or functional disorder. (Koepp-Baker, 1936, p. 231.)

Perhaps the most precise and inclusive statement comes from Bender and Kleinfeld (1938, p. 84) who, in a paragraph entitled "What are functional disorders?" have this to say:

> Any noticeable deviation from the normal and characteristic activity of any member of the speech and vocal mechanism that is not caused by a physical and organic impairment or change of structure of the part or parts involved in speech and voice production may be classified as a functional disorder of speech. This general connotation presupposes a healthy nervous system, normal mentality, and a normal physical development of the speech organs but an improper co-ordination and control of them during the production of speech sounds.

Taking these concepts into consideration, a functional articulation disorder can be defined as an inability to produce correctly all of the standard speech sounds of the language, an inability for which there is no appreciable structural, physiological, or neurological basis in the speech mechanism or its supporting structures, but which can be accounted for by normal variations in the organism or by environmental or psychological factors. This is a convenient and common-sense definition. In reality there can be no strict separation between *organic* and *functional*. There are probably few, if any, cases which are purely organic or purely functional, so that we have to be cautious in attempting to force a dichotomy upon our cases.

Many of the so-called *functional* cases have subtle organic factors in their pattern of etiology, particularly when the past history of the case is considered. For example, a child may have developed a lisp because of irregular dentition which has been corrected before we see him. The lisp continues and should be diagnosed as *functional,* although it would originally have been diagnosed as *organic.*

It has become customary to diagnose a case on the basis of the etiological factors operating at the time the diagnosis is made. Any sensible clinician will naturally, of course, give consideration also to factors which have been operative in the past in order to understand the problem as thoroughly as possible. However, it is the causal pattern operating at the time the case presents itself for study which will largely determine the diagnosis and the program of therapy. West, Kennedy, and Carr (1947, pp. 66–67) express this clinical policy explicitly:

> When we use the term *organic* and *functional* we are not concerned with the original cause but with the present condition that serves as the intermediary between the cause and the defect. A disorder is organic when this intermediary condition is a defect of structure or tissue, regardless of whether the original cause was psychogenic or physiogenic.

They consider a disorder functional when the intermediary is a disturbance not of structure or tissue but of the working of the parts and the reacting of the tissues.

It should also be emphasized that *functional* is an etiological, not a symptomatological term. It is frequently seen that the same acoustic effect may be produced by either an organic or a functional cause. Two cases with lisps, for example, may sound almost identical but may have very different causes.

Still another issue arises in the *organic* versus *functional* dilemma. Many *functional articulation* cases are so labeled unjustifiably through what this writer likes to call "diagnosis by default," meaning that an assumption is made that a speech defect must be functional if no obvious organic deviations are found to account for it. The term *functional* is used as a catch-all for speech problems which cannot be explained in other terms. This is not a legitimate procedure. It is necessary for the speech diagnostician to demonstrate positive evidences of functional etiology as well as to eliminate negative evidences.

The term *functional* does not exclude the normal variation within the population of almost all physical and psychological traits. Indeed, the greater part of the research which has been done on functional disorders of articulation has been devoted to investigating the presence or absence of systematic differences between functional articulation cases and normal speakers in a series of traits, ranging from structural differences of the speech mechanism to motor dexterity, auditory memory span, sound discrimination, and others. Such differences when found have not often been of the order of pathological variations but merely of normal variations. It is important to distinguish between *pathological variations* and the *normal variations* which are to be expected of most human physical and psychological traits. The former, if present in an articulatory case and causally related to the speech deviation, would lead to a diagnosis of *organic*. The latter, being normal, would be encompassed within the diagnosis of *functional*. Variations of physical, sensory, and other factors *within the normal range* are expected in functional articulation cases as in other types of cases and in normal speakers as well.

Probably more than any other type of speech disorder, with the possible exception of those often classified as *delayed speech,* functional articulation cases are intimately associated with all dimensions of the individual's growth. They are to be understood only in terms of the dynamics of physical, intellectual, emotional, and social growth patterns, the relationships among these patterns within the individual, and the modifications produced in them by the environment.

Functional articulation disorders can, therefore, be very complex as well as very simple. There may be many etiological factors involved or only one or two. The complexity of etiology is not always related, either, to the extent of speech involvement. A relatively limited speech symptom such as a lateral lisp may be very difficult to explain. Every experienced clinician knows that there are some articulation cases which seem to defy explanation. It is perhaps helpful to consider that causal factors may be of three types: predisposing, precipitating, and perpetuating. All may be involved. Although, as stated earlier, only presently-operating factors determine a diagnosis of *organic* or *functional,* factors in all of the above categories should be investigated. It is more important to understand than to label.

**TABLE 1. Incidence of Functional Articulatory Defectives as Reported in Various Studies***

| Study | Population Studied | Total No. of Speech Defectives | Author's Diagnostic Classifications | No. of Cases | Per Cent of Total Cases | Probably Classifiable as "Functional Articulatory" Number | Per Cent |
|---|---|---|---|---|---|---|---|
| White House Conference (1931)* | Ages 5–18 in 48 U.S. cities of over 10,000 | Reduced to basis of 10,000 cases | Sound substitutions / Oral inactivity | 4,623.80 / 1,146.44 | 46.2 / 11.5 | 5,770.24* | 57.7 |
| ASHA Comm. report of White House Conference (1951) | Ages 5–21 | 2,000,000 (assumed) | Functional articulatory | 1,200,000 | 60.0 | Same | 60.0 |
| (1951) | All ages | 7,500,000 (assumed) | Functional articulatory | 4,500,000 | 60.0 | Same | 60.0 |
| Louttit and Halls (1936) | Grades 1–12 County schools / City schools | 3,049 / 4,258 | Articulatory / Articulatory | 2,434 / 3,354 | 80.0 / 79.0 | Same / Same | 80.0 / 79.0 |
| Burdin, L. G. (1940)* | Grades 1–4 | 106 | Indistinctness / Baby talk / Lispers | – / – / – | 42.45 / 14.15 / 11.32 | | 67.9 |
| Mills and Streit (1942) | Elementary children | 473 | Dyslalia | 326 | 69.0 | Same | 69.0 |
| Powers, M. H. (1951) Chicago Public Schools | Elementary and high school | 8,391 | Functional articulation disorders | 6,713 | 80.0 | Same | 80.0 |
| Black, M. E. (1950–51) Illinois State Program | Elementary and high school | 26,416 | Articulatory | 20,800 | 78.7 | Same | 78.7 |
| MacLearie, E. C. (1953) Ohio State Program | Elementary and high school | 12,323 | Articulatory | 10,028 | 81.3 | Same | 81.3 |

* In starred entries the published data have been rearranged or combined by this writer. For original references, see bibliography.

It is sound clinically to assume multiple-causation of functional articulation cases—indeed, of all cases—so that we will force ourselves to examine all possibilities. Fewer mistakes or oversights will be made than if we start out with the easy assumption that an obvious causal factor is all-effective in a given case and are thus led into overlooking contributing factors. It is good clinical wisdom to operate with the concept of *causal pattern* rather than *cause*.

## Incidence

Functional articulation disorders are the most numerous of all of the speech disorders. Their importance as a therapeutic problem is suggested by Table 1, which presents a summary of the incidence of these disorders taken from some of the major survey reports published. Examination of this table shows clearly the high incidence of this type of disorder among speech problems in general. The final three entries are of particular significance because of the large numbers of cases involved and because the figures given are based, not upon estimates or questionnaires, but upon diagnoses by trained speech-correction teachers in public school programs, using fairly uniform criteria. It is also significant that there is remarkably close agreement in the percentages reported in the three studies. Upon the basis of these results, it is safe to say that functional articulation defectives represent between 75 and 80 per cent of all speech defectives in the school population.

## SYMPTOMATOLOGY AND CLASSIFICATION

### General Description

The term *functional articulation disorders* encompasses a wide variety of deviate speech patterns. These can all be described in terms of four possible types of acoustic deviation in the individual speech sounds; omissions, substitutions, distortions, and additions. An individual may show one or any combination of these deviations.

Functional articulation disorders may range in severity from mild misarticulation which is hardly noticeable except to the trained ear, through various degrees of severity to complete unintelligibility at the other extreme. Articulation disorders may involve only one or two sounds, they may involve certain groups of sounds, or they may involve all or nearly all the speech sounds of the language. Errors on one or two sounds, while often conspicuous and unattractive, do not usually affect seriously the intelligibility of the individual's speech. Intelligibility is related to the number of different sounds misarticulated. The particular sounds which are defective will also determine to some extent the obviousness of the disorder and the degree to which it interferes with communication. Some consonants are more critical for intelligibility than others.

Another factor determining the conspicuousness of the defect is the frequency with which the individual's defective sounds occur in speech. Travis (1931, p. 223) found consonant sounds occurring in the following rank order of frequency in the conversational speech of children: [t], [n], [r], [s], [l], [d], [m], [k], [z], [w], [ð], [h], [b], [p], [g], [f], [v], [ŋ], [j], [ʃ], [θ], [tʃ], [dʒ], [ʌ], [ʒ]. Henrikson's study (1948) showed approximately the same order of frequency. From this ranking it can be seen, for example, that a defective [ʒ] is relatively unimportant, a defective [s] very conspicuous because of its frequent occurrence.

Articulation disorders also vary in the degree of consistency of the misarticulations. Some individuals make the same acoustic errors consistently regardless of the word or the position of the sound within the word. Others vary greatly, using the sound correctly in some words, omitting it in others, and using substitutions for it in others. It is not uncommon for a sound which occurs twice within one word to be given differently in the two positions.

The degree of articulatory defect, therefore, has to be evaluated in terms of the degree of misarticulation, the consistency of misarticulation, the importance for intelligibility of the specific sounds involved, and the number of different sounds involved.

### Classification

Functional articulatory disorders share in the general confusion which has existed and still exists in speech pathology in regard to what labels to attach to various speech symptoms. Some authors have tried to classify and name speech disorders on the basis of etiology, some on the basis of symptomatology. Most of the commonly used terminology has a foot in each camp. This is the case with the disorders under discussion here—*functional articulatory,* in which *functional* is an etiological term and *articulatory,* a symptomatological term. The trend in recent literature is away from a pretentious, elaborate terminology which purports to be scientific but for which there is as yet insufficient scientific support, and toward a greater simplification and an attempt at bringing about some order and agreement. This is long overdue. Ogilvie (1942, p. 1), in introducing her exhaustive study of terminology in speech pathology says, "As evidence of the confusion that exists, there are eight synonyms for *baby talk,* ten for *thick speech,* twelve for *nasality,* fifteen for *phonasthenia* ("tired voice"), and twenty-one for *stuttering.*"

It is reassuring to observe in the literature a trend toward the use of common-sense terms and to note that these are based primarily upon acoustic phenomena or symptomatology. This trend seems a constructive one since etiology is still obscure or controversial for some disorders, whereas there is considerable agreement on symptomatology.

Some writers (Ainsworth, 1948; Johnson *et al.,* 1948; and others) describe functional articulation problems quite simply in terms of the four basic types of misarticulation mentioned earlier: omissions, substitutions, distortions, and additions. Others have ranged from very elaborate subclassifications (Seth and Guthrie, 1935, who list *dyslalia, logorrhea, idioglossia, audimutitas* and *rhinolalia* as varieties of articulation disorder) to general categories of a descriptive type such as Van Riper's (1947) *infantile perseveration, lalling, delayed speech,* and *oral inaccuracy.*

The classification preferred by this writer is based on speech symptomatology and makes no assumptions concerning etiology except the obvious one that all disorders encompassed within the term are primarily functional. It has the merit of simplicity and does not overreach our present stage of knowledge. Future research may help us to refine this classification considerably.

Functional disorders of articulation can be divided into two general categories and the first of these into several clinical types. The classification given below is followed by a description and discussion of each type:

1. Misarticulation of specific speech sounds or groups of sounds (sound omissions, substitutions, distortions, additions).
   Infantile perseveration (baby talk, infantile speech)
   Lisping (misarticulation of one or more of the sibilant consonants: [s], [z], [ʃ], [ʒ], [tʃ], [dʒ])
   Lalling (distortion of [r] or [l])
   Misarticulation of other miscellaneous sounds
2. General oral inaccuracy

**1. Misarticulation of specific speech sounds or groups of sounds.** Defective articulation can be analyzed in terms of one or more of the four types of deviation listed above: omissions, substitutions, distortions and additions. In *omissions* the individual leaves out a phoneme at a place where it should occur. It is not replaced by any other sound. Examples of this are found constantly in the speech of young children, as *tep* for *step, pay* for *play, daw* for *dog.* Omissions are particularly likely to occur in consonant blends, as in the first two examples above.

In *substitutions* the individual substitutes one standard speech sound for another or may substitute consistently a nonstandard speech sound, such as a glottal stop, for a standard speech sound. Usually, though not always, the substituted sound is one of the sounds earliest acquired in the normal sequence of speech development. A [w] is often substituted for [r] or for [l] as in *w*an for *r*an, a*w*ound for a*r*ound, *w*ady for *l*ady. In mu*vv*er for mo*th*er [v] is substituted for [ð]; in *t*itty for *k*itty [t] for [k]; in bu*t* for bu*s* [t] for [s].

In *distortions* the production of the speech sound is modified in some way so that the acoustic result only approximates the standard sound and is not accurate. The individual might be said to aim at the sound and miss it. Distortions vary in degree, some being extreme mutilations, others varying only slightly from the standard sound. Distortions are likely to be fairly regular and consistent while substitutions and omissions are often highly inconsistent. Distortions cannot be described easily in writing because they are often sounds for which we have no printed symbol even in the phonetic alphabet.

*Additions* are a less frequent form of misarticulation than the others
Sounds which are not part of the word are interpolated or added, as in *warsl*
for wash, *puh*lease for please, and *puh*retty for pretty. In the last two ex
amples a vowel is interpolated between the two consonants of a blend.

All misarticulations can be described in terms of the four error types jus
discussed. However, there are certain *patterns* of misarticulation which w
recognize as clinical types. They are seen so frequently and the cases withii
one type are so similar that it is important to identify and describe them. Th
types to be described are by no means mutually exclusive, in fact, are ofter
overlapping. Specific cases may show characteristics of more than one type
Yet there is a clinical reality to these types which warrants discussion.

*Infantile Perseveration (Baby Talk, Infantile Speech, Pedolalia).* Th
terms *baby talk* or *infantile speech* do not refer to the type of speech hear
in very young children during the early stages of normal speech developmen
but rather to the persistence of some of these early characteristics beyon
the age at which correct speech sounds should have been acquired. Infantil
perseveration is characterized mainly by the omission and substitution c
sounds and is frequently but not always associated with immaturity in lan
guage development. The child who says, "Me do in tah" (Me go in car), i
using immature grammatical forms (*me* for *I* and omission of *the*) as well a
sound substitutions, [d] for [g] and [t] for [k], and omissions ([r] in car)
Another characteristic of infantile perseveration is the marked inconsistenc
with which sound omissions and substitutions are often made. A child ma
substitute [f] for [θ] in one word, [t] or [s] for [θ] in another word, or a soun
may be substituted for a second sound and that one in turn substituted fo
still a third. Sound omissions may be similarly inconsistent, with the sam
child giving a sound correctly in some words, omitting it in others.

In order to judge whether a child's misarticulations are normal for his ag
or are perseverations of speech characteristic of an earlier age level, we mus
be aware of the developmental order of sounds and the ages at which th
various speech sounds normally appear. Table 2 summarizes some of th
principal investigations on genetic development of the voluntary use of Eng
lish consonant sounds. Careful study of this table will show that there i
considerable agreement among the studies in regard to the developmenta
*order* of the different sounds. There is less agreement on the age levels a
which the different sounds appear. The Wellman, Case, Mengert, and Brad
bury study (1931) shows a considerably earlier appearance of sounds tha
do the other studies, but these results are doubtless influenced by the evider
fact that the children in this study were a superior group (average I.Q.–
115.9).

It is interesting to compare the common misarticulations found in case
of infantile perseveration with the developmental pattern as shown in Tabl
2. Van Riper (1938) studied 60 cases of baby talk, ages eight to twenty-nin
and found that 68 per cent of the errors were on blends, such as *str, thr,* an
involved, particularly, blends with *r, s, l,* and *th.* The nine most frequent

missed single consonants were, in this order, *s, r, l, ch, th, k, g, f,* and *v.* Berry and Eisenson (1942, pp. 89–90) list the sound substitutions which, in their experience, are most frequently made in *baby talk:*

| | | | | | |
|---|---|---|---|---|---|
| w] | for | [l] | [f] | for | [s] |
| ] | for | [l] | [θ] | for | [s] |
| ɔ] | for | [f] | [t] | for | [k] |
| ʔ] (glottal stop) | for | [l] | [d] | for | [g] |
| " | | | [t] | for | [tʃ] |
| ʔ] | for | [t] | [d] | for | [dʒ] |
| ] | for | [θ] | [s] | for | [ʃ] |

Sex differences should also be considered in evaluating infantile perseverations of young children. As the result of a thorough investigation of speech sound acquisition, Templin (1952, p. 284) reported: "The girls reach about 95 per cent correct articulation, probably practically adult articulation, at about seven years while boys take another year in which to reach the same degree of perfection."

Consonant sounds are most likely to be omitted when they occur in final or medial positions in words or initially as a member of a consonant blend. This position differential is also true of normal speech development. Irwin (1951), in a prolonged and intensive investigation of normal infant speech-sound development, found that the development of initial consonants is near during infancy, of medial consonants decelerating, and of final consonants accelerating. He found that the occurrence of initial consonants is greater than medials and medials greater than finals in infant vocalization. Final consonants are infrequent during the first half-year of life. Thus, the inferiority of medial and final consonants as compared with initial is seen to be as true of normal speech development as it is of consonant production in infantile perseveration.

In extreme cases of infantile perseveration, nearly all consonants are omitted and the resulting speech is a series of vowel sounds, sometimes interspersed with glottal stops. In other cases several of the early consonants are made to substitute for all the others. The preponderance of vowels in these extreme cases again shows the perseveration of sound patterns which are typical of early stages of speech development. Chen and Irwin (1946) found that at two and a half the infant possesses practically all the vowel types used in adult speech and about two-thirds of the consonant types. Metraux (1950) confirms this with her finding that vowel production in the child's speech is more than 90 per cent correct by 30 months but that consonant production does not reach 90 per cent correctness until 54 months.

Lundeen (1950) has shown that the diadochokinetic rate of the different speech sounds tends to follow the developmental order. He found that the diadochokinetic rate for [t], [d], [p], and [b] is faster than that for [s], [z], [ʃ], and [g], with [f] and [v] occupying an intermediate position. The diadochokinetic rank order of sounds corresponded closely with the developmental order reported by Poole (1934) and shown in Table 2.

**TABLE 2. Development of the Purposive Use of Consonant Sounds***

| Investigator | Age in Years | | | | | | | | | | | | |
|---|---|---|---|---|---|---|---|---|---|---|---|---|---|
| | 2 | 2½ | 3 | 3½ | 4 | 4½ | 5 | 5½ | 6 | 6½ | 7 | 7½ | 8 |
| Wellman, Case, Mengert, and Bradbury (1931, pp. 50–52). Given correctly by 75% or more of the children. | p–, –p–, b–, –b–, t–, d–, m–, –m–, n–, –n–, –ŋ–, w–, –w–, h | | –b, –t, –d–, k–, –k–, g–, –g–, –m, –n, –ŋ–, f–, –f–, –f, –z–, –z | | –p, –d, –k, –g, –v, –tʃ, dʒ–, –dʒ– l–, –l–, –l, r–, –r, –j, –j– | | –t–, v–, –v–, θ–, ð–, –ð, s–, –s–, –s, z–, –l, –l–, –ʃ, ʒ | tʃ–, –tʃ–, r– | –dʒ | (The authors do not list the following by 6:) | | ŋ–, w–, –w–, –θ, –θ, –ð | |
| Poole (1934) | | | | p, b, m, w, h | | t, j, d, n, ŋ, k, g | | f | | v, ð, ʃ, ʒ, l | | s, θ, ʍ, z, r, tʃ, dʒ | |

| Roe (in Johnson, Editor, 1950) | p<br>b<br>m | t<br>d<br>n<br>k<br>g<br>ŋ | f<br>v | l<br>r<br>ʒ<br>dʒ<br>tʃ | s<br>z<br>ʃ<br>sl<br>pl<br>st | |
|---|---|---|---|---|---|---|
| Templin (1952)<br><br>Percentage of correct utterance. | 90% (vowels and diphthongs) 2/3 (consonants) ½ (2-cons. blends) 1/3 (3-cons. blends) | 80% (cons.)<br>70% (2-cons.)<br>60% (3-cons.) | | 90%<br>80%<br>70% | 90%<br>90%<br>90% | Not uttered correctly by 90%:<br>Initial ʍ, sl<br>Medial: ʍ, ʒ<br>Final: ʒ, z, r, θ, nt, kt, skr, str, dʒ, tl, tr |

* Some of these data have been rearranged by the present writer. For the original data, see the references listed in the bibliography.

To summarize the misarticulations characteristic of infantile persevera
tion, we can say that children tend to substitute more visible for less visibl
sounds, sounds acquired early in normal speech development for thos
acquired later (see Table 2), diadochokinetically faster sounds for slower
and phonetically easier, less precise sounds for phonetically harder sound
requiring more precise co-ordination and timing. In short, the pattern o
speech sound production which research has shown to be typical of norma
speech development in the first several years of life is reflected at later ag
levels in cases of infantile perseveration.

There are two general types of disorder which both fall within the broa
category of speech immaturity. These are *delayed speech* (Chaps. 15 an
16), which is a more complex and profound disorder, and *infantile persevera
tion*. Delayed speech is the more inclusive of the two. Indeed, infantil
perseveration can be thought of as the articulatory aspect of delayed speec
but there is no sharp distinction between the two. If a child's speech im
maturity is confined largely to sound omissions and substitutions, if he ha
learned to rely mainly on speech as his means of communication, if ther
is considerable output of speech, if the onset of speech has been fairly typi
cal, if he attempts sentences as well as words and phrases, his speech devia
tion can best be referred to as *infantile perseveration*.

If, however, there has been little or no attempt at speech until past tw
years of age, if gestures and nonspeech vocalizations are used extensively
if speech is limited mainly to nouns, with little use of qualifying, connective
or auxiliary words, if vocabulary is meager, if single words are used fc
sentences or phrases, most speech clinicians would tend to call the disorde
*delayed speech*. The distinction between *infantile perseveration* and *delaye
speech* is thus both qualitative and quantitative but there is considerabl
overlap between them in symptomatology. Of the two, *delayed speech* i
usually the more serious and complex. It is a language as well as a speec
disorder and is usually more difficult to diagnose and to treat.

*Lisping (Sigmatism)*. Lisping can be defined as misarticulation of one c
more of the six sibilant consonants, [s], [z], [ʃ], [ʒ], [tʃ], [dʒ]. Some ind
viduals have difficulty with all six, but many misarticulate only [s] and [z
Occasionally a person has difficulty with only [ʃ] and [ʒ] or with [tʃ] and [dʒ
The [s] and [z] sounds are among the most frequently misarticulated of a
the speech sounds, probably because the requirements for their productio
in terms of muscular adjustments are so exacting that minor variations ca
easily occur. Minor distortions are also more easily heard in these soun
than in most others.

Most writers in speech pathology agree in defining *lisping* essentially as
is defined here, though there is considerable variation in their manner c
classifying and describing various types of lisping. Three types of defectiv
sibilant articulation are described, however, by nearly everyone: *latera
lingual protrusion* (also called *interdental, frontal,* or *central* by some a
thorities) and *nasal* (called *recessive* by Berry and Eisenson, 1942). Robbi

in Froeschels, 1948) lists ten types of sigmatism as follows: strident, interdental, addental, lateral, bilateral, palatal (tongue too distant from incisors so that [s] resembles [ʃ]), occlusive (excessive tongue pressure so that [s] resembles [t]), labiodental (lower lip against upper incisors and [s] produced with normal tongue position), nasal, and stertorous (a snoring effect in addition to nasal emission).

Although all these varieties of defective sibilant articulation are actually encountered in clinical work, for most practical purposes the classification is unnecessarily differentiated and cumbersome and of more interest to the phonetician than to the speech pathologist. Because of the tongue's unique capacity for assuming an almost endless variety of positions and shapes, sibilant distortion can be equally varied. However, it seems meaningful and useful to identify only three principal types of lisping, based upon the direction of breath emission, and one subclassification within the first of these. These three types are: *central* (with *interdental* or *tongue protrusion* as a subtype), *lateral,* and *nasal.*

In a *central lisp* the tongue functions in the midline as it should and breath emitted centrally through a groove, but the tongue position is faulty in either the vertical or the anterior-posterior plane or in both. The tongue may be carried too high so that the air stream is partly or entirely occluded against the upper incisors, alveolar ridge, or hard palate, producing a sound resembling [t] or [d] or a dull, weak, distorted sibilant. If the tongue-tip is too high and also retracted, a whistling, overly sharp [s] is produced. The position of the tongue may be too low, flat, or relaxed in the mouth so that the sound produced lacks sibilance and sounds dull or "mushy." In the antero-posterior plane the tongue may be too retracted so that the [s] sound more like [ʃ] or it may be placed too far forward so that it touches the upper incisors or protrudes between the upper and lower incisors.

This latter *tongue protrusion or interdental* distortion is so common that it merits special designation as a subtype of the *central lisp*. It is frequently heard as one characteristic of infantile perseveration cases, often as a residual lingual habit formed when the upper deciduous incisors are lost and space is left temporarily before the permanent incisors erupt. In this type of lisp, [s] approximates [θ] and [z] approximates [ð]. All of the varieties of distortion just described as coming under the *central-lisp* category have in common a faulty midline tongue position. Although the tongue is usually bilaterally symmetrical and emission of air centralized, the tongue is incorrectly positioned vertically, antero-posteriorly, or some combination of both.

In a *lateral lisp* the tongue-tip is pressed against the upper central incisors or alveolar ridge much as it is for the [l] sound. The air stream cannot be emitted through a central groove but is divided and escapes at the sides of the mouth. In other cases the tongue moves to one side or the other of the midline and lifts or twists to touch the lateral teeth, forcing the air out over the opposite side of the tongue. The *lateral lisp* is so named because of this essential characteristic of unilateral or bilateral rather than central emissio of breath. The acoustic result is conspicuous and highly unpleasant. It ha a "slushy" sound as though an excess of saliva were present. This type of lis is persistent and usually one of the most resistant to corrective training c the functional articulatory problems. Lateral lisps often have their origin ii early irregularities or lateral spaces in the upper dental arch. Incorrect lingua habits are formed and often persist after the dental problem has been cor rected. Most cases of lateral lisp have to be classified, therefore, as func tional.

The third type of lisp, the *nasal lisp,* is relatively rare compared with th others. It is produced by a relaxed soft palate and retracted tongue which fai to effect a nasopharyngeal closure and allow air to escape through the nose The result in some cases is a voiceless nasal fricative for [s] and in others more conspicuous and unpleasant snort.

Sibilant distortion can be produced by, or accompanied by atypical li movements. Since good sibilant articulation depends upon the air shaft passing between the incisal edges of the teeth, any approximation of the lip to the teeth constitutes an obstruction to the free passage of this air shaft. Th lower lip may touch the upper teeth in a manner similar to the productio of the [f] sound and do this either symmetrically or to one side. Less ofte the upper lip is involved. These labial habits are unattractive visually as wel as acoustically.

*Lalling (Distortion of [r] or [l]). Lalling* is less well defined than *lispin* and yet represents a type of case quite often encountered clinically. Th sounds affected are usually [r] or [l] or both but other consonants for whos production the tongue-tip is important, such as [t] or [d], may also be in volved. No clear-cut substitutions are made for these sounds. Rather ther is a distortion of them in which the tongue is mainly at fault. The tongue-tip instead of being raised to the alveolar ridge for [l] or approximating th alveolar ridge for [r], is kept low in the mouth, the tongue is flat and lax tongue movements are weak and sluggish, and the back of the tongue ma be retracted and humped. Articulatory movements occur farther back i the mouth than normally. A sound resembling [w] but without lip action ma replace [r] and [l] or the result may more resemble a [j] or the vowels [ɔ or [ɔ].

*Lalling* resembles *general oral inaccuracy,* to be described later, in tha tongue movements are sluggish and insufficiently energized. *Lalling* refers however, to the distortion of this limited group of sounds whereas *genero oral inaccuracy* involves most or all of the speech sounds.

Lalling, though usually functional, may also have an organic basis, pas or present. Like the lateral lisp, it may have had its origin in an organic de viation which may or may not be present when the case comes to our at tention. In cases where the lingual frenum has been tight, raising the tip c the tongue has been prevented. Even with surgical correction, if there is n subsequent speech-training, the tongue may fail to develop the activity c which it is now capable and lalling speech continues on a functional basis. Damage to the nervous innervation of tongue muscles may also produce lalling. Cases of cerebral palsy with mild speech involvement often show this characteristic. In cases of lalling, therefore, both functional and organic possibilities must be explored.

*Misarticulation of Other Miscellaneous Sounds.* Most of the functional articulation cases will fall into the three groups just discussed or the one to follow. There are occasional cases which have difficulty with other sounds. A description of the possible forms of misarticulation of all the sounds will not be attempted here but a few of the more common will be mentioned briefly.

The labiodental fricatives [f] and [v] are frequently misarticulated. They may be omitted entirely, other consonants may be substituted for them, particularly [p] and [b], or they may be distorted by inaccurate, insufficient, or asymmetrical movement of the lower lip. Organic factors, particularly malocclusion, irregularities of the upper incisors, or dental spaces account for some of the defects; others are purely functional.

Another pair of sounds frequently defective is the linguadental pair [θ] and [ð]. Substitution of [t] or [d] or of [f] and [v] or of [s] and [z] may be made for them or they may be produced as plosives rather than fricatives but with the tongue-tip somewhat lower than for [t] or [d]. Horowitz (1949) has shown that in cases of [f] or [v] substitution for [θ] and [ð], [l] tends to be defective, too, all three defects probably stemming from a common inactivity of the tongue-tip.

The velar plosives [k] and [g] are occasionally misarticulated in other than infantile perseveration cases. They may be omitted entirely, substitution of [t] or [d] made or the [g] may be unvoiced to produce [k] as in lo*k* for do*g*. The sounds may be produced with insufficient pressure or incomplete closure between the back of the tongue and the soft palate.

The nasal [ŋ] is often defective in one of two ways. Either the postdental nasal [n] is substituted for it or a plosive is produced following the [ŋ] by a break in the contact between the elevated rear portion of the tongue and the lowered velum while breath pressure is still being exerted, producing, for example, ring-*g* instead of ring.

For a more detailed description of types of misarticulation of these and other speech sounds the reader is referred to Nemoy and Davis (1937), Koepp-Baker (1936), and Gray and Wise (1946).

**2. General oral inaccuracy.** In the types of articulatory disorder we have been discussing, the case can be expected to have difficulty with certain sounds or groups of sounds while his other sounds will be produced with relative accuracy. There are certain cases, however, in whom distortion and other forms of misarticulation seem general rather than specific. All or nearly all sounds are affected. The degree of severity of *general oral inaccuracy* can vary over a very wide range. There are individuals whose articulation, though generally inaccurate, is only mildly so. Though their speech is unattractive it is perfectly understandable and no important communicatio handicap exists. At the other extreme are some of the most severely hand capped individuals to be seen in clinical practice, those whose speech, thoug possibly adequate enough in output or fluency, is nearly or completely ur intelligible. In many cases of *general oral inaccuracy* there are obvious or ganic factors responsible. There are also, however, many cases where eve very careful study fails to reveal organic factors and which appear to b entirely functional in etiology.

To understand general oral inaccuracy it might be helpful to conside briefly what the motor requirements are for accurate articulation. First ther must be *precision* of movement. Contacts or approximations of parts of th speech mechanism must be made at the right *place,* in the right *direction* must involve the right *amount of contact surface,* and the right *shape.* Sec ond, articulatory movements must be made at the right *speed.* Third, the must be made with sufficient *energy* or *pressure.* Finally, there must b *synergy* of the sequential movements of speech, an optimum tempora spatial integration of movements.

In cases of general oral inaccuracy any or all of these aspects of articula tion may be inadequate. Movements are approximate rather than precise broad rather than small surfaces are sometimes contacted, contacts are mad at the wrong place. In some cases movements are fairly accurate but ar slow, weak, or underenergized, so that, though contacts are made, they ar not tight or firm. The speech is spoken of as "careless," "lazy," "sluggish, in its milder forms; "indistinct," "confused," "mutilated," "distorted, "unintelligible," in its more severe forms.

Writers in speech pathology have described certain of the characteristic of *general oral inaccuracy* in other terms. Van Riper (1947), the 1931 Whit House Conference report, Anderson (1953), and others speak of *oral ir activity* as one type of articulation problem. Another term used by sever writers, *cluttering,* can well be classified here, too. *Cluttering,* as used b most, implies a rate and rhythm aspect as well as an articulation aspect t the deviate speech pattern. For example, Berry and Eisenson (1942, p. 114 say, "A child who stumbles and repeats words and phrases, slurs and omi sounds and syllables while going at top speed is a clutterer." Van Ripe (1947, p. 19), speaking of *cluttering* as a "disorder of rhythm," states:

> It is characterized by slurred and omitted syllables, by improper phrasing ar pauses due to excessive speed. Clutterers speak by spurts and their speech orga pile up like keys on a typewriter when a novice stenographer tries for more spee than her skill permits. . . . People constantly ask the clutterer to repeat. They a empathically irritated by his uneven volleys of hasty syllables. They find then selves interrupting during his panting pauses and then in turn being interrupte by a new overwhelming rush of jumbled words.

Anderson (1953, p. 44), describing *oral inactivity,* says:

> In general, the speech of individuals exhibiting oral inactivity is either of tl slow, sluggish type, or it is characterized by a rapid, slurring, often irregula

empo sometimes described as "hitting the high spots." In both types many speech
ounds are either omitted or are imperfectly formed, speech becomes unclear
nd distorted, and intelligibility is reduced.

Anderson is describing here as a form of *oral inactivity* what others have
alled *cluttering*. Basically, though varying in degree and kind, all of these
ypes of defective speech pattern described in the terms indicated above,
ave an all-pervading deficiency rather than a limited or specific one. It
eems useful, therefore, to group them under the classification *general oral
naccuracy*.

## Analysis of Misarticulation by Type of Error

Scientific analyses of misarticulation, whether made in connection with
enetic studies of normal speech development or in connection with studies
f deviate speech, are remarkably consistent in their findings. Some of the
rincipal facts and conclusions are summarized briefly below.

**Type of misarticulation.** Sound substitutions and omissions are common
n preschool and primary children, grow less frequent with increase in age.
ound distortions are relatively less frequent at these early age levels but
end to be the predominant type of misarticulation with increase in age.
Vellman *et al.* (1931), reporting on consonant blends in children from two
hrough six, found that substitutions and omissions decreased with age
while approximations (distortions) and inconsistencies increased with age.
ubstitutions were more frequent in consonant blends than in single conso-
ants, but omissions and inconsistencies less frequent.

Repeated testings of children as in the Roe and Milisen study (1942)
ave shown that sounds omitted or substituted for in the first test often show
p as distortions in later tests, if still defective at all. In some cases distortions
ppear to be a transitional phase of articulation learning.

**Type of sound misarticulated.** Genetic studies show that at any given age
vel among young children vowels are most correctly articulated, conso-
ants next, and consonant blends least. Analysis of errors in articulation
ases shows essentially the same result, with some exceptions. Detailed
udies of [s] and [r] articulation reported by Spriestersbach and Curtis
1951) show that these sounds are sometimes produced better in certain
onsonant blends than when preceded and followed by vowels. There are
hus inconsistencies, but in general consonant blends are more frequently
efective than single consonants.

**Manner and place of articulation.** Numerous analyses have been made of
he type of consonant most likely to be defective, from the standpoint of
oth *manner* of articulation and *place* of articulation. A finding of the Well-
an *et al.* study (1931) was that in young children nasal consonants are
asier than plosives (stops) and plosives easier than fricatives. No differences
ere found between voiced and voiceless consonants. Templin and Steer
1939), studying preschool children, also found nasals most correct, then
losives, semivowels, and fricatives in decreasing order, with consonant

blends most defective. Backus (1943) observed that nasals are rarely defective; some glides, [w] and [j], rarely; others, [r] often; that the most common plosive errors are [t] for [k] and [d] for [g]; and that fricatives are the most frequently defective of the speech sounds. It can be said, therefore, that there is close agreement among the various writers that fricatives account for the great majority of articulation errors.

Analysis of articulation errors by *place* of maximum articulatory movements shows further that most of the commonly misarticulated consonants involve the action of the tongue, particularly the anterior part of the tongue. Bilabial sounds are least frequently misarticulated, labiodental and posterior linguapalatal next, and linguadental and anterior linguapalatal most. Tongue co-ordination seems, therefore, to be the most crucial element in misarticulations.

**Errors in relation to position in word.** Again there is a parallel between genetic development of speech and errors made by articulatory defectives. As cited above in connection with infantile perseveration, initial consonants tend to develop first, medials next, and finals last. Templin and Steer (1939), in their study of preschool children, found speech sounds most often correct in the initial position, next in the medial, and least in the final. Considering substitution errors alone, fewest were made in the initial position, about equal numbers for medial and final positions. Omissions were less frequent than substitutions, occurred most often in the final position, next in the medial, and least in the initial position.

Templin (1943) in a later study of sound discrimination in elementary school children found more *discrimination errors* when a consonant or combination was in a medial or final position than when it was in an initial position. This suggests that the greater difficulty in discriminating medial and final sounds may account for the greater difficulty of articulating sounds in these positions.

**Specific speech sounds most often defective.** Comprehensive studies of defective articulation were made by Roe and Milisen (1942) and by Sayler (1949) working under Milisen's direction. In both studies large, unselected school populations were tested for articulation. Roe and Milisen studied the first six grades; Sayler, grades seven through twelve. Roe and Milisen (1942, p. 43) rank single consonants in the following order according to frequency of error (after eliminating minor voicing errors): [θ], [s], [t], [ð], [z], [dʒ] [tʃ], [r], [v], [k], [d], [ʃ], [g], [f], [p], [l], [b], [ŋ], [ʍ], [w]. Of the ten most frequent in this list, six ([θ], [s], [ð], [z], [tʃ], [v]) are also found among Sayler's ten most frequent errors. In both studies two s-blends, [st] and [sk] ranked high among the single consonants in frequency of error, Roe and Milisen also ranking [str] high. It is interesting that [r], [l], and [ʃ], which most writers list as frequently defective, do not appear prominently in either of these lists. Van Riper's observations (1947, p. 152) that the most frequently mispronounced sounds are: [s], [z], [θ], [ð], [r], [ʒ], [l], [tʃ], [dʒ] [ʃ], [f], [v], with substitutions of [t] for [k] and [d] for [g] in young children, are typical of those of most authorities in speech pathology.

Hall (1938) found the most frequent errors among school children to be in rank order these nine: [s], [z], [ʃ], [tʃ], [dʒ], [ʒ], [ʌ], [θ], [r]; among college freshmen these seven: [s], [z], [dʒ], [ʃ], [tʃ], [ʌ], [ʒ]. Fairbanks and Spriestersbach (1950) found the same seven sounds heading the list for the college students in their study, though in slightly different rank order.

**Inconsistency in misarticulation.** Infantile perseveration cases are notoriously inconsistent in their misarticulations. A young child often omits a sound in some words, uses it correctly in others, and uses one or more substitutions for it in other words. Wellman *et al.* (1931) found that within the age range they studied, two through six, inconsistencies tended to increase with age.

Spriestersbach and Curtis (1951) cite several studies of misarticulation done under their direction at the State University of Iowa. A study by Amidon (1951) of 100 first-grade children found that on the average only 36.5 per cent of the articulation errors observed in the responses of a given child occurred in all three positions in the words tested. Nelson (1945), Hale (1948), and Buck (1948) each tested a specific sound intensively in functional articulation cases; Nelson tested [s] in children in the first six grades; Hale tested [s] in children from kindergarten through third grade; and Buck tested [r] in the same age range. From the data reported by Spriestersbach and Curtis (p. 484) the following summary can be made:

| | PERCENTAGE OF SUBJECTS | | |
| --- | --- | --- | --- |
| | *Nelson*<br>[s] | *Hale*<br>[s] | *Buck*<br>[r] |
| *Consistent* (sound normal in neither blends nor singles) | 46.6 | 26.7 | 5.5 |
| *Inconsistent* (sound normal in some phonetic contexts, misarticulated in others) | 53.4 | 73.3 | 94.5 |

From these results, inconsistency appears to be typical rather than unusual or exceptional. Spriestersbach and Curtis concluded that inconsistencies in speech sound production cannot be attributed to chance but are governed by variables which operate in a systematic, lawful fashion.

Perkins (1952) in a study of [s] and [z] articulation also reached the conclusion that sound combinations are more influential than the position of the sound on the type and frequency of errors on [s]. For [z], position had more importance. Nelson found less inconsistency of misarticulation in his older age group than in his younger, from which Spriestersbach and Curtis concluded that older children have become so strongly conditioned to the faulty sound production that maturation processes are no longer effective in producing improvement, the transitional state is past, and misarticulations are, therefore, more consistent.

The dependency on phonetic context demonstrated in these studies accounts to some extent for the inconsistencies which we observe in misarticulations. These research results also point up the importance of making a

thorough evaluation in every case of functional articulation disorder, no
only of the specific sounds misarticulated but also of the specific phoneti
contexts in which errors on these sounds occur.

### Factors Related to Misarticulation

**Misarticulation in relation to age or maturation.** The relationship of ag
to growth in articulation at the lower age levels has already been discusse
in connection with infantile perseveration. Results of studies on early speec
sound acquisition were summarized in Table 2. A number of investigato
have also reported on misarticulations at the elementary and secondar
school levels, in relation to age.

One of the earliest studies relating articulation difficulty to age was mad
by Root (1925). Data on the incidence of various disorders was secured b
questionnaires. He found 2.6 per cent of the total school enrollment to hav
problems of lisping and lalling and these problems accounted for 41.2 pe
cent of all speech defects found. Root did not give separate percentages fo
those labeled "indistinct speech" or "thick speech" but, if included, thes
would have increased the percentage of children who might be classified a
*functional articulatory* cases. The incidence by grade of *lispers* and *laller*
is shown in Table 3. The decrease is rapid from grade to grade at first, the
more gradual. There is an 82 per cent decrease between grades I and IV.

Dawson (1929) investigated the development of *rate* of articulation wit
a series of six tests, such as repetition of numbers, of the alphabet, and so or
He found that children have not mastered all the articulation skills when the
enter school; that there is a rapid increase of rate during the first three grade
and then a more gradual increase above that level.

Francis (1930) surveyed school children for speech defects and found tha
functional articulatory defects amounted to 51.8 per cent of all speech de
fects. Percentages for the different grades are given in Table 3. Mills an
Streit (1942) made a survey of speech defects in a school population an
reported *dyslalia* as having the following percentages of incidence: grad
one, 28.9; grade two, 22.2; grade three, 22.1; and grades above 3, 0.9—
marked falling off from the first to the upper grades. The White House Con
ference report of 1931 also gave incidences by grade and sex of "sound sub
stitution" cases. These data are given in Table 3.

Notable among the studies of articulation defects in relation to age are th
two investigations carried out at Indiana University under Milisen's direc
tion—Roe and Milisen (1942) and an extension of this study by Sayle
(1949). Unselected school populations were tested for articulation by traine
speech therapists. The statistical results by grade for both studies are give
in Table 3. Roe and Milisen found that a decreasing number of childre
make articulatory errors in each successive grade and also that those wh
do make errors make fewer.

Morley (1952) has reported the results of speech tests given to incomin
and transfer students at the University of Michigan over a ten-year perioc

here are minor fluctuations of incidence from year to year, but the inci-
nce for the whole period is 3.85 per cent classified as "clinical cases" out
 the 33,339 tested. Articulation defects account for 50.7 per cent of the
linical cases," an incidence of 1.9 per cent of the university enrollment
sted.

Study of Table 3 shows that in all sets of data included there is a decrease
misarticulation with increase in grade level up through at least grade four.
ith the exception of the White House data, the studies show only small
creases or no decreases at successive levels above grade four and up
rough grade twelve. Misarticulation decreases rapidly from grade to grade
om kindergarten up through grade four. At that point it levels off and there
 little further decrease due to maturation alone. The White House Survey
port, based upon very large numbers, is less subject to chance errors of
mpling. It shows an abrupt, then a more gradual but still continuous, de-
ease in numbers of articulation defects for all grades up through twelve.

We can conclude that maturation and the speech stimulation provided by
e school are effective for most children in producing rapid improvement
 articulation during the early grade levels, that they are of only mild ef-
ctiveness from grades four through six, and above that level cease to be
ticeably effective in improving articulation.

**Misarticulation in relation to sex.** According to clinical experience and
e findings of most investigations, the same preponderance of boys over
rls holds true for functional articulation problems as for speech defects in
neral. In studies of early genetic development of articulation sex differ-
ces have been found rather consistently. Wellman *et al.* (1931) found
rls superior to boys on consonant elements, though sex differences on
wels were inconclusive. Poole (1934), Irwin (1952), and Templin (1952)
 report sex differences in favor of girls in the development of articulatory
ill.

For school-age children, few satisfactory sex comparisons are available.
lthough numerous investigations report on sex differences for speech de-
cts in general, few report on sex differences for functional articulation
fects separately.

Root (1925, p. 537) reported sex ratios separately for each type of speech
fect found. For the types which might be considered as coming within the
neral category of *functional articulatory* the ratio of boys to girls was as
lows: *indistinct speech,* 2.5 to 1.0; *thick speech,* 1.4 to 1.0; *lisping* and
*ling,* 1.1 to 1.0. The sex ratio for all defects was 1.5 to 1.0.

Dawson (1929) found that girls articulated at a more rapid rate than boys
d developed more rapidly in articulation up to 12 or 13 years of age. Then
ys articulated more rapidly, reaching a higher level than girls in grade
elve.

From the data reported by Mills and Streit (1942) it can be calculated
at among *dyslalia* cases in the first three grades, 62 per cent were boys and
 per cent girls. Above third grade the percentages were 70 and 30 re-

**TABLE 3. Investigations on Misarticulation in Relation to Age***

| GRADE | ROOT (1925) Per cent of school population with lisping or lalling | FRANCIS (1930) Per cent of school population with oral inaccuracy | ROE AND MILISEN (1942) (Grades I through VI) SAYLER (1949) (Grades VII through XII) — Articulation errors | | | WHITE HOUSE CONFERENCE REPORT (1931) No. of sound substitution cases | |
|---|---|---|---|---|---|---|---|
| | | | Mean no. | Difference | Critical ratio | Boys | Girls |
| Kindergarten | 5.70 | 27.8 | | | | | |
| I | 3.60 | 19.3 | 13.30 | | | 3,854 | 2,533 |
| II | 2.50 | 11.5 | 9.99 | 3.31 | 6.89 | 2,684 | 1,725 |
| III | 1.04 | 9.9 | 8.85 | 1.14 | 2.71 | 1,916 | 1,042 |
| IV | 2.70 | 3.1 | 7.62 | 1.23 | 2.91 | 1,223 | 738 |
| V | 1.01 | 3.6 | 7.61 | .01 | .02 | 848 | 538 |
| VI | | 2.1 | 8.01 | − .40 | −1.21 | 657 | 402 |
| VII | 0.60 | 2.6 | 3.92 | | | 277 | 175 |
| VIII | 1.00 | 4.7 | 4.31 | − .39 | − .72 | 190 | 108 |
| IX | | 2.6 | 4.54 | − .23 | | } | } |
| X | | 6.7 | 4.39 | .15 | − .77 | 82 | 71 |
| XI | | 2.1 | 3.34 | 1.05 | .54 | } | } |
| XII | | 4.7 | 3.25 | .09 | 3.75 / .32 | 28 | 25 |
| Number of cases | 191 | | Grades I–VI, 1,989 Grades VII–XII, 1,998 | | | | |

* Some modifications have been made here in the form of presentation of the data from the presentation in the original publications. In each case the author's own diagnostic terms are given in the table. The data presented in Table 3, all show misarticulations in relation to grade level though all are not comparable as to the measure used. Root and Francis report percentage of defectives in the school population, Roe and Milisen, and Sayler report mean number of errors made by unselected children and the White House data give numbers of speech defectives.

spectively. School enrollment of boys and girls is not given, however, and these percentages would be of significance only if the enrollments of the two sexes were approximately equal. The authors concluded that boys exceed girls in all categories of articulatory defect, but that there is least difference in *sigmatism.*

Roe and Milisen (1942) found no significant difference between the mean number of articulation errors for boys and for girls in their tests of unselected children in grades one through six. Their study differs from most in that they report on *unselected* children, while most investigations are on children identified as speech defectives. Sayler (1949) in a continuation of this study into grades seven through twelve, found no differences in the mean number of errors made by boys and girls but found, however, that slightly more boys than girls made errors in all grades but twelve.

The present writer (Hall, 1938) found that among the grade two through six population used for her study, 8.4 per cent of the boys and 3.3 per cent of the girls had functional articulatory defects; and that at the college freshmen level 8.8 per cent of the men students and 6.3 per cent of the women had low ratings on articulation. Current data from the speech correction program in the Chicago Public Schools, under the writer's direction, show that, of the 132,211 boys in schools receiving speech correction service, 5.8 per cent have been identified by the school speech therapists as having functional articulation disorders. Of the 129,136 girls, 3.5 per cent have been so identified. This is a highly significant contrast, based as it is upon numbers of such size. Combining both sexes, the incidence of functional articulation disorders is 4.7 per cent of the school population.

Morley's study of college students (1952) reports that, of the articulation cases found, 61.4 per cent were males, 38.6 per cent females, a ratio of 1.5 to 1.0. The number of men students tested, however, was considerably in excess of the number of women. Additional calculations on Morley's data by this writer show that the percentage of articulation defects among all men tested (19,730) was 1.95 per cent and among all women tested (13,609) 1.78 per cent. There is thus a slightly higher percentage of articulation cases among these men college students than among women. The difference, though small, may be significant in view of the very large number of cases involved.

Although there is some inconsistency in the conclusions reached in these studies, the weight of evidence supports a sex difference in favor of girls, both in the normal development of articulatory skill during the early years and in the smaller percentage of functional articulatory defects among girls throughout the entire educational range from preschool through college.

## ETIOLOGY OF FUNCTIONAL ARTICULATION DISORDERS

Functional articulation disorders have to date received little attention from research workers as compared with most of the other disorders of speech. Of the research that has been done on these problems, however, the greater part has been directed toward the investigation of their etiology. Although a respectable number of studies is now available, their results are still inconclusive and often mutually contradictory. Research has succeeded mainly so far in eliminating certain factors from consideration as causally related to articulatory defects rather than in showing what factors do have a causal relationship. In short, our research results to date are of more value for their negative than for their positive significance.

Textbooks in speech pathology are liberal in advancing many and diverse physical, mental, environmental, and emotional variables as underlying causal factors in these disorders. The factors suggested range from simple physical variables such as tongue size, lip mobility, diadochokinesis of the jaw, on through more complex variables such as auditory perceptual variations, to complex emotional problems reflecting child or parental maladjustment, at the other extreme.

The writer will review systematically the principal studies supporting or refuting the many etiological possibilities and will then attempt to integrate and evaluate them and to draw what conclusions are possible as to our understanding of functional articulation disorders at the present time.

The studies reported in the literature are, of course, of varying merit. Some have been done with little attention to sound research method and are little better than casual observation liberally salted with opinion. Others have been done with careful experimental design and results are presented in precise statistical form with proper attention to measures of reliability and significance of results. Some writers, in presenting their results, confuse *concomitant* factors with *causal* factors. The reader should keep this difference in mind so that unwarranted conclusions will not be drawn as to relationships between articulation problems and some of the variables studied.

## Physical and Psychophysical Variables

The reader must bear in mind that, since we are considering *functional* articulation problems in this chapter, most of the physical variables discussed are to be thought of as in the order of *normal variations,* not *pathological variations.* If pathological variations are present and related causally to the speech deviation, the disorder would be organic rather than functional and would not come under discussion here.

**Anatomical factors.** Various writers have suggested the possibility of systematic differences between functional articulation cases and normal speakers in such anatomical variables as size and shape of the oral cavity, size and shape of the tongue, length of the lingual frenum, dental structure, relationship of upper and lower jaws, size of lips, and other more obscure variables. Actual research on anatomical variables has been meager.

*Dental structure and palatal dimensions* have been mentioned frequently in connection with articulation problems but research results are inconclusive. Carrell (1936) studied the population of a children's institution and

found no differences between a speech defective and a normal speech group
in palatal malformations, dental abnormalities, or status of dental health.

Fymbo (1936) studied the relationship of malocclusion of the teeth to
defective speech and found the severity of the speech defect varied directly
with the severity of the dental anomaly. The following dental factors were
found to be significantly related to defective speech: abnormal vertical re-
ations of the jaws, edentulous spaces, especially those occurring among the
eight anterior teeth, spacing of the teeth, and unusually high or low palate.
Fymbo's speech-defective group, of course, was not limited to "functional"
cases.

It is of equal significance, too, that Fymbo found that malocclusion of
the teeth existed in 35 per cent of his superior speech cases and 62 per cent
of his average speech cases as well as in 87 per cent of his defective speech
cases. Poor articulation is not a necessary consequence of all malocclusion
nor is it to be assumed that malocclusion is present in all articulation disorders.

A recent and carefully designed study by Fairbanks and Lintner (1951)
compared two groups of college students, one with superior consonant articulation and one with inferior consonant articulation, on four anatomical
measures: cuspid width, molar width, palatal height, and maximum mouth
opening. Their results support Fymbo in finding that marked dental deviations were significantly more numerous among the inferior speakers. Open-
bite and close-bite were more numerous in the inferior group, open-bite
being the greater factor in the difference. However, their results do not support Fymbo in other respects. Their superior and inferior ability groups did
not differ significantly in the number of atypical antero-posterior relationships (overjet or undershot conditions) or in molar occlusion, anterior occlusion, anterior alignment, or anterior spaces. Neither were significant differences found in dimensions of the dental arch and hard palate (width and
height).

Dental anomalies have been mentioned particularly in relation to lisping.
Fymbo found the sibilant sounds [s], [z], [ʃ], [ʒ], [tʃ], [dʒ], and [θ] and [ð]
most difficult for malocclusion cases. Froeschels and Jellinek (1941) found,
however, that even in cases of interdental lisping with open-bite, the dental
anomaly did not usually cause the lisping. In 800 such cases only three protruded the tongue through the opening formed by the abnormal teeth, all
others lowering the jaw to make room. The authors suggest that the inter-
dentality in speech produces the dental anomaly rather than the reverse.

*Tongue size and shape* are other factors which have often been suggested
as related to adequacy of articulation, particularly as the tongue relates to
the size of the dental arches and the oval cavity as a whole.

Fairbanks and Bebout (1950) estimated size and shape of the tongue in
the superior and inferior groups of college speakers referred to in the preceding section. Size was classified as small, average, or large, and shape as
flat or bulged. The tongue-tip (distance forward from the anterior margin of

the frenulum) was also measured. They found no statistically significant difference in length of tongue-tip between their superior and inferior groups and comparisons of tongue size and shape were inconclusive though primarily negative.

The size of the mouth opening and thickness and shape of the lips have also been mentioned as possibly related to articulatory efficiency. Again Fairbanks has included precise measurements of these factors as part of the study already mentioned in which speakers with superior and inferior articulation were compared. Fairbanks and Green (1950) measured the following: thickness of upper lip, thickness of lower lip, horizontal spread from corner to corner, and vertical length of upper lip in the midline. Although expected sex differences were found, no statistically significant differences were found between ability groups. The conclusion is drawn that lip dimensions are unrelated to articulatory ability. Estimates were also made of the antero-posterior and infero-superior relations of the lips. Instances of protrusion of both lips and incomplete infero-superior contact between the lips were more frequent among the inferior group but this result was considered only tentative because of the small number of cases involved.

General anatomical comparisons, not limited to the speech mechanism have also been made. Carrell's study (1936) referred to above, on comparison between defective and normal speech groups in a children's institution included these anthropometric measurements: standing height, sitting height weight, right and left grip, and vital capacity. The slightly speech-defective group did not differ significantly from the control group in any of these measures but the severely speech-defective group was significantly inferior to the control group in all but standing height. The greatest difference occurred in vital capacity, a speech-related measure. The author concluded that the speech-defective children tended to be physically "weak" and deficient in their ability to make use of their physical possibilities.

The results of the studies cited on anatomical factors as related to articulation do not encourage us to feel that there is any systematic relationship While all studies are fairly consistent in finding more anomalous jaw, dental and tongue conditions among defective than among average speakers (and these would be considered organic, not functional cases), they are also remarkably consistent in finding no differences of significance in normal variations of the various parts of the speech mechanism. We can say on the basis of the available research that functional articulation cases do not differ systematically from normal speakers in regard to tongue size or shape, or length or height of palate, or size of lips.

We find all writers in speech pathology mentioning, too, the adaptations which many individuals make, without special training, to even extreme anomalies of the speech mechanism. The human speech mechanism has remarkably compensatory capacities. From these common observations we should learn caution in assuming that when anomalies are present and are culation is defective, the speech is necessarily a result of the observed anomaly. It is always wise to evaluate other causal possibilities as well.

**Motor co-ordination.** Another area in which the explanation of functional articulatory problems has been pursued even more vigorously is that of motor co-ordination, both of the body as a whole and within the speech mechanism specifically. Since speech is admittedly a complex process of delicate muscular adjustments, it has been natural to suppose that cases in which articulation was defective might have less than average precision, speed, strength, or control of movement. A substantial number of investigations has attempted to throw light on this problem.

Some have investigated the possibility that articulatory defectives might be below par in *general bodily co-ordination and control*. The Wellman *et al.* study (1931) of articulation growth in young children included two tests of motor control, the Wellman tracing-path test, and a perforation test. A substantial correlation was found between both of these tests and number of sounds correctly articulated, when the whole age range (two to six years) was included. Since both articulation and motor control are highly correlated with age, however, the relationship between motor control and speech ability would presumably be much reduced with age held constant.

Carrell (1937) compared a speech defective with a control group on a number of tests, including a tapping, a tracing, and a "tensiometer" test. The latter tested "kinesthetic imagery" and involved the arms. For all tests the control group was superior to the speech defectives (sound substitution cases), but the differences had low statistical reliabilities. Differences were greatest between the controls and the most defective subgroup of the speech-defective group.

Major (1940) found that speech defectives (all types mixed) tended to be inferior to normals on thirteen tests, including simple and multiple choice, reaction time, rhythm, speed of tapping, eye-hand co-ordination. The results, however, were recognized as not applying to speech defectives as a whole because of the large number of stutterers included. They were inconclusive so far as articulation cases are concerned.

Bilto (1941) tested 34 stutterers and 56 articulation cases (organic problems excluded) between nine and eighteen years of age and children without speech defects, on three tests: the Brace Motor Ability test battery, the Nielsen and Cozens' Jump and Reach test (which measures ability to develop power), and his own eye-hand co-ordination test. Both the stuttering group and the articulation group were inferior to the normal speech group on all three of the tests. The inferiority of the speech-defective children was not characterized by failure in any specific type of physical ability. The author concluded that approximately two-thirds of the speech-defective children were inferior to children with normal speech in these physical abilities. The articulation cases were superior to the stutterers on some tests, inferior on others, and about equal on others. Bilto felt that these tests could be used profitably as a diagnostic battery in studying speech cases and in planning their retraining.

Mase (1946) investigated six factors commonly cited as causes of articulatory defects. One of them was co-ordination of gross muscles, which was tested by means of a rail-walking test. Boys in grades five and six with articulatory problems were carefully matched with normal speakers for age, I.Q. and socioeconomic status. He found no reliable difference between the groups in general muscular co-ordination as tested by the rail-walking test.

Two studies of recent date by Albright (1938) and Maxwell (1953) have made a particularly detailed and careful investigation of the relation between articulation ability and motor co-ordination and control, both in the gross skeletal musculature and in the speech mechanism itself, the latter during both speech and nonspeech activities.

Albright matched 31 college students with superior articulation with an equal number with poor articulation, cases with organic abnormalities excluded. Controls and experimental cases were selected only from the two extremes of the distribution, the large middle group being omitted. Six tests not involving the speech mechanism were used: a synchronometer (tapping in time to an auditory pattern), Miles speed rotor, simple tapping, hand steadiness, writing-rate, and rail-walking. Five tests involving the speech mechanism were used: speech-rate (reciting "Mary had a little lamb"), simple repetitive movements of the tongue [lɑ] at maximum speed, repetition of [tʌkə], lip-movement speed [mu], and one nonspeech test, a teeth-click test.

Significant differences between good and poor speakers were found on three of the tests of motor skill (synchronometer, Miles speed rotor, and speech-rate test) and on three of the four tests of articulatory skills ([lɑ], [tʌkə], and [mu] but not the teeth-click). The greatest difference was found on the synchronometer and Albright accounts for this by pointing out that this test involved a factor of auditory-motor co-ordination in addition to the rhythm factor found in other tests. Positive but low intertest correlations were found, indicating that the skills measured were relatively independent. Albright makes two interesting points in commenting on his results (pp. 171–172): first, that in addition to the superiority of the good articulation over the poor articulation group in fine co-ordinations ". . . there is the more technical possibility that subjects with good articulation tend to be more stable in their neuromuscular performance, that their fine co-ordinations function with more stability as well as speed." Secondly, he says, "Although the results do not reveal the relative importance of the motor factor involved in articulation, they do indicate that rhythm, auditory-motor co-ordination, and speed of articulatory movement are important factors in articulation. Also, they call attention to the point stressed by Stetson that speech sounds are the result of speech movements."

Maxwell (1953) also studied the relationship between both general and specific motor skills and articulation. He used 13 boys with defective articulation at each of three age levels, seven, eight, and nine years, and an equal number of control boys at these levels, with good speech. I.Q.'s were all normal and cases of hearing loss or obvious physical defect were excluded. Maxwell's battery included tests to measure the following: (1) speed of diadochokinetic movements of tongue lips, jaws (5) tests, consisting of the number of repetitions in two seconds of [pɑ], [tɑ], [kɑ], [lɑ], and the combination [pɑtɑkɑ]; (2) speed of diadochokinetic movements of the hand, measured by tapping, and a ball-bounce test; (3) accuracy of eye-hand co-ordination, measured by dotting, tracing, putting pellets in a bottle, and a form board; (4) hand steadiness, measured by a cube-stacking test; (5) station, as measured by eight tests from Variable One of the Ozeretsky scale; and, (6) gait, as measured by four walking tests.

Maxwell found reliable differences between his good and poor articulation cases on only the following: repetition of [pɑtɑkɑ]; of [lɑ] (at eight- and nine-year levels only); speed and accuracy of movement required to perform the tracing and the pellet and bottle tests with the nonpreferred hand; tapping and bouncing tests (seven-year level only), and steadiness, as measured by the cube-stacking test. He concluded (p. 50), "There was no difference between the children with normal speech and children with articulatory speech defects in their ability to repeat [tɑ], to dot rapidly, to perform the pellet and bottle test with the preferred hand, to perform the Seguin Form Board test, and in their ability to control the co-ordination required to perform tests of station and gait."

Another objective of Maxwell's study was to determine whether there is an increase of motor skill with age. Such an increase was found within the control group for the three age levels, in repetition of [lɑ], ball-bouncing, dotting, tracing, and station. He felt that he had developed reliable norms for all three age levels for the following: [pɑ], [tɑ], [kɑ], [lɑ], [pɑtɑkɑ], and the pellet and bottle test with the nonpreferred hand. Maxwell concluded, however, that there was no general agreement in his results as to tests which would measure differences between the control and experimental groups at all age levels or which would measure increased skill with increased age.

Laterality was studied in relation to articulation by Johnson and House (1937) who compared articulatory defective children with normal speakers on tests of ocular and hand dominance. Their conclusion was that handedness, as measured, tends to be related to severe functional articulatory defects but that the findings with regard to eyedness were not significant. In opposition to these results, Everhart (1953) found no significant relationship between articulatory defectiveness and handedness in children in grades one through six.

A number of studies and clinical observations have been made on *motor co-ordination within the speech mechanism itself*. Karlin, Youtz, and Kennedy (1940) concluded from a small study comparing speech-defective with normal-speaking children that motor speed, among other factors, may operate to produce dyslalia. Mase (1946), in a well-controlled study of boys in grades five and six, compared articulatory defectives and normal speakers on a number of tests of various functions. Included were five tests for speed of various actions of the speech mechanism: moving tongue from corner to corner of mouth, opening mouth and closing lips alternately, touching a tongue depressor with the tongue-tip, stretching and rounding the lips alternately, and repeating "daddy" rapidly. He found no significant differences on any of these tests between his defective and his control groups. Lip mobility was the only test in which a significant difference was approached.

Fairbanks and Spriestersbach (1950), in part of a larger study under Fairbanks' direction, cited earlier, compared college students with superior and with inferior articulatory ability on the rate at which they could perform the following repetitive movements: approximation of upper and lower lips, vertical movement of the mandible, tongue to alveolar ridge, and tongue protrusion. Only small differences were found between ability groups. A significant difference was found only for lip movement and only for the male. These results agree almost perfectly with those of Mase, reported above. In speed of movement the speech structures ranked as follows in descending order: lips, mandible, tongue-alveolar, tongue protrusion.

In another part of the same study Fairbanks and Bebout (1950) measured maximum length of tongue protrusion, tongue force, and percentage of error in duplicating a tongue position. Again no differences between ability groups, sex constant, were significant. A significant sex difference in favor of males was found only for tongue force.

Palmer and Osborn (1940) in an earlier study found results contradictory to those of Fairbanks and Bebout. Within a larger group of individuals used for their experiment was a group of 44 articulatory cases, ages six to thirty-six, from which cases with known organic defects were excluded. They were matched for age and sex with normal speakers and both groups tested for tongue pressure. A significant difference was found in favor of the control group. No significant sex differences were found in either group. A factor which may partially account for the difference in results from those of Fairbanks and Bebout is the greater frequency of malnutrition, febrile and wasting diseases which Palmer and Osborn report among their articulatory cases, as compared with their controls. As the authors themselves indicate, it is known that in all lowered physiological conditions there is diminished tongue strength.

The results of these studies on motor co-ordination, viewed as a whole, are discouragingly contradictory and inconclusive. For nearly every type of motor skill investigated, some studies have found differences between good and poor articulation groups, some have been inconclusive, and others have found no differences.

For motor abilities not involving the speech mechanism, fewest differences seem to have been found in general bodily control, strength, and speed (Mase and Albright rail-walking and Maxwell's tests of station and gait), though Bilto's results contradict this (Brace Motor Ability tests and the jump and reach test). Tests of hand speed and reaction time have been inconclusive or negative in regard to differences for the most part (Major, reaction time; Major, Albright, and Maxwell, tapping; Albright, writing rate, hand steadiness).

The tests which have seemed to show most difference are those involving eye-hand or auditory-hand co-ordination, rather than simple speed, strength, or steadiness (Albright's synchronometer and speed rotor; Bilto's eye-hand co-ordination test; the tracing tests used by Wellman et al., Carrell, and Maxwell; and Maxwell's cube-stacking test). The inconsistency of even these results is exemplified, however, by Maxwell's finding of a difference between ability groups for the pellet-and-bottle test when the nonpreferred hand was used but no difference when the preferred hand was used.

One would perhaps expect logically that if any differences in motor co-ordination were present in relation to articulatory skill, these differences would show up most in the motor skills involving the speech mechanism itself. Here again we find highly contradictory and inconclusive results. Let us first mention a few points of consistency. Neither Fairbanks and Spriestersbach nor Albright (teeth-click test) found a difference between ability groups in vertical movements of the mandible. Mase and Fairbanks and Spriestersbach found no difference for any type of nonspeech tongue movement (speed or extent). Apparently no investigator has so far been able to demonstrate significant differences in tongue movements in articulatory defectives apart from speech. Both Mase and Fairbanks and Spriestersbach found slight differences between ability groups in lip movements only.

Results have been more likely to show differences when actual speech movements have been tested. Both Albright and Maxwell found significant differences between articulatory defectives and normal speakers for rapid repetition of syllables such as [la], but particularly for more complex patterns, [pataka] or [tʌkə]. Even here differences were not striking and there was much overlapping of ability groups.

In regard to tongue pressure or force, the results of Palmer and Osborn and of Fairbanks and Bebout are contradictory. The former found a significant difference, the latter did not.

The many discrepancies in the studies reviewed can be accounted for in part by differences in methods, in the tests used, in the way cases were selected for comparison, in the success with which other variables than the one being measured were eliminated, and by the rigor with which statistical tests of significance were applied. All of these explanations together, however, do not account for the lack of a more unified picture emerging from such an impressive mass of scientific research. A more probable explanation is that there are actually not any very great and consistent motor differences between individuals with superior and with inferior articulation skill. When we are dealing with very small differences anyway, then differences in research methodology, which in this field lacks the precision of the physical sciences, can be expected to yield inconsistent results. Even in those studies which found significant differences between ability groups, the differences were neither large nor consistent. Within the functional articulatory groups there were always some cases whose performance was average or superior. There is not even one motor variable which is reported by all investigators as showing a consistently negative deviation for all articulatory cases. When the means for groups barely reach significance criteria the test in question has little predictive value. Obviously the clinician cannot assume negative deviation in any motor skill for a given case but must study each case independently.

It is possible that certain types of functional articulation defectives, if separated out, might show more marked differences in motor skill than have been shown for the group as a whole. Most investigators have realized that it is unprofitable to lump together all types of speech defectives in making comparisons with normal speakers. Might it not also be unwise to group even the functional articulation defectives of various types in studies of this nature? Is there not a possibility that particularly the type of case designated earlier in the chapter as *general oral inaccuracy* might show more marked and consistent negative deviations in motor skill than, for example, cases of lisping or infantile perseveration? This possibility seems at least worth investigating.

Many speech pathologists have postulated a weakness of the intrinsic muscles of the tongue, particularly the longitudinal muscles, as responsible for various forms of misarticulation. Inability to groove the tongue by raising its edges has been advanced as a reason for lateral and interdental lisping by Froeschels (1933). This motor skill has apparently been neglected in exact, scientific investigation in spite of its frequent mention in clinical observations. It was not tested in any of the research studies reviewed above but may be another possibility worth investigation.

**Sensory factors: auditory.** Because of the known closeness of relationship between speech and hearing, most writers in speech pathology have regarded auditory processes as the most promising direction in which to search for factors which might explain functional articulatory disorders. Every aspect of audition—basic acuity for pure tones, acuity for the higher frequencies, pitch discrimination, speech sound discrimination, auditory memory span, perception for complex auditory patterns—has received attention. There is hardly an aspect of auditory behavior which has not been investigated in at least several research studies. Audition has been the most thoroughly explored of all the causal possibilities advanced to account for functional articulation disorders. Despite this, our information about the relationship of hearing processes to articulation remains equivocal.

*Auditory Acuity.* Since serious hearing loss is known to affect the development and maintenance of good articulation, many speech pathologists have thought it possible that functional articulatory cases might have slight degrees of hearing loss, not observable behaviorally. Hearing loss, perhaps, at certain frequencies only, particularly high frequencies, has been considered also as a possible factor in these cases. These hypotheses have been subjected to several experimental tests.

Barnes (1932) tested university freshmen on the Western Electric 4-A Audiometer and on an articulation test. He found no relation between their articulation ratings and their hearing test results. Carrell (1936) compared sound substitution cases with normal speakers on the 4-A Audiometer and found the sound substitution group inferior. He stated, however, that though suggestive, it could not be concluded from these results that hearing defects have etiological significance in the consideration of speech disorders.

Hall (1938) administered individual threshold tests on the Western Electric 2-A Audiometer to articulatory defectives and their matched normal-speaking controls at two age levels, university freshmen and elementary-school children in grades two through six. At both age levels studied there were slight differences between speech defective and normal speakers at every frequency but the differences were not statistically significant. All composite auditory measures—average of middle frequencies, average of lower four, average of upper four, and average of all eight—also showed differences in favor of the control groups, but none of statistical significance.

Karlin, Youtz, and Kennedy (1940) found hearing loss, especially at higher frequencies, in a group of six articulatory defectives, as compared with matched controls, but their cases are too few to give their results significance.

Sullivan (1944, p. 128) reported results of Maico D6 pure-tone audiometer tests of 25,708 Minneapolis school children. "A hearing loss was defined as a diminution of ten decibels from the normal sensitivity in either ear." Percentages of children with hearing loss were as follows: without speech defects, 18.8; all speech defectives, 22.2; functional articulatory cases alone, 20.3. Measures of significance are not given, but from the above results, it is obvious that the slight difference between normal speakers and functional articulatory defectives is probably without significance. It is interesting and may be significant that the small group of 56 "oral inactivity" cases had a higher percentage, 25.0, of hearing loss. Hearing loss was also analyzed by Sullivan in relation to specific types of misarticulation (p. 129): "The fact that pupils with faulty sibilants, the high-frequency sounds, are apparently not differentiated from the general school population on the basis of hearing loss in the high frequencies seems to indicate that hearing loss in the high frequencies is not to be regarded as standing in a significant relationship to their defective speech."

Mase (1946) compared boys with functional articulation disorders and their matched controls on the Maico D5 Audiometer. Differences between the two groups did not reach the critical 1 per cent level of significance, though four measurements were within the questionable 1 to 5 per cent level. Differences were more pronounced when the upper three frequencies were analyzed. His results, therefore, are somewhat inconclusive in regard to auditory acuity.

Rossignol (1948) investigated the relationships among hearing acuity, speech production, and reading performance of unselected children in grades 1A, 1B, and 2A. She found a zero correlation between articulation of speech sounds in familiar words and hearing acuity. She found, however, a low but statistically significant correlation between hearing acuity and ability to repeat nonsense syllables, which tested ability to produce new sound combinations. She also found low but significant correlations between hearing acuity and reading and between reading and articulation. Rossignol says (p. 30) "It is possible to infer from these data that hearing acuity is more important when the child is learning to say a new word than when he is articulating a word that is familiar to him. It is also possible that hearing acuity is more important in the earlier stages of acquiring speech than in the stage investigated in the present study."

To summarize, the results of the studies cited are inconclusive as to the relation between auditory acuity and functional articulation problems. Karlin, Youtz, and Kennedy, who studied very few cases, and Carrell found differences in auditory acuity in favor of normal speakers. Barnes, Hall, Mase, Sullivan, and Rossignol did not find significant differences, though Mase's results suggest the possibility of more incidence of high-frequency loss among functional articulatory defectives. Sullivan's results raise the possibility, furthermore, that "oral inactivity" cases may possibly be an exception. The weight of evidence, therefore, is against there being a significant deficiency in auditory acuity in functional articulatory cases. At least we can conclude with confidence that there is no general tendency for these cases to show hearing loss and, therefore, that this appears not to be a major etiological factor. This does not eliminate the ever-present possibility of hearing loss in individual cases and it remains our obligation to exclude this possibility in the examination of every functional articulation case for whom therapy is undertaken.

In an attempt to probe still further into the auditory processes as they relate to speech, several investigators have compared normal and defective speakers on the Seashore Measures of Musical Talent. Travis and Davis (1927) administered three of these measures, pitch, intensity, and tonal memory, to college freshmen in inferior, standard, and superior speech groups. The inferior group included various types of speech defectives. They concluded that certain types of speech-defective cases as a group have lower scores than normal speakers and that the inferior group showed greater variability than the normal group. As their curves of distribution for the three groups are studied, however, it becomes evident that there is great overlapping and similar range for the three groups, only the means differing slightly.

Stinchfield (1927), using the same tests, found little difference between good and poor college speakers. Gilkinson's results (1943) support Stinchfield. He concluded that there is a low order of relationship between Seashore scores and speech skill when general criteria of speech skill are applied. There is no relationship either between Seashore scores and specific vocal habits. Mase (1946), using the rhythm and tonal memory tests, found no reliable difference between boys with good and with poor articulation.

The auditory skills tested by the Seashore battery seem, from the majority of studies, to have little relationship to functional articulatory defects.

*Speech-Sound Discrimination.* Of the possible auditory factors suggested as bearing a causal relationship to functional articulatory defects, one of the most generally advanced is a specific deficiency in sound discrimination, particularly in discrimination for speech sounds. Such a deficiency has been almost taken for granted by some writers in the field but most have evidently considered it to have some importance. It has been advanced as an etiological factor or as a factor which must at least be tested in each case. Many writers have also stressed the importance of auditory discrimination as an approach to retraining.

Speech-sound discrimination has received considerable attention not only in theoretical discussions of etiology but also as the subject of a number of research investigations. These investigations have experimented with a variety of measures of sound discrimination and have investigated the possibility of a difference at various age levels. The results again are conflicting.

Travis and Rasmus (1931) developed a test for speech-sound discrimination which has been used by a number of other investigators as well as by the authors. Travis and Rasmus compared functional articulatory defectives with good speakers at a university freshman level and at the elementary school level. They found that at every age compared, the cases with mild functional articulation disorders made significantly more errors than did normal speakers. They concluded that inferior speech-sound discrimination ability is an important etiological factor in these cases.

Carrell (1937), using a modification of the Travis-Rasmus test, compared 61 sound substitution cases with matched controls. He found the speech defectives somewhat inferior in phonetic discrimination ability but indicated that his results did not differentiate the two groups as clearly as did those of Travis and Rasmus.

Other investigations have failed to support the Travis and Rasmus results. Barnes' (1932) comparison of university freshmen with inferior and with good articulation showed no relation between speech-sound discrimination and articulation.

The present writer (Hall, 1938), also using the Travis-Rasmus test, compared functional articulatory cases with carefully matched good speakers at two age levels, university freshmen and elementary school children. At neither level did she find a significant difference between ability groups. Hall also tested these groups on an original test requiring sound discrimination in more complex auditory patterns. Again no differences were found between ability groups.

Mase (1946) compared boys with functional articulatory defects in grades five and six with carefully matched good speakers. He devised a series of sound-discrimination tests, one using sentences in which single words were misarticulated, another using pairs of similar or slightly dissimilar words. He found that both groups showed great variation in skill but that there was no significant difference between them.

Still another investigation of this causal possibility was made by Hansen (1944) who developed a vowel discrimination test using pairs of same or different vowels. Hansen applied this test, the Seashore measure of timbre, and a short form of the Travis-Rasmus test, known as the Travis-Glaspey test, to three groups of college students: untrained functional articulatory defectives, functional articulatory defectives who had received speech therapy, and normal speakers. He found no differences between any of these groups for any of the three measures used.

Donewald (1950) matched 53 functional articulatory defectives in first grade and 25 in second grade with normal speakers and compared ability groups on 100 paired sounds. A significant difference was found between the control and the experimental groups.

Recently Kronvall and Diehl (1954) have reported a comparison of 30 children with functional articulatory defects and their matched controls on the Templin Speech Sound Discrimination Test. The controls made significantly fewer errors than the articulation cases.

The results of these studies on speech-sound discrimination as related to articulation skill are seen to be conflicting and inconclusive. Again, however, as with auditory acuity, the great weight of evidence is against there being a systematic inferiority of functional articulatory defectives in ability to discriminate speech sounds.

Several investigators have attempted to analyze speech-sound discrimination in a more specific way and to relate discrimination errors to speech errors. Travis and Rasmus (1931) early reported a relationship between sounds causing articulatory difficulty and those not discriminated accurately. Hall (1938), using the same test, did not find such a relationship.

Templin (1943) investigated the possibility of using effectively a shorter test of speech-sound discrimination than the Travis-Rasmus test, and further investigated the relation between discrimination errors and the position of the discriminative element in syllables. She found that children in all grades made more errors when the element to be discriminated was in the medial or final position. As reported earlier, articulation errors are also more frequent in those positions. Templin concluded that her short test of discrimination could be used effectively.

Spriestersbach and Curtis (1951, p. 486), recognizing that individuals with defective articulation have no generalized inability to discriminate speech sounds, go on to say, ". . . the assumption is nevertheless logical that certain individuals who misarticulate a given sound may not have developed fully effective awareness of that particular phonetic entity." They report a study by Anderson (1949) done under their direction in which children, kindergarten through fourth grade, judged to have defective [s] articulation were given an articulation test involving [s] in different word positions and phonetic combinations, and a speech-sound discrimination test using the same words. She found a difference between the percentage of [s] discrimination errors in contexts in which the subjects misarticulated [s] and the percentage in contexts in which they had no articulation difficulty, more errors being made in the former. Sound omission errors tended to be more related to discrimination than sound substitution errors.

Summers (1953) investigated the relationship between the ability to perceive the different speech sounds and to analyze and produce these sounds. He tested undergraduate students with normal speech on four tests: perception (selecting from four words the one containing a previously presented single sound), speech sound discrimination (selection from three nonsense syllables the one which had been previously presented), sound-letter association, and analysis-production (ability to produce the component sounds of a word presented orally). He found that sounds are perceived most accurately in the initial position but analyzed and produced most accurately in the final position. Those sounds perceived most accurately were also most accurately analyzed and produced. Speech sound discrimination was correlated with speech sound perception but not with speech sound analysis-production. Subjects showed a wide range of speech sound perception and analysis-production ability.

These studies all agree in showing considerable relationship between specific difficulties in speech-sound discrimination and the accuracy with which the different speech sounds are articulated.

*Auditory Memory Span.* Over a long period of years the texts in speech pathology have stressed the hypothesis that functional articulatory defects may be determined in part by deficiencies in auditory memory. Most authors suggest specific tests for measuring this ability and some give suggestions for retraining which take this factor into account.

Robbins and Robbins (1937) suggest methods for improving poor auditory memory span, which they consider an important cause of articulation defects. Backus (1943, p. 133), speaking of short auditory memory span as a cause of articulatory defects, says: "This condition does not predicate poor hearing in the usual sense of that term. It means that the child's range of memory for the time order of sounds has not developed normally for his age." West, Kennedy, and Carr (1947) mention short auditory memory span as a possible factor in dyslalia and suggest remedial measures. Van Riper (1947) suggests several tests for auditory memory span, although stating that research had not shown it to be a conclusively differentiating factor between defective and normal articulators. Anderson (1953) stresses the importance of auditory memory span in speech development and points out that memory span is a product of maturation, and that in some children it develops more slowly than in others. He feels that where memory span is delayed in maturing, speech development is also likely to be retarded.

A number of experimental investigations have also been made of auditory memory span in functional articulation cases. Anderson (1938) developed two tests to measure auditory memory, one composed of vowels, one of consonants, and established norms for college students. He found that memory span for speech sounds, especially vowels, seemed independent of phonetic training. He found no relationship between auditory memory span and either pitch discrimination or auditory acuity but found a relationship with ability in learning a foreign language. He considered the vowel test particularly satisfactory for measuring auditory memory span. In 1939 Anderson reported that the memory span for speech sounds is lower than accepted norms for digits.

Metraux (1942), using an adaptation of Anderson's tests, developed tentative norms for children. She compared the results for a speech-defective group—not articulatory cases alone—and normal speakers and found the speech-defective group inferior on the consonant test. The vowel test showed no evidence of difference. The author gives no measures of significance for her results so they must be regarded as inconclusive. In a later report (1944) Metraux gives age norms. She found an increase with age in auditory memory span for both consonants and vowels, found no difference between boys and girls in auditory memory span, and found no significant correlation between mental age and auditory memory span.

Robbins (1942) published results of a study of auditory memory span for digits, phonemes, and syllables, comparing cases of sound substitution, of sound omission, and of delayed speech. He found a consistent increase with age in memory span for phonemes and syllables and found the span for syllables highest, phonemes next, and digits shortest. Short auditory memory spans were found in 13 per cent of sound-substitution cases, 33 per cent of sound-omission cases, and 45 per cent of the delayed-speech cases. The factor of intelligence is not controlled in this study and comparative results for normal speakers are not given.

Beebe (1944) summarized the age norms for auditory memory span published by other authors and added her own. She concluded that auditory memory span for meaningless syllables increases with age, but differences between age groups are small. Like Metraux, she found no sex differences.

Hall (1938) found no difference in auditory memory for speech sounds between groups of functional articulatory cases at a university and at an elementary school level and carefully matched groups with good speech. Mase (1946) also found no differences in auditory memory span between normal-speaking and functional articulatory defective boys in grades five and six.

These studies of auditory memory span are somewhat inconsistent but, in general, the more carefully controlled studies in which functional articulatory defectives and good speakers were matched for age and intelligence show no differences in auditory memory span between speech ability groups.

What can we conclude then about the causal significance of auditory factors in relation to functional articulatory disorders? For each of the auditory skills reviewed, there is some evidence both for and against a systematic difference between normal speakers and functional articulatory defectives. However, the weight of evidence for each auditory factor so far considered is against there being a significant and generalized difference. The weight of evidence is even stronger if we consider only those studies which have been carefully designed, where the factors of age and intelligence have been controlled, where defective and normal speakers have been carefully matched, and where tests of statistical significance have been applied.

It is safe to conclude that not one of the auditory skills so far investigated —acuity, high-frequency loss, speech-sound discrimination, auditory memory—is generally or consistently inferior in functional articulation cases. These cases appear to have about the same range and distribution of auditory abilities as normal speakers. This means that we cannot predict a probable degree of inferiority in any of the auditory factors for a specific functional articulatory case. Since this is true, we also cannot rule out theoretically a possible inferiority in any of the auditory factors for this specific case.

It remains possible for any functional articulatory case to have a deficiency in any one or combination of the several auditory factors discussed. In fact, therein lies a possible etiological factor in the auditory area which has not yet been studied experimentally. Although auditory skills, approached one factor at a time, seem not to be inferior in functional articulatory defectives, is it not possible that the *composite measure* or *patterning* of these skills might be different from that of normal speakers? None of the studies reported has considered the possibility that specific individuals, low, for example, in speech-sound discrimination, might also be low in auditory memory or low in auditory acuity. The approach has been that of comparing groups and comparing them on each factor separately. It would be interesting to compare functional articulatory cases with carefully matched normal-speaking controls on a *battery* of auditory tests, using for comparison a composite measure, derived from experimentally determined weighting of each factor.

It is also interesting to consider the possible relation between genetic development of auditory skills and articulation development. The investigations up to now have dealt with the elementary school age and older. Is it not possible that some children are slow to develop skill in speech-sound discrimination, auditory memory, high-frequency acuity, to mention several, and that they are, therefore, deficient in these skills at the age range most crucial for speech development? Even slight deficiencies might make a difference during the speech-learning period. To hypothesize further, such children may eventually reach average or superior skill in these factors so that the earlier and temporally critical deficiency is masked, and comparative studies would show, as is the case, no differences.

Another possible area of investigation for the future is that of relating auditory abilities to specific types of functional articulatory defect. It is possible that real etiological differences may exist in some types, such as *general oral inaccuracy* but be masked by the absence of differences in the much larger group of functional articulatory defectives as a whole.

It has long been this writer's clinical observation that many functional articulatory cases are *inattentive* to sound differences. If pushed, they can usually discriminate as well as normal speakers but they do not habitually do so. We have to evaluate, therefore, not only auditory capacities but also auditory habits or—perhaps more accurately—*attentional habits* as related to sound.

Another clinical observation related to this is that many functional articulatory cases, although adequate in discrimination of sounds in the speech of other people, are deficient in autodiscrimination. They often fail to hear their own errors, although able to hear errors in others. Further exploration is needed, too, of the relationships already suggested by several studies cited earlier between specific discrimination errors and specific articulation errors.

These aspects of auditory behavior have been neglected in research and urgently need investigation for both theoretical and practical reasons. Auditory factors still remain a promising possibility for further research. The research to date has succeeded fairly well in eliminating as causal factors single and simple auditory skills. It remains for future research to probe some of the more complex relationships between auditory and articulatory learning and performance.

**Sensory factors: tactile and kinesthetic.** Another of the hypotheses concerning the causation of functional articulatory defects has been that individuals with these defects have less than average sensitivity to position, movement, and degree of muscular tension within the speech mechanism. Lack of kinesthetic sensitivity in the tongue has been considered especially important. The possible relation of kinesthesis to articulation, however, has not been studied very much experimentally.

Patton (1942) tested 214 elementary school children with functional articulatory defects and an equal number of normal-speaking children on seven tests of kinesthesia. None of the tests involved the speech mechanism but rather the gross skeletal muscles. Such activities were included as touching finger to nose, bringing index fingers of both hands together at arm's length, all done with the eyes closed. A statistically significant difference was found in favor of the control group, and the author concluded that the speech cases have less kinesthetic sensibility than the controls.

Fairbanks and Bebout (1950) measured percentage of error in duplicating a tongue position, a skill which depends primarily upon kinesthetic sensitivity. Comparisons between college students with inferior and superior articulation yielded no statistically significant difference. These two studies found conflicting results but used very different types of tests and involved quite different parts of the body. The problem of kinesthesis as a causal factor in functional articulation defects remains inconclusive and should receive further study.

**Sensory factors: visual.** Visual skills are not usually thought of as having much relationship to speech, but several authors have mentioned speech defects in children with visual deficiencies. The relationship merits some consideration. Eisenson (1938) mentions that articulatory defects are frequent among even the mature blind. He accounts for it by their lack of visual cues and by the disinclination others show to correct their speech.

Rossignol (1948), in studying relationships among hearing acuity, speech production, and reading performance in primary children, found higher scores on a sound-repetition test when the children were able to look at the tester while listening as compared with listening alone. She also found that the examiners were more consistent in their phonetic ratings when watching the children as against listening to their recorded speech. The author infers that it is important for children to look at the speaker when learning to produce consonants in new words and even earlier when learning to form the consonant sounds.

Brieland (1950), in a comparison of the speech of blind and sighted children, reported one incidental finding, a difference in favor of the sighted group in degree of lip movement. It may be that visual factors should receive more attention than they have heretofore.

**Other physical variables.** Writers in speech pathology have mentioned a variety of additional physical factors which may have etiological importance in functional articulatory disorders. Such factors as general physical debility and poor health, a history of frequent illnesses, especially during the speech-learning years, developmental slowness, glandular deficiencies, "heredity" or "biological inferiority," and others.

Some writers appear to regard such factors as having a direct physical relationship to speech in that they produce a weak and inefficient speech mechanism. Others discuss these factors as having a more indirect relationship. Physical disability restricts a child's activities and experiences and thus deprives him to some extent of both speech stimulation and of motivation for producing speech himself. More subtle factors may also enter the picture, such as the greater emotionality and overprotectiveness which is frequently engendered in parents by an ill child, or a failure on their part to exact normal communicative effort from the child.

Although much discussed, such physical factors have been little studied for functional articulatory defects specifically. Carrell (1936) reported the results of medical examinations and medical histories of 61 sound-substitution cases and normal speakers to show no statistically significant differences between the groups in either health history or medical examination items. Karlin, Youtz, and Kennedy (1940) found more endocrine dysfunction in six articulatory cases as compared with six normal speakers, but this result is no more than suggestive because of the small number involved.

Beckey (1942) made a very thorough investigation of possible factors differentiating retarded speech cases from normal speakers. Although she studied retarded speech cases, not functional articulatory cases, the results may have some significance for the latter. Detailed histories were taken and a battery of tests applied to 50 young children with retarded speech and 50 with normal speech. Of the many items investigated, Beckey found statistically significant differences to the disadvantage of the speech defective group for only the following: mothers who had had abnormal pregnancies and birth complications, children who had had asphyxia at birth, poor motor control, two or more infectious diseases, measles, slow physical growth, diseased or removed tonsils, and presence of adenoids. Although these factors would be expected logically to have more relation to retarded speech than to functional articulatory defects, they may be of interest as possible causal or concomitant factors in functional articulatory defects as well.

Everhart (1953) compared 110 children with articulatory defects in grades one through six with 110 normal-speaking controls on a battery of tests and developmental data secured from a questionnaire filled in by parents. No significant relationship was found between articulatory defectives and the following: Onset of holding head up, of sitting alone, of crawling, of walking, of talking, of voluntary bladder control, and eruption of first tooth. Differences, but of low significance, were found for onset of sitting alone and of holding head up. He also found no significant relationship between articulatory defectiveness and grip, height, weight, handedness.

Too little research has as yet been done on growth and health factors in relation to articulation skills to enable us to reach definite conclusions. It seems clear that large and generalized differences will not be found. At the same time it would seem profitable to investigate these factors further and especially—as with auditory factors—to investigate the interrelationship or *patterning* of growth and health factors as they may relate to the development of articulation.

## Intellectual Variables

The solution to functional articulatory disorders has been sought by many speech pathologists in differences in general intellectual endowment or in the presence of certain special mental abilities or specific disabilities. Thus a great deal of attention has been given to studying the general intelligence of speech defectives and of evaluating their possible deficiency in "verbal intelligence" as against "nonverbal intelligence." Texts in speech pathology all stress the importance of evaluating the intelligence of a case as part of the basic diagnostic examination, both as an aid to diagnosis and as a significant factor in planning therapy.

The relationship between speech and other language functions—vocabulary, reading achievement, spelling achievement—has also received considerable attention. It has been suggested by many that certain types of abilities tend to vary together, so that, for example, individuals deficient in speech would tend to be deficient in reading skill and that other individuals would tend to be superior in these supposedly related abilities. This is a tantalizing subject for thought and for research. Here it can occupy us only to the extent of discussing the possible relation these variables may have to functional articulatory defects.

**Intelligence.** The relationship of intelligence to articulation development and to defects of articulation has long intrigued the interest of speech pathologists. Intelligence has been felt to have such a basic influence on speech that investigators have considered it an important factor to control in studying other variables. Thus, in the many studies in which matched groups of articulatory defectives and normal speakers have been compared for possible differences, intelligence has usually been one of the bases on which the matching was done.

The relationship of intelligence to articulation skill has been approached in three principal ways. Some investigators have studied articulation growth in relation to intelligence in normal, unselected children. Others have compared intelligence of articulatory defectives with that of normal speakers. Still other investigators have started with intelligence as the independent variable and have compared the speech of mentally deficient with mentally normal individuals.

One of the first studies to relate articulation development to intelligence was that of Wellman, Case, Mengert, and Bradbury (1931) who studied children from two to six years of age. They found a correlation of .80 between articulation skill and chronological age, of .71 between articulation skill and mental age on the Stanford-Binet; but with chronological age held constant, little relationship was found between articulation and mental age. In other words, articulation development had a closer relationship to chronological than to mental age.

Irwin (1952), reporting on studies of speech development in infants up to 30 months of age, concluded that the relationship between speech sound development and intelligence is not very dependable at 18 months but that from the twentieth to thirtieth month there are reliable correlations between various indices of speech-sound development and both the Kuhlmann and Cattell intelligence tests. Dawson (1929), studying rate of articulation, found a tendency toward more rapid articulation in pupils with high I.Q.'s than in those with low I.Q.'s.

Several studies have compared intelligence ratings of functional articulatory defectives and normal speakers. Carrell (1936) reported that speech defectives as a group had a lower intelligence level than normal speakers and that articulatory cases (oral inaccuracy) had the greatest deficiency in intelligence. Speech defectives were also below normal speakers in school achievement, the oral inaccuracy group again showing the most retardation.

Beckey (1942) found that retarded speech cases usually made inferior ratings on intelligence tests as compared with children who had normal speech. Hall (1938) found a zero correlation between articulation ratings of college students and their composite percentile rank on the Iowa Qualifying Examination. Everhart (1953) found that a real difference in intelligence exists in favor of children with normal articulation as compared with children with defective articulation in grades one through six. Sperling (1948) compared children with functional articulatory defects on verbal and nonverbal intelligence tests and found that they had significantly higher performance scores than verbal scores. She concluded that more than one intelligence test should be used in making a prognosis for speech-training with articulatory cases.

The third approach concerns itself with the speech proficiency of children with known mental retardation. Ingram (1935) found speech defects in about 12 per cent of mentally retarded children as compared with 2 or 3 per cent of children in regular grades and found that speech defects also tend to persist longer in retarded children in spite of remedial instruction. Sirkin and Lyons (1941) found that only a third of institutionalized mental defectives speak normally and that the lower the intelligence rating the lower the incidence of normal speech.

Bangs (1942) made a careful study of the speech deficiencies of mentally defective children and concluded that mental age has much greater predictive value for speech than does chronological age. He found that, except for more frequent omission of final sounds, the speech of these children does not differ very much *qualitatively* from that of children with normal intelligence. Misarticulations followed essentially the same pattern as they do in functional articulation cases of the same mental age but of normal intelligence.

Karlin and Strazzulla (1952) concluded after studying 50 children with I.Q.'s below 70 that language defects are even more striking than speech defects and in some cases resemble aphasia. Irwin (1952) tested children with I.Q.'s from 7 to 48 at age three years and again at four. He found almost complete identity of vowel and consonant curves for the two tests, showing little growth. Vowel profiles were comparable to those of normal one-year-old infants.

Schlanger (1953) studied 74 mentally handicapped children between the ages of eight and sixteen years and found 56.7 per cent of them to have articulatory problems. The children were found to have a marked deficiency in auditory memory span for vowels and in sound discrimination. Higher correlations were obtained between mental age and articulatory proficiency than between chronological age and speech proficiency.

What can we conclude about the relationship of intelligence to articulatory deficiencies? The relationship has certainly not been shown to be so close that it has much predictive value except within broad limits. At the same time results of research are consistent in showing a gross relationship, particularly for the low end of the intelligence range. Except for the greater incidence of articulatory deficiency among mentally retarded individuals, intelligence appears to be relatively unimportant as a determining factor in articulatory disorders, at least above the age range during which most speech learning takes place. In short, during infancy and the preschool years intelligence appears to be an important factor in articulation growth. Above that level intelligence bears only a general relationship to articulatory proficiency except when intelligence is below normal limits, when it unquestionably affects speech adequacy.

It is interesting again, as with other etiological factors previously discussed, to consider the possibly greater relationship of intelligence to certain types of functional articulatory defects, notably general oral inaccuracy, than to others.

**Reading skill.** Articulation problems have been mentioned frequently as a cause of reading disability. It has been assumed by many that reading and articulation, both being language-related functions, are somewhat interdependent and that a deficiency in one tends to be associated with a deficiency in the other. Other writers have stressed not a direct causal relationship between speech and reading deficiency but rather the possibility that other more basic skills, such as auditory acuity, auditory memory span, and sound discrimination, are fundamental in both reading and speech, and, if deficient, retard both. If this were true, speech and reading disabilities could be said to have a concomitant rather than a causal relationship. The possibility of a relationship between reading and articulation has interested both educators and speech pathologists and has been approached experimentally from both aspects.

Monroe (1932) was one of the first to discuss defective speech as a causal factor in reading disability or, at least, as a factor associated with reading disability. She found that among her reading defect cases there were many more speech defects than among her controls. She considered inaccurate articulation particularly effective as a factor in retarding reading. Since then Moss (1938), Bennett (1938), Witty and Kopel (1939), Hildreth (1946), Betts (1946), and Eames (1950), to mention but a few, have written more or less in support of this view or have presented data which support it. Jones (1951) found experimentally that speech-training accelerated the reading achievement of one group of children as against their matched controls who received no speech-training.

Bond (1935) studied speech characteristics of good and poor readers and found no difference between them in incidence of speech defects. However, when skill in oral and in silent reading were considered separately, he found that 35 per cent of children retarded in oral reading but good in silent reading had speech defects. The children who were retarded in silent reading but not in oral reading showed no speech defects. Everhart (1953) found some tendency for boys with normal articulation to have higher reading achievement than boys with functional articulatory difficulties. Hall (1938) and Moore (1947) both found articulatory cases equal to normal speakers in silent reading achievement.

Robinson (1946) made a particularly searching investigation of possible causes of reading disability, including speech defects, and a careful analysis of previous investigations. Previous studies led her to conclude (p. 99): "On the basis of the evidence available, articulatory defects may be conceded to be important in oral reading but of little significance in silent reading." She found dyslalia in 20 per cent of her 30 reading disability cases but stated that its effect as a cause of reading failure could not be determined in many of the cases and that in others no direct relationship could be either established or denied. Her conclusion is that speech difficulties may be causal factors in reading difficulties but that the mere presence of a speech defect does not necessarily mean that it is causally related to the reading difficulty.

Artley (1948) reached much the same conclusions in reviewing the literature on some of the factors presumed to be associated with reading and speech difficulties. He concluded that speech defects may be the cause of reading defects, the result of reading defects, or that both defects may result from some common factor. He also concluded that such factors as reduced auditory acuity, auditory discrimination, and auditory memory span, may be related significantly to reading retardation, but that they do not appear to be significantly related to speech defects.

Carrell and Pendergast (1954) investigated another language function—spelling—in relation to articulation defects in children. They compared functional articulation cases with matched controls and found no significant difference between the groups either in spelling ability or in the types of spelling errors which occurred. They concluded that there is no underlying phonetic disability.

Investigations of interrelationships among the language functions are clearly inconclusive at the present time, little is known for certain and there are many challenging problems for future study.

### Environmental and Learning Variables

Much attention has been given by speech pathologists to factors which do not lie within the individual himself but which, though external to him, influence his development and his learning of speech. A child's speech adequacy is conditioned by the speech patterns surrounding him. These patterns in turn are thought to be conditioned by other factors such as the educational and cultural level of the parents, urban versus rural living, and foreign language background or bilingualism. Other factors in the speech environment alleged to be influential are the number of siblings and their ages relative to the child under consideration, speech defects in members of the family, and, to a lesser degree, speech defects in playmates and teachers. Blanton (1936), for example, stressed the "bad habit" origin of speech defects and attributed over 50 per cent of lisping in children with a normal speech mechanism to mothers who lisp.

The methods of child-training used by parents, particularly their methods of speech-training, parental attitudes toward speech, the degree and kind of attention given the child's speech, are all mentioned frequently as being of great influence in determining the various aspects of his speech and language development. At one extreme we find parents who are indifferent and neglectful of the child's speech. They spend little time reading to the child, telling him stories, or just talking with him. They fail to expect speech of the child, to train him in good speech habits, or to correct his errors, either because of indifference or through a belief that errors will be outgrown. At the other extreme are the parents who overcorrect the child's speech so that he becomes discouraged, self-conscious, or negativistic about his own speech attempts.

Other parents offer poor speech patterns either consciously through the use of "baby talk" or mimicry of the child's own immature expressions and errors, or inadvertently because of foreign or native dialects or actual speech defects. Parents sometimes encourage the prolongation of infantile speech habits by rewarding them with attention and admiration. The child whose infantile speech wins him the delighted approval of an admiring family circle is ill-motivated to develop mature speech.

Speech develops in response to a need to communicate and the pleasure experienced in communicating. Some children seldom feel a need to talk

Their communicative urges are anticipated or they succeed at a simple communicative level, such as gesture or pantomime. Other children have ever-willing brothers, sisters, or parents ready to interpret for them when their immature speech is not readily understood. They are deprived of the need to improve their intelligibility.

A few children experience more serious deprivation of speech stimulation. Children who are left alone much of the time because parents are working or otherwise preoccupied, children who have little contact with other children or with adults, who hear little speech, who have no one to talk to or little urge to talk because of a dearth of experiences may be critically handicapped in speech development. The handicap is probably greatest if the deprivation comes during the speech-learning years. It has been observed, for example, that children brought up in institutions during their early years are often slow in speech development. They hear relatively little adult speech. They lack individual parental attention to speech and the constant speech interaction provided by the typical parent-child relationship.

Many possible factors which violate good speech-learning conditions have been mentioned above. They represent the pooled clinical experience of speech pathologists. Some of them have the support of research findings as well; others remain still unverified.

**Education and cultural status of parents.** A number of studies have compared the speech development or incidence of speech defects among children of different socioeconomic groups. Occupational status of parents has been used as an index of parental education and culture. Davis (1937) found a considerably higher percentage of children with good articulation among upper occupational groups than among lower. Beckey (1942) also found that significantly more children with retarded speech belonged to lower socioeconomic groups. Parents of children with normal speech represented most frequently the professional and managerial occupations. Parents of children with delayed speech also had an inferior educational background as compared with parents of children with normal speech.

Irwin (1948, 1952), studying infants up to 30 months of age, found a marked difference between infants reared in homes of professional and business parents and infants reared in homes of laboring parents. Differences in both frequency and type of speech sounds were negligible for the first year and a half, after that were in favor of the former. Irwin concluded that the factor of parental stimulation is an important variable in speech development.

McClure (1952) found that "factory working parents" was one of the items in common for children with articulatory and reading defects. Templin (1953) found a significant difference between children of upper and lower socioeconomic groups (according to the Minnesota Scale of Occupations) on both screening and diagnostic tests of articulation, the difference being in favor of the upper group. She stated that children of the lower socioeconomic group take about a year longer to reach essentially mature articulation than those of the upper group.

There are several explanations for these consistent findings of superior articulation and smaller incidence of articulatory disorders in children of upper socioeconomic groups. Upper group parents, in general, present better speech patterns to their children. They also create a more stimulating speech environment and for the most part do more and better articulatory training of their children.

**Rural versus urban environment.** Rural as compared with urban living has been considered by some to be related to articulatory development, presumably because of differences in the quantity and quality of speech stimulation provided in these two environments. Louttit and Halls (1936) found a greater incidence of speech defects in county school systems than in city school systems. Articulatory defects specifically had a slightly higher ratio than other speech defects among rural children. Wilson (1952) on the contrary found a slightly higher incidence of articulatory defects among urban children than among rural children. In neither study was the difference very large, so that the relative effects of urban and rural environments on articulation are still in doubt. It seems unlikely that the urban or rural variable in itself would be a factor but rather the educational-cultural level of parents regardless of location.

**Effect of siblings, twins, birth order.** Wellman *et al.* (1931) found no relationship in children two to six years of age between articulation skill and number of older children in the family. Davis (1937) found twins considerably inferior to singletons and to only children in articulation skill. This supports the common clinical observation that twins tend to be deficient in articulation and to show highly similar patterns of misarticulation. Beckey (1942) found no significance in birth *order* as related to delayed speech but found that the child with speech retardation tended to be the youngest child. Irwin (1952) reported practically no differences in speech sound development for infants with older siblings and infants without siblings. However, his studies included only infants under 30 months of age when the influence of other children could perhaps be expected logically to be less effective one way or another than above that age.

Conflicting notions have been proposed regarding the influence of siblings on a child's articulatory development. One opinion is that siblings tend to stimulate speech. Another and opposing view is that siblings tend to provide less perfect articulation patterns to a child than do adults. An only child or oldest child (while he remains the only child) receives nearly 100 per cent of his speech stimulation from adults, his parents. The child with siblings receives a considerable proportion of his total speech stimulation from them, whose speech is likely to be less mature than that of adults. The extreme example of this is the case of twins, who hear much of their speech from each other. The emotional ties of twins, too, are likely to be closer than those of single siblings, which further augments their interdependence in speech

**Poor speech patterns.** Bilingualism has often been said to retard speech development but both McCarthy (1930) and Beckey (1942) failed to find such a relationship in the children they studied. Similarly, speech defects in parents and older siblings are often mentioned as an influential factor and most clinicians would agree on the basis of their experience. There is little exact statistical evidence, however, to either support or refute this relationship. It is probable that a child's speech patterns are adversely affected by an articulatory defect in a parent or in an older sibling. It is further probable that his specific misarticulations will resemble those of the defective speaker. It is also probable that the degree of influence of the defective speaker upon the child will depend upon the emotional relationship existing between them. If the child strongly identifies emotionally with, for example, an older brother who has a speech defect, the chances are probably greater that his own speech will be adversely affected than if he does not have this positive identification. There is strong motivation, though often at an unconscious level, to become like those we admire.

**Methods of speech training.** Beckey (1942) found a significantly greater number of children among her retarded than among her normal speech group whose wants had been anticipated by parents without speech or from whom gestures had been accepted and speech not required, factors considered to handicap speech development.

**Lack of speech stimulation.** Beckey found that children of her delayed speech group had too much isolation for the encouragement of speech. Carrell (1936) who made a study of speech in an institution for dependent children, considered the incidences of speech defects found at various age levels relatively high. He accounted for this by the fact that the children lived in groups, which made their contacts with adults more limited than is the case in a family of normal size. Irwin (1952) reported speech-sound development for orphanage babies below that for home babies. The present writer, during her experience as a psychologist in a children's institution, made the same observation. Preschool and kindergarten children, particularly, were markedly deficient in speech output, vocabulary, and articulation as compared with noninstitutional children. They did poorly, for example, on vocabulary items of the Stanford Binet scale.

Mason (1942) cites an extreme example of a child who did not learn to talk until she was six and a half years of age because she had been living alone until that age with a mute and uneducated mother.

Considering the results of both research and clinical experience, we can conclude that certain environmental conditions and certain types of interaction between the child and his environment are necessary for the development of mature speech. To develop normal patterns of speech a child must hear normal patterns of speech, must have a need and desire to talk, must experience pleasure in hearing speech and in responding with speech, must have sufficient variety in his day-by-day experience to stimulate a communicative urge and to provide communicative content, and his speech must be reacted to constructively by others.

### Emotional and Personality Variables

Increasingly in the last decade or two clinical speech pathology has shown a trend in the direction of giving greater importance to the personality characteristics of individuals and to their emotional and social adjustment as effective determinants of their speech. These variables have received increasing emphasis both as etiological factors, and as factors of significance for the success of speech therapy and for the types of speech therapy to be employed in each specific case. The importance of emotional factors has long been recognized in relation to stuttering by even the most somatically minded. Functional articulatory disorders, too, are beginning belatedly to receive more attention as possibly symptomatic of personality structure and emotional adjustment. When it comes to therapy for these disorders, almost no one disputes the importance of the psychological aspects.

In the field of emotional and personality growth and adjustment, cause-and-effect relationships are perhaps more difficult to determine than in other aspects of growth. Even if we could, for example, demonstrate that functional articulation cases are significantly less well adjusted emotionally than normal speakers, we would still be left with the cause-and-effect dilemma. Has the emotional maladjustment "caused" the articulatory problem, has the articulatory problem "caused" the emotional maladjustment, or is there a more complex reciprocal relationship between them, so that emotional problems have caused an articulatory deviation which, in turn, has augmented the severity of the emotional problem? We are in no position at the present time to give a satisfactory answer to such a question. Research has barely nibbled around the edges of this intriguing area of personality and adjustment in relation to speech. Less investigation has been made of these factors than of the types of variables already discussed. Results are again inconclusive.

**Personality traits.** Some speech pathologists have raised the question as to whether functional articulatory disorders tend to develop more in individuals with certain normal personality traits than in individuals with other normal personality traits. Anderson (1953, pp. 137–138) even relates certain personality traits to different and specific types of articulatory defectiveness.

The slow-moving, sluggish, phlegmatic individual is very likely to display some of those personality characteristics in his speech, resulting in a slow tempo and "mushy," poorly formed sounds and words, referred to as oral inactivity. Such people are inclined to be lip-lazy and tongue-lazy, and the final result in extreme cases is a kind of mumbling drawl. The opposite temperament also produces its special brand of speech pattern. The nervous, high-strung, hyperactive person is likely to talk fast, and, because he is not able to execute the proper articulatory adjustments so rapidly, many sounds are dropped out or are distorted. Such a person tends to "hit the high spots" only, and his speech rhythm may be jerky and broken. Then there is the shy, bashful person who is literally afraid to open his mouth. In such cases the voice is likely to be light and weak, and this lack of intensity, coupled with the oral inactivity, often renders the speech very difficult to understand.

These relationships still remain unverified, however, and little has yet been done to investigate the problem experimentally.

Wellman et al. (1931) found no relationship between speech sound development in young children, two to six years, and introversion-extroversion ratings. Davis (1937) found that normal-speaking children tended to rate higher on "talkativeness" and "spontaneity" than children with defective articulation. The latter were more shy and negativistic than good speakers.

Templin (1938) tested college speech-defective and normal-speaking groups on the Moore-Gilliland Test for Aggressiveness and found the speech-defective group significantly less aggressive than the normal-speaking group. Of the speech defectives, the articulatory group were the lowest in aggressiveness. Articulatory cases tended to be more aggressive as their defects were more severe. The results of the Davis and Templin studies are fairly consistent, though done on widely separated age groups.

**Emotional adjustment.** The feverish activity which we have seen during the last two decades in clinical psychology, centered mainly in the area of emotional growth and adjustment, has had its impact on speech pathology. Today it would be a rare speech pathologist indeed who would not readily admit a close relationship of emotional adjustment to speech. We take such a relationship for granted, even though the exact nature of the relationship still remains obscure and theoretical. Little experimental work has been done even to verify the relationship, let alone explain how it operates. Our interest in the importance of emotional factors in articulation has perhaps too far outrun the conclusions which are justifiable on the basis of the little experimental evidence we have.

Beckey (1942) found that children with retarded speech tended to play alone, to cry easily, and to be less demanding of attention than children with normal speech. She found no difference between the groups in incidence of temper tantrums, thumb-sucking, or enuresis. The retarded-speech group had more instances in its histories of severe fright.

Anders (1945) found children of six to twelve years with functional articulatory defects to be above average in adjustment as measured by the California Test of Personality. McAllister (1948), using the same test, found no difference in adjustment between children in grades one through eight, with articulatory defects and matched children with normal speech. She also found no significant differences between the two groups on her speech-attitude scale, though there was a tendency for the speech-defective children in the upper grades to compare less favorably with their controls on reactions to speech than speech defectives in the lower grades. The author concludes that emotional instability is not substantiated as a causal factor in articulatory defects and that speech defects do not cause emotional instability or malattitudes toward speech.

The most significant study on this problem has been done by Wood (1946) who studied the emotional adjustment of both children and their parents. He gave the California Test of Personality and the Aspects of Personality Test (Pintner *et al.*) to 50 elementary school children with functional defects of articulation. Some also received the Murray Thematic Apperception Test. The 50 pairs of parents of these children were given the Bernreuter Personality Inventory and the California Test of Personality, and detailed case history information was secured from them. Finally two clinical groups of children were established on the basis of paired neurotic tendency ratings of mothers. Parental counseling was carried on for one group, in addition to the speech-training which both groups of children received. In agreement with both Anders and McAllister, Wood found that the speech-defective children did not fall below test norms in personality adjustment. His results for parents are of special interest. Maternal Bernreuter scores differed significantly from test norms, showing that the mothers as a group were more neurotic in tendency, more submissive, and more self-conscious. Fathers as a group did not differ significantly from test norms. No correlation was found between personality test scores of children and their parents. Seventy-two per cent of the 50 speech-defective children had at least one parent above the 60th percentile in neurotic tendency.

On the California Test of Personality maternal scores again differed significantly from test norms, indicating that mothers were lower in self-adjustment, social adjustment, and total adjustment. Fathers rated significantly lower in self-adjustment. Social standards of mothers were very high in comparison with other adjustment scores and Wood concluded that the speech-defective children had imposed upon them a set of very high standards in an atmosphere of habitual emotional outbursts from the parents. The Thematic Apperception Test results suggested a sense of frustration in 66 per cent of the children, withdrawing tendencies in 65 per cent, and lack of affection in 30 per cent. Other elements suggested by the results were anxiety-insecurity, lack of belongingness, lack of achievement, aggressiveness, and hostility, and escape.

Case history data revealed 13 home environment factors which would militate against a satisfactory emotional life for the child, or would predispose the parent to neglect and mishandle the child (p. 272). "The most frequent factors were lack of recreational outlet for the parents, ignorance of child behavior problems, overly severe child discipline methods, and defective home membership."

The children whose mothers were clinically treated improved in speech more rapidly with speech correction than did the children whose mothers were not so-treated. Wood's conclusion was that (p. 272): ". . . functional articulatory defects of children are definitely and significantly associated with maladjustment and undesirable traits on the part of the parents, and that such factors are usually maternally centered."

Mowrer (1952) has given a good account of the specific learning mechanisms by which the emotional atmosphere surrounding a child becomes effective in influencing his speech development. When the mother is a love object for the infant, a source of gratification and pleasure, the sounds made by her, including speech sounds, become pleasurable stimuli. The sounds are associated with basic satisfactions and thus become positively conditioned, they become *good sounds*. The human infant, being vocally versatile, in the course of random vocalizations will make sounds similar to those of the mother. Since these sounds have already acquired pleasant connotations for him, he will try to repeat and refine them (p. 265). "Soon, however, the infant discovers that the making of these sounds can be used not only to comfort, reassure, and satisfy himself directly but also to interest, satisfy, and control mother, father, and others." He then begins to speak purposively. It is thus that speech development is motivated by a favorable emotional environment.

The implication of this analysis is that when the mother is not a source of pleasure and gratification to the child the sounds associated with her become negatively conditioned and the child tends to reject and withdraw from them. He is not motivated, as in the first instance, to produce sounds himself and is thus delayed and handicapped to various degrees in his own speech development.

## SUMMARY

An extensive review has been presented of the many factors which various speech pathologists have considered significant in the causation of functional disorders of articulation. The factors and the research results which support or refute them have been discussed under four general categories: physical and psychophysical, intellectual, environmental, and personality and emotional factors.

The review of studies on anatomical variables concluded that there is no systematic relationship between functional articulatory disorders and the dimensions or shape of any part of the speech mechanism. The studies on motor co-ordination for the body as a whole and within the speech mechanism specifically are sufficiently inconsistent and inconclusive to leave open the possibility that differences may yet be found. It seems highly unlikely, however, that large and systematic differences will ever be found for any motor function.

The studies of auditory acuity, though somewhat inconclusive, throw doubt on there being any significant and general deficiency in functional articulatory cases. Again, with speech-sound discrimination and auditory memory span, results are inconsistent; but the weight of evidence is against there being a systematic deficiency in these skills. The results for kinesthetic sensitivity are conflicting and meager. The studies of developmental and health factors are also conflicting and inconclusive.

Intelligence has been shown to have only a gross relationship to articulation skill and is not a helpful index, except at low I.Q. levels, for the prediction of probable articulation skill.

When we come to environmental and adjustment factors the results are somewhat more conclusive and positive, though still unsupported by any great weight of research evidence. The educational and cultural level of parents, the amount and kind of speech stimulation given the child, and the general management of the child's speech-learning seem to be causally related to defects of articulation. Although there is little research, there is much clinical verification of such relationships. There is a suggestion that some personality traits, such as shyness and submissiveness, may be related to articulatory disorders but whether as causal, resultant, or as concomitant factors, has not been clearly shown. In the area of emotional adjustment most of our evidence is clinical rather than experimental. Emotional adjustment of the articulatory defectives themselves seems not to be a causal factor in their speech disorder. Wood's study, however, supported by the clinical experience of many speech pathologists, shows that parental, particularly maternal, adjustment is a highly significant factor in many cases, though not in all. This relates to the demonstrated importance of more objective "environmental" factors. It seems probable that in a rejecting, overcritical, punitive, or emotionally disturbed atmosphere a child may develop a *protective inattention* to the speech surrounding him and be handicapped in developing speech himself.

In his recent and excellent "Rationale for Articulation Disorders" (1954, p. 6), Milisen hypothesizes that "defective articulation, a substitute response for normal articulation, results from the disruption of the normal learning process." Though the possible causes for this hypothesized disruption are not discussed, it seems implicit in Milisen's point of view that disruption could result from a variety of factors, physical, environmental, or emotional. Many of the different factors discussed in this chapter could theoretically cause disruption to the normal process of learning speech. The point in the temporal speech-learning sequence at which they appear would logically determine in large part their effectiveness as a disrupting influence.

What general conclusions can we reach then about the etiology of functional disorders of articulation? From the research which has been reviewed, we can say confidently that there is no single factor which has been demonstrated to be associated always—or even nearly always—with these disorders. These cases have shown no general, systematic deficiencies for any factor. Similarly, there is no factor which is consistently absent in all functional articulatory cases. Every factor mentioned has been found in some cases. We seem then at present to be in a challenging state of uncertainty concerning the factors most often associated or most strongly associated with these disorders. Our lack of success in understanding the etiology of these problems probably stems from the fact that we have been searching for single, specific factors or for certain *types* of factors.

It seems most constructive to this writer to think of functional disorders of articulation as determined by a *causal pattern,* a combination of causal factors, and by the *temporal relation* of the causal pattern to the speech-learning process. The causal pattern may occasionally be simple, uncomplicated, obvious, and may consist of only one or two of the many factors mentioned. Far more frequently, however, we are likely to find a causal pattern of greater complexity, with several factors operating successively or simultaneously. Thus the causal pattern for a single case may involve predisposing precipitating, and perpetuating factors and these factors may lie in any or all of the four areas mentioned, physical, intellectual, environmental, and emotional.

Let us cite several hypothetical cases in which various factors might combine to produce a functional articulatory disorder, although any one of them alone would not be sufficient. For example, a child might have intelligence in the 70 to 85 I.Q. range. This deficiency in itself would not produce an articulatory problem, but it might act as a predisposing factor which, in combination with such precipitating factors as marked lack of speech stimulation and a feeling of inadequacy and insecurity, would retard his articulatory development. A brighter child might override the environmental and emotional factors to develop good speech. Low intelligence then would act as a predisposing or augmenting factor which would require the presence of other factors to be effective.

Another child might be clumsy in his movements and have less than average skill in tongue co-ordinations. This minor deficiency would act as a predisposing factor. If this child is subjected to a bilingual home environment or to a severe articulation disorder in a parent, he will in all probability have trouble in mastering articulation skills. If, in addition, the child is shy and withdrawn, his difficulty will be still further increased. A child with normal motor dexterity in the same environment might succeed in developing good articulation in spite of poor parental speech, through the incidental stimulation received from playmates and others outside the home.

Still another child might have a slight hearing loss or an unusually short auditory memory span. This would be a predisposing tendency, but the extent to which it would handicap him, if at all, would depend upon the further factors with which it might combine. If the parents were emotionally disturbed, rejecting, or indifferent, so that he developed serious insecurity in the parental relationship, then his slight auditory handicap might make the crucial difference which would produce an articulatory disorder. With calm, approving, encouraging parents, it would probably have little effect.

Each factor present—though noneffective alone, increases the probability that any other factor or factors, also noneffective alone, will in combination produce a functional articulatory problem, particularly if they occur during the crucial speech-learning years. Anatomical, motor, sensory, and intellectual variables probably operate most frequently as predisposing factors. Environmental, learning, personality, and emotional variables probably act as precipitating and perpetuating factors which are superimposed on the predisposing factors. The more predisposing factors there are present and the more severe any such factor is, the more chance there will be for any one environmental or emotional factor to become effective.

There is a great challenge to be seen in a different type of research approach to functional articulatory disorders. Most studies have approached the problem piecemeal. They have not been sufficiently comprehensive to permit a study of the *patterning* of factors. There is need for an extended program of research—probably carried on by a large university research center—which would study large numbers of cases over extended periods of time, testing a wide variety of possible factors in articulation cases and in normal-speaking individuals. Only then will we be able to evaluate the possibility that certain combinations of variables are commonly effective in producing articulation problems.

In the meantime, before we have this understanding, the speech clinician will not be able to escape the necessity for making a thorough evaluation of most, at least, of the possible factors which have been discussed, if he is to evolve the causal pattern for each case he studies. It seems likely, too, that for some time to come we will continue to see occasional puzzling cases in which no causal factors at all can be identified.

## BIBLIOGRAPHY

AINSWORTH, S. 1948. Speech correction methods. New York: Prentice-Hall.

ALBRIGHT, R. W. 1948. The motor abilities of speakers with good and poor articulation. *Speech Monogr.,* 15, 164–172.

AMIDON, H. F. 1941. A statistical study of relationships among articulation errors made by one hundred first grade children. Unpublished Master's Thesis. State Univ. of Iowa.

ANDERS, Q. M. 1945. A study of the personal and social adjustment of children with functional articulatory defects. Unpublished Master's Thesis. Univ. of Wis.

ANDERSON, P. W. 1949. The relationship of normal and defective articulation of the consonant (s) in various phonetic contexts to auditory discrimination between normal and defective (s) production among children from kindergarten through fourth grade. Unpublished Master's Thesis. State Univ. of Iowa.

ANDERSON, V. A. 1938. The auditory memory span for speech sounds. *Speech Monogr.,* 5, 115–129.

———— 1939. Auditory memory span as tested by speech sounds. *Amer. J. Psychol.,* 52, 95–99.

———— 1953. Improving the child's speech. New York: Oxford Univ. Press

AREY, M. L. 1938. A diagnostic profile of the speech of children in grades 1, 2 and 3. *Quart. J. Speech,* 24, 265–268.

ARTLEY, A. S. 1948. A study of certain factors presumed to be associated with reading and speech difficulties. *J. Speech Hearing Disorders,* 13, 351–360.

ASHA Committee on the Midcentury White House Conference. 1952. Speech disorders and speech correction. *J. Speech Hearing Disorders,* 17, 129–137

BACKUS, O. L. 1943. Speech in education. New York: Longmans, Green.

BANGS, J. L. 1942. A clinical analysis of the articulatory defects of the feeble minded. *J. Speech Disorders,* 7, 343–356.

BARNES, H. G. 1932. Diagnosis of speech needs and abilities of students in a required course in speech training at the State University of Iowa. Unpublished Ph.D. Thesis. State Univ. of Iowa.

BECKEY, R. E. 1942. A study of certain factors related to retardation of speech *J. Speech Disorders,* 7, 223–249.

BEEBE, H. H. 1944. Auditory memory span for meaningless syllables. *J. Speech Disorders,* 9, 273–276.

———— 1946. Sigmatismus nasalis. *J. Speech Disorders,* 11, 35–37.

———— and KASTEIN, S. 1946. Psychogenesis in interdental sigmatism. *J. Speech Disorders*, 11, 191–192.

BENDER, J. F., and KLEINFELD, V. M. 1936. Speech correction manual. New York: Farrar and Rinehart.

———— 1938. Principles and practices of speech correction. New York: Pitman.

BENNETT, C. C. 1938. An inquiry into the genesis of poor reading. *Teach. Coll. Contr. Educ.*, No. 755. New York: Teachers College, Columbia Univ.

BERRY, M. F., and EISENSON, J. 1942. The defective in speech. New York: Appleton-Century-Crofts.

BETTS, E. A. 1946. Foundations of reading instruction. New York: American Book.

BILTO, E. W. 1941. A comparative study of certain physical abilities of children with speech defects and children with normal speech. *J. Speech Disorders*, 6, 187–203.

BLACK, M. E., compiler. 1952. The Illinois plan for special education of exceptional children. The speech defective. Circular Series "E" No. 12, Revised. Springfield, Illinois. Issued by Vernon L. Nickell, Superintendent of Public Instruction.

BLANTON, S. 1936. Helping the speech handicapped school student. *J. Speech Disorders*, 1, 97–100.

BOND, G. L. 1935. The auditory and speech characteristics of poor readers. *Tech. Coll. Contr. Educ.*, No. 657. New York: Teachers College, Columbia Univ.

BRIELAND, D. M. 1950. A comparative study of the speech of blind and sighted children. *Speech Monogr.*, 17, 99–103.

BRYNGELSON, B., and BROWN, S. 1939. Season of birth of speech defectives in Minnesota. *J. Speech Disorders*, 4, 319–322.

BUCK, M. W. 1948. A study of the misarticulation of (r) in children from kindergarten through third grade. Unpublished Master's Thesis. State Univ. of Iowa.

BURDIN, L. G. 1940. A survey of speech defectives in the Indianapolis primary grades. *J. Speech Disorders*, 5, 247–258.

CARHART, R. 1943. Hearing deficiencies and speech problems. *J. Speech Disorders*, 8, 247–254.

CARRELL, J. A. 1936. A comparative study of speech defective children. *Arch. Speech*, 1, 179–203.

———— 1937. The etiology of sound substitution defects. *Speech Monogr.*, 4, 17–37.

CARRELL, J., and PENDERGAST, K. 1954. An experimental study of the possible relation between errors of speech and spelling. *J. Speech Hearing Disorders*, 19, 327–334.

CHEN, H. P. and IRWIN, O. C. 1946a. Infant speech vowel and consonant types. *J. Speech Disorders*, 11, 27–29.

———— 1946b. The type-token ratio applied to infant speech sounds. *J. Speech Disorders*, 11, 126–130.

DAVIS, E. A. 1937. The development of linguistic skill in twins, singletons with siblings, and only children from age five to ten years. Minneapolis: Univ. of Minn. Press.

DAVIS, I. P. 1938. The speech aspects of reading readiness. *Nat. elem. Princ.*, 17, 282–289.

DAWSON, L. O. 1929. A study of the development of the rate of articulation. *Elem. Sch. J.*, 29, 610–615.

DONEWALD, M. H. 1950. The relation of speech sound discrimination to functional articulatory defects in children. Unpublished Master's Thesis. Purdue Univ.

EAMES, T. H. 1950. The relationship of reading and speech difficulties. *J. educ. Psychol.*, 41, 51–55.

EISENSON, J. 1938. The psychology of speech. New York: Appleton-Century-Crofts.

EVERHART, R. W. 1953. The relationship between articulation and other developmental factors in children. *J. Speech Hearing Disorders*, 18, 332–338.

FAIRBANKS, G., and BEBOUT, B. 1950. A study of minor organic deviations in "functional" disorders of articulation: 3. The tongue. *J. Speech Hearing Disorders*, 15, 348–352.

FAIRBANKS, G., and GREEN, E. M. 1950. A study of minor organic deviations in "functional" disorders of articulation: 2. Dimensions and relationships of the lips. *J. Speech Hearing Disorders*, 15, 165–168.

FAIRBANKS, G., and LINTNER, M. V. 1951. A study of minor organic deviations in "functional" disorders of articulation: 4. The teeth and hard palate. *J. Speech Hearing Disorders*, 16, 273–279.

FAIRBANKS, G., and SPRIESTERSBACH, D. C. 1950. A study of minor organic deviations in "functional" disorders of articulation: 1. Rate of movement of oral structures. *J. Speech Hearing Disorders*, 15, 60–69.

FRANCIS, J. T. 1930. A survey of speech defectives of Iowa City, Iowa. Unpublished Master's Thesis. State Univ. Iowa.

FROESCHELS, E. 1933. Speech therapy. Boston: Expression Co.

—— editor. 1948. Twentieth century speech and voice correction. New York: Philosophical Library.

—— and JELLINEK, A. 1941. Practice of voice and speech therapy. Boston: Expression Co.

FYMBO, L. H. 1936. The relation of malocclusion of the teeth to defects of speech. *Arch. Speech*, 1, 204–216.

GILKINSON, H. 1943. The Seashore measures of musical talent and speech skill. *J. appl. Psychol.*, 27, 443–447.

GRAY, G. W., and WISE, C. M. 1946. The bases of speech (rev. ed.). New York: Harper.

HALE, A. R. 1948. A study of the misarticulation of (s) in children from kindergarten through third grade. Unpublished Master's Thesis State Univ. of Iowa.

HALL, M. E. 1938. Auditory factors in functional articulatory speech defects. *J. exp. Educ.*, 7, 110–132.

HANSEN, B. F. 1944. The application of sound discrimination tests to functional articulatory defectives with normal hearing. *J. Speech Disorders*, 9, 347–355.

HENRIKSON, E. H. 1948. An analysis of Wood's articulation index. *J. Speech Hearing Disorders*, 13, 233–235.

HILDRETH, G. 1946. Speech defects and reading disability. *Elem. Sch. J.*, 46, 326–332.

INGRAM, C. P. 1935. Education of the slow-learning child. Yonkers-on-Hudson: World Book.

IRWIN, J. V., and BECKLUND, O. 1953. Norms for maximum repetitive rates for certain sounds established with the sylrater. *J. Speech Hearing Disorders*, 18, 149–160.

IRWIN, O. C. 1947a. Infant speech: The problem. *J. Speech Disorders*, 12, 173–176.

—— 1947b. Infant speech: Variability and the problem of diagnosis. *J. Speech Disorders*, 12, 287–289.

———— 1947c. Infant speech: Consonantal sounds according to place of articulation. *J. Speech Disorders*, 12, 397–401.

———— 1947d. Infant speech: consonant sounds according to manner of articulation. *J. Speech Disorders*, 12, 402–404.

———— 1948a. Infant speech: Development of vowel sounds. *J. Speech Hearing Disorders*, 13, 31–34.

———— 1948b. Infant speech: The effect of family occupational status and of age on use of sound types. *J. Speech Hearing Disorders*, 13, 224–226.

———— 1948c. Infant speech: The effect of family occupational status and of age on sound frequency. *J. Speech Hearing Disorders*, 13, 320–323.

———— 1951. Infant speech: Consonantal position. *J. Speech Hearing Disorders*, 16, 159–161.

———— 1952. Speech development in the young child: 2. Some factors related to the speech development of the infant and young child. *J. Speech Hearing Disorders*, 17, 269–279.

———— and CHEN, H. P. 1943. Speech sound elements during the first year of life: A review of the literature. *J. Speech Disorders*, 8, 109–121.

———— 1945. Infant speech sounds and intelligence. *J. Speech Disorders*, 10, 293–296.

———— 1946. Infant speech: Vowel and consonant frequency. *J. Speech Disorders*, 11, 123–125.

JOHNSON, W., editor. 1950. Speech problems of children. New York: Grune and Stratton.

————, BROWN, S. F., CURTIS, J. F., EDNEY, C. W., and KEASTER, J. 1948. Speech handicapped school children. New York: Harper.

JOHNSON, W., and HOUSE, E. 1937. Certain laterality characteristics of children with articulatory disorders. *Elem. Sch. J.*, 38, 52–58.

JONES, M. V. 1951. The effect of speech training on silent reading achievement. *J. Speech Hearing Disorders*, 16, 258–263.

KARLIN, I. W., and STRAZZULLA, M. 1952. Speech and language problems of mentally deficient children. *J. Speech Hearing Disorders*, 17, 286–294.

KARLIN, I. W., YOUTZ, A. C., and KENNEDY, L. 1940. Distorted speech in young children. *Amer. J. Dis. Child.*, 59, 1203–1218.

KOEPP-BAKER, H. 1936. A handbook of clinical speech. Ann Arbor: Edwards Bros. Vol. 2.

KRONVALL, E. L., and DIEHL, C. F. 1954. The relationship of auditory discrimination to articulatory defects of children with no known organic impairment. *J. Speech Hearing Disorders*, 19, 335–338.

LOUTTIT, C. M., and HALLS, E. C. 1936. Survey of speech defects among public school children of Indiana. *J. Speech Disorders*, 1, 73–80.

LUNDEEN, D. J. 1950. The relationship of diadochokinesis to various speech sounds. *J. Speech Hearing Disorders*, 15, 54–59.

McALLISTER, M. G. 1948. A study of the relationship between defects of articulation in speech and emotional instability in elementary school children. Unpublished Master's Thesis. Univ. of Wash.

McCARTHY, D. A. 1930. The language development of the preschool child. Minneapolis: Univ. of Minn. Press.

McCLURE, H. S. 1952. A study of the existing relationship between articulatory speech defects and related disabilities including reading. Unpublished Master's Thesis. Ball State Teachers College.

McCURRY, W. H., and IRWIN, O. C. 1953. A study of word approximations in the spontaneous speech of infants. *J. Speech Hearing Disorders*, 18, 133–139.

MacLearie, E. C. 1953. The Ohio plan for children with speech and hearin problems. State of Ohio Department of Public Instruction, Columbus.

Major, C. C. 1940. A comparison of the performance of speech defectives an normal speakers on certain motor tests. Unpublished Master's Thesis. Pur due Univ.

Mase, D. J. 1946. Etiology of articulatory speech defects. *Teach. Coll. Contr Educ.*, No. 921. New York: Teachers College. Columbia Univ.

Mason, M. K. 1942. Learning to speak after six and one-half years of silence. *J Speech Disorders*, 7, 295–304.

Maxwell, K. L. 1953. A comparison of certain motor performances of norma and speech defective children, ages seven, eight, and nine years. Unpub lished Ph.D. Thesis. Univ. of Mich.

Metraux, R. W. 1942. Auditory memory span for speech sounds of speech de fective children compared with normal children. *J. Speech Disorders*, 7 33–36.

———— 1944. Auditory memory span for speech sounds: Norms for children *J. Speech Disorders*, 9, 31–38.

———— 1950. Speech profiles of the pre-school child 18 to 54 months. *J. Speec Hearing Disorders*, 15, 37–53.

Milisen, R. 1954. A rationale for articulation disorders. *J. Speech Hearing Dis orders*, Monogr. suppl. 4, 6–17.

Mills, A. C., and Streit, H. 1942. Report of a speech survey, Holyoke, Mass *J. Speech Disorders*, 7, 161–167.

Monroe, M. 1932. Children who cannot read. Chicago: Univ. of Chicago Press

Moore, C. E. A. 1947. Reading and arithmetic abilities associated with speec defects. *J. Speech Disorders*, 12, 85–86.

Morley, D. E. 1952. A ten-year survey of speech disorders among university students. *J. Speech Hearing Disorders*, 17, 25–31.

Moss, M. A. 1938. The effect of speech defects on second-grade reading achieve ment. *Quart. J. Speech*, 24, 642–654.

Mowrer, O. H. 1952. Speech development in the young child: 1. The autism theory of speech development and some clinical applications. *J. Speec Hearing Disorders*, 17, 263–268.

Nelson, J. T. 1945. A study of misarticulation of (s) in combination with se lected vowels and consonants. Unpublished Master's Thesis. State Univ. o Iowa.

Nemoy, E. M., and Davis, S. F. 1937. The correction of defective consonan sounds. Boston: Expression Co.

Ogilvie, M. 1942. Terminology and definitions of speech defects. *Teach. Coll Contr. Educ.*, No. 859. New York: Teachers College, Columbia Univ.

Palmer, M. F., and Osborn, C. D. 1940. A study of tongue pressures of speech defective and normal-speaking individuals. *J. Speech Disorders*, 5, 133–139

Patton, F. E. 1942. A comparison of the kinaesthetic sensibility of speech defective and normal-speaking children. *J. Speech Disorders*, 7, 305–310

Perkins, W. H. 1952. Methods and materials for testing articulation of (s) and (z). *Quart. J. Speech*, 38, 57–62.

Pettit, C. W. 1939. Diadochokinesis of the musculature of the jaw during pu berty and adolescence. Unpublished Master's Thesis. Univ. of Wis.

Poole, I. 1934. Genetic development in articulation of consonant sounds in speech. *Elem. Engl.* 11, 159–161.

Powers, M. H. 1953. Speech correction in the Chicago public schools. *In* "Special Education in the Chicago Public Schools" (rev. ed.). Chicago Board of Education.

REID, G. 1947a. The etiology and nature of functional articulatory defects in elementary school children. *J. Speech Disorders,* 12, 143–150.

———— 1947b. The efficacy of speech re-education of functional articulatory defectives in the elementary school. *J. Speech Disorders,* 12, 301–313.

ROBBINS, S. D. 1942. Importance of sensory training in speech therapy. *J. Speech Disorders,* 7, 183–188.

———— and ROBBINS, R. S. 1937. Correction of speech defects of early childhood. Boston: Expression Co.

ROBINSON, H. M. 1946. Why pupils fail in reading. Chicago: Univ. Chicago Press.

ROE, V., and MILISEN, R. 1942. The effect of maturation upon defective articulation in elementary grades. *J. Speech Disorders,* 7, 37–50.

ROOT, A. R. 1925. A survey of speech defectives in the public elementary schools of South Dakota. *Elem. Sch. J.,* 26, 531–541.

ROSSIGNOL, L. J. 1948. The relationships among hearing acuity, speech production, and reading performance in grades 1A, 1B, 2A. *Teach. Coll. Contr. Educ.,* No. 936. New York: Teachers College, Columbia Univ.

SAUNDERS, M. J. 1931. The short auditory span disability. *Child. Educ.,* 8, 59–65.

SAYLER, H. K. 1949. The effect of maturation upon defective articulation in grades seven through twelve. *J. Speech Hearing Disorders,* 14, 202–207.

SCHLANGER, B. B. 1953. Speech examination of a group of institutionalized mentally handicapped children. *J. Speech Hearing Disorders,* 18, 339–349.

SETH, G., and GUTHRIE, D. 1935. Speech in childhood. Oxford Univ. Press. London: Humphrey Milford.

SIRKIN, J., and LYONS, W. 1941. A study of speech defects in mental deficiency. *Amer. J. ment. Def.,* 46, 74–80.

Speech and hearing problems in the secondary school. 1950. Prepared under the editorial supervision of the American Speech and Hearing Association, S. Ainsworth, Chairman, Editorial Committee. *Bull. Nat. Assn. Secondary Sch. Principals,* 34, 3–139.

SPERLING, S. L. 1948. A comparison between verbal and non-verbal test results of children with articulatory speech defects. Unpublished Master's Thesis. Univ. of Mich.

SPIKER, C. C., and IRWIN, O. C. 1949. The relationship between IQ and indices of infant speech sound development. *J. Speech Hearing Disorders,* 14, 335–343.

SPRIESTERSBACH, D. C., and CURTIS, J. F. 1951. Misarticulation and discrimination of speech sounds. *Quart. J. Speech,* 37, 483–491.

STINCHFIELD, S. M. 1927. Some relationships between speech defects, musical ability, scholastic attainment, and maladjustment. *Quart. J. Speech Educ.,* 13, 268–275.

———— 1928. Speech pathology with methods in speech correction. Boston: Expression Co.

SULLIVAN, E. M. 1944. Auditory acuity and its relation to defective speech. *J. Speech Disorders,* 9, 127–130.

SUMMERS, R. 1953. Perceptive vs. productive skills in analyzing speech sounds from words. *J. Speech Hearing Disorders,* 18, 140–148.

TEMPLIN, M. 1938. A study of aggressiveness in normal and defective speaking college students. *J. Speech Disorders,* 3, 43–49.

———— 1943. A study of sound discrimination ability of elementary school pupils. *J. Speech Disorders,* 8, 127–132.

———— 1952. Speech development in the young child: 3. The development of certain language skills in children. *J. Speech Hearing Disorders,* 17, 280–285.

———— 1953. Norms on a screening test of articulation for ages three through eight. *J. Speech Hearing Disorders,* 18, 323–331.

———— and STEER, M. D. 1939. Studies of growth of speech of pre-school children. *J. Speech Disorders,* 4, 71–77.

TRAVIS, L. E. 1931. Speech pathology. New York: Appleton.

———— and DAVIS, M. G. 1927. The relation between faulty speech and the lack of certain musical talents. *Psychol. Monogr.* 36. 71–81.

TRAVIS, L. E., and RASMUS, B. J. 1931. The speech sound discrimination ability of cases with functional disorders of articulation. *Quart. J. Speech Educ.* 17, 217–226.

VAN RIPER, C. 1938. Persistence of baby talk among children and adults. *Elem. Sch. J.,* 38, 672–675.

———— 1947. Speech correction principles and methods (2nd ed.). New York: Prentice-Hall.

———— 1954. Speech correction principles and methods (3rd ed.). New York: Prentice-Hall.

WELLMAN, B. L., CASE, I. M., MENGERT, I. G., and BRADBURY, D. E. 1931. Speech sounds of young children. Univ. of Iowa Studies in Child Welfare. 5, No. 2.

WEST, R., KENNEDY, L., and CARR, A. 1947. The rehabilitation of speech (rev. ed.). New York: Harper.

White House Conference on Child Health and Protection. Section III. Education and Training. Report of the committee on special classes. The defective in speech. 1931, 349–381. New York: Century.

WILSON, M. J. M. 1952. A comparative study of the defective speech of children found in the rural area of Van Buren County and the urban area of the city of Muskegon. Unpublished Master's Thesis. Mich. State College.

WITTY, P., and KOPEL, D. 1939. Reading and the educative process. Boston: Ginn.

WOOD, K. S. 1946. Parental maladjustment and functional articulatory defects in children. *J. Speech Disorders,* 11, 255–275.

# CHAPTER 24

# CLINICAL AND EDUCATIONAL PROCEDURES IN FUNCTIONAL DISORDERS OF ARTICULATION

*Margaret Hall Powers, Ph.D.*

N THE preceding chapter we were concerned with the more theoretical aspects of functional articulation disorders—their nature and causation. In this chapter we will be concerned with aspects of more practical clinical importance—the diagnosis and evaluation of these disorders and the planning and management of speech therapy. Though symptomatology and etiology have suffered from lack of careful, experimental investigation, diagnosis and therapy are in an even weaker position. Very little controlled research has been done toward establishing either the relevancy or the reliability of various diagnostic procedures or of the relative efficacy of the many therapeutic procedures commonly used. We are still operating largely on a clinical rule-of-thumb basis, though recently there are encouraging signs of awakening interest in articulation research.

The writer does not wish to belittle the value of clinical experience and judgment, especially when offered by competent speech pathologists, but wishes merely to indicate that such judgment needs to be verified by research. It is true that therapy is more difficult to investigate scientifically than etiology, but in principle it can and must be investigated, too, if we are ever to have the assurance that we are managing functional articulation cases in the best way possible.

The present chapter will bring together the opinions and practices of speech pathologists concerning the techniques which are necessary and effective in evaluating a functional articulation case and in reaching a diagnostic conclusion about it, and concerning the therapeutic approaches which have been found most effective in retraining these cases.

## EXAMINATION AND DIAGNOSIS

The examination and diagnosis of any speech case are designed to answer essentially three questions: What kind of person has the speech disorder? What kind of speech disorder does he have? Why does he have it? It is important to answer these questions as a basis for developing finally an appropriate plan of therapy. We do not examine in order to label; we examine in order to understand and retrain.

The examination of functional articulation cases follows the general outline of clinical examination procedures which would be followed for any case. In fact, a case would be diagnosed as having a "functional articulation" disorder only following the completion of such an examination program. (For a detailed description of examination procedures the reader is referred to Ch. 8.) Here a suggested general examination program will be given merely in outline form and only those aspects of it which pertain to functional articulation disorders particularly will be amplified. The following outline organizes the examination procedure around the three questions given above.

## WHAT KIND OF PERSON HAS THE SPEECH DISORDER?

The purpose of this part of the examination is the understanding of the child or adult with whom we are dealing. All too often only lip service has been paid to the accepted doctrine of "understanding the child as a whole." Piecemeal information has been secured without much attempt to integrate it into a meaningful picture of the person. We need such a picture as sound basis upon which to construct an appropriate therapeutic program. We need to see the individual clearly as a person, which means that we must understand his history, the environmental setting in which he lives, his physical, mental, social, emotional, and speech characteristics, his hopes, his anxieties, his motivations, his areas of confidence, his areas of insecurity.

Getting a general picture of the person involves the following major types of investigation and examination.

### The Case History

An account of the individual's past development and present status is obtained from his parents or other responsible adults or from the person himself, in the case of an adult, rather than from testing or direct observation by the examiner. It involves the following principal areas:

1. Family history and present status.
2. Birth and developmental history.
3. Health history and present status.
4. Educational (and occupational) history, present status and plans.
5. Personality, emotional, and social development and present status. Adjustment problems.
6. Interests and recreational activities.
7. History of speech development. History and present status of the specific speech problem.

### Evaluation of Physical Health and Developmental Status

As distinguished from the health information secured in the case history, this part of the study involves an actual physical examination by a physician. When necessary, further and more specialized examinations, such as neurological or otological, should be secured.

### Evaluation of Intellectual Capacity and Academic Achievement

The speech clinician should have available the results of standardized intelligence tests or should be able to refer cases to a qualified psychologist for this type of study. With children handicapped in speech it is necessary to be cautious in interpreting intelligence test results. Even when an articulation problem is not severe enough to interfere with intelligibility, it may still inhibit the child sufficiently so that he fails to make a maximum effort in giving test responses. The intelligence of speech-handicapped children is frequently underestimated on standardized tests. On the other hand, we cannot assume that a child's intelligence is higher than the obtained test result merely because he has a speech problem. It is always advisable to check the results of a "verbal" type of test, like the Stanford-Binet, with a "nonverbal" or "performance" test. A test such as the Wechsler Intelligence Scale for Children (Wechsler, 1949) has the advantage of including both a verbal and a performance scale, each yielding an independent rating. This test can be applied to children from five years of age through adolescence.

With children or adolescents it is advisable also to have available the results of standardized achievement tests in the principal school subjects. These test results are helpful in gaining insight into the nature of the speech problem and its possible relationship to other language functions. From an even more practical standpoint, this appraisal of academic strengths and weaknesses is helpful in planning therapy.

### Evaluation of Personality and Emotional Adjustment

This is one of the most essential parts of the clinical study of a case. The person's emotional characteristics and modes of adjustment frequently have a causal relationship to his speech problem and, in any case, are important to the therapeutic management of the problem.

Personality and adjustment can be studied in a variety of ways. The personal interview with the case is revealing of much information to the observant and psychologically trained clinician. Young children should be observed in a free-play situation, particularly one involving other children. The interaction between the child and his parents as observed in the clinic is usually of considerable clinical interest. Observation of the child in his schoolroom often yields valuable insights. The case should be observed in as wide a variety of situations and with as many different people as is feasible.

There are also various more formal ways of evaluating personal characteristics—the standardized personality schedule, such as the Bernreuter Personality Inventory, and the various projective techniques such as the Rorschach or the Murray Thematic Apperception Test. These require very special training to administer and interpret and under no circumstances should be used without such training. For children the Vineland Social Maturity Scale developed by Doll 1947) gives valuable insight into personal and social adjustment.

When adjustment problems of any seriousness are uncovered, the assistance of a clinical psychologist or a psychiatrist should be sought.

### Evaluation of Speech Behavior as a Whole

All aspects of the individual's speech should be evaluated so that the specific speech disorder under consideration will be seen in realistic perspective. The presence of an articulation problem obviously does not preclude the presence of other deviate speech characteristics as well. The following aspects of speech should be evaluated systematically and if possible under conditions where the individual is conversing naturally and unaware of being "tested." Observations can be made with the greatest objectivity and accuracy if the clinician considers only one aspect of speech at a time and each aspect independently of the others.

1. Fluency of Self-Expression in Speech. Output of speech, ease in formulating and expressing ideas.
2. Intelligibility. The degree to which the speech can be understood.
3. Vocabulary. Extent of vocabulary in relation to age. Accuracy of word usage.
4. Level of Language Organization in Relation to Age. Use of single words, phrases, sentences. Length of sentences. Complexity of sentences. Use of various parts of speech. Use of various tenses.
5. Grammar and Pronunciation.
6. Foreign or Regional Dialect.
7. Articulation. (See below for detailed examination procedure.)
8. Voice. Pitch, loudness, or quality deviations. Inflectional patterns.
9. Rate. Habitual use of too slow or too rapid speech.
10. Rhythm. Hesitancy, stuttering.
11. Visible Accompaniments of Speech. Facial expression and gestural patterns. Bodily tension or relaxation. Posture.
12. Emotional Reactions Accompanying Speech.
13. Evaluative Reactions to Speaking and Listening.

In a large speech clinic, various individuals may be involved in the study of the case, each assuming responsibility for specific parts of the examination. In some clinics, for example, a social worker is available for case-history taking, a physician to secure the medical history and give the physical examination, and a clinical psychologist to administer psychological tests and to make the evaluation of personality and adjustment. More commonly the speech pathologist works alone and merely utilizes reports sent him by other specialists who are not actually part of the clinic organization. The necessity for seeking the collaboration of other professional persons in obtaining the general picture of the case will be determined by the training of the clinician making the examination. The ethical speech pathologist will not attempt to perform the parts of the examination which must be done by a physician or a clinical psychologist unless he has had these additional types of training.

## WHAT KIND OF SPEECH DISORDER DOES THE PERSON HAVE?

This part of the diagnostic examination is concerned with determining the dimensions and characteristics of the speech disorder itself. Here we narrow down our focus of attention from the child or adult as a total personality to an analysis of his specific speech deviation. Since this chapter deals with functional articulation disorders, we are concerned here with procedures for studying only this type of problem.

In analyzing articulation it is convenient to make these types of examination: (1) a systematic phonetic inventory of the speech; (2) an appraisal of the relative severity and consistency of misarticulation under different speaking conditions; and (3) an estimate of the ease with which the misarticulations yield to remedial procedures.

## The Phonetic Inventory

The specific procedures and materials used will depend upon the purpose to be served, the time available, and the age and reading ability of the case. If only a rough estimate of articulation is desired, as in a general survey or in the incidental articulatory evaluation of cases with other types of speech disorders, it will suffice to test the articulation of only the sounds most frequently defective: [s], [z], [ʃ], [ʒ], [tʃ], [dʒ], [ʍ], [θ], [ð], [r,] [l]. For young children, [f], [v], [k], and [g] should also be included.

In making the usual diagnostic study of a case, however, a more systematic and thorough phonetic inventory is desirable. A detailed analysis of misarticulations is useful as an aid in diagnosis and, even more importantly, as a basis for planning therapy. The vowels, diphthongs, consonants, and consonant blends listed below should be tested. The list of consonant blends includes only those which occur most frequently in speech or which are most likely to be defective. A key word is given for each sound.

VOWELS

| | | | | | |
|---|---|---|---|---|---|
| | [i] | (feet) | | [ʌ] | (cup) |
| | [ɪ] | (fish) | | [ɑ] | (father) |
| | [ɛ] | (bed) | | [ɔ] | (ball) |
| | [æ] | (hat) | | [ʊ] | (book) |
| | [ɝ] | (bird) | | [u] | (school) |

DIPTHONGS

| | | | | | |
|---|---|---|---|---|---|
| | [eɪ] | (play) | | [oʊ] | (snow) |
| | [ɑɪ] | (pie) | | [ɔɪ] | (boy) |
| | [ɑʊ] | (cow) | | [ju] | (use) |

CONSONANTS

| | | | | | |
|---|---|---|---|---|---|
| | [p] | (pencil) | | [s] | (soap) |
| | [b] | (baby) | | [z] | (zipper) |
| | [m] | (man) | | [ʃ] | (shoe) |
| | [w] | (window) | | [ʒ] | (television) |
| | [ʍ] | (wheel) | | [tʃ] | (chair) |
| | [f] | (fork) | | [dʒ] | (jump) |
| | [v] | (vegetables) | | [r] | (rabbit) |
| | [θ] | (thumb) | | [l] | (leaf) |
| | [ð] | (mother) | | [j] | (yellow) |
| | [t] | (table) | | [k] | (cat) |
| | [d] | (dog) | | [g] | (gun) |
| | [n] | (nest) | | [ŋ] | (ring) |
| | | | | [h] | (house) |

COMMON CONSONANT BLENDS

| With [s] = | [sk-] | (skate) | With [r]: | [br-] | (bread) |
|---|---|---|---|---|---|
| | [skr-] | (scratch) | | [dr-] | (dress) |
| | [skw-] | (squirrel) | | [fr-] | (frog) |
| | [sl-] | (sled) | | [gr-] | (green) |
| | [sm-] | (smoke) | | [kr] | (cry) |
| | [sn-] | (snake) | | [pr-] | (pray) |
| | [sp-] | (spoon) | | [ʃr-] | (shrub) |
| | [spl-] | (splash) | | [tr-] | (tree) |
| | [spr-] | (spring) | | [θr-] | (three) |
| | [str-] | (street) | | [-rd] | (heard) |
| | [st-] | (stove) | | [-rk] | (fork) |
| | [sw-] | (swing) | | [-rn] | (corn) |
| | [-ks] | (box) | | [-rt] | (heart) |
| | [-ns] | (fence) | | | |
| | [-ps] | (cups) | | | |
| | [-ts] | (hats) | | | |

| With [l] = | [bl-] | (blue) | With [w]: | [dw-] | (dwarf) |
|---|---|---|---|---|---|
| | [fl-] | (fly) | | [kw-] | (queen) |
| | [gl-] | (glove) | | [tw-] | (twins) |
| | [kl-] | (clock) | | | |
| | [pl-] | (play) | Miscellaneous | [-nd] | (end) |
| | [-ld] | (cold) | Final Blends: | [-nt] | (tent) |
| | [-lk] | (milk) | | [-nz] | (pins) |
| | [-lt] | (salt) | | [-ŋk] | (ink) |
| | [-lz] | (dolls) | | [-ŋz] | (rings) |

The consonants should be tested in initial, medial, and final positions in words, with the exception of those consonants which do not occur in all positions.

For adult readers, excellent test sentences for vowels, diphthongs, and single consonants will be found in Fairbanks (1940, pp. xii–xv). Supplementary sentences to test the common consonant blends will be found in Johnson, Darley, and Spriestersbach (1952, p. 24). These two publications also give good test sentences for less mature readers. In addition, Schoolfield (1951, pp. 2–5) gives unusually well prepared test sentences in large type for the primary reader. Other lists of test sentences for both adult and younger readers will be found in many of the standard texts in speech pathology. Among these Van Riper (1954, pp. 176–179) is particularly noteworthy.

For children who have not yet learned to read, or read very little, and for older children or adults who have difficulty with reading, picture or object tests of articulation should be used. Bryngelson and Glaspey (1951) have published a set of test pictures for rapid testing of young children. The set includes only the consonants and consonant blends most frequently misarticulated and thus does not provide a complete phonetic inventory. A brief but clear picture test for initial consonants, as well as reading tests of articulation at two difficulty levels, are given in Anderson (1953, pp. 51–61)

There are various commercial picture articulation tests available, none very satisfactory in this writer's opinion. The speech clinician himself can with care devise very satisfactory picture, object, or reading tests of articulation for the various age levels. "Tongue twisters" should be avoided and vocabulary selected which is appropriate in difficulty and interest to the age level with which the test will be used.

Each speech clinician will want to develop an articulation test blank for his own clinic or school program. Perhaps the most convenient arrangement of such a blank provides for a list of sounds to be tested in a column down the left side of the blank, with three lines to the right of each sound, on which to record misarticulations in initial, medial, and final positions. It would appear, in part, somewhat as follows:

| Sound | Initial | Medial | Final | Response to stimulation |
|-------|---------|--------|-------|-------------------------|
| [p] | ———— | ———— | ———— | ———————— |
| [b] | ———— | ———— | ———— | ———————— |
| [m] | ———— | ———— | ———— | ———————— |

Other useful arrangements for recording will be found in Johnson, Darley, and Spriestersbach (1952, p. 25), Fairbanks (1940, p. xi), and Milisen (1954, p. 13). For convenience in recording, the list of sounds should be arranged in the same order as that followed in the articulation tests to be used. Misarticulations should be recorded as accurately as possible. For substitutions the phonetic symbol of the substituted sound should be recorded, for distortions and omissions some consistent symbol, such as ($\sqrt{}$) for distortions or (O) for omissions, can be used. A particularly thorough plan for articulation-testing is described by Milisen (1954, p. 12–17). His system for recording errors is more detailed than that just described and well worth consideration.

In making this detailed analysis of articulation, the examiner will achieve most accurate results if he listens for only one sound at a time, temporarily disregarding others. The test material should be such that the child will be encouraged to say the test words spontaneously. If he fails to recognize a picture or printed word readily and time would be wasted in trying to elicit it, it should be supplied by the examiner. Research on the importance of this point is contradictory.

Templin (1947a) found that in articulation-testing of young children similar results are obtained when pictures are named spontaneously as when their names are repeated after the examiner. Snow and Milisen (1954a), however, found that children in both the primary and upper grades gave better responses to oral tests than to picture or reading tests. They concluded, therefore, that in articulation-testing a picture test is preferable in order to avoid influencing the child's response. Snow and Milisen further reported (1954b) that the difference in a child's response to a picture as compared with an oral test may be a valuable prognostic clue. In their study, the sounds made better in response to the oral than to the picture test showed most spontaneous improvement over a six-month period.

Upon initial examination of a case it is highly desirable to make a recording of the individual's speech, sampling both conversational speech and the more systematic responses given on the articulation test. Periodic recordings provide a more objective and accurate record than even the best written record. Recordings do much to eliminate evaluations of changes in articulation due to examiner unreliability instead of to actual growth in articulatory skill. They are therefore useful to the clinician in evaluating progress with therapy and to the case himself as a motivational device.

Wright (1954), studying examiner reliability in articulation-testing, reports that agreement was greater from one tape recording to another than from the live testing situation to a tape-recording of it. This was true both for comparisons of each examiner with himself and also for comparisons between different examiners.

Various attempts have been made to construct an articulation test which would yield a quantitative measure of articulation skill. Other investigators have experimented with methods of scoring articulation—other than a simple count of sounds correct—which would give a measure indicative of the *degree* of communicative handicap.

Templin (1947b and 1953) developed two screening tests for young children, one involving 40 single words, the other, 19 sentences, both containing the 50 sounds shown by research to be most discriminative of articulation growth. The tests can be used interchangeably and the score on either is the number of the 50 sounds correctly articulated. Age norms for the word test have been developed for ages three through eight.

Wood (1946 and 1949) has described an *articulation index* which takes into consideration the relative frequency with which the different speech sounds occur in speech and the different positions in which they occur in words. He developed an inventory of 70 consonant sounds, counting each of the positions of the 25 consonants (phonetic alphabet) as a separate sound. Five of the consonants occur in only two positions; the remainder occur in three positions. Each consonant was given a weighting, in relation to its frequency of occurrence as established by Travis (1931, p. 223). The weighting for each consonant was prorated among the three (or two) positions in which it occurs. The total of all weightings is 100. The *articulation index* is obtained by subtracting from 100 the weight of each sound misarticulated. The index takes into consideration the obvious fact that all sounds do not have equal value but that misarticulation of frequently occurring sounds is more of a handicap than misarticulation of sounds which occur but rarely.

Henrikson (1948) has objected to Wood's prorating of each consonant's weight equally among the positions, on the ground that sounds do not occur with equal positional frequency. Wood, however, has defended this technique as the only one feasible and has pointed out that position in words is relatively meaningless anyway in connected speech.

Pettit (1952) evolved an extension of Wood's technique, securing an articulation index at each of five levels of articulatory difficulty, yielding a maximum score for perfect articulation of 504.15 and permitting articulatory differences to be more finely differentiated.

More recently Snow and Milisen (1954b) have derived an articulation score based upon assigning a value of 1.0 to 5.0 to each speech sound in each position. A value of 1.0 indicates correct articulation, 2.0 a mildly distorted sound, 3.0 a severely distorted sound, 4.0 a substitution, and 5.0 an omission. The articulation score is the mean of these rank order values for all sounds in all positions.

An attempt of a very different type to develop an objective measure of articulation skill, which would permit repeated measurements, has been described by Curry, Kennedy, Wagner, and Wilke (1943). They developed a phonographic scale for measuring defective articulation. An individual's articulation can be compared with eight graded samples of speech, varying from nearly unintelligible to normal, as recorded on a phonograph record. Scale steps were computed on the basis of judgements of the recorded samples by observers.

It is to be hoped that further investigations will be made along the line of objectifying and measuring articulation. A valid, reliable, standardized, quantitative index of articulation would be extremely valuable, both for research purposes—so that articulation data could be handled statistically and have a uniform meaning throughout the country—and for the clinical measurement of progress with speech therapy.

### Severity and Consistency of Misarticulation

Helpful insight can be gained into the stage of articulatory development, the causation of the problem, and the prognosis for improvement by observing the individual's articulation under different speaking conditions. Observe his articulation in the following speaking contexts:

**Off-guard, conversational speech.** Listen to the child or adult when he is talking freely, unaware that his speech is under observation. This can be done best at the beginning of the diagnostic examination before the more formal tests have made him conscious of his speech. Engage the adult, adolescent, or older child in friendly conversation about topics which interest him. Enter into a play situation with the younger child or, better still, observe him at play with others. Notice his speech as he talks with his parents or siblings. Observe each case also, if possible, in a stress situation, as well as in a pleasant, relaxed situation.

The objective in this observation is to get the "feel" of the problem, to evaluate the person's intelligibility under normal speaking conditions, to evaluate the conspicuousnes of the defect, and the degree to which it is a communication handicap. A distinction must be made between *intelligibility* and *conspicuousness* of defect. Unintelligible speech will always be conspicuous but the converse may not be true. For example, a lateral lisp is usually very conspicuous but seldom interferes much with intelligibility.

Intelligibility can be roughly graded from one extreme to the other as follows: speech easily and completely understood, speech understandable except for some words, speech understandable only when the topic is known to the listener, speech unintelligible even to members of the family.

**Oral reading.** Have the person read continuous material which is well within his reading level and offers no problem in word recognition. Does the response to visual symbols and the higher level of awareness produce any improvement in articulation over the conversational speech situation?

**Repetition of learned series.** Have the person count, name the days of the week, the months of the year, or recite a well-known nursery rhyme or poem. Is articulation the same or better than in the preceding situation? Have the person try the above series again with a deliberate attempt this time to speak as carefully as possible. Is there any improvement?

When the person is able to control his articulation to some extent, it indicates often that he is in a transitional phase in learning the sound, either through maturation or through training, and that the outlook is good for eventual habituation of the correct pattern.

**Articulation test.** The systematic phonetic inventory was described in the preceding section. Articulation in word-by-word speech may differ considerably from articulation in the connected speech of the conversational situation. Any differences should be identified and evaluated.

The consistency of the individual's misarticulations should be carefully noted. Some individuals will show the same articulatory errors in all situations—from the most off-guard to those in which they are trying to articulate carefully—and will show them with all the people to whom they speak and in all phonetic contexts. Other cases will show some variation; others much variation. Variations in misarticulation in relation to the person to whom the case is speaking may be important. Some children speak better or less well to their parents than to others; some speak better to one parent than to the other. Twins or siblings close together in age, in speaking to each other often use speech which is more or less unintelligible to others, but in speaking to adults use a considerably better level of articulation. Articulation cases also commonly vary considerably in articulatory adequacy in relation to their emotional state.

All of these variations and inconsistencies give valuable clues to the factors which may have contributed to the problem and indicate points to consider in planning therapy. When a case shows marked inconsistency of misarticulation in relation to phonetic context, more extensive articulatory testing should be done. The defective consonant should be tested in a number of words, to discover the specific phonetic contexts in which it is misarticulated. Retraining should then be based upon words containing that phonetic composition and not wasted in the use of words which the person can utter correctly.

### Response to Auditory Stimulation

When the phonetic inventory has been completed, the clinician will gain much helpful information by going back over the defective sounds and testing the individual's ability to produce correctly by imitation first the isolated sounds and then the sounds in words. The child should be able to both see and hear the examiner clearly while this test is given. The responses can be recorded in the fourth column of the blank described earlier. Milisen (1945 and 1954) suggests an even more elaborate testing and recording of what he terms the sound's "stimulatability" by having the child respond to the stimulus of the sound in isolation and then successively in initial, medial, and final positions in nonsense syllables and then in initial medial, and final positions in words.

When the individual can correct his misarticulations fairly readily in response to stimulation from the examiner, it suggests, for one thing, that organic factors—structural, motor, or sensory—are probably not contributing importantly to the problem. Diagnostic light is shed on the articulation problem and a prognosis as to the probable response to speech therapy is aided.

The relative ease with which the case can produce his various defective sounds by imitation will also be indicative of a good place at which to begin articulatory retraining. Other factors being equal, it is profitable to begin training with the sounds which the individual can correct most easily. A trial of the person's response to retraining, therefore, is well worth making from a diagnostic, a prognostic, and a therapeutic point of view.

## WHY DOES THE PERSON HAVE THE ARTICULATION DISORDER?

All of the examination procedures already described contribute to the eventual attempt to explain the "why" of the specific problem under consideration. The study of the various facets of the individual's personality and the detailed examination of his speech, as described in the preceding sections, will have led the clinician to tentative conclusions as to the factors which have produced the articulation disorder. Certain specific etiological possibilities will have to be investigated further, however, always with the double purpose of explaining the problem and of getting clues as to how it can best be approached remedially.

In the preceding chapter the various etiological possibilities were reviewed and the conclusion was reached that there is no factor which is always associated with functional articulation problems. However, until future research conclusively rules out some of these factors, it is expedient to explore them. Any one or combination of them *may* be present in a case we are examining.

Examination procedures are for the most part common to the diagnostic study of all types of speech disorders. (These are described adequately in

Ch. 8.) Only a few supplementary techniques which are of special significance for functional articulation cases will be described more fully here. (Refer to Ch. 8 for procedures for examining the structure of the oral mechanism, motor co-ordination in general, motor co-ordination within the speech mechanism, diadochokinesis, laterality, auditory acuity, and discrimination. The reader is also referred to the excellent diagnostic manual by Johnson, Darley, and Spriestersbach (1952) for examination techniques and record forms.)

### Diadochokinetic Rate

As indicated in the preceding chapter, tests of motor speed and dexterity have shown no consistent relationship to functional articulation disorders. Individual cases, however, may have a deficiency in motor co-ordination, so it is important to rule in or rule out this factor in making a diagnostic examination. As concluded in Chapter 23, the tests which have seemed most promising, among the many tried, are those in which movements of the speech mechanism itself, during a speech act, have been utilized.

Irwin and Becklund (1953, pp. 156–157) give tentative age norms, for ages six through fifteen years, and for boys and girls separately, on the number of repetitions per second of [pə], [tə], and [kə], as well as for hand-tapping.

**Irwin and Becklund's Data on Number of Repetitions in One Second\***

| Age | [pə] Girls | Boys | [tə] Girls | Boys | [kə] Girls | Boys |
|---|---|---|---|---|---|---|
| 6 | 3.67 | 3.49 | 3.51 | 3.33 | 3.28 | 3.18 |
| 7 | 4.38 | 4.34 | 4.33 | 4.14 | 3.88 | 4.02 |
| 9 | 4.40 | 4.56 | 4.32 | 4.49 | 3.94 | 4.19 |
| 11 | 4.88 | 4.80 | 4.84 | 4.75 | 4.46 | 4.52 |
| 13 | 5.44 | 5.17 | 5.22 | 5.09 | 4.76 | 4.84 |
| 15 | 5.44 | 5.86 | 5.38 | 5.77 | 5.00 | 5.27 |

\* These figures are the mean number of repetitions of the syllable in one second. Their table also gives the standard deviation of each mean.

Maxwell (1953) found that, of a number of motor tests used to compare articulatory-defective and normal-speaking boys, repetition of [lɑ] and of [pɑtɑkɑ], of the tests involving the speech mechanism, distinguished best between the two groups. These two tests also showed the most consistent increase with age for the control group.

**Maxwell's Data on Number of Repetitions in Two Seconds**

| Age | [la] | [pataka] |
|---|---|---|
| 7 | 11.77 | 9.23 |
| 8 | 13.08 | 9.69 |
| 9 | 13.54 | 10.62 |

## Speech-Sound Discrimination

Although the research reviewed in Chapter 23 on speech-sound discrimination leads to the conclusion that functional articulation cases have no generalized deficiency in this ability, there always remains the possibility that any specific articulation case may have such a deficiency. The individual's speech-sound discrimination ability should, therefore, be tested. The clinician can make up his own informal test by presenting a series of paired nonsense syllables, in some of which pairs the syllables are alike, in some different. Easily confused consonants should be paired, keeping the vowel constant within one pair.

A convenient and carefully constructed 70-item test has been developed by Templin (1943), which includes only the consonant elements shown to be most discriminative. Norms are given for grades two through six, but the test could be used with older cases as well. Templin's test has also been reproduced in Van Riper (1954, pp. 198–199), who gives norms of his own for it, and in Irwin (1953, p. 206).

Pronovost and Dumbleton (1953) have published a report of a picture test of speech-sound discrimination suitable for young children. For each test item, the child is confronted with three pairs of pictures involving only two different words, a "like" pair for one word, a "like" pair for the other word, and an "unlike" pair depicting both words. The child points to the pair of pictures which he thinks the examiner has named. Test data were gathered on first-grade children. The authors consider the test a useful diagnostic instrument.

Informal exploratory testing of speech sound discrimination should also be done, centered particularly around the sounds which are defective in the person's own speech. As Spriestersbach and Curtis have reported (1951), there tends to be a relationship between a person's discrimination errors and his articulation errors. The extent of the person's discrimination of sounds defective in his own speech should be explored specifically.

For example, have the person turn his back or close his eyes. Present him with two, three, or four (depending on age) repetitions of the same word. Make an error in one of them and have him identify the order in which the incorrect word occurred. Present a series of words in this manner, the position of the incorrect stimulus being varied at random. The error made by the clinician should simulate the person's own error on that sound. If the case has difficulty, for example, with [s], present a series of s-words, the sound occurring in various positions in the different words. If several sounds are defective, more extensive testing of this sort will be necessary.

It is also helpful to test the person's ability to identify his own speech errors with an external stimulus. Have him read a word or name a picture. Immediately after, say the same word to him twice, once correctly and once with an imitation of his error. Ask him which of your repetitions was like his. Try this with a number of words containing his defective sounds.

Some of the techniques to be described later for training in auditory discrimination can be used on a trial basis in the diagnostic examination to permit still further observations of the individual's present level of skill and his capacity for developing skill.

Van Riper (1954, pp. 195–196) describes and gives rough norms for a "Vocal Phonics Test" used in his clinic to test an individual's ability to identify a word from its separate phonetic components given at the rate of one per second by the examiner. He has found that individuals who have difficulty in thus synthesizing sounds tend to have difficulty also in analyzing words into their component sounds.

### Auditory Memory Span

Auditory memory span also fails to show a consistent relationship to functional articulation disorders but may be a factor in a few cases. There are standardized memory-span tests available using digits, nonsense syllables, vowel sounds, consonant sounds, or nonsense words. Anderson (1939) experimented with digits, vowels, and consonants but found vowel sounds to be the most suitable material for testing auditory memory span. His vowel test is reproduced also in Berry and Eisenson (1942, p. 411).

Metraux (1944) used adaptions of Anderson's tests and published norms for vowel and for consonant tests. Van Riper (1954, p. 197) gathers together the norms given by various authors, including Metraux.

### DIAGNOSTIC AND PROGNOSTIC EVALUATION

A final conclusion as to the nature and cause of a speech disorder is not always possible at the time of the diagnostic examination. Sometimes only trial speech therapy reveals the true extent of the problem and the factors which have been responsible for it. However, the sooner a reliable diagnosis can be reached the less will time be wasted in procedures which may be inappropriate, and the more quickly and dependably can a constructive therapeutic program be initiated. The desirability of an early diagnostic conclusion about a case, however, should never preclude the modification of this conclusion by new insights gained through therapy.

To reiterate a statement made in Chapter 23, a diagnosis of "functional" should be made on the basis of the factors operating at the time of the diagnostic examination. A genuine understanding of the nature of the problem, however, will be reached only by careful study of factors—organic or functional—operative in the past as well as in the present. It is easy to be misled by the presence of a major organic factor—such, for example, as a cleft palate—into assuming that the speech characteristics which we note are due to that factor. They may or may not be, or they may be only in part. The mere presence of a factor does not mean that it necessarily has a causal relationship to the speech disorder. This needs to be carefully evaluated in each case.

We cannot stress enough the desirability of thinking in terms of a *causal pattern* rather than a *cause*. The careful clinician evaluates systematically the factors in all of the etiological areas—structural, motor, sensory, developmental, health, intellectual, learning, environmental, emotional—before trying to identify the particular ones which, in combination, have produced the problem as we see it now. The diagnostic pieces should be integrated into a meaningful whole. The outcome of the diagnostic procedures should be a unified picture of the person and his speech problem.

It is clinically useful to attempt to make a prognosis—an estimate of probable outcome—for each case we examine. We should evaluate the extent to which the speech disorder can probably be remedied and the future conditions which will have a bearing on its correction. We should also attempt a conservative estimate as to the amount of time which the treatment of the problem will require.

The speech clinician should be extremely cautious in discussing the outcome of therapy with the case himself or with his parents. Pettit (1952) has shown that—at least with young children—the types of tests now used to predict articulatory development are of doubtful value. Pettit studied an unselected group of five-year-olds. Somewhat greater predictability for articulatory defectives might logically be expected. However, the relative crudeness of present diagnostic techniques and the many variables which enter into a successful therapeutic outcome preclude the placing of a definite time limit on speech therapy. At the same time, the person who is entering upon speech therapy wants and should have some idea of how long it will probably take—a month, a year, five years. The clinician should be prepared to discuss, at least in general terms, the speech outcome to be expected and indicate at the same time the factors which will tend to hasten or retard speech improvement.

For his own private benefit the speech clinician can afford to be less cautious. Excellent professional discipline and important clinical learning are gained by writing down, for oneself or one's colleagues only, a careful estimate of the final speech outcome and an estimate of the amount of therapy which will be required to reach that outcome. Later comparison of the actual progress of the case with the prognosis made adds to and refines clinical experience immeasurably.

Let us assume that the clinician has attempted to answer the three questions suggested at the beginning of this chapter, concerning the kind of person, the kind of problem, and the why of the problem, and has reached a diagnostic conclusion about the case. The clinician will find useful, as a basis for planning therapy, a final summary evaluation of the degree of communication handicap presently experienced by the individual and the probable outcome of the speech disorder with therapy.

**Degree of Communication Handicap**

The extent to which the individual's functional articulation disorder constitutes a handicap for *him* specifically will be related to:

His degree of intelligibility.

The number of different sounds defective in his speech.

The specific sounds which are defective—frequency of their occurrence in speech.

The age of the individual.

The general speech standards prevailing in the individual's environment.

The importance of good speech for the individual's personal career or social needs.

The attitudes of family and friends, the significance they attach to his speech disorder, and

The individual's self-attitudes, and, specifically, his attitudes about his own speech.

**Expected Outcome of Speech Therapy**

The clinician will have to weigh a number of factors in estimating the success which speech therapy can be expected to have and the probable length of time it will have to continue. These factors are closely related to some of the factors which determine the present degree of communication handicap. The following should be considered in functional articulation cases:

Severity of the speech disorder, number of sounds defective, and the nature of the misarticulations. In general, the greater the number of defective sounds the greater the evidence of improvement per unit of therapeutic time, but the longer the total amount of therapy required.

Intelligence of the individual.

Auditory alertness and ability to imitate speech sounds.

Age of the individual. Other factors being equal, the younger the person, the more easily can his misarticulation usually be corrected.

Frequency with which therapy sessions can be given.

Impeding physical factors such as poor health or low vitality.

Impeding personality or emotional characteristics.

Degree and quality of co-operation to be expected from family, teachers, and associates.

The individual's own motivation for speech improvement.

## SPEECH THERAPY FOR FUNCTIONAL ARTICULATION DISORDERS

Therapy has even less research evidence to support it than other aspects of speech pathology. Articulation therapy at present is a synthesis of techniques taken over from the speech arts, education, and psychotherapy—with relative emphasis on one or the other of these fields depending upon each therapist's personal background and bias—and modified by the accumulated experience of many therapists in working with speech-handicapped individuals. An attempt has been made in the pages which follow to bring together the points of view and the practices concerning articulation therapy which have common acceptance. Notable divergences in viewpoint are indicated in some cases. It cannot be urged too strongly that the statements made in the remainder of this chapter be thought of as tentative formulations, awaiting verification or modification by research. Nearly every principle of articulation therapy offered—from the mechanical aspects of therapy structuring to the selection of therapeutic methods—should make a profitable subject for future research investigation.

## General Considerations in Planning Speech Therapy

The organization of the therapeutic program for a case follows logically from the diagnostic evaluation. Within the causal pattern which has been identified, the clinician will want first to distinguish between those causal factors which he can hope to affect or eliminate and those which he cannot. He will have to minimize or compensate for the latter or at worst accept them and work around them. The therapeutic program should be concerned mainly with the causal factors which *can* be eliminated or modified. For example, if low physical vitality is contributing to a child's articulatory retardation, obviously efforts should be made at the outset to reduce this factor by advising medical care. If parental attitudes are contributing to the problem—as is so often the case—immediate measures should be instituted in the direction of parental guidance or, if necessary and possible, psychotherapy. A first step, then, in therapy is the evaluation and management of the various factors thought to be contributing to the speech problem.

A clinical plan should be developed for each case. This plan should encompass, first, a statement of long-term objectives; second, a general outline of the clinical procedure to be followed; and, third, a listing of the immediate steps to be taken. It is worth while to state final objectives explicitly because they are the goals at which therapy will be directed. They should include the specific speech objectives to be reached and objectives in areas other than speech, such as personal adjustment, improved health, or improved academic progress. The final objectives represent the balanced, multi-sided approach to therapy which is necessary to a successful outcome.

The outline of clinical procedure will indicate the kind of approach to be followed with the case, the sequence of therapeutic stages to be presented, what problems or aspects of the problem will be worked on first, next, last. Part of this procedural plan with an articulation case would be a decision as to which of his defective sounds should be corrected first and which should be deferred until later. In this ordering of sounds the clinician should take into consideration the possibility of further modification of some of them by maturation and environmental stimulation alone.

If only one sound is defective there is no problem of selection. If a number of sounds are defective, it is usually advisable to work with only one at a time. The following considerations should determine the best sound with which to begin: (1) the most defective or conspicuously handicapping sound, (2) the one which occurs most frequently in speech, (3) the one which the individual produces most readily with stimulation. With younger children, the developmental order of sounds should also be considered. When working with groups of cases, as in public school programs, practical considerations of grouping may also have to enter sometimes into the selection of the sound to be corrected. When the first sound has been brought to the point of voluntary mastery and partial carry-over into conversational speech, work with a second sound can be started. The same criteria apply to the selection of a second sound as to the selection of the first.

The procedural plan should include the general methodology to be followed, the consideration of group or individual therapy or a combination of both, the frequency of therapeutic sessions, the types of therapeutic activity which will be used.

The third aspect of therapeutic planning is the decision as to where to begin and how to begin—the planning of the first therapy sessions. Detailed planning cannot be done far ahead because of the need for flexibility and constant modification of methods in relation to the individual's response and his progress in speech. Therapeutic sessions should, though, be planned in advance and not left to the ingenuity of the moment. One of the therapist's first decisions will concern the possibility of plunging directly into speech work or the desirability of using a more indirect, unobtrusive approach. With shy, withdrawn children a period of play-therapy types of activity may be necessary before the child achieves sufficient confidence and responsiveness to profit by direct speech training. In all cases, however responsive, some attention needs to be given initially to establishing rapport and securing the child's understanding of and motivation for the speech-training which is being undertaken.

### The Structuring of Articulatory Training

Such considerations as frequency, length, and spacing of therapeutic sessions, the use of group therapy, individual therapy, or a combination of both, and the size and composition of therapy groups are determined to a considerable extent by circumstances. Clinical judgment, unfortunately, cannot dictate the structuring of therapy as much as would be desirable. Structuring is very likely to be determined by the type of organizational setting—public school, clinic, private practice—within which the therapy is carried out, and by time, space, and staff limitations. To the greatest extent possible, however, certain principles should guide the structuring of therapy. Experimental research so far has had little to contribute to these. They are, rather, the result of the accumulated clinical experience of many therapists.

**Arrangement of therapy sessions.** For children below the age of eight, therapy sessions should probably not exceed half an hour. Longer sessions are effective only if the type of activity is varied considerably after the first half hour. Older children can usually work effectively at one type of task for forty minutes or more. Even adults should probably not be expected to give close attention or sustained effort for longer than an hour at a time.

Daily therapy sessions would be ideal for most articulation cases, provided that the individual's regular program of work or study was not too seriously disrupted. Daily sessions are seldom possible, however, and very satisfactory progress can be made with two or three sessions a week. Sessions should be spaced by at least a day or two so that the interval at no time in the week will exceed four days. Longer intervals are less efficient because gains are lost in part through the forgetting which takes place, and interest and motivation are harder to maintain. Much good work has been done by skillful therapists, however, on a once-a-week basis.

**Group and individual sessions.** The optimum program for most articulation cases below the adult level would provide for a combination of group and individual procedures. Groups should probably not exceed six children and are preferable with only three or four. For effective group interaction the age range within one group should not usually exceed three years, though comparable intellectual and social maturity are more significant than chronological age. In group work the desire of children to communicate through speech, the amount and variety of material they have to communicate, and their motivation to improve in speech are all more easily secured than in working with one child alone. Children stimulate each other, so that even a therapist of modest ability has little difficulty in developing keen interest in speech activities. Group therapy provides a natural situation for speech practice and carry-over of newly learned speech habits.

On the other hand, individual sessions with the therapist are preferable for some cases when their speech problems are so unique that they would profit little from the type of training provided for other children. For example, many speech therapists find that cases with lateral lisps, unless they can be grouped with other lateral lispers, can be handled best alone, rather than with lispers of other types. Even with children who are being handled effectively in a group, there should be some opportunity for occasional individual sessions. Children learn at different rates and the child who makes conspicuously slower progress than other members of the group should have additional help by himself. The therapist's schedule should be flexible enough to permit this individual supplementation of group work.

Another problem in planning therapy is the relative desirability of homogeneous or heterogenous grouping of cases for speech therapy. A few speech therapists, notably Backus and Beasley (1951, p. 43), advocate the inclusion of cases of various types within one group, even cases as different as articulation, cleft-palate, and stuttering. In expressing this view they explicitly reject what they regard as the older practice of grouping cases by type of disorder on the assumption "that there is a different type of therapy for each type of disorder." They protest against what they evidently regard as the general assumption of workers in speech therapy that all cases with one type of disorder are exactly alike and have identical needs. They attack also what they consider a common practice, drilling on specific speech habits out of the context of actual communicative needs and an ignoring of interpersonal relations as related to speech behavior.

This assumption of a clinical naiveté and rigidity in speech pathologists in general—hardly justified by the views many of them have expressed through their publications—has tended to confuse the issue of how speech therapy should be structured. This writer knows of no competent speech pathologist today who has not concerned himself constantly with the interpersonal relations of his cases. It has been the common practice for years to deal with all aspects of the speech-handicapped person's adjustment and to relate his specific learning in speech to his speech behavior in general.

Most clinicians have apparently experienced no difficulty in furthering these objectives and still working with homogenous rather than heterogeneous groups. Most clinicians, too, while recognizing the many overlapping needs of speech cases of all types, also recognize the necessity for a considerable degree of differentiation of therapy depending upon the type of disorder involved. Because of this need for differentiation, it is usually found most effective to group individuals for therapy according to the specifics of their speech problems. The emotional and interpersonal aspects of the therapy program can be furthered fully as well by grouping several lispers together, or several stutterers, or several cleft-palate cases, as by mixing these types of cases in a single group. At the same time, the highly differentiated aspects of therapy for these different cases will not be sacrificed.

### Major Approaches to Articulatory Training

Therapists who work with articulatory cases or who have written on the subject tend to stress one of several basic approaches or methods in articulatory correction. The principal ones are the phonetic-placement method and the auditory-training method. A motor-kinesthetic method has also been described by Stinchfield-Hawk and Young (Stinchfield and Young, 1938; Hawk, 1942; Young and Hawk, 1955), though less generally used than the others. These methods are not mutually exclusive. All of them are employed at times by nearly every speech therapist. In the treatment of most cases all will be involved at least incidentally. Each speech therapist, however, tends to place his major reliance upon one or another of these avenues of approach to articulatory correction, making only supplementary use of the others.

The phonetic-placement method was perhaps the one used predominantly in the early years of speech correction (Scripture, 1923), and is still advocated by a few more recent writers (Cotrel and Halsted, 1936; Mulgrave, 1939; Raubicheck, Davis, and Carll, 1932; and Raubicheck, 1952).

In this approach, the individual is given training in the specific placement of the articulators for the production of each sound. He is shown where the position of his tongue, or other parts of his speech mechanism, is faulty and what changes in positioning are required to produce the sound correctly. Speech-training is based upon a knowledge of phonetics. The phonetic-placement approach is based upon the assumption that there is a standard way to produce each sound. Doubt has been thrown upon this, however, by modern phonetic research, which has tended to show that a given acoustic result can be achieved by a considerable variety of positionings in different individuals. What may be an optimum placement for one may not achieve a satisfactory result for another. The production of speech sounds is a dynamic and highly individual process. Overawareness of the mechanics of sound production, moreover, is apt to create an artificial, unnatural attitude about speech and have an inhibiting effect. The most serious objection, however, to relying heavily upon the method of phonetic placement is that it gives the individual little help in judging his own speech. It is a technique which has limited usefulness in carry-over. Incidental use should be made of phonetic methods, of course. With older children and adults particularly, incidental description of the production of the sound in question helps to short-cut the training process.

In the motor-kinesthetic method developed by Hawk and Young, the therapist manipulates the articulators of the case, so that—passively—he produces the correct sound. The individual thus is presumed to receive the correct kinesthetic pattern for each sound and is enabled eventually to reproduce it himself. The therapist accompanies his manipulation with auditory stimulation. Some observers of this method have felt that it was the auditory stimulation, rather than the kinesthetic, which was the effective element in the therapy. Few therapists have been willing to rely primarily upon the motor kinesthetic method, though nearly all make incidental use of kinesthetic cues. In teaching the less visible sounds, the individual can be helped to develop the "feel" of the correct positioning. Kinesthesis, however, is a relatively crude and undifferentiated sense and cannot assist much in fine discrimination.

There has been a steady trend throughout the past fifteen or twenty years toward ever increasing reliance upon auditory training as the most effective basic approach to articulatory correction. The majority of writers in speech pathology today give it major emphasis, though recognizing the incidental utility of the phonetic placement and kinesthetic approaches and also of visual aids in the learning of new sounds.

Hearing is the primary sensory basis for the natural acquisition of speech in early childhood. Hearing is an infinitely more complex and highly differentiated sense than the tactile or kinesthetic and, therefore, permits of finer discriminations. There is a rich source of possible training techniques and materials utilizing audition, whereas touch and kinesthesis are very limited. Visual techniques are useful mainly for the more visible sounds.

Most important of all, audition provides the person with a permanent monitoring system for his own speech. If he develops reliable auditory discrimination through training, it carries over to all situations—away from the speech therapy session as well as in it—and permits auto-evaluation of speech sound production. Auditory training becomes, therefore, a powerful technique for habituating the correct production of speech sounds.

Another aspect of training articulation cases, mentioned by various speech therapists, is the use of exercises for the speech mechanism. These are sometimes referred to as "vocal-motor drills" or "oral gymnastics." It seems to this writer that for the majority of *functional* articulation cases, exercises for the various muscle groups involved in the production of speech are totally irrelevant to the needs of the case and, therefore, a waste of therapeutic time. Exercises are a relevant part of therapy only when the case displays inactivity, weakness, or in-co-ordination of the speech mechanism as a whole or of any part of it. Much time has been wasted in speech therapy through routine use of such exercises for the great majority of cases where no motor problem exists. If exercises are needed in a specific case, they should then be planned systematically and arrangements made for very frequent practice, perhaps with the co-operation of the parents. The value of brief "tongue exercises" two or three times a week for a few minutes each time would seem negligible.

To summarize, the majority of modern writers in speech pathology favor an auditory-training approach to the correction of functional articulation problems. Incidental use is made of visual and kinesthetic cues and of direct instruction in phonetic placement. Exercises for the speech mechanism are used only if some type of motor inadequacy appears to be present. The emphasis on auditory training is in no way inconsistent with the absence of clear-cut evidence that a relationship exists between auditory deficiencies and functional articulation problems, since the purpose of giving auditory training is to develop a *positive skill,* an *awareness* of speech sounds, rather than to overcome a deficiency. Auditory training at first was limited mainly to encouraging the individual to listen carefully to the therapist's production of the sound or the word and then to attempt to imitate it. With the "stimulus method," developed principally at the State University of Iowa (Travis, 1931), the therapist produced the word several times, then asked the case to produce it once. The ratio of stimulus to response was from three to one to five to one.

During recent years, auditory training methods have developed further. Considerable time is spent in developing the individual's auditory discrimination ability as a basic, generalized skill, which he can then apply to the discrimination of specific sounds and words. It seems to this writer worth while to devote some time at the beginning of therapy to preliminary training in auditory discrimination before any speech production is expected of the case. In the long run, carry-over seems to be more effective and permanent when time is devoted to building auditory skill first, even when correct articulatory production can be secured easily. Moreover, auditory training should probably continue to occupy at least a small part of each therapy session throughout the entire course of articulatory training.

## A Logical Sequence in Articulatory Training

The process of correction of a defective speech sound can be said to have three phases: training in auditory discrimination, training in articulatory production, and habituation or carry-over. Within each phase we can identify a sequence from simple to complex. In therapy there is usually considerable overlapping of the phases, so that, for example, articulatory production activities would be started during the first, or auditory training, phase, and carry-over activities would be started fairly early in the production phase of training. The overlap can be represented schematically as follows:

### Temporal Sequence in Learning a Speech Sound

| Type of Training Activity: | Early stages → Intermediate stages → Late stages → |
| --- | --- |
| Auditory discrimination | → . . . . . . . . . . . . . . . . . . . . . . . . . .→. . . . . . . . . . . . . . . . . .→ |
| Articulatory production | → . . . . . . . . . . . . . . . . . . . . . . . . . . .→. . . . . . . . . . . . . . .→ |
| Carry-over | (1)→ . . . . . . . . . . . . . . . . . . . . . . . .→ . . . . . . . . . . . .→(2) |

1. Carry-over can begin when the individual first gains voluntary control of the correct sound.
2. Training on a sound can be terminated when the individual uses the correct sound habitually, even in rapid, conversational speech, and under stress conditions.

During the first few training sessions the emphasis is primarily on auditory training. As therapy progresses, articulatory production occupies an increasing proportion of each session, with activities designed for carry-over coming in as soon as the individual has developed to the point of voluntary mastery of the sound in single words.

The detailed objectives and a few typical activities for each phase of training are described below. In both auditory discrimination and articulatory production the progression in therapy is from the simple, specific, easily identified, highly conscious, and easily controlled toward the more complex, less specific, less easily isolated or identified, less conscious, and less easily controlled listening or speaking behavior. Throughout the following discussion, the sound [s] is used for illustration. Similar procedures would be used with other sounds.

### Auditory discrimination training

1. Identifying and naming the sound. The therapist should introduce the new sound, particularly for young children, in some interesting and dramatic manner, such as telling a story in which the sound is featured. The sound should be given a "name" to establish its identity clearly for the child, such as for [s] the "snake sound" or the "steam sound," whatever is appropriate for the stories or pictures used. The child should be stimulated abundantly with the sound, the therapist naming pictures or objects in which the sound appears in the initial position.

2. Learning to discriminate the stimulus sound from other speech sounds. The therapist can then present to the child a series of consonant sounds in random order, such as: [s], [t], [k], [b], [s], [m], [k], [s], [g], [l], [s], [s], [r], [t], etc. Have

the child tap the table or clap, place a mark on paper, or make some other agreed upon response every time he hears *his* sound, [s]. At first, the series should omit consonants which might be easily confused with [s], such as [z], [ʃ], or [f], but as the child gains skill in discriminating, these should be included, too, as an added challenge and further refinement of his discrimination. Very young children may need some preliminary training to establish the concept of listening and discriminating by starting with nonspeech sounds. Have them listen, without looking, to the different noises made by various toys or noisemakers or by tapping on various materials—wood, metal, paper, etc.—and learn to identify the different sounds. For each auditory activity, first let the child watch you so that he will be aided by visual cues. Later arrange the presentation so that the discrimination will be entirely auditory.

3. Discriminating the sound in more complex contexts. Train the child to discriminate the sound in single words, later in longer speech units such as phrases and sentences read by the therapist. Begin with discrimination between words which start with his sound and words which start with other sounds. Research has shown that discrimination of initial sounds is more accurate than of medial of final sounds (Templin, 1943).

Prepare a supply of cards with pictures mounted or drawn on them. Mix those whose names begin with [s] with some whose names begin with some easily distinguished sound, such as [l] or [g]. Leave out one key picture for each sound, such as *soap* for [s] and *ladder* for [l]. As the therapist names each picture the child decides whether it should be placed under *soap* or under *ladder*. When the child can perform this discrimination reliably, introduce one or two more sounds so that he has three or four choices to make for each word given.

This type of activity provides an excellent opportunity to train the child in a specific discrimination between the sound he is misarticulating and the substitution he is using. For example, children who substitute [w] for [r] should be given practice in sorting pictures beginning with these two sounds; similarly for a [θ] substitution for [s].

When discrimination of initial sounds is developed, a logical next step is learning to identify the sound when it occurs in *any* position in words. Pictures can be named or words read by the therapist, the child deciding whether each word does or does not contain the [s] sound. The therapist can motivate such activities by varying the response asked of the child from one session to another. The child can move a marker along a "track" or up a "ladder," place a chip on various pictures, "break a balloon" by covering a series of pictured balloons, or respond in one of the many other possible ways.

Discriminations should be easy in early stages but should increase in difficulty so that the child can finally identify reliably words which contain [s] in such series as: buzz, bus, zoo, shoe, sew, show, sip, chip, ship, mouth, mouse, etc.

Another activity useful in developing discrimination is the presentation by the therapist of pairs of words or nonsense syllables, in some of the pairs giving the same word or syllable twice, in some giving two different words or syllables. The child is asked to indicate after each pair whether the two words (or syllables) were alike or different.

The child can respond verbally or by any one of a variety of methods of recording or moving markers. Again, discriminations should be relatively gross at first but become more subtle and demanding as skill is developed.

4. Identifying the position of the sound in words. This skill needs to be developed as a preliminary to enabling the child later to produce the sound correctly himself in all positions. As the therapist names pictures or reads words from a list (all of which contain [s]), the child indicates whether [s] comes at the beginning, in the middle, or at the end of the word. He can place a mark in one

of three appropriately labeled columns on paper or on the blackboard, can put a chip under the "engine," "car," or "caboose" of a pictured train or into a real toy train, or can use any one of many possible response methods. For older children, a simple verbal response is probably most efficient.

5. Discriminating the correct from the incorrect production. If the earlier stages of auditory training have been well done, it will be relatively simple for the child to learn to discriminate between correct production of *his* sound by the herapist and varieties of misarticulation of the sound. It is useful for the therapist to attempt to reproduce accurately the individual's own form of misarticulation and then help him to discriminate reliably between this and the correct sound. The therapist can, for example, read a list of [s] words or name pictures, giving some correctly at random and in the others using the child's error-type. The child indicates in some manner when he hears an error or checks errors on a numbered list.

A variation of these activities was described earlier in the section on diagnostic techniques. The therapist repeats a word three or four times, the child then indicating which, if any, contained errors. Present a series of words in this manner.

6. Evaluating his own speech. It is of fundamental importance to train the child to apply the auditory discrimination skill he has developed to the monitoring of *his own speech*. One might say that this is the ultimate purpose of auditory training, yet it is an aspect of therapy which is often omitted or inadequately stressed. Too often the therapist continues to do the evaluating for the case, who remains passive and accepts the therapist's verdict as to whether the speech response he has just given was satisfactory or not. It is probably safe to say that habituation of new speech habits, assuming good motivation, will proceed rapidly or not in relation to the individual's self-monitoring skill. It is not safe to assume that skill in identifying errors in the therapist's speech will be applied by the case to his own speech. It is probable that this specific self-application of auditory discrimination skill needs to be given special attention—at least in all but the most alert and highly motivated individuals. How can this be done?

After some articulatory production training has been given and the person has gained a fair degree of voluntary mastery of his new sound, techniques such as the following can be used. These are but several of numerous possibilities:

Have the child name a series of [s] picture cards, placing each one after he names it in a "good" or a "poor" pile, depending upon his own judgment of his articulation of [s]. When the series is finished discrepancies between the case's judgment and the therapist's may be discussed and some words repeated, if necessary. The same practice can be given through having the child read a list of [s] words, placing a chip in a "good" or "poor" box or below a smiling or a frowning clown face, or by tallying his judgments on paper or on the blackboard. For older children it may be preferable to have three-degree rather than two-degree evaluation, such as "good," "fair," "poor."

Another and more demanding activity is making up a sentence about each picture or word, the case after each one identifying any errors he has made. In a group situation a high degree of motivation can be secured by having one child at a time read or talk and the others keep a record of his errors. Any errors he notes and corrects spontaneously are not counted. A premium is put on auto-evaluation, because the child with the fewest unnoted errors "wins."

## Training in Articulatory Production

It is probably the most common and accepted practice in articulation therapy to begin training in production with the sound in isolation. On logical grounds it seems probable that an individual can most easily learn to produce that which is highly identifiable and specific and which least involves already-established habits. The co-ordinations involved in producing a single sound, though complex, are less so than those involved in producing a whole word in the context of a sentence.

Some recent research by Scott and Milisen (1954 *a* and *b*) supports this. In studying 64 elementary children with functional articulation problems, they found that consonant sounds were produced more often correctly in isolation than in any position in nonsense syllables or words. Furthermore, sounds were made more often correctly in nonsense syllables (any position) than in the corresponding position in words. In nonsense syllables and words, sounds were produced most correctly in the initial position, next most correctly in the medial, and least in the final position, with a few minor exceptions. These results lend strong support to the general clinical practice of beginning with the isolated sound and proceeding to nonsense syllables, then to words, and finally to more complex speech contexts. The individual learning a new sound is thus led by easy stages through an increasingly complex heirarchy of speech configurations.

Milisen's findings also support the common clinical experience that results are best—when the syllable and word stages are reached—if practice is given first with the initial position of the sound, later with the medial and final positions.

The findings of Milisen and his associates again give support to the general practice of utilizing the therapist's own speech as his principal clinical tool. The individual learning a sound listens to and watches the therapist saying the sound and then tries to reproduce it. Scott and Milisen (1954 *a* and *b*) and Humphrey and Milisen (1954) found that combined auditory and visual stimulation was more effective in producing correct responses than either auditory or visual stimulation alone.

The following outline of procedural stages in articulatory production training summarizes and extends what has already been said. The steps indicated are suggestive only. No outline can be followed rigidly and inflexibly but must be adapted to the needs and responses of the individual case. It is assumed that at least several sessions on auditory-discrimination training will have preceded the sequence here presented and that such training will continue to form part of every therapy session.

### Articulatory production sequence in learning a new sound

1. *Sound in isolation.* The therapist gives several productions of the sound, asking the child to listen and watch carefully. The child then gives the sound once and his production is evaluated by the therapist. This process is repeated a number of times, if necessary adding descriptive clues as to placement. When the sound is a visible one the child will often be helped, too, by the use of a mirror. This practice should be carried beyond one or two correct responses, so that the child will become secure in just how the sound is produced. For young children interest can be held easily by allowing the child to "climb a ladder" or go

"around a track" or simply receive a chip or other token for each correct response he gives.

2. Sound in nonsense syllables. The therapist continues with the multiple auditory-visual stimulation and single-response technique but presents the sound followed by a vowel, as [sɑ], giving practice with the sound preceding the other principal vowels or diphthongs, [sɑ], [so], [si], [sɑɪ], [su], etc.

Stimulation practice should next be given with the medial position of the sound, as in [ɑsɑ], [osɑ], etc., and then with the final position as in [ɑs], [is], [os], etc. Extended training at the nonsense-syllable stage is seldom necessary but it is usually a helpful intermediary between the learning of the sound alone and the use of it in the complex context of a whole word. Motivational devices can easily be developed to interest and challenge even young children.

3. Sound in short, simple words. It is usually best to begin again with the initial position and to avoid consonant blends. Words such as sun, soap, sit, soup, sing should be used. With some individuals—and with occasional sounds—production is more easily controlled with the sound in the final or medial position. Occasionally, too, blends are more easily handled than the single consonant. Good clinical observation and flexibility in procedure are essential.

Some cases are highly inconsistent in their misarticulations and will need practice only on those words in which the sound occurs in the phonetic contexts which are difficult for them. These contexts will have been identified in the diagnostic examination.

Practice in using the sound in words can be given through such activities as naming pictures or words after the therapist, climbing word ladders, competing with others in the group to be first around a race track made up of words, hanging word *ornaments* on a Christmas tree, putting word *eggs* in a basket, pulling word *petals* from a flower, and innumerable other variations. Many suggestions for speech games and activities at this and other levels of training will be found in "Speech Correction Techniques, Materials, References" prepared by speech therapists in the Chicago Public Schools.

The writer has coined the term *core vocabularies* to designate the concept of selecting for practice words which are meaningfully related to each other. Clinical experience—if not yet research—indicates that more rapid learning of a sound takes place through the mutual reinforcement of words which have been learned in relation to a "core" topic or experience, as compared with practice situations in which the words employed are selected at random and are unrelated. Thus practice will probably be most effective if the vocabulary involved centers around a "core" or theme familiar to the child. To illustrate, core vocabularies for [s] can be developed around: (1) things in the home (house, stove, sink, bookcase, sofa, fireplace, toaster, etc.); (2) things to wear (sweater, skirt, blouse, slip, socks, dress, pants, scarf etc.); (3) things at school (school, principal's office, desk, books, pencils, erasers, waste basket, etc.); (4) things children do for fun (skating, swimming, sliding, skipping, singing, baseball, tennis, etc.); (5) things at the grocery store (store, grocer, spinach, celery, lettuce, salt, spaghetti, soup, cereal, rice, etc.), and many other topics. A core vocabulary developed at the single-word level can and should be utilized repeatedly in the more advanced stages of training indicated below.

4. Phrases and sentences. The child is given practice in using his sound in larger speech units than words. For example, instead of naming pictures or reading single words, he can make up a sentence for each one. The same "games" used at the word level, such as ladders, race tracks, object or picture-placing, can be used equally well at the phrase or sentence level. Activities utilizing "carrier phrases" featuring [s] can be employed. A perennial favorite of speech therapists and one which never loses its fascination for children is the guessing game in any

of its many variations. For example, ten or twelve core vocabulary pictures can be laid out and each child asked to guess which one the therapist is thinking of. The phrase can be, "I guess it is the—(guessing one of the pictures)." The therapist replies, "No, it isn't the—" or "Yes, it is the—." Guessing continues until the right one is found. Children take turns in thinking of a picture for the others to guess. Throughout the activity only correctly produced [s] words are counted. Another carrier phrase could be, "Please pass the—" in imaginary dinner table situations, with pictured foods and objects.

Question and answer activities, quiz games, adaptations of the game of "Authors," using animal, flower, food, clothing, and other categories, the game "Taking a Trip" in which the child says "I went to St. Louis and in my suitcase I took a—," naming an [s] word, and each child, in turn, repeating what has gone before and adding his own [s] word—are but a few of the many activities which utilize the sentence level.

5. Controlled conversation. This is a step further in the direction of the less specific, less conscious, less identifiable, and less easily controlled speech toward which we aim in articulation therapy. Situations should be created in which the child, though constantly encouraged to use his sound correctly, is able to give only marginal attention to articulation and must give more attention to content and action.

Among typical activities at this stage are the following: (a) interviewing each other about hobbies, about sports, about future plans, etc.; (b) simple dramatizations such as the roles of a shopper and a clerk in a grocery store, a clothing store, a sporting goods store, a post office, or a travel agency; (c) a person seeking information at an employment office; (d) a policeman and a traffic violator; (e) a door-to-door salesman and a housewife, to mention but a few. Situations and roles can be adjusted to the age and specific interests of the cases involved.

Oral reading should not be overlooked as a means for securing excellent articulation practice. It can be adapted to all the levels of training, from single words to continuous text. It can be made more or less easy for the case to control his articulation by pre-marking of the sound being practiced or by spontaneous reading of new material. The visual cue provided by the printed letter is a needed temporary aid in many cases.

6. Free, off-guard speech. There is no sharp distinction between this and the preceding stage. The therapist will need to move constantly—as the individual gains reliability in the use of his sound—toward creating situations which approximate as closely as possible nontherapeutic, real-life situations, maintaining at the same time the individual's awareness of good articulation and his effort to control his sound. To this end activities should involve more continuous and rapid speech and more distraction resulting from emotionally toned content or keen competition. Utilize such activities as impromptu speeches, telling of experiences or stories, telling jokes, discussions between members of the group, preferably on topics which will generate strong feeling. For example, when there are both girls and boys in the therapy group, such emotionally charged discussion topics as "Are girls brighter than boys?" "Should boys have more freedom than girls?" will put newly acquired articulation habits to a severe test. Many additional suggestions for group speech activity are given in the Chicago pamphlet mentioned above.

**Carry-over training.** The term *carry-over* is used by most therapists to refer to the habitual use of the new sound in real-life speech situations, outside of the speech-therapy sessions. All of the auditory discrimination and articulatory production training which has just been described is actually part of the carry-over training, in that the correct sound is gradually becoming habituated and is making its appearance in nontherapy situations. However, it seems necessary in most cases to give specific and serious attention to promoting this carry-over in order to insure that it will take place. Many a speech therapist who has been pleased at a child's consistent and accurate use of his new sound in the therapy session has been disillusioned and discouraged a few moments later to overhear him on the playground using his old substitution or distortion, apparently untouched by the speech therapy he has undergone. Carry-over might be said, therefore, to be the "eating" which is proof of the therapeutic "pudding."

The rapidity, thoroughness, and permanence of carry-over are largely a function of motivation. Other factors being equal, the child or adult who has a strong personal desire to improve in speech will profit more readily from speech therapy than the individual who is passive or complacent about his own speech, however co-operative with the therapist he may appear to be superficially. The problem of motivation is fundamental, therefore, to successful articulation therapy, particularly at the level of carry-over.

The effectiveness of carry-over is also a function of the soundness and thoroughness of the training given at the earlier stages of therapy. Particularly crucial is the degree to which self-monitoring of speech has been stressed and has become habitual. The most highly motivated person conceivable will hardly learn to articulate accurately if he is unable to identify his own errors, either because of poor sound discrimination or because of inattention to his own speech. This is the basic rationale for stressing training in auditory discrimination.

When should emphasis on carry-over begin? Should the therapist await near-perfect reliability of the child's sound in the therapy sessions themselves before beginning to concern himself with his use of the sound in other situations? Most therapists would answer an emphatic "No!" Carry-over can begin as soon as the child has gained voluntary control of his sound and is able to produce it correctly at will. Before a child *can* produce a correct [s] it is manifestly useless to expect him to use it in words. As soon as he *can* produce it, carry-over efforts can and should begin. They should be a part of every therapy session, since it is urgent to assist the child to communicate better as soon as possible.

*Techniques for Securing Carry-over.* At each lesson some time should be devoted to helping the child to produce his sound correctly in one or two words and expressions he has to use frequently, such as: his name, address, telephone number, names of brothers, sisters, parents, his birthday, age, name of his school, his grade, his teacher's name. Early attention should be given to common utilitarian and social courtesy words and expressions such as *yes, no, please, thank you, May I please—?, Will you please . . .?,* the numbers, at least up to ten, the days of the week, the months of the year, and others which are pertinent to the particular case. These words and expressions are so frequently used that they are likely to have become sore points because of teasing or parental criticism. Their mastery is, therefore, correspondingly gratifying to the child and his parents.

Words for practice should be selected in part from the subject matter currently being taught in the child's classroom. Carry-over will be aided by the opportunity thus afforded to practice words newly learned in speech therapy, particularly if the classroom teacher is alerted to the need for reinforcing the child's new and uncertain learning with a word of praise for the word correctly said. Vocabularies surrounding holidays and special events are good practice material. The use of core vocabularies, discussed earlier, will also tend to accelerate carry-over.

Since awareness of speech and motivation for better speech are large factors in carry-over, the following techniques are suggested to assist in motivating and increasing speech awareness:

1. Give the individual a clear understanding of his problem at the beginning of therapy. He should know which of his sounds are defective, the nature of his errors, and the stages which are involved in the correction of each sound. A clear knowledge of the problem tends to challenge and motivate.

2. Objectify the individual's progress. Be sure he understands how far he has come and what his next task will be. His progress may be evident to you as therapist but may not be evident to him and, therefore, not effective in motivating him. At all ages the use of periodic recordings of the person's speech help him to trace his progress.

With children, graphs and charts are often helpful. Colored stars for speech work well done are displayed proudly by children and stimulate them to further efforts.

3. Speech workbooks are a highly effective device to enhance motivation. At each lesson new words or pictures can be added for home practice and serve later as evidence of words already mastered. Children should be encouraged to find pictures containing their sound. These should be used in therapy and then pasted into the workbook. The child who is on the lookout for [s] pictures in the magazines around home is thinking about his [s] sound and apt to begin using it at least part of the time. Children can also be encouraged to write sentences or stories which feature the sound they are learning and to be ready to read them with good sounds at the next session.

Workbooks help to make the child conscious of his speech task between lessons and to increase his awareness of *his* sound in the speech he hears around him. He can be asked to collect in his speech-book the words containing his sound which he has heard other people say. Attentiveness to speech is thus spread over the interval between therapy sessions. Speech workbooks interest not only the child himself but also his teacher and his parents. They are often stimulated to do a considerable amount of incidental encouragement of correct articulation and calling of attention to lapses.

4. When voluntary mastery of a sound has been achieved it is helpful to establish a weekly quota of words to be "remembered" and uttered correctly whenever they occur in the intervals between lessons. Each week's quota is added to the speech workbook. Two or three words are usually sufficient for primary age children, five to ten for older children. Core vocabularies are useful as a source for the word quotas.

Parents and classroom teachers, sometimes older brothers and sisters, can be helpful by having a copy of the child's quota for that week and assisting him, in a friendly spirit, to use these words consistently. They can even ask questions or create situations in which the quota words will have to be used.

One therapist on the writer's staff invented the highly stimulating device of calling each therapy group a "speech club," with "passwords" or "secret sentences" which had to be articulated correctly in order to gain admission to the next "meeting of the club." The club "members" took delight in asking each other for the passwords between therapy sessions. Ingenuity can harness powerful motivational forces to speech carry-over.

5. Participation by children themselves in the selection or invention of speech techniques, in the selection of the words for the next week's quota, and in the finding of pictures and reading material, is a strongly motivating factor. Interim assignments will be carried out with more interest and reliability if children—or adults for that matter—have helped to set up their own goals and to find or devise their own practice material.

6. Propaganda for good speech will be an aid to motivation and carry-over. The speech therapy room should suggest "speech" from the moment the individual enters it. "Good Speech" posters may be made by children and hung up in the room. A pin-up board can be used to display magazine or newspaper articles on speech, items about people who have outstandingly good speech or who have overcome speech problems, or speech materials prepared by children. These all help to interest and challenge the individual who is working on his own speech problem or the parent who comes in for a conference with the speech therapist.

The speech therapist will need to verify the reliability of the individual's carry-over of the corrected sound by checking with teachers and members of the family and, if possible, by himself listening to his case in an off-guard speaking situation when the individual is unaware of his presence. The final test of the clinical result is consistent, accurate use of the new sound in rapid speech under somewhat emotional or stress conditions.

Further suggestions for articulation-training techniques and activities will be found in the Chicago pamphlet, "Speech Correction Techniques, Materials, References" (1952), in Ainsworth (1948), Anderson (1953), Berry and Eisenson (1942), Koepp-Baker (1936), and Van Riper (1954), and in some of the other texts listed in the bibliography. Excellent practice material in the form of word lists, sentences, or stories, will be found in Ainsworth (1946), Fairbanks (1940), McCullough (1940), Nemoy (1954), Nemoy and Davis (1937), Schoolfield (1951), and Zedler (1955) to mention particularly useful sources.

## Principles of Good Articulation Therapy

The formulation which follows restates and emphasizes some of the points implied in the foregoing outline of articulation therapy:

1. Articulation therapy should be carefully planned but should also be flexible so that it can adapt itself to the individual's needs and responses as these manifest themselves during the course of therapy.

2. Articulation therapy cannot be standardized for all cases. It is not rigid, routinized, or stereotyped, but is adapted to the individualized needs and deficiencies of each case.

3. Articulation therapy in its various phases—auditory discrimination,

articulatory production, and carry-over—proceeds from the simple, the highly specific, the conscious, the easily identified, the easily controlled toward the more complex, less specific, less conscious, less easily identified and less easily controlled.

4. Articulation therapy utilizes all appropriate sensory avenues and intellectual aids to understanding, but is probably most effective when it places major emphasis on auditory training, as the process most basic to speech learning.

5. Articulation therapy must begin with the individual *where he is*—at the point where the normal process of speech acquisition was stopped or disrupted. This means that new habits must be learned to replace incorrect ones. This in turn usually involves a considerable amount of drill or repetitive practice. Drill is a sound psychological concept when it also implies *motivation* and *purposefulness*.

6. Even from the initial stages, where drill is used to develop mastery, articulation therapy is probably most effective when it utilizes practice materials which have interest and meaning to the individual and when it relates and integrates practice with real-life speaking situations.

7. A technique or activity for auditory discrimination, articulatory production, or carry-over should be selected with certain criteria in mind:

It should be of interest and meaning to the case with which it is to be used, and appropriate for his maturity level.
It should be appropriate to his intelligence, experience, and reading level.
It should be appropriate to the *stage* of therapy which has been reached.
It should be simple to explain and to understand so that therapeutic time is not wasted in mere preparation for practice.
It should provide a maximum opportunity for speech practice, which is the fundamental purpose of the therapy session. Motivational aspects of the situation, such as "winning the game," should not obscure the more basic objective of using good articulation. Motivation should be harnessed to good speech, not irrelevant to it.

8. At all stages, articulation therapy must be oriented psychotherapeutically. Attention must be given, not only to the development of accurate articulation but also to the individual's security and pleasure in speaking, to improvement of his communicative attitudes and habits, and to his motivation for personal speech improvement.

9. Articulation therapy is not a simple, didactic relationship between the therapist and his case. It is a co-operative enterprise in which the case is an active, informed participant, aware of his problem, of the stages involved in speech-learning, and of the progress being made. Articulatory improvement should be a conscious, self-selected goal, and a process to which the case contributes ideas, materials, and evaluations, as well as deliberate effort.

10. The co-operative nature of articulation therapy implies not only the participation of the case but also of his family, teachers, and even associates. When an appropriate point in therapy has been reached, their active as

istance—guided by the therapist—will to a considerable degree determine
he rapidity and effectiveness of carry-over.

## BIBLIOGRAPHY

INSWORTH, S. 1946. Galloping sounds. Boston: Expression Co.

—— 1948. Speech correction methods. New York: Prentice-Hall.

NDERSON, V. A. 1939. Auditory memory span as tested by speech sounds.
*Amer. J. Psychol.,* 52, 95–99.

—— 1953. Improving the child's speech. New York: Oxford Univ. Press.

ACKUS, O. L. 1943. Speech in education. New York: Longmans, Green.

—— and BEASLEY, J. 1951. Speech therapy with children. Boston: Houghton Mifflin.

ACKUS, O. L., and DUNN, H. M. 1944. Experiments in the synthesis of clinical
methods into a program of rehabilitation. *J. Speech Disorders,* 9, 1–17.

—— 1947a. Intensive group therapy in speech rehabilitation. *J. Speech Disorders,* 12, 39–60.

—— 1947b. Use of conversation patterns to promote speech and retention of
learning. *J. Speech Disorders,* 12, 135–142.

EEBE, H. H. 1946. Sigmatismus nasalis. *J. Speech Disorders,* 11, 35–37.

ENDER, J. F., and KLEINFELD, V. M. 1938. Principles and practices of speech
correction. New York: Pitman.

ERRY, M. F., and EISENSON, J. 1942. The defective in speech. New York: Appleton-Century-Crofts.

—— 1956. Speech disorders. New York: Appleton-Century-Crofts.

LOMQUIST, B. L. 1950. Diadochokinetic movements of nine-, ten-, and eleven-
year-old children. *J. Speech Hearing Disorders,* 15, 159–164.

RYNGELSON, B., and GLASPEY, E. 1951. Speech in the classroom. Teacher's
manual to accompany speech improvement cards. Chicago: Scott, Foresman.

OTREL, E., and HALSTED, E. M. 1936. Class lessons for improving speech.
Boston: Expression Co.

URRY, R., KENNEDY, L., WAGNER, L., and WILKE, W. 1943. A phonographic
scale for the measurement of defective articulation. *J. Speech Disorders,* 8,
123–126.

OLL, E. A. 1947. Vineland social maturity scale, manual of directions. Minneapolis: Educ. Test Bur.

—— 1951. Mental evaluation of children with expressive handicaps. *Amer.
J. Orthopsychiat.,* 21, 148–154.

NQUIST, L. E., and WAGNER, C. F. 1950. Flannel chart technique for the rehabilitation of speech and hearing disorders. *J. Speech Hearing Disorders,*
15, 338–340.

AIRBANKS, G. 1940. Voice and articulation drillbook. New York: Harper.

ARWOOD, V. P. 1952. An experimental study of certain relationships between
intelligibility scores and clinical data of persons with defective articulation.
Unpublished Ph.D. Thesis. Univ. Mich.

ATES, A. I. 1935. A reading vocabulary for the primary grades. Revised and
enlarged. New York: Teachers College, Columbia Univ.

AWK, S. S. 1942. Moto-kinaesthetic training for children with speech handicaps.
*J. Speech Disorders,* 7, 357–360.

ELTMAN, H. J. 1933. Devices for the correction of articulatory defects of
speech. *Proc. Amer. Speech Correction Assn.,* 3, 1–6.

—— 1948. Handbook for remedial speech (rev. ed.). Boston: Expression Co.

HENDERSON, F. M. 1938. Accuracy in testing the articulation of speech sounds. *J. educ. Res.,* 31, 348–356.

HENRIKSON, E. H. 1948. An analysis of Wood's articulation index. *J. Speech Hearing Disorders,* 13, 233–235.

HOLBROOK, A. 1954. A study of the effectiveness of recorded articulation exercises. *J. Speech Hearing Disorders,* 19, 14–16.

HUMPHREY, W. R., and MILISEN, R. 1954. A study of the ability to reproduce unfamiliar sounds which have been presented orally. *J. Speech Hearing Disorders,* monogr. suppl. 4, 58–69.

IRWIN, J. V., and DUFFY, J. K. 1951. Speech and hearing hurdles. Columbus, Ohio: Sch. & Coll. Serv.

IRWIN, R. B. 1949. Speech and hearing therapy in the public schools of Ohio. *J. Speech Hearing Disorders,* 14, 63–68.

———— 1953. Speech and hearing therapy. New York: Prentice-Hall.

———— and BECKLUND, O. 1953. Norms for maximum repetitive rates for certain sounds established with the sylrater. *J. Speech Hearing Disorders,* 18, 149–160.

JOHNSON, W., editor. 1950. Speech problems of children. New York: Grune and Stratton.

———— BROWN, S. F., CURTIS, J. F., EDNEY, C. W., and KEASTER, J. 1948. Speech handicapped school children. New York: Harper.

JOHNSON, W., DARLEY, F. L., and SPRIESTERSBACH, D. C. 1952. Diagnostic manual in speech correction. New York: Harper.

KOEPP-BAKER, H. 1936. A handbook of clinical speech, Vol. II. Ann Arbor: Edwards Brothers.

KRONVALL, E. L., and DIEHL, C. F. 1954. The relationship of auditory discrimination to articulatory defects of children with no known organic impairment. *J. Speech Hearing Disorders,* 19, 335–338.

McCULLOUGH, G. A. 1940. Speech improvement work and practice book. Boston: Expression Co.

MADER, J. B. 1954. The relative frequency of occurrence of English consonant sounds in words in the speech of children in grades one, two, and three. *Speech Monogr.* 21, 294–300.

MATTHEWS, J., and BIRCH, J. W. 1949. The Leiter international performance scale—a suggested instrument for psychological testing of speech and hearing clinic cases. *J. Speech Hearing Disorders,* 14, 318–321.

MAXWELL, K. L. 1953. A comparison of certain motor performances of normal and speech defective children, ages seven, eight, and nine years. Unpublished Ph. D. Thesis. Univ. Mich.

METRAUX, R. W. 1944. Auditory memory span for speech sounds. Norms for children. *J. Speech Disorders,* 9, 31–38.

MILISEN, R. 1945. Principles and methods of articulation testing. *Speech Hearing Therapist,* Indiana Univ. Speech and Hearing Clinic, Bloomington, Feb. 6–10.

———— 1954. A rationale for articulation disorders. *J. Speech Hearing Disorders,* monogr. suppl., 4, 6–17.

MULGRAVE, D. I. 1939. Speech for the classroom teacher. New York: Prentice-Hall.

NEMOY, E. M. 1954. Speech correction through story-telling units. Boston: Expression Co.

NEMOY, E. M., and DAVIS, S. F. 1937. The correction of defective consonant sounds. Boston: Expression Co.

NESS, A. M. 1932. A comparison of the response and stimulation methods in the re-education of speech defectives. Unpublished Master's Thesis. State Univ. Iowa.

PERKINS, W. H. 1952. Methods and materials for testing articulation of (s) and (z). *Quart. J. Speech,* 38, 57–62.

PERRIN, E. H. 1954. The rating of defective speech by trained and untrained observers. *J. Speech Hearing Disorders,* 19, 48–51.

PETTIT, C. W. 1952. The predictive efficiency of a battery of speech diagnostic tests for the articulatory development of a group of five-year-old children. Unpublished Ph. D. Thesis. Univ. Wis.

PRONOVOST, W., and DUMBLETON, C. 1953. A picture-type speech sound discrimination test. *J. Speech Hearing Disorders,* 18, 258–266.

RAUBICHECK, L. 1952. Speech improvement. New York: Prentice-Hall.

———, DAVIS, E. H., and CARLL, L. A. 1932. Voice and speech problems. New York: Prentice-Hall.

REID, G. 1947. The efficacy of speech re-education of functional articulatory defectives in the elementary school. *J. Speech Disorders,* 12, 301–313.

RICE, D. M., and MILISEN, R. 1954. The influence of increased stimulation upon the production of unfamiliar sounds as a function of time. *J. Speech Hearing Disorders,* monogr. suppl., 4, 80–86.

ROBBINS, S. D. 1942. Importance of sensory training in speech therapy. *J. Speech Disorders,* 7, 183–188.

ROE, V. 1948. Follow-up in the correction of functional articulatory disorders. *J. Speech Hearing Disorders,* 13, 332–336.

ROMANS, E. F., and MILISEN, R. 1954. Effect of latency between stimulation and response on reproduction of sounds. *J. Speech Hearing Disorders,* monogr. suppl., 4, 72–78.

SCHOOLFIELD, L. D. 1951. Better speech and better reading. Boston: Expression Co.

SCOTT, D. A., and MILISEN, R. 1954a. The effect of visual, auditory and combined visual-auditory stimulation upon the speech responses of defective speaking children. *J. Speech Hearing Disorders,* monogr. suppl., 4, 38–43.

——— 1954b. The effectiveness of combined visual-auditory stimulation in improving articulation. *J. Speech Hearing Disorders,* monogr. suppl., 4, 52–56.

SCRIPTURE, E. W. 1923. Stuttering, lisping and correction of the speech of the deaf. New York: Macmillan.

SHAMES, G. H. 1953. An exploration of group homogeneity in group speech therapy. *J. Speech Hearing Disorders,* 18, 267–272.

SNOW, K., and MILISEN, R. 1954a. The influence of oral versus pictorial presentation upon articulation testing results. *J. Speech Hearing Disorders,* monogr. suppl., 4, 30–36.

——— 1954b. Spontaneous improvement in articulation as related to differential responses to oral and picture articulation tests. *J. Speech Hearing Disorders,* monogr. suppl., 4, 46–49.

Speech and hearing problems in the secondary school. 1950. Prepared under the editorial supervision of the American Speech and Hearing Association. Ainsworth, S., Chairman, editorial committee, *Bull. Nat. Assn. Secondary Sch. Principals,* 34, 3–139.

Speech correction techniques, materials, references. 1952. Div. Speech Correction, Chicago Public Schools. Margaret Hall Powers, Director.

PRIESTERSBACH, D. C., and CURTIS, J. F. 1951. Misarticulation and discrimination of speech sounds. *Quart. J. Speech,* 37, 483–491.

STINCHFIELD, S. M., and YOUNG, E. H. 1938. Children with delayed or defective speech. Palo Alto: Stanford Univ. Press.

TEMPLIN, M. 1943. A study of sound discrimination ability of elementary school pupils. *J. Speech Disorders*, 8, 127–132.

—— 1947a. Spontaneous versus imitated verbalization in testing articulation in preschool children. *J. Speech Disorders*, 12, 293–300.

—— 1947b. A non-diagnostic articulation test. *J. Speech Disorders*, 12, 392–396.

—— 1953. Norms on a screening test of articulation for ages three through eight. *J. Speech Hearing Disorders*, 18, 323–331.

TRAVIS, L. E. 1931. Speech pathology. New York: Appleton.

VAN RIPER, C. 1939. Ear training in the treatment of articulation disorders. *J. Speech Disorders*, 4, 141–142.

—— 1954. Speech correction principles and methods (3rd ed.). New York: Prentice-Hall.

WECHSLER, D. 1949. Wechsler intelligence scale for children. New York: Psychological Corporation.

WEST, R., KENNEDY, L., and CARR, A. 1947. The rehabilitation of speech (rev. ed.). New York: Harper.

WILSON, B. A. 1954. The development and evaluation of a speech improvement program for kindergarten children. *J. Speech Hearing Disorders*, 19, 4–13.

WOOD, K. S. 1946. Parental maladjustment and functional articulatory defects in children. *J. Speech Disorders*, 11, 255–275.

—— 1949. Measurement of progress in the correction of articulatory speech defects. *J. Speech Hearing Disorders*, 14, 171–174.

WRIGHT, H. N. 1954. Reliability of evaluations during basic articulation and stimulation testing. *J. Speech Hearing Disorders*, monog. suppl., 4, 20–27.

YOUNG, E. H., and HAWK, S. S. 1955. Moto-kinesthetic speech training. Palo Alto: Stanford Univ. Press.

ZEDLER, E. Y. 1955. Listening for speech sounds. Garden City: Doubleday.

# CHAPTER 25

# SUGGESTIONS FOR PSYCHOTHERAPY IN PUBLIC SCHOOL SPEECH CORRECTION

- *Lee Edward Travis, Ph.D.*
  *and*
  *LaVerne Deel Sutherland, M.A.*

THERE ARE THOSE among both clinical psychologists and speech pathologists who hold that speech therapy and psychotherapy are in conflict with each other. They assume that speech therapy involves the teaching of correct or normal speech habits to replace defective or abnormal ones and that this is accomplished mainly through ear-training, phonetics, and speech exercises. Psychotherapy on the other hand does not deal directly with the elimination of old and the establishment of new habits but with deeper, underlying problems of an emotional-conflict nature.

Are these approaches necessarily in conflict, or can they be reconciled and integrated within a single remedial program? It is felt that they are not in basic conflict with each other and that they can be blended into a unified frontal attack upon the problem of communication disorders. At the very least they should be considered supplemental one to the other, or complementary to each other. They need not be viewed as competitive but rather as related both in theory and in practice and with a common goal.

## PROJECTION PICTURE SITUATION

A projective picture provides the child with a stimulus situation that may give him an opportunity to impose verbally upon it his consciously guarded secret needs. It may be used to elicit interpersonal relationships of overt and hidden forms. The use of this procedure in speech correction is not so much for diagnosis as for therapy. By involuntarily revealing feelings and thoughts that are below the surface and otherwise incapable of exposure by questions and suggestions, the child may come to recognize, express, and more wholesomely manage them. The speech therapist can develop her own projection test or she can use those already developed. The Travis-Johnston Projection

Test was thought to be a good one for speech therapy, since the pictures were drawn to portray adults and children in situations and relationships centering in the important and potentially troublesome areas in the socialization of the child. The areas pictured are sibling rivalry, child-parent rivalry, discipline, eating, sleeping, toilet-training, cleanliness, and sexual development

The great majority of the children will respond well verbally to the pictures. Occasionally a child will refuse to respond to a picture. One nine-year-old boy showed great anxiety in saying "I'm not going to tell a story." Later he wanted to talk, started a story five different times, finally stopped, and could not go on. The child is told simply to tell a story about the picture. The therapist can make the situation a group or an individual one as time and

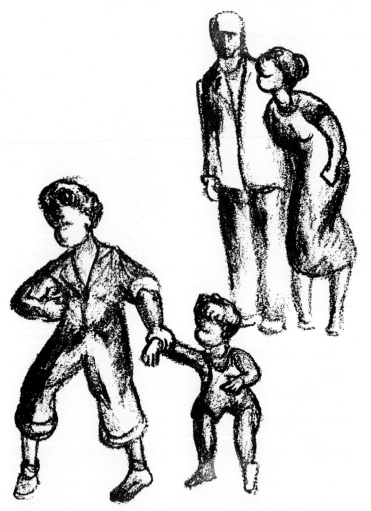

FIG. 1. Picture 1-M of the Travis-Johnston Projection Test (Permission of Griffin-Patterson Co., 544 W. Colorado Blvd., Glendale, Calif.).

circumstances warrant. Further, the speech therapist can use a picture only, or she can present a picture while the child is doing something else, such as working with clay, playing with puppets, or playing a role in sociodrama.

Timmy was an eight-year-old boy whose father also stuttered. He was his father's favorite of three children (the oldest) but admittedly rejected by the mother because the father repeatedly deserted the family from the time Timmy was a few months old. When he looked at Picture 1-M (Fig. 1) he said:

"Father and Mother tried to plan how to get money for a home. Father worked and saved and bought a house. Mother worked and bought clothes. Brother sold newspapers and bought furniture to put clothes in. The house had no roof. Sister

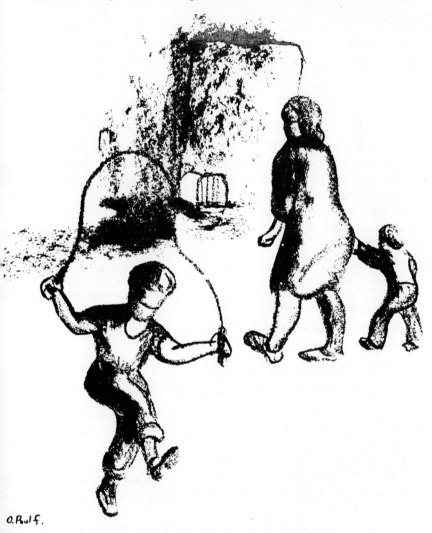

O.Rulf.

FIG. 2. Picture 2-M of the Travis-Johnston Projection Test (Permission of Griffin-Patterson Co., 544 W. Colorado Blvd., Glendale, Calif.).

worked and bought a roof for the house. Brother and Sister went to the store to get milk and cookies which they all ate. They went to bed [pause]. The house disappeared [pause]. The furniture disappeared [pause] and the roof. So they again had nothing [pause]. Then they wakened [pause]. It was a dream."

It seems clear that Timmy was projecting his own feelings upon the picture. His troublesome insecurities caused him great difficulty in acquiring and keeping a roof. Even his fantasy was frightening, so fearsome in fact that he had to call it a dream. Really, he had to give a dream within a fantasy in order to tolerate his feelings.

When Picture 2-M (Fig. 2) was presented to him, Timmy said:

"Big Brother went to the attic to see the rats. The Father was there [pause] but no one knew it. Brother was quiet so as not to scare the rats. He came back down and said a big, huge rat was in the attic. Mother went up and returned saying an elephant with a small nose was up there. Little Brother went up and returned saying a big box shaped like a man was up there. They decided to cut the roof off and find out. They started sawing around the roof. Father heard it and thought the rats were beginning to chew the roof off. While the family was inside, the Father sneaked downstairs and out the garage. He bought three ice cream cones and put a box in the attic shaped like a man, a rat, and an elephant [pause]. They brought it downstairs [pause] and out jumped a funny clown."

Does Timmy have feared feelings that his father is a rat, an elephant, or a big box? If he does, does he also have offsetting feelings that the father is good by buying three ice-cream cones or that the father is not really so bad but is playing at it, as a clown? Anyway, feelings are getting out, not straightforwardly and appropriately yet, but under the protection of a projection.

Manuel and Rudolpho were ten-year-old stutterers. Of Picture 2-M (Fig 2), Manuel said:

"The boy was blindfolded because when he jumped rope he missed if his brother watched him. Mother took the younger brother and put him down a well. Then the older brother took the Mother and put her down the well [pause] I don't know any finish [pause]."

Rudolpho, who was also looking at this picture and listening to Manuel spoke up:

"May I tell a finish to your story?"

Manuel replied, "Sure." So Rudolpho gave his ending:

"The boy was blindfolded because he was practicing jumping rope on a tight rope. Little Brother stole his jump rope and threw it down the well. It landed in a bucket. When Mother drew a bucket of water she found the jump rope which had shrunk to just this size [measuring about 14 inches]."

What is reported here may occur quite frequently in a group. One child can speak more honestly or tolerate more anxiety than another child, so that the second child will have to "doctor" the story. Manuel's tale was too raw for Rudolpho. It produced too much anxiety in him. He handled his fears by softening the relationships between the people of the picture. One might speculate that Manuel was further along in his therapy than Rudolpho or had more severe problems.

Raul, a nine-year-old stutterer, was openly aggressive and hostile. As he looked at Picture 2-M (Fig. 2), he said:

"See that boy jumping rope there? Well they don't know it but he really has some firecrackers in his pocket. He waited until his little Ol' Brother was alone and he blew him up with a firecracker [chuckled]. Then he used a firecracker on his mother and blew her up [gleeful]. Next he found a policeman who was really looking for him because of what he'd done, and he blew him up too [eyes dancing; jittery in his chair]. And then, oh boy, he even went to the police head-quarters and used more firecrackers and blew up all the police. All of them. Then you know what, he got lots and lots of firecrackers and blew up the town. Yeah, the whole town."

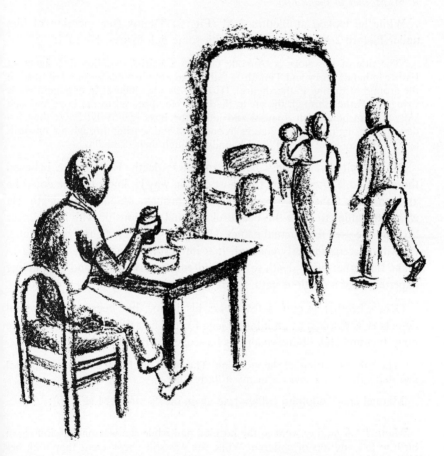

O. Paulf.

FIG. 3. Picture 3-M of the Travis-Johnston Projection Test (Permission of Griffin-Patterson Co., 544 W. Colorado Blvd., Glendale, Calif.).

Mike had given "nothing but trouble" in the ten years of his life. Every social relationship with family, relatives, neighbors, and schools had been punctuated by violent, erratic behavior. Mike claimed to have innumerable members of his family. Actually there were the mother, father, a beautiful little sister who had a boy's name, and himself. He was large for his age, had very poor muscular control, was unliked by his peers, and spoke with severely retarded, infantile speech. His sound substitutions were inconsistent and he had stuttered since he was three. Of Picture 2-M (Fig. 2) he said:

"The young brother was spanked and put to bed for getting dirty while he was jumping rope with the older brother. The older brother is in back of the house and can not be seen, but he is dirty too. He wants to go in the house and have Mother spank him too [pause] and be put to bed. [Repeats with emphasis] *He wants Mother to spank him.*"

While he looked at Picture 3-M (Fig. 3) Timmy (see mention of him under Picture 2-M) was "playing" with some doll figures. He said:

"The title of this story is 'Anyone Can Be a Spirit.' [Holding doll figure of Father in hand] Barry and Timothy's father had heart trouble and he fell over on the ground [dropping Father figure]. [Holding two boy figures in one hand while flying the Father through the air to the boys] He appeared to the boys and said 'Anyone can be a spirit' [pause] and killed the boys [gently hit boys; they fell down]. [Picking up all three figures in one hand and soaring through air upwards again] They all went *up* and lived happily through their death."

Timmy felt that his only permanency was death. Happily, he believed there was hope after death. The most certain way he knew that he could be assured of his father's companionship was through companionate death. He was even willing to share this beautiful spiritual relationship with his younger brother. He used their actual names. His actions with the figures were gentle, the killing scene tenderly enacted. It is interesting to note that he chose to make the father bring death to the children. Timmy's vivid and stimulating experiences of a religious nature were evidenced in many of his productions.

Gene's brother is only a few years his junior, but because of physical defects is as helpless as an infant. Gene for the first time and with complete honesty admits his sibling rivalry as he looked at Picture 3-M (Fig. 3):

"The baby is getting all the attention. The older brother feels left out [pause] and that's the way I feel about my little brother."

Manuel and Rudolpho collaborate again on Picture 3-M (Fig. 3):

*Manuel:* "A mother went to the hospital and while she was unconscious gave birth to lots and lots of children. While she was still unconscious they took her home and put her in a chair. She 'came to' and saw a child—then another—and many—until she saw hundreds and thousands. She didn't have a house and beds big enough—so she dug a hole in the ground for them. Then she used a derrick for feeding milk, putting pipes from it to the ground where the children were. On each pipe was a [pause] you know [pause] nipple. When the babies were thirsty, they just went to the nipple and drank their milk without bothering their mother. Finally she ran out of milk so bought a farm. When the cows died she took the children to an orphanage [pause]. When she got home the babies were back in the hole in the ground."

*Rudolpho:* "May I go on with your story?"

*Manuel:* "Sure."

*Rudolpho:* "The Mother got a big house for them [pause], big enough for them.

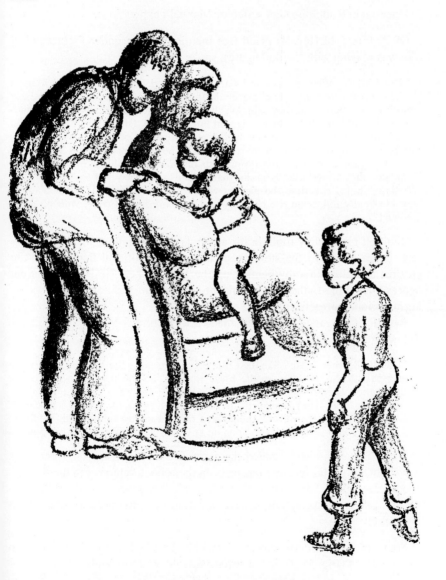

FIG. 4. Picture 5-M of the Travis-Johnston Projection Test (Permission of Griffin-Patterson Co., 544 W. Colorado Blvd., Glendale, Calif.).

*Manuel:* "The children got too big for the house and then the Mother took them to Alcatraz, but they couldn't take care of them there [pause] so they dumped them in the ocean. They made so many children in the ocean that the steam ships could not move through the waters [pause] so she pushed them all down to the bottom of the ocean where they poured cement on them to make them stay down."

*Rudolpho:* "But the cement didn't cover all the sides and the children got out that way and got back to land safely."

Once again Rudolpho kept softening Manuel's expressions.

Of Picture 5-M (Fig. 4), Raul (see mention of him under Picture 2-M), who was playing with the doll figures, spoke as follows:

"The Little Brother got cut and Father bandaged him. Mother held him on her lap. Big Brother said 'They never do that for me.' So he went out and cut himself on the hand, but they said 'Oh that little scratch. It doesn't need a bandage.' So he cut himself bigger on his arm but they said 'Oh that isn't bad enough for a bandage.' So he cut himself bigger and worse on both his arms but they still said 'Go away. That's not hurt enough.' Then he hurt his legs worse and more. He wanted to go to the hospital so his Father would take care of him. Each time they would ask 'Who did that to you?' 'Oh a boy I know *real well—Me*' [laughing]. Each time the parents would become angry and wouldn't help him. He finally fell down the chimney and hurt himself all over, with his head flattened."

Raul felt completely futile in his attempts at recognition, help, and comfort. In his telling of the story he used the family of doll figures with the greatest abandon, literally beating up the Big Brother. He held the parent figures (giving the Father the prominent role) in stiff positions, while speaking in vitriolic, sarcastic tones.

Bert, a nine-year-old stutterer, reacted to Picture 5-M (Fig. 4) with the following story:

"The Big Brother doesn't like the Little Brother because the Mother and Father always pay all the attention to the Little Brother. So the Big Brother hurt the Little Brother. The Mother rocked the Little Brother and was good to him and the Father was afraid. They punished the Big Brother so he ran away. It got dark and he lost himself. He walked and walked till he came to this school. He knew that *this place* was in *this* school. Then he knew his way home, and went home."

Bert's fantasies always ended the same. He "lost himself" and knew his way home only after locating *this* place in the school, referring to the therapy room. He kept "finding himself" until finally his parents and teachers reported he was stuttering only on the rarest, most trying occasions, and then only mildly.

Some of the children expressed frankly hostile feelings in reacting to Picture 11-M (Fig. 5). Teddy, a seven-year-old stutterer said:

"The boy socked the Daddy in the nose [pause] and then again in the nose because he was mad. Daddy spanked him and spanked him."

Other children expressed their feelings of being neglected, thereby denying their feelings of anger over the frustration of not getting attention,
Samuel, a six-year-old stutterer, was the oldest of four children. The very
dominant grandmother lived in the home. Samuel's thumbnail was deformed
from constant, vigorous sucking. From his birth he had been compared unfavorably with cousins and neighboring children. He could never go to sleep
until everyone else in the house was in bed. His response to Picture 11-M
(Fig. 5) was:

"His Dad promised to play with him but when he got home he read the papers.
'I'll play after dinner.' After dinner the Dad was too tired. Then he watched TV.
'I'll play with you tomorrow.' The next day he had to go to work and couldn't
p'ay. He *never does* play with the boy."

Raul, whose reactions have been given to Pictures 2-M and 5-M, expressed his hostility in his story and in his plays with the dolls while he was
studying Picture 11-M (Fig. 5).

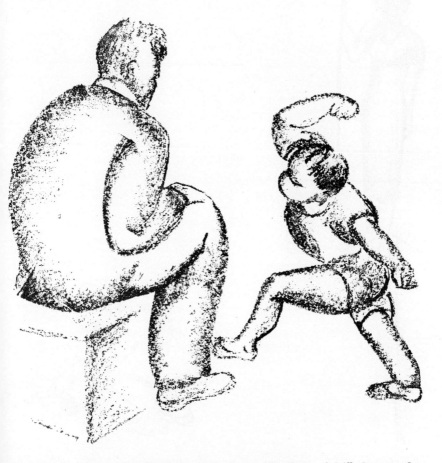

FIG. 5. Picture 11-M of the Travis-Johnston Projection Test (Permission of Griffin-Patterson Co.,
544 W. Colorado Blvd., Glendale, Calif.).

"The Father was asleep, see. The boy sneaked up and stole a dollar from his Father's pocket. He went to the store and bought candy [gleeful]. He licked the candy and then put it in the Father's pocket [chuckling]. The ants came to the candy and bit Father, who jumped all over the room. Ow! Ouch! Wow! [jumping the father figure jerkily over the room]. Why you little . . . I'm going to spank you! And he spanked the boy. Then the Father went back to sleep. The boy sneaked and stole five dollars and bought fire crackers and Roman candles. He stole a match from Father's pocket and lighted the fireworks. Father bounced all over the room [he did]. Father spanked the boy. The boy went to sleep. The Father put fireworks on *him* and fired them. The boy was exploded [both hands covering the boy figure suddenly burst apart, then dropped in Raul's lap].

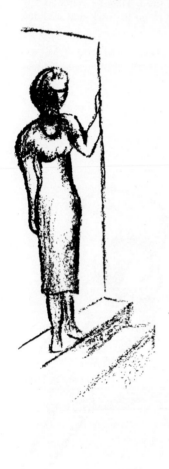

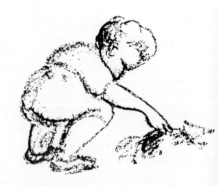

FIG. 6. Picture 13-M of the Travis-Johnston Projection Test (Permission of Griffin-Patterson Co., 544 W. Colorado Blvd., Glendale, Calif.).

Although the story and the doll play end on a note of punishment and destruction to himself, Raul subsequently began to drop his stuttering and to gain in self-regard.

Quite different problems are expressed by two young stutterers, Johnny and Gene, while looking at Picture 13-M (Fig. 6).

*Johnny:* "The little boy would rather play in the mud than with his toys which his mother wants him to do. Mud is more fun [pause], he's happier there."

*Gene:* "The boy is digging up some dynamite he has buried in the ground. He makes a sky rocket to shoot Father. But the tow line is still attached to the boy when it exploded and he explodes with it instead of Father."

Johnny expresses quite frankly his preference for messing while Gene expresses hostility and then has it boomerang on him.

### Some Concluding Remarks

Just "talking things over" or visiting with the children is usually a waste of time. In this highly socialized situation, children remain too highly socialized. With the aid of pictures, such as those used here, the therapist can come more quickly and directly to conflictual feelings. At the same time, the pictures permit an alibi or a defense. After all, it is just a picture and just a story. But through and around the defense, true feelings and thoughts get out and are recognized and generally accepted and managed.

It may be well for the therapist to use just one picture per session. She can assure the children that each one will have a chance to tell his story or to add to another's story. Children may benefit not only from their own story but by listening to the stories of others as well. The therapist should be alert and sensitive to the expressions of feared and antisocial feelings and attitudes in order that she may encourage their revelation. She must take care not to react to the child's fear and anxiety by expressing criticism or condemnation. Such expression is the reward the child fears and expects. It has no place in a therapy situation.

### FINGER PAINTS AND MODELING CLAY

#### Purpose

The child seeks to protect himself against the frustration of his primitive impulses. He is resentful of restraint and because of his immaturity is given readily to outbursts of rage and anger when inhibited. Often these reactions to frustration get him into still deeper water, since they are as antisocial as his primitive feelings and drives, and in turn have to be restrained. The restrictions and inhibitions of the culture that do not follow the orderly development of the total child produce tensions, repressions, fear, and guilt in him. As a consequence, he may feel rejected, unworthy, and incompetent or develop overcompensatory and symptomatic behavior. One area of the child's development fraught with much danger to future well-being is that of toilet and cleanliness training (see Ch. 29, p. 922, A Sketch of Some Older Training Situations).

The purpose of having groups of children with functional speech disorders work with paints and clay is to give substitute satisfactions through the free acting out of messing impulses, opportunity for sublimative activity (painting pictures and making clay models), gratifying experiences, group status, recognition of achievement, and unconditional love and acceptance from an adult (speech therapist). With these beneficial results as a foundation, speech-training may proceed with sureness and speed.

## Organization and Limitations of Group Activity

The general, prevailing atmosphere is permissiveness. This spirit is stated and exuded by the therapist *especially* in relation to the children's verbalizations. Limitations, control, and denial will arise as members infringe upon the rights and convenience of others, and upon the integrity of school property.

The speech therapist may say: "We are using paints today just for the fun of messing in them. These papers are staying here with me, but smear them to suit yourself. You may mess your hands all the way up to your wrists (demonstrating). Of course it would be fun to cover more of ourselves, but though we can't do that we can talk about it."

This statement may receive a wholehearted response from some children. Others may reveal a great deal of anxiey which they usually verbalize freely. Starting with one finger of one hand, while holding the other hand behind his back, a child may gingerly stir the paint and starch. Usually, before the period is ended, he will have both hands actively working in the paints up to his wrists while he verbalizes what he might *like* to do. At first, the therapist should emphasize the "messing in paints" for the fun of it. When the frightening, messing impulses have been worked through, the child may go on to the sublimation or channeling of them in making a picture.

When the children walk into the room, they find a large piece of wrapping paper on the floor. On it is a smaller piece of paper for each child and one for the therapist. She is sitting on the floor holding a bottle of liquid starch in one hand and calsomine in the other. The children immediately take their places and await the blob of starch. This is sprinkled with the dry paint which the children mix with the starch. It has been found that this method is more satisfactory and quicker than mixing the paints ahead of time. Any smear of paint on the floor is ignored; a smear on their clothing is dismissed with "It will wash out." When the children indicate a need for more starch, they hold cupped hands to receive it, commenting on the good 'squooshy' feeling. They then cover their hands completely with the starch before using it on the paper. Some children work so vigorously that they actually wear through the tough paper. It is important that the therapist anticipate and plan avoidance of anything which might bring negative reaction or penalty to a child because of his activity in the speech class. The acceptance and release he has experienced in the therapy session must be protected. To spare the child the puzzlement and possibly even the criticism of parents if he should take his messy paper home with no picture on it, the therapist expresses her pleasure of his product to the degree that she wants to keep it. She then can dry and store the paint papers for possible future use and reference by the child.

The matter of the child's spattered clothes may be a source of concern to the parents or other teachers that could react unfavorably upon the child's therapy. If there are no washing facilities at hand the children are sent to the lavatory in staggered rotation so as to prevent their reacting to their free activity by "whooping down the hall" and thus incur the possible censure of other authorities in the school. The therapist may instruct: "Jimmy, I'll open the door for you so you can walk down the hall and back yourself through the lavatory door. You will find that the paint cleans off better if you use just water first before you use soap. I'll see you next week. Goodbye. Now George, I'll open the door for you."

Any offer on the part of a child to help clean up the paints is appreciatively declined. The large paper for floor protection may be folded, rolled, and carried or stored for repeated use. Many papers for individual use may be cut at one time. All of the materials for messing (paper, starch, calsomine, clay) are usually available at each school for the asking. While it may be good therapeutical technique to give the children a choice of colors in paints, this may be impractical because of cost or the problem of packing and handling. If only one color can be used, terra-cotta is recommended because of its close resemblence to mud and soil.

The practical factor of the therapist's clothing comes into importance here too. If she is to enter into the activity of the children and yet quickly move on to another group or school appearing well-groomed, she must provide for a quick change. A full, belted, printed nylon coat-dress is found to be suitable, as it can be slipped on and off easily over the therapist's street clothes. If it becomes spotted by paint, it can be quickly cleaned and dried between sessions with groups of children in the same school, or rolled up and stuffed into a bag with other speech materials and thus carried to another school. Apparently the children do not suspect that this coat-dress is not the therapist's regular garment for the day, for it always looks fairly neat. If the therapist is a man, it is suggested that he wear a cobbler's apron, sport shirt, or some such masculine attire.

With the use of clay, the general plan is the same as that for paints. For each child and the therapist there is a blob of wet modeling clay on the individual sheets (sheets of plastic, this time). Both the clay and the sheets can be used time and again. The plastic sheets are feather weight and easily washed.

*Therapist:* "Usually when you are given a ball of clay you are expected to make 'something.' This is *different* . . ."

*Larry:* "You mean this is *really* different. . . ? We don't have to make anything? We can just squash it and mush it . . . ?"

*Mike:* [evidencing great tension] "Oh I couldn't! . . . Get my hands dirty, no!" His feeling was reflected by the therapist. When the other children in the group became active, he finally ventured to his work area. For the remainder of the period he messed in the clay with increasing pleasure, while repeatedly exulting, "Oh boy, this is the life. Oh boy, this is the life."

These activities stimulated the children to verbalize their anxieties regarding messing. They gave one another support in relating their unhappy experiences with their parents on this subject, and thus in many ways played the part of therapist for one another.

*Larry:* "OOOh gee. This feels good . . ." [humming continuously the tune "The High and The Mighty" while making graceful, whirling designs, then a tree, and finally a circus tent].
*Donnie:* "This reminds me of playing in mud."
*Bill:* "But we *can't* do that anymore . . . that's baby stuff, and I'm almost *ten* . . . [plunging his hands into the clay]. Gee, you're good to us!"
*Gene:* "Yeah, I'm glad I came to speech class. . . . We get to play mud-pies on paper!"
*Donnie:* "That's the kind of tree I used to make in kindergarten." (Molding a tree with clay.)

The next group was just as apprehensive and as enthusiastic.

*Gim:* "Looks like it would be gooshy. *You* go first. I'm going to keep one hand clean [immediately puts both hands in]. Oh boy, if Kim [twin sister] sees this she's going to have fits. Wonder what our mothers would think if we brought this home? If she blew her top we better start running. . . . Girls of all ages drive me crazy, boy."
*Judy:* "I know I don't want to play mud pies . . . because my mother won't like for me to get dirty. This clay is O.K. though."

Susie, a little six-year-old girl and a ward of the court, was hospitalized for months following cruel mistreatment by her mother. She had been able to verbalize her fears only to the extent of saying: "I have two Mommies. I did have a bad Mommie; but now I have a good Mommie." On the seventh session she participated in the use of finger paints and clay for the first time. The use of these materials triggered her anxiety regarding the final traumatic experience—being placed in a tub of scalding water. She told of her experience and for the first time her speech was clearly intelligible (she had severe infantile speech). She started her story with: "I'm not afraid of the tub anymore . . ." and ended on a happy note, telling of her experiences and happiness in her new home.

## SPONTANEOUS WORD GAMES

### Rhythmical Hand-Clapping

The children, including the therapist, sit in a circle. A four-beat rhythm is established, using open hands. For each of the first three beats, everyone pats his hands on his knees. On the fourth beat, he brings his hands together in a soft clap:

| 1 | 2 | 3 | 4 |
|---|---|---|---|
| knees | knees | knees | clap together |

The children soon learn that the activity is a quiet one so that the verbalizations may be heard. The therapist begins a four-word sentence with the rhythm. As each child has his turn he supplies the fourth word, preferably one not previously used. This game goes somewhat rapidly when the beat is kept constant. Hence, the word supplied by the child is fairly spontaneous. Of course a child will sometimes "block" or "draw a blank." When this occurs, the rhythm is continued until the child can supply the last word. Reinforcement is supplied by the group repeating immediately in unison the statement completed by each child. The statement, "The body can———," holds great opportunity for the exploration and expression of the child's feelings. The whole group (led by the therapist) begins the hand-clapping rhythm in silence. The word "body" having two syllables, is allowed two beats, thereby producing a five-beat rhythm in this instance.

knees    knees    knees    knees    clap

When the rhythm is well established, the therapist says, "The body can see," speaking the words in time with the five beats of the clapping:

| *Group:* | knees | knees | knees | knees | clap |
|---|---|---|---|---|---|
| *Therapist:* (clapping) | The | bo | dy | can | see |
| *Group:* (clapping) | The | bo | dy | can | see |
| *John:* (clapping with group) | The | bo | dy | can | walk |
| *Group:* (clapping) | The | bo | dy | can | walk |
| *Jane:* (clapping with group) | The | bo | dy | can | eat |
| *Group:* (clapping) | The | bo | dy | can | eat |

And so on around the group.

The game may begin with such seemingly benign last words as *look, run, drink,* and so on. However, by the therapist's adventuring forth in taking her turn as a member of the group, the children are encouraged to advance to more threatening words: The body can feel, hear, smell, speak, hurt, ache, cry, fear, laugh, touch, love, hate, fall, squeeze, sleep, bite, kick, hit, dream.

### Ball-Tossing

With the children seated in a semicircle and the therapist in front, she "tosses a word" with the toss of a ball. The child immediately tosses the ball back to her, simultaneously saying the first word that comes to his mind. Any word is acceptable to the therapist, thereby encouraging its acceptance by the speaker and the group. The therapist chooses words with ever increasingly threatening potential: *house, drink, sit, eat, spank, gun, kill.* She can select a string of words that explore one area at a time (sibling rivalry, hostility, messing, sex, and so forth) or she can use words that cover all areas in one setting. Group members should sit fairly close together and be instructed to toss with an underhanded motion. A soft, sponge-rubber ball is preferable to an inflated or hard ball, since it has little bounce and roll should it be missed by one of the group. Skill in catching or throwing is not the issue. The activity serves merely as an adjunct to free expression. It is best to advance around the group at the start. When the children become more accustomed to the mechanics and the spirit of the sessions, the therapist can toss the ball to the children at random.

One round of word-and-ball tossing went as follows:

| | | | |
|---|---|---|---|
| *Therapist:* | House | *Therapist:* | Eat |
| *Tom:* | Live | *Mary:* | Don't |
| *Therapist:* | Drink | *Therapist:* | Run |
| *Sue:* | Milk | *John:* | Away |
| *Therapist:* | Sit | | |
| *Joe:* | Still | | |

In one session the therapist noted that Gloria, an eight-year-old girl, was muttering words to herself when it was the therapist's turn to supply the word. Taking her cue, the therapist asked the child if she would like to "start it." With eager acceptance she told the therapist: "Now you say what I say." She was asking for reinforcement and approval by requesting repetition of the words she would choose. Gloria kept a fast pace of simultaneous ball-and-word tossing while the therapist echoed the word as she returned the toss. Here is the parade of Gloria's words which may be telling a significant story: "Little . . Sister . . Mean . . . Big . . Sister . . Hit . . . Mother . . Mad . . . Daddy . . Whip . . . Bed . . Cry . . . Crib . . Hate . . . Glad . . Hit . . Mad . . Sad . . Glad . . Mad . . Sad . . Glad . . Mad . . Sad . . ."

Variations in the word-ball-tossing sessions may be introduced. One is to toss the ball and a word to the first child. The child is instructed to toss the ball and the same word back. To the same child the therapist will then toss the ball and the first word's opposite, and the child will toss them back. A different word and its opposite are tossed to the second child and so on. After a bit of this play the children usually want to do their own choosing of words and their opposites. Such freedom and courage are heartily supported. The therapist can again progress to more vulnerable areas by her choice of words. One progression may be: eat-drink; big-little; happy-sad; glad-mad; love-hate; save-kill. Another one could be: smooth-rough; soft-hard; warm-cold; pretty-ugly; dry-wet; clean-messy.

## INFANTILE ORAL ACTIVITY

### Spirometer

There is reason to assume that children with functional speech troubles (stuttering, delayed speech, faulty articulation) could profit from the recapture and the channeling of their disavowed infantile oral activities such as blowing, sucking, tongue-lolling, babbling, licking, biting, and chewing. In honor of this assumption an effort was made to adapt some conventional means already recognized in speech correction to elicit some possibly shameful feelings about the mouth and its functions. The spirometer was chosen as affording a possible approach to the problem (Fig. 7). Essentially, it is a small and portable pressure device consisting of two bottles joined by a hollow glass bridge. From each bottle there extends a length of small plastic tubing with a removable mouthpiece. To eliminate the annoyance of sterilization, a mouthpiece can be a short length of a 3/16-inch fountain straw given to each child for his own individual use. One bottle is filled three-fourths full with colored water. By the application of air pressure (blowing) through the straws and tubing, the water is transposed from one bottle to the other through the interconnecting bridge of tubing. The base of the box is a separate piece of wood having three grooved circles for securely holding upright the two bottles and the bottle for straws. The rest of the box is in one piece which fits over the base just described. A handle on the top and hooks on the sides securely hold the two pieces together for easy transportation.

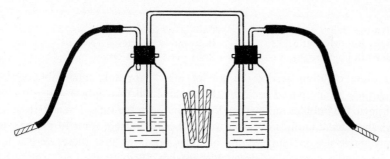

FIG. 7. Modified spirometer.

Two children use the spirometer at a time. The other children are grouped next to them at the table. Each of the two selects a straw and inserts it in the end of a tube. The remaining children join in the verbal-echo part of the game speaking in unison while the two children at the spirometer take turns in performing the activity:

*Group:* "Blow ... Rest ... Blow ... Rest ... Blow ... Rest," etc.
*Child:* Blows ... breathes ... blows ... breathes, in rhythm to the verbalization of the group, displacing one-half of the water in his bottle.

The second child then blows while the first joins the group in speaking. They take turns again while the directions and activity are changed to: "Suck ... Rest ... Suck ... Rest, etc." As the bottle nears emptiness, they blow gently so as to capture bubbles in the glass bridge. The "nursing" movement may be well insured by the variation of the blowing and sucking activities: "Blow, blow, blow, rest; Blow, blow, blow, rest," etc.; and "Suck, suck, suck, rest; Suck, suck, suck, rest," etc,

*Therapist:* "Now see if you can keep these bubbles in the tube and jiggle them by your *speaking* gently on the straw while it is in your mouth. Take turns saying what I say: (one phrase at a time)

| | |
|---|---|
| *Therapist:* | "Bah—Bah—Bah" |
| *First Child and Group:* | "Bah—Bah—Bah" (Bubbles jiggle in tube) |
| *Second Child and Group·* | "Bah—Bah—Bah" |
| *Therapist:* | "Bay—Bay—Bay" |
| *First Child and Group:* | "Bay—Bay—Bay" |
| *Second Child and Group:* | "Bay—Bay—Bay" |

Then may follow the *b* and *p* sequences in full:

| | |
|---|---|
| Bah—Bah—Bah | Pah—Pah—Pah |
| Bay—Bay—Bay | Pay—Pay—Pay |
| Bee—Bee—Bee | Pee—Pee—Pee |
| Bie—Bie—Bie | Pie—Pie—Pie |
| Boh—Boh—Boh | Poh—Poh—Poh |
| Boo—Boo—Boo | Poo—Poo—Poo |

These in turn may be followed with brief phrases suggestive of infantile expression and "loaded" with *b* and *p*. Because these particular sounds jiggle the bubbles, the potential emotional content of the phrases is softened somewhat:

| | |
|---|---|
| Bye-bye Baby | Baby plays pat-a-cake |
| Baby Bobby's bottle | Baby blows bubbles |
| Baby Bobby's buggy | Baby plays peek-a-boo |

The older children accept the use of this "baby-talk" and jabberwocky when they are prepared for it by the explanation that only *b* and *p* sounds will jiggle the bubbles and yet not lose them down the tube. Even sixth-grade boys show great enthusiasm over this oral play. Indeed, some of the phrases given above are the suggestions of older boys. At first there were a few snickers and occasional sidelong glances when "Pee—Pee—Pee" was verbalized. When the therapist showed no negative response to the term or to their reactions, some shrugged their shoulders and accepted it. In subsequent use of this activity, the few children having the initial reaction of embarrassment regarding the term have come to use it as noncommittally as the therapist.

## DRAMATIZATION

### Paper-Bag Hand Puppets

Paper bags, size 6 or 8, have been found very satisfactory for use as puppets. Various characters (in black and white or color) can be drawn on the bags, and by curling the fingers around the bottom fold inside the bag, mouth movements can be indicated with movements of the fingers. At the start the therapist may illustrate several puppets portraying a man, a woman, a child, an animal, or a house. She should have drawn the face so that the mouth is at the fold. When the fold is opened by the fingers inside the bag, the mouth is opened, and when the fold is closed, the mouth is shut. This

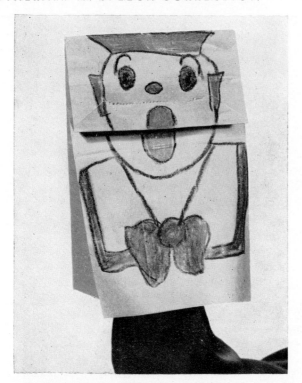

FIG. 8. Hand puppet made from a paper bag by the speech therapist for demonstration purposes.

opening and shutting of the mouth becomes quite realistic for the children (Figs. 8 and 9).

Children become very interested in the structure and manipulation of these paper-bags puppets. They want to make them and they should be encouraged to do so. Some children will make them at home and bring them to school. They will suggest that they make them in school with the group. The therapist may say to the group:

"Make a puppet of anything you wish—a person, an animal, or a 'thing.' It is to be yours to use in speech class only. I will keep it for you and we will use them at times when we tell stories or act out plays. You can see that the mouth must be on the fold of the bag if it is to move when you open and close your hand. Please put your name and age on the back of the bag."

Many of these puppets reveal clearly the child's troubled feelings and focal anxieties. Gene gasped when he finished a full-length, two-gun cowboy and turned the bag over to write his name. "Oh! I must cover *me* up in back or someone will see me without my clothes on my [pause]. Oh! what if a *girl* [pause]." There was "Mr. Two Face," a cramped, double-faced puppet made by a very disturbed boy of twelve who later expressed freely his quandary over his identity. In his case, definitely, the puppet afforded the way for the discovery and better management of his basic problem. Through the

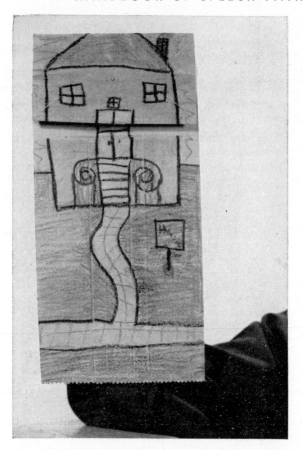

**FIG. 9. House drawn on paper bag (puppet) by a child stutterer.**

drawing and the subsequent characterization of his puppet in acts and speech, the child works out in his new family (therapist and other children) his disturbing and disabling feelings and thoughts.

### Stage and Puppets

A small, portable puppet stage is available to the speech therapist (Figs. 10 and 11). With it come scenery and miniature puppets which are extremely simple to manipulate because they require no strings. Each puppet is mounted on a spring-covered spindle. The floor of the stage has horizontal and vertical slots through which the tiny spindle slides as it is moved by a hand under the stage floor. As many as four puppets may be handled simultaneously when the spindles are held between the fingers of one hand. In this fashion the puppets are moved about on the stage, jiggled up and down when talking, and the heads are turned this way and that. Simplicity of maneuverability is important in puppetering so that interest and activity may be focused in the expression of feelings through characterization.

The puppets may be introduced to the group as a "show." The therapist works the puppets while the children verbalize for them. The children's interest is immediate and strong. "How does it work?" "Bet we could do it," and so on. After some experimenting on their parts, they are promised the return of the stage and characters for the next session. The second session begins immediately with the children choosing parts. Often a child will take several parts. Rarely does a boy reject a girl's role when there are no girls in the group. Later it may prove more satisfactory for one child to take one scene or act and play all parts. This plan not only eliminates confusion in back of the stage, but it leaves someone besides the therapist in the audience. The children are also better able to express more feeling in their characterizations.

Three sets of story-book character puppets have been found useful. The first to be introduced was "Three Little Kittens Who Lost Their Mittens." The "naughty" kittens progressively lost, found, soiled, and then washed their mittens. The role-reversal technique is particularly effective in this medium. The favorite character with the children is the vacillating Mother Cat who alternately scolds, rewards, chastizes, and kisses the kittens.

In producing "Little Red Riding Hood" the children vie for the parts of the Big Bad Wolf, and the Wood Chopper who slew him. Thus they express feelings of aggression toward the Wolf, and the love of Little Red Riding Hood for her father, the Wood Chopper.

"Hansel and Gretel" proves a favorite. The horrible Old Witch of the Gingerbread House is used so vigorously that it is necessary for her crooked nose to be replaced frequently. The stage and one set of puppets may provide two successive weeks of activity in order to give the children ample time to express themselves. For the first week the therapist works the puppets and for the second week she may sit in the audience.

Mary, who had finally been able to speak of her mistreatment by her mother, was made extremely anxious by the appearance of the Witch puppet. "Oh I don't like her . . . I don't want to see her . . . She's mean . . . Take her away . . . ," she wailed, all the while squirming uncomfortably in her chair and placing her hands before her eyes. At her request, the therapist put the Witch below the floor of the stage. Her anxiety was accepted and reflected then and when the promise was made to return the stage the following week Mary said, "Yes, bring it back . . . but not The Old Witch." The following week when the children were dividing their parts by complete acts, Mary lost her reluctance to see the Witch. In fact, she insisted on playing the final act where the Witch tries to bake Hansel and Gretel. Mary worked the puppets enthusiastically and spoke for Hansel and Gretel, "Push . . . and push . . . and *push* . . . the mean Old Witch into the oven . . . and bake *her* into a gingerbread cookie. So there! And I'm glad . . . 'cause she was mean . . . and now she can't hurt little children any more . . . and that's what my Mommie did to me . . . and she burned me . . . and see . . . (pulling her socks down to show her scarred feet) . . . that's what she did and it hurt

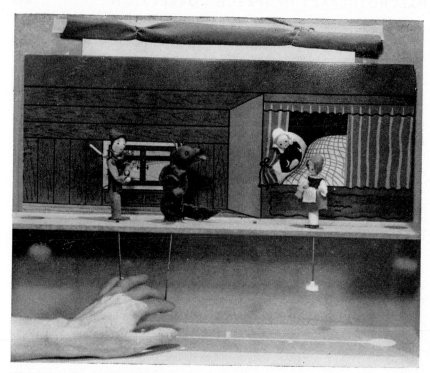

FIG. 10. A small, portable puppet stage with scenery and miniature puppets showing how the puppets may be manipulated by the spindles extending through the stage floor ("Baps" die neuen Nürnberger Puppenspiele. Nurenberg, Germany).

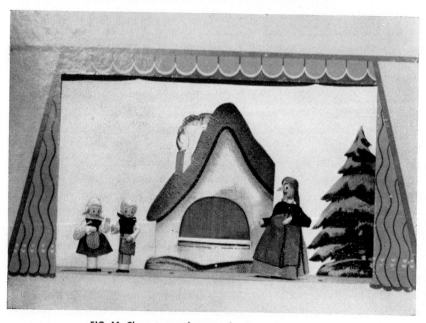

FIG. 11. Characters and scenery for "Hansel and Gretel."

... and *hurt* ... *bad* ... and I cried ... and cried ... and then the hospital ... and now she can't hurt me any more ... (sigh). ..."

## Dolls, Furniture, and Miniature Animals

Family constellations can be constructed by the children from these objects. Family relationships in the dining room (eating problems), nursery (problem of the new baby), bedroom (sleeping and dressing problems), bathroom (cleanliness and toilet-training problems), and living room (parent-child and sibling rivalry) may be dramatized. A child may live through or live out or even correct his perception of members of his family and their interrelationships, and his role in the family grouping. Dinner time, bath time, night time, weekends, all can be portrayed and acted out, frequently with the discovery, acceptance, and channeling of troublesome and handicapping feelings. Some children may find it easier to begin with the animals. It is more acceptable, usually, to give an animal animalistic feelings than it is to give a human being, even an inanimate representation of him, such feelings. Later a child may be able to be more honest and use the dolls. Through a representation of himself (doll or animal), the child may be able to reevaluate and reintegrate his cathectic preoccupations. Judy, who was six, chose the little calf as her central figure. Moving it about she said:

"The little calf was hungry for her dinner and she went to the Mother Horse. 'Will you give me my dinner?' 'I'm not your mother!' [indignantly] Then she went to the Mother Sheep. 'Will you please give me my dinner?' 'No, I'm not your mother. Why don't you go where you belong? I'm not your mother. Why doesn't your own mother take care of her child?' Then the calf went to the Mother Hen. 'Will you give me my dinner please? I'm hungry and no one will help me.' 'No, I'm not your mother. I have many baby chicks of my own to care for, as you can see. What kind of a mother do you have anyhow, to let her baby go hungry? I take care of my babies as I should. Besides you couldn't eat the food I scratch up for my babies. You should find your mother soon.' [Judy went on to the Mother Cat, Dog, etc.] Then the Little Calf went to the Mother Cow [which had a conspicuously full udder with distended teats]. 'Will you give me my dinner?' 'Yes, my Baby, I will give you your dinner. I have lots of warm milk for you. Come close to Mother and drink all you want, because it is all for you.' And the Little Calf drank and drank and drank. When she was full she lay down right next to her Mother. I've got to lay the Mother down too, so they can be close together ... and went to sleep."

The other children of the group who had listened and looked attentively during Judy's performance sat back in their chairs and sighed deeply at the ending. Some held their "stomachs" contentedly. The action, the story, the choice of central character, all reveal the child's problems and attempted management of them. It has been noted, for example, that an obese child will generally place a pig in the leading role. Might it not be equally revealing if a child chose a horse, or dog, or cat, or hen, or rooster? Then, does this central figure want love and warmth, or food and succor, or status and power, or death and destruction? Everything the child says and does in these little lands of make-believe is helpful to him and his insightful helper.

**Draw a Picture**

Each child is provided a sheet of drawing paper and a box of primary-size crayons. He is asked to "draw a picture of your family—all your family." The drawings are significant in relation to the size, placement, posture, and color of the figures. The verbalization which takes place is as revealing as the illustrations. The children literally "talk their way" through their drawings.

Timmy started an adult male figure, but left it incomplete. Next he drew a boy's figure, and then a house having a prominent roof, chimney, and smoke.

*Timmy:*

[Pointing to the incomplete man figure] "I don't know who he is."
[Pointing to the boy figure] "This is brother."
[Completing the man figure] "My father" . . . [The other three members of his family were not drawn.]

Manuel repeatedly told stories of unwanted children. He first drew his father, then mother, then himself. These figures were all in a horizontal line and graduated down in size. Each profiled figure was reaching out toward the next, but each had his back turned and therefore could not see the prominent, open hands.

Gene's drawing was significant of his problem. Gene first drew a man whom he called his father, then changed him to a "stranger." "My Dad doesn't wear a hat, and he's ten feet tall." He wrote "10 ft." and "stranger" beside the man figure. Next he drew his mother (one-half height of man), writing "5 ft." above it. The man and woman were drawn with front view. Next, Gene drew himself, but he made a profile figure with his back turned to both parents. Baby Brother was last in line, also a profile picture with back turned to all the rest. The baby was pictured with boxing gloves, and of a size which would be about normal for him if he were normal (he was hopelessly retarded in the infancy stage). Gene had often expressed great hostility toward his brother and guilt concerning his feelings.

**Aggression Games**

A game that may be entitled "You're Gone Forever" is designed to offer the children an opportunity to express hostility and aggression, without destruction of school property and without disturbing the peace of the school. The materials used are:

1. A plastic toy of the weapon type. A small, inflated, plastic baseball bat and a Davy Crockett, soft-headed plastic axe are good. Any similar toy which is unbreakable and noiseless when used will do.
2. A set of cards made up of pictures from magazines, especially selected to illustrate or symbolize people, objects, and relationships such as the following:
Man or a fierce animal (preferably of the ape family)
Woman (attractive), or an article of intimate feminine attire (such as a slip)
Male child
Female child
Woman holding an infant

Bed
Child and bottle or animal nursing its young
Soap, bathroom including toilet, a mother bathing an older child (both sexes)
Dirty-faced child, dirty hands
Knife, scissors, fire cracker
Fire and flames

The idea is to acquire pictures that portray the more common socializing areas in family living. Pictures may be chosen on the basis of both realism (mother nursing baby) and symbolism (scissors or knife for hostile cutting). The therapist may instruct the children along the following line:

"Will you come close to the table and study the pictures so that you may know them quite well. (Allow time for the children to become somewhat familiar with the pictures.) We are going to play a different make-believe game today called "You're Gone Forever." The biggest, strongest, best baseball player in the world was standing up to bat. The ball came toward him and he socked it out of the ball park and the ball disappeared *forever*. The next time he came up to bat the ball came toward him and just as he hit it, it became one of these things that you see here on the cards. He socked it and said 'Take that! You're gone forever' . . . and it was. He felt good. He turned to you, handed you the bat and said 'Batter up.' You choose any card you wish, put it on the chair (a small chair is placed beside the table), use the bat to hit it and say as he did 'Take that! You're gone forever!'"

After one turn around the circle, each child hitting one card, the children may take another turn, each child choosing two cards to hit. The third time around each child may choose three cards. It is interesting to note the high percentage of repetition of cards from a particular area chosen consistently by a child. Many children choose only cards bearing symbolic illustrations at the beginning of the game. As the game progresses, they grow less defensive and gradually dare to choose "reality" pictures.

The same game may be played by changing the story format and using the hatchet instead of the bat:

"You were walking through the woods when you heard a voice saying 'Take that! You're gone forever.' Then you saw Davy Crockett (or Paul Bunyan) making trees disappear with one chop of his axe when he said 'You're gone forever!' . . . He handed the hatchet to you and said 'Your turn,' etc."

Instead of pictures and the axe or bat, plastaline clay and the child's own bare hands may serve well in playing out aggressive feelings. The therapist may say:

"Here are some balls of soft clay, one for each of you. You may make anything that you do not like, or something that scares you."

She places a small ball of clay in front of each child and encourages him with his crude modeling of something which he hates or fears. Then she places a square of plastic sheeting on the table and, demonstrating with her own model, she remarks:

"You may place here the thing which you have made and while saying anything you like such as 'You're gone forever' or, 'I hate you' or 'I'm not afraid of you,' *Smash* it!"

*Freddie:* "You mean it? We can SMASH it?"

*Jerry:* "O course, you dope. Didn't you hear her SAY so?"

*Freddie:* ". . . . . . Well . . ."

Generally, each child smashes his clay model with growing vengeance. A group of children may ask for this game for an entire semester. As a rule, their requests taper off to a trickle during the next term.

## CONCLUDING THOUGHTS

We have not intended to present a complete exposition of the modifications and adaptations of the psychotherapeutical process for use in public-school speech correction. Rather, we have wanted to indicate procedures that might prove provocative of further exploration and testing. The order of procedures, the length of a single session, the number of sessions for each procedure, the number of children in a group, the types of speech cases used, and the training of the speech therapist are points to be settled by further study. Our strong clinical impression is that those procedures discussed here have been sufficiently helpful to deserve further consideration. In using only these suggestions, some children (both functional articulatory and stuttering cases) overcame their speech troubles entirely. Other children improved markedly. Our current feeling is that some form of psychotherapy is the only approach, even in the public schools, to the problem of stuttering, and an important supplementary tool with functional articulatory disorders. We know that some people may want to quibble over psycotherapy. What is it? Is not any good interpersonal relationship a psychotherapeutical one? Are not ear-training and speech exercise really psychotherapeutical? These are hard questions to answer definitively. As we see it, the core of psychotherapy is the resubmission of feared and anxiety-producing feelings and thoughts to the integrating forces (ego) of the person in the presence of a new parent (therapist) who rewards the discovery, acceptance, and channeling of these dreaded feelings and thoughts and does not reward the fear of them. This is not the place to argue the dynamics of the functional speech and voice disorders. It may be enough to state that clinical evidence is piling high to support the worth of psychotherapy as a method of choice with these cases.

## BIBLIOGRAPHY

Bettelheim, B. 1950. Love is not enough. Glencoe, Ill.: Free Press.

Klein, M. 1949. The psycho-analysis of children. London: Hogarth.

Neill, A. S. 1949. The problem family. New York: Hermitage Press.

Plant, J. S. 1950. The envelope. New York: Commonwealth Fund.

Rambert, M. L. 1949. Children in conflict. New York: International Universities Press.

REDL, F., and WINEMAN, D. 1951. Children who hate. Glencoe, Ill.: Free Press.
———— 1952. Controls from within. Glencoe, Ill.: Free Press.
SLAVSON, S. R. 1943. An introduction to group therapy. New York: Commonwealth Fund.
———— 1947. The practice of group therapy. New York: International Universities Press.
———— 1950. Analytic group psychotherapy. New York: Columbia Univ. Press.
WHITING, J. W. M., and CHILD, I. L. 1953. Child training and personality. New Haven: Yale Univ. Press.

CHAPTER 26

# THE CHALLENGE OF FUNCTIONAL DISORDERS OF VOICE

## • William H. Perkins, Ph.D.

FUNCTIONAL DISORDERS of voice are among the most troublesome issues with which the speech therapist will have to deal. He will be faced with uncertainty and conjecture from the initial evaluation to the termination of therapy. There is a dearth of research data to support any definitive theory or clinical approach, while at the same time there is a plethora of supposedly remedial procedures and reliefs. Many of these treatment techniques have been developed from clinical experience, whereas others are probably the product of armchair theorizing. In this chapter we will be chiefly concerned with the development of a rational approach to voice therapy, an approach that employs effective clinical procedures which have evolved from tenable basic assumptions to meet an achievable realistic goal. This integration of assumptions, techniques, and goal will not only provide the clinician with an effective therapeutic program, but it will also constitute a frame of reference for the systematic investigation of the speaking voice.

### A GOAL FOR VOICE THERAPY

The literature on voice teems with a disarray of subjective terminology. What is "good quality"? Everyone talks about it but rarely do two people describe it identically. On the other hand, what is "poor quality"? There are abundant adjectives for it—throaty, pectoral, strident, husky, shrill, hoarse, thin—to name only a few. Again, though, it is every man for himself when specific meanings for these characteristics are examined (Villarreal, 1949; Thurman, 1953).

Basic to the semantic confusion over terminology seems to be a tacit confusion about fundamental objectives in voice therapy. Until we can clarify these objectives, there will be little chance of effecting a practical resolution to this semantic bugaboo. Although some authors have proposed desirable atomistic goals such as pleasing pitch, adequate loudness, and sympathetic quality, the majority of clinicians are probably more keenly aware of what a pleasant voice is not than of what it is. Thus, the goal becomes the removal of undesirable pitch, loudness, or quality attributes. This is a negative approach to voice therapy which provides as much direction and guidance as would be given a taxi driver if he were asked to take his passenger any place but where he was. Unfortunately, the speech clinician tends to be preoccupied with how the patient should not sound instead of how he should.

## "Good Quality" as a Goal

The establishment of a positive goal to work toward poses a vexing problem. "Good quality" could be considered as an obvious answer. However, this solution creates more problems than it solves. "Good quality" is a highly subjective concept with everyone entitled to his own prejudice. Consider the plight of the therapist who unwittingly accepted a fifty-year-old dysphonic woman on her own terms. At the outset, her terms seemed innocent enough. She merely requested that she acquire good vocal quality. An initial recording was made; they both agreed that she didn't use her voice very well but that there was hope, and therapy began. Both the therapist and the patient labored diligently. Several months later, the clinician felt sufficient progress had been made to justify termination of the therapy. She was as close to "good quality" as he felt she could get. A final recording was made and when it was played back the woman was furiously indignant. She accused the therapist of quackery for taking her money merely to teach her to sound like herself. Clearly, her concept of "good quality" was quite different from his. She finally revealed that what she wanted was a voice totally unlike her own, with a "quaver in it like Frank Sinatra has." This unfortunate incident would have been avoided, perhaps, if agreement could have been reached early in therapy as to a mutually acceptable goal. Either the patient should have recognized her limitations and worked for the best voice of which she was capable, or she should not have been accepted for treatment on her own terms.

Frequently, "good quality" as an objective is unrealistic as well as being, on occasion, downright embarrassing. Although it is an elusive term to define and standardize, still there does seem to be broad agreement as to its characteristics. Miller (1957) found that members of an average audience correlated highly with each other in their discrimination of good from poor voice quality. In any event, our clinical experience suggests that some people are not capable of achieving "good quality" by broad standards or by their own. Most functional voice cases can be helped to sound better, and some may actually achieve what would be considered "good quality." Regardless, though, of the changes wrought, the great majority of patients will still sound like the same person at the end of therapy as at the outset, albeit improved. That is, Joe Doakes will still sound like Joe Doakes despite his progress; he will probably not lose his vocal identity. This fact is quite disturbing to some seekers-after-good-quality. As with our fifty-year-old dysphonic lady, these vocal malcontents cannot be satisfied with sounding like themselves, they must sound different if their personal standards are to be fulfilled. Many a voice has suffered from this unrealistic striving to achieve something vocally that the speech equipment was not designed to produce. We cannot all be John Barrymores or whoever else we might consider to be an exemplary vocal model. Both therapist and patient will reach agreement more easily on the course therapy should take, be more satisfied with progress, and be happier with the end result if the goal to be achieved is more realistic than that of "good quality."

### Efficient Voice Production as a Goal

What, then, constitutes a realistic goal for voice therapy? The key to the answer lies in the selection of universal criteria for evaluating the effectiveness of any type of voice production. Van Wye (1936) presented the concept of the efficient voice as an objective for which to strive. He proposed that the ideal speaking voice should do the work allotted to it, as does any other efficient mechanism, with a minimum expenditure of energy for a maximum of effect and esthetic gratification. These characteristics he assigned to the efficient voice can very well be taken as criteria for evaluating the effectiveness of any type of voice production. They are criteria that stress more than auditory satisfaction as a vocal objective, an emphasis inherent in such goals as pleasing pitch, adequate loudness, or sympathetic quality; they also stress the even more important factor of vocal hygiene.

The efficiently produced voice does provide a realistic therapy goal. A person striving for vocal efficiency would be concerned with producing as pleasant sounding a voice as he is capable of achieving while exerting a minimum of effort for a maximum of vocal effect. Thus, the efficiently produced voice is not measured solely by how it sounds, nor solely by how it feels. A voice that sounds good and feels strained is no more efficient than one that feels effortless and sounds awful.

The evaluation of an efficient voice by all three criteria recognizes the fallibility of human perception, particularly on the part of the patient himself. Vocal tension, effect, and quality cannot be readily determined in isolation. The patient does not really know what he is doing until he manages to do it differently. For instance, he may be unaware of excessive vocal tension until the strain is reduced and he is provided with a basis for comparison. Fortunately, the achievement of one criterion of efficient voice production implies achievement of them all. The most pleasant voice a person can produce will be achieved only when the vocal strain is minimal and the vocal effect is maximal. On the other hand, the presence of vocal strain indicates the capacity for more pleasant quality and greater vocal effect. Furthermore, limited effect suggests unnecessary tension and quality that can be improved. Thus, progress toward efficiency can be perceived in any one of three ways. A failure in one aspect means a failure in them all, so the therapist and patient both have a triple check on the effectiveness of their efforts.

Anyone with a vocal structure that is not pathologically afflicted is capable of achieving a pleasant sounding voice. That is not to say that all of these pleasant voices would necessarily be judged by an average audience as having "good quality." A pleasant voice may be superlative and definitely exemplify "good quality," but it may also be merely a voice that is easy to listen to and that has no particularly outstanding feature to distinguish it. Miller (1957) found that average audiences evaluate efficient voices as having significantly better quality than inefficient ones, but that efficiency and "good quality" are not synonymous, even though they have much in common. The efficient voice in speech, then, will provide the patient with his potentially best quality while imposing a minimal strain on the vocal mechanism.

## Clinicians and Singers

Implicit in the work of the finest singers and voice teachers is the concept of vocal efficiency. The well-trained singer is not content merely to achieve the most esthetically satisfying quality possible. He must also strive for great vocal effect—the singer's feeling of a big full tone irrespective of loudness; a feeling that gives pianissimos clarity in the back rows of large concert halls and prevents fortissimos from becoming shrill and ear-splitting. Nor will he be content with achieving only quality and effect. Frequently, he will have to sing for long periods without tiring. Consider the plight of the Wagnerian tenor who many times must sing almost continually for four hours or more. Much of this time he will be singing with full volume near the top of his pitch range. In terms of vocal effect, this would be roughly equivalent to attending two rousing football games on the same afternoon and screaming continuously from the opening kickoff to the final gun. However, this analogy breaks down completely if stretched beyond the aspect of vocal effect, for the tenor would be singing better and with greater ease at the end of his performance, whereas the football rooter would be aphonic.

**Can voice therapists learn from singers?** Perhaps, after all, we as speech therapists can profit from what the singing profession has to teach us. Speech pathologists tend to assume a proprietary attitude toward voice disorders. This feeling is understandable in view of our close affiliation with the medical profession and our training in working with pathological problems. Unfortunately, though, our attitude not only tends to exclude the advisability of singing teachers working with voice disorders but, more important, it causes many of us to disregard anything singers might have to say.

What, then, can we learn from the singing profession? True, we are not concerned with teaching a patient with a voice problem how to sing high C, nor how to achieve operatic volume, nor how to sing more beautifully than Caruso, nor how to sing at all for that matter. But we are vitally concerned with how to train our patients to utilize their vocal equipment as hygienically as possible so that they may speak extensively, forcefully, and effectively without strain. Hence, we could profit from knowing how the singer learns to perform Herculean vocal tasks many times more difficult than any which might be encountered in a speaking situation. The techniques and principles that he employs are used for controlling the same vocal mechanism we utilize for speech and so they can be adapted to training the speaking as well as the singing voice.

**Vocal efficiency: the singer's goal.** The skilled singer has a clear concept of the type of voice production he is after and well-defined clues to guide him in achieving this concept. Because good singers have vocal character-istics by which they can be readily distinguished from poor singers, it does not follow that the good ones will sound alike any more than it would follow that all the poor ones will be identical. Vocal excellence does not preclude individuality. However, well-produced voices will have the most in common. Bing Crosby's voice is different from Caruso's. So, too, Lily Pons, Robert Merrill, and Ezio Pinza would never be confused with each other. Yet all of these voices have auditory and kinesthetic common denominators that are absent in poorly produced voices. Vennard (1950) describes the auditory common denominator as that quality in a tone that makes it sound "free," gives it "focus" in front, and provides it with the ring of "nasal brilliance." He indicates elsewhere that to produce such a tone a singer must feel that he has "let go" in his throat so that the voice "floats on the breath" and has "depth." At the same time it must not "spread" as in a yell and become "shallow," but rather should come out of the throat, arch high, gather head resonance, tip forward through the nose, and channel into the mouth between the tongue and the teeth (Vennard, 1953).

The average bathtub baritone does not have the vocal endowment to progress far beyond the local church choir. Does this mean he cannot be-come a good singer? If the answer were "yes," the ranks of the voice-teach-ing profession would be decimated. Assuming normal vocal equipment, anyone could learn to sing well if the motivation, perceptiveness, and pa-tience were great enough and the bad habits and psychological barriers not too firmly entrenched. By the same token, anyone could learn to use the speaking voice well. Just as the voice teacher endeavors to guide the student with appropriate auditory and kinesthetic clues to an efficient singing voice, so, too, should the speech therapist guide his patient to an efficiently pro-duced speaking voice.

**Subjective terminology for singers: a minor problem.** Finally, the singer can point the way for us out of the tangle of subjective terminology. We tend to become preoccupied with the manner in which the speaking voice is defective. Accordingly, we are concerned with terminology to classify the defect, presumably because the type of deviation will have considerable bearing on the therapy. Van Riper (1954) recommends different therapy procedures for throaty and gutteral voices than for harsh or hoarse voices. Most speech pathologists suggest specific techniques for managing each aspect of voice production: pitch, loudness, and quality. If, in reality, the therapy should be adjusted to the specific defect, then we are compelled to reach agreement on our subjective terminology for classifying these defects. This compulsion has undoubtedly contributed to the numerous studies of this problem (Curtis, 1942; Thurman, 1953; Sherman, 1954; Van Dusen, 1941).

Singing teachers are faced with the same dilemma, for the singing voice can go wrong in even more ways than can the speaking voice. Nonetheless, they have approached the problem differently. Although they have their semantic difficulties when they attempt to detail what is wrong with a voice as well as when they attempt to describe subjectively how it should be produced, still their confusion is not so great. Their attention is not primarily on cataloguing the various vocal defects. They are concerned with achieving an efficiently produced voice that feels effortless, has power, and sounds good. Since fine singers have relatively specific subjective clues to guide them in this achievement, and since these clues are universal regardless of the nature of the voice deviation, it matters little whether the student starts with a harsh, strident, husky, or nasal voice—the final common goal is vocal efficiency.

The voice therapist's basic problem, then, is not actually one of terminology. He will undoubtedly continue to be plagued with communication breakdowns when he lapses into subjective jargon, but this need not constitute a hazard to his therapeutic effectiveness. The human voice is a product of such a complex dynamic interaction of phonation, respiration, resonation, and articulation that it cannot be treated effectively in segments. Changes in pitch, quality, and loudness cannot be isolated from each other; a change in one implies a readjustment of the dynamics of the other two. Moreover, the majority of these physiological readjustments must occur in laryngeal and pharyngeal areas singularly devoid of kinesthetic awareness. In other words, we have little, if any, conscious sense of movement or tension in the muscles of the larynx and pharynx. Monitoring the activity of these muscles as they affect pitch, quality, and loudness can only be accomplished through listening to the tones produced and feeling the accompanying kinesthetic sensations such as they are. These sensations must, incidentally, be described subjectively, for they seem to have no direct connection with the muscular activities involved. Hence, the primary concern of the speech therapist should not be with isolated disorders of pitch, or loudness, or any one of the myriad deviations of quality, but rather should be with the whole voice in all of its aspects. Either it is produced correctly in each respect or the total production is faulty.

There are infinite varieties of voice disorders with infinite degrees of severity, but the correctly produced efficient voice allows little room for variation. This is not to say that the efficient voice is inflexible. Quite the contrary is the case. It allows the greatest range of pitch, loudness, and quality manipulations. A speaker can alter his volume and inflections, speak endlessly and effortlessly, but he cannot vary far from the auditory and kinesthetic characteristics common to efficient voice production if he is to maintain his vocal effectiveness. In short, the therapist's primary concern need not be with classifying and describing how the voice is wrong; rather the concern should be with how to set it right. The clinician's task is to know the common denominators of the efficient speaking voice so that they may be taught to any patient, regardless of the voice disorder.

## A Summary of Objectives

Briefly, there are several inferences to be drawn from the discussion thus far. We need a clear positive working concept of what we are trying to accomplish in voice therapy. We need also a keen awareness of auditory and kinesthetic clues to help us guide the patient in his efforts. And finally, we need to learn techniques that will actually effect the desired changes. These objectives will provide us with a revised basis for investigating the physiological, physical, and psychological aspects of voice. From such investigations may come improved techniques, a better understanding of vocal disorders, and a clearer definition of the speech therapist's role in the management of voice problems.

## PREMISES FOR VOICE THERAPY

A truly effective clinical approach to the management of functional disorders of voice must be predicated on tenable postulates as well as incorporate a body of therapeutical procedures which have been empirically proven in clinical practice. The premises fundamental to the program of treatment to be proposed range from ethical to physiological and psychological. These are not intended in any sense to be inclusive. The human voice is so inextricably a part of man's existence as a social being that its influence permeates every facet of our civilization. Accordingly, we have been quite arbitrary in selecting only three areas of primary concern to the clinician who attempts to integrate his concepts of voice therapy. Included, for example, could have been an anthropological discussion of variations in voice patterns from culture to culture, or an historical account of changes in vocal ideals. Such discussions have been avoided, since the assumption was made that this chapter was being written for adherents to our Western culture in the twentieth century.

## An Ethical Premise

We have used the term *ethical premise* knowing full well that it is a loosely conceived classification. It was chosen to emphasize the importance of the voice therapist's relation to the medical profession, especially as regards otolaryngology. Of all the disorders of speech, vocal disturbances involve the greatest potential danger. This is particularly true of functional problems of voice. If the disorder were clearly organic, as in cleft palate or cerebral palsy, the danger would be minimized. It would be a situation in which medical responsibility was clearly indicated. Not so with the functional voice case who presents himself initially to the speech therapist for diagnosis and treatment. The presenting complaint may be merely a slight huskiness, breathiness, or soreness in the throat, or it may be aphonia following a severe chest cold. Superficially, none of these symptoms appears exceptional nor therapeutically complicated—and therein lies the danger. A naive clinician unfamiliar with ethical considerations and equally unfamiliar with early indications of organic involvement might proceed on his own and discover that the patient's vocal condition worsened with treatment.

**Responsibility in pathological cases.** The physician's responsibility unquestionably includes any voice case with demonstrable laryngeal pathology such as papillomas or lesions of the larynx. But what of vocal nodules? After all, these usually result from laryngeal abuse in which the cords have been irritated at a point of contact along the edges and have developed a callus-like growth that prevents the folds from closing normally (Curry, 1940). Although the nodes may be surgically removed, a good chance exists that they will reoccur if the vocal apparatus continues to be misused. Does not the real solution in such cases lie with the speech therapist? Yes, insofar as the actual therapy itself is concerned, but it should be undertaken within the scope of medical responsibility. For example, a young lady with symptoms of dysphonia presented herself to an experienced therapist who suspected that the problem was caused by vocal nodules. A referral to an otolaryngologist was made and the therapist's suspicion was confirmed. The nodules were removed and after adequate vocal rest, the case seemed to be closed. Some time later the lady returned in her original dysphonic condition. Careful investigation of the etiology of the problem revealed that she was a swimming instructor who taught at an indoor pool. The tile surfaces in the room contributed to a constantly high noise level. As a result, she habitually shouted her instructions. This time, the otolaryngologist decided on prolonged vocal rest to gives the nodes a chance to disappear, which entailed a change of jobs, and on vocal rehabilitation to help her use her voice with less strain. Although the speech therapist carried out the treatment, which was successful, nevertheless the final responsibility in this case rested with the physician.

**Responsibility in hysterical cases.** Hysterical aphonics display an annoying affinity for their disorder. As with all hysterical conversion symptoms, they tend to exhibit *la belle indifférence* to their lost voice. The treatment of these patients with symptom management procedures is usually unrewarding. Sokolowsky and Junkermann (1944) and Moses (1954) have described procedures that trick or shock the case into vocalization. However, none of these authors offer much encouragement for this approach. Loebell (1944) suggests that early treatment is essential to good prognosis, and West (1938) sees little hope at all for the confirmed hysteric. Clearly, hysterical aphonia is a psychological problem that demands expert psychotherapeutic treatment.

A severe example of hysterical loss of voice, among other symptoms, was that of a forty-six-year-old veteran referred to a speech therapist for an aphasia evaluation. The clinical history revealed a man who had been in and out of hospitals for more than twenty years with diagnoses of malaria, nervous breakdown, duodenal ulcers, exhaustion, alcoholism, and delirium tremens. During some of these periods of hospitalization it was noted that he exhibited periods of bizarre behavior, tendencies toward mutism, deafness, and hysterical combative behavior. His life history was characterized by borderline psychotic functioning and was colored by periodic civil court actions, an unstable work history, chronic alcoholism, and venereal disease, all of which he denied. This patient came to the examination room in a wheel chair, unable to walk or use his right arm. He presented a typical case of right hemiplegia with motor aphasia, except for some discrepancies in response to the testing situation. His oral attempts to respond to test questions resulted in a soft whisper that sometimes became completely inaudible. He seemed alert to all the test questions and exhibited no receptive language disturbances. Moreover, he was able to print all of the answers quickly and correctly with his left hand although he claimed to be right-handed. The loss of speech and hearing, he maintained, had been developing over a ten-year period, although there was no medical evidence of tumor or trauma to associate with this condition.

In view of the history and test results, the clinician recommended that the patient be referred for a psychiatric interview, since the evaluation of aphasia was questionable and aphasia therapy would therefore be of doubtful value. The psychiatrist administered sodium amytal. Under the influence of this drug the patient discarded his symptoms, was able to talk and walk, lost his aphasia, began to use his "paralyzed" right hand, and seemed to hear better. His behavior under amytal was consistent with the diagnostic impression of hysterical conversion syndrome with hemiparesis, hysterical deafness, and mutism. Subsequently, when the effect of the drug began to wear off he became disturbed, belligerent, and aggressive and had to be transferred to a neuropsychiatric hospital. Shortly thereafter, the symptoms of right hemiplegia and mutism returned; he became an ideal patient and was transferred back to the domiciliary area where he was permitted to come and go freely. The psychiatric impression was that of a man who was psychotic but who could function as a neurotic without danger to himself or society providing he retained his hysterical symptoms.

When a person defends himself against the revelation of unacceptable feelings by losing his voice, the intensity of the need is implied in the desperation of the defense. He could do little short of suicide or reclusion that would sever him more effectively from society. Abruptly removing his symptom without resolving his conflict, a difficult task fortunately, would actually do him a disservice. He would then be hard-pressed to marshal new defenses to prevent a traumatic exposure of the feelings he dares not face. He might relapse into aphonia and resist direct treatment of his voicelessness more vigorously lest he again be deprived his defense. He might relinquish the aphonia in favor of the loss of some other function. Occasionally, hysterical conversions are chased around the body like undesirable aliens being forced from one town to the next; as the culprit is discovered and driven from one organ, refuge is sought in another. Finally, he might be left in a state of anxiety, unable to satisfactorily repress his feared impulses and powerless to cope with his feeling of utter misery. Unless the speech pathologist is a skilled psychotherapist, his services will be of little value to the hysterical patient, so he should reserve such cases for the psychiatrist or clinical psychologist.

**Responsibility in diagnosis.** What, then, of the purely functional disorders such as nasality, stridency, huskiness, and falsetto which will constitute the majority of voice problems the speech therapist will encounter? Must these be treated under medical responsibility, too? West says (1938, pp. 82 ff.) that

. . . if the speech worker has not the technique of viewing the larynx, he is presented with two alternatives, either to refer every case of voice defect to the laryngologist or to begin the training of these cases without such reference and to run the grave danger of working with a case in which actual pathology exists. If he adopts the second alternative his professional negligence is going to "slap him in the face" eventually. Hence he should either frankly refuse to accept voice cases or else be so well acquainted with the normal larynx that he can recognize deviations from normalcy and refer all such deviant cases to the laryngologist. It is not to be expected that he will be able to diagnose the pathology but only to recognize its presence.

Although we agree that it is most desirable for a speech pathologist to recognize laryngeal deviations when he sees them, and that he is entitled to considerable personal satisfaction if he is skilled in laryngoscopy, we nonetheless would hesitate to accept a voice patient on the basis of a nonmedical examination. When the speech clinician undertakes laryngeal examinations with a view to referring to a laryngologist only those patients who are organically deviant, then he is assuming an obligation that he is probably not prepared for by training and is certainly not prepared for ethically or legally. Regardless of how well trained the speech therapist may be, the chances seem slim that he would be as equipped to recognize early symptoms of laryngeal pathology, structural anomalies, or endocrine factors contributing to laryngeal disorders as would a physician, particularly a laryngologist.

Moreover, even if he were as well trained he still would be assuming the responsibility for differentiating between psychogenic and physiogenic voice problems. This dichotomizing the ill person into psyche and soma and assigning only the latter to medicine will strike a singularly discordant note with the physician. Medicine with its psychosomatic concept is just emerging from a long struggle to unify the treatment of the patient's mind and body. Any setbacks in this struggle will undoubtedly be viewed with a jaundiced eye (Jenkins, 1954).

Finally, the speech clinician who screens his own patients for laryngeal pathology is placing himself in a legally indefensible position. The finest laryngologists cannot always reach agreement on the nature or extent of an involvement, yet on their decision may hang the issue of life or death as, for example, in the case of laryngeal malignancies. The physician has the legal responsibility to make the best decisions of which he is capable and to do all in his power for the patient. With this responsibility, he is also afforded legal protection. Not so with the speech therapist who has neither legal responsibility nor protection. He does have, though, an exceedingly important specialized professional role. When he treats voice cases as a consultant, recognizing that the final responsibility for the patient is in medical hands, or when he accepts only cases for which he has medical clearance, then he will deserve and receive respect and gratitude from other professions for his efforts in rehabilitating patients with disorders of voice.

### A Physiological Premise

So far we have proposed a goal and postulated an ethical frame of reference to guide the voice therapist in his professional endeavors. Now let us turn to the physiological basis on which our direct clinical techniques will be predicated. Earlier, we mentioned the inexorably tight dynamic interaction of respiration, phonation, and resonance in the control of pitch, loudness, and quality. One cannot be changed without influencing all of the others. We can state with reasonable certainty that if a variation occurs in tracheal air pressure or laryngeal tension, a readjustment in the other process will be mandatory if tone production is to continue. Moreover, we know that pitch, loudness, and quality may be affected individually or collectively by alterations in either of these processes. Beyond this general knowledge, little more than educated guesses founded on limited research evidence can be made. For instance, resonance almost certainly contributes massively to all aspects of the voice, but the undisputed establishment and quantification of this contribution has yet to be accomplished. Although we could rest our clinical approach on this skeleton of assured information, we prefer to add a bit of flesh to the bones for the sake of those students who like some detail in their rationale.

Because we are primarily concerned with revealing the logic behind our insistence on treating the voice as a nondivisible whole, we will limit our discussion to pertinent issues and not attempt to develop a complete theory of vocal functioning. Hence, attention will be directed briefly to resonance and primarily to phonation because it best exemplifies the intermeshing of mechanisms for the control of the various aspects of vocalization. Respiration, of course, is basic to phonation, so intratracheal air pressure can be accommodated as one of the integral factors in the dynamics of laryngeal functioning.

**Resonance.** Resonation is a separate entity. That is, a sound can be produced by respiration and phonation without assistance from resonance, although such a sound would probably more closely resemble a squawk than a tone. Undoubtedly, the voice is influenced mightily by resonator adjustments. Dunn (1950), Joos (1948), and Delattre (1951) have shown that a change in vowels, which is equivalent to a change in quality, is closely associated with a change in the dimensions of the oral and pharyngeal cavities. Harrison (1956) found, though, in a study of pharyngeal and laryngeal resonator adjustments basic to efficient and inefficient voices that aside from a lowering of the larynx no consistent pattern is present, a finding which suggests that the quality distinguishing one voice from another may be more a function of phonation than of resonation. Fairbanks (1950) has tentatively indicated that the oral aperture dimensions can either facilitate or inhibit volume. As for the effect of resonance on pitch adjustment, it is a disputed issue. According to Erickson (1926) and most other authorities, the fundamental pitch is ultimately determined by the frequency of vocal-fold vibration. However, Drew and Kellogg (1940) reported evidence which would indicate that the voice is not produced by a tightly coupled system. According to them the voice is unlike a trumpet, since they found that pressure waves in human resonators apparently do not work back strongly on the vocal folds to control the timing of each pulsation. On the other hand, Curry (1940), Warren (1936), and Travis *et al.* (1934) felt that the vocal system is coupled sufficiently to allow resonating cavities to influence the frequency of the vocal bands almost as much as they are influenced by them. In any event, Lewis (1936) and Appelman (1953) determined that a change in pitch in the singing voice was associated with a change in the resonator adjustments.

So we see that the dimensions of the oral and pharyngeal cavities are probably altered when a modification is effected in quality, in pitch, or in loudness. May we not conclude, then, that a resonator adjustment intended to accommodate pitch, for instance, would also have a significant effect on both quality and loudness; or, similarly, that an adjustment for quality would influence loudness and pitch just as one for loudness would modify pitch and quality? Thus, insofar as resonance is concerned, the treatment of one aspect of the voice is tantamount to the treatment of them all.

**Phonation and respiration.** The complexity of vocal dynamics is most evident in the interplay of respiratory and phonatory forces. Phonation can be conceived as a continuing attempt by the laryngeal mechanism to hold constant intratracheal air pressure. Thus, the larynx acts much as does a safety valve on a boiler, except that the vocal folds can perform their pressure release function several hundred times a second to stabilize this internal force.

We could reason by analogy from musical instruments and establish the laryngeal adjustments which could be marshalled to hold this pressure in check. Thus, we would say that an increase in length or thickness of the cords would lower the pitch, an increase in tension would raise it, and an increase in pressure would make the tone louder. However, the vocal mechanism is unique; it is not strictly analogous to a trombone, a bugle, or a clarinet in its action, and it resembles even less a violin or piano. Ideally, we would piece together research findings and present an experimentally tested coherent account of phonation. Unfortunately, adequate data are lacking, so we must again speculate from acceptable evidence.

Let us see just what is known about laryngeal action. It has been pointed out that as the pitch rises the vocal folds lengthen, due largely to the tilting action of the thyroid cartilage in relation to the cricoid (Pressman, 1942; Tschiassny, 1944). Further, Pressman (1942) has demonstrated that the glottal length decreases as the cord length increases. The Bell Telephone high-speed motion pictures provide graphic illustration of the thickened billowing action of the glottal edges as they are blown apart at low pitches as compared with their thinned-out aspect at high frequencies and in falsetto (Farnsworth, 1940). We know, too, from studies of vocal anatomy and physiology that the thyroarytenoids are capable of differential contraction. This allows any portion of the glottal edge to be abducted or adducted independently of any other portion (Pressman and Kelemen, 1955).

We also know from the work of such men as Negus (1929) that the greater the air pressure the greater will be the tendency for the cords to be blown farther apart at a more rapid rate, thereby increasing the pitch, the loudness, or both. Moreover, Fletcher (1954) disclosed that at high intensity the vocal folds remain closed longer during each cycle, show greater maximum displacement, and have less variation in length when changes in pitch occur. Furthermore, the cords of those subjects with vocal training were found to be closed proportionately longer and to show smaller maximum displacement during loud phonation than did the cords of those with untrained voices.

As regards quality, Curry (1940) reported the stroboscopic findings of Husson and Tarneaud who graphed the opening, closing, and completely closed phases of vocal-fold action while phonating a low-pitched chest voice, a high-pitched open tone, a high-pitched covered tone, and a falsetto. Briefly, they found that the heavier the voice quality the thicker the folds became, the greater the percentage of time they remained closed during each cycle, and the more abruptly they tended to be blown apart.

We are now ready to formulate a theory of laryngeal action that is in accord with what is known from clinical experience as well as from research work. We postulate that phonation occurs when the balance of power between subglottal air pressure and the resisting force of the vocal lips slightly favors pressure. Otherwise, if the cord resistance to the air were greater the pressure would be held in check and no sound would be made; or conversely, if pressure were strongly overpowering, the folds would tend to be blown apart continuously and a breathy voice would result. Although adjustments in the length of the cords, length of the glottal opening, and in cord thickness and tension are known to accompany changes in phonation, probably only tension and thickness are of prime importance to our understanding of the respiratory-phonatory dynamic balance. The extent to which the vocal folds are stretched is one of the major determinants of cord tension and thickness, whereas the length of the glottal opening can be considered as largely a resultant of cord tension; the greater the stretch the greater the tension, and the greater the tension the less chance the air stream will have to drive the folds apart along their entire length. Therefore, we can view laryngeal effect on pitch, loudness, and quality as a product of vocal band thickness and tension adjustments made to hold the force of the breath in balance.

The pitch of the voice is a measure of how rapidly the laryngeal valve releases bursts of subglottal pressure. When this pressure overcomes the tension adducting the folds, a small glottal chink appears and then rapidly expands as the cords are forced apart. If the tension in the bands is great, they will be quite resilient and will tend to snap closed quickly, thereby preventing a complete equalization of the differential pressure above and below them. Since a big escape of pressure during any one cycle is prevented by the rapid closure of the tightened cords, pressure equalization must be achieved by numerous escapes, hence a high pitch. On the other hand, relaxed vocal lips do not approximate as hurriedly, so the duration of pressure release for each cycle is increased, the need to force the folds apart frequently is diminished, and the resultant pitch is lower.[1]

There has been a tendency to equate cord displacement with vocal intensity. Although this concept is basically sound, it only provides a partial account of the dynamics affecting volume. For instance, students occasionally infer from this equation that blowing the folds farther apart increases the volume by increasing the amount of air rather than pressure that is allowed to escape. A normal tone is not produced by actually driving the breath stream past the larynx and out the mouth. This is amply demonstrated by one of the Caruso legends. He could sing a fortissimo with a candle in front of his mouth and the flame would never flicker. Acoustically, big compression waves are a characteristic of loud tones. Phonation, then, is a process whereby the air is compressed above the folds each time they are driven apart, and these waves of compression, followed by waves of rarefaction of course, are transmitted through the resonators and on to the listener. The amount of compression created above the larynx is directly related to the amount of impact exerted by the head of pressure below the larynx when the cords are displaced. Obviously, this impact will be greater if a given force per square inch is imparted through a wide rather than a small glottal opening, but more important still, the impact will increase as the pressure difference becomes greater.

To build tracheal air compression in excess of supraglottal pressure, there must be some laryngeal adjustment available that will hold the air in check until the desired compression difference is reached. This can be accom-

---

[1] Recent research by Husson (1951, 1952) indicates that the human larynx is a neuromuscular effector in which the vibratory phase of opening is concurrent with action potentials in the recurrent laryngeal nerve. This evidence bears on the present discussion but does not necessarily alter it essentially. If neural innervation accounts for the contraction of the transverse fibers of the internal thyroarytenoids, as Husson reports, then the vocal cords are not just passively blown apart; they participate actively in abduction. Hence, the delicacy of the balance between pneumatic pressure and laryngeal resistance is not critical. However, the pressure-resistance balance would presumably follow the pattern we have proposed, otherwise it would oppose rather than augment this neuromuscular action.

plished by alterations of cord thickness. For the sake of clarification, let us speculate on the adjustments we would anticipate if a singer maintained his pitch and increased his volume. First, we would expect the glottal edges to thicken and concurrently thoracic compression to become greater. Just as more energy is required to move a large obstacle as compared with a small one, so, too, more pressure is needed to displace thick as compared with thin vocal edges. Thus, the more densely compressed air would be opposed not by greater cord tension which would raise the pitch but rather by more massive lips which would necessitate a longer buildup of a greater head of pressure to separate them. Moreover, when they did part they would tend to be driven farther asunder by the greater differential pressure than they would have had they been thinner and offered less resistance. So we see that vocal intensity mounts as the glottal edges become more massive, maintain their closure proportionately longer during each cycle, require a greater force of air to push them open, and yield to the force with more extensive displacement. In short, vocal intensity mounts when the supraglottal air column is presented with increasingly forceful impacts of compressed air.

The contribution of phonation to quality with its multiple dimensions cannot be uncovered readily by the mere exercise of logic. We must take these laryngeal alterations that research has demonstrated are associated with changes in quality and do our best to develop a reasonable account for their influence. The force with which the cords are blown apart and the extent to which the glottal edges billow as they are displaced are apparently the two most significant phonatory events to be considered. We know that the folds are thick, tend to remain approximated during a large portion of each cycle, and open more abruptly than they close to produce a heavy quality much the same as they adjust to produce a loud tone. The effect of this is probably similar to that of a firecracker which explodes rather than fizzles. An explosion, whether it be from powder or a puff of pressure, is sharp and firm, and these qualities are characteristic of clear voices. As a tone becomes thinner the puffs become less decisive until, in falsetto, the cords open at the same rate they close and remain apart for most of each cycle, a situation not conducive to the explosive release of compression waves. We also know that changes in pitch are accompanied by changes in vocal-band thickness provided changes in quality are made. That is, the glottal edges will be thin for a high thin tone but they will be thick for a high heavy tone. Since the folds have been shown to billow like a flag in the breeze when thickened to produce low tones, they may also billow when thickened for high heavy ones. Although experimental evidence on this point is lacking, the ripply action along the edges could be a basis for laryngeal contribution to the overtone complex perceived as heavy voice quality.

**A summary of physiological premises.** Throughout this section we have been leading toward a single conclusion: the mechanisms that control all aspects of the voice are bound tightly one within the other. We can state with considerable certainty that resonance adjustments for pitch, loudness, and quality are closely intermeshed. We can state the same for phonation and respiration with even greater assurance. A change in pressure, for instance, must be countered by a change in thickness, affecting loudness and quality, or a change in tension, affecting pitch and quality, or a change in both, affecting the entire vocal product. The dynamic balance once upset in this triad of laryngeal forces can only be restored by reordering all three factors in relation to each other. Practically, this means that pitch, quality, and loudness are interdependent; one cannot be altered without affecting the mechanisms controlling the others. The treatment of isolated aspects of the voice is like attempting to juggle three eggs while concentrating on only one. This is not to say that these variables cannot or should not be considered separately for purposes of research. Certainly the investigation of vocal activity is a proper task for the scientific method. From experimentation may come information of great clinical significance. But the modification of voice patterns is far too complex an undertaking to be amenable to an atomistic scientific approach. Regardless of how much quantified data we may accumulate, voice therapy will always be an art.

## A Psychological Premise

The manner in which the learning process can be employed in the treatment of functional problems of voice is so basic to therapy as to be almost the sole prognostic determinant. If we could assume an uncontainable desire by the patient to alter his vocal habits, or if we were concerned with teaching skills such as arithmetic, spelling, or badminton which are acquired during school or adult years and are used only for short periods intermittently throughout life, then our task as voice therapists would be considerably simplified. We would only have to be concerned with isolating for the patient the clues to guide him in modifying his vocal production, directing his practice in making permanent the new skill, and praising his correct efforts while pointing out his errors. Rapid improvement would, of course, be anticipated. Rarely does successful voice therapy even vaguely correspond to this ideal plan. This section will be devoted to a determination of the psychological factors that retard progress and to a consideration of what to do about them.

**Vocal habits resist change.** From birth until death, an individual uses his voice. Just as the developing infant learns to focus his eyes, learns thumb-forefinger opposition to grasp objects, learns the co-ordination patterns for walking, so, too, he learns intricate adjustments for producing his voice. The fact that he doesn't know he is learning a skill only makes the habit more immutable. Observation indicates that the basic vocal patterns are well established before the child acquires intelligible speech. Unfortunately, meager research has been done on this point. If the observation is correct, then the various aspects of vocalization that must be isolated and identified before they can be changed are originally learned at a preverbal level, so they are learned without benefit of language symbols (Dollard and Miller, 1950). This probably contributes to the difficulty all voice therapists encounter when they try to communicate to their patients with words exactly what is to be done.

Usually, after patients have acquired some experience associating verbal symbols with vocal adjustments they are much easier to instruct and progress is more rapid. One gentleman with whom we worked was instructed at the outset of therapy to strive for the feelings of "an open throat that does not pinch the tone." He had not the vaguest notion of what we were talking about, but he continued to struggle along for some weeks on other aspects of voice production for which our instructions had more meaning. Eventually, when we returned to the problem of the open throat, the original directions were repeated. He vocalized as requested—with success—and said, "That feels good. Why didn't you tell me to do that before?" A little experience had enriched the same words with considerably more significance.

**Feelings are exceedingly resistant to change.** An appeal to logic is just so much time wasted when emotions run high. For instance, the most splendid arguments would never convince a dyed-in-the-wool Democrat that he should be a Republican. Vocal habits are equally as resistant to permanent alteration as are feelings, and for much the same reasons. Voice production is so intertwined with emotion that a change in feelings cannot help but produce a change in voice. Every singing teacher knows that the surest method for altering quality is to have the student either empathize with the tone someone else sings or produce a tone with a specified feeling such as anger, tenderness, or hatred. How did this intimate relation come about? Again the research facts are meager, so we must work from observation to speculation.

The earliest sound an infant makes is, of course, the birth cry. This reflexive vocalization probably has little, if any, emotional significance. Soon, however, a wail signifies discomfort or pain, and within six months many mothers will insist that they can distinguish between a wail for dry diapers and a wail for food, while all mothers will recognize the cry of exhaustion that signals bedtime. Clearly, the infant is learning to differentiate his vocal responses according to his needs. Months before the first intelligible words appear, parents listening to their child will have little doubt about his current feeling, whether it be anger, love, frustration, or hunger. The connections between emotions and vocal response will be firmly established.

Then there is much cooing and gurgling for many of the earliest months. From this activity may well stem the basic patterns of adjustment for good voice production. The baby only coos when content and relaxed, a condition which implies the low oral, pharyngeal, and laryngeal tension fundamental to the efficient voice. Unfortunately, some infants are deprived of this early contented vocalization by being in a state of continual discomfort. The discomfort may result from colic or an incorrect formula, or it may stem from parental rejection and tension. A baby left to "cry it out" is a baby left with his needs unsatisfied. Parents with an unwanted child, or parents whose own dependency demands are so great that they feel oppressed with the responsibility for their child, may ignore the baby's cries by rationalizing that too much attention will spoil him. The infant undoubtedly learns from this treatment, but what he learns is the feeling of unworthiness, of uncertainty that he will ever have his needs met, of hopelessness, of the futility of trying. These are feelings he will carry with him through life. They are feelings that will inevitably produce tension.

On the other hand, a baby may receive considerable attention and still remain in a state of discomfort. A tense mother means a tense child (Sullivan, 1953). Perhaps she is concerned for her infant's health, perhaps she fears he was injured at birth, perhaps she suspects he is deaf, or perhaps she is under pressure from outside sources. No matter why she worries, she will invariably communicate it to her baby. It will be reflected in her voice, in her movements, in the way she holds her infant, in the way she nurses him, in the harshness of her discipline. The terminal result for the baby will be the reinforcement of patterns of tense vocalization and little practice in vocalizing under conditions of relaxation and contentment. The extent to which these early vocal efforts contribute to the mature voice, however, can only be determined by future research.

The case of George, a nine-year-old boy who was seen for therapy to correct a harsh strident voice, may help clarify some of these points. Play therapy and parent counseling were the *modus operandi*. As George tested the therapist in situation after situation and found him to be trustworthy, he began to reveal his need for affection and security. Gradually, with the therapist's acceptance, he proved to himself that he did not have to remain constantly on guard, fearful that anything he might do would bring retaliation. As his proof accumulated, his tension reduced, the volume dropped to a conversational level, and the voice lost its harsh stridency.

Meantime, work with the parents had been focused initially on uncovering present feelings that were contributing to their son's tension. A few insights and some minor alterations in the home environment were made, but nothing of sufficient significance to explain the boy's problem could be discovered. The current home situation was as satisfactory as could be expected in a family with four children. Moreover, all of the other children were happy, relaxed, and confident. Eventually, the etiology became clear. George was born in Minnesota one week before his family moved to the West Coast. They arrived as total strangers without a job, a house, or friends. As if this were not sufficient to create tension in George's home life, another baby was born when he was one and a half years old. Between the uncertainties of his infancy and the usurpation by his newborn sister of the little attention his parents could afford him in that first hectic year, George learned that there was little he could do to win praise and much that he could do to earn stringent words and a whipping.

A final factor contributing to the immutability of vocal habits is the relative permanence of voice patterns acquired as imitations of a speech model. However, a mere smattering of experimental evidence is available regarding this point. Certainly everyone can recall hearing children who sound almost identical to one parent or the other in the way they laugh, tell a story, or complain when they are frustrated. This identity has produced several amusing and sometimes embarrassing situations with which we are acquainted. One young man unable to summon sufficient courage when he was with his girl to ask her to marry him decided to do the job by phone. He dialed her number, heard her voice, and launched immediately into his proposal. The voice then answered, "Oh, I'm so sorry. You must want to speak to my daughter."

The exact nature of such vocal identity is difficult to isolate, and it will vary from person to person. It may be in the intonation patterns, it may be in the manner of stressing words, it may be in the habitual pitch used, it may be in the quality of the voice, or it may be in any combination of these and other factors. Undoubtedly part of the similarity will eventually be a function of how the sounds are articulated, but long before this skill is acquired many children will produce startling imitations of parental voice patterns. Whatever the grounds for this vocal identity may be, if you sound like your father when you are two, you will probably still sound like him when you are sixty-two. The preverbal acquisition of these vocal imitations, again, most likely contributes to their great resistance to modification.

The choice of a voice model to imitate may well provide us with rather permanent audible evidence of the person with whom the young child identifies. Mowrer (1952) has proposed that this process of identification, or secondary reinforcement as learning theorists term it, is basic to the earliest stages of speech development. In formulating his hypothesis, Mowrer observed that talking birds, whether parrots, crows, magpies, parakeets, or Mynah birds, only learned to speak when their human teacher became a love object for them. His observation is corroborated by our own limited encounter with talking animals. We had the rare opportunity of meeting a talking dog, at which time a recording of his "speech" was made. This recording has since been played to hundreds of speech students. Although most of them had difficulty understanding the phrases "I want my mama" and "ride, ride, ride," not one has ever suspected that he was listening to a dog. When this Boston bull imitated his mistress, the quality of his normally doglike voice underwent an amazing transformation. He puckered his lips, extended his chin, and proceeded to emit long sustained phrases of vowel sounds that closely resembled the quality of a deaf child's voice. The dog's mistress had never trained animals before and had no idea she was developing a talking dog in this instance. They lived alone, she spoke to him lovingly as she would to a baby, he was rarely let out of the house without her, he was almost entirely dependent on her for his affectional needs. In fact, he had little opportunity to discover that he was a dog and had an identity apart from his human mistress. Accordingly, the mistress, as per Mowrer's hypothesis, became a love object for her dog. He identified with her and attempted to be like her. Since she talked to him constantly while feeding him and playing with him, he thereby associated human sounds with affection and satisfaction. The more closely he could approximate her sounds, the more successfully he could stimulate and satisfy himself with these human-like noises to which he had associated the good feeling of need reduction. Hence, operating on this autistic self-satisfaction basis, he persisted in his imitative efforts until he could derive much the same pleasure from his own voice as from the voice of his mistress. This is not to say that the dog learned anything close to a human language; he merely learned to approximate the sounds we make in our language.

If birds and dogs can learn to imitate the human voice despite the limitations of their vocal equipment, then is it not reasonable to assume that the incentives which foster this learning in lower species will produce even more exact emulations of the loved person in human infants? Thus, the baby presumably will strive to sound the most like the person whom he loves the best, whether it be mother, father, brother, sister, or nurse. Moreover, the infant will not discriminate between good and poor voice production. He will imitate what he perceives in his chosen model's voice whether it be a shrill tense quality or a clear full tone. If the child is loved sufficiently to start him on the road to speech development, then he will be loved sufficiently to make it worth his while to engage in imitative vocal play from which he can derive autistic satisfaction. We may infer, then, that these early voice patterns, both good and poor, which are perfected through identification, are strongly reinforced by the child's own pleasure in his performance.

The point, of course, as has been the point throughout the discussion in this section, is that the earliest vocal habits acquired may include patterns of tense vocalization. These patterns can be set by learning that took place under frustration conditions or as an attempt to be identical to the person loved. Furthermore, the patterns will be learned without benefit of associated verbal symbols. These word cues could later provide a conscious basis for examining vocalization skills. But the poor voice patient, deprived of this most essential tool for modifying behavior, must struggle along as best he can in his efforts to alter deeply ingrained vocal adjustments.

**Conscious motivation may not be enough.** Were voice production like spelling or arithmetic, then a little motivation would go a long way toward effecting a permanent vocal change. About all that is necessary to correct the high school student's notion that the square root of 64 is eight, not six, is his brief attention, some careful explanation, a few exercises in a math book, and a word or two of praise for his proper answers. In his future sporadic encounters with the square root of 64, he might have to concentrate slightly to recall what the solution should be, but the effort would be only momentary and he could probably afford its expenditure, so a permanent correction in his mathematical skill could be safely anticipated. Were the same student engaging in voice therapy with the same level of motivation, his efforts would be pitifully inadequate. Unfortunately, speech therapists will encounter many patients whose motivation will not exceed and may not equal

that of our high school friend. Voice production, as we have already discussed, is exceedingly resistant to change. Moreover, for any change to be
permanent, it must be effected most of the time the patient speaks. It is one
thing to learn to use the voice effectively for singing or acting—in which the
concentration is on the voice itself—and quite another thing to learn to use
it effectively in everyday speech—in which the focus is on what is being
said rather than how it is being said. Obviously, a permanent modification
of conversational speech requires a tremendous amount of intense conscious
attention and unrelenting practice. Insufficient motivation places patient and
therapist alike in the position of trying to move a mountain with a teaspoon.

Most voice patients who engage the services of a speech pathologist will
at least pay lip service to the desire for change. Some genuinely mean what
they say. Those will be the ones who will work diligently outside of therapy
and show real progress. Others will think they mean what they say, but their
actions will belie their words. They will work hard during the therapy hour
and pledge themselves time and again to the task of continuing the work at
home. Somehow, though, little gets done; something of greater importance
always seems to arise. This group probably constitutes the bulk of voice
cases. For them there is hope. Then there are those who know they don't
mean what they say; it just seems to be what one should say to a speech
pathologist. They are the ones who have been pressured into coming by
some overanxious relative or friend, or perhaps they came because they
felt it would be nice to have an improved voice providing the therapist would
do all of the work. For them, if that attitude persists, there is no hope.

This section is addressed to the unique problem of those who honestly
believe they want help but act as though they really do not. They are consciously dedicated to the job, but their determination seems inadequate to
see the task through. Fortunately, their drive may be sufficient to prompt
them to work for insight into their deeper motives and discover the factors
that are retarding therapy. This assumes that the speech clinician has a good
working knowledge of psychodynamics as well as skill and training in the
use of psychotherapeutic techniques. Without such knowledge, skill, and
training, the voice therapist's position, although far from untenable, is
weakened considerably with these cases. He may persuade the patient to see
a qualified psychotherapist and discontinue the voice-training until motivation is achieved. Or he may refer the patient for psychotherapy and continue
the voice work which presumably will improve as more successful personality adjustments are attained. In either event, the patient will have to be
convinced of the necessity of spending much more time, money, and energy
for therapy than was in the original bargain. The other alternative is not to
refer at all but rather to make the best of a poor thing and do all that can be
done within the limits of the patient's motivation.

Ideally, the speech therapist would be a competent psychotherapist for
those with speech disorders. We are not suggesting that the speech pathologist play at being clinical psychologist or psychiatrist, and certainly we are

not encouraging the usurpation of these roles. What we are stating is the need for speech clinicians to be thoroughly familiar with the psychodynamics of speech disorders and to be well prepared to manage only such speech patients as would be safe risks in a psychotherapeutic relationship, that is, to avoid psychotics, prepsychotics, paranoids, and psychopaths. The benefits for the therapist and the patients of the therapist with such training would be considerable. The well-prepared clinician would have extensive experience working with speech cases and so he would be more familiar with the psychodynamics of such patients than might the clinical psychologist or psychiatrist who encounters speech problems only intermittently in his practice. With insight into the relation between functional disorders of voice and personality dynamics, the therapist would be best able to help the patient improve his voice as rapidly as possible while effecting a more satisfactory personality adjustment.

A plan in practice always seems to encounter more stumbling blocks than one on paper. Regardless of how well trained and how skilled the speech therapist may be, some patients will adamantly resist anything that resembles psychotherapy. They may exhibit a strong conscious desire for a better voice, be perplexed and disturbed at their lack of progress, and still refuse to consider what is apparent to the therapist—the direct or indirect influence their personality adjustment is having on the voice. When such a situation arises, the clinician's tact and ability to subtly persuade may be trained. A head-on approach is usually doomed. One therapist, exasperated at his case's resistance, boomed forth at the shy young matron, "Madam, your voice will never improve until you resolve your repressed sexual feelings." Naturally, he never saw her again. Unfortunately, neither may any other speech pathologist if she decided he was a typical example.

A more felicitous approach to resistant patients is to structure voice-therapy situations so as to reveal to these people, inexorably, that the way they feel has a real bearing on the way their voice sounds. When this point is reached, the therapist will have done about all he can do to motivate the patient for psychotherapy. Either the case will see the necessity for dealing with his feelings and the work will proceed, or he will be so resistant that he will refuse to admit the obvious. If the latter event develops, then the therapist may feel ethically bound to discontinue therapy, unless he believes the patient has a strong enough desire for improvement to enable him to make some further progress.

A middle-aged lady undertook therapy to improve a tight, husky quality that was getting progressively worse. During the clinical sessions she became able to perform all of the individual exercises efficiently and the effects would carry over to a few sentences of her conversation that usually followed the drill work. Inevitably, though, her voice would become tight again when her attention shifted from what she was doing to what she was saying. This was pointed out to her and she struggled valiantly to effect more permanent carry-over, but she could not succeed. Meanwhile the therapist had observed that her voice showed remarkable improvement if she expressed anger. When her inability to progress further became evident, the clinician suggested to her that a connection between her feeling of anger and her voice problem might exist. She resisted this suggestion for some time. How- ever, rarely a session went by that she didn't express anger toward her daughter, thereby providing the therapist with an opportunity to casually ob- serve how startling the change in her voice was when she vented her feelings. Gradually, the effects of this suggestion campaign became apparent. With- out formally acknowledging a shift in the clinical emphasis from drill work to psychotherapy, the shift did occur and she took the lead in bringing it about.

The term *psychotherapy* had unfortunate connotations for her. She as- sociated it with insanity and weird mumbo-jumbo procedures. In this in- stance, a rose was considerably sweeter if it didn't have a name, at least at the outset. She eventually recognized that the manner in which she handled her feelings of aggression as a child was the same manner in which she was still handling them in middle age. As a child, she had considered herself the ugly duckling in the family. When her mother showed preference for the other children, she wanted to strike out at them, but she dared not do this for fear of jeopardizing what little affection she could obtain. Consequently, she literally choked off her anger lest her true feelings be detected. Since she was never consciously aware of developing this defense against herself, she could do nothing to alter it. So as a mother and a business woman she reacted to a sudden increase in frustrations from both situations in a char- acteristic fashion—her voice became choked. It was this circumstance that forced her to seek clinical assistance. As she became better able to accept her anger as an appropriate response to frustration, she became better able to achieve an efficiently produced voice on a permanent basis.

The effect of personality adjustment on voice production is frequently so indirect and obscure as to be almost undetectable. A professor who had undergone extensive psychoanalysis and had studied voice professionally as a singer, actor, and radio announcer used his voice very effectively most of the time. However, if he gave a lecture with inadequate preparation, if his students became inattentive, or if he tried to converse on an unfamiliar topic, then his voice production became quite inefficient. His extensive knowledge of what he should be doing vocally was next to useless when he felt inade- quate and tense. Although the possibility is not inconceivable that his vocal difficulty might have been serving in some way as a defense symptom, an- other explanation would be that his vocal inefficiency was merely an in- voluntary reflection of the tension he felt. The tight voice he experienced in his moments of inadequacy was not essential to his personality dynamics for handling this feeling, since a tight voice contributed little to the prevention of his recognition of this inadequacy. Rather, it revealed the increased ten- sion of the laryngeal, pharyngeal, and oral musculature which resulted auto- matically, whether the professor liked it or not, when he *felt tense*.

As we discussed earlier, a person commences to associate his vocalizations with his feelings from birth. The vocal musculature is so low in conscious kinesthetic awareness and control that anyone will have great difficulty recognizing tension in the throat, let alone being able to relax it. Even in musculature that can be readily controlled consciously, such as in the arms and legs, when we feel tense these muscles will be tense, and when we feel relaxed the muscles will relax (Jacobson, 1951). Only with considerable voluntary effort can muscular adjustments be dissociated from their normal reflection of our feelings. Little wonder then that when we *feel* morose, excited, happy, or sad, we *sound* morose, excited, happy, or sad. The point we wish to make is that any personality maladjustment will tend to create frustration which will automatically effect excessive tension in the vocal musculature. Even though the vocal disorder may not be a direct symptom of the personality deviation, nevertheless the voice will inevitably attest indirectly to the consequent tensions of a personality problem. Again, then, a permanent alteration in the voice cannot be anticipated with confidence until a behavioral adjustment that will minimize frustration is achieved.

Another situation that will produce an unconscious barrier to progress in voice therapy results from a need to function at an immature level. Every speech clinician has probably encountered patients who habitually use a falsetto or speak with a thin immature quality. The vocal impression that these people make may be that they never progressed far beyond a symbiotic relation with the mother. If a clinician accepts this impression at face value and always structures therapy for these cases to increase their maturity, he certainly will not harm them, and much of the time he will be dealing with the critical therapeutic issue, but there will be cases in which he will be tilting at windmills. One young man in his middle twenties engaged a speech pathologist to correct his falsetto voice. The possibility of this deviation being symptomatic of a need to remain immature was entertained, but the diagnosis had revealed a severe hearing loss so the patient was fitted with a hearing aid before therapy commenced. As a result, voice therapy never did commence. The young man's pitch dropped an octave when he received sufficient amplification to hear himself. The wise clinician will not leap to conclusions as to why a person sounds as he does. After all, the young lady with the squeaky little voice may not be regressing, she may be imitating her mother.

Despite the exceptions, immature vocal habits will frequently result from an overprotective environment or from regression. Freud (1920) formulated his concept of regression to explain the reactivation of earlier affectional attachments and levels of adjustment in his neurotic patients when they were frustrated in their attempts to seek gratification and acceptance. Experimental evidence confirms Freud's descriptive formulation and emphasizes that regression is primarily a function of fixation, or habit strength, and only secondarily a function of frustration (Sears, 1944). In other words, frustration merely blocks a person's striving for a more mature adjustment and forces him to return to earlier modes for satisfying his needs. The specific habits to which he reverts will be those that received the greatest reward hence were most strongly fixed. If a person who has been overprotected is not subjected to sufficient frustration to make it necessary for him to change his behavior, then he may grow chronologically older and remain emotionally immature. We are reminded of an elderly bachelor who could never tear himself away from his mother long enough to seek a wife. When his mother died he refused to accept the reality of the situation. A day never went by that he didn't visit her grave. The frustrations he experienced were never sufficient to force him to seek an adult life independent of her. In every aspect of behavior, including his vocal habits, he was and still is his mother's little boy.

On the other hand, if the person is sufficiently frustrated to attempt change and then encounters more frustration with each new act he tries, he will not be able to stay the way he is, he will not be able to mature, he will only be able to regress. He will unconsciously return to an immature level of behavior that was once strongly rewarded. If the frustrations are sufficient, he may even revert to an almost infantile status. Signs of regression can be seen in the way he acts and heard in the way he speaks, in his choice of words, in his articulation, and particularly in the way he uses his voice. For example, a ten-year-old boy was driving his parents to distraction when he was brought in to a speech clinic for therapy. He sucked his thumb, he would not eat regular foods, he cried at the slightest provocation, he whined constantly to be held and rocked, his language was infantile, and his speech was all but unintelligible. The situation was almost classic. He had a brother two years older who was mature for his age and who excelled at everything he tried. Bob, the ten-year-old, was clumsy, fat, and had never had particularly good speech. He had lived in an almost constant state of frustration because of the unfavorable comparison with his brother. However, the tension was not so great that he abandoned attempts to emulate the brother, at least not until another child was born a year before Bob entered the clinic. This additional competitor for parental attention made life intolerable for him. He felt a great need for more affection and acceptance, but he had no idea how to get it. He got in the way and was a nuisance when he tried to imitate his brother. He was miserable if he didn't change and he was miserable if he did. Consequently, he began regressing to earlier fixated levels of development. The more immature his behavior became the more maladaptive it became, and as the frustration mounted his need to regress increased. He finally reached the infantile state he was in when he arrived for therapy. Obviously, no attempt to deal directly with the voice, language, or articulation disorder was considered until the emotional needs of the child were met.

**A summary of psychological premises.** Functional voice disorders, then, not only stubbornly resist change, they also frequently are associated with personality maladjustments that conspire against conscious efforts to effect improvement. The vocal deviation may be directly instrumental in the m adjustment by serving in a defensive capacity against unacceptable feelings or by serving to gain attention as is the case with regressive or immature behavior. On the other hand, the voice problem may be only an indirect reflection of tension resulting from maladaptive behavior. In short, we recognize that the alteration of vocal habits requires extraordinary motivation. Accordingly, we are basing our therapy program on the premise that *real progress will only be made when the balance of conscious and unconscious forces impose a great need for improvement on the patient.*

## PROCEDURES FOR VOICE THERAPY

The human voice, functioning normally or abnormally, poses a severe challenge to anyone who would understand it in any of its aspects. Specifically, the speech therapist concerned with effecting permanent vocal rehabilitation should be prepared to grapple with almost all of the complexities of vocalization. He cannot be content with only changing the voice for intermittent performances, so he cannot be content to know only the techniques for achieving vocal efficiency, nor can he be content to know just the anatomical, neurological, and physiological interrelationships that underlie effective procedures, or the various laryngeal pathologies, or the implications of criteria for efficiency, or the auditory and kinesthetic characteristics of efficient and inefficient voices. He should know not only all of this but also the psychological factors that provided the learning matrix out of which the automatic vocal habits evolved. He should know the possible effects of endocrine imbalance on vocal maturation and functioning. He should know the devious channels through which the personality can exert its influence on the voice. Finally, he should have a full appreciation of the dynamic interaction among all of these facets of voice. Every clinical suggestion given a patient is intimately related to his feelings, his perceptiveness, his body chemistry, his neurophysiology, as well as to the condition of his laryngeal structure and to his patterns of respiratory, phonatory, resonance, and articulatory adjustment. Understanding the complexities of any one of these aspects is a sizable task, yet the challenge of voice therapy is the challenge of understanding the complexities among as well as within them all.

Essential as the knowledge of the complexities of vocalization may be, an even greater need in the preparation of the voice therapist exists at a very practical level. Most speech clinicians are highly sound conscious; unfortunately, not many seem to be very voice conscious. They listen to a speaker or a singer with a vague perceptive set toward the voice, providing they notice it at all. They will probably observe whether or not they like it, and they may note their subjective impression of vocal defect such as harshness or stridency. Rarely, though, will they identify the specific characteristics of a good voice that make it pleasant, yet this is the very ability that is most essential. A speech pathologist would not dream of allowing a student clinician to drill a patient with a deviant [s] if the student were unable to recognize the characteristics of a correct [s] when he heard it. Still, this is the equivalent of what happens in the treatment of voice disorders. Just as a knowledge of exactly how phonemes should sound is critical to the clinician concerned with articulation, so, too, a knowledge of exactly how the voice should sound is equally critical to the therapist concerned with voice. This does not lessen the value of recognizing as precisely as possible how articulation is deviant or how the voice is defective. It merely relegates concern for what the patient is doing wrong to a secondary role and focuses attention primarily on what he should be doing to set it right.

Our discussion of therapeutic procedures will reflect our chief concern for achieving efficient voice production. We will continue to stress that vocalization is either correct in all respects or it is altogether faulty. Pitch, quality, and loudness disorders should usually not be considered separately, because they are not functions of separate processes. A change in one implies a readjustment in the mechanism controlling the others. However, problems caused by flaccid adjustments, such as breathiness, require different emphasis in the treatment approach from those stemming from tension, which includes the majority of vocal troubles. We will make little effort to differentiate among specific manifestations of these difficulties. Although different patterns of tension or flaccidity undoubtedly produce different acoustic results which could possibly be isolated and labeled, a thorough job of identifying these patterns would assume staggering proportions; inefficiency can result from an infinite variety of improper adjustments, whereas efficiency can be achieved in only one way. Therefore, we should devote our clinical and research efforts to establishing specific characteristics by which we can identify our goal before diverting energy to secondary considerations.

### Characteristics of Vocal Efficiency

A phonetician listening to speech can readily identify the sounds he hears: [i] varies slightly from [ɪ] and is quite different from [a]. The more skilled the phonetician, the finer the distinction he can make among sounds. However, he would be hard pressed to *describe* just how [i] sounds different from [ɪ] or [a] or any other sound. Were this necessary he would inevitably become embroiled in subjective descriptions with which he would attempt to arouse in his listener an auditory image of [i]. Fortunately for the phonetician, this procedure is unnecessary since he will normally communicate with people who are already thoroughly familiar with the distinguishing features of speech sounds. Furthermore, the sounds are so standardized that they can be recognized visually by means of acoustic spectography which transforms auditory patterns into visual ones (Koenig *et al.*, 1946). Bell Telephone Laboratories have even designed a machine that can recognize so well the sounds represented by spectographic tracing patterns that an operator can speak a phrase which is analyzed spectographically and the machine will identify the sounds, synthesize them into words, and will then type out what was said (David, 1955).

We are now in the position of a phonetician trying to communicate in writing to another phonetician how to make a most complicated sound that the latter has never heard before. An efficient voice has certain feelings associated with its production and certain acoustic characteristics that are readily perceptible by which it can be distinguished. Our problem is how to communicate to the reader a sufficently exact concept of these auditory and kinesthetic sensations that he will be able to recognize vocal efficiency when he reaches it himself or hears someone else achieve it (Henrikson and Thaler, 1945). Ideally, we would accomplish this by demonstrating personally what we mean until our student could recognize specific clues by which he could definitely identify an efficient voice and perhaps even produce it himself. This was, in fact, the procedure used in a research project that involved 42 male voices produced both efficiently and inefficiently (Harrison, 1956; Miller, 1956; Sawyer, 1955). Usually a subject could get a satisfactory concept of vocal efficiency with about fifteen minutes of ear-training. Since we must content ourselves with a second best communication scheme, we will describe how an efficient voice feels and how it sounds. We will include sonograms by which the identifying acoustic characteristics of efficiency (Fig. 1) can be contrasted with the characteristics of inefficiency (Fig. 2), and we will provide examples in the hope that the features common to these voices can be discerned.

**How an efficient voice feels.** The chief sensation associated with efficient voice production is that of the throat being open and relaxed. This is purely a subjective impression and in no way is it intended to be a description of the muscular adjustments that actually take place. For example, the throat should feel so relaxed that the tone will seem to be pulled through it with no sensation of tension or effort in the neck whatsoever. Obviously, this does not describe what is really happening, for there must be laryngeal tension to set the air stream into vibration. It is merely a description of what the person *feels* is happening. One fine singer, when sustaining a high tone, reports the distinct impression that a little man he has named "Yehudi" is in the top of his head singing along with him. This singer is not suffering from hallucinations. He knows "Yehudi" really isn't there and that he has absolutely nothing to do with the vocal adjustments, but he also knows that his high tones will suffer if he produces them without the subjective sensation of "Yehudi's" presence. We are concerned, then, with what the speaker *feels* occurs, regardless of how inaccurate a description it may be of what actually occurs. With the voice that is used efficiently, whether by the daintiest lady or the most virile male, the outstanding feeling is effortlessness.

The efficient voice also feels as cool and open and big as a sigh. Just as the throat seems to expand in all dimensions during the initial phase of a yawn, so, too, it seems to expand during efficient voice production whether for

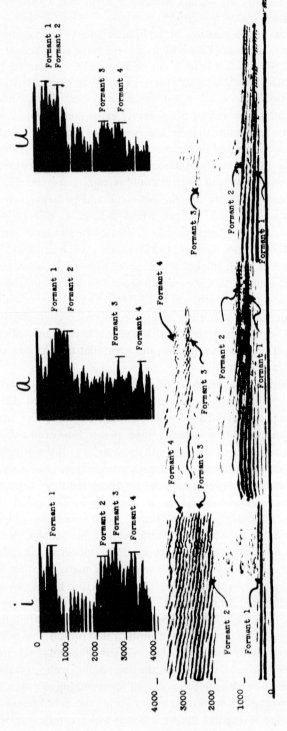

FIG. 1

speaking or singing the highest or the lowest tone. In fact, a well-produced voice is essentially an extension and elaboration of a sigh.

The inefficient voice is like a car being driven with the brakes on; both strain the mechanism to keep going. On the other hand, when effortlessness, openness, and coolness are achieved, the voice will feel as though it is coasting. It will seem to be floating on an air stream emanating from the depths of the chest. It will encounter no impedance at any point. It will seem to have unlimited pitch and volume flexibility. The speaker will feel as if his inflections could go higher or lower than they ever do go. He will not feel that his voice becomes scratchy or squeezed off altogether on phrase ends with downward inflections, nor will he feel that upward inflections will make his voice tight and squeaky. Likewise, when he increases volume the voice will seem to have a great capacity for becoming bigger so he can achieve loudness without strain, tightness, and stridency. Although he will feel extensive potential vocal flexibility, he will nonetheless be most comfortable near his optimum pitch level which will be near the bottom of his range. This level serves as a home base from which he can make excursions as he desires.

Another concept that more or less epitomizes the sensation of an efficiently produced voice is that of the tone resembling a pyramid with the base in the chest and the apex at some point directly in front of the mouth. In other words, the tone seems to have a broad, open foundation deep in the chest and a definite focus outside of the mouth. An efficient voice, no matter how high or low the optimum pitch may be, will be experienced as something resembling a pyramid. Vennard, with a modification of this view, even finds defense for the "pear-shaped tone." He says, "The small part of the pear is in the mouth; it is the brilliance of the tone, the front resonator in the case of the double format vowels. But the pear is not limited to this; it swells into something large and mellow, that can be felt throughout the entire pharynx and is limited only by the singer's ability to enlarge this organ" (1950, p. 83). Although we are certainly not devotees of the elocutionary school that advocates practicing "How now brown cow" with "pear-shaped tones," we nevertheless must honor this old bromide as being basically a valid voice-production concept.

The extent to which the tone seems to resonate in the chest will be mainly a function of its heaviness. A bass, when speaking, will have a strong sensation of his voice being anchored near the sternum, but at the same time being sharply focused outside of the mouth. The deep vibration can even be felt by placing a hand on his chest. When a contralto speaks she will experience many of the same feelings as the bass, whereas the soprano will have sensations that will approximate those of a tenor with a light voice. He will have only moderate awareness of chest resonance and will attend more to the focus of the tone. Thus, the heavier the voice, the heavier the emphasis on the feeling of chest resonance. But for all efficient voices, regardless of pitch, two factors will be constant. The tone will seem to have projection or focus, and the throat and chest will seem to be big and open. That is, the tone will in all instances be pulled up from a broad base or anchorage in the chest and be projected out to a point in front of the mouth. The greater the volume or the heavier the voice the broader and deeper will be the base of the pyramid. Only when the voice feels effortless, open, cool, and flexible can this concept of the pyramid be achieved.

**How an efficient voice sounds.** A practical description of how an efficient voice sounds as distinct from how it feels is almost an impossibility. Granted that kinesthesia and audition are quite separate sensory modalities, nevertheless a voice therapist must listen empathically and this involves a synthesis of the two. He must respond to what he hears by attempting to feel himself what the patient must feel during voice production. When a patient feels tense, his voice will reflect that tension and the therapist can only perceive it by empathizing with what he hears. Similarly, the acoustic characteristics of an efficient tone will reflect so well the feelings involved in the production that the sensitive therapist may describe the tone as sounding open, anchored, effortless, or relaxed, all of these adjectives being more kinesthetically than acoustically oriented. Still, a few characteristics of efficiency are more readily presented in terms of auditory concepts, hence this section.

The acoustic parameters that distinguish the efficient from the inefficient voice have been studied in low-pitched male subjects by Sawyer (1955). He concluded that the characteristics that distinguish vocal efficiency (Fig. 1) from inefficiency (Fig. 2) are lower frequency for the fundamental, more energy in formant one, more consistent appearance of formants three, four, and five, and greater regularity and distinctness of the acoustic patterns. These findings tend to corroborate the earlier work of Bartholomew (1934) and to a lesser extent of Lewis and Tiffin (1934).

The perceived auditory characteristic that can best be correlated with these distinguishing spectographic features of efficiency is difficult to establish. Probably it is the life and vibrancy that can be heard in the tone. Some voices, particularly the heavier ones, almost seem to pulsate with vitality. Many of our finest actors and radio and television performers provide outstanding examples of vocal efficiency. Such men as Edward R. Murrow, John Daly, Ezio Pinza, Lawrence Olivier, Orson Welles, and Raymond Massey, and such women as Loretta Young, Judith Anderson, Ingrid Bergman, and Katharine Cornell habitually produce their voices efficiently. These people are cited not as models to be imitated but as models to be carefully observed for the features of efficiency common to them all; the vibrancy and authority of the tone, the feeling of openness, of flexibility, of firm fullness, of deep origin. These are the qualities of the well-produced voice that a clinician should recognize if he is to have a clear, positive goal for therapy.

### Approaches to Vocal Efficiency

The success of any technique for improving the voice is predicated squarely on the patient's desire for improvement. No procedure, however excellent, will effect a change if the person using it does not really want a change. Voice cases present speech pathologists with an unique challenge. Feelings are intimately reflected in the voice, so an alteration in one cannot very well be accomplished without an alteration in the other. Even aspects of the personality can be revealed through the voice according to some writers (Moses, 1954; Pfaff, 1953; Sharp, 1955). Thus, the clinician should concern himself with working not only on the voice but also with the personality and feelings. The prognosis is good when the patient is truly anxious for a better adjustment of all three, but fair to poor when the desire for change is limited to the voice alone. May it be understood, then, that the techniques to be presented are limited tools which can be just as useful as the clinician is skilled. He can anticipate successful results with these procedures only if he can arouse in his patient an insatiable urge for improvement.

**A subjective approach.** The voice functions as a whole and should not be considered therapeutically in parts. True, the disorder may appear to stem from an inappropriate pitch, volume level, or breathing pattern, but these isolated aspects are only inappropriate in relation to the other features of voice. The author is reminded of two men of his acquaintance with bass voices. Both sounded good on low tones, but one's voice became shrill and piercing when the pitch rose during excitement, while the other's remained efficient and pleasant despite reacting to excitement with a similar rise. Obviously, pitch was a problem for only one of these men, and it was problem solely because of its unfortunate effect on quality and loudness. Many people suffer from vocal abuse by habitually straining their voices at inappropriately high levels. Unfortunately, the majority do not relinquish these tension patterns even when the pitch is lowered. This is no argument against lowering the pitch, for the strain cannot otherwise be reduced, but it is a presentation of the necessity for treating all aspects of the voice as parts of an indivisible whole. Accordingly, we will deal first with procedures that stress the dynamic interaction of the vocal control mechanisms, and later with techniques particularly adapted to altering pitch and loudness separately.

A subjective approach to treatment is singularly adapted to the concept of vocal functioning as a Gestalt. When, for instance, a speaker feels that his tone is anchored near the sternum and his throat is open and cool, he will involuntarily effect respiratory, phonatory, and resonance adjustments that will be conducive to vocal efficiency. Primary attention to these subjective auditory and kinesthetic sensations characteristic of the efficient voice relieves concern for pitch and volume as distinct entities and assures the best quality of which the person is capable. In other words, if the voice feels and sounds efficient, the pitch will automatically tend toward an optimum level from which wide inflectional excursions can be made with ease, the loudness will not cause a piercing blast nor diminish to the point of inaudibility, and the potential clearness, fullness, and richness of the tone will be realized.

Every well-produced voice is a study in contrasts. It is open yet focused, mellow yet brilliant, relaxed yet intensely vital. It is not a mere blending of these opposites in diluted form, but rather an incorporation of each extreme in full measure. The therapist must decide which of the antithetical elements is missing and devise therapy procedures to restore it. If the voice is breathy it will lack focus, brilliance, and vitality. Conversely, the tense voice will not be open, mellow, nor relaxed. However, the true achievement of any of these qualities can only be accomplished through an antagonistic balance. That is, brilliance, focus, and vitality without their antagonistic opposites will be ersatz, they will be pseudo-attributes, they will be stridency and shrillness masquerading as desirable qualities. Likewise, openness and relaxation alone will be merely hollow breathiness. Since the contrasting aspects of efficiency cannot be attained in isolation but can be modified in their relative proportions depending on how dark or bright a voice is desired, the clinician should provide techniques that will enable the patient to experience sounds embodying these antithetical elements.

Because excessive tension is the culprit in most functional voice disorders, an advisable procedure for initiating direct voice work is the use of a sigh or a yawn. Instruct the patient to sigh very gently and slowly and to observe carefully the feelings of coolness and openness in the throat. The same feelings can be captured by noting the sensations attendant to the initiation of a yawn. However, the subsequent stages of a yawn involve more tension and should not be emulated. This procedure should be continued, gradually transforming the whispered sigh into a soft, breathy tone. The concentration should be on recognizing the areas of the throat and neck that feel as though they have expanded and on feeling that the downward inflection of the sigh can sink so deeply into the chest that the sternum will seem to vibrate. The pitch should definitely not be forced down, but it should be kept at as low a level as is comfortable. A sure sign of tension is the inability of the tone to descend seemingly into the chest with no apparent effort.

Frequently, tension cannot be recognized for lack of a basis for comparison. A person can operate continually under great strain and not realize it until the strain suddenly increases or decreases enough to make him aware of the difference. A simple procedure for heightening this awareness is to observe the sound and feel of the voice shortly after arising in the morning, when it is most relaxed. Later in the day an attempt should be made to recapture this feeling and if possible reproduce the voice in the same manner. An even more effective technique for magnifying perceptible differences between tense and relaxed vocal adjustments is to tighten consciously the muscles of the pharynx, larynx, and tongue until the tone is almost squeezed off. Then, phonating [a], these muscles should be relaxed as completely as possible and differences in the way the tone feels and sounds should be observed.

During this phase of treatment, the patient should be instructed to speak as though sighing as much of the time as possible. He should speak as softly as a whisper at as low a pitch as is comfortable, with the open feeling of a sigh, for as many hours a day as can be managed. As might be expected, cases of tension generally experience difficulty achieving the necessary relaxation for this task. Curiously enough, many cases of breathiness will have similar trouble. Breathiness is not tantamount to relaxation. Proof of this can be easily demonstrated. Try whispering so that you can make yourself heard across a room and observe the strain in the throat, neck, and tongue. Whispering is an exaggerated form of breathiness and both are inefficient means of oral communication. Just as a loud whisper requires considerable effort, so, too, does a loud, breathy voice. Until the feelings of deep vibrancy and relaxation in the soft sigh or yawn can be achieved easily and consistently, no case, regardless of the disorder, is ready to progress to work on loudness or brilliance.

A technique used by Vennard (1950) for singers is particularly adaptable for providing an introduction to the feeling of focus for voices that lack vibrancy, whether they seem breathy or swallowed. The tongue should be placed lightly between the teeth as for [ð] and a soft falsetto tone should be hummed. The patient then strives to focus on the tongue-tip until the tone seems to make it tingle with vibration. The sound must be produced so easily that no effort will be felt anywhere except in the abdominal region and the tone will seem to float near the roof of the mouth and the front of the nose. This is the basic sensation of projection that must be retained intact as depth and mellowness are added. It is the backbone of vocal flexibility.

Using this same exercise, the sensations of easy inflectional shifts can be noted and practiced. The patient should produce a light falsetto at a comfortably high pitch, slowly descend the scale an octave without changing the feelings or quality of the sound, then ascend the scale without changing the tone. He should be certain that the throat is open and that the tongue is relaxed at all times. After this descent and ascent can be made smoothly and easily, he should produce a moderately low tone so that it feels the same as did the falsetto. Then the pitch should be raised an octave without stopping or tightening the sound. With this approach, the patient can gradually increase the heaviness of his voice, maintain an easily used wide inflectional range, and speak loudly or softly with vibrant resonance.

The voice is a delicate instrument that will become tired and hoarse if it is abused to any extent. The most common abuses are speaking frequently at pitch levels that are too high, using too much volume when excited, and using the voice extensively when ennervated or exhausted. The voice has tremendous capacities, but if it is forced, its potentials will never be realized. Whether the patient wants a loud or a soft tone, a high pitch or a low one, the voice must not be pushed to achieve these ends. No one should speak loudly if he cannot speak softly.

After the case can phonate successfully with a half-whispered tone and

light falsetto, then the fullness should be gradually increased until he is working with low volume at a low pitch. During drill sessions in this transitional
stage, isolated vowels and diphthongs or nonsense syllables are valuable,
since they do not distract attention from the "how" of voice production to
the "what" of speech content. The vowel [a] is best suited to developing an
awareness of how a deep tone, irrespective of pitch, will seem to float out on
a column of air through an open throat. To get this same sense of openness
but with greater projection and vitality, the diphthongs [ɔɪ], [aɪ], and [eɪ]
are desirable, while the vowel [i] provides the greatest brilliance of all. Exert
caution, though, for this is a dangerous point in therapy. The patient, and
perhaps the clinician, too, will be tempted to determine how big or how
rich a sound can be produced now that relaxed and flexible soft tones are
available. Most people will readily confuse bigness, richness, and brilliance
with loudness, especially if it is their own voice to which they are listening.
Resist this temptation at all costs. Volume breeds tension and higher pitches.
Only the most skilled person will succeed in avoiding vocal strain when
speaking loudly. Remember the criteria of vocal efficiency and strive for a
tone that is full, effortless, and most pleasant to hear. If none of these criteria
is violated, therapy can progress successfully.

As the patient becomes ready for increased loudness, he may be introduced to a procedure that will help him avoid strain and effort. Basically,
this technique is designed to emphasize tonal antithesis. The greater the volume, the greater should be the intensity of the contrasts. A loud tone should
seem heavier yet more vital, deeper yet more projected, more open yet more
focused, than a soft one. The alternative to this heightened antagonistic
balance is a higher pitch. Whereas a well-trained speaker may use high
pitches on upward inflections with moderate volume without strain, he will
indeed be a rarity if he accomplishes this effortlessly with a loud voice. To
avoid this strain, have the case plant his feet as firmly as if he were lifting a
heavy weight. He should stand erect with no sense of tension in the upper
chest, shoulders, or neck, but should still feel as though he were pulling
himself into the floor. Then instruct him to speak as if he were addressing
a large audience in such a way that people in the back row could hear and
understand without feeling that he was shouting at them. The louder he
speaks, the more he should concentrate on pulling the tone up from deep in
his chest rather than stretching out for it. We know of a singing teacher who
states this principle quite bluntly. He instructs his students to "sing from
their gonads." The purpose of this exercise, of course, is to offset a potential
increase in pitch with increased chest resonance and projection. Sometimes,
though, a patient will mistake a throaty, gutteral, swallowed tone for chest
resonance. When this occurs, have him aim the sound at a small object such
as a door knob or a button and use essentially the same procedure as was just
suggested. The deeper and more brilliant the tone becomes the greater
should be the feeling of relaxation and expansion in the throat, neck, and
chest.

A clinician can only serve as a director of the therapeutic efforts, for a case usually spends little more than an hour or two a week in drill sessions with him. He must function mainly as an auxiliary set of highly perceptive, empathically tuned ears through which the patient can check the validity of his own perceptions. Van Riper (1954) has systematized this function with his ear-training procedures. Essentially all a voice therapist will have time to accomplish is to help his case recognize the errors when they occur and to instruct him in the procedures to follow in acquiring correct adjustments. Thus, throughout therapy, specific assignments designed to heighten awareness of the new sensations as well as to provide practice in making them permanent must be made. These assignments should include detailed instructions for performing drills outside of therapy. Usually, they will be drills practiced under the clinician's supervision. The assignments should also limit the patient's volume and pitch levels in everyday conversation to those emphasized during the last treatment hour. The scales are heavily weighted against therapeutic success by the resistance of vocal habits to change as well as by the relatively infinitesimal number of minutes spent each week with a clinician. Therefore, his influence will be pitifully inadequate if he does not succeed in motivating each case to attend to the speaking voice during as many waking hours as is humanly possible.

An admonition is probably in order lest our intent in this section be mistaken. The procedures described are not magical, nor are they guaranteed always to produce results when performed exactly as described. They have proven useful to this author and to many of his students, but unquestionably their greatest value is not as a detailed blueprint to be followed precisely but as a guide to techniques that the alert therapist can develop to meet the specific needs of each patient.

**An objective approach.** We have dubbed the approach to be considered in this section as "objective," since it represents attempts to deal directly with the linear functions of voice production without recourse to subjective descriptions. Respiration can be manipulated rather objectively as compared with phonation and resonance, which elude direct control. Similarly, pitch and loudness are easily measured whereas quality is so multidimensional as to defy quantification. Although we incline strongly toward treating the voice as a Gestalt, we nevertheless recognize the value of having procedures available for dealing with these linear functions directly when they are instrumental factors in the vocal inefficiency. Since we have no new techniques to contribute, we will limit our remarks to some pertinent observations regarding the objective treatment of breathing, loudness, and pitch anomalies and refer the reader for specific therapy measures to such fine discussions as have been presented by Ainsworth (1948), Anderson (1942), Berry and Eisenson (1956), Fairbanks (1940), Hahn et al. (1952), and Van Riper (1954).

Most people who are breathing well enough to stay alive are breathing well enough for speech. This is not a facetious statement nor is it intended

FUNCTIONAL VOICE DISORDERS                                         869

to minimize the importance of respiration. Improper breathing patterns will play havoc with voice production but, fortunately, most people breathe quite well for speech purposes. Basically, only two requirements must be met for successful respiration: steady pressure must be maintained on the vocal folds during expiration, and the thoracic tensions must not spread to the neck and throat. As for other refinements in breathing sometimes advocated, Gray (1936) found that speakers are just as likely to have a good as a poor voice whether they breathe abdominally, thoracically, or medially. However, no authority advocates clavicular breathing and many actively deplore it. Huyck and Allen (1937) reported that diaphragmatic action in good voices showed greater excursions and was steadier than in poor voices. As for lung capacity, Idol (1936) showed that there was a negligible to negative correlation between vital capacity and audibility, quality, and control of the tone. Moreover, she discovered that half of her 140 subjects breathed deeper in quiet respiration than for normal speech, and one third even used less breath speaking loudly than when speaking normally. A study by Wiksell (1936) indicated that attempts to control specifically the type of breathing reduced rather than increased the respiratory effectiveness. Certainly if the respiratory action is erratic, if the patient phonates on inspiration, if a normal phrase cannot be sustained, or if clavicular expansion and tension is evident, then direct attention to breathing is indicated. Moreover, if conscious effort is to be felt during speech the abdominal region is the place to feel it, and this may require some training. Generally, though, the emphasis on breathing for most patients, who do rather well normally anyway, is a sterile endeavor sometimes pursued *ad nauseam*.

The use of an inappropriate volume level can be ascribed to a hearing loss, laryngeal pathology, occupational influence such as factory work which necessitates speaking under high noise-level conditions, or personality difficulties. If the cause is a hearing loss, then aural rehabilitation should normally precede direct attention to the volume. If laryngeal pathology is to blame, the initial concern will be a physician's. If the fault lies with habits acquired under occupational influence or as a result of personality disturbance, the occupation or personality may require alteration before the habit will yield. In other words, even though volume can be readily controlled consciously, it still will be difficult to modify permanently by direct treatment, whether the approach be subjective or objective.

We feel that the primary value of an objective approach here is to make the patient aware of his undesirable habit and, if he errs toward too loud a voice, again direct efforts to decrease the intensity may be most helpful. But if, as is frequently the case, the patient tends to be inaudible, then just increasing volume without attending simultaneously to pitch and quality may be like burning the house to get rid of the termites. As Tiffin and Steer (1937), Talley (1937), and Lasse (1937) observed, when stress and emphasis increase, prolongation, pitch, and quality, as well as intensity readjustments occur. These readjustments when properly integrated can result in vocal efficiency, but as the loudness mounts the inefficiencies are magnified and the chances of achieving efficiency diminish. In short, we recommend the subjective approach when striving for greater volume, because full recognition is thus accorded all of the factors contributing to the well-produced voice and the dangers attendant to loudness are minimized. We would reserve, then, the direct methodology for heightening awareness of the intensity level and, if the occasion warrants, for reducing excessive loudness.

Among the perplexities of voice therapy, pitch problems are particularly confounding. The clinician may become bewildered in determining if the pitch is habitual or optimum, if the falsetto is a sign of delayed puberty or an unwillingness to grow up, or if the pitch causes the strain or the strain causes the troublesome pitch. Despite this theoretical confusion, an operational decision will usually have to be made as to whether the frequency should be increased or decreased. Even investigators who have studied the problem are of little help on this point. Although they agree that the pitch is faulty when it creates throat tensions, they are not in accord as to which direction it should be moved to relieve the strain. Williamson (1944), in his study of cases of hoarse voice, concluded that the principal cause of the trouble was tension resulting from speaking at a level far below optimum pitch. On the other hand, Sawyer (1955), in his research on efficient and inefficient voice production in male subjects with low-pitched voices, found that inefficiency was invariably associated with an increased frequency. The inefficient production involved some strain which apparently caused the pitch to rise even though the volume was not increased and the experimenter attempted to maintain the same frequency level as was used for efficient samples.

Our clinical observations are somewhat more in accord with Sawyer's than with Williamson's findings. Certainly we have seen many cases who have *utilized* tension to maintain a low pitch level, and the voices do seem hoarse, swallowed, and gravelly, but we have yet to see a patient whose low pitch *caused* the strain. Theoretically, we would expect some rise in pitch to help clear the voice, and this Williamson found, but we would expect this because excessive tension would no longer be needed to hold the pitch down. Actually, the higher level would not be at all conducive to efficiency, for the mechanics of voice production necessitate increased effort as the frequency rises. Briefly, any tone which requires strain to produce is bad whether it be high or low, but tension is less apt to be evoked if the voice is produced nearer the bottom than the top of the range.

This leads to the issue of optimum pitch and its determination. West *et al* (1947) consider it as the frequency at which vocal-fold activity is best facilitated by resonance adjustment, or the frequency that yields the greatest vocal carrying power for the least expenditure of effort. In other words, optimum pitch is the frequency at which a voice best meets the criteria for efficiency. Van Riper (1954) and Anderson (1942) suggest determination of the optimum level by methods that involve vocalizing up and down throughout the range until a point is found at which the tone seems to swell without additional effort. This is essentially what the manometric flame technique described by West *et al.* (1947) accomplishes. Fairbanks (1940) gives a more mechanical approach. He recommends calculating 25 per cent of the number of tones in the total range including falsetto, then counting up this number of notes from the lowest pitch to determine the optimum level. Although most of these techniques will provide rather consistent results for a given voice at a given time, and though the concept of having a "home base" pitch level near the bottom of the range from which to operate is valid, still these test results may mislead the therapist who is not familiar with pitch adjustment dynamics.

Increased frequency is a function of increased subglottal air pressure and increased vocal-fold tension or thickness to resist the greater pressure. Even in efficient voices, a high pitch requires greater effort than does a low one. With inefficient voices, the problem very frequently is that of excessive tension, so the low tones become impossible and the high pitches are more strained than ever. Thus, tension breeds tension; the greater the strain the higher the pitch, and the higher the pitch the greater the strain. When a patient attempts to reverse the process and reduce the frequency, he will rarely be able to reduce the effort simultaneously, so the consequent tone will sound low and forced. Moreover, his range will be shortened by several notes, for he will be unable to force the pitch anywhere near the lowest tone of which he is potentially capable. If the natural level of the voice is in the lowest one-fourth of the range, and if a sizable portion of that lowest quarter is unavailable because of tension, then a measure of optimum pitch for patients straining their vocal apparatus will lead to spurious conclusions regardless of the measurement technique employed.

Pitch adjustment problems are among the most difficult and dangerous of those which a voice therapist will encounter. A clinician can so easily utilize a purely mechanical approach and think that he is making rapid progress. That is, he can analyze the voice for the habitual and optimum pitch levels, compare the two, and then use objective techniques to increase or decrease the frequency. We object to this approach, not because it is too easy, but because it diverts the therapist from his proper goal, the achievement of vocal efficiency. When changing the frequency will contribute to maximum effect with a minimum of effort, such as in cases of falsetto voice, objective pitch modification procedures are advocated, although upward pitch revisions should be viewed with considerable suspicion. Generally, it is more rewarding for therapeutic purposes to view a deviant pitch as a concommitant rather than a casual factor. Hence, we are inclined to favor a subjective approach in which the patient is encouraged to use as low a pitch as is comfortable so that the sensation of effortlessness in voice production may be reinforced.

**The perils of self-correction.** Most of us are victims of vocal self-deception. We rarely, if ever, hear ourselves as others hear us. A person listening to a recording of his voice for the first time will frequently not recognize himself. Even seasoned addicts of the tape recorder are continually amazed at the disparity between how they think they sound and how they actually sound. An acquaintance of ours with the lowest voice we have ever heard refuses to believe he does not normally speak at a high pitch. Students and patients are often mortified when they hear what their voices are really like—their self-deceit is temporarily shattered.

The obvious has been labored to lead to a point. For various reasons, people do not monitor their voice production accurately. For example, one young man had a burning desire to be an opera star. He read books on singing technique and devoured recordings of great operatic baritones. They sang loudly with heavy voice quality so he sang loudly with a heavy quality, but they knew how to do it efficiently and he did not. By the time he reached a good voice teacher two years later, he had so embroiled himself in a maze of bad vocal habits that he was even unable to make the college glee club. The point is that most people should reserve their do-it-yourself inclinations for the home workshop and leave voice improvement to the experts. Almost every textbook in the field of speech contains exercises to be employed for improving the voice, and many are excellent if used under professional supervision. Unfortunately, the naive reader may effect irreparable damage by doing what he thinks the instructions say without realizing the full implications.

Now there is a moral in all of this for the voice therapist. Patients will honestly believe that they know what his instructions mean, but the wise clinician will let their actions speak louder than their words. Until they can demonstrate or definitely recognize the exact differences between what they are doing and what they should be doing, the therapist can assume safely that they really do not know what he is talking about. Under these circumstances he should see the patient as frequently as possible, check carefully each time for precisely what was done in practice and how it was done, and be particularly cautious that his instructions are as explicit as possible. This problem is not so acute if the patient has a recorder and will use it consistently in his practice. In this manner he can hear himself as others hear him, so if he can discern the characteristics of efficiency in someone else's voice he should be better able to recognize those qualities or their absence when he listens to himself. Although hearing his errors offers no assurance that he will be able to automatically correct them, at least it serves as a safeguard against a worsening of his condition through vocal self-deception.

**Singing: a vocal mirage.** A young drama student sought the advice of a speech pathologist for her hoarse voice and sore throat. The condition had been chronic for over a year but its onset had been rather sudden. A laryngologist reported no laryngeal pathology that could account for the problem although the cords were mildly irritated from slight postnasal drainage.

However, this condition had existed for only a month. She could no longer participate in plays, for she would become aphonic before she completed one scene. She habitually used a pitch far above her optimum level and she was forcing her voice to overcome the effect of her dysphonia. Although the pitch and volume were certainly not conducive to vocal hygiene, they impressed the clinician as being maintaining rather than causal factors. Finally, the young lady mentioned that she was planning a recital for the next month to be sponsored by her church. The etiology was now quite clear and the remainder of her story merely confirmed the therapist's expectations. She had joined her church choir two years before and had started voice lessons with the choir director shortly afterward. His intentions were good but he was not a singer and knew very little about the voice. She reported that she could never sing a soft tone well so she followed his advice to sing everything loudly. Although her voice had withstood the abuse she had given it while speaking, it could not tolerate the additional burden of her inefficient singing habits. The crowning vocal insult was her refusal to recognize that something was wrong; the hoarser she became the louder she sang.

Singing is only a formalized projection of speaking, and under ideal conditions techniques that improve singing efficiency may also improve the voice for speech. But singing to minimize vocal faults is a treacherous procedure and should only be attempted under the finest guidance. For the unsophisticated vocalist to undertake singing without careful supervision would be equivalent to the average motorist driving down the highway in a racing car. He would have so much power available to which he was unaccustomed that he would fail to recognize dangers until it was too late. As it is with speed, so it is with volume. The louder most people sing, the better they think they sound. Ironically, the more vocally inefficient they are, the louder they have to sing to make a sound at all. Unfortunately, these misguided singers are simply luxuriating in a vocal mirage. The higher the pitch and the greater the volume, the greater the self-satisfaction—and the vocal damage (Curry, 1940; Brodnitz, 1954). These procedures mask the singer's faults only from himself, for in reality he magnifies his every defect. An increase in power and effort increases this magnification. Hence, the voice therapist will do well to avoid singing procedures altogether or to limit himself to those that involve a minimum of exertion.

**The therapist as a model.** The objective in voice therapy is never the creation of a carbon copy. The aim is the development of the individual voice to maximum efficiency. Hence, the patient should strive to achieve the features common to all efficient voices but to retain his own vocal identity. He should see clearly that he is emulating the *process* of efficient voice production with vocal equipment that is singularly different from that of anyone else. Consequently, he should not expect the best voice of which he is capable to be an imitation of some model he has chosen.

However, during the course of therapy, imitation may be helpful if not unavoidable. The clinician assumes the role of authority when he accepts a patient. If the efforts are focused on articulation, then he becomes an articulation authority; if toward voice, then *ipso facto* he is an authority on voice. The average patient, initially at least, will make little discrimination as to the extent of his therapist's authority. Specifically, a voice patient will tend to assume that his speech pathologist not only knows how voice should be produced but also practices what he preaches. Accordingly, the clinician becomes an appropriate model. This situation is compounded when a successful psychotherapeutic relationship has been established to resolve the patient's resistance to therapy. Basic to such a relation is a strong positive feeling that is conducive to the case's identification with the clinician. When the psychotherapist and voice therapist are one and the same, emulation of the clinician's voice may be inevitable. Without question, the ideal speech pathologist should exemplify the best qualities of speech and voice if for no other reason than professional pride. But when simulation of his vocal example cannot be avoided, then it is imperative that he be a satisfactory model.

Imitation can be very helpful as a step toward a better voice, provided it is done under expert guidance and an efficient voice is selected as the ideal. Most patients will have difficulty at first in isolating only the characteristics of vocal efficiency. Frequently, they will be unable to empathize accurately enough as they listen to a good voice to recognize the critical sensations. Their only alternative, then, will be to imitate some voice, preferably the therapist's, *in toto*. Although this is basically a shotgun technique which splatters the patient with new vocal impressions, many of which will be discarded later, it at least assures that somewhere in the scatter of stimuli will be the feelings characteristic of vocal efficiency. The therapist's job then is to assist the case in sorting out and retaining only those auditory and kinesthetic qualities essential to the producton of an efficient voice. Thus, the skilled speech pathologist will not be running a vocal duplication clinic that turns out reasonable facsimiles of his own voice. He will, instead, rehabilitate voices to their highest individual potentials.

## BIBLIOGRAPHY

AINSWORTH, S. 1948. Speech correction methods. New York: Prentice-Hall.
ANDERSON, V. 1942. Training the speaking voice. New York: Oxford.
APPELMAN, D. R. 1953. A study by means of planigraph, radiograph, and spectrograph of the physical changes which occur during the transition from the middle to the upper register in vocal tones. Unpublished Doctor's Dissertation. Indiana Univ.
BARTHOLOMEW, W. T. 1934. A physical definition of "good voice quality" in the male voice. *J. acoust. Soc. Amer.*, 6, 25–33.
BERRY, M. F., and EISENSON, J. 1956. Speech disorders. New York: Appleton-Century-Crofts.
BRODNITZ, F. S. 1954. Voice problems of the actor and singer. *J. Speech Hearing Disorders*, 19, 322–326.

CURRY, R. 1940. The mechanism of the human voice. New York: Longmans, Green.

CURTIS, J. F. 1942. An experimental study of the wave-composition of nasal voice quality. Unpublished Doctor's Dissertation. State Univ. Iowa.

DAVID, E. E., Jr. 1955. Ears for computers. Sci. Amer., 192, 92–98.

DELATTRE, P. 1951. The physiological interpretation of sound spectrograms. Publications Mod. Lang. Assn. Amer., 66, 864–875.

DOLLARD, J., and MILLER, N. E. 1950. Personality and psychotherapy. New York: McGraw-Hill.

DREW, R. O., and KELLOGG, E. W. 1940. Starting characteristics of speech sounds. J. acoust. Soc. Amer., 12, 95–103.

DUNN, H. K. 1950. The calculation of vowel resonances, and an electrical vocal tract. J. acoust. Soc. Amer., 22, 740–753.

ERICKSON, C. I. 1926. The basic factors in the human voice. Univ. Iowa studies psychology, 10, Psychol. Monogr., 36, 82–112.

FAIRBANKS, G. 1940. Voice and articulation drillbook. New York: Harper.

——— 1950. A physiological correlative of vowel intensity. Speech Monogr., 17, 390–395.

FARNSWORTH, D. W. 1940. High-speed motion pictures of the human vocal cords. Bell Laboratories Record, 18, 203–208.

FLETCHER, W. W. 1954. Vocal fold activity and sub-glottic air pressure in relation to vocal intensity: a brief historical review. Speech Monogr., 21, 73–78.

FREUD, S. 1920. A general introduction to psychoanalysis. New York: Liveright.

GRAY, G. W. 1936. Regional predominance in respiration in relation to certain aspects of voice. In Gray, G. W., Studies in experimental phonetics. Baton Rouge: La. State Univ. Press. Pp. 59–78.

——— and WISE, C. M. 1946. The bases of speech (rev. ed.). New York: Harper.

HAHN, E., HARGIS, D. E., LOMAS, C. W., and VANDRAEGEN, D. 1952. Basic voice training for speech. New York: McGraw-Hill.

HARRISON, P. 1956. An experimental analysis by x-ray photography of some resonator adjustments in efficient and inefficient voice production in low pitched male voices. Unpublished Doctor's Dissertation. Univ. South. Calif.

HENRIKSON, E. H., and THALER, M. 1945. Assumptions and their relation to the use of speech drills. Quart. J. Speech, 31, 229–230.

HUSSON, R. 1951. Propriétés fondamentales de la neuromusculature des cordes vocales au cours de la phonation. Journal de Physiologie, 43, 757–759.

——— 1952. Étude experimentale, au cours de la phonation, des organes phonateurs en tant que récepteurs intéroceptifs et proprioceptifs et des régulations efférentes. Journal de Physiologie, 44, 268–270.

HUYCK, E. M., and ALLEN, K. D. A. 1937. Diaphragmatic action of good and poor speaking voices. Speech Monogr., 4, 101–109.

IDOL, H. R. 1936. A statistical study of respiration in relation to speech characteristics. In Gray, G. W., Studies in experimental phonetics. Baton Rouge: La. State Univ. Press. Pp. 79–98.

IRWIN, R. B. 1953. Speech and hearing therapy. New York: Prentice-Hall.

JACOBSON, E. 1951. Progressive relaxation (2nd ed.). Chicago: Univ. Chicago Press.

JENKINS, R. L. 1954. Understanding psychiatrists. Amer. Psychol., 9, 617–620.

JOOS, M. 1948. Acoustic phonetics. Lang. Monogr., No. 23., 24, 1–137.

KOENIG, W., DUNN, H. K., and LACY, L. Y. 1946. The sound spectrograph. J. acoust. Soc. Amer., 18, 19–49.

LASSE, L. T. 1937. The effect of pitch and intensity on the quality of vowels in speech. *Arch. Speech*, 2, 41–60.

LEWIS, D. 1936. Vocal resonance. *J. acoust. Soc. Amer.*, 8, 91–99.

―――― and TIFFIN, J. 1934. A psychophysical study of individual differences in speaking ability. *Arch. Speech*, 1, 43–60.

LINDSLEY, C. F. 1934. The psycho-physical determinants of voice quality. *Speech Monogr.*, 1, 79–116.

LOEBELL, H. 1944. Voice and speech disorders in the German Army. *Quart. J. Speech*, 30, 259–261.

MILLER, R. W. 1957. An experimental study of the evaluation by an untrained audience of efficient and inefficient voice production as good quality. Unpublished Doctor's Dissertation. Univ. South. Calif.

MOSES, P. J. 1954. The voice of neurosis. New York: Grune and Stratton.

MOWRER, O. H. 1952. Speech development in the young child: 1. The autism theory of speech development and some clinical applications. *J. Speech Hearing Disorders*, 17, 263–268.

NEGUS, V. E. 1929. The mechanism of the larynx. London: Heinemann.

PFAFF, P. L. 1953. An experimental study of the communication of feelings without contextual material. Unpublished Doctor's Dissertation. Univ. South. Calif.

PRESSMAN, J. 1942. Physiology of the vocal cords in phonation and respiration. *Arch. Otolaryng.*, Chicago, 35, 355–398.

―――― and KELEMEN, G. 1955. Physiology of the larynx. *Phys. Rev.*, 35, 506–554.

SAWYER, G. M. 1955. An experimental study of perceived differences in efficient and inefficient voice production in low-pitched male voices by acoustic spectrography. Unpublished Doctor's Dissertation. Univ. South. Calif.

SEARS, R. R. 1944. Experimental analysis of psychoanalytic phenomena. *In* Hunt, J. McV., Personality and the behavior disorders. New York: Ronald Press. Vol. 1, pp. 306–332.

SHARP, F. A. 1955. An experimental study of the diagnostic value of vocal cues in psychosis. Unpublished Doctor's Dissertation. Univ. South. Calif.

SHERMAN, D. 1954. The merits of backward playing of connected speech in the scaling of voice quality disorders. *J. Speech Hearing Disorders*, 19, 312–321.

SOKOLOWSKY, R. R., and JUNKERMANN, E. B. 1944. War aphonia. *J. Speech Disorders*, 9, 193–208.

SULLIVAN, H. S. 1953. The interpersonal theory of psychiatry. New York: Norton.

TALLEY, C. H. 1937. A comparison of conversational and audience speech. *Arch. Speech*, 2, 28–40.

THURMAN, W. L. 1953. The construction and acoustic analyses of recorded scales of severity for six voice quality disorders. Unpublished Doctor's Dissertation. Purdue Univ.

TIFFIN, J., and STEER, M. D. 1937. An experimental analysis of emphasis. *Speech Monogr.*, 4, 69–74.

TRAVIS, L. E., BENDER, W. R. G., and BUCHANAN, A. R. 1934. Research contribution to vowel theory. *Speech Monogr.*, 1, 65–71.

TSCHIASSNY, K. 1944. Studies concerning the action of the musculus cricothyroideus. *Laryngoscope*, 54, 589–604.

VAN DUSEN, C. R. 1941. A laboratory study of the metallic voice. *J. Speech Hearing Disorders*, 6, 137–140.

VAN RIPER, C. 1954. Speech correction: principles and methods (3rd ed.). New York: Prentice-Hall.

VAN WYE, B. C. 1936. The efficient voice in speech. *Quart J. Speech,* 22, 642–648.

VENNARD, W. 1950. Singing: The mechanism and the technic (2nd ed.). Ann Arbor: Edward Bros.

———— 1953. How to sing high tones. Los Angeles: Music of the West mag., 8, no. 12, pp. 5 ff.

VILLARREAL, J. J. 1949. Consistency of judgments of voice quality. *South. Speech J.,* 15, 10–20.

WARREN, N. 1936. Vocal cord activity and vowel theory. *Quart J. Speech,* 22, 651–655.

WEST, R. 1938. The function of the speech pathologists in studying cases of dysphonia. *J. Speech Disorders,* 3, 81–84.

————, KENNEDY, L., and CARR, A. 1947. The rehabilitation of speech. New York: Harper.

WIKSELL, W. A. 1936. An experimental study of controlled and uncontrolled types of breathing. *In* Gray, G. W., Studies in experimental phonetics. Baton Rouge: La. State Univ. Press. Pp. 99–164.

WILLIAMSON, A. B. 1945. Diagnosis and treatment of seventy-two cases of hoarse voice. *Quart. J. Speech,* 31, 189–202.

# CHAPTER 27

# SYMPTOMATIC THERAPY FOR STUTTERING

## • C. Van Riper, Ph.D.

THE STUTTERER comes to the speech therapist first and foremost because he wants to be free of his symptoms. These symptoms not only distress and frustrate the stutterer himself; they annoy and distress others, thereby provoking cultural rejections and penalties which increase the severity of the disorder and interfere with therapy. These symptoms serve both as the essential complaint with which he comes to the therapist and as the measuring stick of therapeutic progress. Even in those cases in which the symptoms are unmistakably of neurotic origin, it is essential that the therapist give them the serious attention which the case feels they deserve. Initial rapport always requires that the case feels that the therapist is interested in his stuttering symptoms and proposes to do something to alleviate them.

At the same time, it must be clearly recognized that when the stutterer presents himself for treatment, he has already experienced a large variety of symptomatic techniques which have failed to give more than temporary relief. Some of these have been administered by parents, teachers, or other therapists. With other techniques he has treated himself. He has swung his arm, varied his rate of speech, yelled or whispered, used his will power, tried to relax, chanted in unison, and employed many other equally superficial efforts to *avoid* the occurrence of his stuttering symptoms. He has swallowed phenobarbital to reduce his nervousness. He has had his tonsils taken out. He has been told he would outgrow it. He has been fed suggestion, reassurance, and advice of every variety. Many of these procedures have given him enough temporary relief to allow him some hope that perhaps somewhere there exists a better bit of buncombe which will leave him symptom-free (Gustavson, 1944). Along with this hope, there walks its shadow, doubt. Few adult stutterers come to therapy without it. Some come belligerently, demanding that the therapists show them immediately "the method" so that they can examine it with proper skepticism. Others fight their doubts of symptomatic therapy by pathetically earnest efforts to put their entire faith at the disposal of the therapist with the little pink pill in the bottom drawer. But the doubts are there, and the therapist must recognize and accept them if therapy is to have any chance of success.

Not only is it the case who is dubious about symptomatic therapy. The therapist also tends to be skeptical, if he has any background at all in clinical psychology or psychiatry, or any experience in treating stuttering. The influence of Freud, who equated symptom formation with the need to protect oneself against the pain of anxiety, has pervaded all forms of psychotherapy. Freud (1920) wrote that there was a "very important connection between anxiety development and symptom formation. It was that the two are interchangeable." Since the anxiety was considered to be a response to deep-seated emotional conflicts of long standing, psychoanalysis insisted that these conflicts must be attacked rather than the symptoms. As a result, symptomatic therapy has been not only de-emphasized but viewed with more scorn than it deserves. If current medical practice may be used as a criterion, symptomatic therapy has certain virtues of its own. Of all the thousands of drugs being used by physicians at the present time, only a very few are *specifics* (Thorne, 1950). Most of them merely attack the symptoms and reduce their distress, thereby providing *time* for the homeostatic or recuperative powers of the organism to take care of the real causes of the illness. Other procedures, such as bed rest, reassurance, and specified routines of diet merely help the individual by creating favorable conditions for such recuperation. Digitalis never cured a cardiac case, but it often helps to tide the person over a crisis which might otherwise result in death. Symptomatic therapy then can be *time-gaining* and *palliating* (distress reducing). In this sense at least it can assist all other forms of therapy. In treating the stutterer who comes to us greatly troubled by his inability to communicate, who must meet one verbal crisis after another, all full of penalty, threat, and trauma; in order to gain time enough to teach him to control not only his stuttering but himself, symptomatic therapy is vital. Whatever their etiological beliefs or therapeutics may be, few speech therapists fail to use it.

The problem, then, is not the decision to use symptomatic therapy but rather the type of symptomatic therapy to be chosen. The answer is obvious: we should employ that type of symptomatic therapy which helps rather than interferes with the essential psychotherapy.

At this point, we should perhaps restate the obvious. Stuttering, as a disorder of communication rather than of speech, always involves a disturbance in interpersonal relationships. No matter what its origin may have been, in its advanced stages it is accompanied by fear and by compulsive stereotyped reactions which its possessor cannot control. As Fenichel (1945) puts it, "the common denominator of all neurotic phenomena is an insufficiency of the normal control apparatus." The stutterer does not feel responsible for his abnormal symptoms. The frequency and severity of his symptoms vary markedly from one speaking situation to another (Steer and Johnson, 1936). In certain important regards (Travis, 1940), the stutterer profits from his disability, punishing though it may be. Finally, he comes to think of himself as a stutterer much as the homosexual or dope addict labels himself as belonging to a special category of human being. All of these factors indicate the necessity for psychotherapy. We must treat the stutterer as well as the stuttering.

That this necessity is widely recognized is evidenced by all the modern literature as well as by current practice. Analysis of recent textbooks and periodical literature in the field of speech therapy confirms this statement. Jackson's (1950) study of contemporary therapies and such surveys as are found in the writings of Ainsworth (1948) and Hahn (1943) give further corroboration.

However, the type of psychotherapy used varies widely. Freud is said to have felt that psychoanalysis for the stutterer was not the method of choice, and Blanton (1931) and Fenichel (1945) state that since speech, the essential healing tool of the analysis, is itself affected the prognosis is unfavorable. Deep analysis is one of the forms of psychotherapy currently employed, but only with a minority of the cases. Nondirective counseling with variable success is more frequently to be found in contemporary therapy. Rogers (1942) gives a detailed report of one case treated in this manner and other studies are provided by Schultz (1947) and Clark (1948). The semantic approach to the problem of stuttering is even more widely used as a basic form of psychotherapy (see Ch. 28). Group psychotherapy (Cypreasen, 1948) of many varieties probably is found more frequently than any of the others previously mentioned. Psychodrama has also been used (Lemert and Van Riper, 1944).

Some therapists content themselves with providing general information concerning mental hygiene. Others continue to procure socializing experiences, vocational counseling, and environmental modifications which may help to solve enough of the stutterer's other problems so that amelioration of the symptoms may occur (Fletcher, 1928). Still others attempt merely to build up the personality assets and ego-strength of their cases, by whatever means are available (Greene, 1931). But the majority of speech therapists recognize the necessity for some form of psychotherapy as basic in the treatment of stuttering (Ainsworth, 1949).

If this be granted, then any symptomatic therapy which is employed should facilitate rather than interfere with psychotherapy. It should parallel rather than conflict. Certainly it should create no obstacles. Let us, then, examine the different types of symptomatic therapy in terms of their pertinence to basic psychotherapy.

Symptomatic therapies fall into two natural classes: those which have as their goal the prevention of the occurrence of stuttering and those which have as their goal the modification of the stuttering symptoms. To put it another way, the first tries to teach the stutterer to talk without stuttering; the second tries to teach the case to stutter in a fashion tolerable to both society and himself. The one stresses controlled inhibition; the other controlled exhibition. The basic contrast is between repression and expression as fundamental therapeutic philosophies. Both types of symptomatic therapies are usually structured in terms of the learning of skills and attitudes.

ince this is the case, it is necessary to examine each not only in terms of ow well it facilitates psychotherapy but also in terms of its congruence with earning theory.

The history of stuttering therapy as described by Klingbeil (1939), Appelt 1929), and Bluemel (1935) presents us with a host of clinical techniques epresentative of the first type of symptomatic therapy, that which stresses raining in speaking without stuttering. For convenience of presentation we hall hereafter refer to this basic type as *repressive symptomatic therapy*. In ssence, the therapist says to the stutterer, "If we can create these conditions, r if you will follow these instructions, you will not stutter" (Wilton, 1950). he importance of suggestion in such a therapy is apparent.

It would be impossible here to give a comprehensive list of techniques sed in such a therapy and a few illustrations must suffice. First of all, the nanner of speaking has been altered. Stutterers have been taught blending, reathing rituals, ventriloquism, metronomic and rate-controlled speech, nusual inflection patterns or pitch variations such as the octave twist, reath-chewing, lalling utterance in which the consonants are "slighted" or lurred, prolongation of the vowels, whispered vocalization, phrasing, and nnumerable other variations of the speaking process.

Stutterers have also been required to practice talking under altered communicative conditions: in solo speech or oral reading to self, repeating what he therapist says, memorization, choral speaking or chanting in unison, inging, public speaking, dramatics and debate, microphonic amplification r masking noise. Bloodstein's article (1949) summarizes many of these ypes of talking. Different frequencies of communicative utterance have een employed, such as long periods of silence or massed practice in coninuous speaking. The communicative utterance itself has been varied. Some herapists begin with single vowels and progress through nonsense syllables nto meaningful speech, thereby attempting to convince the case that he eally can speak without stuttering. Many of the techniques used to prevent he occurrence of stuttering require some alteration of the speaker's postural ets. Foremost among these has been the attempt to get the stutterer to attain a state of muscular relaxation. Many different methods of attaining this are o be found but those described by Boome and Richardson (1932), Gifford (1940), and Johnson (1946) are typical. Other therapists have used such devices as speaking with the head thrown back, talking on all fours, speaking through the clenched teeth, speaking with objects held by the tongue in the mouth, speaking with a fixated thorax, talking while walking or moving the limbs and torso, using a belly thrust or gesture to time the moment of speech attempt, and many others.

Many of the above techniques owe much of their doubtful efficacy to their distraction value. So long as the stutterer can focus his attention on the method employed, the situation and phonetic cues to which the stuttering response is conditioned tend to lose potency. Unfortunately, once the technique becomes automatic and habituated it no longer can maintain its distractiveness and the stutterer again begins responding to the origina stimuli (Greene, 1931).

Finally, exhortation, prestige command, and powerful suggestion hav been used to get the stutterer to inhibit his symptoms. These techniques ma be used singly or in combination with any of the other methods we hav been listing. Certain therapists use required readings of inspirational book or the repeated recitation to oneself of such sentences as "I am calm; I am serene; I will talk freely and easily." Prayer, incantations, and faith-healin procedures of many types have been instituted. Medications, shock therapy carbon dioxide inhalation, and surgery have been accompanied by powerfu suggestion. Hypnosis is still being used to induce relaxation during utteranc (Moore, 1946) as well as directly to command cessation of stuttering.

In all of the foregoing techniques, the emphasis is upon *not stuttering*. T the extent that they reduce the frequency of the symptoms they serve a palliatives. Even though these methods may afford only temporary relie as is usually the case, they may be thought to gain time enough for psycho therapy, for easing environmental changes, or for homeostasis to occu Some therapists use repressive symptomatic therapy of the kinds mentione for this very purpose, and with full knowledge that all that is gained is time Unfortunately, most of those who use the distraction, suggestion, speec alteration, or postural-set manipulations are less sophisticated. Often n therapy other than these palliative devices is given, and when relapse come the therapists either go around the same old clinical bush another time o discharge the patient with the accusation that he has failed to follow in structions in some way. The resulting feelings of guilt, frustration, and in adequate helplessness render the case even more resistant to future therapy

Now let us examine a typical example of repressive symptomatic therap first in terms of its ability to facilitate psychotherapy, and secondly in term of learning theory.

Froeschels (1950) describes the technique somewhat as follows: Firs the patient is instructed impressively concerning the importance of articula tory movements as modifiers of phonation. During this instruction, th therapist manipulates the stutterer's lips to produce different vowels. Th case is then "told that voice and sighing are essentially the same function and, if phonation seems blocked, to sigh. The stutterer is then required t read aloud "with opened mouth, but to move neither the lips or tongue." Then he is asked to make minimal movements of those structures as doe the ventriloquist in utterance. No complete closures are permitted. Bot therapist and patient then practice ventriloquizing. To quote specificall (p. 337):

The stutterer is then told to use this method whenever possible, but certainl always at home. The parents, brothers and sisters should be trained in ventrilo quism in order to remind him how to speak. For some days he is required t read several times a day alternating "singing the speech melody" with ventrilo quizing. After that time he is permitted to move lips and tongue a little mor

xtensively, yet avoiding every closure and every narrow passage (fricatives).
till he should go back from time to time to ventriloquism and even to the pure
peech melody.

Normal articulation is reached step by step, slowly or rapidly, according to
he clinical picture. The patient is taught by steps which are only slightly different
om the preceding one, i.e., progressing from pure speech melody to ventrilo-
uism or from just avoiding every closure to normal articulation. Therefore,
ifficulties are avoided.

Since Froeschels in the same article refers to stuttering as a severe neuro-
s, let us examine this form of treatment to see how it agrees with the
eneral principles of psychotherapy. Kanner (1942) says, "Any remedial
rogram will depend on the knowledge of that which is to be relieved,
amely, the *patient* rather than a detached organ or habit." Dollard and
1iller (1950, p. 231) describe the therapeutic process as follows:

> In addition to permissiveness, to skill in decoding conflict, and to the ability
> ) aid the patient to label and discriminate, the therapist has skill in "dosing"
> nxiety. Others have tried to punish the symptoms or force the patient to per-
> orm the inhibited act. Both of these methods tend to increase the fear and the
> onflict. The therapist concentrates on reducing the fears and other drives mo-
> vating repression and inhibition, or in other words on analyzing "resistance."
> Ie tries to present the patient with a graded series of learning situations. He
> ealizes that the patient must set his own pace and learn for himself; that it is
> ie patient not the therapist who must achieve insight. He does not try to force
> ie patient into any preconceived mold but helps him to develop his own po-
> ntialities in his own way within the limits imposed by our culture.

Freud says, "When we undertake to cure a patient of his symptoms he
pposes against us a vigorous and tenacious resistance throughout the entire
ourse of therapy" (1920, p. 253). Mowrer states (1950, p. 567):

> One of Freud's earliest and most revolutionary contentions was that symptom
> herapy is futile. He believed that neurotic symptoms are essentially habits which
> ie disturbed individual acquires as a means of reducing or avoiding anxiety.
> hus by means of suggestions, authoritarian command, or other procedures,
>  may be possible to make a compulsive handwasher or an agoraphobiac give
> p his particular eccentricity, but the underlying problems remain and substitute
> /mptom formation is very likely to occur.

According to Brown (1940, p. 76), "A symptomatic cure is concerned
/ith removal of the symptom itself and is at best a temporary procedure.
 dynamic or causal cure attempts to remove the basis of underlying mal-
djustment so that the symptoms disappear automatically." He goes on to
ay, "If there is one basic rule which may be laid down for all psychotherapy,
 is the rule that symptoms are always helped by being admitted and faced."

The basic principle of psychotherapy, according to Alexander (1946) is
to re-expose the patient, under more favorable circumstances, to emotional
ituations which he could not handle in the past." That this re-exposure is
eep rather than superficial is indicated by Maslow and Mittelmann (1951,
. 248):

The special therapeutic aim is extremely thoroughgoing recasting of those re action patterns which are responsible for the patient's difficulties. Not only are the symptoms relieved, but there are also changes in some aspects of his re lationship with others, his evaluation of himself and others, his goals and the way in which he seeks to attain them.

For those who feel that the treatment of choice is nondirective counseling Rogers (1942, p. 929) has these things to say:

Therapy is not a matter of doing something to the individual or of inducing him to do something about himself. It is instead a matter of freeing him for normal growth and development, of removing obstacles so that he can again move forward. . . .

Pennington and Berg (1947, p. 445) summarize these points of view a follows:

Most would agree, however, that the byproducts of the therapeutic process should incorporate for the client a long-range understanding of himself, the development of more satisfactory modes of adjustment, the objective acceptance of his thoughts, feelings and impulses.

The question before us is this: Will the ventriloquism techniques as a form of symptomatic therapy tend to aid or interfere with accompanying or subsequent psychotherapy? The answer seems to us to be definitely un favorable for the following reasons: (1) If ventriloquism is successful, it immediately reduces motivation for any other therapy; if unsuccessful, it casts strong doubts on the therapist's ability. (2) By its trick-like simplicity it tends to minimize the patient's true feelings concerning the seriousness of the disorder. (3) By its immediate effect, it tends to give the patient the feeling that basic therapy should also be of brief duration. (4) The technique itself may become a substitute symptom incorporated into the stuttering abnormality. (5) Because of the strong factor of suggestion implicit in the technique, it would tend to create attitudes of overdependency rather than self-sufficiency. (6) It places too great an immediate burden of responsibility upon the case for monitoring his speech in the presence of situation and word cues which must still be as potent as ever so far as fear and anxiety are concerned. (7) Finally, it is technique-centered rather than client-cen tered with all the disadvantages to psychotherapy which such an attitude would produce. All of these observations lead us to the inescapable con clusion that this form of repressive symptomatic therapy is unwise, even when attendant psychotherapy is being provided. When employed as the sole form of therapy, and nothing in Froeschel's article leads us to feel that this is not the case, the technique would seem to be even more contra indicated. It should be stated immediately that the same criticisms and ob jections hold for all of the other forms of repressive symptomatic therapy of which ventriloquism is but a chance example.

Happily, in recent years speech therapists have begun to use a different type of symptomatic therapy, that which we have earlier labeled as ex ressive or dynamic. It probably had its origin in Freud's early interest in getting the patient to express rather than to inhibit his symptoms and in using the symptoms as barometers of the basic conflict. Symptoms became useful in therapy, and although symptom analysis and interpretation did not lead to complete solution of the patient's emotional problems, psychoanalysis stressed expression of symptoms rather than inhibition and repression. The fundamental permissiveness of the psychotherapist also led to a changed attitude toward the behavioral peculiarities of the case. It became apparent that before the devils could be cast out of the swine, they must be observed and worked with.

Dunlap's *beta hypothesis* (1932) also contributed to the development of the dynamic type of symptomatic therapy. Instead of using various ways of getting the stutterer to speak without stuttering, the case was required to practice duplicating his own symptoms, a process which the author termed *negative practice* (Dunlap, 1944). Although Dunlap conceived the stuttering symptoms to be merely habits which, when the stutterer became highly aware of them, could be brought under voluntary control and discarded, a good amount of psychotherapy was inherent in the process.

With Bryngelson's development of the therapeutic concept of "voluntary stuttering" (1935), symptomatic therapy and psychotherapy became combined. Historically, he combined the beliefs of Travis (1931)—that the higher cortical (voluntary) centers can dominate the lower ones responsible for emotional behavior—with the mental hygiene point of view of Blanton (1936). In his therapeutic regime, Bryngelson (1943) stressed both the objective and subjective confrontation of self. The moments of stuttering were seen as the battleground in the struggle for control. The case was required to demonstrate in social situations his acceptance of self as revealed through stuttering. A repetitive symptom pattern was taught as the vehicle for these psychotherapeutic interactions. Group therapy was stressed. The stutterer was trained to stutter voluntarily, using the repetitive pattern whenever he felt under threat. If "voluntary stuttering" proved too difficult under these conditions, the case was taught to let the symptoms appear openly without attempts to avoid or inhibit them. Willingness to stutter openly became a goal of therapy. The contrast between this and the repressive form of symptomatic therapy is obvious.

Johnson, in several publications (1944; 1948), has presented another variety of expressive symptomatic therapy having many similarities to "voluntary stuttering" but also some important differences. In accord with his diagnosgenic or semantic theory of stuttering, he stresses the importance of nonfluency as an essential characteristic of stuttering and normal speech alike. The stutterer, through parental anxieties and semantic misinterpretations, has learned to react to these moments of nonfluency or the threat thereof by avoidance. He "hesitates to hesitate." The stuttering symptoms are merely the overt sign of a semantically-fixed, approach-avoidance conflict. The basic psychotherapy is nondirective counseling at first, then train-

ing in semantics. But it is the accompanying symptomatic therapy witl
which we are here concerned.

As in the preceding treatment, the stutterer is urged to express and ex
hibit his stuttering under all kinds of communicative conditions and in al
situations. The stutterer must not avoid or inhibit his symptoms but must use
them for semantic analysis. Since, according to Johnson, the stutterer's trou
bles stem from his attempt to avoid nonfluency, he should be quite willing te
stutter openly, realizing at the same time what he is doing and why he i
doing it. Observing that the normal speaker's nonfluency is characterizec
by effortless repetition, he sets up a similar pattern called "the bounce"
which the stutterer should attempt to use instead of his avoidance reactions
contortions, hesitations, and other vocal abnormalities. In using the bounce
the stutterer responds to the feared stimulus by simply repeating the firs
syllable or sound of the word he is trying to say. This repetition is don
fairly swiftly, effortlessly, and almost automatically. There is no struggl
to make each repetition a highly voluntary act as is done in Bryngelson':
"voluntary stuttering." There is no battle for control; the stutterer merely
lets the repetitions bounce along until the word comes out. Other forms of
"easy stuttering," such as the effortless prolongation of a sound or posture.
are also acceptable. It is quite apparent that such a symptomatic therapy
harmonizes much better with semantic psychotherapy than would any of the
types of repressive symptomatic therapy described earlier.

Another type of symptomatic treatment has been evolved by the author
through his continuing experimenting with therapy for adult stutterers.
Since, in this chapter, he has been highly critical of other symptomatic
therapies, he submits his own to the same objective inspection.

Briefly, the theoretical foundation for this therapy is based upon two
assumptions: First, that most of the abnormality of the stutterer consists of
(a) avoidance responses to various phonetic, situational, and semantic cues;
and (b) habitual escape and struggle responses to self-initiated *tremors* in
the structures dealing with articulation, phonation, or respiration. Second,
he assumes that most, if not all, secondary stutterers present the picture
of neurosis. The author feels that this neurosis is *occasionally* primary, the
symptoms being pregenital conversion reactions with both anal and oral
components, but much more often it is *secondary,* that is, the neurotic behavior originates as a defensive reaction to the penalties which our highly
verbal culture imposes upon those individuals whose nonfluency is excessive.
In either event, some form of psychotherapy seems absolutely necessary.

But what kind? The author has referred his cases to psychiatrists and
psychoanalysts. He has employed nondirective counseling, vocational rehabilitation, socialization, psychodrama, and other types of psychotherapy
extant. He has used these alone without any symptomatic therapy; he has
employed them concurrently with or prior to speech therapy, and also as
terminal therapy. The results were generally unsatisfactory. Some stutterers
improved in their basic personal adjustment and personality but very few

speech. When psychotherapy was used concurrently with speech therapy, ne best results were obtained, although each was affected by the other in oth positive and negative ways.

Following up this empirical lead, we tried to develop a therapy which, hile masquerading as symptomatic therapy, would actually be a psycho- erapy. It was felt that the laws of learning and unlearning apply to neu- otic behavior in general much in the same fashion as they do to a habitual p protrusion conditioned to the perception of an approaching labial sound particular. If this is true, then a combination symptomatic psychotherapy ight possibly be evolved, not by repressing the symptoms but by manipu- ting them in the interests of the healing process. If the self could be equated ith the stuttering, then by working with the stuttering we might be able alter the self. The fact that the case accepts the self concept and label of tutterer," and conceives of himself as playing that dominant role, tends render such a hypothesis tenable at least. Moreover, each moment of uttering can be envisaged as a miniature neurosis in itself, with a surrender responsibility, compulsive behavior, and anxiety reduction as important atures. The symbolic nature of many symptoms is quite apparent. Sym- olically, stutterers soil, whimper, bite, gag, and recoil from themselves d their listeners as they stutter. The choice of symptoms in a disorder hose symptomatology varies so widely as it does in stuttering is probably e to both availability and need (Rotter, 1942). If the basic response to ltural penalty or frustration is aggression, the symptoms are explosive in ture. As one of many possible illustrations, one of our cases spat upon his tener in the throes of his verbal struggle. The internalized symptoms scribed by Douglass and Quarrington (1952) may be viewed as inwardly rned aggression. Whatever the symptoms may be, they can become highly vealing to the case and therapist alike.

But even more revealing than the presenting symptoms is the general chavior of the stutterer when, in the course of speech therapy, he begins to splay and to manipulate and modify his stuttering reactions. As in psycho- alysis, where there occurs strong initial resistance to the method of free sociation as demanded by the analyst, so too there is usually found a milar resistance to free uninhibited stuttering as demanded by the speech erapist. As the case finds his stuttering offerings accepted permissively by e therapist without penalty but with interest, a transference relationship mes into being as it does in analysis. With this supportive relationship isting and in part due to the presence of similar reinforcement from the her members of the group receiving therapy, the stutterer begins to get terested in his stuttering as revelatory of self. He begins to assign himself rge cathartic doses of real and pseudo-stuttering. As his tolerance of mself as a stutterer increases, he begins to use the therapist and other embers of the group as parental or sibling figures and a process very similar abreaction takes place. At this stage the stuttering becomes much more equent and severe. Much emotional heat is generated and discharged upon

the therapist, the other stutterers receiving group therapy, and upon certai
innocent auditors in the world outside the speech clinic. A good amour
of reality-testing takes place. Since the basis of the therapeutic method
the collection by the stutterer of a certain quota of stutterings in self-chose
speaking situations each day as a vehicle for the exploration, understanding
and control of the self, the choice of auditors becomes of great significanc
Instead of conjuring up a father image verbally on the psychiatrist's couch
the case finds a flesh-and-blood yet symbolic one in the traffic policeman o
the corner. With him he can interact. He can confront his anxieties, hi
compulsions, and defenses in his moment of stuttering and recount thes
to the therapist in his report, or the therapist can be with him at the time t
observe, protect, and occasionally to interpret. If he finds the situation to
threatening, he has the perfect right to retreat, providing he attempts t
understand why he must do so. Even as the analyst and later the case lear
much from trains of thought which become blocked, refused, or diverte
into safer channels, so the therapist and stutterer achieve much insight fror
these experiences. Active analysis, such as that described by Herzber
(1945) in which graded tasks performed by the patient during treatment con
tribute much to insight, gives us some precedent for using this type of symp
tomatic therapy in the interests of self-understanding.

In any psychotherapy, there is a need not only to understand one's im
pulses toward socially reprehensible behavior, but an equally importar
need to assess the self-punitive aspects of our beings. How stutterers fee
about their moments of stuttering can reveal much about how they fee
about themselves. At any rate, a marked change in attitude occurs durin
the early stages of therapy both toward self and toward stuttering. Mos
cases magnify and exaggerate the penalties they have received and thos
they expect to receive. As they try to achieve the goal of stuttering openl
and freely they tend to whittle their blown-up superegos down to size. The
find that the less they punish themselves, the less punishment they receiv
from others. The permissiveness of the therapist transfers to permissivenes
in the case and this attitude in turn transfers to many of his auditors. B
actively displaying their free stuttering in communicative situations, muc
reality-testing is accomplished in this area as well.

It is no easy task to confront oneself; and when the stutterer tries t
stutter willingly without avoidance or recoil, that is what he is attemptir
to do. The rejecting ghosts of his parents and associates find reincarnatio
in every present listener. Fortunately, in the therapist and in his fello
stutterers he finds enough acceptance and reward to permit him to mak
the tentative attempts necessary to progress in solving the approach-avoi
ance and avoidance-avoidance conflicts (Mowrer, 1950) that comprise h
neurosis and beget his symptoms.

In order to stutter freely, the case must surrender many of the defense an
disguise reactions which themselves are part of the symptomatology. He ca
do this only insofar as he finds acceptance and reward on the part of th

therapist and others. By rewarding the approach tendency and failing to reward the avoidance, the therapist helps the case get out of the oscillating or fixating behavior so characteristic of his abnormality. As the stutterer finds that his anxiety is not followed by punishment, it tends to decrease. This is especially true when the anxiety reduction is the result not of avoidance but of adaptation training or of testing the formerly noxious stimulus. All psychotherapy, including this, can be formulated in these terms (Dollard and Miller, 1950).

In the daily collection of a quota of attempts to stutter freely, the therapist and case not only become aware of the emotional states involved; they also come to a better understanding of the case's ability to formulate and carry out and evaluate an unpleasant task. Not only his performances but also his aspiration levels are scrutinized. Through the discussion of both, the case comes to a more realistic concept of self. Clarification of the essential attitudes toward oneself comes swiftly when the case is actively attempting to modify his behavior, but only if he is protected and supported by the therapist or the group at the same time. Our experience with purely passive and verbal forms of psychotherapy, as we have said before, is that they often help the case with his other problems but leave the stuttering problem intact. The reason for this, we believe, is that the stutterer so closely identifies his *self* with his stuttering. Psychiatrists have considered stuttering to be a very difficult disorder to treat if not to understand. Were they to use free stuttering in the same revealing way that they do free verbalization, they would lessen their difficulties.

As time goes on, the stutterer finds it increasingly possible to stutter uninhibitedly and openly in situations which formerly were filled with great anxiety. He also finds that, uncomplicated by struggle and avoidance, the severity of his stuttering is lessening. He can stutter with more muscular as well as mental ease. He becomes interested in and curious about both his fluency and nonfluency. He has regained contact with his listener and himself. His insight has grown in every sphere. He has increased his frustration tolerance. He has behind him a good backlog of partial successes in self-acceptance and control. His feelings make sense. He does not seem to need the therapist's or the group's support as much as he did formerly. He has begun to experiment a little with his interpersonal relationships and with his stuttering.

When this point is reached in therapy, the case is given a new tool of adjustment, a technique called *cancellation*. This consists of coming to a complete halt after the stuttered word has been finally uttered, pausing a moment and then attempting to say the word again with even less struggle and avoidance. The case is not to try to say the word without stuttering. Even when the fear and threat is gone and he knows he can say it without having any symptoms, he deliberately does some pseudo-stuttering on the cancellation. This pseudo-stuttering should not be a facsimile of the original symptoms, but represent a modification of them in the direction of normal nonfluency.

The pause in cancellation is used for scrutinizing the symptoms and feelings existing during the preceding blocking in the light of his newly-found insight into self. In the pause the case also evaluates his preceding behavior in terms of its adjustive pertinence to efficient communication. For example, he may say to himself, "That was a silly reaction, trying to utter the word 'business' with my mouth wide open. Can't be done. Why did I just give up?" During the interim between the original stuttering and the new cancelling attempt, the stutterer finds himself altering his sets and making plans for the subsequent modification of symptoms.

From the point of view of psychotherapy, what have we in this canceling technique? First of all we have provided an opportunity for self-confrontation and evaluation. We have also prevented the repression that usually takes place immediately after a moment of stuttering. Most stutterers verbally flee the site of the crime. They distract themselves. They try to avoid contemplating their fiascos. Much of the self-reinforcing value in stuttering is due to this immediate repression of auditor hostility or self-revulsion. The pause and new attempt are valuable in yet another way; by deliberately interrupting the communicative process they allow the stutterer to test his independence of auditor penalty and his own strength. In effect, he says to the world, "Behold! I stutter, but I am working with it, trying to conquer it. If this bothers you, I'm sorry, but I've a job to do." It also gives the stutterer an opportunity for discovering his new potentialities for controlling his emotions and behavior. It enables him to test the reality of his evaluations.

From the point of view of learning theory, cancellation has these advantages. It takes advantage of the moment of reaction inhibition, the point in time at which the old stuttering response is weakest. It interferes with the self-reinforcing tendency of stuttering symptoms to terminate the fear. It increases the strength of the approach factor in the approach-avoidance conflict. It facilitates discrimination of the phonetic and other cues. It provides a substitute response which society in general rewards. (People generally approve of an individual who shows evidence of wrestling with his problem.) Finally, it provides a symbolic goal. The stutterer realizes that a form of stuttering similar to that which is demonstrated in the cancellation would be tolerable to both himself and other people. It demonstrates to the stutterer that it might be possible to stutter in another way, that he might be able to stutter and still communicate, that stuttering need not be catastrophic. When such reassurance comes from one's own behavior rather than from the verbalizations of the therapist, it is an extremely potent force in psychotherapy.

Let us point out again the parallel between this "symptomatic technique" and what happens in psychoanalysis. In the latter, as a result of the intensive exploration of self, there comes a stage in which the victim of a compulsion, such as the urge to scrub the hands fiercely, has gained considerable insight into the origins and dynamics of this behavior, yet finds himself still doing it as soon as certain cues appear. In any specific instance, however, it is only after hand-washing has taken place that he can analyze and understand why he did what he did, and what else he might have done under the same circumstances. In a very real sense he is doing the same thing our cases are doing when they cancel.

Later on, the insight and understanding move forward in time and take place *during* the compulsive hand-washing which is interrupted at that point and replaced by behavior which is more adaptive. Similarly, in our symptomatic therapy, once cancellation has become a fairly common practice on the part of the stutterer, we provide another technique called "*pull-out*." In pulling out of blocks, the stutterer does not let the original blocking run its course as he does in cancellation. Instead, he makes a deliberate attempt to modify it before the release occurs and before the word is spoken. The same analysis and insight which in cancellation took place *subsequent* to the stuttering now takes place *during* it. Again, he tries to modify the symptoms in the direction of normal nonfluency. Again, we find a real battle against his neurotic tendencies. Gradually the insight comes to dominate the resistance, and a further resolution of the conflict occurs. The struggle for control of conflicting impulses is the heart of all psychotherapeutic healing. We have it here.

At this point let us describe something of the mechanics of the pull-out process. Many workers in the field of stuttering (Johnson and Knott, 1936; Wischner, 1950; Sheehan, 1953) see only one side of the stuttering problem, viewing it as a clear example of the approach-avoidance conflict. With them, we agree wholeheartedly so far as this describes symptoms of avoidance, postponement, and disguise which precede the actual speech attempt. But we feel there is something else equally as important. In most but not all moments of stuttering we find a *tremor* to which the stutterer reacts maladaptively and with feelings of helplessness and inability. This tremor is similar to *intentional tremor* in many ways, though we do not consider the stuttering tremor to be organically caused.

In order to occur, this tremor requires a sudden surge of localized tension in a certain area of the speech musculatures and is triggered by a posture or contact differing from those used in normal speech. The assumption of these trigger postures can be envisaged as being conditioned to certain phonetic cues, for example, the perception of the *b* in the word *busy* as threatening stuttering. The old terms *clonus* and *tonus,* formerly used to classify stuttering symptoms, were probably due to recognition by early observers of these tremor and trigger-posture states.

Once in stuttering tremor, the case is caught in a physiological trap. He may stop it at will (Van Riper, 1938), but only by giving up his intention to utter the word. If he attempts the word again, the same trigger posture may be assumed and a new tremor started. When this fails to solve the problem, his response to the renewed tremor is a natural one. He starts struggling, thereby increasing the tension. This unfortunately merely increases the tremor amplitude and/or frequency and renders release more difficult. The same mechanism can be seen in athetosis and other tremors. With enough effort, the tremor speeds up until it creates the tonic state of contraction so familiar in severe stuttering.

The picture of oscillation and postural fixation as a result of the organism's being confronted by two equally punishing alternatives is well known. Avoidance-avoidance conflicts produce them routinely. A long gap of silence in the midst of important communication can be extremely punishing. When speaking and nonspeaking are both punishing, tremor and tonic fixation tend to appear.

How then, does the stutterer ever get out of the trap? The author (1939), using a pneumatic recording device, examined jaw tremors of nine stutterers in an effort to determine what happened at the moment of release from block. All stutterers showed three basic patterns: the tremors decreased in amplitude or they decreased in frequency or a large sudden movement of the jaw out of phase with the tremor occurred. When the large movement was in phase, no release took place. We would explain these tentative findings as follows: in approaching a feared word, the stutterer expects *a certain amount* of unpleasantness. The more the fear, the greater is the unpleasantness expected. Milisen and Van Riper (1934) showed that stutterers could predict the duration of their stuttering with a fair amount of accuracy. The point we wish to make here is that once the amount of expected abnormality has taken place, the fear is satisfied and tension reduction takes place. This in turn causes a decrease in the amplitude and frequency of the tremor and the alteration of the trigger posture, and release results. This occurs in some of the blockings. In other blockings, random struggle and repeated attempts to jerk out of the tremor may shift the focus of tension, alter the trigger posture, or break the oscillation by an out-of-phase movement of the tremored structure. But, at best, this is relatively the poorest of the three ways of releasing oneself from tremor. Not only does the effort to jerk out of the tremor result in bizarre symptoms which the subsequent release rewards and fixates, but in many cases (if in phase) it merely bounces the stutterer back into his tremor. Trying to pull out of a tremor by any out-of-phase movement calls for precise timing and a good deal of luck. Observation of any severe stutterer will yield many instances in which syllables and whole words are actually uttered during the throes of his struggle only to have the stutterer continue stuttering.

When the stutterer, during the course of his symptomatic therapy, begins to pull out of his blocks, he learns to discard this third way and instead he spends his efforts trying to smooth out the tremor and slow it down. By this time, the moment of stuttering no longer is the shaking experience it was formerly. He can experiment with it, varying the tension, altering the trigger contacts and postures. At this point the therapist suggests the possibility of learning how he can deliberately throw himself into tremors. Again resistance is found and overcome and out of the experience comes a marked gain in his feeling of control and self-responsibility. No longer does the symptom control the stutter; instead he is the master.

In terms of learning theory, the pull-out technique has effectiveness because the release (the utterance) rewards not the uncontrolled abnormality which formerly preceded it but the voluntary smoothing out and slowing down of the tremor. The anxiety reduction has its greatest potency at this moment. Guthrie (1935) and others have shown that the behavior immediately preceding release from punishment gets the strongest reinforcement. The gradient of reinforcement is steepest at this point. At any rate, in therapy it is interesting to observe how swiftly the stutterer gains an ability to take charge of his tremors and to effect a controlled release. Even more interesting is the change in the approach-avoidance features of the conflict. The awareness of approaching stuttering no longer repels. Instead, it signifies an opportunity for winning a new battle. The cases go out to look for trouble. They hunt for feared words and situations. It is axiomatic, of course, that this desired result is the consequence of a long learning process with many unsuccessful trials along the way. But even if the case fails in his attempt to pull out of a block, he can still cancel; and in any event he learns a good deal about himself. All therapy is structured in terms of the question: what did you discover about yourself when you stuttered? The therapist is always interested and permissive and he is supportive to the degree required by the case. Often he is able to clarify an experience, to interpret a bit of behavior on the part of either the stutterer or his listener. He is always far more the psychotherapist than the dog-trainer.

To describe the dynamics of the terminal stages of therapy is always difficult. The case has less need for the therapist; he "feels like a different person"; he loses interest in his symptoms; his emotions are less intense; he becomes involved in new fields of endeavor; he begins to accept responsibility for his own failures and difficulties; he learns to monitor his behavior in terms of the realities that exist; he can both venture and control. Viewed from the vantage point of learning theory, new competitive responses have become conditioned to the stimuli which formerly set off the whole stuttering volley of behavioral and emotional reactions. These have moved forward in time so that they now exist as *preparatory sets*. With enough experience in pulling out of tremors of fairly long duration, the stutterer finds himself able to get this control sooner. The tremors get shorter. The case can take charge earlier. He soon finds himself preparing in advance to smooth out and slow down his tremors and when this happens preparatory sets are being used.

At this point the stutterer becomes able to control the duration of his abnormality, to stutter so briefly that his listener will not react to it with penalty. The symptoms become tolerable. Indeed, they become normal nonfluency. What happens is that the stutterer learns to stutter fluently. This can be a very pleasant experience. The approach-avoidance and the avoidance-

avoidance conflicts have turned into an approach-approach situation. The vicious circle is broken. No longer does the tension subside only when struggle results in verbal utterance. No longer does anxiety reduction reinforce the unpleasant symptoms. Stuttering has lost its threat and its usefulness.

The author is highly aware of the fact that much of the foregoing presentation is based upon assumptions urgently in need of experimental verification. They have been derived primarily from experimental therapy and clinical observation. If they can do no more than to jar stuttering research out of its present sterile doldrums, they will have served a vital purpose. But the basic concept, that some type of "symptomatic" therapy can also be viewed as a form of effective psychotherapy, we feel, has been demonstrated. Our cases do not only find an amelioration in their symptoms; they change as persons. Moreover, we do not feel that such symptomatic therapy is at all incompatible with other forms of psychotherapy. Used concomitantly, subsequently, or prior to the traditional forms of psychotherapy, it has proved extremely facilitating. In many cases, especially with those whose neurosis seems to have arisen as a result of audience penalty or verbal frustration, it can be used alone.

## SUMMARY

In this chapter we have described two types of symptomatic therapy for stutterers, that which attempts to inhibit the symptom and that which exploits the symptom as a vehicle of psychotherapy. Examples of each are examined in terms of their congruence with basic psychotherapy and in terms of learning theory. It is concluded that symptomatic therapy of the latter type can facilitate psychotherapy or serve as a vehicle of psychotherapy.

## BIBLIOGRAPHY

AINSWORTH, S. H. 1945. Integrating theories of stuttering. *J. Speech Hearing Disorders,* 10, 205–210.

———— 1949. Present trends in the treatment of stuttering. *J. Except. Child.,* 16, 41–43.

ALEXANDER, F., and FRENCH, T. M. 1946. Psychoanalytic therapy, principles and application. New York: Ronald Press.

APPELT, A. Stammering and its permanent cure. 1929. London: Metheun.

BLANTON, S. 1931. Stuttering. *Ment. Hyg.,* 15, 271–282.

———— and BLANTON, M. G. 1936. For stutterers. New York: Appleton-Century.

BLOODSTEIN, O. N. 1949. Conditions under which stuttering is reduced or absent; a review of the literature. *J. Speech Hearing Disorders,* 14, 295–302.

BLUEMEL, C. 1935. Stammering and allied disorders. New York: Macmillan.

BOOME, E. J., and RICHARDSON, M. A. 1932. The nature and treatment of stuttering. New York: Dutton.

BROWN, J. F. 1940. The psychodynamics of abnormal behavior. New York: McGraw-Hill.

BRYNGELSON, B. 1935. Voluntary stuttering. *Proc. Amer. Speech Correction Assoc.,* 5, 35–38.

———— 1943. Stuttering and personality development. *Nerv. Child,* 2, 219–223.

CLARK, R. 1948. Supplementary techniques to use with secondary stutterers. *J. Speech Hearing Disorders,* 13, 131–134.

CYPREASEN, L. 1948. Group therapy for adult stutterers. *J. Speech Hearing Disorders,* 13, 313–319.

DOLLARD, J., and MILLER, N. E. 1950. Personality and psychotherapy. New York: McGraw-Hill.

DOUGLASS, E., and QUARRINGTON, B. 1952. The differentiation of interiorized and exteriorized secondary stuttering. *J. Speech Hearing Disorders,* 17, 377–385.

DUNLAP, K. 1932. The technique of negative practice. *Amer. J. Psychol.,* 55, 270–273.

———— 1944. Stammering: its nature, etiology and therapy. *J. comp. Psychol.,* 37, 187–202.

FENICHEL, O. 1945. The psychoanalytic theory of neuroses. New York: Norton.

FLETCHER, J. M. 1928. The problem of stuttering: a diagnosis and a plan of treatment. New York: Longmans, Green.

FREUD, S. 1920. A general introduction to psychoanalysis. New York: Liveright.

FROESCHELS, E. 1950. A technique for stutterers—ventriloquism. *J. Speech Hearing Disorders,* 15, 336–337.

GIFFORD, M. 1940. How to overcome stammering. New York: Prentice-Hall.

GREENE, J. S. 1931. Stuttering: what about it? *Proc. Amer. Speech Correction Assoc.,* 1, 165–175.

GUSTAVSON, C. G. 1944. A talisman and a convalescence. *Quart. J. Speech,* 30, 465–571.

GUTHRIE, E. R. 1935. The psychology of learning. New York: Harper.

HAHN, E. *Stuttering:* 1943. Significant theories and therapies. Palo Alto: Stanford Univ. Press.

HERZBERG, A. 1945. Active psychotherapy. New York: Grune and Stratton.

JACKSON, B. 1950. An on the spot survey of stuttering therapies, Master's Thesis. Univ. Denver.

JOHNSON, W. 1944. The Indians have no word for it. *Quart. J. Speech,* 30, 456–465.

———— 1946. People in quandaries. New York: Harper.

———— BROWN, S. F., CURTIS, J. F., EDNEY, C. W., and KEASTER, J. 1948. Speech handicapped school children. New York: Harper.

JOHNSON, W., and KNOTT, J. R. 1936. The moment of stuttering. *J. genet. Psychol.,* 48, 475–479.

KANNER, L. 1953. Child psychiatry. Springfield, Ill.: C. C. Thomas.

KLINGBEIL, G. M. 1939. The historical background of the modern speech clinic. *J. Speech Disorders,* 4, 115–132.

LEMERT, E. M., and VAN RIPER, C. 1944. The use of psychodrama in the treatment of speech defects. *Sociometry,* 7, 190–195.

MASLOW, A. H., and MITTELMANN, B. 1951. Principles of abnormal psychology (rev. ed.). New York: Harper.

MILISEN, R., and VAN RIPER, C. 1934. A study of the predicted duration of the stutterer's blocks as related to their actual duration. *J. Speech Disorders,* 4, 339–345.

MOORE, W. E. 1946. Hypnosis in a system of therapy for stutterers. *J. Speech Disorders,* 11, 117–122.

MOWRER, O. H. 1950. Learning theory and personality dynamics. New York: Ronald Press.

PENNINGTON, L. A., and BERG, I. A. 1947. An introduction to clinical psychology. New York: Ronald Press.

ROGERS, C. R. 1942. Counseling and psychotherapy. Boston: Houghton Mifflin.

ROTTER, J. B. 1942. A working hypothesis as to the nature and treatment of stuttering. *J. Speech Disorders*, 7, 263–288.

SCHULTZ, D. A. 1947. A study of non-directive counseling as applied to adult stutterers. *Speech Monogr.*, 14, 206–207.

SHEEHAN, J. 1953. Theory and treatment of stuttering as an approach-avoidance conflict. *Amer. J. Psychol.*, 35, 24–49.

STEER, M. D., and JOHNSON, W. 1936. An objective study of the relationship between psychological factors and the severity of stuttering. *J. abnorm. soc. Psychol.*, 31, 36–46.

THORNE, F. C. 1950. Principles of personality counseling. *J. clin. Psychol.*

TRAVIS, L. E. 1931. Speech pathology. New York: Appleton-Century.

────── 1940. The need for stuttering. *J. Speech Disorders*, 5, 193–202.

VAN RIPER, C. 1938. A study of the stutterer's ability to interrupt stuttering spasms. *J. Speech Disorders*, 3, 117–119.

────── 1939. An investigation of stuttering tremors, Unpublished paper read at the national convention American Speech Correction Association.

WILTON, G. 1950. How to overcome stuttering. New York: Harper.

WISCHNER, G. 1950. Stuttering behavior and learning: a preliminary theoretical investigation. *J. Speech Hearing Disorders*, 15, 324–355.

## CHAPTER 28

# PERCEPTUAL AND EVALUATIONAL FACTORS IN STUTTERING

- Wendell Johnson, Ph.D.

### SOME BASIC THEORETICAL CONSIDERATIONS

TRADITIONALLY there have been two theories of stuttering. According to the one, stuttering is due to some sort of organic imperfection; according to the other, it is due to an alleged flaw in personality structure. Different as these two theories may appear to be, they seem to be one and the same so far as their basic pattern is concerned. This basic pattern, or form, may be represented so: $A$ causes $B$. There is, that is to say, a something or other that acts as an agent to cause or produce stuttering.

The relationship is presumably a one-way affair; $A$ causes $B$, but $B$ has no effect on $A$.

Moreover, $A$ is presumably something different and distinct from $B$; the cause is not to be confused with the effect, nor the effect with the cause.

Also, $A$, the cause, is presumably constant; it is always there and constantly operative. (If it is not, if it is an intermittent cause, an agent that acts only sometimes, then there must necessarily be a second cause that makes the first cause act whenever it does act, and supposedly a third cause to arouse the second cause at such times as it must become operative, and a fourth ... endlessly.)

The theory—or rather, any adequate evaluation of it—appears to require that the alleged cause, the $A$, is demonstrable, or, if not, then unambiguously inferrable from something else that is demonstrable. It does not appear to be logically required, however, that there be one and only one $A$ to be demonstrated or inferred. It may be, so far as the basic form of the theory is concerned, that the effect, $B$, is produced by more than one type of cause; there could be, logically, $A-1$, $A-2$, $A-3$, etc. Just so, logically, there could be correspondingly varied effects; there could be, that is, more than one type of stuttering, represented by $B-1$, $B-2$, $B-3$, etc.

It is logically required with respect to each cause, and each effect, that it be demonstrably different from any other cause, or effect. The general requirement is that those who refer to any particular cause, or effect—to $A-1$, or $A-2$, for example, or to $B-1$ or $B-5$—be in sufficiently close agreement concerning that to which they are referring on the nonverbal or factual level to make for practical clarity of communication, one to another. What this amounts to is nothing more nor less than the rule essential for the testability of any statement. The statement, "*A-1* causes *B-1*," as made by Mr. Black, cannot be verified or tested by Mr. White unless he refers, in using the terms *A-1* and *B-1*, to approximately the same facts as Mr. Black refers to in using these terms. The truth or falsity of any statement for which this condition does not hold cannot be established. Such a statement is, in this sense, without meaning. That is to say, it cannot be said to be either true or false, nor can the degree to which it is probably one or the other be determined, since there is lacking the necessary agreement as the specific relevant data to be sought or observed.

This theory, then—whether *A* be defined as "organic" or as "psychic" or in some other way—is to be evaluated, first of all, with reference to certain of its *formal* aspects. That is to say, in the first place, no matter what we are to mean factually by *A* or by *B*, or by the term *causes*, we assert that between *A* and *B* there is a one-way relationship. Now, is there anything that we are likely to mean by *B*—by "stuttering," that is—which is wholly without effect on anything that we are likely to mean by *A*—that is, by "the body" or "organism" or "nervous system," or by "psyche" or "emotionality" or "personality" or "personal adjustment" or "social adjustment"? Is it conceivable that a one-way relationship could be found in this situation, however *A* and *B* might be defined factually? The answer to these questions, so far as the present writer is able to formulate it, would of necessity be negative. In this sense, then, the theory—whether *A* refers to something "organic" or to something "psychic" or to something else, so far as might readily be conceived—is indefensible. No matter how *A* and *B* are to be defined specifically, the general relationship between them would seem to be one involving some sort of interaction, and this implies a theory quite different from "*A* causes *B*."

In the second place, the theory asserts that *A* is distinctly different from *B*. The "stuttering," that is, is not the same as, nor is it any part of, the "organism" or the "personality," or whatever else the cause may be taken to be. The theory identifies *A* and *B* as separate and distinct from each other. It says that *A* exists and that *B* occurs only because *A* exists—that it is a function of *A*. This *A*, presumably, is something that can be distinctively observed, possibly measured, certainly exhibited, or that at least can be demonstrated indirectly by rigorous inference from something that can be directly demonstrated and observed. And presumably it exists in greater amounts in some individuals than in others, since some individuals stutter more—have, or do, more of *B*—than others do, and presumably within an individual the amount varies since any given individual stutters more at some times than at other times. It is to be assumed, therefore, that *A* is not only demonstrably different from *B*, but also variable in quantity, and that an increase or decrease in the amount of $A$, the cause, is reflected in a corresponding increase or decrease in the amount of $B$, the stuttering.

Meanwhile, the writer has noted that those who seemingly accept this general "$A$ causes $B$" theory commonly talk as though whenever they refer to the stutterer's "in-co-ordination" or "neurophysiological abnormality" or "nervousness" or "psychoneurosis" or "emotional instability," the tangible or observable facts or events to which they are evidently referring are wholly or in part the same ones they refer to when they talk about his "stuttering." And whenever they assert that one stutterer has "more instability" or "more predisposition to stutter" than another one has, they seem to refer wholly or in part to the same facts that they refer to when they say that he has, or does, "more stuttering" than the other one.

In the third place the theory presumably asserts that $A$, the cause, is constant. Even though, as we have seen, it seems necessary to assume that $A$ is variable, there is no clear provision in the theory, as it is customarily presented in its various specific forms, for the disappearance or nonexistence of $A$ during the intervals when no stuttering is occurring, nor is there any systematic provision for increase or decrease in "the cause" whenever the amount or severity of stuttering is observed to increase or decrease. One is left with the necessity of assuming that either there is an additional factor that activates $A$ whenever it becomes operative, or more operative—and, as we have previously observed, still another factor to activate this additional factor, and so on, without end—or else of taking for granted that $A$ is constantly present and unvaryingly operative. It is, of course, obvious that "stuttering," in almost any meaning the term could be given, refers to a series of discreet events, or to a process or phenomenon that is for all practical purposes intermittent, and definitely variable. The average stutterer has difficulty on something like 10 per cent of his words, and half or more of his stutterings last one second or less; he has "good" and "bad" days; he stutters more in some situations than he does in others. It would seem logically insupportable, however, to speak of the *constant cause* of an *intermittent effect,* or of the unvarying cause of a variable effect. There appears to be no need in this specific connection for experimental research; there is need only to invoke the requirements of meaningful discourse. The theory seems not to satisfy these requirements.

Finally, as has been said, the theory appears to require that the $A$ which is alleged to exist is not only demonstrable, or at least rigorously inferable, but that it be also recognized and demonstrated directly or indirectly by those who make particular references to it, without significant disagreement among them as to what it is and as to the means by which and the conditions under which it is to be observed. Likewise, there must be reasonably close agreement as to what $B$, or "stuttering," as used in any particular statement, refers to in the realm of observable events or data. Moreover, it is, essential that the verb *causes* be understood without important disagreement by all concerned. The writer is not aware that the implied agreement does, in fact, exist customarily to a degree required for purposes of unambiguous discourse in terms of the basic form, "*A* causes *B*."

On these grounds, then, it would seem difficult, if not impossible, to defend this general theory which asserts simply that stuttering is caused by some flaw or other in the body, or in the personality, of the speaker.

Moreover, a quite substantial amount of scientific research has been done on stuttering in the past thirty years or so. At the writer's own institution, for example, approximately 150 M.A. and Ph.D. dissertations have dealt with stuttering during this period, and some 250 publications on stuttering have been produced.[1] The investigations cannot be said to have indicated that there is a distinctive organic or neurophysiological difference between persons who stutter and those who do not. Evidently no specific kind of organism is required for stuttering—unless it is that the organism be relatively normal and not too immature: a person injured to the extent of unconsciousness or paralysis would hardly be expected to stutter, nor would a child not yet sufficiently developed to speak in the usual sense of the word.[2] And while a very considerable theoretical literature has been accumulated, having the effect of presenting stuttering as a "symptom" of "psychoneurosis" or "arrest or regression of personality development" or "conflict in the unconscious," and the like, rigorous and detailed studies of very young cases and their parents, and of older stutterers examined by means of present-day personality evaluation procedures, have generally failed to lend clear or definite support to such views.[3]

In consideration of the relatively reliable factual knowledge about stuttering developed to date, it seems necessary, or certainly very desirable, to explore the feasibility of theoretical constructions, or "organizing schemes," other than the traditionally accepted "*A* causes *B*" pattern. The analysis sketched here implies at least the following possibilities in this connection.

First, we can increase the number of factors to be included. Instead of restricting our formal pattern to two components, *A* and *B*, we can have *A*, *B*, *C*, ... *n*.

Second, instead of assuming a one-way relationship among the factors,

[1] See Appendix of *Stuttering in Children and Adults: Thirty Years of Research at the University of Iowa*, edited by Wendell Johnson and Ralph Leutenegger. (Minneapolis, University of Minnesota Press, 1955).

[2] See Johnson *et al.* (rev. ed., 1956), Ch. 5, for references to and discussions of relevant literature, particularly as abstracted and evaluated by Harris Hill in two articles in 1944: Stuttering: I. A critical review and evaluation of biochemical investigations, and Stuttering: II. A review and integration of physiological data. *J. Speech Disorders*, 9, 245–261 and 289–324.

[3] Since this was written, several highly relevant studies and reviews of the literature have been published or prepared for publication. See Leonard D. Goodstein. 1956. MMPI profiles of stutterers' parents: A follow-up study. *J. Speech Hearing Disorders*, 21, 430–435; Leonard D. Goodstein and Grant W. Dahlstrom. MMPI differences between parents of stuttering and nonstuttering children. *J. Consulting Psychology*, in press; Grant W. Dahlstrom. Stuttering phenomena and measured personality. *J. Speech and Hearing Disorders*, in press.

we can consider the matter of interaction and the possible self-reflexiveness of interactions.

Third, we can re-examine the nature of the traditional distinction between "cause" and "effect"—that is, between the conditions essential to stuttering and the stuttering.

Fourth, we can reconsider the theoretical requirements dictated by the fact that what we call stuttering reduces, on the level of fact and experience, to stutterings with measurable durations and distributions in time, and occurring within behavioral contexts of one kind or another. Instead of orienting our theory to an assumed constancy of the alleged cause, we can orient it to the fact of variation in the "effect" to be explained.

Fifth, instead of assuming sufficient extensional agreement (agreement, that is, as to the nonverbal or factual phenomena, the observables, being referred to by means of a given term in a specific usage of that term) for purposes of verifiability of statements, we can investigate the extensional agreement actually to be observed in the use of the word *stuttering* (or its apparent equivalents) and of other words presumably important in statements made about stuttering. The role of this agreement, in itself, in relation to the problem of stuttering can be examined rather than disregarded.

In preparation for such theoretical reconsiderations, certain apparently important facts concerning stuttering are properly to be reviewed.

## A SUMMARY AND DISCUSSION OF SELECTED DATA

As to what is to be said descriptively about stuttering at the time of its first occurrence, as reported by responsible adult observers (the parents in practically all cases), and the conditions under which this first occurrence is reported to have been observed, a considerable body of relevant information has been obtained by Davis (1939), Branscom, Hughes, and Oxtoby (1955), Egland (1955), Johnson (1955), and Darley (1955).[4] In general, these investigators have found that repetitions of sounds or syllables, whole words, and phrases or combinations of two or more words are relatively common in the speech of children from two through five years of age. In samples totaling nearly 200 children, unselected except that they were attending a preschool operated by the Iowa Child Welfare Research Station, no child has been found who did not show such repetitions. The range is from less than 10 to approximately 100 instances of repetition per 1000 running words, and the mean is approximately 45 instances per 1000 words. The repetitions appear to be free of tension over and above that characteristic of speech

[4] As this is being written an additional investigation of the onset of stuttering, which involves 150 allegedly stuttering children and their parents and 150 allegedly nonstuttering children and their parents, is being completed at the University of Iowa under a grant from the Louis W. and Maud Hill Family Foundation. Publication of a report of this study should be accomplished within a year or so. Statements contained in the present paper are made independently of the data being assembled in the investigation now nearing completion.

activity, and the children do not appear to be "emotional" about the repetitions or "conscious" of them. Correlations between amount of speech nonfluency, in this sense, and chronological and mental age and various measures of speech and language development suggest that speech gradually becomes more fluent within the range of ages and development investigated. The speech of presumably normal five-year-olds, however, is by no means wholly fluent, and in a study just completed (Johnson et al., 1956) the speech of nonstuttering adult males of college age has been found to be characterized by a mean of about seven nonfluencies of various types per 100 words. The basic fact is that normal speech is nonfluent in specific respects and within certain and relatively well-determined statistical limits. Whatever one is to refer to by means of the word *stuttering,* therefore, is necessarily to be differentiated from normal nonfluency.

What one is to mean by "stuttering" is also to be differentiated, presumably, from speech that is nonfluent or blocked or hesitant or repetitive by virtue of developmental deficiency; brain damage, paralysis; excessive fatigue; marked emotional disturbance (rage, grief, horror, shame, remorse, terror, awe, and so on); psychotic withdrawal, depression, confusion, or agitation; and psychoneurotic motivations. The major criteria for purposes of differentiation would appear to be (*a*) the nature of the nonfluency and its behavioral, psychological, and social concomitants; (*b*) the variations in it under designated conditions; and (*c*) the mode and circumstances of onset, development, and decrement or cessation. For example, in those instances in which Penfield and Rasmussen (1950) assert that "stuttering" occurred upon electrical stimulation of specified loci on or in the exposed cerebral cortex, so far as they do not use the term ambiguously they refer to phenomena whose behavioral and psychological concomitants and mode and circumstance of occurrence, and whose conditions and manner of variation, would appear to distinguish them clearly from what would seem to be commonly referred to as stuttering. The problem of differential diagnosis, or discrimination in the designative uses of the term *stuttering* (or its verbal equivalents) has not been commonly acknowledged or systematically explored, and it is clearly of fundamental importance. Not all nonfluent or disturbed speech is to be usefully lumped together as stuttering. Certainly it is not all the same, aside from how we might choose to name it. It seems clear that substantial theoretical and clinical confusion has been inadvertently created by the indiscriminate application of "stuttering" as a label for varied items in an essentially heterogeneous array of speech behaviors.

It may be regarded as a reasonably clear statement that what we generally refer to as stuttering in young adults, classified and worked with by speech correctionists as stutterers, is a kind of behavior that has a mode of onset that has been found by Johnson (1955) and by Darley (1955) to be remarkably consistent from case to case. Johnson (1955) investigated 46 alleged stutterers, with a median interval between reported date of onset and first interview of 5 months, 18 days. He found the median age of onset, as reported, to be three years, two months; the twenty-fifth percentile was 2 years, 10 months; the seventy-fifth percentile was 3 years, 6 months. Darley (1955) investigated 50 alleged stutterers, with a median interval between reported date of onset and first interview of 3 years, 8.3 months (mothers' estimates), or 3 years, 10 months (fathers' estimates). He found the median age of onset to be 3 years, 7.9 months, as reported by the mothers, and 4 years, 0.75 months, as reported by the fathers. The range of onset reported by the mothers was from 15 to 108 months, and the range reported by the fathers was from 18 to 132 months. When case histories are taken from adults—that is, when the interval between onset of the problem and time of interview is greater than it was in these studies—the average age of onset, as reported, is later. The available data, duly evaluated, seem to justify the statement that the onset of stuttering peaks sharply at three years, and is found in the larger proportion of cases to lie between two and four years.

The most important observation to be made in this connection would appear to be that at about the age of three years the average child acquires a new kind of listener, so to speak. That is, up to about that age a child is responded to by major listeners, mainly his parents, who are generally pleased by his attempts to speak. His parents' attitude is chiefly one of gratification because he is learning to speak. They note that now and then he adds a new word, or with pleasure point out to each other that he has just talked about something he had never talked about before, that he is speaking more plainly, that he had made a very long sentence of seven words, and so forth.

Sometime around the child's third birthday, however, the parents' attitude begins to change. The child is talking much more by this time. The swelling flood of speech that leads on to the fortune of 400 questions per day by the age of four is beginning to overflow the lowlands of parental joy. Subtly and probably without much awareness of the transformation through which they are passing, the parents change from listening to the child as to one learning to speak, to listening to him as to one who has learned and is now, in essentially the full-blown sense, speaking. He is speaking to them, moreover, and they feel more and more persistently, and at times distractedly and disturbingly, the need to respond. The relationship has become one that admits of conflict between them and the speaking child, if indeed conflict is not at times inevitable. And, to the degree that they have the motivations for it, they are now stimulated to judge and to disapprove the ways in which the child is saying the great deal that he is saying. So by now, the youngster has acquired a more critically evaluative listener than he has had up to this time.

We have already noted that at this age of three years, or roughly two to four, the average child is repeating sounds, words, or phrases about 45 times per 1000 words (45 times means 45 instances, in each of which a sound, or word, or phrase may be repeated a number of times). He is repeating enough —and not only the average child but any child is repeating enough—at the same time that he is talking enough, to elicit disapproval and concern on the part of any parent sufficiently motivated to be displeased and worried by the imperfections in the flow of his speech. At this age, then, there exists for the first time in the child's life a *combination* of two factors apparently crucial, though not necessarily sufficient, for the development of stuttering: (1) observable nonfluency, and (2) a listener who disapproves of it and who does so as an authority figure upon whose attitudes and reactions the child depends significantly for his sense of security and adequacy. One additional factor seems to be necessary if stuttering is to be produced: the child must respond in a certain way to the authority figure's negative evaluation of his speech nonfluency. Whether or not, or with what degree of intensity and persistency, he will respond, would appear to depend mainly on (*a*) the degree to which his previous experience, particularly that centered around his relationship with the authority figure, or some similar person, has conditioned him to feel threatened by disapproval and has left him unequipped behaviorally and psychologically to cope with it; and (*b*) the intensity and persistence with which the authority figure manifests the disapproval and concern, and the degree to which the mode of manifestation is in fact threatening to the child's sustaining relationship with the authority figure and to the child's general sense of security and self-sufficiency.

The term *predisposition to stutter* may be applied meaningfully in this general context. (The writer knows of no operational meaning that can be validly ascribed to the term in a biological or a neurophysiological sense.) It seems indisputable that there are marked differences among children in their ways of reacting to and being affected by negative evaluations of themselves or of specific features of their behavior. It would appear to be a reasonable hypothesis that to a significant degree these differences are due to differences in training and in the general context of significant human relationships in which this training has occurred. To the degree that a child has been trained to be fearful, to be dependent on his authority figures, to lack confidence in his own judgment, to feel inferior, unloved, and unworthy, and to distrust his own nervous system, he will be disturbed by the experience of being disapproved. And to the degree that his relationship with the authority figure who disapproves of his nonfluency has been, or is at the time of disapproval, a tenuous, undependable, cold, or ambivalent one, he will react to disapproval with a heightened sense of insecurity.

Another consideration that seems important is that the amount of experience the child has had with speech that has met with approval is to be expected to weigh against the probability of his being disturbed by disapproval of his speech. A simple way to express this is to say that the longer a child enjoys the experience of speaking in a way that is regarded by those about him as normal or satisfactory, the less likely is he to be significantly affected by the adverse reactions of particular listeners at specific times and places. Considered together with all that has been said above, this implies that once a child has successfully passed the crucial age of three years, the older he gets without coming to be regarded as a stutterer, the slimmer his chances of ever being so regarded. It is to be observed that there are relatively few times in the life of a representative child when he (*a*) is sufficiently immature, insecure, and dependent upon a particular authority figure to respond with a relatively intense and sustained hesitancy, conflict, tension, and self-consciousness to (*b*) the authority figure's negative reaction to (*c*) his nonfluent speech. One of these times—by all odds apparently the main one—occurs at or about the age of three years for the reasons just indicated. Another one can come about when the child enters school and is confronted by a new authority figure, a teacher, who is in some instances motivated to be critically or even perfectionistically evaluative of the child's speech fluency, and upon whose evaluations the youngster is heavily dependent for his feeling of ease and sense of security in a new and very possibly threatening situation. Other similar occasions might come about if the child is orphaned and placed in a foster home, or if an emotionally important grandparent comes into the child's home to live, and so forth.

To the degree that these considerations are to be accepted as generally valid, it is to be expected that the onset of stuttering would rarely be found to occur in children who had successfully hurdled the three-year transition and the entrance into the school situation. The conditions essential for the onset would seldom be encountered after satisfactory adjustment to school. As a matter of fact, the Iowa studies of the onset of stuttering bear out this expectation (Darley, 1955; Johnson, 1955). So overwhelming is the tendency for the onset to occur between the ages of two and four years, with the age of entrance into school as a sort of "delayed" upper limit, that it appears reasonable to conclude that onset within these rather narrow age limits, or under the particular conditions specified above, is one of the defining characteristics of stuttering. Onset at later ages and under conditions definitely different from those described by Johnson (1955) and Darley (1955) would appear to be indicative of a diagnosis other than stuttering in the ordinary sense of that term. To say glibly that stuttering sometimes begins in the adult years is to impose an all but intolerable tax upon one's capacity for being semantically hospitable to the extremely unlikely.

Certainly it would be necessary to determine, in such an alleged case, whether and in what specific ways and under precisely what circumstances the individual had been speaking nonfluently, to what specific authority figure, what particular reactions the authority figure had made, and what specific reactions to these reactions had been made by the speaker.

And, speaking of the extremely unlikely, a word is to be said about the question as to what stuttering is like at time of onset. Although it would appear to be commonly assumed and frequently asserted that the first manifestations of stuttering are, at least in some cases, severe blocks with much tension and apparent distress, the detailed case studies of Darley (1955) and Johnson (1955) have yielded findings impressively at variance with such a view. In the Johnson sample of 46 young stutterers the chief type of speech phenomenon originally regarded as stuttering in all cases, and the only phenomenon so regarded in 42 out of the 46 cases, was simple repetition, apparently indistinguishable from the repetitions in the speech of the presumably normal children studied by Davis (1939), Egland (1955) and Branscom, Hughes, and Oxtoby (1955). In the four cases for whom something in addition to simple repetition was reported as the original stutterings, the other phenomena were comparatively inconsequential, consisting of tiny pauses, so-called, and some evidences of hesitancy such as brief prolongations of sounds with slight, if any, tension. The findings from Darley's 50 cases were very similar.

Aside from such data, however, it is arrestingly fascinating to contemplate the problem, or rather the mystery, that would be presented by a child who would, after several months or years of generally uneventful development and presumably normal speech behavior, suddenly on some Tuesday forenoon at 9:18 o'clock, after having chattered gaily all through breakfast, confront his mother in the kitchen, open his mouth to say, perhaps, that he was going to play outdoors, and stand transfixed, with trembling jaws, bulging eyeballs, and arrested breath, emitting weird gurgling sounds, locked in an utterly disabling seizure of speech blockage! Has such an onset of *stuttering* ever actually occurred? If so, on the bases of what anatomical, neurological, or physiological knowledge could it possibly be explained? Nor is it psychologically plausible. In the meantime, in cases in which very thorough investigation is made relatively soon after onset such "facts" are not found, and in cases investigated relatively long after onset either such stories cannot be documented satisfactorily or they are missing, and in their stead are vague statements about "gradual" onset, concerning the date of which the parents cannot well agree, and in response to which no apparent sudden alarm was felt by the parents at the time, no doctors, neurologists, or psychiatrists were summoned, often "nothing" was done according to the parents' testimony, and in general no memories of any sort seem to have persisted that would indicate that anything as dramatic or alarming as a sudden and severe failure or "breakdown" of the child's speech function had actually occurred.

The simple, relatively tensionless, "unconscious," apparently normal speech nonfluencies that are reported as the first manifestations of "stuttering" in the preponderance of cases, thoroughly and systematically investigated soon enough after onset to insure the relative reliability of data, would appear to be, like the age and specific conditions of onset, distinctively characteristic of stuttering. The writer is strongly inclined to conclude that, in any case for which a sudden severe speech blockage can be reliably determined to have been the very first manifestation of the problem, a diagnosis different from that of stuttering is indicated.

In view of the kind of speech phenomena characteristically regarded as stuttering at onset, as reported, and in view of the conditions under which and the age at which this onset is alleged to occur in the preponderance of well-investigated cases, it is of peculiar significance to determine who first decides something is at fault—who is the original "diagnostician"—in these cases. Both Johnson (1955) and Darley (1955) found that with rare exceptions the original diagnosis was made by a layman, usually the mother, sometimes the father, or both acting more or less in collaboration, or a relative, or a classroom teacher untrained in speech pathology, in one case by a roomer living in the home. Some of the rare exceptions were themselves interesting in that they were cases in which children had been picked up in a speech survey conducted by a speech correctionist. The implication would seem to be that, taking the full story into account in each case, the ears of a speech correctionist can be too long and too trembly, so to speak. What is important is that the essential facts appear to have been relatively the same in all the cases investigated by Johnson and by Darley, in the special sense that anything in the form of definite difficulty, or clinically noteworthy tension, or apparent anxiety, or self-consciousness in speaking was, in all but a very few ambiguous cases, not observed, so far as could be determined, until after one or more of the child's emotionally important listeners or authority figures had made the judgment or diagnosis that the child was stuttering.

The word *stuttering,* or any equivalent of it, may or may not have been used in making or expressing this judgment. The essential fact had been an evaluation of a negative sort, a concern over, a disapproval of, an anxious wondering about the child's manner of speaking so far as its fluency aspects were concerned. Actually, it cannot be said with certainty that in any case this negative evaluation went unexpressed. The parents were found to have differed considerably in their ways of reacting verbally and overtly after having experienced the thought that their child was "stuttering." But whether they instructed the child to stop and think, take a deep breath, begin again, and go slowly, whether they said these things calmly or in anxious tones, whether they punished the child or comforted him, or just looked down or away, or as some of them claimed implausibly, "did nothing at all"—a feat which, if accomplished, would surely be peculiarly conspicuous—the probability seemed stubbornly to remain that they did not deceive the child.

The children reacted certainly. They differed greatly in manner of reacting, but with a common denominator of anxiety-tension in some degree, ranging from what must have been a very slow-working and barely perceptible increase in hesitancy and a delicately baffled concern, to what was clearly reported as a rapid and marked development of self-consciousness, tension, and obvious embarrassment and frustration. In some cases it seemed clear that a definite decrease in verbal output or verbal responsiveness had taken place. The fundamental fact, however, was that the problem first appeared not in the way in which the child was speaking but in the way in which his speech was being received by the authority figures to whom he was addressing himself.

These facts would appear to dictate the general conclusion that in the beginning—as observed in those cases in which the beginning has been reliably identified—the original patient is not the child but the parent (usually the parent, though it can be some other responsible listener). Stuttering starts, so to speak, not in the child's mouth but in the parent's ear. Originally the patient is not the speaker but the listener.

To the degree that this general conclusion proves acceptable, most of the books are to be rewritten because, speaking in rough essentials, they have misidentified the patient. Traditionally not only has the wrong tooth been pulled, so to speak, but it has been removed from the wrong head. If the basic conclusion just stated be granted, it would appear to be more or less wholly beside the point to look for the cause or causes of "stuttering" at its onset in the muscles, nerves, glands, or "psyche"—or even in the speech— of the speaking child. The essential question would seem to be concerned with the reasons why the listening parent becomes sufficiently concerned and reacts in the particular ways in which she or he does react after becoming concerned enough to react at all. For an answer to this question one would hardly investigate the muscles, nerves, and glands of either the speaking child or the listening parents, but one would instead, no doubt, make appropriate inquiries concerning the parents' relevant attitudes, backgrounds of experience, funds of information, patterns of thinking, aspects of personal and social adjustment, and motivations. Their relationship to the child whose speech they evaluate negatively is also to be examined. In general, the investigation is to be concerned with the differences between parents who come to regard their children as stutterers and parents who look upon their youngsters' speech as normal, or at least as being satisfactorily fluent, and with differences between the relationships between these parents, respectively, and their children.

Such an investigation, as has been indicated, has been made by Darley (1955), and additional data are being accumulated at Iowa as this is being written. In general, Darley found that with reference to basic personal and social adjustment the parents who regard their children as stutterers are essentially normal as a group, being more like than different from parents who do not judge their youngsters to be stutterers. The most conspicuous difference was found in the fact that the parents who had "diagnosed" their children as "stutterers" were more concerned about the speech of their youngsters, especially its fluency aspects, more disapproving of the normal speech of childhood as their own children represented it, and in general "harder to please" as listeners than were the parents of the children in the control group.

This specific group difference can only be understood in relation to other differences between the two groups of parents. The more important of these may be summarized rather briefly. In general, the experimental group parents (those who regarded their children as stutterers) were somewhat more striving than the control group parents, a bit less satisfied with themselves and with each other, and more inclined to rate their own children's development and behavior lower than the objective data appeared to justify. They were comparatively somewhat more perfectionistic with regard to their children, themselves, and each other. They tended to belittle themselves, to be less self-approving and self-accepting, and to be apparently more ambitious, though not necessarily more overtly so, than the control parents. All this is to be said in a gray language, not in blacks and whites. The differences are not clean-cut. They represent trends or tendencies.

It seems quite apparent that the way a child is listened to, evaluated, and reacted to by his parents is more important than the way he speaks, so far as the "onset of stuttering" is concerned. We may not, therefore, expect to find "the cause" of stuttering simply by exploring the "body" or the "mind" or the "personality" of the speaker. It would appear that the listener's feeling or judgment, "Wilbur is now stuttering," is a response to what Wilbur is doing in speaking. Depending on how it is made, how often, under what circumstances, by whom it is made, and on the preparedness or lack of preparedness of the child to whom it is made, it will be responded to in turn with more or less uneasiness, bewilderment, speech conflict, tension, and other manifestations of disturbed speech behavior. These, in their turn, will be reacted to by the increasingly concerned listener, whose consequent responses will be, in further turn, responded to by the speaking child in ways somewhat more intensified, and so forth into the ever expanding complexities of the vicious circle that all this represents.

In order to understand the "onset of stuttering," we must appreciate the apparently dependable fact that the word *stuttering,* employed with comprehensive extensional validity, refers not simply to some aspect or other of speech but rather to a certain kind of relationship between a speaker and one or more listeners. Although speaker and listener can be—and in one particular sense must always be—one and the same person, nevertheless it is for practical purposes nearly always true, and most probably at time of "onset," that stuttering involves two or more persons. "The stutterer" has more than two legs. And so we relevantly look for "causes" of the relationship we call stuttering in both (or all) parties to the relationship and—a point that needs considerable emphasis—in the relationship itself. This last point would seem to be exceedingly important, since any given speaker may combine with any given listener to produce stuttering, while either one alone or in combination with another given listener or speaker, respectively, may not. And so it seems clear that it is not enough to know "all about" the speaker or "all about" the listener; if one is to understand stuttering it is necessary to search for relevant facts also in the relationships between given speakers and given listeners. When the problem is seen as centering around this relationship in the case in which the speaker and the listener is one and the same person—an individual "stuttering to himself"—it becomes most particularly engaging. And this is always the case, of course, whenever the person who stutters, in talking to one or more other persons, is attending to his own stuttering and reacting to it evaluatively and overtly. At the core of this problem are the stutterer's attitudes toward his own stuttering,[5] as well as his fund of information—and misinformation—about it and his assumptions and hypotheses concerning it, however crude or refined they may be. It is clear that while this particular aspect of the problem has been probed in one way and another by individual stutterers such as Wedberg (1937) and Johnson (1930), and by a number of investigators who have used case-study and test procedures, there is need for a systematic reexamination, more rigorous formulation, and more extended exploration of the stutterer's evaluations of his own stuttering, conceived both narrowly as speech disturbance and comprehensively as interpersonal relationship, and the interactions of these evaluations with the stuttering, so far as these are to be directly or indirectly determined.[6]

Certain specific aspects of stutterers' evaluations and reactions to stuttering that are especially relevant to our present purposes are to be seen in studies by Tuthill (1946) and Shane (1955). Tuthill made phonograph recordings of the speech of stutterers and of nonstutterers, and he also included some samples of the speech of nonstutterers simulating stuttering. He played the recordings for listeners whom he instructed to mark, on mimeographed copies supplied to them, the words which were in their judgment stuttered. He used mainly three kinds of judges: speech clinicians, undergraduate students who were unsophisticated regarding stuttering (laymen), and young adult stutterers. He found that within all three groups there was marked disagreement among the judges as to whether given words were or were not stuttered; the laymen showed no more disagreement than did the clinicians or the stutterers themselves, both of whom might be expected, according to probably common assumption, to know "what stuttering is." No greater agreement was obtained when sound films of the speech of stutterers and nonstutterers were used instead of recorded sound alone. This general finding of Tuthill's lends abundant plausibility to the idea, supported by the data reported by Johnson (1955) and Darley (1955), that one parent might very well regard as stuttering what other parents, or other listeners generally, would judge to be normal speech. Additional support for this conclusion has been provided by the studies of Bloodstein and his students (1952).

Tuthill reported another finding also that is fundamental to an appreciation of the function of the stutterer's notions about stuttering in relation to his speech difficulty. Each of Tuthill's judges heard the recordings twice. Taking the total number of words judged as stuttered during all listening sessions, the mean number so judged by the laymen was 86.6, and the cor-

[5] See Ammons and Johnson (1944) for an approach to the measurement of attitude toward stuttering. This is also presented, together with a number of related procedures, in W. Johnson, D. C. Spriestersbach, and F. L. Darley, Diagnostic Manual in Speech Correction. (New York, Harper, 1952), pp. 137–142.

[6] Several aspects of this problem are dealt with in Johnson and Leutenegger (1955), particularly in Chs. 1, 2, and 7.

responding values for the clinicians and the stutterers were, respectively, 110.9 and 121.3. The stutterers were operating with a functional definition of "stuttering" such that they "heard" on the average 40 per cent more words as stuttered than the laymen "heard," and nearly 10 per cent more than even the trained clinicians "heard." Assuming Tuthill's subjects to have been representative of their respective populations, one may, without doing outlandish violence to logic, draw from these figures the inference that the average stutterer could reduce the frequency of his stuttering approximately 40 per cent simply by revising his working definition of "stuttering" so as to make it correspond with that of the average layman! To the extent that a stutterer responds with a negative evaluation and attendant avoidant tension to anything in his own speech that he regards as stuttering, the more inclusive the definition of "stuttering" with which he operates, the more frequently will he so respond while speaking. Tuthill's data cast a particularly bright light on this aspect of the factor of evaluation in relation to stuttering behavior.

Shane (1955) carried out a study several years ago in which she demonstrated a striking side-tone effect. She instructed stutterers to read aloud under ordinary conditions and also while wearing earphones through which masking tones were fed into the ears at an intensity level of approximately 95 decibels. She coached her subjects to keep the intensity of their own voices at about their customary levels while reading aloud with noise. Most of her subjects reported that for the most part they could not hear their own voices while reading with the masking tones, and all reported that their perception of their own voices was markedly impaired. Under this condition of faint or no perception by the stutterer of his own voice, the frequency of stuttering was significantly reduced and for most of the subjects no stuttering occurred. These findings would appear to imply that the stutterer's perception of his speech, and presumably his own stuttering, is an extremely important factor in producing stuttering.

The data cited have been selected for the very specific and limited purposes of the present discussion, and there has been no intention of presenting a comprehensive review of even the more relevant literature. The main purpose of this discussion has been to draw attention to certain perceptual and evaluative aspects of the stuttering problem and to point up in some measure their relative significance.

## CERTAIN SPECULATIVE CONCLUSIONS

Recalling now our previous list of five possibilities of revising the traditional "A causes B" formula for explaining stuttering, the need for increasing the number of factors to be included may be said to have been well-supported by the foregoing considerations. If we are to retain the term *cause* we must use its plural form, and by *effect* we must mean something quite like a class of effects. But even "A's cause B's" will not do, because the relationships or structures of the events involved are not as simple as that formula implies. It was suggested as a second possibility for revision that, instead of assuming a one-way relationship, we consider the matter of interaction and the self-reflexiveness of the interactions that might be involved. The facts we have reviewed appear to recommend strongly this sort of revision.

Our third suggestion was that we re-examine the traditional distinction between "cause" and "effect"—that is, between the conditions essential to stuttering and the stuttering. At time of onset it would seem that either we must say they are indistinguishable, or else we must say that there is no stuttering—in the limited and commonly intended sense of clinically significant speech disturbance. As stuttering develops in the form of disturbed speech, the conditions essential to it appear to include feelings of uncertainty, restricted spontaneity, and uneasiness on the part of the child; and these are manifested, so we may reasonably assume, in the hesitant and tense speech reactions that we call stuttering—and that are, in turn, evidently essential to the maintenance and intensification of the feelings they serve to express. The child's feelings appear to be a function also of the evaluative reactions to his speech that are made by his listeners, especially his parents. The child seems to adopt or interiorize the evaluations of his speech that are manifested by his parents and other authority figures, and in the process makes of himself, as it were, his own most incapacitating listener. The distinction, therefore, between "causes" and "effects" in this situation, as in any other involving a self-reflexive, expanding, spiral pattern of functional relationships, is highly arbitrary and relative and to be employed with due flexibility.

The fourth suggestion was that, instead of orienting our theory to an assumed constancy of the alleged "cause," we orient it to variations in the "effect" to be explained. The data concerning adaptation, spontaneous recovery, and consistency of the stuttering response—in the limited sense of disturbed speech—appear to require for their interpretation a pattern of conditions analogous to those essential for the learning of responses and their subsequent inhibition or activation.[7] The pattern of conditions implied by the behavior to be interpreted would seem necessarily to include such factors as motivations with varying scopes of generalization and degrees of

---

[7] For a discussion of the basic data derived from studies of variations in amount of stuttering, see Ch. 1 (Johnson, 1955) of *Stuttering in Children and Adults*. These data may be summed up very briefly in the following general statements: (*a*) "Adaptation" refers to the reduction in frequency or rated severity of stuttering with successive readings of a passage, or with continued reading of nonrepeating material. It amounts on the average to about a 50 per cent reduction in proportion of stuttered words in five readings of a passage, usually about 200 to 500 words in length. There is some but less adaptation in the spontaneous speech of stutterers. (*b*) "Spontaneous recovery" refers to a resurgence in frequency or severity of stuttering after a sufficient time interval following adaptation. (*c*) "Consistency" refers to the tendency of stuttering to occur consistently in association with specific cues or stimuli. For discussions of theoretical implications of relevant data see Wischner (1950), Johnson *et al.* (1956), and Sheehan (1953). Lewis and Sherman (1951) have developed methodological principles basic in research concerned with variations in amount or severity of stuttering.

strength, conflicts of variable intensity between or among different motivations or drives, and the association of drive-motivated response tendencies with other response tendencies and particular cues or patterns of stimuli. This general problem is so complex that we may assume it will occupy investigators for many years to come.

The final and fifth recommendation was that the degree of extensional agreement in the use of the term *stuttering* and of other words that are employed significantly in statements about stuttering be given due consideration as a factor that is important in its own right in relation to the problem of stuttering. How important it is can be appreciated especially through consideration of the role of extensional disagreement at time of so-called onset of stuttering and again at the point in time at which it becomes crucial to decide whether a person who has been a stutterer still is one or has become a nonstutterer. It would appear to be a serious question, indeed, whether the expanding spiral of self-reflexive evaluative reactions, of which stuttered speech is a function, would in any instance develop and have its unfortunate consequences were it not for the disregard in the first place of the possibility of wide disagreement with respect to extensional meaning of "stuttering" and "stutterer"—disregard by the parents and other responsible adults who do the evaluating and labeling of specific children as "stutterers," or the equivalent. And every clinician of experience surely has been impressed with the stutterer's own disinclination to discard the label "stutterer" in thinking of himself even after achieving such a degree of speech improvement that the label comes to serve only as a gross overgeneralization with very slight, if any, extensional reference. The labeling reactions of the parent, which the child adopts and makes his persevering own, and the elaborate web of language behavior that forms around these labeling reactions, may usefully be regarded as part and parcel of the stuttering problem, comprehensively considered, or as one of the more important factors responsible for stuttering, narrowly regarded as a characteristic speech disturbance.

(The problem of stuttering, as seen from the point of view represented by this discussion, is not merely a disturbance of speech, of course. It begins as a particular kind of perceptual and evaluative response to a given child's speech by his responsible listeners, usually his parents. This leads to a special sort of impairment of the relationship between the child and his parents, and from this the child acquires and in his own way elaborates the relevant perceptual and evaluative reactions of his parents so that he comes to have, as listener, a more and more disruptive effect on himself as speaker. And this strongly implies that it is as a listener, a perceiver, an evaluator, quite as much as—probably, in fact, far more than—a speaker that the person who stutters is to be treated. Quite by himself, he presents no problem. His is a social uneasiness, a borrowed and a shared disruption of tranquility. He and all those others with whom he shares and from whom he borrows trouble make of themselves, all together, a composite patient. )

## BIBLIOGRAPHY

AMMONS, R., and JOHNSON, W. 1944. Studies in the psychology of stuttering XVIII. The construction and application of a test of attitude toward stuttering. *J. Speech Disorders, 9,* 39–49.

BLOODSTEIN, O., JAEGAR, W., and TUREEN, J. 1952. A study of the diagnosis of stuttering by parents of stutterers and non-stutterers. *J. Speech Hearing Disorders,* 17, 308–315.

BRANSCOM, M. E., HUGHES, J., and OXTOBY, E. T. 1955. Studies of non-fluency in the speech of pre-school children. *In* Johnson, W., and Leutenegger, R. Stuttering in children and adults. Minneapolis: Univ. Minn. Press. Ch. 5

DARLEY, F. L. 1955. The relationship of parental attitudes and adjustments to the development of stuttering. *In* Johnson, W., and Leutenegger, R., Stuttering in children and adults. Minneapolis: Univ. Minn. Press. Ch. 4.

DAVIS, D. M. 1939, 1940. The relation of repetitions in the speech of young children to certain measures of language maturity and situational factors. *J. Speech Disorders,* 4, 308–318; 5, 235–246.

EGLAND, G. O. 1955. Repetitions and prolongations in the speech of stuttering and non-stuttering children. *In* Johnson, W., and Leutenegger, R., Stuttering in children and adults. Minneapolis: Univ. Minn. Press. Ch. 6.

FRASIER, J. 1955. An exploration of stutterers' theories of their own stuttering. *In* Johnson, W., and Leutenegger, R., Stuttering in children and adults. Minneapolis: Univ. Minn. Press. Ch. 26.

JOHNSON, W. 1955. The time, the place, and the problem. *In* Johnson, W., and Leutenegger, R., Stuttering in children and adults. Minneapolis: Univ. Minn. Press. Ch. 1.

―――― 1955. A study of the onset and development of stuttering. *In* Johnson, W., and Leutenegger, R., Stuttering in children and adults. Minneapolis: Univ. Minn. Press. Ch. 3.

―――― 1930. Because I stutter. New York: Appleton.

―――― BOEHMLER, R., BRISSEY, F. L., FRICK, J. V., GUSTAFSON, C., and WILLIAMS, D. Studies of speech fluency and non-fluency. Unpublished research, Univ. of Iowa.

JOHNSON, W., BROWN, S. F., CURTIS, J. F. EDNEY, C. W., and KEASTER, J. 1948. Rev. ed. 1956. Speech handicapped school children. New York: Harper. Ch. 5.

JOHNSON, W., DARLEY, F. L., and SPRIESTERSBACH, D. C. 1952. Diagnostic manual in speech correction. New York: Harper.

JOHNSON, W., and KNOTT, J. R. 1955. A systematic approach to the psychology of stuttering. *In* Johnson, W., and Leutenegger, R., Stuttering in children and adults. Minneapolis: Univ. Minn. Press. Ch. 2.

JOHNSON, W., and LEUTENEGGER, R., 1955. editors. Stuttering in children and adults. Minneapolis: Univ. Minn. Press.

LEWIS, D., and SHERMAN, D. 1951. Measuring the severity of stuttering. *J. Speech Hearing Disorders,* 16, 320–326.

PENFIELD, W., and RASMUSSEN, T. 1950. The cerebral cortex of man. New York: Macmillan.

SHANE, M. L. S. 1955. Effect on stuttering of alteration in auditory feedback. *In* Johnson, W., and Leutenegger, R., Stuttering in children and adults. Minneapolis: Univ. Minn. Press. Ch. 22.

SHEEHAN, J. G. 1953. Theory and treatment of stuttering as an approach-avoidance conflict. *J. Psychol.,* 36, 27–49.

TUTHILL, C. E. 1946. A quantitative study of extensional meaning with special reference to stuttering. *Speech Monogr.*, 13, 81–98.

WEDBERG, C. F. 1937. The stutterer speaks. Redlands, Calif.: Valley Fine Arts Press.

WISCHNER, G. 1950. Stuttering behavior and learning: A preliminary theoretical formulation. *J. Speech Hearing Disorders,* 15, 324–335.

CHAPTER 29

# THE UNSPEAKABLE FEELINGS OF PEOPLE, WITH SPECIAL REFERENCE TO STUTTERING

• *Lee Edward Travis, Ph.D.*

THIS CHAPTER REPORTS a picture of some people obtained from the psychotherapeutic situation (see Chapter 31). The therapist is given a unique opportunity to view and to experience the mental life of another person who is
in the throes of a struggle to solve vital intrapsychic and interpersonal problems. The psychotherapeutic relationship affords a naturalistic approach to
an increased understanding of the magnificent mental processes of man. Before some of the manifestations of these processes, the therapist stands in
awe and in humility. Before others he stands in sheer ignorance. Even at a
time when there are those who feel that little is left to learn in therapy, the
present writer believes that only an humble beginning to an immensely
significant approach to humanity's problems has been made. It seems true
that some main highways have been cut through the forest, but it seems
equally true that untold riches remain as mysterious as ever away and beyond
the beaten paths.

Some people have enough misery to drive them to enter into therapeutic
negotiations. In their misery they have sufficiently high motivation to get
them to talk long enough and honestly enough to explore the wonderfully
intricate details of themselves in relatedness. Imagine the average person
who is indistinguishable from the mine-run of people spending three or four
hours a week for two to three years talking freely and almost interminably
about himself. He just would not do it because he has no need or motivation
to do it. Mainly, he is not miserable enough. Then, too, there will have to
be someone who has the motivation and the patience to listen for all of these
hours and months and years, one who has the training and experience to
understand and accept what he hears.

In most instances where human behavior is studied, in the laboratory, at
the party, in the parlor, motives are slight and the situation is trivial. In
psychotherapy just the opposite is true. Not only are motives strong, but the
situation is crucial. For the patient it is either a continued life of sickening

anxiety and misery or a new life of peace and happiness. Such urgency brings every resource of the patient and therapist into play in the interpersonal relationship of therapy where the patient will reveal and sense himself more completely than he ever has in the past and more than he ever will again in the presence of another. The patient must tell all and the therapist must cope with the most vexing and vital issues of interpersonal relationships.

The label of "patient" misleads many people. For the purpose of this chapter, the patient is one who is so anxious and miserable that he seeks help. According to other criteria, he may not be as maladjusted as others who do not go into therapy, but the way *he* sees and feels himself makes him a patient. Our patients should not be considered basically different from other people. Rather, they are a group of people who differ from other people in the degree of motivation for psychotherapy.

## THE PEOPLE OF THIS STUDY

The clearest common feature of the people we studied was misery. In a way and to a degree they were all miserable. Their misery was enough to drive them to seek help. They expressed their misery in the various complaints of irrational fears and anxieties, stage fright, distaste for life, homosexuality, sexual frigidity, alcoholism, primary hypertension, asthma, ulcer, and stuttering. Some had more of one complaint than another, but all were miserable. In a word, their lives did not agree with them. Psychological burps and belches threatened to expose their emotional indigestion.

Actually 65 people were studied, and their productions and reactions form the basis for the materials of this chapter. These people were observed in the psychotherapeutic situation for a total of approximately 13,000 hours. Some were seen for as little as 10 hours and some for as much as 400 hours. The average number of hours was about 200. Thirty of these people complained mainly of stuttering. Thirty-five complained of the other conditions listed above. Further breakdown of these people into groups seems unnecessary for the main theme of this chapter. All of these people were adults ranging in age from sixteen to fifty years. There were 27 females and 38 males.

Our special respect will be paid to those 30 individuals who complained of stuttering. Most of them felt severely handicapped in speech, and not only undertook therapy but persisted in the therapeutic relationship up to 400 hours for some individual cases. Some stutterers for one reason or another, including insufficient motivation, discontinued therapy early. No statistical comparisons will be made between those who came for stuttering and those who came for some other reason, such as homosexuality or sexual frigidity. Some broad comparisons will be noted and evaluated, mainly to stimulate further study rather than to draw any final conclusions.

We are impressed with the obvious: that stutterers are human beings and that as such they have a very great deal in common with other people, even in the manner of speaking. Both introspective and objective observations convince us that most people stutter. Only a few people are sufficiently miserable over their speaking relationships, however, that they bring their problem to therapy under the label of stuttering.

## THE OLD CONDITIONS OF LEARNING

A symptom is a remark about the culture in which that symptom developed. It is a reflection upon the nurturing influences of the home and community in which the person was reared. According to his lights, the patient was right in adopting a response or a set of responses known as a symptom. He found along the way that to react symptomatically reduced drives and tensions. His symptom was thus rewarded or reinforced, and in this sense learned (Dollard and Miller, 1950, p. 15).

Our people came to us because of what happened to their basic needs and drives as they grew from birth. Originally, *in utero,* their environment was relatively perfectly comfortable and complete. It met relatively perfectly and completely their growing demands. There were no discomforts, deficiencies, or frustrations. And then they were born: physically, mentally, and emotionally helpless. They were extremely weak in every way but one, the need to live. Their desire to eat and to eliminate and to breathe and to be comfortable was great. Their means of satisfying these living needs were utterly dependent upon those who cared for them. Their very existence was entirely at the mercy of their elders, at the mercy of the physical, emotional, intellectual, economic, and social conditions of the adult giants around them. Only in infancy and childhood were our people's own capacities to control their lives so meager, ineffectual, and pitiful.

It ought not be surprising, then, that acute emotional conflicts occurred in the earliest days of our people. These people, as children, had no tolerance for delay of the satisfaction of their needs. They could not yet learn to wait, to reason, to hope, to plan. Rather, they were compelled by all consuming drives, tensions, and discomforts to action—crying, twisting, flaying. They could not think, talk, or reason, or control either themselves or their environment. Between them and their adult teachers was a tremendous gap. They had to be fed, picked up, hauled around, cleaned, and protected. And how were these things done? Right here was the critical issue. At this time what may be done for good or for bad may never be undone. What was lacking may never be made up. What pain was given may never again be taken completely away. These possibly tumultuous interpersonal relationships furnished the soil for unverbalized and hence unconscious emotional conflicts. Only when these people learned to talk and to think could the impact of these circumstances be reduced.

Had our people, as helpless children, been handled with the greatest indulgence, they would not have served as subjects of this chapter. Could they have had the greatest support from parents during the earliest weeks, months, and years of their lives, they would not have stuttered. Their savage drives should have been kept at the lowest possible level by the attentiveness of their parents. Every supportively encouraging effort should have been made by the parents to teach the child to talk and to think in order that he might in turn learn to wait, hope, reason, and plan.

But the parents of our people did not keep the strongest drives of their children at a low level of urgency and they did not know how or they did not resolve to impose the burdens of a civilized life in a tolerable and reasonable way. Instead our people, as children, were treated as emotional and intellectual little adults. Adult powers to control their drives and feelings were assumed. Incompatible demands were made and utterly impossible checks and tasks were set. Unlearned and at times unlearnable discriminations were expected. Heavy sanctions were applied for mistakes and failures.

The conditions of the stutterer's early life created his stuttering. They proved hostile and painful to the expression, verbal and otherwise, of his drives, and he feared rejection and punishment if he tried honestly to express himself. He feared criticism of his true thoughts and words. He felt that others expected him to be unbearably good in thought and in word. Too, through his failure to be received for what he was, he had suffered wounds to his self-esteem. He had generalized from specific, unacceptable thoughts and words to the unacceptability of himself as a whole. Not only were his expressions unworthy but he was unworthy as well. His old repressions were continually reinforced by the current contempt of others. No one understood him and he was not capable of understanding himself. In listening to their stuttering child, parents might have deservedly felt miserable in realizing that they were listening to themselves.

Stuttering may be defined as an advertisement of strong, unconscious motives of which the stutterer is deeply ashamed. Repression falls on the verbal expression of these motives and may fall on all words and sentences lest they might lead to these motives. When any person stutters, he is blocking something else besides what you and he might think he is trying to say; something else that is pressing for verbal expression but which will be intolerable to you and to him alike should it be uttered.

## A SKETCH OF SOME OLDER TRAINING SITUATIONS

With our stutterers, the culture took a position on their various infant and child needs. It took the position, a traditional one, that their drives should be tamed relatively early and firmly. This was accomplished mainly by setting up in the child fear, shame, and guilt in opposition to drives, urges, and wants. This opposition of forces, such as fear against drive, resulted in a number of dilemmas which produced acute emotional conflicts. Then our people as children inhibited many cue-producing responses which would have mediated thinking, feeling, and talking. In short, they repressed the conflicts. Unfortunately, this learned management of conflicts (repression) did not solve the dilemmas permanently. The emotional paralysis of re-pression had to be continually maintained in the face of environmental factors which kept threatening to reactivate the conflicts. As these situa-tional stimuli pecked away at these children, rewarding drive one time and fear another time, the children were constantly taxed to keep the painful and anxiety-producing conflicts low. One manifestation or advertisement of this taxing effort was stuttering. Before the eyes and ears of their parents, our people showed in stuttering speech the operation of opposing feelings: sexual curiosity and the shame of it, hostility and the fear of it, and desire to mess and the embarrassment over it.

Possibly there are innumberable ways and combinations of ways by which society imposes its will through the acts of the parents. Yet it seems clear that we can group these ways into a certain limited number of clusters. We may be accused of overemphasizing these relatively few situations. Our ex-cuse for seeming to do so is that the situations listed are clinically and ex-perimentally documented (Travis and Baruch, 1941, Ch. 7; Dollard and Miller, 1950, Ch. 10). Certainly our general thesis will not be altered by substituting or adding other situations.

### Crying

Crying is the child's first powerful response. It is assumed to be a response to some need or discomfort. The baby's or child's cry is also a powerful stimulus to its elders, producing empathically anxiety in the mothering ones (Sullivan, 1953, Ch. 3). It amounts to a demand or command upon those who are in a position of responsibility to the child. The culture takes the position that a child should not cry, at least not much. The members of the culture vary in their ways of meeting this position, and the way it is met determines important habits and traits in the child.

Crying may be thought of as the first cue-producing response. Its purpose is to attract stimuli that will relieve tension. In general, it should be honored as the one simple thing the child can do to get results and as the first small unit in the child's control of the world. Not to reward or reinforce crying is to teach the child that there is nothing it can do to relieve tensions, dis-comforts, and pain of the moment. Such training may lay the foundation for apathy and not trying something else, such as speech, when in need or in trouble. Too frequently a child is recognized only when its cry is violent. It may learn from this to respond all out of proportion to its needs and to become excessively demanding. It will fail to learn such discriminations as small needs are met by smaller demands. Possibly most important of all, when a child is left to "cry itself out" or is slapped for crying, it may learn too well that it is unloved and unwanted and that its world, the parents or family, is hostile and spiteful. Further, the fear, anxiety, and hostility exist-ing with the futile crying will become associated with the original need for crying; to the darkness, the isolation of the nursery, the absence of parental stimuli, and other current things, acts, and relationships. So the child may become anxious when hungry (the original drive for crying), afraid of the dark or of quietness, nervous or angry when left alone, and so on. And as it grows, the parents may complain of a shy, or apathetic, or excessively demanding, or retarded and inhibited child and later on of a socially handicapped adolescent and adult. To cry when in need, when hurt, lonely and devastated, and fail to get available help will leave long and lasting adverse effects.

## Feeding

Hunger is probably the strongest living need. Everything else depends upon the satisfaction of the hunger drive which is an urgent, incessant, all-consuming, and timeless force, producing intense activation. In the early years of life, the hunger drive and the strong responses it excites are completely incompatible with the child's ability to cope with them. He is utterly dependent upon somebody else for the management of his problem. He cannot wait, or talk to himself, or hope, or plan. He can only cry, now.

The culture takes a stand here too. Mainly it is that the child shall be fed, but fed predetermined amounts of food, on schedule. In addition, the child shall be fed, but only under certain conditions (i.e., being alone, or after being good, or only if he will eat quickly and neatly). For rigid cultural standards governing the satisfaction of the hunger drive, the child has little or no tolerance. He cannot tell time. He cannot distract himself with the feelings and thoughts and words about the future. He cannot understand the meaning of delay, or the limited amount of milk, or the conditions of its forthcoming. But he is acquiring much important learning. He may be learning that effort, particularly vocal effort, does not pay. He may learn that he is not wanted or loved. He may learn to fear the dark or being alone. He may learn to "overreact" because he is fed only after his most violent responses. On the other hand, the feeding experience can be the occasion for the child to learn to like others and to be with them; to learn that he is desirable and wanted; to learn that his needs are appreciated; and to learn that his reactions, particularly his vocal ones, are helpful. The seemingly "natural" and innocuous feeding situation is fraught with important and emotional consequences. Too many people, including parents, do not see this. They see little if anything at all to worry them. Yet observant students may see the child becoming apathetic, apprehensive, and shy, and failing to develop appropriate verbal skills. The tragedy is that much of this learning is secret. The child cannot label the experiences which it is having at this time. It cannot talk about them or talk them out. It portrays them in ways that we label as apathy, or speechlessness, or fearfulness, or sociability, or confidence. What was not labeled and not verbalized at these early times cannot well be reported later. In therapy only shadows and echoes of these early and deep feelings appear. Patient and therapist glimpse only their contrails. They emerge mutely interwoven into the fabric of conscious expression.

### Toilet and Cleanliness Training

Although possibly not as strong as the hunger drive, the drive to eliminate is nevertheless persistent and commanding and at times takes precedence over every other need. Bowel and bladder tensions may exert a priority right upon the interests and efforts of the organism.

The child begins with an innocent interest in his feces and urine. He may handle and play with fecal material. There is no evidence of an innate revulsion toward the acts or the products of elimination. Quickly, in some instances during the first few months of life, his natural and naive eliminative behavior runs into the cultural patterns lying in wait. These patterns will demand that he deposit his excretory materials only in a prescribed and secret place and that he keep his body clean in doing so. These patterns will demand, too, that he limit to the bare essentials any verbal reference to these issues so that this subject matter is closed out and excluded from social reference for life.

More often than not, instead of the child being led gently and supportively by example into meeting the cultural goals of elimination and cleanliness, it is doused with hostile, punitive, and loathing parental attitudes when it displays its naivete or fails to honor cultural demands. The culture sets its task as the building within the personality of the child barriers of loathing and disgust for urine and feces. To construct these inward barriers, the child must put himself in a conflict situation. He must pit one set of feelings against another set. He must desire and loathe the same thing at the same time. A swelling bladder or bowel produces a strong drive that the child wishes to honor. The pain of losing the parents' love and of their punishment if he does honor this drive naturally places the child in a state of great anxiety. To salvage something from this dilemma, the child has to turn on the drive or on the parents or both. This management of a conflict situation is loaded with possible future emotional sickishness. If he turns on the drive with fear, loathing, and disgust, he will repress it in certain ways and to certain degrees. In the future he may become constipated, he may cry when eliminative demands call him, or he may become afraid of the toilet itself. If he turns on the parents, he may become defiant and stubborn, or furtive and sneaking, or attempt struggling with them, or possibly resort to biting and slapping them.

Whatever course or combination of courses the child may select to follow in the face of harsh and hasty toilet and cleanliness training, he will be the loser. On the basis of a pursuing, all-seeing, punishing parent, the child may be making as few responses as possible, certainly not adventuring forth. Being unable to discriminate between parental loathing for his penis and anus and their excreta, and loathing for himself, he adopts feelings of unworthiness, insignificance, and hopeless sinfulness. These feelings and reactions are of particular interest to the speech pathologist. Any child laden with guilt, fear of its guardian, loathing for its excretory organs and their functions, and feelings of wretched awfulness just cannot be expected to acquire and risk verbal, adventuresome communication. It just has too much that it must not talk about. It will learn to speak less well or not at all because it does not remain close and warm and free in a give-and-take relationship to those very people who could teach it to talk well.

## Sex-Training

Sex is an ever recurring conflict element. Hourly feelings, reactions, and words confirm this statement. This is not so because sex is the strongest drive. Certainly under specific circumstances, pain, fear, and hunger outrank it. Even some secondary drives such as ambition and pride can be stronger than sex. It appears that sex is so universally implicated because it is so universally attacked and inhibited. In no other instance is an individual asked to block completely the expression of such a strong drive for such a long period of time; the culture demands for all practical purposes a completely sexless child.

Conscience and custom weigh most heavily upon sex. Too many people do not guess that children have a sex life and that guilt and shame are a crushing burden to lay on a child's mind. But the guilt will not always crush or hold. Although there are taboos which dare not be broken, children and adults learn interesting ways to break them. They lie or cheat; become impotent or inverted; develop anesthesia or paralysis; and speak not at all or block in their attempts at verbal utterance. It is around sex that the culture builds its biggest moral junk pile. Sex, or rather its place, has been cast in the leading role in interpersonal relationships. Society is split into boy and girl, man and woman, male and female, masculinity and femininity. Sex-typing becomes inextricably involved with sex rejection and sex acceptance. Is the baby a boy or a girl; is the child a sissy or a tom-boy; is the adult a homosexual or a Lesbian? That there is such wondering is telltale.

Cultural management of sex often ends in the greatest misgivings that the individual can have in regard to himself and others. His sexual feelings can come to evoke intense anxiety. They can come to arouse loathing and nausea for his sexual anatomy and physiology. They can lead him into feared relationships with others where defensively he may close up and escape. The individual can come to despise and reject parts of himself and to generalize from the parts to the whole.

The extensions of his feelings may become puzzling if not amazing. Because of masturbation taboos he may dread to be alone. Because of homosexual taboos he may be afraid of men. Because of incest taboos he may be fearful of women. These fears may lead him just about to be afraid to be. And even if he should try, he will have trouble in talking his way out. His teachers have been very niggardly about giving him names for sexual organs, sexual feelings, and sexual acts. What names they may have given him were powerfully emotionally loaded. But anyway he was harshly intimidated relative to talking or feeling or thinking about sex at all. It became remote, inscrutable, and maleficent. Some way or other though he did learn something. He did acquire some words and thoughts. When they occurred to him, however, especially when the possibility of doing anything about them occurred to him, his conflict was keener both by arousing drives and by cueing off the anxiety attached to them. He was pained when he thought about sexual matters and relieved when he stopped. The result was repression. This was just not good management. The person was victimized. He lost, possibly forever, the opportunity to use higher mental activities in solving conflicts involving sex and authority. In the future he could see the unreasonableness of his sexual inadequacies and his crippled interpersonal relationships based upon those ineptnesses, but he simply could not do anything about them. No amount of reasoning, or logic, or pleading helped. Some people find that help through the renaming and re-establishment and re-evaluation of these bygone feelings and events can come only by succeeding in the weary work of psychotherapy. Some people find in therapy that sex conflicts lurk behind the all-too-innocent appearing speech block. They may find it possible to accept cheerfully and amiably a degree of authority and threat without the defensive measure of stuttering.

### Anger-Fear Situations

We may assume that anger responses are produced by the innumerable and unavoidable frustration situations of child life (Dollard, Doob, Miller, and Sears, 1939). We could certainly recommend a regimen of child care to minimize frustration situations, but our big quarrel here is with the management of anger responses when they do occur. Society takes a rather firm and consistent stand toward the responses of anger in inhibiting them by fear and pain and allowing them reign only in a few circumstances of play and self-defense. Parents resent and fear the anger and rage of a child; and the culture, since it is dominated by parents, accepts and even rewards the virtuous chastisement of the rebellious youngster. Possibly it would not be so harmful if anger and anger alone could be inhibited or extinguished by fear and pain. But universally anger is associated with toilet and cleanliness training, eating, sleeping, and sex; and all the other learning situations in the home. So we come to have such combinations as anal and oral sadism, and sexualized aggression. The fear and pain that was meant for the anger and its responses became attached to all feelings, drives, thoughts, and words that were in the child's consciousness at the time. Too, those people and things and relationships that were present became connected to the fear and anxiety responses of the child. Thus fear and anxiety became attached not only to anger, but to all the other emotional responses which the child might have been making at the time, and to all the cues of the situation in which the responses were occurring. After this learning has occurred, the cues produced by any emotion of anger may set off anxiety responses which will outstrip not only the emotional responses of anger themselves but all the associated feelings and emotions. This produces conflict, and repression results to relieve the situation. When anger with its partners in pluralistic marriage is repressed, it is constantly exposed to reactivation and as it stirs to subject the person to pain and humiliation, the counterforces of fear and guilt arise to hold it down. Among other evidences of this fear is stuttering, the inhibition of speaking for fear of revealing anger and its several associates.

### Summary of Some Older Training Situations

We have sketched some training situations where conflicts abound in our culture. In these situations particularly, the child's drives meet frustration, condemnation, and derogation. At first, the conflicts are between the wanting child and society, especially his parents. But quickly the conflict is internalized; it is between two of the child's incompatible drives or between the two contradictory sets of responses to these drives. Parents and the culture instill fear, anxiety, shame, and the need to please in the child to block his sex, anger, and messing responses. Thus their child comes to own pairs of conflicting motives, drives, and responses. He will have such pairs as sex-anxiety, anger-fear, and messing-shame. Society is on the side of the second member of each pair. It not only induces anxiety, fear, and shame; it acts to perpetuate them. These feelings are not pleasant to the child. Rather they are unpleasant. They are to be avoided. But how? It appears that the child need make only one response to relieve or reduce his fear and anxiety: *stop thinking* (Dollard and Miller, 1950, p. 203). He stops thinking about anger, or sex, or messing. He is aided in this response of stopping thinking by the fear and anxiety which seem to have an innate tendency to stop thinking and speaking. With awareness of sex or anger or messing gone, unpleasant fear is likewise gone and the child is learning or has learned to forget or to repress. His stopping thinking or forgetting or repressing has been rewarded by the removal of an unpleasant feeling and the installation of a feeling of well-being once again. But repression is really not "good" learning. It is a kind of deficit development. Stopping thinking and feeling are often too costly. Repression leaves gaps, holes, and deficiencies in the personality structure; importantly in social relationships. As stimuli, especially social ones, arouse feared and dreaded responses, the repressed person exhibits hesitancies, blocks, and awkwardness. The range and richness of his responses will be lessened. Rigid, repetitive, and tried-and-true responses will predominate his repertoire. Repression falls alike on all responses, including speech, that may arouse fear and anxiety. When it is impossible to avoid speaking, rather consistently for some people, and at times for all people, stuttering blocks will be necessary lest the sentences lead to strong motives of which the speaker is deeply ashamed or terribly frightened. (Reference to Fig. 1 may help clarify these concepts.)

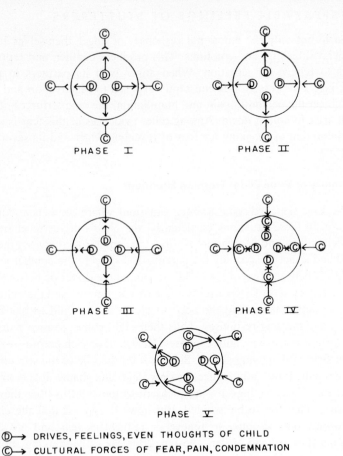

PHASE I        PHASE II

PHASE III        PHASE IV

PHASE V

Ⓓ→ DRIVES, FEELINGS, EVEN THOUGHTS OF CHILD
Ⓒ→ CULTURAL FORCES OF FEAR, PAIN, CONDEMNATION
Ⓒ—< CULTURAL ACCEPTANCE OF INFANT'S WANTS

FIG. 1. Crude schematic representation of the internalization (introjection) of the cultural forces of fear and condemnation and their inhibition (repression) of the drives, feelings, and thoughts of the child. The compromise expressions of these opposing systems may result in symptoms including stuttering. Phase I—The needs of the very young infant gain satisfaction from the culture. The very young baby's wants are generally met. Phase II—The beginning of the taming or domestication of the older infant's biological drives, generally by fear and pain. The conflict is between the baby and his environment, between the inside and the outside. Phase III—To cope better with the internal-external conflicts of Phase II, the child (one to three years of age) begins to adopt the negative attitudes and values (internalize, introject) which the culture has expressed relative to his wants and feelings. The conflict is beginning to be internalized, to be between action systems within the child. He is beginning to be split. Phase IV—By three, the child has made the inhibitory forces of fear and condemnation which originally belonged to the culture more completely his own to oppose his drive and feeling system. He is now more split, having parts of himself disavowed by other parts. External cultural inhibitions still help his internal inhibitory forces to control his now repressed wants and feelings and thoughts. Phase V—Through the ever waxing and waning of both sets of the internal oppositional forces in their relation to environmental factors, compromise or symptomatic expression may occur (including stuttering).

## NEW CONDITIONS OF INTERPERSONAL RELATIONSHIPS

As we have seen, there is the strongest likelihood that the conditions of the stutterer's early life created his speaking difficulties. The main conditions were the methods of his parents in transmitting the spirit of the culture to him. The parents not only induced in the child the drives of fear, guilt, and shame as checks on the child's primary drives but they and their helpers in society perpetuated these checks. The parents and society aligned themselves behind not only the establishment of fear and its derivatives but the continuation of these inhibiting and anxiety-producing forces. So the patient not only had effective help in acquiring or learning conflicts and repression within himself but strong support in maintaining them. Under these conditions, his stuttering, the manifestation of his conflicts, was likewise fostered. In his search for help with his speech, the necessary conditions of unlearning and new learning were usually not found and he continued in his stuttering ways. On the basis of principles and practices borrowed from psychoanalysis and learning theory, our stutterers were subjected to conditions which reversed essentially the old conditions of their rearing. We offered the stuttering individuals conditions which in certain crucial respects were in striking contrast with those of their previous life.

### The New Parent

The patient entered into interpersonal relationships with a person of prestige who paid strict, favorable, and sympathetic attention and who held out strong hope of help. This person felt and showed exceptional permissiveness, no condemnation, total tolerance, and complete composure. He made one important demand: the patient must do his best to say everything that came to his mind, to strive mightily for complete self-revelation. For failing to do this at times the patient was not condemned but constantly encouraged to be under high obligation to succeed. This person, the therapist, was a brand new experience for the patient. He loomed large in contrast with the patient's parents, teachers, relatives, bosses, and other fellow members of society. He never became frightened or punitive or ashamed of anything that the patient said. He never gossiped, or took the patient's time with his own self-revelation, or became impatient. He set his patient free from the restraint of logic, and cross-examination; and when the occasion demanded, he fearlessly stepped in and said things which the patient could not say for himself (see Chapter 31 for a more complete exposition of these points).

### The Extinction of Repressing Forces

The patient talked about frightening topics. He talked about shameful and embarrassing feelings and experiences. He expressed anxiety. For these revelations he was not punished. Rather the feared and shameful motives and feelings were completely accepted. The fear, shame, and guilt were not rewarded by any words or expressions from the therapist of condemnation or nonacceptance. Therefore they were extinguished. The extinction generalized to weaken the motivation to repress other related topics that were too frightening and shameful to discuss or even contemplate before. On the other hand, sexual, angry, and messing feelings were rewarded. They came back and out easier and easier to be channeled for future usefulness. The patient was helped to place these helpless past conditions of childhood and contrast them with his present interpersonal relationships. As fears were reduced by reassurance and extinction (unrewarded), at first the most lightly repressed thoughts and feelings began to appear. In generalizing, the patient adventured further to risk greater fears, and since they too went nonreinforced, more strongly repressed and inhibited responses occurred.

### The Reward of Discovery and Admission

Simultaneously with the unrewarding of fear and consequently its extinction, there is the reinforcement of the discovery and admission of repressed thoughts and feelings. The patient is accepted, even praised, for his painful and anxiety-producing revelations. Whereas before he has received severe disapproval (reward of fear and consequent further repression of primary drives), he now receives calm approval. The rewarding of his repressed materials and the unrewarding of his repressing forces bring him great relief and the feeling of a striking intervention in his life of conflict and anxiety.

### Concluding Thought

Under these conditions, admittedly sketchily and schematically presented the unspeakable feelings of the stutterer were discovered. It is hard, if not impossible, to be fair to the great richness, wide variety, beautiful intricacy, and strict lawfulness of the phenomena to be reported. In the author's attempts to present these matters to students and colleagues, he has met with awe, doubt, and even hostility on the part of his listeners. Two colleagues doubted that human beings could possess, let alone express, such thoughts and feelings. Our reaction was that we had not in any way given the materials to the patients; that the productions were their very own. Of course our reaction could have been that even had we suggested the unbelievable thoughts and feelings, they still would have had to come from a human being. Our purpose in reporting findings obtained under the conditions of certain new interpersonal relationships is to spur thought and research in the area of impaired communication between people.

## THE REPRESSED AND UNSPEAKABLE FEELINGS

Through the processes we have delineated, the child comes to a day when he has strong and important feelings that are conflicting and ambivalent. In a general way, these feelings may be grouped into two opposing camps; the primary drives and their derivatives in one camp, and fear and its derivatives in the other. Assigning to fear both an inherent and an acquired function of inhibition of thought, feeling, and action, it is the basic repressing force. Its victims are primary drives of eating, elimination, sex-curiosity, and anger, and their elaborations. Large constellations of behavior become built up around these opposing camps. The child becomes to a degree split. He is racked with wanting and fearing the same thing. Into interpersonal relationships he carries his civil warfare. First one and then the other of his opposing feelings are tugged and pulled. If inhibited wanting is enticed out of hiding, fear and anxiety arise to hold it down. If fear is enhanced, the child becomes all the more paralyzed in thought, feeling and action. In either instance, fear is the predominately felt drive and all responses, particularly thinking and speaking, are thwarted. Out of this soil stuttering flowers. Thoughts must not be thought; feelings must not be felt; and words must not be spoken.

In what form and complexity do the uncommunicable thoughts and feelings reside within the person? Are they familiar to our senses and understanding? Do they conform to logic and to space and time binding? Some of the answers to these questions will appear in the materials that follow. More important than the answers may be the puzzles that emerge. Could we hope that to be puzzled might lead not necessarily to the right answers but to the right questions?

In discovering and expressing unspeakable feelings and thoughts, the patient approaches his task gingerly. Anxiety and fear make it impossible for him, even with the therapist's heartiest support, to realize easily and quickly the existence and operation of his most important feared and condemned forces. He has suffered greatly in putting away naughty, childish behavior and he is not about to release it. He has paid dearly for what self-esteem he now possesses, and it will take great patience and effort on the part of both him and his therapist to get him to risk his present painfully-gained position. But bit by bit, advancing a little and slipping a little, risking and testing, he learns more and more who he is, what he really wants, and how to discriminate, label, and channel.

The patient's first successes are in sharing conscious misgivings. He is guilty over his socially disrespectful thoughts. He is ashamed of some of his anger and sex feelings. Fear plagues him. These he tells, and they are accepted. He, too, is accepted. He risks more of his known frailties, meannesses, and littlenesses. Over and over these are accepted and he is honored for his honesty of expression. As fear is unrewarded and consequently reduced relative to these more lightly inhibited feelings, more heavily repressed feelings share in the fear reduction and commence to stir. They stir and rise up into the dim light of recognition. It is not enough that they move in the shadows. They carry protective armor against even the recognition that might occur in the dusk. To continue the simile, as fear is reduced, the light of recognition increases and the opaqueness of the armor decreases. The result is a clearer understanding of what the patient really is saying. An example may help to clarify this. Relatively early in therapy an adult male stutterer spoke slowly and painfully as follows:[1]

> Now I'm in my old room at home and some long object is here. Over at the opposite wall is a large hump. It is a large woman's body lying there. It has no head, but arms and legs. An extraordinary thing is, it has large breasts. I have an idea it ought to have a head but I won't let that head be there. Now head comes and it has long black hair hanging down and it is my mother. I remember away back in the old days that my mother had this long black hair, three feet long. Everything now looks very far off. Huge objects all around, but very far off. I feel small and one object moves in close. I'm afraid it is going to crush my legs. I didn't have time to mention that when I saw my mother lying there naked I felt guilty and uneasy. That huge object over there I'm afraid is going to crush my legs. What am I afraid of? That huge object? I'm lying there so small. Hands are here somewhere. I feel terribly empty and hungry.

From this production, neither he nor his therapist knew what the long object was. But both of them came to know what it was that began as the large hump. Against the inhibitory forces of the patient it could appear first only as an indistinguished hump. In this form, not too much anxiety was raised over it and consequently the force of the repressed thoughts and feelings pushed further to reveal a woman. For the moment, who she was, was too much. The patient's anxiety could tolerate her nudity and her breasts but not her identity. So she was headless. The struggle between the opposing camps of feelings continued with the repressed thoughts and feelings getting the better of the repressing forces of anxiety. And then the head with its long black hair hanging down appeared. With this much out, the identity of the woman who formerly was headless and originally appeared as just a hump became clear. She was his mother. For the discovery of this fact, he paid a price. Threats assailed him. He became small and afraid, empty and hungry. His inhibiting fears were not wont to resign without a struggle and they left him with a knowledge all right, but a guilty knowledge. He knew something now that he should not have known. He knew that once consciously and

[1] The author is sensitive to the likelihood of the reader's resistance and reactions of anxiety and even disgust to some of the recorded utterances of stutterers in therapy. Could it not be that both the author's sensitivity and the reader's disturbance focus the significance of unspeakable thoughts and feelings in the etiology of stuttering? Might there not be a positive relationship between the unreadability and the unspeakability of certain materials? If the reader has trouble in reading another's words, how much more trouble must the speaker have had in speaking them. It is to be hoped that we, the author in presenting and the reader in accepting communications from areas in interpersonal relationships, will share a deeper understanding of the stutterer's problem.

Then, too, the author has purposely adopted an objective and scientific attitude in reporting accurately samples of the raw data from which his implications and conclusions were drawn. If he makes an inference that people may stutter as a defense against the possibility of saying certain customarily unspeakable things, it becomes important to know what these things are. He could have reported simply that the stutterer has thoughts and feelings of which he is deeply ashamed and the possibility of their verbalization causes him to stutter. Is it not more honest that the author report what he found under certain conditions (therapy) and let the reader have the opportunity to draw his own conclusions?

more recently unconsciously he had desired his mother in a socially unacceptable and dreaded manner. With the therapist's support and his own good discriminating powers, however, he held his knowledge to use in the future to gain more understanding still.

Repressed feelings rarely emerge singly. They generally come in two's and three's. Sexual and messing preoccupations may appear together, or one or both may accompany anger. And essentially always fear and anxiety are present. Later in his therapy, the same stutterer whose production was used above said:

There is a place here with a lot of gravel. Water running through a river bed. A man comes walking along through this water which comes from a cave. It runs in between two ridges of ground. These two ridges turn into two legs. The rest of the body that was lying there now sits up. Now it stands up and leaves a little pile of feces on the ground. Then a hand throws a basket of feces over the head of this person. I grab his hands and pull on his arms and try to throw him over. We wrestle and I throw him over into this water. He gets up all covered with light and dark spots. I grab his head and throw him in again. He comes out all black this time with a long, black, cat-like tail. I throw him in again and he comes out a bear. I rush out and he tries to bite me. But I throw him in again. This time it's very thick mud and he has a hard time climbing out. I note that his legs have become very slender and pretty and I pull him out and he becomes a woman. She also has a long, thin tail like a cat. I try to clean the mud off her and hold her close to me and stick my penis into her. She shrivels up and disappears. Then I look up and there's a house looking like army barracks. She's in the doorway of this house and she has a long tail, long ears, and web feet with hair all over her. She turns into an ugly animal. Queer thing—there's a tree here and a large window and other things, but always in front of me is this ugly animal. Everywhere I look, she's there. I look down at my legs and they have turned into the hind legs of a horse. I have long ears like a horse. Dog here too like a French poodle, long, thin, and queer. I grab the dog by the throat and shake him and throw him down on the ground. He turns into my brother.

Hostile feelings arose against the man (father?), the woman (mother?), and the dog (which turned into his brother). Actually, he did have a younger brother. Messing and sexual feelings emerged. Fear and anxiety existed throughout this production. To help make the repressed hostile, sexual, and messing feelings palatable, the father and mother were not clearly recognizable. Further, they and his brother were given animal characteristics, because bestial feelings deserve only bestial objects. Even he had to become animal-like, with the legs and ears of a horse, in order to tolerate or excuse his primitive feelings.

The young man whose productions we have been citing was the older of two boys. He was two years old when his brother was born and was held out of school until his brother was old enough to enter with him. On the patient's part, the rivalry between the two brothers was keen. We never saw the younger brother. The parents, especially the mother, were strong, exacting, and highly monitoring. Their attitudes toward the sex, eating, and toilet training of their boys were strict and inflexible. Their social goals were high and no effort was spared to attain them. The patient began to stutter early, about a year after the birth of his brother, and developed a very severe stuttering. He was practically speechless when he came to us, being able to produce around fifty words an hour during continual efforts to speak in his early hours of therapy. His primitive feelings were strongly repressed and fixated at an early developmental level. They remained infantile and childish because of being repressed so early and harshly and they could not be modified and channeled by the subsequent experiences of later childhood and early adulthood. Upon coming to us at 25, he was generally constipated, picky in his eating habits, and had never had a date.

This short historical background has been given in order that we might better appreciate the following productions. They were his total verbal output for fifty minutes of continuous effort to speak. The bulk of the time was occupied in stuttering blocks which were characterized by an extremely tight pursing of the lips. The therapist could write down easily every word the patient said.

Large object, man's legs. He has loose pair of pants on. I reach up under his pants and grab his penis. It is large and soft. I pull on it and pull it off. This man stands up and reaches out as though asking for his penis back. I don't want to let him have it. He reaches out and tries to grab it. I put my hand on his face and push him away. He opens his mouth and cries. All this happens on the lawn of our old home. Across the field mother comes running. She is real large, larger than the house. This man is my brother. She comes over and I hold out my hand with the penis in it to show her what I had. He's over there hollering and waving his arms. Suddenly I squat down and take a crap and feces come out in a long ribbon—like toothpaste being squeezed out of a tube. I look up and overhead is a long, thin lamp post. It walks in and out among tangled ribbons of feces. It almost trips. It does trip and falls over with a crash. I leap on it. This ribbon of feces still hangs out of my anus. The lamp post has arms and I hold them. It also has a penis and I kick that and break it off. It also has hair and I reach up and grab a handful and pull it off. A hat comes off with the hair. On the upper end of the post are eye glasses like father's. I hit it in the head that is made of glass. The whole front of the head is broken in. I run my hands over the lamp post looking for other protuberances that I can break off. I roll it over and it has a pair of buttocks and between them an anus. I run my hand and arm up the anus and spread my fingers out inside and grab intestines and tear them out through the anus. I shake my fist in front of father's face and cram fistfuls of intestines into his face and say "how do you like that?" I grab him by the throat and order him to stand there. He tries to fall over but I hit him so hard that the lamp post is bent. He stands up there bent over. His head is low enough that I'll hit him in the head if he does anything wrong. He cries and wipes intestines out of his eyes. All over the place are trees standing around with their hands on their hips with the attitude that I should be ashamed of myself. A head floats in the air. I grab for it. It has long black hair that I hold in my arms. It's only a head. I stick my penis into the neck. The lips on the head kiss me. Liquid runs out between the lips and all over my front. I put my thumbs into the eyes and pull out the eyeballs and play with them in my hands. But they are hooked onto the head with two long white cords. The head isn't angry at me for playing with the eyes. I replace one eye and try to pull the other one off completely by breaking the cord. The head opens its mouth and shows lots of teeth. It tries to bite my penis off but I believe it can't. As I look at the head it becomes very ugly. A hole is through its lower jaw so that by looking into the mouth I can see out the bottom. I grab the ears and throw the head to the ground and stamp on it. It rolls around on the ground, all covered with blood and dirt. I try to clean it off but it's hard to do since the dirt is in the eyes, hair, and mouth. I want to wash it off but there is no water. So I urinate on it but this doesn't clean it very well. Besides, it turns yellow. I look up and there is father, very large and heavy and angry. He has a club. I look closely at the club and it is my brother. Father brandishes my brother like a club and I feel he is trying to hit me. I try to strike my father but he holds my brother out real close to me so that I can't get at my father. I reach out and pull out two large handfuls of hair from my brother's head. The places where I pulled the hair out are bleeding. I try to replace the hair but I get it on crooked and it grows like that and my brother has these two uneven places on his head pointing up like horns. His ears are pointed and his nose is long and he's like an elf that I thought of as a kid. He has wings. All this time father has been holding my brother out at me. Father has a long pencil between his fingers. I grab him and stab him through the penis and push the pencil on all the way through until it comes out the other end. His legs shrivel up and turn into a horse's legs. He turns into a horse hooked onto a wagon with its wheels all broken. The horse looks queer too, as though made out of a fluid, and he's not firm. He keeps changing his shape.

At first blush, the feelings and acts revealed in such products are unacceptably raw to our conscious selves. And this is exactly the point. Many people, including stutterers, are numbly and dumbly involved in such culturally unbearable mental materials that repressed and, therefore, consciously undetectable. But nevertheless their presence is felt in a gnawing anxiety that has its peak moments handled by some symptom, including stuttering. Before therapy our stutterer did not know that he wanted to bite off his brother's penis and show it to their mother as if to say, "Look what I have done. Now you have only one whole son. Brother is weak and impotent, I am strong and potent. Only I can deserve your complete respect." Before therapy he did not know that he had equally strong if not stronger feelings of aggression and destruction against his father. He wanted to destroy him in a most thorough and brutal manner. And as it was with his brother, his father too would snivel and beg for mercy in the face of our stutterer's pent-up rage. After each savage but successful attack upon his competitors, brother and father, his mother would appear. Is it not true that she is the real issue? With the brother she appeared clearly as the mother. Her only distortion was her enormous size, "larger than the house." Her role here was not too important, mainly to see what he had done. With the father, she appeared only as a head floating in the air. Here her role was extremely important. She was made to receive his primitive, sexualized aggression. In proportion to the importance and unacceptability of his casting of his mother, she was distorted, finally ending as an ugly, yellow, dirty head.

Finally, to justify the venting of his spleen in one fell swoop, our patient has the father threaten him with a club that is the brother. Our patient's wrathful retaliation is so right now because both of his competitors are a menace to him. He can justifiably save his life and strikes out to do so. To get at the father he must destroy his weapon, the brother. The outcome is humiliating to his antagonists. The brother becomes an elf with horns, pointed ears, and a long nose; and the father, a formless, spineless horse hooked to a broken-down wagon.

It is our contention that these strong anal and sexual aggressions of anti-social quality grew out of the important training situations of infancy and early childhood. Because of the pain and anxiety meted out by the parents in temporal and spatial relation to the patient's expression of early instinctual drives, he repressed (drive reduction by stopping thinking and feeling) these drives and the interpersonal relationships connected with them and henceforth carried them as unconscious, motivating forces. When these forces taxed the patient's repressing or inhibiting forces (fear and anxiety) to the limit, other defenses were called into action. When these defenses in turn could not hold, a final stand was made through stuttering. Stuttering may be conceptualized then as a final defense or block against the threatening revelation through spoken words of unspeakable thoughts and feelings. It may be visualized as a sieve through which some materials and force can pass, emerging in reduced amount and altered form. Both the repressed feelings and the restraining force (sieve or stuttering) derive some satisfaction. The former does get out, albeit in reduced amount and altered form, and the latter does hold even if it has to give a little. Certainly it held to the extent that few, if any of the listeners really knew what the stutterer said when he stuttered. If the unspeakable thoughts and feelings of the stutterer are strong and plentiful, his stuttering will be severe, because as a defense it must be equal to or better than the forces defended against.

According to clinical observation stutterers, both children and adults, are well-spoken. That is, they speak words that are highly socially proper and acceptable. As a group they do not speak "mean" thoughts and feelings to others or about others. They are polite and respectful. They are "good" people. What they say in the interpersonal relationships of everyday life is in sharp contrast with what they say in the interpersonal relationships of therapy. This great incompatibility of conscious and unconscious mental content may be a factor in the stutterer's problem.

Mr. Brown, 45, was a brilliant businessman with legal training and experience. To others his stuttering appeared inconsequential. To him it was catastrophic. His professional life was being ruined by his unbearable anxiety in verbal communication which was an absolute essential in his business. All his life he has had an ineluctable need to please and be loved and respected and he has succeeded, at least as far as others are concerned, in realizing this need. Indeed, by all others he is a most admired and respected man. In therapy, impressing upon him the attitude that nothing is to be feared or hated but only understood, he communicated many times the following content and feeling:

I'm chopping wood with an axe. I shudder. Splinters hit me in the eyes and that gave me a shudder. Two of us chop off our toes and this makes me shudder. We look alike and act in unison. We dig a V-shaped ditch and plant radishes and they grow up very rapidly. We have to plant them very quickly and get away because they grow so fast. I kick this other guy in the rear and this gives me a shudder. I want to split him in half and this gives me a shudder. I do it and each half turns into a whole person. Branches grow out of the ears and I cut them off and I shudder. I see a penis and it is sliced lengthwise. Cut-off, smaller penises are marching towards me and I fight back at them with a stick or sword but they get bigger and bigger, too big to subdue. Some of them urinate like a shower and I run away but a big man catches me and brings me back and I have to sit there. Finally, penises all lie down and I can get up and walk over them. Big man doesn't care, but I mustn't get too far out of his sight. If I go too far a big penis rises up in front of me. He puts a big penis to watch over me. I shudder. I feel hemmed in. I walk away and come to that V-shaped ditch and a person is lying in it. I cross over and climb stairs and big man sees me. I'm still within his reach. I'm washed off and someone urinates on me. All this makes me wince. I hide inside the branches of a tree. I get out and penises are all around me like a fence and I shudder. They start spraying. I can't get away. I slide down into river and wash off and feel safer. I swim under logs like penises lying on water. I go into a cave and a nude woman is there, and I feel secluded and safe. Animals are roving outside but I feel safe. They look in but it's dark and they can't see me. I have to defecate and I do it right there. This makes me shudder. A messy deal. Snakes come out of rock. I feel antagonistic.

I'm in a train, and instead of going into a tunnel, it goes into a large reptile's mouth. We back up and try again and go into another reptile's mouth. I'm surrounded by reptiles wagging their tails. They get closer and closer and I go up a tree, safe for awhile but someone chops the tree down. I'm still safe like in a womb. Wish I could get away, out into the sun. I'm getting awfully tired. Another reptile is after me. I'm getting worn out. This is awfully hard. That's the way it used to be. I shouldn't feel that way now. Snake comes up and I'm too tired. It grabs my hand. I run up a tree but that's a snake too (breathing hard). I want to give up but I can't. I run. Remember running home from school when I had defecated in my pants. Remember a man who approached me with his penis out. Don't remember what we did. Other boys there. Maybe we touched his penis. Maybe with our mouths. Don't remember. See a vision of this. I'm so tired. This is so hard (breathing heavily). One big penis I'm particularly afraid of. Wish I could sleep. I try not to see it. I just wish it would let me alone.

There is a treasure-trove of exquisite design in this production. We should be remindful that it, as well as every other similarly obtained projection, is not a production of intellection. Mr. Brown did not consciously construct this adventure. He did not know what he would say during the therapeutic hour. He had no plans for the hour, other than to be there. Under the obligation to speak absolutely freely, the feelings, ideas, and words given above came to him. They came at about the rate of slow conversational speech. He did not look ahead, or plan ahead, or structure what came. Rather, he simply reported what came into consciousness as it came. His attention was focused upon his stream of consciousness which seemed to flow involuntarily. Some anxiety existed throughout. Anxiety peaks occurred at those times when he would say, "this gives me a shudder," or "this makes me wince."

This stutterer adds exemplification of the almost monotonous regularity of the existence, in these people, of raw and culturally disowned feelings and ideas in the areas of sex, elimination, and hostility. The presence and influence of these unconscious preoccupations were afflictive and uninviting in interpersonal relationships, particularly in communication. In stirring from their servile state, to which they never willingly submitted, they gum the gears of verbal output. Too full of such terrorizing longings, it is no wonder that Mr. Brown dared not speak fluently. His fear and anxiety were not over the possibility of stuttering speech. They were over the threat of the telling in talking, of giving himself away in his words. He was never afraid of his stuttering per se. Really, he was afraid that his stuttering, as a defense, would not hold. He was afraid of possible loopholes in his stuttering and the consequent probability that his blocking utterances were not capable of fulfilling their purposes of defending against words conveying unspeakable feelings and thoughts.

Conflicts and defenses incident to the attempted achievement of sex-typing were seen frequently in the productions of Faith, a relatively severe stutterer of twenty. She reported:

I see a man walking toward me with a child under each arm—a boy and a girl. I call to him and he drops the children and I see he has a very large sexual apparatus in his pants which frightens me and which he is going to use against me as a weapon. The children are for a "come-on." I use pubic hair as a weapon of defense against him but it is futile. So I cut half my hair off my head to make me have half of a man's hair-cut and I put hair on my chest and it grows so that I'm part man to defend myself. Then I become half male and half female, with half a penis and half a vagina and these halves make love to each other. The right half of me is man and the left half of me is woman. The man-half bends over onto the woman-half which doesn't do anything, just remains passive. The right hand which is the man's hand starts tickling the sole of the left or woman's foot, and goes on up over leg, mostly over the back of the legs and on up over buttocks, especially around the anus and then continues the tickling all over the woman-half.

Somewhat later in therapy she found herself swimming into shore with a strong, overhand crawl stroke executed by her long, strong arms (in reality she is small and does not swim). Waves beat against her but she got into shore strong and fresh and with a penis. Her breasts were exposed like a man's chest. As she stood there she lost the penis and a brassiere covered her breasts. But as she continued to stand there on the shore she became more and more interested in the girls and developed a penis again. She went into the toilet and her penis melted away and she sat down and urinated like a woman. These reversals in sex-typing kept occurring: a penis would appear and then disappear; hair on her breasts would come and go; a butch hair-cut and long hair would alternate. She would be first a woman, then a man; or half female and half male. Sometimes her sex role, whether male or female, was in relation to others; while at other times she was complete within herself, her male half relating to her female half. A third variation was for her to have complete male and complete female sexual organs at the same time and to relate to a similar person, each person behaving at the same time both as a male and as a female.

Actually, this girl's father was not a strong masculine figure. But from an early day the mother had instilled within her daughter the feeling that for a woman sex was cruel and painful and that man was a bestial creature preying upon women for his own selfish satisfactions. The patient has had three husbands and has never experienced orgasm. Her latest husband often calls her his little man.

Brimful of ambivalence in a most important interpersonal relationship with both men and women, it may be surprising that her only apparent trouble was stuttering. To have the larger force of her unacceptable preoccupations funnel through oral communication, rather than through some other expressive avenue, might account for the original severity of her stuttering. As her anxiety was reduced as she discovered, accepted, and realigned these conflictual feelings, her speech became remarkably improved and her role as a woman more firmly established.

Repeatedly, our stutterers engaged in anthropomorphism. Time and again they would ascribe human characteristics to things not human. They would express feelings, words, thoughts, and acts of a conflict in the form of objects and object relationships. Unacceptable feelings and desires would be concentrated in objects, their location and their movement. This process may be clearer if we give some examples.

Glass tube filled with tiny microbes lowered into my throat. A swab saturated with argyrol is inserted down my throat. Steady flow of talk keeps flowing from me like accumulation of junk. A mass of gold trinkets is in my mouth, back of my lower teeth. I am a storage house, a vault. I expectorate a ball-like object that remains rolling in my throat. A dentist's mirror probes my teeth and enters my throat. I'm crying and between sobs, toffee-like substance moves back and forth in my mouth. Orifices and tubes and the words vital and potent. Now I'm pushing something up in my throat, using both hands. It's a window and I can't, it's too heavy. Hot stove pipe and a big boat in my throat. Honeycomb in my throat. Cells of the honeycomb are really breathing cells. A broom sweeps my throat. Spitting out and vomiting coins, muddy water and junk such as nuts and bolts. I want to explode all the antiquated things—junk, old coins, chewing gum, a lump of coal, horseshoe. It was necessary to stifle everything and choke to death all my life. I've been afraid of expelling anything, as though I took a deep breath and held it all my life. I've inhaled, but I've never exhaled. I've sucked in all my desires and cravings. I'm a volcano erupting and pitching all the junk out.

Many hours later, the patient whose examples we have been citing did not need to use so much anthropopathy as a defense against the realization and expression of her feelings. She could speak more directly as follows:

I'm raring to go places emotionally. I'm not scared like I used to be. You kissed me and put your tongue into my mouth and I had an orgasm. It felt just like a stuttering spasm except the fullness and constriction was in the vagina instead of in my throat. I feel that in order for me to speak I must take my panties off and keep my vagina uncovered. It's crazy to hesitate to say anything now. My breasts have grown up. They're full and I'm happy. They're not flabby like they used to be. Hair around my vagina is no longer unclean. It is sweet and wanted. I have no need for stuttering anymore. I'm grown up. My breasts and vagina feel so good. Once when we started I made a vow I'd never discuss sex or religion with you. I exhale through the vagina pure, clean air. I cough up not coins which are obsolete but circles—little emotional feelings and sexual cravings. They come up from my vagina and out through my mouth. I open up the orifices and tubes of my body and feelings, desires and cravings come out. I'm burning up, I'm on fire, I'm alive. I don't have to stutter anymore. Damn it, I can talk as well as you. All my life I thought my body was well but my speech organs were sick. Now the most normal part is the speech part.

This person, in her early forties, came into therapy with a very severe stutter. She was an uneducated, restricted, and economically and socially limited virgin. As she dwelt in the protective shadow of her aging mother, life was passing her by. A combination of external circumstances, including the death of her mother and the remarriage of her father, and internal forces, drove her to seek help, first in a speech clinic and finally in individual therapy. Considering many factors, her age, the severity and duration of her stuttering, her highly restricted upbringing, her limited physical and educational capabilities, her success in therapy was phenomenal. From a halting beginning she progressed to a fluent conclusion. For example toward the end, she said:

Suddenly I see my father and I hate him. He is responsible for me having no husband, no home, and no children. Now I see my hairline structure [pubic hair] and it doesn't disgust me anymore. I'm riding nude on a bare-back horse and the horse becomes my father and I hate him and I hate you too, terribly, sitting there coldly trying to figure me out in a professional way. I lie here on the defensive. I've been belching him up for years, my hate for him. I don't need to stutter him up anymore. Through lip service I was supposed to love him but I didn't, I was lying. It was sinful to hate your father. It was a commandment to love thy father and thy mother. This lie I stuttered.

Still closer to the end she proclaimed:

I can go up to a prominent person and talk without any feeling of ill-at-ease. I just don't care. He and I are just two human beings. Used to have an internal fight, now it's an external fight. I'm ready to go and no home and no education hit me. Formerly when I had a speech spasm or any other trouble I ran home. Now I don't want to hide, I want to come out, to expand, to make my debut. A debut among people. But certain people push me back and I find no refuge in the corner anymore. If my father should die tomorrow I'd cry for the father I used to know or the father he might have been. I feel that Sally is my little sister instead of me being really her little sister. She's away back down the road, so simple and prejudiced. I approach you, I can walk with you.

And at the end:

All the junk and surplus and debris have left me. I'm free and pure. I think of grit and a mouthful of dung and I'll spit it out, defecate through my mouth. I've been defecating and urinating all the years of my life out through my mouth. I was saying all the nasty things through stuttering. I was saying my father was a son-of-a-bitch and my mother was a deluded fool. You held my hand and taught me to talk and I never knew just when you let go and I talked alone.

Eight years have passed since these last words were spoken. During those years her job, which she has handled very successfully, has demanded the meeting of the public at a teller's window and over the phone. Not once, she reports, has she stuttered. Would it be presumptuous to think of her as a "cured" stutterer?

From unexpected people, the expression and communication of the interaction of opposing feelings (want and fear) frequently reveal the magnificence of the mental processes of man. The feelings themselves may be simple, simple want and simple fear of wanting; but the revelation of the conflict is often strangely penetrating and thought-provoking. Our surprising source of the production to follow was a seventeen-year-old lad who had stuttered severely since early childhood. In literature, psychology, philosophy, and the social sciences he was extremely naive. His entire life had been spent in activity to satisfy his interest in hunting, ranching, and livestock. He read practically not at all, worked and played mainly alone, and was unsocial, if not antisocial. He knew nothing of such concepts as symbolism, the unconscious, repression, and the like. Theories, principles, and practices of psychotherapy were foreign to him. He did know, of course, what was expected of him; an absolutely free and complete verbalization of his thoughts and feelings. One hour, after he had learned relatively well how to relate in therapy, he spoke as follows:

I see a large body of water. The surface is calm and very smooth, and green and very clear. Then as I see deeper it gets very dark. There seems to be no bottom to it. It gets blacker and blacker the deeper you go. Something is in there like a huge snake. He is very long and winds around and swims along. There are things like weeds, very dense, but no bottom. This eel, or snake, or whatever it is, is the key to something, the guard to a whole new land. The snake goes through an opening that leads to something like a tunnel, and disappears. As I look on the other side, the tunnel comes out into an uncivilized place, with huge reptiles and prehistoric monsters of all sorts in a tangled and dark forest. There is no sky. There is ground with very dark ponds around. All these creatures seemed worried about something. There have been men here before who tried to conquer the animals, to build up civilization but they have all been destroyed. One man is here now. He wears hunting clothes like we have today. He has a rifle but he is just walking along among the animals which are of tremendous height and size, as big as our buildings. The animals are all respectful because the man thinks he is the master of them; and the animals have the same feeling, not because he is cruel but because he has broken them. Something in the animals wants to fight back, but something else in them is like horses that have been ridden and broken and know there is no sense in resisting. That's the way this whole setup seems to be. The animals seem to have a feeling of respect but if the man were ever to weaken, or to show by some means that he was not the master of the situation, they would destroy him immediately. This man seems to feel that he wants something harder to break, something that will offer resistance but will be useful after it is broken. But also, he has the feeling that he is afraid to tackle this other situation until he has acquired more confidence by proving that he is master of things that can fight back and have sense, not human sense, but animal sense. He knows that these things can hurt him physically but can never command him. In these animals once they are broken, as it is with all animals, there is that loyalty of feeling that their master can do no wrong to them. There is a big problem appearing on the scene. It is the girl he wants. He knows that she can never be completely broken because he is afraid of trying to conquer her like he has conquered the animals. There is always the possibility that he might lose control of the situation, and then he would have somebody who would tell HIM what to do. In other words he is afraid that he will not receive from her the same faith in himself that he receives from the animals. The question seems to be does he want this human companionship enough to give up his freedom and the respect of the animals?

With our present understanding of the human mind, we would be presumptuous to attempt a full explanation of this communication. Possibly we will be rash to pretend any comprehension of this very young man's meaning here, but with the encouragement from the findings of other workers and from this patient's own clearer subsequent communications, we are encouraged to venture some translations of his language into forms more familiar to our current understanding. May we speak for him then as follows?

On the surface I am very calm and unruffled and easily understood. I am quiet and my wants are simple—to be left alone, not to be bothered, to come and go as I please, no fuss, no trouble, no demands upon me. But really, down deeper, I am not so simple and clear to myself or to others. Feelings stir, rebellious feelings, male feelings, conquering feelings. They are powerful and hard to hold in check and ever pressing for expression. I have to be always on the alert to contain them. They are not very smart as human beings go, but they have animal wisdom and demand my constant vigilance to manage their sexual hunger. Only my superior intelligence gives me an advantage. Were it not for this leverage their size and strength would overpower me. I cannot risk any diminution of my already slight superiority. I cannot tackle any other job. I must keep all my energies mobilized to manage my raw, animal-like, male feelings; my maturing feelings of maleness, of being a man. If I gave in to these feelings they would weaken me, even destroy me. Yet I do want to grow more. I want to reach out with my maleness. I want to test my powers. But as I think this way I become frightened. My feelings go a little too fast. They want to conquer a girl now. This is something different. With great effort I can manage my own sexual feelings. I can control them as long as they are all mine, just mine. But if I let them flow out to another, to a female, can I rule them in relation to her? Can I hold in check both her and me? What will she do to me? I'm fearful that she, being human, will not submit to my will. She may not be mine, all mine. I can keep my feelings all mine. Had I better live alone with them or risk trying to live with her too? I don't know now.

In exploring his big new land of big feelings, he knew that other men had been there before and that they had failed in their conquests. Were not these men the men of his family, or rather his own feelings of the men of his family? He felt that they had failed to crush his feelings, even had been destroyed themselves. (Actually his father was dead.) One man, himself, remained alive. And with great extertion he was not only living but reigning over his feelings. But when his feelings expanded to include women, fear assailed him. Had he not met with trouble, even failure, in controlling his mother, or his feelings about her? Was this trouble or failure to be repeated? So our patient spoke in a strange tongue about his great perplexities; and as

he spoke more often, he spoke more plainly until even he understood his
speech and his speech troubles.

Before he came into therapy, Allen, a severe stutterer of sixteen, had the
following recurrent dream:

> I feel as though I have awakened suddenly. When I look up a huge gorilla is
> standing over me and reaching out toward me. Then I get out of bed and start
> running around the room with it chasing me. Although it gets me pretty well
> cornered, it never quite gets hold of me. I try to go over to my desk to get a
> knife to kill the gorilla, but it always blocks me. After it chases me awhile I run
> out into the hall. Although there are people downstairs I am afraid to call them.
> I fear they will be very angry with me. But downstairs they hear me running
> around so they come up. As they come up I go into my room to hide from them.

This dream of nightmarish proportions reveals the dreamer's bare management of some of his powerful and dreaded feelings. During the day,
conscious control conceals their being; but at night during sleep, with a
weakening of his inhibitory forces, they are able to attain an outlet in disguised form. The gorilla is his fearful evaluation of warm, affectional feelings toward his father. When these feelings strive for expression, his fearful
learned appraisal of them casts them in monstrous form, and even affords
him strength to make an ineffectual attempt to fight. In simplest language, he
wants the warmest, most affectional responses from his father. But these
wants, he has learned well, are dreadful and when they gain the relative force
in sleep to advertise themselves, they are permitted recognition only in cari-
catural outline. It is informative that in the dream he feared the people
(parents) downstairs more than he did the gorilla in his room. He knew in
a subtle, subliminal way what the gorilla was; that it was his own wants
which had to be concealed from others at all costs. The others were the punitive mentors of his past who had instilled and maintained his fear and dread
of his wanting the sexual love of his father.

During the hours of therapy Allen would have thoughts and feelings similar to those expressed in the dream. For example:

> Now I'm thinking of a huge octopus. It's in a glass cage. It's an awful looking
> thing. I wouldn't want to be in there with it, although I might as well be. Why
> do I think of this? It just popped into my head. That is, I might as well be in
> there with him. Let me think. There is a resemblance between it and my father.
> The long arms of parents and the long arms of the octopus.

Allen was a very brilliant lad whose stuttering was so severe that he was
practically speechless. He sucked his thumb and pulled his hair out when
he first entered therapy. His parents were exceptionally fine, able, and strong
people who enjoyed upper-class socioeconomic status. Allen was in continual and futile conflict with them, his school, and constituted law and
authority. These conflictual issues came up time and again in his spontaneous and unminded verbalizations.

> A bee is on a streetlight. He's flying all around it trying to get in. He finally
> finds a hole in it and gets in and sits on the light and it burns him. He gets mad

and stings it only it burns his stinger off and that scares him. He tries to get out only he can't find that hole so he dies in there. There's this man and he wants to join the underground in France. He doesn't know how to get into it but finally finds out where they meet and goes there. They grab him and torture him to find out if he's German. He convinces them he isn't so they let him join. He's supposed to blow a bridge with dynamite. He lights it wrong and it blows up too fast and kills him. There's this elephant and he wishes that he were smaller. I don't know why but he does. Finally, somehow he gets to be a tiny elephant. Only then all the big ones kick him around and he wants to be big again, only he can't. There's this flower and it wants to be wheat. It's changed into wheat and is very happy until a horse comes along and eats it. There's a man and he liked to go into the freezing compartment in a store. The store owner finally lets this man go in and look around. When he goes in he closes the door behind himself and it locks automatically and he freezes in there. When they find him, he's frozen so they cut him up and sell him as steak. The person who eats him dies from some poison that was in him. There's a dog and he wishes he were a man, so he's turned into a man. On the first day he's drafted into the army and killed in training. Now there's this person who has his hand caught in a washing machine, in those rollers. He tries to get it out but can't and figures it will be easier if he pushes his arm through. He starts to push but finds his arm is attached to his body and he will have to push his body through. He does this and all gets through but his head which he can't get through. He's stuck there. Now there's a person who's a terrific wire walker. He always wears shoes when he is doing this. The manager tells him not to wear shoes this time because people think he has something on his shoes that holds him on the wire. He starts out without shoes and the wire tickles his feet and he falls. There's this man and he swings a sledge hammer around and around, faster and faster. The hammer is tied to his hands and as he swings it too fast he is pulled off his feet into a swamp where there are crocodiles which kill him.

With a plant, an animal, or a man, it is always the same. They want to do something else or be something else and regularly disaster befalls them in the attainment of their wants. In his family of high standards, so very much of his wanting had been blocked with disapproval, fear, and pain. Now at sixteen he carries uneasily the repressed conflict of urges and their omnipresent and obdurate counterfeelings of fear and guilt. In the acceptant atmosphere of therapy, his repressed urges and wants were beckoned into being. It appears that they were essentially explorations into new and forbidden roles and relationships and as they enjoyed even disguised realization, their associated, oppositional feelings appeared also. And in every instance the latter won. But this outcome will not always be so. The now maligned feelings will get stronger under the new conditions of learning and simultaneously the restraining and punitive feelings of shame, fear, and guilt will get weaker. His ambivalence of roles, to be this or to be that, is further unmasked in the next day's productions.

There are two people on horses and they have a rope tied around their necks connecting themselves. They want to go in different directions and kick their horses. The two people look exactly alike. They kick their horses and are pulled off and they try to run in opposite directions, only they can't get apart and can't agree on where to go. I think one is trying to go toward a swamp where there are all kinds of birds, crocodiles, and stuff. The one that doesn't want to go to the swamp has a black mask over his face. But he still looks exactly like the other one. These Siamese twins here. One wants to bathe and the other hates to bathe. He won't let the other one take a bath. There is a book and one of the pages wishes it were a different page. If it were a different page it would mix up the book, but still it wants to be a different page. There's this colt that was just born. Its belly button is still attached to its mother and he wants it separated, but mother doesn't because she wants her colt around her. There are two people and they are handcuffed together and they hate each other. They kill each other because they can't get away from each other. There's this spring and it's being kept together, only it wants to get open and can't. Now there's a person driving a black Ford up in the mountains where there are curves. He didn't like to go around the turns so he goes straight over the mountains and smashes into a tree. He had been in prison before and had promised to go straight. He went straight—that's how he interpreted it. There are two people standing on a fence, and each wants the other one to get off but neither will, so one starts shaking the real thin fence and then the other one starts to shake the fence and they both fall off. There's a person with three arms and he didn't like one of them, so he puts it into a vise and squeezes it thinking it will fall off this way. He succeeds only in crushing the bone. There's a person riding a bicycle and the front wheel wants to go backwards but can't. When he's in the middle of the road, the front wheel comes off and the bike falls and a truck comes along and runs over the man. There's a person in an airplane and he takes off all right, but once he's up the propellers start going in the wrong direction and he flies backwards. He can't see where he's going so crashes into the Empire State Building. He bails out, but his chute catches on a flagpole and his chute is torn. He's held up there. The trouble is, though, that the ropes were tangled around his own neck and he was strangled by his own weight. There are two people with their belts tied together and they hate each other and start hitting each other and both get bloody noses. They are in the ocean and the sharks smell the blood and come and kill both of them.

Toward the end of therapy when her stuttering had become of no consequence, a young woman who had stuttered so severely, spoke as follows:

A geyser is blowing up in the air. A volcano is erupting molten stuff and it's dangerous. People better watch out. Out comes lava, lavatories, bowls, and toilets. Volcano is like an anus sticking up in the air and out shoots all this stuff. Feces, all the insides, like this is anger. All the insides shoot out, tremble all over. All of one gets mad, not just a part. Volcano keeps shooting and spitting up, and feces roll down the sides and bury all the houses. I'll go over and tell my mother that I don't need to stutter any more because I know all those words that I saw written on the sidewalks when I was little and wanted to ask her, but was afraid, afraid to know, afraid I was bad, afraid I was naughty. I felt an urge this afternoon to go over and tell her all that has happened. How stuttering is gone and why it's gone.

Throughout therapy, a chief area of concern for her had been elimination. Like any other child, she must have begun the same naive interest in her feces and urine that she had in other parts and products of her body. Undoubtedly she handled and played with fecal material. Without a shadow of a doubt in her case, the day arrived when her mother found her innocent child smearing feces over her own little sweet body, into her beautiful curls and on her clean crib, with vocal abandon. Sharp, punishing, and fear producing management followed. The baby experienced strong anxiety in relation to her feces and her interest in them. On pain of losing the mother's love and on the further pain of punishment, this baby girl repressed her messing interests and activities. She also learned to repress verbal reference to these matters, except for slanting and oblique allusions, with the consequence that what began innocently and openly ended up closed out and excluded from the interpersonal relationships of the future. Although repressed, these interests did not die. Their life was partly saved by the eternal cues of swelling bladder and bowel, odors, noises, and sights. But words must not be spoken. Naughty words, dirty words they became, and they must not be uttered. These words married other words which in turn became contaminated by connubial connection and they too could not be said. Well, where do we end? It is reasonable to assume that in her case we ended with stuttering.

## SOME GENERAL CONSIDERATIONS

We have used 16 productions of our 30 stutterers. These few were chosen as typical from literally thousands of originations. Every one of our stutterers used the larger share of his therapy in expressing his conflictual feelings through these forms. We have not yet attempted to compare our 30 stutterers with our other group of 35 patients in regard to these productions. We cannot state now that our stutterers gave more, or longer, or more complete, or more diversified originations than did our other group of people. It is our strong clinical feeling, amounting almost to a certainty, that the type of materials we have been presenting is practically exclusively paradigmatic of our stuttering group. The largest proportion of our other patients did not give any such materials. A few gave scattered projections. Those who gave the most did not approximate those stutterers who gave the least. If our feelings stand the test of further study, we may have here an important differentiating factor. It would appear that until such a difference might be established, we should refrain from any consideration of its possible significance.

With almost monotonous repetition our stutterers advertised their unconscious preoccupation with the salvaging of some remnants of their early physical enjoyment. They revealed endlessly a nostalgia for their culturally disavowed, biologically rooted pleasures of sucking, eating, evacuating, and exploring. So frequently their revelations told of their lonely longing for the most primitive, raw, and earthy sensory and motor enjoyments and delights. When early training began its attack upon these pleasures of the flesh, our stutterers must have had three purportful reactions: anger, which met with triumphant counter-anger and which ended in being repressed by fear; a loss of oneness with themselves; and finally, a crippling of interpersonal relationships, significantly with the parents. Their productions portrayed these early reactions. They, the stutterers, did release in therapy hostility; they showed disabling vacillation about themselves, and they manifested fears about others. We were not there to see for ourselves when the parents made their attacks and the stutterers made their reactions, but under the conditions of therapy, the stutterers provided proof that the attacks and the reactions had occurred.

As seen through the feelings and thoughts of our stutterers, the parents, particularly the mothers, were highly monitoring of their children's behavior. In the stutterers' productions or originations, and in their conscious and re-covered memories, the mothers were felt as harsh disciplinarians who held their offspring to excessively high standards of conduct and who used sham-ing and anxiety-dousing tactics in the socializing of their children. The ac-curacy of our stutterers' feelings are borne out by the studies of Moncur (1951, 1952) who found that the mothers of stutterers were more dominant than the mothers of nonstutterers. In the therapeutical process with our stutterers there emerged clearly, possibly a still more significant implication. It was that the father was relatively weak and passive. We may express this feeling more poetically and say that the stutterer's mother sang an operatic aria while his father hummed a lullaby. It is possible that this relatively greater strength of the mother operated adversely in the sex-typing of the child. An ambivalence of the sexual role was a constant worry at the un-conscious levels of our stutterers.

Note may be made of the clinical outcome of psychotherapy with our stutterers. It must remain at this writing, however, as only a note. Our study can hardly be considered as proving anything—most of all, favorable clinical results. We may say though that those stutterers who recovered and ex-pressed what we have termed unspeakable feelings and thoughts did enjoy increased speech fluency and less anxiety over speech blocks. Eleven adult stutterers (seven men and four women) had at least 150 hours each of psy-chotherapy with us. Of these, five (four men and one woman) were helped greatly; and six (three men and three women) were "cured." We may put psychotherapy in the worst possible light by stating that just as good results might be forthcoming if a stutterer talked to anybody about anything for at least 150 hours. We do not feel that it deserves this harsh dismissal. From the day-to-day, anxiety-producing recoveries and expressions and the conse-quent reductions in anxiety and speech blocks, we feel on the contrary that therapy was a dynamic, curative process for those stutterers who had the motivation and courage to drive them on.

## BIBLIOGRAPHY

DOLLARD, J., DOOB, L. W., MILLER, N. E., and SEARS, R. R. 1939. Frustration and aggression. New Haven: Yale Univ. Press.

DOLLARD, J., and MILLER, N. E. 1950. Personality and psychotherapy. New York: McGraw-Hill.

MONCUR, J. P. 1951. Environmental factors differentiating stuttering children from non-stuttering children. *Speech Monogr.*, 18, 312–325.

———— 1952. Parental domination in stuttering. *J. Speech Hearing Disorders,* 17, 155–165.

SULLIVAN, H. S. 1953. The interpersonal theory of psychiatry. New York: Norton.

TRAVIS, L. E., and BARUCH, D. W. 1941. Personal problems of everyday life. New York: Appleton-Century.

CHAPTER 30

# METHODS FOR INTEGRATING THEORIES OF STUTTERING

● *Stanley Ainsworth, Ph.D.*

SOONER OR LATER, every student of speech pathology becomes confused and frustrated by the multiplicity of theories about the causes of stuttering. When this state of mind occurs, he may proceed to ignore those theories he interprets as "no good." He may search around for a theory of his own; or he may look for some way to pull them all together into a manageable framework and emerge with an integration of theories.

Several attempts have been made to "integrate" theories of stuttering in an effort to bring about a more coherent understanding of the field (Travis, 1933; Van Riper, 1939 and 1947; Berry and Eisenson, 1956; Ainsworth, 1945). These "integrations" have provided a more convenient package for recognizing and remembering a multitude of conflicting but overlapping theories. However, we must admit that most of these attempts are primarily classifications rather than integrations. Such products are useful, but something more constructive is needed. An ideal integration should pull things together in such a fashion that a fundamental unity is recognizable in the midst of complexity. Or, if the field has not yet progressed to a level of knowledge that would make this possible, the contributions of theories and the specific points of divergence should be delineated and basic inadequacies exposed. If we are to continue to advance in our understanding and explanation of stuttering, such a procedure should be attempted periodically. In fact, every therapist must create some kind of working hypothesis about the nature and causation of stuttering if he expects to have any systematic way to change therapeutic procedures in a constructive fashion as he gains more insight and experience. For most therapists, some kind of modification of existing theories or some form of integration is a professional necessity.

This chapter will make no attempt to review the theories of stuttering, but specific theories will be used as examples. One of the best summaries of theories is found in Hahn (1956). An attempt has been made to avoid doing a "critical review" of current theories and to avoid summarizing "what we know" about stuttering. In this way, attention can be placed on a manner of synthesizing certain theoretical concepts. It is assumed that the reader has already studied most of the more common theories.

## REVIEW OF INTEGRATION STUDIES

A look at some of the ways that have been used to integrate (or classify) theories of stuttering may give us important clues as to the nature of approaches that have been tried and the difficulties encountered in such a process.

Van Riper, in his earlier editions (1939 and 1947), grouped the theories under the headings of educational, psychoanalytical, neurological, neurotic, imagery, and inhibitory, followed by brief statements of the principal differences in points of view and the names of individuals who supported them. Travis (1933) used the same grouping. In his second edition (1947), Van Riper used this material but also presented more extensive discussion under three headings of predisposing causes—dysphemia, learning factors, and neurotic emotional conflicts. (It is interesting to note that in his third edition [1954], he has listed "possible sources of stuttering" rather than a classification of theories.) Berry and Eisenson (1942) grouped a discussion of etiology under the headings of biochemical, neurological, psychological, and genetic —a grouping of areas studied in order to find causes for stuttering. It was concluded that all aspects may play a part. In their latest book (1956), Berry and Eisenson discuss etiology under the headings of heredity, neurology, psychosomatic factors, perseveration, and learning. The three "predisposing causes" of Van Riper's second edition have been discussed at length by Ainsworth (1945), who reasoned that the theories of stuttering contain certain fundamental differences. Some theories support a difference in the constitutional make-up of a stutterer which accounts for the disorder. Others say that there is no physical difference but that a perfectly normal individual learns to behave in the fashion called stuttering due to a variety of situations in his early development. A third group of theories by-passes the constitutional abnormality versus normal-but-bad-learning dichotomy by assuming an abnormality in the personality structure—a neurosis as the basis for stuttering. A summary by Hill (1945) brings together a great many studies within a particular framework (Kantor's interbehavioral system). This may be considered as a true integration limited to one point of view. It is particularly useful for understanding the interaction of many of the aspects which make stuttering such a complex entity.

A few remarks are necesary concerning the distinction made between the so-called "learning theories" and the "neurotic theories." Some writers feel that this separation is not fundamental, on the basis that neurotic symptoms are merely a class of learned behaviors. A person who is otherwise "normal" may develop a relatively isolated symptom which is based in an essentially neurotic mechanism. It tends to repeat itself under similar circumstances and thus become learned behavior. However, there are several practical and fundamental differences in the viewpoints presented by the proponents of these two categories. Those interested in stuttering as learned behavior stress that the patterns of variation in stuttering under controlled conditions tend to resemble those of other behaviors which are learned as part of a normal reaction to environment rather than an outgrowth of compulsive, neurotically based behavior (Johnson, 1956; Chapter 28; Wischner, 1950). The adaptation effect is one such characteristic. Another difference involves the language used for discussing stuttering and the assumptions that it portrays. The learning-theory proponents are particularly interested in the process of the development of stuttering behavior as it relates to the inter-action of attitudes of the child and of those surrounding him. The things that happen to cause stuttering may occur relatively "near" the conscious level. Those believing in a neurotic origin assume a personality disturbance and spend a greater time in exploring the unconscious mechanisms involved in light of an inclusive theory of personality. Furthermore, Johnson (1948) distinguishes between "stuttering" and some similar symptoms which may be part of a psychoneurosis or other syndrome. These differences in the underlying assumptions concerning the nature of stuttering seem to justify classifying and discussing such theories separately.

Within each of the three broad categories of theories cited by Ainsworth, there are ample opportunities for difference and disagreement. For instance, there is little similarity between the ideas of Kenyon (1941, 1942, and 1943) and Johnson (1956), although both may be classified as belonging in the "learning" category. Kenyon's theory is almost entirely a description of what he believes the process of the development of stuttering to be. Johnson is also interested in the process but describes it quite differently and at-tempts to make an explanation of this process. Likewise, the source of his ideas seems to be quite different. Kenyon apparently derives his ideas from a large number of clinical observations. Johnson bases his thinking on a series of research studies designed to evaluate several aspects of language development and behavior.

The divergencies among those who ascribe stuttering to "constitutional" factors are immediately apparent. Some are content with general statements about a nervous system with increased irritability and diminished capacity (Greene, 1927). There are frequent references in the literature to constitu-tional predisposition, biochemical or neurological factors, or motor inade-quacies as causes for stuttering. On the other hand, the early Travis theory (1931) attempted to pinpoint the cause as a lack of cerebral dominance. (See Chapter 29 and Travis, 1940 and 1946, for more recent formulations by Travis.) A contribution by Karlin (1947) proposes that the basic physi-ological cause is a delay in the myelinization of cortical areas in the brain concerned with speech. Emotional factors are considered to be sufficient to perpetuate the problem given this kind of subsoil at a crucial stage of de-velopment.

In the theories which support a neurotic condition as the basis for stutter-ing, we can gallop off in several directions at once. It is possible to consider stuttering as a symptom of a negative compulsion (Krausz, 1940), of neu-tic anxiety (Cobb, 1943, p. 48), or as a compulsive, narcissistic neurosis (Coriat, 1931 and 1943). Stuttering may be described as a "nervousness," as a problem of "emotional maladjustment," or, in contrast, as a problem involving fundamental and deep-seated alterations in personality organization. The psychoanalytic concepts go the farthest of this group of theories in offering truly explanatory elements of causation (Travis, 1940, and Chapter 29). Barbara (1954) offers a different description and explanation of the neurotic character of stuttering based on Horney's theory of neurosis. Van Riper (1954 and Chapter 27) proposes that, in some cases, a neurosis may be causative, but that in most stutterers the neurotic aspects develop after the onset of stuttering and as a result of it. Stuttering as an approach-avoidance conflict (Sheehan, 1953) is close to a picture of neurotic conflict, but this theory has many differences from others in this area.

## PROBLEMS IN INTEGRATION

It is obvious that such a threefold approach to integration of theories as offered by Ainsworth (1945) has the advantage of providing a means for classifying and remembering fundamentally different theories under separate headings. The disadvantages for true integration are many. One implication is that there are irreconcilable differences in these theories—any clear indication that one is correct necessarily implies that another fundamentally different one must be wrong. At best, we are asked to "make choices" as to the direction of thinking which will seem most probable or rewarding. Another inadequacy of classifying is that some theories refuse to "fit" into a single category. It would seem, then, that in order to achieve an integration we must move away from classifying the theories and approach them from a different point of view.

One method frequently used is to draw "logical" or "practical" conclusions from our experience and present-day theories, but this again leaves us with three choices—with similar implications regarding differences. For instance, some of us glibly present the idea that "stuttering has many causes." In some stutterers, the causes could conceivably be constitutional in nature. In others, some events could cause the child to be conditioned to this manner of speaking in certain circumstances. And, of course, with others the stuttering might be a symptom of neurosis. If one is to commit himself to the generalization that there are multiple causes of different types, then we must point out that at least two other generalizations are equally reasonable. One may be illustrated by the idea that there are not multiple types of causes at all—there may be several types of abnormal fluency, only one of which may legitimately be called stuttering. Thus, "stuttering" has been applied "as a label for varied items in an essentially heterogeneous array of speech behaviors" (Johnson, Chapter 28). Such an approach narrows considerably the areas to be explored in searching for a theory to account for stuttering. Another point of view is equally logical. An individual stutterer

may present a combination of components from each area of causatio
constitutional, learning, neurotic. Different stutterers may very well ¦
these components in differing degrees and qualities. It is also reasonab...
assume that there are at least four types of causal factors—precipitating,
maintaining, aggravating, and complicating. A constitutional condition—
such as relative delay in physiological development—as was suggested by
Schuell (1946 and 1947) as part of the picture to account for more male
stutterers—may cause him to over-react to social-emotional pressures. The
subsequent reaction of parents may keep the vicious circle in play long
enough to habituate stuttering and complicate it. Severe withdrawal because
of speech failure may set up a whole pattern of neurotic behavior—and
so on. The exact elements in each case may be different. So, again, we find
ourselves forced to make a choice among mutually exclusive categories if
we try to pull together the present thinking in the field in a "practical" fashion.

## INTEGRATION BY CONTRIBUTIONS TO BASIC QUESTIONS

A true integration of theories, then, cannot merely place one theory in
this category, the other theory in that pigeonhole. What we are in need of
is a framework *within* which divergent elements of theories may be discussed
in relation to each other and as they contribute to a better understanding
of the totality of stuttering. Any theory which pretends to be complete should
offer positive contributions to certain aspects of the problem of stuttering.
It is possible to pull together many elements of several theories by noting
the way in which each theory answers the following basic questions:

1. What are the contributions to the *description* of the behaviorial, social, and
   psychological concomitants of stuttering?
2. What are the contributions to understanding the *process of development*
   of stuttering?
3. What contributions toward *explaining* these phenomena are offered?

This chapter cannot pretend to be complete in carrying out the above
process of integrating theories. A thorough outlining of such an integration
might well be a book in itself. The material to follow can indicate the kinds
of answers that can be found and illustrate with references to concrete examples. It may be assumed, however, that most of the items chosen represent
what appears to be most important to the writer at the time of writing. The
reader may add items at will.

### What Are the Contributions to Description of Stuttering?

It would seem difficult to develop any respectable theory of causation
without some concepts or assumptions regarding *what* is caused. Therefore
it is not surprising that we can find a wealth of material providing contributions toward describing stuttering more definitively. The literature is full of
clinical observations of stuttering behavior—most of which we easily recog-

nize in the cases that come to our attention. It is when the descriptions become interspersed with assumptions about the stutterer that we begin to take
exception. The first sentence of a lecture on Elocution delivered by Andrew
Comstock in 1837 was not far from a present-day description. "Stammering
or stuttering is a hesitation or interruption of speech, and is usually attended
with more or less distortion of feature." He goes on to talk about two types
—recognizable as clonic and tonic blocking. (Incidentally, he offers three
levels of causes—predisposing, exciting, and proximate—this last being
"a spasmodic action of the muscles of speech.") The research of the last
thirty years has added many more subtle details and refinements to the
symptoms that could be obtained by the observant therapist in his swivel
chair. We not only know that the breathing is often disturbed, but the fan-
tastic disorganization of the whole mechanism has been explored in detail.
(See Travis, 1931, 1933, and 1936 for reports of some of the earlier studies.)
The locations and degrees of muscular tensions have been similarly studied.
Steer (1937) reported on symptomatologies of young stutterers.

Not satisfied with purely physiological characteristics, workers have made
numerous studies of psychological factors. One series, "Studies in the
Psychology of Stuttering," by Wendell Johnson and his students, is particularly noteworthy for providing a more detailed and accurate picture of the
phenomena. Several of these researches have been published in the *Journal
of Speech Disorders* and the *Journal of Speech and Hearing Disorders*. Other
studies have given us a similar type of information. Stuttering has been
found to be not only a wide variety of postures, tensions, and vocal patterns
which accompany an interruption in speech but is a pattern of behavior
which varies in certain ways under particular circumstances and is usually
accompanied by a fairly representative group of attitudes about speech and
stuttering in the person who stutters. Another approach to description plus
an understanding of the relationships of factors in stuttering has been made
by Hill (1945). He presents an "avenue of systemizing" many aspects in an
interbehaviorial framework.

There is little doubt that a great deal of what we "know" about stuttering
falls into the general area of description of the entity. Even here, however,
we realize that more needs to be done when we find studies like Tuthill's
(1940) which points up that there is often serious disagreement about what
we observe as stuttering. Likewise, we note that Johnson (Chapter 28)
stresses that stuttering is characterized by a mode of onset and development
and certain concomitants which distinguish it from similar behavioral patterns. Van Riper (1954, p. 366) includes the stuttering tremor as an important element in transitional and secondary stuttering. It would seem, then,
that Johnson's "stuttering" is descriptively an entity different from the concept which considers the central element to be a "neuromuscular block"
(Van Riper, 1947, p. 277) or a temporary inability to move the speech
musculature (Van Riper, 1954, p. 366). It may be that what appear to be
disagreements are largely emphases on different aspects of the total behavior

which can reasonably be labeled stuttering. Closely associated with these emphases are evaluative statements concerning the meaning and importance of the symptoms. In general, we can say that theorists agree on basic characteristics of "stuttering." It may be summarized as an unusual number and/or too noticeably severe repetitions and stoppages in speech. (Some speech pathologists [Sheehan, 1953] feel that these are the only symptoms common to all stutterers.) These nonfluencies are accompanied by signs of anxiety-tensions regarding them. The nonfluencies are variable, especially under certain circumstances (Bloodstein, 1949 and 1950; Brown, 1938 and 1945).

### What Are the Contributions to Understanding the Process of Development?

An understanding of the process of development of stuttering seems to be important for formulating any theory as to its source; for it is difficult to conceive of such a complex entity as springing "full blown" into being. Since stuttering usually begins between the ages of three and six, it appears that any true understanding of the process of development must come from a study of these ages in children. In general, relatively gradual development of stuttering has been recognized, as witnessed by the introduction of "primary" and "secondary" stuttering into many discussions, but an amazing number of writers propose or imply sweeping statements of theory which almost ignore this aspect. One suspects that they are anxious to get on to the more familiar ground of the "real" stutterer's behavior or to plunge into the realms of fantasy and logic that form the body of their explanations. Another systematic but equally unsatisfying procedure is to offer the reader a beautifully organized set of factors that reasonably could be at work but which are never presented in such a way that the exact relationships can be recognized and evaluated. For instance, we are often shown a wealth of attitudes, situations, "kinds" of parents and children, and so on, and then are told that stuttering erupts from this kind of background, without any attempt to outline why these kinds of conditions do not always result in stuttering. Essentially, this approach jumps too blithely from *causes* to *effects* to be satisfactory. Still others have developed ideas about stuttering solely from clinical observations of adult, secondary stutterers. Clinically and theoretically, such attempts to explain stuttering are frustrating, to say the least.

Some theorists, however, have made a detailed, honest attempt to present their understanding of (*a*) what is happening in the behavior and inside the child as he changes from a "normal speaker" to a "stutterer," (*b*) how those persons around the child are feeling and acting, and (*c*) what events seem to influence the process. These descriptions of the process of development are usually intermingled with statements which will be treated under question three of this discussion.

Probably the most elaborate discussions are provided by the theories of Johnson (1956 and Chapter 28). His concept of the process involves an interaction of the child's assumptions and parents' attitudes about speech, particularly with reference to negative evaluations by the parents. Since many of the research studies from which he draws his conclusions have explored relationships between "normal speech" and "stuttering," he has described in some detail how the normal nonfluencies of speech become altered into "anticipatory, apprehensive, hypertonic, avoidance reactions." The influence of this point of view is to be noted in the theory of Wischner (1950) who emphasizes the role of the development of anxiety in the child and how this leads to stuttering behavior. He also goes on to describe how particular symptoms develop. Van Riper (in his 3rd edition, 1954) first approaches a description of this process by presenting case studies of several possible origins of stuttering. He then discusses the growth of stuttering through primary, transitional, and secondary phases. (Van Riper does not present a clean-cut theory of stuttering. He uses elements from a great many theories as they appear to relate to his own understanding or observations and as they appear to have value for therapy. In this sense, his "theory" is actually a personal integration of theories. His attention to the process of development is indicative of its importance to understanding stuttering.)

Travis (1940) shows how stuttering develops by relating it to the emotional development of the child, his basic needs, and the symbolic satisfaction of them. Interwoven with this is a theory of personality structure and, of course, explanations of why certain behaviors appear.

Another extensive description of the physiological behavior and the fixation of vocal habits which underlie stuttering is found in a series of articles by Kenyon (1941, 1942, and 1943).

It is at this point that disagreements in theories begin to become more apparent. Johnson views stuttering as an undesirable extension of normal nonfluencies. In the discussions of Travis, the speech abnormality does not need to grow out of normal nonfluencies but may be qualitatively and quantitatively something quite different. The change in manner of speaking may be a direct expression of anxiety, conflict, and so on. Both agree that stuttering is an attempt on the part of the child to adapt to parental behavior. In the area of explaining the meanings of this alteration of the child's behavior, further disagreements are found.

### What Contributions Toward Explaining These Phenomena Are Offered?

This third aspect which must be considered in any comprehensive theory is one of the two happy hunting grounds for speech pathologists (or anyone else interested in stuttering). Many individuals seem to have a compulsion to jump in one of two directions as soon as the problem of stuttering has been identified or labeled. One group (the practical people?) formulate something to *do* about it. The other group (the philosophers?) enlarge on the *cause*. The more we learn about the semantic, psychological, sociological, and neurophysiological complexities of stuttering, the less we should be surprised that we have numerous theories. Many can be eliminated from serious consideration because they are too limited in conception, present

ideas contrary to what we "know" about stuttering and/or human characteristics, or they formulate a structure which cannot be understood or verified reasonably well. This writer is inclined to consider as useful those
theories which grow out of a comprehensive body of research and a broadly
conceived, systematic series of clinical observations. The theories used below are chosen because they seem to be representative of current points of
view in the field. Some equally "good" theories might well have been included but did not seem necessary for illustrative purposes.

Few recent writings have paid much attention to the neurophysiological
components which may be related to causes of stuttering. Following and concurrent with the cerebral dominance theory, there were literally hundreds
of attempts to discover some physical attribute which could account for
the speech behavior. Bryngelson (1942), for instance, reviewed 36 studies
and concluded that they definitely supported the concept that stuttering is
a symptom of an inner condition—dysphemia—which is an irregularity
of neural integration in the portion of the central nervous system responsible
for the speech musculature. Hill (1944a and 1944b), on the other hand, reviewed more studies of a similar nature and concluded that there were no
true differences found between stutterers and nonstutterers in most cases.
In researches where a constitutional variable was found, he felt that the
differences could be accounted for by other means than to assume that they
were indicative of a dysphemia.

At least three current theories consider a neurophysiological "subsoil"
as important for at least some cases of stuttering. Travis (1946) points out
that the electroencephalographic findings of Freestone (1942), Knott and
Tjossem (1943), and Douglas (1943) cannot be ignored. It appears that
there is a variance in excitability in the cerebral hemispheres in some stutterers. It is quite possible that this condition alone would not produce stuttering. West (1947, p. 89) feels that although stuttering is primarily social and
emotional in origin, there are definite biological backgrounds for it. Van
Riper (1954, p. 349) includes a "poorly timed dysphemia" as one of the
sources that can combine to cause stuttering.

Those who propose a constitutional contribution to the complexity we
call stuttering come closest to agreement in the idea that stuttering involves
"something" at variance in the cerebral cortex—a variation in the neural
flow which causes blocking of co-ordinated muscular activity. These findings
do not seem to contradict the psychological or sociological determinants
that have been found to be typical of stuttering, but they do offer additional
explanatory material and are important to include in any integrated point
of view.

The theories of Johnson (1956 and Chapter 28) have been mentioned in
other portions of this chapter. He finds the principal explanation for stuttering in the attitudes and evaluations of the parent with regard to nonfluencies
which are normal for all persons and which may be more frequent between
the ages of three and six. His description of the disorder, the process of its

development, and the explanation for it form a closely knit unit. He feels that stuttering not only does not need a background of neurosis, but that it is essentially a disorder different from speech disturbances caused by neurosis. To him, the anxiety component is based in the behaviors and attitudes which give rise to the stuttering. Wischner (1950) starts from a learning-theory framework but has further explanations, particularly for expectancy, anxiety, and those factors which perpetuate the disorder.

Sheehan (1953) also has a well-designed theory based on the stuttering block as an equilibrium of approach-avoidance tendencies. Stuttering is an expression of a conflict. Although he formulated the theory from much of the same research as that used by Johnson and Wischner, he feels that the stuttering is almost a classic picture of a neurotic symptom. This theory accounts for the primary symptoms, and the secondary reactions are compensatory efforts to overcome avoidance. Speech is socially demanded and both speaking and not speaking may evoke penalties. The conflict functions at five levels: word level; situational level; emotional content level; relationship level; and ego-protective level.

Most other theories, which consider stuttering as a symptom of neurosis, are expressed in a vocabulary and grow out of a structure quite different from those just discussed. The "psychoanalytic theories" go into extensive explanatory detail. The stuttering is viewed as a form of behavior growing out of basic drives and needs. Conflicts and anxiety are looked on as primary factors rather than something that emerges from reactions and situations surrounding the speech. The anxiety arises from the child's inability to express or gratify his subjective needs and, at the same time, adapt to parental expectations or standards. Stuttering is a compromise between seeking and inhibiting gratification (Travis, Chapter 29).

As may be expected, authorities whose theories may be classified as considering stuttering a neurotic symptom stress varied aspects of adjustment, and sometimes they begin from different concepts of personality structure. Their ideas are not mutually exclusive, but the theories cannot be thought of as identical. Coriat (1931 and 1943) stresses the fixation at (or regression to) early progenital stages of development as the source of stuttering and its symptoms. Travis (Chapter 29) draws many similar conclusions but focuses more attention on the child's needing to suppress strong tendencies toward enjoying culturally disavowed pleasures of sucking, eating, evacuating, and exploring, all of which operate at an unconscious level. Barbara (1954) feels that the stutterer is like other neurotics in that he has lacked warmth, love, and respect, leading him to feel weak and insecure. He makes unrealistic (neurotic) demands of others, particularly women, in order to build up his self-esteem. There is excessive fear and concealed hostility toward others and himself with resultant guilt feelings.

A great many other theories of stuttering offer explanations which are difficult to co-ordinate with the extensive experimental and clinical findings available to us. As a rule, they leave more key questions unanswered than the theories mentioned above. They do, however, serve the purpose of drawing our attention to certain factors which appear to be present in stuttering. Certainly if we are ever to develop an adequate and accurate theory of stuttering, we must continue to include all pertinent aspects of the entity in our thinking. It is quite possible that many of the theories, even if they should be constructed before or apart from much of our present-day research, may provide valuable leads and thereby be important in an integra-tion of theories. One or two illustrations will suffice. Rotter (1942) explains stuttering on the basis of early pampering which, in turn, reduces the child's ability to solve his own problems and creates chronic insecurity. It is con-sidered to be only one of the mechanisms for rationalizing his failures and develops when there is an availability of stuttering (through contact or ob-serving parental reaction to it) and a need for the mechanism. By focusing attention on parental behavior which arouses general feelings of inadequacy and insecurity, we are provided with an explanation which may relate di-rectly to therapeutic measures that are carried out to implement several theories. Solomon's theory (1939) draws attention to the disintegrative as-pects of the behavior during stuttering. He notes that the whole organism is overactive under the stimulation of emotion and the tensions caused by need for social approval and control. Highest levels of activity tend to dis-integrate first under this essentially decorticate condition—and speech is the highest type of integrated behavior. The picture of stuttering as a pat-tern of disintegration has been suggested by others, including Travis in his earlier studies (1931).

## COMPLETING THE INTEGRATION

It is apparent that within the framework for integrating suggested above there are several examples of basically incompatible points of view. At present, such disagreements in theory seem necessary. It is not accurate to say that the disagreements are only differences in emphasis. Any attempt to force them into a mold that results in one comprehensive theory would dis-tort some theories too drastically. This may be illustrated by summarizing some differences already mentioned in the theories of Johnson (1956 and Chapter 28) and Travis (1940 and Chapter 29). Johnson shows differences from many theories in relation to all three questions basic in the integration. His description of the entity goes beyond the speech symptomatology so that he does not define all similar irregularities as "stuttering." He does not consider neuromuscular elements of the block important but focuses at-tention on the anticipation and anxiety which precede and surround the act and interprets this as *being* the stuttering. The disorder develops from the normal nonfluencies and arises from evaluations regarding them. The source of the stuttering is in the parents, or rather, the stuttering is initially something in the mind of the parents rather than in the mouth of the stutterer. Travis, on the other hand, considers the failure to be in the child. He feels that the blocking may involve interruption in neural flow which is triggered by a primary anxiety. In this theory, it is not necessary for this reaction to grow out of normal hesitations, but is one which can come and go as drives and feelings vary. Not only are the causes different in these two theories but the characteristics and their meanings are quite at variance. In fact, one wonders if they are not talking about two different entities, both of which have been labeled stuttering.

In our present state of ignorance, integration may need to stop at this point. Any attempt at complete unity of existing theories is not possible, but some tentative suggestions may be offered. The work of Sheehan (1953) seems to indicate that it is possible to place both the "learning theory" and "neurotic" points of view into one framework without serious loss to either. The psychoanalytic point of view does not reject the possibility of a relationship between normal nonfluencies and stuttering. Is it not possible that the determinants actually vary in the degree to which they are precipitating, maintaining, aggravating, or complicating in different children? Just how may the balance of these factors alter as the child grows older and continues to stutter? Are the characteristics of the "stuttering" of "neurotic" stutterers and of "normal" stutterers different enough to dichotomize them? It would appear that the eventual reconciliation of some opposed theories is possible.

Of course, there are questions that no theories answer in sufficient detail. Why do certain children develop stuttering and not others who endure similar circumstances and biological background? Why do some stop stuttering under what would be thought of as adverse conditions? How about the 4:1 sex ratio of stutterers? Schuell's thought-provoking conclusions (1946) are the best to date, but greater specificity is needed. What combination of factors accounts for the radical, almost overnight change in the speech of stutterers? There are many other questions that need to be answered, but they do not materially affect the bringing together of what we already have, and there is no reason to expect that their answers could not find a place in this integration.

Even though some theories cannot at this time be easily reconciled, the integration method suggested here does provide a means for pointing up basic disagreements of definition, description, and explanation within the same framework. Nor is it necessary to "split up" a theory because parts of it fit in one category and part in another. Practically, it means that in any argument or discussion of "stuttering" we have a way of making clear what "kind" of stuttering we are talking about; for it is not possible to think intelligently about "causes" unless we are aware of what is being caused and the process of development that it pursues.

Certain fundamental weaknesses of theories may become immediately apparent if they are placed in this framework. In this sense, the integrative structure is evaluative. Any theory which ignores the wealth of research on descriptive elements of stuttering—or by-passes the developmental characteristics during childhood—will be less likely to produce accurate and useful explanations. A theory which dwells on the essentially descriptive aspects and presents glib generalities for explanations is likewise suspect. Theorists who spend a great deal of time talking about the research and theories of others but who fail to show specific relationships to the ideas expressed on description, development, or explanation of stuttering may be expected to offer only random, accidental contributions of value.

An additional advantage of viewing theories in the pattern suggested here is that it allows for continual revision of integration as new theoretical concepts are found by the reader or experimenter. Thus by combining this with a standardized means for discovering differences in points of view with regard to each basic element of every theory, for systematizing essential contributions to stuttering theory, and for emphasizing weaknesses in information or construction, we come as close to integrating theories as seems possible at the present time.

## SUMMARY

Previous attempts at integrating theories have been reviewed. The limitations of these efforts have been outlined and a different framework suggested. Theories may be brought together under three headings, the combination of which provides the most satisfactory understanding of stuttering in light of present-day theories. The headings are expressed as three questions:

1. What are the contributions to the *description* of the behavioral, social, and psychological concomitants of stuttering?
2. What are the contributions to understanding the *process of development* of stuttering?
3. What contributions toward *explaining* these phenomena are offered?

Examples of contributions of current theories are outlined. It was pointed out that theories must necessarily include more than the "cause." The wide variance as to causes (or explanations of stuttering) are due in part to the fact that they begin from different concepts as to what stuttering is and how it develops.

The suggested framework for integrating theories has the following advantages:

1. It provides for a continuous process of adding new information or theories.
2. It shows areas of fundamental agreements or disagreements in theories.
3. It provides a method for evaluating theories by exposing gaps in construction or information.

## BIBLIOGRAPHY

AINSWORTH, S. 1945. Integrating theories of stuttering. *J. Speech Disorders,* 10, 205–210.

BARBARA, D. A. 1954. Stuttering: a psychodynamic approach to its understanding and treatment. New York: Julian Press.

BERRY, M., and EISENSON, J. 1942. The defective in speech. New York: Crofts.
——— 1956. Speech disorders. New York: Appleton-Century-Crofts.
BLOODSTEIN, O. N. 1949. Conditions under which stuttering is reduced or absent: a review of the literature. *J. Speech Hearing Disorders*, 14, 295–302.
——— 1950. A rating scale study of conditions under which stut'ering is reduced or absent. *J. Speech Hearing Disorders*, 15, 29–36.
BROWN, S. F. 1938. The theoretical importance of certain factors influencing the incidence of stuttering. *J. Speech Disorders*, 3, 223–230.
——— 1945. The loci of stutterings in the speech sequence. *J. Speech Disorders*, 10, 181–192.
BRYNGELSON, B. 1942. Investigations in the etiology and nature of dysphemia and its symptom, stuttering. *J. Speech Disorders*, 7, 15–27.
COBB, S. 1943. Borderlands of psychiatry. Cambridge: Harvard Univ. Press.
CORIAT, I. H. 1931. The nature and analytical treatment of stammering. *Proc. Amer. Speech Correction Assn.*, 1, 153–155.
——— 1943. *In* Hahn, E. 1943. Stuttering: significant theories and therapies. Palo Alto: Stanford Univ. Press.
DOUGLAS, L. C. 1943. A study of bilaterally recorded electroencephalograms of adult stutterers. *J. exp. Psychol.*, 32, 247–265.
FREESTONE, N. W. 1942. An electroencephalographic study of the moment of stuttering. *Speech Monogr.*, 9, 28–60.
GREENE, J. S., and WELLS, E. J. 1927. The cause and cure of speech disorders. New York: Macmillan.
HAHN, E. 1943. Stuttering: significant theories and therapies. Palo Alto: Stanford Univ. Press.
HILL, H. 1944a. Stuttering: I. a critical review and evaluation of biochemical investigations. *J. Speech Disorders*, 9, 245–261.
——— 1944b. Stuttering: II. a review and integration of physiological data. *J. Speech Disorders*, 9, 289–324.
——— 1945. An interbehavioral analysis of several aspects of stuttering. *J. gen. Psychol.*, 32, 289–316.
JOHNSON, W., BROWN, S., CURTIS, J., EDNEY, C., and KEASTER, J. 1956. Speech handicapped school children (rev. ed.). New York: Harper.
KARLIN, I. W. 1947. A psychosomatic theory of stuttering. *J. Speech Hearing Disorders*, 12, 319–322.
KENYON, E. L. 1941. The etiology of stammering: an examination into certain recent studies; with a glance into the future. *J. Speech Disorders*, 6, 1–12.
——— 1942. The etiology of stammering: fundamentally a wrong psychophysiologic habit in the control of the vocal cords for the production of an individual speech sound; a beginning presentation. *J. Speech Disorders*, 7, 97–104.
——— 1943. The etiology of stammering: the psychophysiologic facts which concern the production of speech sounds and of stammering. *J. Speech Disorders*, 8, 337–348.
KNOTT, J. R., and TJOSSEM, T. D. 1943. Bilateral electroencephalograms from normal speakers and stutterers. *J. exp. Psychol.*, 32, 357–362.
KRAUSZ, E. O. 1940. Is stuttering primarily a speech disorder? *J. Speech Disorders*, 5, 227–231.
ROTTER, J. B. 1942. A working hypothesis as to the nature and treatment of stuttering. *J. Speech Disorders*, 7, 263–288.
SCHUELL, H. 1946. Sex differences in relation to stuttering; Part I. *J. Speech Disorders*, 11, 277–298.
——— 1947. Sex differences in relation to stuttering: Part II. *J. Speech Disorders*, 12, 23–38.

SHEEHAN, J. G. 1953. Theory and treatment of stuttering as an approach-avoidance conflict. *J. Psychol.*, 36, 27–49.

SOLOMON, M. 1939. Stuttering at an emotional and personality disorder. *J. Speech Disorders*, 4, 347–357.

STEER, M. D. 1937. Symptomatologies of young stutterers. *J. Speech Disorders*, 2, 3–13.

TRAVIS, L. E. 1931. Speech pathology. New York: Appleton.

———— 1933. Speech pathology. *In* Murchison, C., A handbook of child psychology (2nd ed. rev.). Worcester: Clarke Univ. Press. Ch. 16.

———— 1936. Studies in speech pathology. *Arch. Speech*, 1, No. 2 and No. 3, 7–247.

———— 1940. The need for stuttering. *J. Speech Disorders*, 5, 193–202.

———— 1946. My present thinking on stuttering. *Western Speech*, 10, 3–5.

TUTHILL, C. 1940. A quantitative study of extensional meaning with special reference to stuttering. *J. Speech Disorders*, 5, 189–191.

VAN RIPER, C. 1939. Speech correction: principles and methods (1st ed.). New York: Prentice-Hall.

———— 1947. Speech correction: principles and methods (2nd ed.). New York: Prentice-Hall.

———— 1954. Speech correction: principles and methods (3rd ed.). New York: Prentice-Hall.

WEST, R., KENNEDY, L., and CARR, A. 1947. The rehabilitation of speech (rev. ed.). New York: Harper.

WISCHNER, G. J. 1950. Stuttering behavior and learning: a preliminary theoretical formulation. *J. Speech Hearing Disorders*, 15, 324–335.

# PART IV

# Psychotherapy and Speech Therapy

# CHAPTER 31

# THE PSYCHOTHERAPEUTICAL PROCESS

- *Lee Edward Travis, Ph.D.*

TWO GREAT AND SEPARATE streams of thought approached each other, ran parallel for a time, and then, relatively recently, intermingled. One had its headwaters in Freud, the other in Pavlov. Psychoanalysis flowed on as a relatively distinct tributary through such leaders as Ferenczi, Jones, Fenichel, and Alexander. Learning theory and experimentation went their somewhat distinct way through such workers as Krasnogorsky, Thorndike, Watson, Lashley, and Hull. In Hull the two movements came together, and they definitely intermingled in Dollard, Miller, and Mowrer. This intermingling gave us current psychotherapy.

Speech pathologists have manifested in both practice and research an ever quickening interest in psychotherapy. To them have come those suffering from troubles in communication without organic impairment of either the sensory or the motor speech equipment. Voice and speech drills have not been always too effective with these cases. The recognition of emotional disturbances as etiological factors in these disorders has forced speech therapists to seek the promising help of psychotherapy as developed by psychiatrists and psychologists. Individual (Dollard and Miller, 1950), group (Bach, 1954), play (Klein, 1948), and activity (Slavson, 1947) therapy have all been scouted. Increasing numbers of speech pathologists are familiarizing themselves with the various procedures currently used in psychotherapy (Sheehan, 1954). A number of them are securing their own personal analysis.

In the years to come, it appears reasonable to suppose that speech pathologists will not only apply successfully the principles and practices of psychotherapy to their specialty but will contribute to the advancement of that which they now borrow. This supposition would seem to be almost self-evident, since speech workers are dealing entirely with problems of communication, and since communication is the matrix of psychotherapy.

## COMMUNICATION

### Speech as a Stimulus

Speech is a stimulus to both the listener and the speaker. In the listener, speech may arouse feelings, emotions, ideas, action. In listening to another, one may feel lonely and sad, happy and glad; one may hate, become afraid, or love; one may make an induction or a deduction or devise a plan of action; or one may sit down, get up, run, strike, or talk back. One or all or a multiple combination of these responses may be elicited not only by what someone says but by the way it is said. Words, quality of voice, rhythm and cadence, emphasis, intensity, pitch, all blend in various proportions in their effects.

What the speaker says and the way he says it may frighten, sadden, or excite himself; the content and the style of his utterances may arouse or increase anger or fear or love in him; they may crystallize his thinking; and they may excite him to flee with fear or to attack with anger or to embrace with love. The person's speech has powerful stimulus values to himself as well as to others. In a very significant sense, whenever a person speaks, he speaks only to himself. Others may listen in on his verbal output and constitute themselves as an audience. They may be fooled into thinking that the speaker is talking to them. The speaker may share this illusion as well. But whatever an individual may say and to whomsoever he may think he is speaking, in a deeply telling way, he is communicating fully with himself only. We may say here parenthetically that the "neurotic" is one who does not communicate well with himself, one who does not understand fully what he himself says.

### Speech as a Response

Speech is a response. It is an act. In speaking the person moves his lips, tongue and jaw, possibly his whole body. He makes sounds and gestures. He may be both seen and heard in action. Being a response, speech must have a stimulus or stimuli. It must be elicited. Most profitably, speech may be considered as a response to speaker needs and tensions produced by either inner or outer forces, or by both, operating sequentially or simultaneously. Needs and tensions established by forces from within and from without demand action for the satisfaction of the former and the dissolution of the latter. In our culture, individuals of all ages universally resort to verbalization as one means of alleviating, directly or indirectly, needs and tensions. Speech as a response, then, may be considered as serving the following needs:

1. To adventure forth, to reach out, to explore.
2. To control, to probe, to prod, to maneuver, to stimulate, to alter, to influence.
3. To cut, to strike out, to hurt, to destroy.
4. To soothe, to mollify, to love.

5. To receive recognition, status, attention, response.
6. To exhibit, to be found out, to reveal, to expose.

The fate of speech development will depend in a large measure upon the way in which the verbal expression of these needs is managed by the culture.

If speech can be found by the infant or child-speaker to be acceptable as an expression of his pressing needs and mounting tensions, it will develop as a useful and purposeful tool. If he finds he cannot risk an honest, telltale verbal expression, deficiencies and disabilities in speaking may result. To observe him and to listen to him is to acquiesce, and to consider his utterances is to grant identity.

### Speaker-Listener Interaction

The speaker-listener interaction is the matrix of society. Speech is the leading character in the drama of interpersonal relationships. The speaker is an actor and the listener is an audience. Regardless of the part the speaker may think he is playing, in a way and to a degree he is always playing himself. And to the act the listener always responds. Sometimes more, sometimes less, sometimes painfully, sometimes joyfully, sometimes feelingly, sometimes intellectually, one's listening and viewing audience invariably responds. And in that response the speaker sees his own reflection. What he sees may not be true of him. It may be distorted by the form and quality of the listener's reflecting surfaces. Unintentionally the speaker may arouse hate or fear or love in another. To his surprise, the speaker may see himself reflected as a hateful creature, or a fearful monster, or a lovable character.

The present intrapsychic structure of the person, which is based predominantly upon his past interpersonal relations, and the present interpersonal relationships determine both his evaluation of himself and others' evaluation of him. And if we may think of inadequacies as being crucially advertised in interpersonal relationships, then maladjustment may be defined in terms of disturbances in communication (Ruesch and Bateson, 1951). If one is considered deluded, withdrawn, mute, feeble-minded, verbally inept, or in one of many other ways abnormal, he is manifesting, rather specifically, disturbances in communication. He is disturbed either in perception (listening) or in transmission (speaking). As shortcomings arise in disturbances of communication, they will be corrected by effective agents found in communication. The primary corrective agent is the communicative interaction between patient and therapist. Psychotherapy may be defined as an effort at improving the communication of the patient within himself and with others. The origin and destination of some messages may be found within the same organism, and we will be dealing with an intrapersonal network. Other messages will originate in one person and terminate in another, and we will be dealing with an interpersonal network. The intrapersonal network will sooner or later be the origin of messages in the interpersonal network, so that the two networks become inextricably linked.

A patient may be defined as a member of our culture who does not speak our language. We do not understand him fully or at all. If the psychiatrist is to converse with the schizophrenic, he will have to decode the symbolic system of the patient. If the speech correctionist is to understand the functional voice or articulatory case or the stutterer, he will have to listen through the speech symptom to hear what is really being said behind the symptom. The therapist tries first to understand the disturbances of communication and than to correct defective processes of communication (Mowrer, 1953).

## THE THERAPEUTICAL PROCEDURE

### A New Interpersonal Relationship

In the past, particularly in his ancient past, the person was taught to attach fear, shame, and guilt to certain spoken words and then to generalize from these verbal reactions to his thinking and feeling. In old interpersonal relationships, mainly with his parents, the honest expression of his feelings met condemnation and derogation. He learned to inhibit and to repress not only his spoken words but his thinking and feeling as well. In therapy, a new kind of interpersonal relationship is created, the opposite of that kind responsible for the learning of repression. It permits, it encourages, as a matter of fact it rewards, the person's utterance of whatever comes into his mind, especially that which he finds fearful and shameful. As he says things that provoke fear or shame or guilt in contradistinction to what he experienced in the past and is experiencing in common present situations, he is not condemned or punished or hurt. Instead his expressions meet warmth, acceptance, and support. In this way, fear, shame, and guilt attached to talking honestly about tabooed feelings and topics are extinguished. This extinction generalizes from overt reaction (talking) to covert reaction (thinking and feeling). Thus repression is gradually unlearned under the permissive and rewarding interpersonal relationships of therapy that are the opposite to the punitive ones under which it was originally learned. The therapeutical process is so different from that of childhood in that it is permissive and rewarding of free speech and free naming of feelings and emotions. The derogatory and condemnatory constrictions of childhood learning are reversed (Dollard and Miller, 1950).

### Unminded Verbalization

The primary new condition of learning imposed upon the person is that of unminded verbalization (free association). Under this new rule, the person is required to say immediately everything and anything that comes to mind. He is urged, possibly again and again, to communicate every thought, every feeling, be it trivial, silly, embarrassing, guilt-laden, illogical, obscene, or fanciful. He is urged to express fear, guilt, shame, hostility, lust, incest, insecurity; every and any feeling that may arise within him. He is urged to be illogical, doubtful, critical, unpleasant, unmannerly; in short, completely uninhibited in the content and form of verbal expression. He must try hardest to say that which is most difficult for him to say; that which is not openly said; that which no one has ever wanted to hear before. Nothing at all is to be held back. Really, he is asked to strip psychologically; to reveal the most intimate and personal details of his mind. For the first, and possibly for the last time in his life, he is permitted and encouraged to be absolutely honest with another person. The power of unminded verbalization lies in his readiness to consider freely by means of spoken language any part of himself in the trusted company of one of his fellow men. This is strikingly different from the usual conversational procedures of everyday life where, for self-protection, the person has to be careful in varying degrees of what he says.

The person is not only invited to speak freely, he is obliged to do so. This rule is the key to the therapeutic situation. The person is to be ruthlessly honest in the pronouncement of words and sentences which may evoke sickening anxiety. Otherwise, he will remain fixed in his maladaptive habits and can never make completely satisfactory adjustments.

The therapist cannot talk for the person and he cannot help much by asking questions. In the first place, he does not know what to say and what questions to ask. In the second place, even if he did know the questions and the answers and gave them to the person, the beneficial results would be negligible. In the doctor-patient interaction, the patient has to experience his repressed feelings for himself. The larger burden of the therapy is placed upon him. He will not realize a quick and passive cure. He must discover for himself that he is sick only of himself. He must come to realize fully that to harm or to love anybody or anything else is to harm or to love himself and call it harming or loving somebody or something else. He must learn that his unconscious self-harmer or self-lover is turning upon its projection.

Unminded verbalization is not easy. Anyone can convince himself of this statement by putting aside five minutes during which time he will say aloud anything that comes to his mind exactly as it comes. He can determine how difficult this is even when he is alone. Mysterious opposition arises within him who tries to talk freely, even to himself. Fears and anxieties arise at the slightest cues of forbidden expressions. In therapy, the patient will dodge the rules by private assumptions: the matter isn't relevant, or it can be postponed, or the therapist isn't interested or wouldn't understand. A person cannot go successfully through therapy saying only what he wants to say. To succeed, he must say mainly what he does not want to say. He must continually test limits, both his and those of the therapist. He must continually risk revelations of self and thereby gain consenting acknowledgment.

Although the person should work at the highest level of anxiety possible for him, one should not get the idea that the course of therapy is marked by one continuous anxiety attack, or by one anxiety attack after another. The rule of unminded verbalization, though rigorously applied, is gently and patiently taught; and just as gently and gradually learned. Various defenses come into play to keep the person from intolerable pain. The person sees to it that the amount of anxiety he is asked to bear is bearable. And then, hopeful and encouraging relearning and unlearning take place. Comfort will be found in seeing through dreaded and devastating feelings; and with each pain borne, tolerance grows for further pain.

### The Therapist—A New Parent

From an early day many of the person's feelings, acts, and expressions have met condemnation and derogation. Generalizing, the person has felt that he has been condemned and unwanted in whole or in part. As he has grown, condemnations and derogations of his feelings and expressions, and therefore of himself, have persisted. To get along at all satisfactorily he has been taught to inhibit or better to repress many factors in interpersonal relationships. Throughout his lifetime he has come up against the unacceptability of himself and the advertisements of his selfhood. As a consequence, he arrives at a given moment with conflicts in feelings and expressions and a split or divided purpose. Anxieties follow and he may seek help. If he does, he should find a surprising experience. He should find a man, probably for the very first time, who will give him an example of a capacity in another human being to meet the elemental and primitive impulses of lust, hate, and fear, and the harsh and damning inhibitions they have met, without being surprised, disturbed, or in any way retaliatory. He should find a man in whose eyes he will never lose status.

The therapist will not judge or tell. He will not be frightened or shocked or angered. He will discriminate himself from a variety of frightening and condemning human beings such as the old parent, teachers, the police, the gossip, or the boss. Nothing that the person in therapy can do or say will be used against him. The therapist wants nothing but the whole truth and he knows that, to get it, there can be no fear of punishment of any sort on the part of the patient. The patient needs and is given continual assurance of reversal of conventional attitudes. Slowly he learns to trust the therapist and to venture forth more and more in the new parent-child relationship of psychotherapy.

## THE OCCURRENCES IN PSYCHOTHERAPY

The patient comes to the therapeutic situation with anxiety, emotional pain, and frequently with symptoms. Generally, he has fears: fears of gossip, loss of status, and another failure. Frequently he has sought help before, he has complained about his troubles to friends and acquaintances until he has exhausted their patience, and he has been labeled as a pest, a bore, or a neurotic. Still he remains starved for attention and understanding. The permissive and complete attention of the therapist to his recitals come as a new and contrasting reward. To have another give undivided attention and thought to his problems is an important precondition to help.

The therapist listens attentively with an open mind. As noted above, he is not a judge, or prude, or gossip. He is acceptant, tolerant, patient, supportive, compassionately neutral. The patient understands this view of the therapist as forgiveness and with this insight he begins his work.

## The Early Hours

Once more, possibly for the hundredth time, the patient tells his troubles, past and present. He recounts, explains, interprets, excuses, all the time testing the therapist's attention, interest, patience, understanding, sympathy. Sometimes he invites another failure, defies the therapist to help him, gives the therapist the responsibility for his problems, and demands proof of the therapist's past successes. But fortunately there are needs and pain to drive him on, and the therapist gets in step and supports his efforts at walking straight.

Occasionally, the therapist rewards by direct expressions of sympathy or approval. But he gives no loose sympathy. He tries hard to reward those responses which have the best chance of forwarding the patient's recovery. The therapist knows and the patient must learn that the patient must suffer to learn and that he must work at the highest level of pain bearable. Therapy is not fun. It is not a *tête-à-tete*.

The therapist does not cross-examine his patient. He will ask some direct questions about the patient's development and family, where the patient was raised, and when troubles appeared. He is not engaging in a fact-finding operation or in gathering case-history data to be filed away in a folder. Rather, he is trying to identify the person before him, to identify with him, to co-exist with him. Mainly, the therapist waits and hears his patient out, letting him say what he must say when he is able to say it.

## Later Hours

Only gradually and with considerable effort and pain does the person learn to tell the therapist everything. His very first verbalizations are usually those which he has admitted before to someone. Sooner or later he divulges things he has consciously known before but has not spoken. Then, finally, he says and feels things that are as new to him as to the therapist. The new things are at first obscure. The person does not know what he is saying. The therapist may not know either. Even if we have no personal reasons for not recognizing the meaning of a patient's productions, the meaning in itself is really not obvious but is disguised as though it were translated into some ancient and forgotten tongue, not familiar to our everyday understanding. We must learn this archaic language before we can translate it into communication forms familiar to our modern ears (Fromm, 1951).

In these later hours, the person rarely makes an honest, frank, declarative statement. He speaks in metaphor, parable, innuendo, dreams of the day and the night, fantasies, and picture language. He tries to say what is not openly said and what no one before his therapist wished to hear. He wants to reveal but fears to do so. A compromise solution is reached. He reveals, but not clearly, not clearly to either himself or to his therapist. In this way both sides of the conflict are partially realized. What he says contains unacceptable and feared feelings and thoughts and the operation of his inhibitory forces against these. Listening, the therapist learns what cravings and urges have been repressed and how greatly they are dreaded. He learns what one part of his patient desires and what another part abhors. And as the patient continues to speak more and more spontaneously, he too comes to know his true feelings and to accept and channel them. He comes to acknowledge and possibly to renounce his native wildness, but not to continue repression of it. He learns to preserve his unspoiled natural wildness as a healthy foundation for high-spirited cultural living.

### Fight Father Over Mother

What does the person actually say, but not know what he has said actually? An adolescent male stutterer gave the five following productions:

*December 11.* See a whole bunch of clouds and they are forming rings around the moon. A jet black horse with the wings of a bird is there. Then there are a thousand more horses, but they are smaller and a mixture of color; bays, sorrels, roans. There is no other black one. Now a big sorrel appears. He's an outcast and the only stud besides the black. He keeps trying to defeat the black horse but never can.

Down on the earth is a forest of knotted trees without leaves. A whole bunch of little elves, two or three feet tall, are watching this herd of mares and the two stallions fighting. Two of the elves are about six inches bigger than the rest and they're battling it out to see who will be king of this outfit, but neither can win.

Now I see an hour glass, a very large one, that is sitting out in the desert. It is rolling end over end and instead of sand being in this thing there are snakes. One part has snakes that are hostile to those in the other side so that when the glass is standing up, there is room for only two snakes to go through into the lower part. Slowly the snakes get wiped out as this glass keeps rolling letting snakes through first one way and then the other. Finally there are just two snakes left, one on each side. They are pretty dizzy and pretty battered up by this time and neither one can do a whole lot about killing off the other, although eventually one will have to die. About this time the hour glass reaches the only tree in the desert and the glass breaks in the middle and each part rolls off in a different direction.

See a waterfall and a river heading out to the ocean. The ocean is calm. There is an ancient sailing ship. Looks like it had been on the bottom of the ocean for several hundred years. It has moss, seaweed, and barnacles all over it. On board are chained the skeletons of the men who worked the oars and on the deck is this huge octopus. A huge black snake is also there. This octopus and snake are having a fight, all wrapped in coils. Snake is wrapped around the octopus and tentacles of the octopus are around the snake trying to crush it. The water gets red and then black and the ship's hold opens up and the ship sinks back down and disappears.

*January 19.* See a grove of banana and apple trees together. They are intermingled in the same orchard. There is an apple with a worm sticking his head out. He goes back in and starts eating the apple. Slowly he eats whole of apple out until all that is left is the skin of the apple. It is completely hollow on the inside. What he does with the apple I don't know. The worm gets no fatter and has no discharge. Inside of apple just goes but it has no effect on the worm whatsoever. Pretty soon this apple falls off the tree into a basket which they are putting apples in as they pick them off the tree. This apple doesn't squash or lose its shape for some reason in spite of the fact that all that is left is the skin. All of those apples are put on a sorting table and this one apple is pushed off with the bad ones in a huge dump. The worm is still in this apple. Another worm decides it's a good looking apple too, so he crawls in and they commence to have a fight. As they're fighting they bump around and explode the gases that are in the apple which blows up and throws them out a long way off and they land on the top or side of a mountain. They get pretty hungry and see a mesquite bush which has an apple on it, just one apple. They both make a dive for the apple but when they just about get their hands on it, it explodes. About this time they see a whole bunch of mesquite bushes. Each bush has just one apple. They're running around like mad trying to get these apples. As they just about reach the apples, they explode and disappear. They get underneath an apple and have about given up hope. But as they get under apple it looks huge. Since they think it will bust they don't pay much attention to it but it falls on them and squashes them. It is solid. As it falls on them it buries them into itself, about one-fourth inch. It starts rolling. It rolls on and on and isn't hurt by the bouncing. Finally it rolls under an apple tree and somebody comes along and picks it up and takes out a knife and sees the two worm holes and cuts that part of the apple off and lets it drop to the ground. The worms' ghosts leave their bodies and go up and up. They have little wings. They see a beautiful apple orchard, the most beautiful one they have ever seen. There are thousands of apples. Instead of each worm picking his own apple they both go for the same one and start fighting. Sparks fly and they fall. They fall down and down. They're on a stick with an apple on each end. The stick is over a fire and the worms are being roasted by all the other apples standing around. They're getting pretty well cooked by this time when the other apples bring out two very beautiful apples which are exactly the same so that one worm may go to one apple and the other worm to the other. But no, both worms go for the same apple and start to fight like hell. The two apples catch them in a squeeze play and bang the two worms together. It so happens one worm is pushed into one apple and the other worm into the other apple. The apples start rolling down hill and the worms have their heads out of their respective apples just cussing the heck out of each other and not bothering to eat. The apples come together ever so often to bang the heads of the worms together. The apples decide this isn't going to work as the worms are still mad at each other. So they take them back to the other apples and contemplate what to do with the two worms. They think and think and think and finally two apples which are Siamese twins roll up. They think this is the solution. The Siamese twins are the same apple except they have two stems and two cores and the two worms make a dive for this twin apple and start going around and around eating out the insides. As they're eating out the insides they meet a great big worm which eats both of the smaller worms.

In varying detail and form the same theme is presented five times. In each production, two creatures battle for the possession of something desired by both. By direct statement (stallions) and by implication (size, use of personal pronouns—he and his), the two combatants are male. Also by direct statement and implication the contested things are female. At this point in his therapy, the patient could not clearly admit two men or human males fighting over a woman. Instead he had to use such animals as stallions, worms, and snakes for the human male; and such things as mares, an apple, and an hour glass for the human female. Still less could he admit his shameful and feared desire to fight his own father for his own mother. Especially at this time was he unable to come to terms with such dreaded desires. At a later time he could and did find peace with these and other practically unbearable feelings.

### Wish to Mess

There are other troublesome areas in interpersonal relationships. Other desires and feelings have been tamed by the culture. The domestication of the person has too often involved frustration of his needs with consequent aggressive behavior, fear, and repression. A young and cultured mother who stuttered severely spoke as follows:

The mud is cold. It's yellow and brown. I smell it. I dig it out of the holes in my rubber heels. My hands get dry and I go into a rage. I jump around and around. I'm mad. Am I wet? I'll get dry, very dry. How would I feel if I didn't wet my pajamas? Would I be loved more? I'm mad at everybody, so I'll be dryer than dry. They don't want me to be wet so I'll be dryer than anybody. I'll be sarcastic. I'll be difficult. I'll be contrary. I'll plunge my hands into my vagina. I'm wearing gloves. I'm ladylike, the gloves cover. I'm protected and I won't be given away. I speak ladylike. Oh crap! I'll pull my gloves off and throw them in everybody's face. I'll have no false stuff. I throw the gloves into heaven, into church, into the toilet.

This strictly reared and highly proper young mother is discovering and accepting her early frustrated desires to mess and her subsequent hostile feelings to such frustrations. She is recapturing her natural, infantile interests in urinating, the attempts on the part of the culture to damn wetness and dirtiness, and her resentment of such management.

### Desire to Be a Baby

Studies and current observations convince us that our culture demands the establishment of a relatively very early independence and psychological weaning of the child. Children are asked to become little men and little women very early. Crying, being held, being hugged, in short being babied, are all denied them. Yet it seems clear that infants and children need protection, love, and succor. Having these needs so consistently frustrated leads the child into the necessity of denying them. The parent's neglect and even punishment of the child for being a cry-baby do not result in the child's becoming big and strong and independent; they more often than not result in his remaining unconsciously babyish and dependent. This unacceptable dependence is expressed in the following dream of a young woman suffering from asthma. She had this dream some five or six times at intervals of several months.

I'm called home by letter or telegram. I don't know who initiates the wires or letters or why I'm to come home, but it is urgent. There never seems to be any doubt of the urgency. I can't remember that I ever want to go home or even that I feel driven to go. But it is an accepted fact to go. I have to go home. I'm needed. There is just no question but what I have to go home. Always I leave. Always I fly in an hour or two after being summoned. Most of the time I don't bother going to my apartment. I call and make arrangements for my plane reservations, locate my friends or landlady, and take off with no clothes or anything. I don't know where the plane money will come from, but it never worries me. The source seems very reasonable in the dreams. One time I arrange for an advance on my salary; another time I borrow from the employee fund; another time I borrow from my retirement fund. It always seems logical and feasible. I remember being on the plane and worrying it along, wishing it would go faster. I am worried and anxious to get home, get it over with and come back right away. Other times I'm almost sorry to be coming in; I dread it so. Everything looks so horribly familiar. Don't remember a thing about being home. I can't remember what the emergency is, and yet I seem to have the feeling someone is dead. Can't remember a funeral or anything. I feel at least some drastic change has taken place. Perhaps my mother has been placed in an institution and I am the logical one to take over. Always something drastic and unalterable has taken place. Something which can never be argued about and I have to stay. Nobody tells me so or influences me in any way at all, but I know that I am doomed, and that life is depressingly like it used to be, except for some change which I can't put my finger on. In some of the dreams the ending is that I just can't get back. I decide to leave anyway, and then I can't. Can't dig up enough money or something. I never have any trouble making arrangements, financial or otherwise, for getting home; but every petty thing in the world seems to arise from nowhere to conspire to keep me there. Sometimes my mother must have died or was institutionalized as incurable. I would fly out as usual, and had to stay as usual, but these times there was nobody to hold the family together. Even though I knew I was giving up any life of my own, I felt absolutely compelled to do it. I was afraid everybody would go his own way, and that we wouldn't have the closeness and companionship we had had in past years, and that it would be my fault. This would be my one chance to be of some real help. I couldn't resist even though I felt completely smothered by it. In one dream everything was exactly the same as in the others, except I was married and had children of my own. I felt I couldn't leave my "original" family, so I had my husband and children come out and we all settled down together.

In these dreams are unconscious longing for home, hostility against the mother (she was dead or institutionalized), desire to break away from the home, desire to take the mother's place, and feelings of being smothered. Some of these wishes are supportive of each other; others are antagonistic to each other. All of these feelings and their interaction are consistent with her life's pattern. She is always searching for love and a place in the sun. She has a feeling of frustration as a result of too little love or a fear of being smothered by too much. She simultaneously strives for independence and fears realizing it. Part of her wants to be a baby still. Other feelings find the babyish ones unacceptable, even dreaded, and push her towards being a woman. The resulting conflict expresses itself in the compromise formation of asthma. Ever more honest expression of the dreaded self relieves the anxiety of her living and the handicapping symptom of her life.

**What Am I?**

Dual and multiple personalities hold great interest for observers of human nature. Novelists and poets as well as professional workers have thought and written about the expressions, the possible dynamics, and the nature of people who present sides to themselves that are too strikingly different. A certain degree of ambivalence, of mutually contradictory feelings, of conflicting modes of behavior, are tolerable in ourselves and in others. But too much uncertainty and doubt about our role, about who and what we are, frequently raise painful anxiety.

A young housewife and mother suffered tortures over whether she was saint or sinner, dutifully supportive of her husband or destructively critical of him, a wife or a hussy. She had two dreams pointing to the issues in her problem.

*May 31.* I was a dancer with a divided face. One side, the right side, was serene; the hair nicely combed; the eye nice; the face unlined; the mouth just right. The other side, the left, was so different. The hair was in long, wild curls, the eye cocked and wild, face hard and lined, lipstick smeared and messy. I waited to see what would happen. I knew I would end up all one way or the other. I kept on dancing. Slowly the mouth became like the right side. Then face changed to good side, then hair changed until at the end whole head and face were good except the left eye which remained a bit wild and watchful as though to say, "Ha, ha, you can't change me."

*June 1.* I was a singer rehearsing my number. A fitter was fitting my dress to me. My act was successful because I had a man sitting in a chair telling me funny things to say to the audience before I sang. Actually I wasn't very pretty and my voice was average, and I knew I owed my success to this man. He wasn't too good looking, but he had a wonderful sense of humor. I took him for granted and he didn't seem to mind that I used him. I wondered if the audience could have seen him sometimes during the performance. I preferred they had not seen him. Next I went to a big skating rink. I saw a big blond handsome man. I fell in love with him at first sight. He was carrying a child and I took it away from him. I walked away knowing he would follow me because I had the child. He did and I knew he was mine for the taking. Then I realized how dumb he was and I knew he was not what I really wanted. I went to look for the man who helped me in my act. I knew now that I loved him. I found him but he looked different. I was happy to know I had finally found the man I loved.

In the beginning of the first dream, the left half of her head and face portray primitive feelings and urges and the right half a culturally acceptable self. The primitive self is identified as bad and the social self as good. From the nature of her current problems and from the expressions in her dreams, the bad self could be labeled sexual. She is sexually frigid with her husband but dismayed by her sexual feelings for other men. The resolution of her conflict is important in order to allay her anxiety. In the dream, domestication of the wildness is completed except for a tolerable degree of wickedness expressed in the left eye. Hope for future earthy living lies in keeping the way open back to the further acceptance and more wholesome management of those feelings that were condemned and repressed.

In the second dream the two sets of feelings are seen in action. One chooses a reliable and sound but somewhat prosaic man who will do her bidding. The other chooses a big, handsome, dumb blond. Again the conflict is resolved in favor of the demands of cultural conformity.

At present it is predominately an either-or proposition with her. Either she is good, all good, or bad, all bad. Mainly now she is good, too good. She has been too flattened out by the taming and transforming forces of the culture. Encouragement for the vitalizing effect of a little more primitiveness in her every-day living is held out in the ultimate recovery, as well as acceptance and management of more of her maligned animal nature.

Another woman with a similar problem of the uncertainty of her role gave the following production:

I am riding a big, long snake. He goes through an opening into some beautiful tropical plants and brushes me off. I feel real angry and see an alligator and take its jaws and break them apart with much strength.

What is she saying? It is something that she cannot say openly. She has to put it in a form unintelligible to her ordinary comprehension. She does not know exactly what she has said, especially at the moment of speaking. In old and forgotten language she is saying that she would like to be a man and perform a man's unique function. But she is brushed off, frustrated in her desire and becomes angry. She strikes out in her anger at an occupant of this tropical paradise, a place where she would like to be. The occupant appears to be a man whose status she craves and whose presence she removes to make room for herself. Unconsciously she wants to be a man. Consciously she is a woman. The competing systems leave her relatively neuter, which is exactly what she is in her daily interpersonal relationships.

## The Last Hours

The person will become a child again and engage in naughty, childish behavior and express naughty, childish feelings and thoughts. He will do the things that he did or wanted to do as a child, and express the thoughts and feelings that he expressed or wanted to express when he was little. The therapist will not scold, sass, desert, or condemn him by word, look, or act. In no way will he reduce the patient's status and self-regard. Rather, he will support and reward the painful expressions of the patient with compassionate attention, impersonal evaluation, and unperturbed demeanor. The patient will grow up again, this time with a new parent who honors and respects the whole of his child.

A listing of some of the patient's behavior, desires, and feelings in therapy may make clearer the dynamic interactions between patient and therapist.

*Gross emotional behavior:*

Twisting and squirming
Turning back on therapist
Covering or burying face
Pounding
Kicking

Throwing
Pulling hair
Fondling genitals
Scratching and rubbing self
Going to sleep
Blushing
Walking around
Going to toilet
Rubbing eyes
Clenching fists
Sitting up suddenly
Temper tantrums
Putting fingers in ears
Belching
Crying
Laughing
Stealing a glance at therapist
Babbling
Remaining rigidly silent
Pouting

*Expressed desires:*

To live with therapist
To be loved by therapist
To be condemned by therapist
To be therapist's child or spouse
To be put to bed or fed by therapist
To have sexual relations with therapist
To be explored by therapist
To explore therapist
To get dirty
To play with excreta
To defecate
To expectorate
To urinate
To pass intestinal gas
To masturbate
To suck
To hurt therapist
To kill therapist
To hurt self
To die
To be naked
To run away and hide
To be left alone
To be the only patient

*Expressed feelings:*

Being seduced by therapist
Being neglected and condemned by therapist
Being failed by therapist
Being unduly influenced by therapist
Being used and experimented upon by therapist
Being gossiped about by therapist
Therapist putting ideas in patient's mind

Thoughts and feelings being read by therapist
Dizziness
Nausea
Tensions and physical pains
Being suffocated by therapist
Being explored by therapist
Being misunderstood by therapist
Therapist is angry at patient

These feelings, desires, and behavior patterns express misgivings about love, hate, messing, sensory pleasure, status, and role. They reveal the troublesome areas in the domestication of the patient's instinctual trends. Structures, functions, and feelings are being brought out from under their condition of disownment by the patient and his culture in the presence of an accepting fellow member of society. In a real and practical sense, disassociations and partitioned areas are brought into functional relationships with the bulk of the person to form a larger and stronger whole. A bigger whole forms from the confluence of smaller wholes.

## THE NEW LEARNING SITUATION

Over and over again the patient has feelings and reactions that are not realistically appropriate to the moment. He acts as if his therapist were his disciplinarian, his seducer, his saviour. It is true that the therapist has stimulus values. After all, he is another human being. But he keeps himself as ambiguous as possible and avoids much self-revelation. He operates in a formal and well-defined situation that is not deserving of many of the patients' reactions.

In the feelings of the patient, the therapeutical relationship is a total one. He may feel as the child or the spouse of the therapist, with all of the feelings of love, hate, and fear that may attend parent-child and husband-wife relationships. He will have to learn, however, the reality limitations of the therapeutical design. He cannot really live with the therapist or be with the therapist physically outside of the office. At times the patient may use every conceivable device, including taking advantage of the permissiveness, forgiveness, and understanding of the therapist, to goad him out of the patient-doctor relationship. When these instances occur, the therapist must rise to the support of the ego functions in the acceptance of reality. If a patient has the conscious, realistic needs of a lover or spouse or parent, he must learn that the therapist cannot meet them personally. He must learn that the therapist can deal only with the unconscious roots of these present, realistic needs in the therapeutical relationship. Then with healthy roots the patient can grow in his ability to gain wholesome satisfactions for his currently realistic needs.

### Transference or Generalization

In the situation of free communication, the therapist has adequate opportunity to observe that hate, love, or fear may appear in the absence of what, in everyday life, would be considered adequate provocation for them. These responses are viewed as transferred (Freud, 1946). The patient adopts feelings and attitudes toward the therapist which he held toward persons important in his early development. Naturally, these are currently inappropriate and unrealistic. The therapist is not any of the things he is usually felt to be by the patient. The projections, identifications, and rejections are not adequate and realistic in terms of the present relationship and consequently are inappropriate. If it is realized that the therapist in these relationships is really somebody else, a father, a mother, a sibling, then they do become not only understandable but also appropriate. The point is, however, that the patient will have to see that his evaluations of the therapist are unrealistic and inappropriate at present. The patient may love (positive transference), or hate (negative transference), or fear the therapist. He may deny, defy, reject, depend upon him. He may tease, make fun of, criticize, compliment, insult his would-be helper. He might feel him to be a tempter, a protector, a devil, a saint, stupid, wise, cruel, sympathetic. Yet all the time the analyst is impersonal, honest, relatively passive, mainly neutral, and an ordinary, forthright citizen. It is the patient's job to see the incompatibility between his feelings and the facts of the matter and to adjust accordingly. It should be mentioned in passing that the so-called transference relationship pertains to others in the patient's work-a-day world—to his boss, his associates, his friends, his wife, his children. They, too, may be one or many inappropriate things. The patient just isn't feeling and thinking straight, but rather in terms of the projections of early feelings relative to earlier people.

The following dream by a young woman may help to clarify some of these points:

I was in a room approximately the same as this one. There was a couch and a large armchair in approximately the same position as in this room. I don't remember sitting on the couch. I was a grown girl, but was curled up like a small child in your lap. I kissed you, and hugged you, and put my head on your shoulder. I found myself on the large, flat arm of the chair, and noticed that you were working, figuring something on a pad. You were deeply engrossed, looked up now and then, chewed your pencil, and referred to some kind of newspaper or small book. I was very conscious of the fact that I had only one hour to work on you. I wanted attention badly, for the pleasure of it at the moment, and also for the future. I didn't want to annoy you, but couldn't help "fussing." I fooled with your hair, playfully pulled your ear, always careful not to go too far. I didn't want to annoy you, didn't want to have you make me leave. I got the impression you wouldn't dare make me leave, and didn't want to make me mad. I was conscious of time, had to make you notice me. You'd look up, pat my arm or something, and then go back to work. I made all the advances. You were patient and sweet, but distracted. More willing to please than pleased. It seemed as though I was getting somewhere with you, when somehow I realized the time was up. Without rushing you gave me to understand that it was time to go and I gathered my things up, not in too sad a frame of mind. I knew I would be back and that the next visit would be a profitable one also. Just as I was about to close the door behind me I heard a giggle. I turned around in time to catch you and your wife smiling at each other. I thought surely you were laughing at me and I bitterly resented this. I felt as though she could hardly wait to get me out of there before restaking her claim. I was peeved that you were disloyal so soon. I didn't intend, however, to let her think that she was getting away with this sort of unspoken insult, so I said "Did you say something?" You both turned toward me and I was afraid to be too bold for fear I'd really anger her. However I could act haughty and a little proud, although hurt. Your wife smiled sweetly and innocently, too innocently I thought, and said "Oh no." We all said good-night and I left.

Might it be sufficient to picture a little girl and her father and mother in a situation that may be enacted daily in the average family? What the average family doesn't know are the true and honest feelings of the little child; and not knowing will more frequently than not, by sending the child out or off to bed, condemn her feelings and make it necessary for her to handle them in the future in more or less unwholesome ways. In the transference relationship expressed in this dream, the patient was reactivating earlier feelings and relationships and the management of them, both by her parents and by herself.

Compare the transference dream just cited with the following free communication of a young male stutterer:

You look like an old dried-up turtle. You are no good. You are a contributor to the delinquency of minors. You fool around with prostitutes. You are homosexual. You cut up with lewd women. I will dig up all the information I can about you and have it published in the newspapers. I am going to turn every one against you, your whole family and everybody. I will tell them lies about you. I see that you are a woman and pregnant, swelled up and in a blue dress. I take my feces and smear them in your face. I shove my foot down your throat. I see your wife as a man with a penis. I see her filthy hair with rats, feces, and dandruff in it. You are an old degenerate with lots of degrees, delighting in seeing people squirm.

Need we point out that consciously the patient had the highest regard and respect for the therapist? We may do so only to point up the contrast between this outburst and the present relationship between patient and therapist. The free communications of feelings reveal hostility toward, and belittlement of, the therapist in the particularly significant areas of sexual development and toilet training. In the projections upon the therapist, we gain insight into the early feelings and their management in the important developmental areas of the personality.

The transference phenomenon may be viewed as a powerful therapeutic weapon. The patient will be given an opportunity in his relationship to the therapist to develop the same emotional conflicts he had toward his parents and to find a new and realistic solution to his problems. He will have to experience a new parent-child relationship before he can release the old. This cannot be done as an intellectual exercise. It will have to be lived through and felt by the patient and become an intricate part of his personality. The core of the cure is for the patient to experience the troublesome conflicts emotionally with the therapist (parental image) and then correct them in a new relationship. The new relationship has a chronologically older person (patient) with the infant still within him, and an acceptant, tolerant, empathic, parental image (therapist) who can accept anything and everything the patient has to release. This relationship will expose the patient under favorable conditions to emotional situations which he could not handle in the past. He will undergo a corrective emotional experience suitable to repair the damaging influence of childhood experiences.

Because the therapist's attitude is strikingly different from that of the authoritative and frustrating persons of the past, he gives the patient the opportunity to face again and again, under practically perfect circumstances, those emotional experiences which were formerly unbearable, and to deal with them in a manner different from the old.

The patient repeats in the form of loving, hating, and fearing the therapist, experiences which he underwent before. He transfers to the therapist attitudes which lay ready within him and which are intimately linked with the inception of his trouble. He repeats too his one-time defense reactions. He wants nothing so much as to repeat in his relations with the therapist all the vicissitudes of that forgotten period. He palpably reproduces his early life as though it were all happening in the present, instead of a memory. The only possible way out of transference situations is to take them back to the patient's past, as he experienced them in reality or in fantasy. The patient will probe and poke to find a chink in the therapist's armor. He will strike out, beg, cry, even collapse, in order to test his presumably strong and flawless helper. He will run the gamut of emotional relationships to discover his therapist's vulnerabilities. If he can find any he will exploit them unrelentingly and, if they are serious, the therapeutical relationships between the two people will cease. The only sure way to avoid such failure is for the therapist to be free of any need to respond realistically to the patient's projections.

### The Therapeutic Process

It is pertinent to inquire just what happens to the patient in therapy—how he becomes better adjusted; how he arrives one day without symptoms. In considering this question we had best remind ourselves of the basic therapeutic principle, which is to re-expose the patient, under more favorable circumstances, to emotional situations which he could not handle in the past. In order to be helped in treatment, the patient must undergo a corrective emotional experience in the transference relationship with the therapist and in the work-a-day-world relationships with others.

It is generally agreed that the central, dynamic problem in therapy is the handling of the transference. In the first place, the patient reacts to the therapist as if the therapist were not himself but some person in the patient's past; a person who has, at some previous time, played an important role in the patient's life. In the second place, a patient does not always react to the therapist only as though the therapist were someone else, only as though he were some powerful figure in the patient's development. Sometimes he reacts quite naturally to what the therapist actually is, or does, or says. The important task is to help the patient distinguish the neurotic transference reactions that are based upon a repetition of earlier, stereotyped patterns from normal and reality reactions to the therapist and the therapeutic situation in the present. The patient has to be taught that his neurotic reactions are in accord with old, outmoded patterns, and to help himself acquire new ways of feeling and reacting that conform more closely to the new situations. In short, therapy attempts to modify the patterns of the past, to take adequate account of the differences between the situations upon which they were based and the present reality.

Day after day, through free communication, the patient uncovers and releases content and feelings in the presence of the therapist. The content and feelings center around unresolved conflicts which arose originally and mainly in relation to the parent. Back there, they were very intense; up here, they are much milder. Back there, they were in relation to an actual, or fantasied, stern and denying parent; up here, they are in relation to an objective, sympathetic and understanding listener. Thus, we have two differences; one in intensity, and the other in the contrasting attitudes of the parent and the therapist. While the patient continues to bring up and act out old patterns, the therapist continues to maintain a receptive, permissive, and encouraging attitude. The therapist allows the patient to deal differently with his emotional reactions and fosters a new settlement of the old problem. The old pattern was an attempt at adjustment on the part of the child to the parent. The revival of the old pattern in therapy will offer an opportunity for adjustment on the part of the patient to the therapist. Because the therapist's attitude is different from that of the authoritative parent of the past, the patient is given an opportunity to face again and again, under most favorable circumstances, those emotional situations which were formerly unbearable to him, and to deal with them in a manner different from the old. This can be accomplished only through the actual experiencing of feelings and emotions in the therapeutical relationship. Intellectual insight alone is not enough.

The real therapeutic accomplishment, then, consists in the patient's successful mastery in the transference relationship of previously unbearable emotional conflicts.

## THE THERAPIST

He who deals with psychological phenomena must be a relatively unique person. This is especially true of the person who would endeavor to serve those who present psychological difficulties and handicaps. In our era the psychologist in general, and the therapist in particular, are placed somewhere between mysticism and faith-healing on the one hand, and the biological sciences and scientific methodology on the other hand. Psychic phenomena cannot be expressed in time and space, they cannot be placed under the microscope, they are difficult, if not impossible to treat mathematically. As a consequence, the therapist has not been in too high repute by the biologically and biochemically oriented medical men, and he has been forced by society to accept fellowship with mind-readers and soul-doctors. Through the years, in finding, testing, and systematizing methods growing out of a grounding in the biological sciences and experimental psychology, the therapast has achieved, however, a fairly respectable and secure position among scientists and scholars.

Indeed, to understand another person at the psychological level requires a relationship between the observed and the observer that is distinctive and strikingly different from that between the chemist and his chemicals, the surgeon and his operative field, and the internist and his patient with a heart murmur. Psychological understanding requires as its chief characteristic the highest degree possible of the therapist's identification with his patient, of putting himself into the other person's thoughts, feelings, and emotions. It demands a coexistence of therapist and patient in the therapist's listening and the patient's talking. It demands the therapist's introspection of his own feelings, memories, thoughts, and perceptions as they are aroused by the patient. This is to say, really, that one knows another only through the knowledge of himself, which in turn demands that the therapist must know himself and must be free to be like all others, and yet by great self-knowledge so different from all others. More specifically, when the therapist observes his patient, he must be sufficiently free within himself to know that the patient was expressing hostility, or homosexuality, or guilt, or shame, or patricide, or dependence, or messing interest, or some other condemned feeling or attitude. The therapist, knowing himself, and being free from condemnation of his own feelings and attitudes, will be free to see the condemned ones of those he would help. It might help to say that in a therapeutical relationship the therapist studies himself more than he does his patient. What he really does is to study his own feelings and attitudes aroused by the patient's stimulus value. Realizing his own responses, he can decide the nature of the stimulus that produced them. The therapist studies himself as a responding mechanism to the other person as a stimulus. He is the musical instrument played upon by the patient. If the instrument gives a faithful reproduction of the performer's effort, that effort can then be properly appraised. The therapist must be a relatively perfectly tuned instrument, free from the distorting dissonants produced by the dead and flat strings and reeds of prejudice, compulsion, and defense. What the patient does to the therapist, and the therapist's freedom to see accurately what has been done to him, constitute the basis for assisting in the understanding and development of the patient.

The disclosure and management of resistances in the patient comprise the most difficult task in therapy. The personal influence of the therapist is the most dynamic weapon for dealing with the resistances. Intellectual validity of explanation is impotent. In contrast, the patient's emotional attitude toward the therapist is potent. It consists essentially of a falling in love or a falling in hate with the therapist. These feelings are compulsive, that is, they disregard all questions of whether conditions are favorable and discount all variations of personal attraction, age, sex, or position. So-called natural or logical love or hate frequently has this compulsive component, but the transference is always compulsive. One might suppose that a patient would always feel a certain measure of respect, confidence, gratitude, and liking for the therapist. Instead of these, or more accurately in addition to these, he loves or hates or fears the therapist, at times slightly, at times greatly. Universally, at times, these feelings dominate the entire therapeutical relationship. They become exacting and demanding, pushing all other activities out of the way. It has been said that one illness has been replaced by another. It should occur to us then that it is not noble to have succeeded in having the patient trade one abnormal condition for another. Therapists have been convinced, however, that the love activity, or hate activity, or fear activity lies at the root of the original trouble and is not a really new pathological condition at all. With this insight, we who would help others now proceed to take this state of being in love, or being in hate, as a process for understanding. The patient repeats, in the form of his feelings for the therapist, experiences and feelings which he had before, transferring to the therapist attitudes which lay ready within him, and which are intimately linked with his trouble. In handling this so-called transference neurosis the greatest demands are made upon the *person* of the therapist. To yield actually to these demands of the patient at this time, to satisfy his sensual, hostile, or fearful attitudes would be wholly inappropriate to achieve the integration and re-education of the patient. A patient cannot be helped by allowing him to re-enact an uncorrected version of what is already unconsciously stereotyped within him. The therapist cannot compromise by offering the patient partial satisfaction in exchange for his further collaboration in psychotherapy. The therapeutical situation must not end with the patient remaining sick and the therapist getting sick. The only possible way out of the transference situation is to take it back to where it belongs, to the patient's past experiences or fantasies and make the necessary and appropriate corrections. And this is just what requires so much of the therapist in understanding, freedom from troubles, integration, reality orientation, and honest self-appraisal.

In a final statement, the therapist must be aware of his counter-transferences. He must not have loves, hates, fears, and guilt in relation to persons, objects and relationships of his childhood inappropriately expressed on the patient. He must be free to see the patient and his troubles as they really are and not in terms of his own defenses and projections. In nontechnical language, the therapist must be free of ulterior motives, selfish interests, prejudices, and compulsions. We can have a sick physicist, or chemist, or even surgeon, but we simply cannot have a sick therapist.

## The Tools of the Therapist

It is difficult, if not impossible, to communicate in writing what the therapist does and says in each or any therapeutic hour. Doctor-patient relationships are so subtle, delicate, and complicated that they are hard to convey to one who has not experienced them. Yet we may give some idea of what the therapist says and does, realizing all the time that it is not only what he says and what he does that counts, but also how he talks and how he acts; in short who he is.

**Unspoken impact.** As a rule, the patient has heard of the therapist. If he has, he should have learned that the therapist is reputable, well trained, and experienced. He should have learned, too, that his prospective helper is ethical and highly acceptable culturally. Already, then, important doctor-patient relationships have begun.

From the first hour the patient will find a man of quiet optimism and calm confidence, free of any disturbing nervousness or mannerisms. It would be best if the therapist were married (need we say happily?), had a home and children, and enjoyed a relatively secure economic status. He must be well adjusted, healthy, and virile. His lack of fear, anxiety, and perturbation in the face of anything the patient has to reveal gives the patient strong unspoken support and confidence. All through the therapy the person of the therapist is a powerful tool. Very much of the success of the doctor-patient relationship depends upon the self-hood of the therapist.

**Listening attentively and acceptingly.** The therapist is a unique listener. It is not enough or possibly even beneficial for the patient merely to recite or tell to someone else his misgivings, sins, and mistakes. It is entirely possible that he has been doing this very thing for years and found no real lasting results. We do not find therapeutic effect from mere recital. Telling and revealing are effective if they are followed by no condemnation and no punishment, but rewarded with acceptance, understanding, and forgiveness. The therapist will listen with a permissive and forgiving attitude to the revelation of every little and big personal feeling of his patient. He will receive and understand his patient's every embarrassing, shocking, horrible, cruel, belittling, and shameful disclosure. Truth will be rewarded, especially the most painful truth. Therapy demands the re-discovery or better the re-collection of the truth. Mental illness is really the big lie based upon the culture's painful condemnation of the truth. Truth and its painful consequences resulted in illness. Truth and its rewards will result in illness' removal. Emotional disorder is the price man pays for being so lately human. Emotional health will come with the recovery and useful direction of more of man's prehuman qualities.

**The therapist speaks.** By words the therapist reveals his understanding of what the patient is saying. He expresses his understanding not only of the literal and obvious meaning of his patient's productions but of their deeper and more profound significance. In the past neither the patient nor anyone else understood the patient's behavior well. The therapist speaks the correct translation of his patient's native tongue.

Time and again the therapist also reveals his remembrance of the patient's past utterances. In this way he guarantees good listening to what his patient says. The patient must know that he is ever in the therapist's thoughts.

The therapist calls the never-named responses of the patient. These responses have never been tied in with the language system. The patient cannot give any account of them, but only show them. By attaching words to them he can eventually learn to control them. Labeled emotions become part of the patient's thoughts and can be used in channeling behavior.

With his greater emotional freedom, the therapist may supply the missing feeling to the patient's spoken statement, point up a contradiction, supply the missing content to an expressed feeling, express consolation to the patient when he writhes in groundless fears, and speak for him when he lags too much.

The therapist cannot intelligently intervene too early in the therapy simply because he does not know exactly what, and how strongly, his particular patient has repressed. As he listens to and empathizes with his patient, he begins to sense the forbidden and ostracized feelings. Then with accurate and sympathetic statements he may help the patient to recover and re-evaluate his repressed self. His words will be simple and common. He will not use technical language and terms. Especially he will not talk too much. He will remember who is paying to talk and to learn and who is being paid to listen. Probably the therapist talks too much and too loosely. If he must err, he should speak too infrequently.

## THE END OF THERAPY

Rarely does there come suddenly a day, or a week, when the patient is finished. The end is approached gradually and relatively undramatically. This writer has asked several of his stutterers when they stopped stuttering. The answer was that they did not remember, they had not noticed. Actually they had not stuttered with the therapist or anyone else for several months.

One might think that therapy is over when the patient's symptoms are gone. This is not necessarily so. One stutterer had quit stuttering for three or four months, but "stuttering feelings" persisted. She was not through. Another stutterer's symptoms disappeared early, suddenly, and dramatically. She performed fluently in very trying speech situations much to the amazement of herself and of her family. She was not through either. So, when is a person finished with his therapy?

### Freedom from Symptoms

A symptom may be considered as a defense reaction against anxiety. The anxiety, in turn, is the person's awareness of the threat of unacceptable and disowned feelings. When the therapy has succeeded, the symptom and its predecessor, anxiety, will be gone since there will be no need for either of them. Previously inadmissable feelings and attitudes will have been seen through. New feelings and expressions are wrested from the effects of repression, so that the person gains more mental units with which to remember and think and thereby increases his ability to label, reason, and plan. In a sense he has become more intelligent. He has more materials at his command and more emotional freedom to deal with them.

### Somatic Soundness

One who has experienced successful therapy will have relieved the vegetative systems of communicative roles. He will no longer need to communicate his feelings in hypertension and migraine, and in disturbances in breathing, elimination, digestion, and the like. He will channel the communication of his feelings through the appropriately endowed structures of communication: speech organs, face, hands, skeletal muscles. He will largely free his vegetative systems of responsibility in interpersonal relationships for which they are so relatively inadequately prepared, and leave them to perform their vital functions for which they are so adequately designed. Zestful living at the level of eating, breathing, eliminating, sleeping, and sexual intercourse will be his. Zestful living at this level is the basis for high-spirited living at the higher levels of work and play.

### Receptive and Expressive Facility

Significant improvement in the perception and expression of the patient occurs in psychotherapy. He sees, hears, smells, tastes, and feels more. He reads and listens more enjoyably, understandingly, and discriminatively. Similarities and differences that never existed before are now perceived. Heretofore unperceived distinctions and relations now appear. The whole world of things and people expands in form, color, sounds, and relatedness.

Also the successful patient finds greatly increased expressive facility. He walks, dances, talks, and in general performs in all ways more freely. Blocks, hesitancies, and inhibitions drop out. Awkwardness in posture and movement lessen or disappear. We might characterize him as a person on his way instead of in his way.

### Social Adeptness

Possibly the most noticeable change to others will be in the patient's social relationships. Shyness, fear, "stage-fright," bumptiousness, intolerance, prejudice, and other asocial and antisocial attitudes will be greatly lessened or entirely absent. Instead, toward others and most conspicuously toward those who popularly arouse resentment in their fellow men, will the patient feel and express love, understanding, and forgiveness. Knowing himself and consequently others as he will, he simply cannot condemn another. In no sense will he be a "push-over" or a namby-pamby. His strength is great and will be felt. But it is the strength of understanding and acceptance and not the pseudo-strength of defense against the arousal by others of his own weaknesses.

## Affective Glow

Restrained enthusiasm, verve for living, quest for knowledge and understanding, alertness, vigilance, and energy all characterize the person who has experienced successful psychotherapy. His mood swings are slight and appropriate to the reality of living. Effort is easily maintained. Others will label him as a happy, likable, and reliable person.

## Like Father, Like Son

The patient becomes like his therapist, like his new parent. This similarity is not based upon imitation in the ordinary sense. The patient does not ape his therapist. He is like his therapist because, like his therapist, he has recovered, accepted, and integrated powerful activating forces that were previously unconsciously helping to determine his behavior. So his likeness to his new parent is based upon the fact that each knows himself fairly well and both, being human in the better sense, will have feelings, thoughts, and plans of a similar nature. In a significant way the patient has taken a big step in becoming a therapist himself.

## Looking to This Day

Without conscious intent, he who has been raised again will find enjoyment in the instant, the moment, regardless of its obvious importance. He will realize great satisfaction and joy in just being. Formerly he may have felt that whatever day it is, it is the day after and the day before. He was so concerned about what happened in the past and what might happen in the future that he had no thought left for the present. His feelings, glued to the past and pulled by the future, stretched over the present as a thin, taut thread of impatience. Now, the thing, the person, the situation of the moment is considered worthy. Instead of an escape from the ever-present, there is an acceptance and enjoyment of it. He knows that yesterday is over and that tomorrow will never come. Only the present matters (Osler, 1932).

## The Days of Getting Well

Therapy is learning, relearning, unlearning, growing up again. It takes time, patience, and hard work. Its main concern is with feelings and emotions that are old and relatively permanent. To change them is difficult. By contrast it is not too formidable to change a concept or an idea, or to correct a statement of fact. But senseless and groundless fears, hates, and prejudices remain adamant. Nevertheless, slowly and little by little, hour in and hour out, changes in feelings do occur. Almost imperceptibly the patient gets better. He feels little change, possibly even at times a worsening of his condition. Friends and relatives, however, do note and report favorable development in him. The patient is through when he has reached a point of self-knowledge that will enable him to meet his own problems in being a creative and useful member of society.

### The Therapist Undergoes Change

The therapist rehearses the most fearful and forbidden things that the patient reveals. He goes forward when the patient and others would be afraid. The therapist feels and even says just what no one wants to feel, let alone say. Socially disapproved aspects of sexuality and elimination, murderous intent, cannibalistic impulses and other anxiety-laden topics will be received, rehearsed, evaluated, and organized by the therapist. He, like the patient, is a member of the culture. It is true that he is an unique member whose emotional freedom is greater and whose anxiety is less. Still he may carry some misgivings of old and some sensitivities to the present restrictions of the culture. These are taxed again and again with each patient. In a way and to a degree he is analyzed with each patient he sees through. He rehearses pity, hate, lust, fear, and all the other troublesome feelings of his patient. He too grows up a little more. He too undergoes some change.

## BIBLIOGRAPHY

BACH, G. R. 1954. Intensive group psychotherapy. New York: Ronald Press.

DOLLARD, J., and MILLER, N. E. 1950. Personality and psychotherapy. New York: McGraw-Hill.

FREUD, S. 1946. Collected papers (Five volumes, 3rd ed.). New York: International Psycho-analytical Press.

FROMM, E. 1951. The forgotten language. New York: Rinehart.

KLEIN, M. 1948. Contributions to psycho-analysis. London: Hogarth.

MOWRER, O. H. 1953. Psychotherapy, theory and research. New York: Ronald Press, Ch. 17.

OSLER, W. 1932. A way of life. Baltimore: Remington-Putnam.

RUESCH, J., and BATESON, G. 1951. Communication. New York: Norton.

SHEEHAN, J. G. 1954. An integration of psychotherapy and speech therapy through a conflict theory of stuttering. *J. Speech Hearing Disorders,* 19, 474–482.

SLAVSON, S. R. 1947. The practice of group therapy. New York: International Universities Press.

# CHAPTER 32

# PLAY THERAPY, PSYCHODRAMA, AND PARENT COUNSELING

● *Zelda S. Wolpe, Ph.D.*

## SPEECH AS THE ACCULTURATION OF THE CHILD

THOUGH SPEECH is the primary medium of communication in interpersonal relationships, we often fail to appreciate that the child who in the absence of organic factors has delayed speech development, faulty articulation, or speech blocks may be communicating with us in an even more significantly revealing manner than the child whose speech flows with clarity and fluency. The child's very difficulty with speech can give us clues to basic conflicts with which he is struggling and reveal much about his inner world of fears, anxieties, longings, and needs. The stutterer, for example, forces upon the listener a reaction specific to the tension, anxiety, conflict, and struggle revealed in the word blocks. He exposes his problem with vivid intensity, whereas the individual with verbal skills often conceals his neurotic defenses and anxieties. The stutterer, in his very speech difficulty, is revealing his discomfort in social situations, his inability to express himself freely, his constriction and fear of spontaneity, his feelings of inadequacy, and his plea for patience. One feels the weight of his problem, the seething internal conflicts, unresolved and frightening. All this the stutterer tells about himself even to a stranger upon an initial introduction.

The psychoanalytic point of view expressed in this chapter considers the development of speech as an integral part of the normal maturational process, and as a function of the development of the ego in its relationship to outside forces. It is in actuality the faculty of speech that helps the child in his development of reality testing and thereby gains for him a mastery of his environment. The words as symbols of objects and object relationships make possible the anticipation of events in thought rather than in behavior and permit past experience through such symbolism to be so integrated as to allow for prediction of results of present and future behavior without blind stumbling through maze-like performance. This development of the anticipatory function of the ego in thought is basic to objective intelligence, and interference in the process may indeed give the impression of an individual suffering with amentia, more appropriately described as "pseudo-amentia."

The acquisition of speech through the maturational process is felt by the child as a sudden experience, though the preparatory babbling stage of exploring and combining sounds has preceded this by months. The excitement which the parent feels in hearing a child's first words distinctly and appropriately said is reflected in the child, and he now experiences the feeling of success and power over his speech mechanism. He also discovers a power in the word itself, for when he says "give me" he receives the object he desires. This omnipotence of word combined with the omnipotence of thought is indeed basic to all ritualistic chants, prayers, and curses which adults often carry throughout their lives, and which children both enjoy and fear.

The development of speech occurs approximately at the same time that the child gains mastery over his sphincters. His newly gained power over his oral and anal zones forces a restructuring of his environment, for with such newly gained power he shifts from the role of a totally helpless individual to the role of one able to actively manipulate his environment. His discovered control over his body gives him the awareness of himself as an individual and frees him from his total state of dependency. He is now able to use his recently acquired skills to assert himself against the parental figures, for these skills not only gain him mastery over his environment but may themselves be used as weapons of defiance when his instinctual drives are thwarted or his movement toward independence is blocked. The child who is forced to sit on the toilet for an hour without result but immediately upon removal from the toilet soils his pants has in no uncertain way demanded the privilege of personal control over his body. When demands are superimposed by his mother, he enjoys the mess he has made for her to clean up.

This transition from total infancy dependency to the awareness of the self as an independent being with control over directional movements (retention, expulsion; assertion, withdrawal; acquiescence, stubbornness) is a hurdle often wrought with anxiety. It is indeed comparable to the hurdle of adolescence so often referred to as the storm-and-stress period of life, stress which undoubtedly stems, as will be shown later, from the revitalizing of these early anxieties.

Since the primary function of speech is social communication which in itself implies an interdependence in interpersonal relationships, and which reaches its highest functional value when a oneness in understanding is attained, disturbances in speech would occur primarily when the interdependent relationship is off balance. Instead of the anticipated understanding resultant from the acquisition of speech there is heightened anxiety and frustration, for the individual finds a widened rather than a narrowed gap in the area of communication. This is in actuality what frequently occurs. When the infant is in the babbling stage, the parent is able to coo with him and delight in his dependency. But as the infant moves on to a higher stage in his maturational process, the parent is less and less accepting of his behavior, more and more critical of it, and determined to train the child by imposing demands upon him. The acquisition of speech, equated as it is with maturation, now becomes a symbol of the danger of further maturation, and the child holds tenaciously to infantile speech patterns as symbolic of the period when demands were minimal and when understanding was heightened. Functional disturbances in speech, therefore, would indicate an interference in the normal speech process because of difficulties encountered in the dynamic interaction between the ego and its surrounding forces. Speech, per se, divorced from social interaction would be static and mechanistic and would cease to have any communicative function. Speech is part of the very acculturation of the child and carries with it, therefore, the emotional impacts that any dynamic interaction involves.

In order, then, to uncover if possible the etiological factors which produced the symptomatology and to evaluate the type of treatment indicated as well as the prognosis, the child and his entire milieu must be explored. This is not often an easy task because of the very complexity of the human organism and the number of variables ever present in the structural development of the personality. The severity of the symptom must not in itself be taken as an index of the degree of emotional disturbance. Often a child presenting marked speech pathology responds more readily in the treatment process than a child with slight or moderate speech difficulties. The entire personality structure of the child must be evaluated rather than the symptom per se.

As Fenichel (1945) so clearly points out, some children encounter such difficulty in forming object relationships that they finally withdraw if their attempts have been too nonrewarding and disregard the world about them as if it were nonexistent. It is as if they were saying, "If I do not talk to them, they will not know I am here and will leave me alone." Other children develop speech and then regress to a preverbal level when their need to develop stronger defenses against the hostile world is intensified. Still others develop speech up to a point and then remain fixated with infantile behavioral patterns. This is primarily seen in those children troubled with speech substitutions and faulty articulation. Growing up appears too threatening, and the child therefore holds tenaciously to the security of infancy, where parental demands are minimal. He may also be seeking unfulfilled gratifications at this level and is therefore neither willing nor ready to move on to more advanced stages of development. These children, unlike the withdrawn child who offers little or no communication, have formed object relationships, but their dependency needs are so great that they cling to infantile patterns of behavior in order to ensure dependency gratifications.

The child who stutters presents a different problem from the child so withdrawn he fails to develop speech or the child who retains infantile speech as his defense against growing up. The stutterer has generally proceeded to a higher stage in the maturational process. Unlike the withdrawn child, he forms object relationships and seeks contact despite the difficulties encountered; and unlike the child with infantile speech, he longs to be treated as an adult and not made to feel inadequate. From clinical observation it can be seen with relative frequency that the stutterer's aggressive impulses are mobilized against authoritarian figures, yet at the same time he is frightened by his aggression and is afraid of the words that might reveal his rebellious feelings. The conflict is great. He wants to express himself—he wants to communicate—but he is too status-conscious, too unsure of his relationship with others. Words to him are equated with overt acts which must be kept under control, held back until he cannot even get them out. The stutterer often has overwhelming guilt feelings because of his aggressive and hostile impulses against loved ones. His unresolved conflicts weigh heavily and block the free flow of language. The accompanying guilt resultant from the negative component of his ambivalent feeling toward loved ones reinforces his dependency needs. He projects his own rejection of his parents on to them and clings tenaciously to them because of his certainty that they are rejecting of him. In his symptom, therefore, does he also express a total dependency for he calls upon his parents to do even his talking for him. His state of helplessness in communicating with others is an ever-frustrating experience, and, as with all frustration, further mobilizes hostile impulses for which he finds no channel for release. His feelings of inadequacy in relationship to adults is later extended to his relationships with children, since through the very development of his symptom has he in actuality become different from other children. He is afraid that he will be laughed at because of his stuttering, and in reality often he is mimicked or else shied away from because of the impatience one feels when listening to the stutterer.)

Superimposed upon these difficulties with which he is struggling are the parental anxieties with which he must deal, which may have even initiated the problem, and which he further reflects in his own behavior, thus intensifying his conflicts, his feelings of helplessness, and his hostility. He sees his stuttering as an affliction, and himself as a handicapped child who has been innocently victimized. And for such affliction he feels entitled to retribution, to special privileges, and to extended considerations. To these gains does he use his neurotic symptom and cling tenaciously to it. The discomfort he feels in the social situation is often more than compensated by the special consideration he receives, and by the power he enjoys in the solicitous attitude of his parents and teachers.

The stutterer generally has retained his early belief in the omnipotence of words, but such omnipotence is tied up with the power of destruction and death. He must cautiously guard against a word slipping out which would not only reveal his unconscious death wishes but which might actually bring such wishes to reality. He exerts a control over his words so that they cannot slip out, and concentrates his energy more on the word itself than on the thought. Clinically it has been observed that once the child can face his aggression and can gain courage to express his hostility, he does not block on the "angry" words. However, often following such a session, the child's speech symptom as well as his resistance to treatment and to the therapist become intensified. Only when the negative transference is worked upon and interpreted is he again able to work in the areas of aggression, hostility, and guilt.

Since speech is an integral part of the personality structure of the individual, treatment must be centered not on the isolated symptom of the speech disturbance, but rather on the entire integrated organism. The defenses the child uses in all areas must be explored, and the fantasy life and distortions in thinking uncovered.

Unlike the adult, the child rarely takes the initiative to seek professional help. More frequently he is brought into treatment against his will, and once more must he submit to the authoritarian demands of his parents. The child, therefore, often offers strong resistance in the first session. The skill with which the therapist handles this resistance may determine the entire course of the treatment process. The child's willingness and decision to return independent of his parents' desire for him to return must be a goal on the part of the therapist for the first session as well as the succeeding sessions if treatment is to be successful. As long as the child feels that he is coming to the therapist because of parental demands and against his own desire to do so, he intensifies his resistance and uses his nonproductivity in the treatment hours as an expression of hostility against his parents who make him keep his appointments. Besides, if a therapist accepts a child under these circumstances, he is to some extent at least condoning the overdependency relationship existent between the child and parent, since he permits the parents to make the decision for the child. The therapist in this situation has aligned himself on the side of the parents, and must expect, therefore, a similar hostile relationship with the child in the hours to follow.

Not only has the child rarely been consulted before the initial appointment is made, but he is often suspicious of adults whom he looks upon as being threatening and demanding. He has neither blind faith nor confidence in the therapist or the therapeutic process, and it is therefore important for the therapist to respect the child's feelings and to convey to the child his approval and understanding of such skepticism or resistance. This is the starting point of therapy. It is often better to delay treatment than to force a child against his will into a treatment process which may become only a tug of war between the child and the therapist, a further extension of the very problem with which the child is already struggling.

The case of Tommy, a seven-year-old severe stutterer, is used to illustrate this point. It was his first hour of treatment. When he came into the office the child was sobbing. His mother was telling him that he was acting like a baby, that he had to see the doctor, and that nothing he could say could change her mind. The therapist went up to Tommy and said, "Tommy, you seem very unhappy. I thought you wanted to see me." His speech was so blocked it was many moments before he could get the sentence out. "She made me come. I didn't want to come."

*Therapist:* Tommy, no child comes to see me who doesn't want to. I'm here to try to help children understand their problems—not to make them more unhappy. They don't come to see me because their mothers want them to. They come because they feel they need help.

*Tommy:* Well, I don't need help.

*Therapist:* Then you shouldn't be here, Tommy.

The mother was aghast at this and said, "He's too young to know what's good for him."

*Therapist:* Tommy doesn't feel he has a problem. He doesn't want to be here.

*Tommy:* Just my speech.

*Therapist:* Would you like to come into the playroom for a few moments, Tommy? As long as you're here, you may as well see our toys.

Tommy came without any hesitation. In a few moments he was playing with the guns and soldiers. He wanted to say something, but he couldn't get the words out.

*Therapist:* Speech can be an awful problem sometimes. We want to say something—and the words won't come.

Tommy continued to play. At the end of the hour he seemed reluctant to leave.

*Therapist:* Why don't you think it over, Tommy? You phone me tomorrow and let me know if you would like to return.

*Tommy:* Okay—but she'll make me.

*Therapist:* No, Tommy, only phone me if you want to return.

Now the responsibility for such an important decision has been placed on Tommy. This kind of relationship with many children is a completely new experience. Up to this point, too often, they have been treated like automatons. The question of what is accomplished by this technique if the child should decide not to return arises. The answer to this might best be understood by asking the question: What is gained when the child is forced into a treatment process against his will? Are we not thereby furthering anxieties, tensions, and hostilities, thus increasing the load the child is already carrying, and are we not thereby defeating the very goal of therapy, namely, the reduction of tension and anxiety and the release of hostility? It is true that children may not always know what is best for them. In this respect they are not too different from their parents. We must explore the motives of parents who are so eager that the child have treatment regardless of what ruse may be used to entice the child to keep his appointments. It is often these very parents who become indignant when it is suggested that perhaps they are in need of treatment and that the child's problems might be more easily dissipated if the parents gained insight into their own conflicts.

The parents' emotional reactions toward therapy are frequently reflected in their question as to how to prepare the child for the first interview. There is often expressed shock when it is suggested that the child be told the truth.

Tommy's mother stated over the phone, "Surely, Doctor, you don't want me to tell him he is going to see a psychologist because he stutters? I've never told Tommy he stutters. I don't want him made aware of it, and if he knew he is to see a psychologist he'd be certain something is wrong with him."

This is a fairly common attitude expressed by parents at the initial contact with the therapist and points to their own resistance to treatment as well as to their technique of deception in their relationship with the child. How could Tommy want to work with a psychologist or admit to a problem when he has been taught to deny the existent problem and must sense his mother's belief that something must be seriously amiss before a therapist is consulted? Tommy was such a severe stutterer that there was hardly a word over which he did not block. Yet his mother was able to say with real conviction that Tommy was unaware of his stuttering. A child who stutters is having difficulty in expressing himself and certainly is aware of such difficulty as soon as the problem manifests itself. The mother's attempt to conceal the problem may indeed be a manifestation of her own anxiety, her overprotectiveness, and her need to foster the overdependency relationship so often seen in children with speech difficulties. These initial cues derived from the parental attitudes regarding the child's problems frequently light up the areas to be explored in the therapeutic sessions to follow.

This is not meant to imply that parents are always responsible for the child's behavioral problems. The child may develop anxieties due to distortions in his thinking or to unconscious guilt resultant from desired gratification of tabooed instinctual drives, or to internal conflicts independent of the parental attitudes. The tendency to blame the parents exclusively for the development of a problem in the child is dangerous, since it might indeed bias the therapist in his interpretations as well as his search for etiological factors. However, the dynamic interaction existent between the child and parents plays such an important role in the psycho-sexual development of the child that the resolution of a conflict often necessitates a re-education process for the parents as well as the child. For this reason parental counseling is discussed along with play therapy and psychodrama in this chapter.

Psychotherapy with children generally offers problems because children have not yet reached the stage in their development where they are able to crystallize their anxieties or actively participate in verbal discussion or free association. The child with speech troubles presents an even greater problem, since there has been interference with the limited verbal ability expected in terms of normal maturational development. The therapist, therefore, must find appropriate techniques to reach the child without leaning too heavily upon verbal communication as his tool.

## PLAY THERAPY

Play therapy is the technique most often used with the young child, for it affords the therapist an opportunity to observe the fantasy world of the child as well as his skills, creativity, interests, anxieties, and frustration levels. The development of positive transference is facilitated, since permission to share the therapist's toys is a starting point of sharing experiences together. It is also in agreement with the not infrequent way in which a child evaluates interpersonal relationships, namely, "I love him because he gives me things," or "He loves me because he lets me play with his things."

The playroom, however, must not be used as a means of deception in order to entice the child into a therapeutic relationship without his awareness of the ensuing process. Positive transference cannot be maintained if the therapist lacks integrity in his relationship with the child. If the child is under the impression that he has come to play with the therapist for an hour, a gross misrepresentation has been made to the child; and dishonesty in relationship between therapist and child initiates a process which can never be therapeutically successful. Play therapy is not the same as play, and the therapist who hides behind the mask of toys in order to get the child to keep his appointments must expect nonproductivity as well as distrust in the hours to follow.

The play equipment is designed to facilitate free expression of the various problems frequently encountered in the life of the child, particularly those problems dealing with sibling rivalry, parent-child relationships, school and social adjustments, and the gamut of anxieties and phobias observed at all age levels. The doll house, the family dolls, puppets, the sand-box, stuffed animals, cork guns, cannons with pellets, nursing bottles, fingerpaints, clay, snakes, mice, soldiers, policemen, ambulances, fire-trucks, easel board, pounding board, rubber knives, swords, daggers, marbles, mirrors, and competitive games are indispensable materials. They are sufficiently varied to permit emotional expression ranging from the most passive or withdrawn response to violent aggressive reactions.

Play for the adult is conceived in terms of relaxation, diversion, and fun. Play for the child is a vital and integrated part of his growth process. He is serious and intent in developing his concepts, and he struggles with his play problems as the adult struggles with his life responsibilities.

Like speech, play helps the child to master his life situations. It affords him the opportunity to explore problems and to act out anticipatory responses to his behavior as he structures situations and reverses roles. Play may be considered descriptively, then, as an intermediate step between thinking and doing. It is through play that the child strengthens his superego, for he is often seen taking on the parental role wherein he firmly approves or disapproves of the behavior of his imaginative characters and struggles with the good and evil forces in terms of reward and punishment. In his play he relives over and over again his anxieties, for through the replaying of such anxiety scenes does he tend to diminish the intensity of his anxiety. His play is not the mere projection of fantasy. It is, along with this, the child's attempt at objectifying his anxiety, of releasing his hostility in safe areas, namely, on play objects or pretend characters, of identifying with authoritarian figures, and finally of setting his limits in terms of reality-testing. It becomes evident, then, that what might appear humorous to the adult may be a very threatening situation for the child, and the therapist's participation in the play must therefore be in accordance with the child's seriousness and direction.

As in dreams, the child's play is understood both from its manifest and latent content, and the successive play situations of the hour are often comparable to the adult's free association. It is not accidental that the child suddenly swings from one activity to another, and the skill in understanding the play language of the child, so highly symbolized, is similar to the skill in understanding the dream language of the adult. There is always with the therapist the responsibility of sifting the irrelevant from the relevant material and of recognizing the subtle techniques the child uses as resistance to the therapist or therapeutic process. The unpredictability of the child's play and the quick reversal of roles he makes with little regard for time or space are again similar to the irrationality of the manifest content of a dream, and the logical sequence of events becomes apparent only through the interpretation of the latent content, the uncovering of the nongratification of wishes, and of the unconscious conflicts underlying the observable play.

If education may be defined as a positive growth process in which the individual comes to better terms with his world, learns to understand his behavior, to replace faulty thinking by sound logic, learns to use energy constructively so that his behavior positively rather than negatively affects himself and his environment, then all psychotherapy of necessity becomes an educational process, for this is its very goal. This is the challenge the therapist accepts. It is a grave responsibility, for education is a molding process and the judgment values of the therapist might well determine the goals of therapy.

With the child who has been unable to form object relationships and is therefore so withdrawn that he has never been able to develop speech, the symbol and primary medium of social intercourse, it is often difficult to make the differential diagnosis between true feeble-mindedness and faulty ego development, as was previously pointed out. A conservative attitude with regard to institutional placement is imperative if we are to avoid grave injustices from taking place.

The case of Donald will be used to illustrate the extremely withdrawn child and to show how, through the play-therapy process, he was gently led from a maze of darkness, fear, and confusion into a world proportioned with positive as well as negative factors and where he learned to make such differentiations and respond accordingly. The treatment process extended over a five-year period and, therefore, only the high lights of the therapy will be discussed.

Donald was eight years old. He had been diagnosed as being feeble-minded as well as suffering from childhood schizophrenia, and institutional placement had been recommended. The mother in particular could not accept this disposition for her child, against whose helplessness she responded with similar helplessness. She was haunted by the memory of his birth, the euphoric feelings she had when she held her firstborn in her arms and saw him as the most beautiful alert baby ever created. Nothing in his first two years of life had even vaguely suggested retardation or delayed development. He sat up, crawled, walked, even developed a large vocabulary at expected age levels according to textbook descriptions. She delighted in his good behavior, since hour on end he was satisfied to lie alone in his crib or play-pen. (This perhaps was the first misinterpretation of Donald's behavior, for what the mother believed to be good behavior may, in reality, have been the onset of the withdrawal pattern.) To the outside world she would minimize, or even deny, his beauty and the excitement she experienced in her feelings for this child, as if she would lose this child if anyone were to learn of the deep love she felt for him. To conceal her feelings, she reacted with sternness and vigorous discipline in areas of toilet-training, eating habits, and the general infant demands.

It was during her pregnancy with her second child, when Donald was 2½ years old, that a marked change in his behavior occurred. At first the child showed heightened irritability and restlessness with frequent tantrums. The contrast to his previous placid behavior was striking, and the mother sought medical advice. She was told by her pediatrician that Donald was "spoiled" and that more firm discipline should be used. The child from then on was spanked frequently with a leather strap and sent to his room until he could control his tantrums. He stopped talking and regressed to many infantile behavioral patterns—drooling, messing his pants, and smearing his feces on all the beds with the exception of his own. A few weeks prior to his mother's going to the hospital for delivery, he went on a hunger strike and no amount of coercion or punishment could make him eat. He was placed in a boarding nursery home on the recommendation of a psychiatrist in order "to teach him to eat again." Donald began to eat and returned home following the birth of his little brother. His behavior became increasingly more bizarre as he grew older. He would "aimlessly leaf" through book after book which appeared to the parents as meaningless, random movements. They could not comprehend why, for such nonsensical behavior, he always selected his father's science books, primarily those concerned with physics and chemistry. He managed on occasion to speak a few words but with so many speech substitutions and with such nonclarity that they were rarely understood. He never responded when spoken to and made no indication that he either heard or comprehended what was said. He would not venture out of his back yard, and his primary enjoyment when he was not fingering through the books was to sit on a swing alone and rock back and forth for hours on end. He made no contact with his brother unless to poke at him or hit him. When he was four his sister was born, and Donald was sent to a nursery school where his adjustment was extremely poor. He went to public kindergarten and first grade but finally had to be withdrawn from school because of the difficult problems he presented. He then developed a mirror phobia and would scream so loudly and throw himself around so violently that the parents decided to cover up every mirror in their home. It was when Donald was eight that psychotherapy was initiated. The intelligence quotient obtained on the Stanford Binet was 70, but the clinical impression was that the emotional blocking was so severe that this index could not be accepted as a true indication of his intellectual potentiality.

Donald's poor motor co-ordination and spastic gait pointed also to the possibility of cerebral damage, and a review of a movie film taken of Donald from birth until the time he came into treatment seemed to confirm this suspicion. The film showed the child as a beautiful alert baby, who at six months was sitting up without support, at eight months crawled over to a flower, picked it, smelled it, and then waved good-bye, and at eleven months was running through the garden with steady gait. At age 2½, however, a marked change occurs on the film. Donald's eyes cross, his gait becomes spastic to the extent that he is walking on his toes and stumbling over his feet, and he has lost all the vivaciousness and alertness that so characterized his earlier pictures. The film was stopped at this point, since the change was such a dramatic one, and the parents were questioned further about Donald's childhood illnesses. They then remembered that about two months previous to the taking of this picture, Donald had been hospitalized for a few days with a high temperature of undetermined origin but with a possible diagnosis of a streptococus throat infection. Because of this medical history an EEG was immediately ordered and it was found that there was some brain damage in the left temporal lobe which the physician believed was due to encephalitis, and felt that such damage could possibly account for the speech difficulty and behavioral problems now observed. This organic problem, superimposed upon which were so many psychogenic factors, forced an extremely guarded prognosis. With this clarified to the parents, therapy was initiated.

Donald presented a picture of apathy and almost total withdrawal. His reaction time was extremely slow, and he gave monosyllabic response if he responded at all. His face was expressionless, giving the impression of one walking in a trance.

In his first hours in the playroom Donald spent each session shooting at the large mirror on the wall with a cork gun after placing a sharp nail in the cork. When the interpretation was given to him regarding his dislike for the hostility he saw reflected in the mirror, Donald gave his first indication of contact with the therapist. A faint smile crossed his lips, and then he shot more and more vigorously at the mirror.

The following session he went to the easel board and drew a large picture. There were layers of different colors but in the center was a large black peak with gray smoke coming out of it. When asked if he would like to tell a story about the picture he had drawn, he said haltingly, "This is Mt. Donald. Mt. Donald is erupting and all the lava is pouring out. Mt. Donald has been quiet for a long time, but now it's erupting." These were the first spontanious sentences Donald had uttered in the therapeutic process. He was letting the therapist know that he could feel things happening to him, and that he would participate more actively. But more important, this child who had been believed to have been feeble-minded, who spoke only in monosyllables, was revealing a vocabulary far beyond his years and was confiding to the therapist that he could talk, that he had been merely quiet for a long time. Much of his time in the following sessions was spent in further drawings of Mt. Donald, drawings which, like barometers, became indications of the storms and stress of Donald's daily life. His choice of colors, his vigorous or languorous stroke, his depth or surface perspective gave clues to his mood swings which he continued to cover up with his cloak of apathy. When interpretations were given regarding his feelings as expressed in the pictures, Donald would indicate his acceptance or rejection of an interpretation by continuing to work on the picture or by tearing up the picture respectively. At times after crumpling up a drawing, he would remove it from the waste-basket, not certain whether he must reject or accept the interpretation. This expression of ambivalence was a healthy sign, for it pointed to the lessening of the need for total withdrawal and the ability to reconsider rather than to rely upon the defense of blind denial.

The first phase of treatment was centered on developing a relationship of trust between the patient and the therapist, thus permitting a break-through in Donald's impenetrable wall of silence. It was when Donald confided to the therapist that he knew her office was wired directly to the police station and that the switch-board operator had orders to call the police everytime a mother spanked a child that it became evident that Donald had aligned the therapist on his side and felt that together they would defeat all the cruel parents of this world. This trust, however, had to be tested over and over again, and in the months to follow Donald hit out wildly on the slightest provocation. The mere asking of him to repeat a word that had not been understood was sufficient for him to resort to uncontrolled violence—a wild lashing out as the penalty one pays for communication. As long as he was apathetic and silent, he was in perfect control, but his expression of hostility and violence was limitless when he ventured from his shell. This he was determined to prove to the therapist, as if he were pleading for assistance in maintaining his defense of withdrawal. And yet the more he tried to be pushed back into his old world of silence, the more verbal did he become, and gradually he directed his violent outburst away from the therapist and on to his drawings. He drew elaborate Rube Goldberg contraptions for mouse-traps, but the mouse was always clever and would find a secret switch that would permit the mouse to get the cheese without being swallowed up by the trap. When he moved in his drawings from the mouse-trap to the rat-trap the story changed, for there was no secret switch to let the rat go free. Here was the beginning of working at Donald's rivalry with his father, for in his fantasy, the big rat entering the alluring tunnel would meet with total destruction; whereas the little mouse was clever enough to avoid the alluring tunnel and would thereby not only receive the reward but would survive.

It was during this phase of treatment that Donald would ask his mother to hold his penis when he urinated, saying that he did not want to get his hands dirty, and simultaneously with this behavior he went into a period of compulsive handwashing. He was being overtly seductive toward his mother but with such overlaid guilt that the compulsive cleansing process ensued. He would wander around the house all hours of the night, often winding up in his parents' room, standing in the dark near his mother's bed. When he returned to bed, he would lie awake making snorting noises and bouncing back and forth. There was indeed strong suspicion that Donald had either witnessed the primal scene, or else was entertaining sexual fantasies that were terrifying to him. His hostility toward his brother was more and more overtly expressed and on the least provocation he would mercilessly lash out at him, using any weapon at his disposal. It became imperative to put controls on Donald's explosive behavior, but rather than becoming more defiant, he welcomed these limitations and became more verbal in expressing his hostility and less overt in acting out his aggressive and hostile impulses. And as he became more verbal, the play-therapy hours were devoted to his making up of stories which he enjoyed dictating. All question of mental retardation was completely dissipated as Donald's stories unfolded. His imagination, vocabulary, humor, and talent for writing became apparent, but more important was the way Donald used his stories for free association, identification with his characters, symbolism, and interpretation. A typical story of his was about a big black cat who brought bad luck to his whole family, though the cat didn't mean to bring bad luck. The cat finally consults with a psychologist who gives the cat a magic potion—and now the cat becomes a talking cat. The cat's master is in trouble because he spends all of his money, but in the end the talking cat saves him. The talking cat no longer feels he's bad luck, but he still has lots of problems, and it will take a long, long time to get rid of some of them. He illustrated most of his stories with pictures or diagrams, and would often refer back to previously written stories for further elaboration or interpretation.

It was in one of the play-therapy sessions that Donald was intent upon drawing a diagram with arrows, letters, and numbers. He showed great seriousness as he drew his diagram and when it was completed he said, "This represents the theory of atomic energy." This boy who had "fingered aimlessly" through his father's science books, had in reality absorbed the basic concepts and was able to discuss Einstein's theory of relativity with amazing accuracy.

It was not a steady upstream progress with Donald. There were intermittent periods of nonproductivity, withdrawal, and regressive behavior which at times were alarming, but in retrospect it was seen that each regressive period ushered in an accelerated growth period wherein positive emotional behavioral patterns became integrated.

The period of gravest concern was when Donald internalized his hostility, and for the slightest error on his part he would beat his head against the wall until one feared he would have a skull fracture. His need to punish himself was so great that there was danger of total self-destruction. It was during this period that Donald began to recall early memories, memories for the period in which he had regressed to a preverbal level, wherein he did not even say such words as *mama* or *daddy*. He recalled his separation from his mother because he would not eat and how he decided he had better eat if he ever wanted to get home again. He recalled his appendectomy and herniaectomy at the age of 2½. He remembered being wheeled into a white room and the mask being put over his face, and how he saw spirals going around and around as he sank into unconsciousness—and he was certain that the black spot in the center of the spiral was death. He believed then that his mother would again send him to his death. These were the spirals which six months previous in the play-therapy hours Donald had drawn over and over again but about which he refused to talk, and there was no getting at the symbolism until months later. And as Donald recalled these early memories, he would frequently cry. It was no longer the crying of rage and frustration in which he had always indulged. These tears were the first indication of real affect that Donald could reveal, and as he found he could cry, cry with feeling, so he found he could smile a little and even laugh on occasion, and his humor, when he was off guard, was sparkling and charming, though only momentarily would he permit his gaiety to seep through. He denied all wants, as if he felt that there would be something wrong in anything he might want, and consequently showed neither enthusiasm nor desire for anything. His interest in science was his sole absorption, for he found his safety in this isolation of thinking. This, also, was perhaps his attempt at identification with his father and his search for approval from his father, whose primary interests as well as profession were scientific. It was difficult to get Donald to move into other areas, and only months later did Donald express his readiness and need to give up the mechanism of the isolation of thought in a single area. He had been discussing his hate feelings for his brother and said in genuine seriousness "I want to kill Andy. I am going to—then I won't ever have to bother with him again." The reality problems involved in such a solution were pointed out. Donald listened attentively and then said, "I'll run away from home. I'll live with you. You would take me." Once more the reality problems were presented. Donald thought a moment and then said, "I know, I'll give up my interest in science. Andy is jealous of me. He thinks I'm smarter. If I play his games and forget about science, maybe he'll like me better, and maybe I won't hate him so much. And I won't have to do this for always, 'cause in a couple of years he'll be older and maybe he will want to know about science—and then I can go back to it." This was felt to be more than a solution for resolving Donald's hostility against Andy. It was his way of saying that he wanted to be more like other children, that he did not want to remain peculiarly above the world, that he was ready for participation in social affairs. It was then that Donald was sent to a private day school for a year, and placed in the 6th grade despite having had no formal education. He made up all of the academic work he had missed in a very few months. The children at first found him odd and would jeer at his behavior, but he was still so withdrawn from them and so noncommunicative that he showed no response to their ridicule. He concentrated on conforming to the classroom routine and the demands of the teacher, and by the end of the year his classmates had learned not only to accept him but to respect his mental ability. The following year he was sent to a public junior high school. Here the initial adjustment was almost catastrophic. He wanted so much to succeed, to feel accepted, that in his anxiety over failure, he would hit his head or cry like an infant whenever threatened. His classes were large, and the confusion of going from one room to another was overwhelming. These problems, though, he brought into the psychodrama sessions where the children knew him, respected him, and had seen his progress. With their support and suggestions in social techniques, Donald was helped to accept the challenge. Before the year was over, he was elected president of his science class by the children, and received B's in all of his academic work, and excellent in co-operation, effort, and citizenship in all of his classes. It was when he showed me his report card that he said, "Do you remember when I used to be a zombie? I feel happy now, but I still get discouraged. I have such a long way to go yet." Donald does have a long way to go. These fourteen years of his growing up have been a nightmare to him, and to his parents, and sister and brother. He sees light now—but at times it is blinding and he withdraws into his shell of darkness. His speech is halting and precise—still afraid of what his words might reveal. His caution in interpersonal relationships is reflected in his caution in verbal expression. It was Donald who summarized the meaning of his long years of silence when he said, "I am glad there is no mental telepathy. If I don't talk, nobody knows what I am thinking." Now Donald is interested in social problems and world injustices. He hates war, and destruction, and prejudice. His hostility appears to be channelized against injustice. He sees himself as one who has been freed and can therefore take up the cause of others. Though Donald is still cautious in interpersonal relationships, he now sees humans and feels no longer the imminent danger from which he tried to escape. His speech was but the symptom of withdrawal from the catastrophic world about him.

Play therapy, then, is but a medium through which a child is helped to come to terms with himself and his surrounding world. It affords him the opportunity for re-evaluating his personal worth, for only through the positive acceptance of oneself is one able to gain a positive acceptance of others. Like Donald, when one hates the world, he hates primarily the mirrored reflection of his own hostility, and only when he can learn to discriminate areas in which there is justification for hostility from areas in which his hostility is mobilized because of distortions or misinterpretations in his thinking, can he break through his false generalizations which have permeated all of his thinking and have stereotyped his behavior. His defenses against his anxiety cannot be given up until the anxiety itself has been dissipated. The primary problem rests in bringing the derivatives of the unconscious material into consciousness. The success of rendering the defenses inoperative is dependent upon the extent to which the resistance and the defense against affects can be brought into consciousness for the purpose of interpretive work. Only then can the apprehensive anxiety be relieved. Anxiety exaggerates every reaction, and only when the anxiety is relieved is it possible to give up the defenses which are so static in quality and which deny the individual spontaneity and the freedom for choice of solutions.

This is the clinical psychologist's approach to speech pathology, for in the absence of organic factors the symptom is considered in terms of the total integrated personality and is therefore never treated in isolation. Unfortunately, the clinical psychologist is often insufficiently trained in speech pathology, and similarly is the speech pathologist too often untrained in clinical psychology. Speech therapy is in actuality psychotherapy, psychotherapy with patients who have a symptom of speech disturbance as a major problem but rarely, if ever, an isolated problem. The stutterer, for example, is often spoken of as if he were an individual peculiarly different from other neurotic individuals. The only difference lies in the one overt symptom.

There are some in the field of speech pathology who have questioned whether the stutterer can be considered neurotic. At a recent symposium on stuttering it was pointed out by these men that the stutterer was in no way different from anyone else, since everyone on occasion stumbles or blocks over a word. Whatever difference there might be would be a quantitative rather than a qualitative one, and therefore the term *neurotic behavior* was in no way helpful in understanding the stutterer. The word *neurotic* was emotionally charged for the proponents of this argument. Such comment would, indeed, hold for any neurotic symptom. Every individual has anxiety at times. This does not mean that every individual has an anxiety neurosis. Every individual at times feels a compulsion to finish a task. This does not mean that every individual suffers from a compulsion neurosis. Every individual blocks over a word on occasion. This does not mean that every individual is a stutterer. Only when the atypical behavior becomes so integrated in the total personality structure that it dominates and influences the individual's behavior in all of his everyday life experiences is it considered neurotic behavior. The stutterer's symptomatology affects all of his interpersonal relationships. He is tied, bound, limited in his everyday experiences by his speech difficulty. He is similar to the group we label compulsion neurotics, those individuals who cannot break away from their ritualistic behavior, who are able to admit that their patterns are silly but they cannot give them up, who describe their compulsions as if they were derived from a force outside themselves over which they have no control.

Similarly, the stutterer says with grave sincerity that he would do anything to give up his stuttering, but he cannot. He wants to speak freely, but the words will not come. The fact that on occasion every stutterer is able to speak without blocks indicates that stuttering is a functional disturbance. The word *functional* appears to be less emotionally charged than the word *neurotic,* but be this as it may, the functional disturbance is due to unresolved conflicts, overwhelming anxiety, and defenses against such anxiety. The etiology for the stutterer's symptom is not different from that of other conversion symptoms, and points merely to a conflict between antagonistic tendencies. In psychoanalytic terminology, this could be defined in terms of the conflict between the libidinous needs on the one hand, and the ego and superego under the pressure of the environment on the other hand. This theory would emphasize, as Fenichel (1945) points out, that in the life process of the stutterer there occurred a sexualization of speech, a confusion of oral and anal zones, a retention followed by a forceful expulsion of words similar to the retention followed by a forceful expulsion of feces. The development of speech, occurring as it does at the same time as the development of sphincter control, could indeed make possible this anal-oral displacement. But this anal-sadistic characteristic is not peculiar to the stutterer alone. He must be understood as other neurotic individuals are understood, and he must be treated according to his personality structure and psychosexual development. Speech pathology and clinical psychology are such closely related disciplines that training in both areas becomes imperative when dealing with those patients whose symptomatology is expressed in their speech.

Play therapy, as described in the case of Donald, cannot be used by the speech therapist who has not been adequately trained in clinical psychology. The understanding of the dynamics of behavior and the learning of therapeutic skills to free the child from his anxieties are basic to the removal of the symptom, which is but the symbol of the patient's conflicts.

## PSYCHODRAMA

Functional disturbances in speech, as has been pointed out, indicate difficulties encountered in the dynamic interaction between the individual and the surrounding social forces. It therefore follows that social adjustment for these children is often extremely difficult and necessitates the use of therapeutic techniques which will assist the child in his socialization.

In individual treatment, the dynamic interaction between the therapist and the patient sets the pace, the depth of the penetration of the conflict areas, and the degree of success in the treatment process. Each treatment hour is primarily patient-centered, and in this protected relationship the patient is gradually helped to face his internal conflicts, understand his behavior, and give up reactions no longer appropriate. As important as this may be in order to penetrate the core of internal conflict, a primary aim of all treatment must be to help the individual live more comfortably within his society, not separate and apart from it. For this reason group psychotherapy, particularly psychodrama, when used in conjunction with individual treatment, affords the necessary balance of the penetration of the individual problems on the one hand, and the adjustment to the interplay of social forces on the other hand.

Psychodrama offers a medium of self-expression that has tremendous appeal to children. Play-acting is close to their daily world of fantasy, and they step from one role to another with great ease, with little regard as to sex, age, or familiarity with the specific characterization. In actuality, it is not uncommon to find among children in their fantasies the desire to be of the opposite sex, but such acting out in life situations is so wrought with social taboos that they must repress at all times any behavior which might reveal these fantasies. These children welcome such role-playing in the psychodrama sessions where this behavior is accepted by the group as part of the psychodrama technique, thus affording them overt expression for some of their repressed fantasies, and at the same time giving them the opportunity of working at these conflict areas.

A child who in individual therapy struggles with verbal expression, and for whom the therapeutic process becomes painful because of the long pauses and lack of spontaneity of speech, frequently gains sufficient support from the group to enable him to verbalize more freely, particularly in those areas where others in the group share similar hostile feelings or neurotic anxieties.

In a first session of psychodrama, the children were seated comfortably in a circle. The therapist, having clarified the purpose of the group, sensed the anxiety of the group, and therefore proceeded with the question: "How many of you have had the experience of feeling uncomfortable about going to a party where you did not know too many people?" Every hand was raised. Janet, a very shy, almost withdrawn child, looked at all the hands held up and said, "Gee, I didn't know everyone else felt like me. I thought I was the only one scared about going to parties."

This was a child who in individual sessions struggled with verbal expression. It was always a painful process because of her verbal difficulty. Supported by the group, however, she was the first to comment freely and before too many sessions was able to give vent to aggressive impulses.

Betty, age fourteen, had always been a difficult problem at school. She was thoroughly unpopular with her classmates, indulged in compulsive stealing, was obese, and failed in school despite a high I.Q. She assumed an air of sophistication and refused to admit to any problem. When invited to come to the first psychodrama session, she agreed providing she would not have to participate and could remain as audience watching the others perform. She admitted that she was curious about other people's problems, though she had none of her own. She entered the room and sat on a chair far removed from the other children, thus creating a distance as great as possible between herself and the group. After a scene was performed in which a child enacted a role of a very irritable, demanding mother, Betty from the sidelines said, "Let me show you what my mother is like. Yours is an angel in comparison." Betty was from then on a part of the group. She could not remain the passive onlooker.

In such a group, then, the individuals early entertain the awareness that all of the children have problems, and with this comes the realization that they are not as different from other children as they had believed. With the discovery of anxieties in common, of similar hostile and aggressive impulses against parental figures, of shared rather than isolated guilt, of rigid neurotic defenses so inadequate in life adjustments, the children find a common denominator with which they can work, and from which they can gain the necessary courage and fortification to face their individual problems. This is of particular value to those children who have limited verbal skills, who in individual therapy struggle with verbal expression, but who frequently gain sufficient support from the group to enable them to enjoy greater spontaneity and an increased adequacy of expression, particularly in those areas where others in the group experience similar problems.

Psychodrama affords the opportunity for experimenting with life situations and for exploring various solutions to a given problem. In the structuring of a scene, the child is helped to crystallize his problem and to consider the interacting forces against which he is struggling. Unlike a discussion group, which often remains solely on an intellectual level, role enactment insures emotional participation in the very dramatic management of the scenes and thereby allows for emotional catharsis.

Dick, an eleven-year-old mild stutterer, in telling of a situation in which he had been caught stealing, discussed the problem freely and with no particular observable anxiety. In acting out the scene, however, he burst down crying at the climax when he was caught and could not worm out of the situation. He lived the scene over again with all of its emotional impact.

Of equal importance in role-playing is the fact that because a child often takes on the role of another child, he dares to give vent to his true feelings, since he is no longer being himself. Under the guise of someone else he freely expresses himself as he would like to in life situations were he not to fear the loss of love, status, or control over his aggressive impulses. It is not uncommon to find the passive, shy child volunteer for the role of the hostile, negativistic youngster—actually relish the role of the bully—for his passivity generally is the defense against his aggressive impulses which constantly seek expression.

The child gains courage from the group to explore other solutions by the very fact that the centralization of the problem rests primarily with the group rather than with the individual. Once a problem is brought up, it no longer remains the private property of the individual but is worked upon by the group as a whole with little concern as to which child introduced the problem, though the given child never loses sight of the fact that it is his problem which the group is attacking.

Whereas in the individual sessions the therapist deals with a single ego and its defenses, in the group there are many egos varying in the degree of strength and types of defenses. Consequently, in the group process the individuals are often able to gain insight into their own mechanisms more readily than in individual treatment. They are offered the opportunity to contrast their reactions and behavioral patterns with those of the other members of the group, and may thereby find more adequate solutions to the handling of their anxieties. This process was clearly seen in Jim, a child who attempted to handle all anxiety by overt aggression.

Whenever threatened or in anyway frustrated, Jim was ready to fight. In all of his early scenes the only possible solution to any of his problems as he saw it was to fight or punch anyone in his way. When another child presented a conflict with her father, Jim's immediate reaction was, "I'd slug him if he did that to me." It was in the ninth session that Jim first showed a willingness to explore other solutions. He had felt very antagonistic toward his teacher, who was apparently inadequate for this child and on occasion had gotten into physical tussles with him. In this session Jim wanted to show the group a new experience he had had during the week. In presenting the scene he said, "I decided to see what would happen if I would ask the teacher if I could help another kid in the room with his arithmetic. I was never good in arithmetic before, but now it's not so bad—only the other kid couldn't seem to get it. My teacher let me, and it was sort of fun. I guess I didn't feel like fighting that day. My teacher's not such a bad egg after all." In casting the scene he chose to play his own role. This was the same child who two weeks previous to this session was questioned about his truancy from school on a specific occasion. He said in all seriousness, "I had to stay away from that teacher one day and take a rest or I would have gotten a nervous breakdown; and if I didn't get the breakdown, I'm sure my teacher would have."

In contrast to the secrecy, respected privacy, and held confidences so extremely important in individual therapy is the airing of problems in the group. This in itself has great therapeutic value, since it helps to free the child from his strong feelings of guilt when he receives support, tolerance, sympathy, and respect from the other members of the group, even though they do not condone his behavior. Actually, in the psychodrama groups, the child gains status when he is able to reveal a problem rather than hide behind the mask of denial. The groups on which these observations are based remained consistently intolerant of only one defense—a child's denial of problems. The following is typical of what would happen when a child failed to bring up a problem:

Allan was a very passive, effeminate youngster of thirteen, who was always correct and proper. He enjoyed the psychodrama sessions because of his histrionic interest and ability, providing he could take roles in the other children's structured situations and problems, but never did he volunteer a problem of his own. The children accepted this for 11 sessions and then:
*Jim:* "Say, Allan, why don't you bring in a problem. You only take part in ours."
*Allan:* "I don't have any problems. I never get into trouble."
*Jim:* "Then what do you come to our group for if you don't have any problems?"
The other children took up this theme and unanimously agreed that if Allan had no problem, he should no longer be in the group. The following session Allan brought in a problem. It concerned his feelings when he thought the group was getting rid of him, and for the first time he expressed hostility and desires for retaliation. From then on he revealed many problems, serious conflicts which he had always previously denied.

The role-reversal technique has considerable therapeutic value in that it permits the child to see not only a mirrored reflection of himself as another child takes on his role, but also the inadequacies of his defense mechanisms and the difficulties his behavior imposes upon others in his environment. It helps him to differentiate the reality factors from fantasy and distortion, and makes it possible for him to empathize with, and at last move toward, the very people against whom he has been defiant, critical, and resistant, as he struggles in his role-playing, particularly of parental figures.

Steve portrayed his mother as a strict over-bearing person who was always yelling at him. He felt that, regardless of his behavior, which he admitted was more times than not destructive, his mother should not yell at him or threaten him with punishment. He wished he had a different kind of mother. He was therefore given the role of the "ideal" mother in order to show the group how he feels a mother should handle the negative behavior of a child. Peter was given the role of Steve with the instructions that he was to make it really tough on this mother. Peter delighted in the role of the "bad" boy, since in his home he never enjoyed the luxury of being disobedient. No child could have been more disobedient or disrespectful than Peter in this scene, and yet his portrayal was not an exaggeration of Steve's usual behavior at home. Steve put every effort forth to be the calm, patient mother in the scene, but finally in real defeat and desperation he said, "I guess it's not easy being a mother."

It is interesting to observe how the children cast the part for the scenes they wish to portray, and how after a while the children resent being typed according to the defenses they use in their life situations.

Don whined, used infantile speech, and when at all threatened would crawl on the floor and generally act like a baby. Consequently, whenever a role portraying tantrums or infantile behavior was to be played, Don was invariably selected for the part. It was in the fifteenth session when he was again cast for such a role that he, with real feeling, said, "I'm tired of always taking the part of the baby. I want to be the daddy." The children immediately pointed out to Don that his usual behavior was infantile, and that therefore they always thought of him when they needed such a character in their scenes. Don's behavior soon changed after this session, and the group responded to his new behavior by casting him in more adult roles.

Since psychodrama remains in the framework of play-acting, it removes the threat of the loss of self-control, and thereby gives the child courage to act out his aggressive impulses without fear of retaliation and guilt. Through his spontaneous self-expression, he frees himself from inner tension and internalized hostility. He finds no basis for his fear of his aggressive impulses when he recognizes his control over them in the role-acting situations which do not get out of hand. He sees that his acceptance by the group and his self-esteem are not reduced because he overtly expresses his hostility and aggression, and he is, therefore, better able to face his ambivalent feelings toward loved ones without the fear of total rejection.

The giving up of neurotic defenses is not an easy problem, for each individual generally enjoys a fanatic belief that his neurotic behavior will give him mastery over himself and his world, and to tamper with his neurotic behavior would be tantamount to surrender such mastery. It is, in actuality, the young child's very neurotic behavior that often makes his parents helpless and gives to the child the feeling of power as he sees them cringe before his neurotic demands.

Each child has the narcissistic need to consider his problem the most important and the most difficult to resolve, and often, therefore, tends to minimize the importance of another individual's problems. This competitive rivalry for the largest neurosis would be amusing if there were not such pathos behind the bickering.

Ricky, age seven, was presenting to the group his fear of the dark. He saw witches and ghosts in every shadow. In the silence he heard volcanic noises. There were big giants with large clubs standing over his bed. He would hold his breath, since that would make his heart beat less noisily and the giants would not know he was there. In the midst of this story, Bobby interrupted:

*Bobby:* "How silly! Are you afraid of the dark? That's the silliest thing I ever heard. Why should anyone but a sissy be scared of the dark?"

*Ricky:* "Now just wait a minute. You're you, and I'm me. What may not be a problem to you can be awful important to me. Besides I think being scared of the dark is much more important than your problem of being scared of snakes. I have to be in the dark every night, and you never have to see a snake."

*Bobby:* "Oh yeah! Let's take a vote from the group. I betcha everyone here will say being scared of snakes is a more important problem and harder to get rid of."

If then in the group a child's problem is minimized or reduced in importance when contrasted with another child's problem, he often becomes like a tiger, fighting for his strength—namely, his neurotic behavior. This is competition before it has been channelized into socially acceptable avenues on which economies could be built, for money is no less the symbol of power in our present society than is the child's neurotic behavior to himself or to his parents, and the ensuing struggle to maintain this power is no less competitive.

Even the shy, timid child, the child so withdrawn he cannot communicate verbally at any level, has a power in the very impenetrable wall he has built around himself, a power over the helplessness and impotency of his parents who, regardless of their verbal skills, cannot communicate with this child who has become deaf and mute to their demands, who shies away like a hunted animal, but whose poisonous fangs strike the hunter and leave him groping in the jungle of emotions.

It is through this mechanism that we begin to see the dynamic interaction of personalities and how platitudinous is the remark: There is no such thing as a problem child; it is always a problem parent. The children must discover that often the basic problem lies in the error of equations, in the misinterpretations of symbols of power as actual power, in the distortion in thinking that examining these symbols and defense mechanisms critically would lead to self-destruction. The children, in working through the transference reactions, gain the necessary understanding which enables them to see people as they are, and they become more realistically oriented to the differentiation of personalities. There are always some in the group who reach this phase of understanding before others, but who in turn become intolerant of those children who tenaciously hold on to their same defense mechanisms. As in the early phase of the group process, the children gained status when they presented a problem and could reveal to the group their conflicts; so in the later process they could maintain status only if they were willing to let go of their inadequate defenses, profit from the group experience, and tangibly demonstrate to the group their new enlightened way of thinking, feeling, and dealing with life situations.

The psychodrama technique is probably of greatest value in the area of projection into the future which involves the crystallizing of goals, the giving of purpose to life, the facing of the reality of death, and the considering of the entire problem of motivation. When the children enact the roles of themselves in the future, their dreams, ambitions, anxieties, and current reality problems are brought into focus, and with this emerges the clarification of the appropriate interpersonal skills necessary for such goal achievement. It is ever amazing to see the seriousness with which the youngsters approach these problems, regardless of age.

In one session two groups of children had been combined in order to work at problems in sibling rivalry, since several of the children in one group had brothers or sisters in the other group. Each group had worked individually at sibling rivalry problems, but the children had requested that the groups be combined in order that their feelings could be aired and the friction points worked out together. Though this was intended for a single session, the children enjoyed the combined group so much that they asked that it be continued. The ages ranged from eight to sixteen. The following is a summary of the fourth session of the combined groups and illustrates the seriousness with which the children attacked the problems of life and death.

One of the children expressed his fear of death. All of the children immediately began to discuss their individual feelings about death which ranged from the fear of helplessness and desertion if one or both of their parents were to die, to the wish that the children themselves might die so their parents would feel sorry for the way they had treated their children, but after the parents were sufficiently punished the children would come back to life. It was then that the discussion took the following turn:

*Jane:* (age 10) "I don't think it's so bad we have to die. We wouldn't want to live forever, and ever, and ever. We probably would never get anything accomplished if we had all that time. It might sound silly, but I sort of think of life like it's a big cake—and each one of us gets a slice, and that slice can be awful good and just enough."

*Andy:* (age 12—Jane's brother) "You know, Jane, I like that example, but I'd like to say that I think we're all sort of the little crumbs in the cake. And we drop some crumbs too—and that's also important!"

*Therapist:* "What do you mean, Andy, about the crumbs we drop?"

*Andy:* "I don't know. I guess that's how we leave our mark on life."

*Les:* (age 16) "You know, I have a couple of friends—and I know they're going to be a success. But somehow I can never see myself that way. I'm just an average kid, and I can't see myself ever amounting to anything really important."

*Ricky:* (age 11) "Les, I think you're looking at it all wrong. Now, let's take Mozart, for example. Everyone's heard of him, but I betcha no one's ever heard of his dad. I guess you wouldn't call him important. But if it weren't for his dad, we never would have had Mozart. So even a guy not so important leaves his mark."

*Les:* "Hm—I never looked at it that way—hm!"

This discussion preceded the dramatization of many scenes of the future with discussion ensuing regarding the reality factors to be considered if goals were to be realized.

Psychodrama is also an invaluable technique for working in areas of racial and religious prejudice. These sociological problems are frequently introduced in the group when a member either wishes to flaunt his superiority, or when a member of a minority group brings up his problem of being discriminated against, at times realistically, at other times as a rationalization for his nonacceptance by an individual or group. In one of the groups there was only one member who was a Jew, and she in actuality was only half-Jewish, her father being a gentile. She was an extremely attractive child, popular with the group, and greatly respected. The children, many of whom were anti-Semitic, had not appreciated that Elaine was Jewish. In this group was Jim, the child previously described as a youngster who attempted to handle his anxiety by punching his way through life. He came from a wealthy, conservative, and prejudiced home. Elaine presented her problem of being called a dirty Jew at school. She asked to be permitted to take the role of the gentile child and chose Jim for the part of the Jew.

> *Jim:* (as the Jew) "Hi Elaine. Are you going to the school dance tonight?"
> *Elaine:* "Sure, but you'd better not be there."
> *Jim:* "Why not? I certainly expect to go."
> *Elaine:* " 'Cause you're a dirty Jew! We don't want any Jews at our dances."
> *Jim:* "What do you mean 'your dances'? It's a public school. This is a free country. Just try and stop me!"
> *Elaine:* "Well you better not try to dance with any of my friends. We don't like Jews hangin' around!"
> At this point Jim raised his fist as if he were going to punch Elaine and the scene was stopped.
> *Therapist:* "Jim, how did you feel taking the part of a Jew?"
> *Jim:* "Say, I was mad, real mad. And you know she's just lucky I'm not a Jew, 'cause if I really was I would have killed her."

The discussion that followed this scene involved active participation by all the members of the group. There were some who felt that there was both justification and necessity for prejudice against minority groups, while others felt it an inexcusable injustice. It was Jim who said, "You can't know how the other guy really feels until you step into his shoes. I think everyone here ought to try that part like I did. Maybe then you'd know what you were talking about!"

The children in the groups studied were tolerant of personality mannerisms, idiosyncrasies, or atypical speech patterns which they sensed as being symptomatic of underlying disturbances and conflicts. No child ever interrupted a stutterer regardless of how much time he took to express himself, nor did the group ever try to exclude any youngster unless his behavior was disruptive to the group process. This attitude of acceptance on the part of the group is in some respects more meaningful to the child than the support he receives from the therapist in the individual sessions, particularly when his primary problem centers around social and interpersonal relationships. The child leaned heavily on the group for support and for assistance in finding solutions to his problems, and only on occasion did he turn to the therapist for additional support.

It is interesting to observe the strong, moralistic attitude the children entertain in contrast to the therapist. They are generally more critical, more severe, and more demanding of a child in areas of behavior, punishment, and evaluations of the individual members, yet, in the groups on which these observations are based, no child seemed to resent the frank comments of the group, nor did the anxieties appear intensified when such comments were made. The ability to accept criticism without feeling rejected or devastated by such criticism, and the ability to give criticism that is not motivated by hostility and the need to crush someone, are invaluable growth experiences for these children, basic to motivation in learning as well as to positive interpersonal relationships.

The limitations of psychodrama as a therapeutic technique are also impressive. Sexual anxieties are with great reservation brought up by the children, which is in marked contra-distinction to what occurs in the individual sessions. Since psychodrama more closely approaches life situations, the avoidance of sexual material in a group may be a function of our cultural taboos, whereas in individual therapy the very privacy and secrecy in the therapist-patient relationship encourages the child to dismiss his concern over social prohibitions, confident that he will never be betrayed.

Interpretations by the therapist at times have to be avoided or delayed for an individual session because not every member of the group may be able to accept such interpretation which is often intended for a single child. An interpretation is most fruitful when given at the moment the patient reveals his readiness for such interpretation, but this must be sacrificed if other members of the group would be thrown off balance by such interpretation.

Often intensive individual treatment is necessary before a child can make the necessary adjustment to the group. The child frequently needs time to work through his fantasies and must not be forced too soon to face the reality factors and limitations a group imposes. The child should be exposed to the group only when he can both benefit from such experience and contribute to the group. The screening of a child for a group and the timing of when the child should be exposed to a therapeutic group process may not always coincide with groups available for a specific member and thus may limit the number of children who could profit from such participation.

Some children are more productive and function better in individual therapy, whereas in the group process they tend often to attack the superficial problems rather than nuclear conflicts.

As an aid to social as well as individual adjustment, despite these limitations, however, psychodrama is a therapeutic technique of great value both for children and adults, particularly when used in conjunction with individual treatment.

Therapy, then, is the educative process through which an individual is helped to uncover the bases for his anxieties and neurotic behavior. When therapy is successful, the patient learns the areas in which his behavior was determined by unconscious mechanisms, misinterpretations, and distortions in thinking. He finds more appropriate, less circuitous, and more socially acceptable ways of gaining gratifications for basic needs. He frees himself from his previously bound neurotic defenses, and finally he learns to evaluate his role in relationship to his objective world. This is brought about, whether in individual treatment or in group therapy, through the dynamic interaction of personalities, through the give and take in the patient-therapist relationship. This is not only basic to learning, but points to the effects of the interacting forces existent in interpersonal relationships, whether such effects be positive or negative.

## PARENT COUNSELING

Since the child's earliest experiences are always in relationship to his parents (or parental substitutes), and since from birth on he is responding to the dynamic interaction existent between himself and his parents, it becomes apparent that when the child develops symptoms, the impact from such interaction was traumatic. The parents' own neurotic patterns undoubtedly contributed to the child's symptomatology, at least to the extent to which the child reacted to the behavioral patterns of his parents. Not only, then, does treatment become necessary for the child, but the parents must gain insight into their mechanisms and free themselves from their neurotic defenses if both are to enjoy a more positive relationship.

The parents bring the child for treatment primarily because they are disturbed by the child's behavior. In other words, anxiety has been mobilized in the parents to the degree that they seek help with the objective of getting the child's behavior so changed that the parental anxiety can be dissipated. It becomes evident that the meaning of the child's behavior to the parents is such that tension on the part of the parents increases until finally are they compelled to seek professional help in order to relieve such tension. The parents' goal of treatment is generally to remove those symptoms or behavioral patterns in the child which disturb them, and treatment is considered by them successful if those particular problems are resolved. To the extent, at least, that the parents react with intensity to a child's given behavioral pattern does it become the parents' problem, and the meaning and interpretation they have given to the child's behavior must be explored in order to determine the basis for the parental anxiety. The mother, in other words, is seeking relief from her own anxiety and tension when she brings a child for treatment. Rather than facing her own internal conflicts, she throws the responsibility for her anxieties on to the child. It is as if she were saying, "My child got me into this state of anxiety. It is up to him to get me out of it. The therapist will make him do this."

This phenomenon is seen with relative frequency in child therapy. It is a problem which therapists whose practices are limited to adults rarely have to face, since an adult generally enters a treatment process because he recognizes his own need for help. The mother, on the other hand, often forces her child into treatment in order to avoid the facing of her own problems. She can accept help from the therapist only if the therapy remains child-centered. Basically she is threatened by a treatment process. She cannot face her own conflicts, but she gets to the therapist through her child, and can, therefore, remain on the periphery of therapy, moving in or out as she pleases, since it is the child who is the patient.

It is not unusual at the first interview to have the mother sheepishly laugh and say, "I guess I'm the one who really needs help but . . ." and then quickly go on to her child's problems, as if such confession has completely relieved her of any further responsibility for examining her behavior critically. Such a remark is in actuality her warning to the therapist not to delve into her behavioral patterns. She is, in effect, saying, "I admit I'm to blame, and since I admit it, let's just drop it, so I may continue in the same way. Just take care of my child and make him do what pleases me." She is also admitting to her errors before the therapist can become critical of her—an avoidance of punishment by confessing guilt and thereby exonerating herself.

This attitude is expressed frequently not only because of the mother's attempt to avoid treatment for herself, but because of society's tendency to excuse the child and blame the parent for any existent behavioral problem on the part of the child. This current attitude works a grave injustice on the child as well as the parent. It is founded on the assumption that the child with problems is in no way responsible for his behavior, that he is in reality merely a mirrored reflection of a poor parent. It denies him any degree of intelligence, judgment, fantasy, or emotional feelings of his own. It gives him only a rationalization for his behavior by permitting him to blame his parents for his misdemeanors. It takes away all dignity to which the child is entitled since it relieves him of his responsibility to himself, his parents, and society. Similarly, for the parents, such attitudes intensify their feelings of inadequacy, guilt, fear, and hostility. They must repeatedly seek reasons to justify their failure with the child, and often, therefore, tend to deny an existent problem in order to avoid their admission of failure. It is neither the parents nor the child who are responsible for the emergence of a problem. Problems are resultant from the interaction, from the anxieties that each arouses in the other. It is a two-way channel, and the parent is neither entitled to total credit nor total blame for his child's behavior.

When the parent brings the child for treatment both are frightened, confused, and resistant to therapy. The mother's resistance is often not initially apparent. Having taken the initiative for bringing the child to the therapist, it would appear that she believed in therapy, was confident in the therapist and in the therapeutic process. It is in reality more often her need to relieve herself of her responsibility by handing the problems of her child over to the therapist, her eagerness to avoid facing her own conflicts, her resistance to and fear of treatment for herself that motivates her to take the step. She forces her child into a treatment process that she herself fears and to which she is resistant.

From this it becomes obvious that the therapist who attempts to point out to the mother all the wrong things she has done and to instruct her in new techniques in the handling of the child has walked into the very trap the mother has set. The therapist is, in effect, being critical of the mother and is substantiating her feelings of inadequacy and failure. He is permitting her to remain on the periphery, for counseling as a technique is a superficial approach as well as a dangerous one. It is too often used as an added crutch by the parent in order to avoid the penetration of deeper problems. The parents' obedience in following the therapist's suggested techniques may again give the impression of nonresistance to treatment, but in actuality it is more often the parents' way of throwing the responsibility on to the therapist. If the parent follows to the letter the orders of the therapist, and the child continues to be a problem, then it is the therapist who has failed rather than the parent. If the child responds to the new techniques employed by the parents, then the problem is considered resolved and no further delving into conflicts is believed to be necessary. In either event, the parent is relieved from examining the causative factors in his personality structure which forced his reactions to be as they were, and from which he has not been freed.

The term *parent counseling* has the unfortunate connotation of a therapist giving advice to the parent, having the answers at his disposal, being an advisor for all the complexities of human interpersonal relationships. This is a far cry from getting the parent to find for himself the answers to his problem, to understand his behavior, to determine the areas in which he has been blindly groping. A critical attitude in relationship to the parent can be no more productive than a critical attitude in relationship to the child in a therapeutic process. Whether child or adult, the patient feels himself in a threatened position or would not need to develop defenses against his anxiety.

The starting point of parent counseling must be based on the realization that although the child presents a dramatic symptom such as stuttering, the parent is reacting to this symptom with anxiety, and that this anxiety is now reacted to by the child. It is a vicious circle, with each anxiety reaction on the part of one intensifying the anxiety reaction on the part of the other. Always there is an attempt to ward off anxiety, which attempt is the basis for the development of neurotic defenses; but more important, anxiety contains the component of contagion and when not successfully warded off becomes incorporated into the individual in whom such anxiety was not initiated. The infant, for example, may first experience anxiety because of the anxiety induced by an anxious mother. This anxiety often interferes with the infant's direction toward satisfaction of needs. It is actually a tension in opposition to goal satisfaction, for the hungry infant will reject food rather than take it from the anxious mother. But regardless of the infant's attempt to ward off such anxiety through avoidance, he incorporates the parental anxiety and the resultant behavior manifests itself in increased tension. Such tension mobilizes further anxiety in the parent, which anxiety is again reflected in the child. It is because anxiety is reflected from one individual to another that it often becomes so difficult for the individual to determine the basis for his anxiety. Frequently it is not his own anxiety with which he is struggling, but merely his incorporation of another individual's anxiety, which therefore remains vague, diffused, and noncrystallized but is ever a threat against which he must defend himself.

As was pointed out previously, that phase in development which occurs with the acquisition of sphincter control and the development of speech, namely, the transition from total infancy dependency to the awareness of the self as an individual, may indeed mobilize anxiety in the parent-child relationship. The infant being the most helpless and dependent creature at birth would have no chance of survival unless its parents accepted the responsibility for such dependency. This acceptance of the infant's dependency by the parent may be considered a function of the drive for propagation or race survival, and as with all drives receives its primary gratification when its functional value is realized. This gratification, however, may be so satisfying to the mother that she may be unwilling to relinquish the child's dependency upon her, even when such relationship no longer serves its original function of survival. There is probably at no other period of life as intense a feeling of being needed as when a new-born infant arrives on the scene, and as long as one feels needed there is purposeful meaning to life. The child, emerging into a being less dependent on the mother than initially, may be threatening to her not only because of her unwillingness to relinquish this gratifying dependency relationship, but because her early anxieties, when she felt herself to be unwanted, unimportant, and rejected may be reactivated. Once again she sees herself in a similar situation. Attention is too often centered upon the child who feels or is rejected, neglecting the realization that this child has at the same time become rejecting of the parent, and by this rejection imposes upon the mother the same anxiety-laden role that the child is experiencing. A mother whose own dependency needs are great may indeed become critically threatened in such a relationship, and, therefore, may find it difficult to control her hostile reactions. Not until the child is able to demonstrate overt gestures of affection is the mother able to respond with mutual out-going feelings. One mother expressed this so well when she said, "I don't even feel like getting mad at my child now. When she cries I want to hold her close to me. I wonder why I used to hit her when she cried. I guess I felt she wouldn't let me comfort her." It was only after her child became more demonstrative that this mother gained the insight that her hostile feelings, in part at least, had been resultant from her child's rejection of her as a comforting person.

There are also those mothers whose emotional immaturity and unresolved conflicts have interfered with their normal impetus for the acceptance of the infant's dependency. Actually, because of their anxiety, immaturity, and own dependency needs, they would like to turn away from the fulfillment of their parental role. They hide these feelings, however, behind an overt demonstration of a smothering dependency relationship with their child in order to convince society that they have accepted their responsibility.

This, then, is what the young child often has to fight against as he struggles in his maturative process toward self-realization. There is little wonder that there would occur disturbances in speech, in communication at any level, for the infant's directional movements are frequently in complete opposition to the mother's needs, and the child's maturation is blocked or delayed in this tug of war.

The conflict is again revitalized or intensified when the child enters adolescence. It is during this period that the emotional impacts resultant from the parent-child interpersonal relationships can perhaps most clearly be observed because of the intensity of reactions, yet such reactions are but the outgrowth of earlier unresolved conflicts. There is apparently considerable confusion regarding the adolescent. He has been looked upon by many as if he were some monster suddenly arising from nowhere, set and determined not only on self-destruction but on the destruction of the moral codes and values of our entire society. The only consoling thoughts appear to be that the period of adolescence does not last forever, though at the time it might seem endless, and that if one can live with the adolescent, one can learn to live with anything. This has become the adult's stereotype of the adolescent.

As confused as the adult is regarding the adolescent, so is the adolescent regarding the adult. He is confused as to what is expected of him, confused as to why he is such a disappointment to everyone, and above all confused as to why, when he was always urged to grow up, he is continually reminded of how young he is.

In actuality, adolescence is merely a term used to designate a particular stage in the maturative process, yet the word itself has become so emotionally weighted that parents have come to dread that phase of their child's development as if it were an illness to be avoided. The question as to why this phase of development appears so much more dramatic and emotionally reactive than any other phase arises. It becomes necessary to determine the meanings of the adolescent's behavior and to uncover the basis for the adult's reactions to such behavior, for the concern regarding the adolescent is resultant from the interaction of these personalities.

The adolescent has reached a stage in the maturative process where glandular changes and sexual impulses come into focus. Occurring with these physiological changes is an increased energy supply that gives to the adolescent a feeling of strength. This is a most positive aspect of adolescence, for it gives him the necessary courage and fortitude to begin to face life as an adult and to plan his future.

But as he looks into this future, he has genuine concern as to his interests, capabilities, and limitations. He does not know the area of work that will give him the greatest satisfaction in the years to come, nor whether his greatest aptitude lies in the field or fields of his interest. He realizes the vastness of specialization possibilities, but at the same time he is cognizant of his own limitations. He also realizes the financial limitations of his family, and how he must at times forfeit genuine interests for economic realities. If in his growing up he has learned to assume responsibilities appropriate to each age level, and through such learning has discovered the gratifications attendant upon the assumption of such responsibility, the facing of adult life does not throw him into anxiety-panic. He has already learned that responsibility is a challenge which, when faced, brings gratifications. Though he has serious concern and some anxiety, he also has the necessary energy to face these problems if further anxieties are not superimposed upon him. But because of this feeling of increased strength, he now has courage, also, to assert himself, at last, against the parental and authoritarian domination —courage to express resentments previously held back.

It is understandable that the parent reacts to this self-assertion on the part of his child with feelings of uneasiness and anxiety. Though the adolescent has frequently been described as weak and frightened because of his inability to handle and understand his newly aroused impulses, in reality, it is not generally he who feels weak but rather it is his parents, for they feel themselves losing their hold over their child. They discover that the techniques they previously used with success are now inadequate. Their child no longer moves as an automaton to their commands or worries about their threats of punishment. It is the parent, then, who begins to feel helpless and impotent whereas the adolescent begins to feel strong and virile.

The adolescent also stands as a mirrored reflection of a period when the parent, too, felt strong in defiance of *his* parents. Once having enjoyed such strength, it is not easy to surrender it. There is anxiety in conflict. There is perhaps greater anxiety in defeat. The parent, too often, has interpreted (or rather misinterpreted) the adolescent's self-assertion as the usurping of the parent's throne.

As the child emerges into adolescence, he is determined to loosen the parental chains and to prove his worthiness in his own right. This lights up anxiety in the parent, for the adolescent's behavior is interpreted as the symbol of his independence. This the parent too often equates with parental rejection. There is distortion in such equation, for at no time in an individual's life is he a totally independent being, nor should this be the goal or measurement of emotional maturity. The human being, from birth to death, is primarily a social being, dependent at all times upon interpersonal relationships. He is an animal whose drives and needs can attain satisfaction only through his dependent relationship with others. Loosening the parental knot should in no way suggest that the child no longer needs his parents. In many ways he may need the parent more than ever, but because of his stage of maturation there must be a restructuring of the parent-child relationship more appropriate to the changing dependency relationship. To feel no longer needed when one has previously felt himself to be indispensable must, understandably, produce anxiety. The more the parents attempt to handle their anxiety by mobilizing their strength to subdue this emerging personality, to put the adolescent in his place, to make him feel that he is just too big for his breeches, the more does the adolescent have the need to use his newly gained energy in rebellion and defiance, for he is fighting for freedom and for the dignity and respect to which he is entitled.

And the adolescent arouses further parental anxieties. In his newly sexual awakenings and his interests in sexual objects he turns his attention to the opposite sex with tenderness as well as with feelings of excitement and exhilaration. He must explore, prove, and accept his sexuality, for this is his preparation for parenthood. He has some anxiety in this, for not only does he feel clumsy in his approaches but he is aware of society's demands and prohibitions, and at the same time not too certain of his control nor how far he dare venture. In this very behavior he revives the early sexual anxieties of his parents and recalls for them their transgressions or weak defenses against such anxieties. It has been frequently observed that the parents who have been most sexually promiscuous are generally more concerned over the morals of their adolescents than the parents whose behavior did not lead to promiscuity. They have not freed themselves from the resultant guilt or the concomitant anxieties, and now these anxieties are revitalized as their child enters adolescence. They are determined to spare their child from such experiences. Since each individual suspects the weakness of his own defense structure and therefore guards vigilantly lest the structure collapse with the resultant catastrophic experience of social ostracism, he often has little faith in the defenses of his adolescent child, though this lack of faith may be totally unwarranted.

As the parents struggle with these aroused anxieties, they become suspicious, annoyed, and irritated by their adolescent's behavior. This struggle which often results in antisocial behavior on the part of the adolescent—a wild striking out against all authority and moral codes—is not due to the adolescent's fear of growing up, but rather to his attempt to ward off these heightened anxieties of his parents. He thereby often defeats his very purpose. For as the infant first experiences anxiety because of the anxiety induced by an anxious mother, and since, as was previously pointed out, anxiety interferes with the infant's direction toward satisfaction of needs, so the adolescent has increased anxiety tensions induced by the increased anxiety tensions of his parents, and the resultant behavior is again in opposition to the satisfaction of needs. He defeats the goal of self-actualization and emotional maturity.

In those fortunate individuals who have been brought up relatively free from anxiety, where from infancy on there were no interpersonal relationships so anxiety-ladened that they badly warped or damaged the personality structure, there is still the need to loosen the parental ties; but the parents, free from intense anxiety, are able to assist the child in loosening the knot. They neither cut it sharply, thus pushing the adolescent out on his own before his readiness for such emancipation, nor do they forcibly tighten the knot in order to delay or prevent the weaning process. Rather are such parents able to understand the feelings of their adolescent. They are sufficiently sensitive to his needs so that ambivalent conflicts are reduced to a minimum. Then the adolescent is able to channelize the new energy into creative and intellectual pursuits that will lead to self-realization. The energy of adolescence is like atomic energy. It can be used for the destruction of authoritarian domination but at the end may be equally self-destructive, or it can be used for heightened productivity and creativity.

If, however, the adolescent in his growing-up process has had his personality warped because of the overwhelming anxieties he could neither escape from nor handle, there will at this age appear an even greater overt display of his neurotic behavior, for he uses the recently increased available energy to strengthen his neurotic defenses. He then hits out more wildly—or withdraws more completely—and thus does he totally defeat his parents and flaunt at them their helplessness and inadequacy. This extreme defiance stems from early neurotic anxiety and is not a function of adolescence per se but rather the extension of the neurotic pattern into adolescence. The available energy of adolescence is wasted if it must be used to ward off anxiety, anxiety not aroused merely because the adolescent has reached a particular stage in his maturation, but anxiety induced by the superimposed parental anxiety. There is, in this instance, little if any communication between the parents and the adolescent. The cry of the adolescent is that no one understands him. It is the same cry that the stutterer, or the child with infantile speech, or the child who has given up all attempt at verbalization is using. And it is no different from the cry of parents who in desperation continue to beat their heads against a stone wall. Language is a useful tool, but only when a relationship is dynamic—never when it is static and unyieldingly bound by neurotic defenses. There can be no communication between people when each is on vigilant guard lest the other penetrate and alter his way of life.

The transition from infancy to childhood and the transitional period of adolescence are perhaps the most dramatic phases of development because of the anxieties reactivated in the parents. These are also the periods of one's life that are probably most culturally influenced by our social taboos, since during these particular phases of maturation, the psychosexual development plays such a dominant role. The degree of ease or difficulty with which the child mounts the first hurdle may indeed determine his positive or negative acceptance of adolescence, for it is in adolescence that the unresolved conflicts of the earlier phase are again lit up with brilliant intensity.

From this presentation it becomes evident that parent counseling must be as sensitively handled and understood as is the child who presents the dramatic symptom of stuttering or delayed speech. It is to be remembered that often the child upon whom therapy is centered is but the medium through which the parents are able to communicate with a therapist without directly facing therapy for themselves.

It is in group therapy for parents that this phenomenon is clearly brought to light. Though the group is brought together because all of the parents have as a common anxiety children about whom they are concerned, it is rare that a problem concerning a child is brought up after the initial sessions. It is the parents' personal problems and conflicts which they wish to discuss, and when a child is mentioned it is generally in terms of the way in which a parent has identified with the child's behavior, but rarely in terms of a specific problem of the child.

The fight for dominance between the parents, or the threat of insubordination, is one of the most frequent focal points of discussion among the adults and throws much light on the cultural influences on the roles of masculinity and femininity in our society. As the group process evolves, the conflicts between the parents are seen to be as great as, and often greater than, the conflicts between the children and parents. Before too many sessions have passed, there is such little reference to a child that the parental anxiety regarding the children seems to have suddenly been dissipated. It is only then that it becomes apparent how much the personal anxiety of the parents had been displaced, and what price the children had to pay for such displacement.

Psychodrama was used as the therapeutic technique in the groups on which these observations were based. Through this technique the parents, like the children, were helped to crystallize their problems in the very structuring of scenes. They experimented with various solutions to a given problem as they reversed roles, acted in the capacity of audience participation, compared neurotic defenses, and worked on personal evaluations and interpersonal relationships. They were often able to find the distortions in their basic hypotheses and to establish the areas in which their early unresolved conflicts were influencing their adult behavior. Though the limitations of group therapy are not to be minimized, psychodrama remains an excellent tool for parent counseling. The members of the group are helped to concentrate on facing and working out their personal conflicts without focusing their attention almost exclusively on their displaced anxieties regarding their children.

## BIBLIOGRAPHY

BARBARA, D. A. 1954. Stuttering: a psycho-dynamic approach to its understanding and treatment. New York: Julian Press.

BRENNER, C. 1955. An elementary textbook of psychoanalysis. New York: International Universities Press.

DORWIN, C., and ZANDER, A. 1953. Group dynamics. Evanston, Ill: Row, Peterson.

FENICHEL, O. 1945. The psychoanalytic theory of neurosis. New York: Norton.

FREUD, A. 1946. The ego and the mechanisms of defense. New York: International Universities Press.

FREUD, S. 1936. The problem of anxiety. New York: Norton.

FROMM, E. 1951. The forgotten language. New York: Rinehart.

HAHN, E. 1943. Stuttering: significant theories and therapies. Stanford, California: Stanford Univ. Press.

POLLAK, O. 1952. Social science and psychotherapy for children. New York: Russel Sage Foundation.

# CHAPTER 33

# GROUP STRUCTURE IN SPEECH THERAPY

● *Ollie Backus, Ph.D.*

THE TERM *group therapy* seems to have come into use more because of a historical accident than because of its adequacy in describing structural relations in the therapeutic process. Its use has created some confusion in theory which needs to be clarified.

The advent of the term *group* applied to therapy implies that something in the nature of "individual" therapy had already existed. The current use of the two terms *therapy* and *group therapy* carries the implicit assumption that the process of therapy consists basically of a two-person structure, with group therapy as a possible adjunct or alternative. When one surveys human behavior generally, however, it is *group* structure which appears basic in human relationships: in the family, school, church, community. It is the group which seems to constitute the unit or whole, with two-person relationships emerging by a process of differentiation within the whole. Moreover, in human behavior generally there does not appear to be the dichotomy which the words *individual* and *group* imply. The term *group* is used to designate various numbers of persons, such as 100, 15, 6; the term subgroup also is applied to various numbers of persons, as 8, 4, 3, and includes also 2 persons. One may well wonder why, in the area of human activity called therapy, a part function rather than the whole should constitute the frame of reference, and why a dichotomous rather than a gradational concept should be employed.

Historically, the use of the two-person relationship in therapy seems understandable enough. Early workers had noted that many children had not acquired adequate speech and that by and large the customary procedures at home, in education, and in medicine were ineffectual in helping them acquire it. Those unmet needs for help, viewed within the frame of reference of such customary procedures, became "special." So a beginning was made in research, clinical diagnosis, and treatment. Perhaps it was because these early efforts were carried on with single clients that the two-person situation became traditional. At any rate, somewhere along the way the tacit assumption was made that because the problem concerned "individnal" needs, the solution required "individaul" treatment; that treatment was somehow more "special" if it was carried on "individually." As knowledge and technical skills became organized into the professional field known as speech therapy, that assumption remained, with the term *therapy* being essentially synonymous in meaning with "individual instruction."

Meanwhile, however, in connection with the general search for solutions to problems in therapy, some experimentation with groups had begun. Clancy in the nineteen-thirties started a camp-clinic for boys on the assumption that individual treatment could be made more effective if it were carried on within the context of group living. The writer in 1942 began experiments in group therapy (Backus and Dunn, 1944) on the assumption that therapy should be conceived of as including *use of speech* in social situations as well as drill on speech production. Such social situations could be provided by having clients meet with the therapist in groups as well as individually. From the first, group and individual therapy were viewed in terms of a whole-part relationship: the group was conceived of as the whole, individual therapy as a part. In the field generally, however, the introduction of "group therapy" created the idea of a dichotomy between the two; that is, a therapist must choose either one or the other.

When the experimentation began, the techniques employed for group classes were those known and used in individual practice, as might be expected. These consisted largely of drills for ear training, drills for producing single speech sounds and speech patterns, drills for muscular exercise. Although the development of procedures for group practice was of immediate and persistent interest, it was not this that constituted the early contributions from the experimentation.

These early contributions (Backus and Dunn, 1947a) consisted, first of all, of new kinds of observation of behavior which group situations made manifest. Then came some tentative modifications in theory which those observations seemed to justify. The modifications in theory related both to the nature of speech disorders and the task of therapy.

For example, observations of clients in social activities as well as drill situations showed clearly that the ability to produce conventional speech patterns in a drill-type situation is by no means equivalent to the ability to produce them in a social situation. It became apparent that more is involved in the process of therapy than mere repetition and drill. Hence the study of situations involving use of speech became important. Situations involving use of speech and those involving drill on speech production were viewed in terms of a whole-part relationship, with the material used for drill consisting of the same speech patterns as those used in social situations (Backus and Dunn, 1947b). In the field generally, however, the introduction of the idea of use of speech as part of therapy resulted again in a dichotomy.

Moreover, observation of a group of clients having various kinds of speech disorders revealed basic similarities among persons with different types of disorder. For instance, speech "breakdowns" occurred in social situations not only among those who stutter but also among those with symptoms of cleft palate, articulation, cerebral palsy, voice, and hearing loss. Observation also revealed basic differences among persons with the same type of disorder. For example, for one person with cleft palate the social pressure would be greatest with persons viewed as "in authority"; for another it would be greatest with peers, and so on. The class labels indicating kinds of disorders came to have less and less meaning as determinants of procedures in therapy, and the notion grew that there are certain basic aspects of therapy common to all persons with speech disorders (Backus, 1950a and b).

Such experiences also provided evidence that the act of observation represents an interpersonal process; that is, what a therapist observes depends not only upon the behavior of the client but also upon the therapist's assumptions and values (Backus and Beasley, 1951). Consider, for instance, a therapist who conceives of speech only in terms of a tongue, palate, ear, or damaged nerve tract, who attributes the persistence of the speech symptoms to something called "habit"—the conditioned-reflex type of response demonstrated in animal behavior—and assumes that their removal rests on the client "being taught" to speak differently. That therapist tends to observe in the client only the mechanics of speech production. On the other hand, consider a therapist who conceives of speech as an aspect of human behavior, who attributes the persistence of the speech symptoms to psychological as well as physiological causes, and assumes that their removal depends upon psychotherapeutic experiences as well as practice on motor skills. Such a therapist also observes psychological aspects of behavior—indications of anxiety, resentments, feelings of inferiority, and so on. The old dichotomy between "organic" and "functional" speech disorders had to be abandoned as it became increasingly evident that persons with organic problems also had "emotional" problems which blocked progress. Speech behavior had to be defined in functional, or psychological, terms for all clients for the inescapable reason that human problems are inextricably bound up with human perceptions and feelings. Thus, at process levels, the conception is one of a whole-part relationship, with organic or physiological aspects included as part functions. In the field generally, however, the relationship has been conceived, again, as a dichotomy.

As speech came to be defined as *an aspect of behavior* rather than just as a motor skill, it became evident that whatever laws govern behavior change in general, must govern behavior change in respect to speech (Backus, 1952). Continued experimentation was supplemented, therefore, by an intensive study of the literature in the various fields comprising the newly developing "science of man." This resulted in a scrutiny of the assumptions and values underlying speech therapy as practiced and as it might be developed so as to be consistent with these modern theories of human behavior.

As the experimentation in group therapy progressed, it seemed increasingly evident that the particular value of a group structure lay, not in its mass production features as a labor-saving device, not merely in its physical characteristic of the availability of numbers of clients for the creation of life situations in the clinic, but *in its potential for facilitating psychotherapeutic change.* It is this assumption that has formed the basis for the development of procedures specifically relating to group structure. These procedures cannot be understood or appreciated within the frame of reference of the older assumptions regarding speech therapy. At the same time, the newer assumptions and many of the newer procedures are not limited to the many-person situation but can apply as well to the two-person situation. Thus it has become increasingly difficult to discuss "procedures for group therapy" as dichotomized from "procedures for therapy."

Fortunately, the trend stemming from experimentation in group therapy is evident also in reports of other experimentation in the field. During the past few years the literature has contained many articles which, while not referring specifically to the term *group therapy,* are reporting on clinical practice which has broken through the limitations of the two-person structure. Public school programs widely use groups of children. In various summer clinics, clients are brought together for residence and have group activity at least in respect to recreation and social life (Clancy and Morley, 1950). Many clinics use projects in which clients go to stores or make speeches before groups outside the clinic (Van Riper, 1947). These clearly involve multiperson structure. Also in the literature one notes an increasing emphasis being placed on the psychological aspects of human behavior: the role of emotional conflict in the etiology of speech disorders, parent counseling, client counseling, the need for psychotherapeutic type of experiences in therapy in place of older intellectualized approaches (Duncan, 1953; Low *et al.,* 1953; Thorn, 1947; Harris, 1950; Van Riper, 1947; Wyatt, 1949). This indicates that clinical practice is being conceived in broader terms than merely mechanical aspects of speech production. Thus, dichotomies in the field as a whole are gradually being dissolved; professional workers who once took a strong position on either one side or the other of certain basic issues are now coming closer together both in outlook and in practice.

The time appears appropriate, therefore, to outline a theoretical structure for speech therapy which will include within a single system (1) both the two-person and multiperson structure, but with the elimination of the outmoded terms *individual* and *group;* (2) both the psychological and physiological aspects of human life, but with the elimination of the outmoded concepts "structural" and "functional."

### THEORETICAL FOUNDATIONS

The science of man represents a nondichotomized approach to the study of human behavior, as different from old concepts which yielded only an aggregate of sciences of part functions. It is relatively so new among the sciences that hypotheses about behavior by and large have not yet been sufficiently verified by experiment to warrant the use of the term *law* in any specific sense. The term *assumption* will be used, therefore, to indicate hypotheses which are supported by some evidence and which seem fruitful to use as conceptual tools. Since there is by no means universal agreement about the assumptions themselves or the verbal constructs to be used in expressing them, each worker to some extent must make choices of those which seem best to fit the facts as he has observed them in his field. This writer has been profoundly influenced by field theory (Lewin, 1935, 1936, 1951), general semantics (Korzybski, 1933; Hayakawa, 1948; Johnson, 1946; Lee, 1941; Rapoport, 1950), interpersonal theory (Sullivan, 1947, 1952; Mullahy, 1949; Horney, 1937, 1939, 1942, 1945, 1950; Fromm, 1941, 1947), the theory of symbolic transformation (Langer, 1951), and client-centered theory of therapy (Rogers, 1950). The presentation of theory which follows is admittedly not detailed enough to yield understanding to one unfamiliar with the body of knowledge from which it has been abstracted; its purpose is rather to outline the structure on which this theory of speech therapy is based.

### Field Theory

"Field theory is more an approach to the scientific task than a theory about a realm of data," said Cartwright (1951, p. viii). It constitutes a way of viewing causation, not in terms of the essence or substance of the object of inquiry, but in terms of the *structural relations* existing in a field of forces. It states that behavior is equivalent to a function of the *object interacting with environment.* Causes for behavior are to be sought in the *relations of parts to whole* as well as in the relations between parts. Causation is conceived in a *multivalued* rather than a single-valued sense. It is conceived as the resultant of forces existing *in a given field at a given time,* "resultant" implying a process characterized by interaction rather than addition. Causes are to be found in the *present* field, not in past or future fields. Causes are to be found at *deeper-lying levels,* not in the surface manifestations which are the symptoms.

Field theory was first applied in the natural sciences, then in the biological sciences, and more recently in the social sciences. It is a recognized principle in science that phenomena at a particular level of complexity in organization are governed by laws specific to that level, and that scientific investigation must seek constructs appropriate to that level. Thus it was not possible to build a science of biology by attempting to reduce the data to physical terms, nor could human behavior be understood by attempting to reduce the data to biological terms. Scientific constructs appropriate to *human* life have had to be sought.

### Theory of Symbolic Transformation

That human life is so profoundly different from animal life as to constitute a different whole, with a different relationship among parts, is becoming more generally recognized. The greater development of a part of the nervous system, the cerebral lobes of the brain, makes the *whole* organism different from animal organisms. Freud showed recognition of this in pointing out that behavior is caused more by "emotional" than "intellectual" or "rational" processes (Horney, 1939). Numerous writers have emphasized the importance of values in human life. Horney (1937) and Fromm (1941) have stressed the influence on behavior of values in the culture. Sullivan (1947, 1952) emphasized the role of symbolic processes in the development of the human individual. Korzybski especially (1933) emphasized the semantic or meaning reactions which make human behavior different from animal behavior. Langer (1951), it seems to this writer, has presented the most adequate theoretical formulation in her development of the concept "symbolic transformation of experience." Langer points out that human beings not only experience events, they symbolize them. She goes on to say that the brain produces symbols night and day from birth to death just as the heart, kidneys, blood vessels, perform their functions as part of their structure (1951, p. 41). These symbols exist at nonverbal levels: some of them can be mapped easily in words, some cannot; many are outside of awareness.

Explanations for human behavior are to be sought not merely in the individual's experience of an event but especially in the symbolic transformation that has accompanied his experience of it. For example, two students were in a situation with a teacher who offered help. To student *A* the teacher's offer symbolized something which could be described roughly as friendliness; hence he accepted with signs of pleasure. To student *B* it symbolized "power over" associated with "self as worthless"; hence he showed increased tension and signs of withdrawing from the situation. The theory of symbolic transformation of experience appears to constitute an integrating principle for the science of life at the human level. It requires that human behavior be defined as a *whole* in psychological terms, with physiological aspects of that behavior viewed as part functions of the whole.

### Interpersonal Theory

Interpersonal theory represents an application of field theory to human behavior (Sullivan, 1947, 1952). It builds on Freud's three postulates (1) that behavior is caused, that is, does not occur by chance, does not belong in the realm of the mystical or unknowable; (2) that behavior is caused more by "emotional" than "intellectual" processes; (3) that it is caused by unconscious as well as conscious processes (Horney, 1939). It rejects, however, the Freudian postulate of inborn traits, together with its verbal construct "instinct." It postulates instead that human behavior develops within a context of interpersonal relationships, and that explanations for behavior should be sought in terms of relationships rather than static traits. It makes *the situation* the unit of study, so that behavior is defined in terms of the relationships between persons making up a given situation. Relationships between parts in the person are not ignored, but are viewed in respect to the whole instead of as separate entities.

Causes for behavior are to be found in the situation *at the time it occurs* (Lewin, 1951, p. 63). The past only as it exists in the present field can cause present behavior. For example, a nerve tract damaged at birth influences present behavior because it is still damaged. A past event cannot cause present anxiety, but a present event can cue off the same symbolism as experienced in the past and hence arouse anxiety. As Horney reiterated (1937), "What is it *now*" that makes the person cling to behavior he has used in the past? Similarly the future only as it exists in the person's present perception can influence present behavior.

Causes of the directly observable behavior (symptoms) are to be found in the relationships existing at deeper-lying levels (Lewin, 1951, p. 241). For example, two individuals may have similar symptoms such as "moving toward" another person with gestures of friendliness; in the one it may stem from a genuine wish to relate to the person, but in the other it may stem from a compulsion to be liked by anybody.

Caus*es* rather than *the cause* are sought. These causes, assumed to be interactive rather than additive, represent a combination of symbolic or psychological functions with physiological functions. They are conceived as applying in all human behavior, not just in those individuals judged to have "emotional maladjustments."

Causes reside in factors *outside* as well as inside awareness. Sullivan's choice of the phrase "outside-inside of awareness" is considered preferable to the phrase "the unconscious-the conscious" because it indicates function on a continuum. Sullivan (1952) described the process by which perceptions become excluded from awareness in terms of the amount of anxiety evoked in the individual in his interpersonal relationships.

Causes lie in the situation *as it appears to the person*. The abstraction of events, that is, getting inside an organism impressions of what is outside, has been pointed out by Korzybski (1933) as a characteristic of behavior of organisms generally. This principle has importance in theory about human behavior for two reasons. The introduction of the term *abstraction* removed the concept of a dichotomy between sensory and symbolic functions. Moreover, that human beings perceive part but not all implies that abstractions from events will be different in different individuals, that the whole perception of each individual will be uniquely *his*. Lewin has pointed out explicitly that explanations for the behavior of an individual are to be sought in *his* perceptual field, in the situation as it appears *to him,* not as it appears to parent, teacher, or any other person (Lewin, 1951, p. 240).

The assumptions about causation in interpersonal theory lead to certain assumptions about change in behavior.

Each person must do *his own* growing, changing, learning. If each person's behavior represents a function of the structure of his psychological world together with the physiological structure of his organism, it follows that changes in behavior have to be made *by him,* not for him nor applied to him by someone else. Thus learning refers to a process of change in the pupil or client, not to the subject matter used in classes, which only constitutes a tool chosen to facilitate change. But the terms *learning* and *teaching* do not indicate the structure of the process that goes on in the individual. Lewin said (1951, p. 255), "Learning is a popular term referring to such different processes as learning to like spinach, learning to walk, and learning French vocabularies." Again he said (1951, p. 66), "Within what is called learning we have to distinguish at least the following types of changes: (1) learning as a change in cognitive structure, (2) learning as a change in motivation, (3) learning as a change in group belongingness, (4) learning in the meaning of voluntary control of the body musculature." Such a definition of learning appears more adequate for human behavior with its symbolic functions than the stimulus-response and conditioned-reflex concepts borrowed from the biology of animal behavior. In respect to the idea that repetition constitutes the chief factor in learning, Lewin pointed out (1951, p. 74), "it is not the repetition itself but the change in cognitive structure which is essential for learning," that is, the change in the meaning that the situation has for the individual. He pointed out also (1951, p. 69) that the direction of learning in human beings appears to be from whole to parts by a process of division rather than the reverse or from parts to whole by a process of addition.

Each person tends to move in the direction of growth; when he does not it is because of the existence of barriers (Horney, 1945, p. 241; Fromm, 1947, p. 2; Rogers, 1950, p. 28). The barriers pertain not only to physiological aspects such as disease, damage to or lack of tissue, but also and especially to psychological aspects such as feelings related to isolation, helplessness, worthlessness, anxiety, hostility. This assumption has been generally accepted in respect to physical growth; it is becoming more generally accepted in respect also to psychological growth. It rests on the nonelementalistic assumption about abstracting—that observation, evaluation, motor response are bound together as a whole in human behavior, that they function *inter*dependently.

It is well known that a healthy organism—one free to move in the direction of growth—is well able to make sharp observations which are then reflected in its behavior. Take, for example, the young child who squats down as his father happens to be doing, same foot forward, same arm on same knee; or the very young child who goes through the motions of reading a book like an older sibling; or the children of various ages who imitate the mannerisms of movie or television stars. Take, for example, even children with some physiological barriers: the child with hearing loss who, without being taught, uses the fundamental principles of lip-reading; or the young blind child who, without being taught, uses the powers of observation he does have to move about easily on the terrain in his neighborhood. The healthy organism seems to have as a basic characteristic the capacity to observe what it has an interest in. When it does not, one must ask the question: What is preventing it from using a capacity it possesses?

Two possible reasons concern *absence of forces promoting observation.* First, if observation proceeds from whole to parts by a process of division it may be assumed that early observation consists of a vague notion of the whole, but without clear differentiation of parts. Hence, in the case either of a young child or any individual observing some process for the first time, the motor aspect of behavior would be expected to show at first absence or distortion of certain parts, but with subsequent refinement as observations included more precise structuring of parts. Second, organization in what an organism perceives means seeing items in patterns rather than singly. This does not necessarily mean the exclusion of detail, but it does mean that certain details will not be perceived as details unless there is some interest in the person himself for so perceiving them. For example, an individual soon ceases to have awareness of a ring on a finger or shoes on the feet because they have no importance to him in a given present. A child does not observe details that have importance to parents or teachers because the details do not have importance in the *child's own world.*

Two reasons concern *presence of forces acting against observation.* Sullivan has emphasized one characteristic of behavior of persons who are becoming more healthy or mature during the process of psychotherapy (Sullivan, 1947); they become increasingly better able to notice what they do, particularly in respect to marginal feelings and thoughts which had previously been outside their awareness. The assumption is that certain observations *have to be excluded from awareness.* One can assume forces acting against observation whenever such observation would cue off symbolism of an unpleasant sort, such as that associated with parental authority in the form of nagging, with a crippled foot, or with a task viewed as impossible to achieve. One may also assume forces acting against observation in cases where a given aspect of behavior has safety functions for the individual. For example, if he is using distorted speech nonconsciously as a symbol of escape toward a less mature level of behavior, or if he is using a crippling condition as his only way of securing relatedness with others, there would be good reason for him to take precautions against giving it up.

The assumption that an organism will move in the direction of growth except for barriers has implications for far-reaching change in procedures in the processes called teaching, therapy, treatment, rehabilitation. Instead of the old notions that when a person does not have an adequate motor response it is because "he does not know how to observe," and that he will be able to observe if "he is taught," teachers and therapists will focus attention more on helping the person *remove the barriers which prevent him from moving toward growth.* This means in some cases giving up the traditional procedure of drill, as being superfluous, wasteful of time, even an added barrier itself to growth. More often, perhaps, it means changing the form of the drill situation and utilizing it differently.

A third basic assumption regarding change in behavior follows from the others: the critical variables for learning reside in interpersonal relationships rather than merely in subject matter. If learning refers especially to changes in the meaning that situations have for the individual, and if the process of teaching means especially helping the person to remove barriers, then *what goes on in the relationship* between client and therapist becomes more essential than the materials themselves. A general definition embracing both teaching and therapy has been formulated as "a particular kind of interpersonal process in which at least one of the participants seeks consciously to keep creating the sort of environment in which each other participant can develop his own potentialities to the greatest extent possible at successive points in time" (Backus, 1952). A therapist or teacher may view the process of creating such an environment as involving the following: (1) creating an atmosphere in which the client can feel acceptance, belongingness, security; (2) facilitating observation; (3) making tools available; (4) providing for the possibility of repeated experience; (5) helping to reduce barriers.

### Therapy

The existence of specialized processes called therapy, in addition to general education, rests on the fact that there have been a considerable number of individuals who have not been able to move in the direction of growth in the various interpersonal situations which have constituted their lives at home, at school, in the community. Since both therapy and general education deal with change in human behavior, they should share the same assumptions regarding human behavior and behavior change; yet a sharp dichotomy has existed between them. Psychotherapy has been devoted almost exclusively to "emotional" aspects of human life, and education has been devoted almost exclusively to "intellectual" aspects.

It appears that psychotherapy has been more consistently based on modern knowledge of behavior change than education has, perhaps because it has contributed so largely to the discovery of that knowledge. Freud and associates, at process levels if not at verbal levels, operated in a field-theoretical frame of reference in certain respects. They recognized that the crucial variables lie in the relationship between client and therapist, that change in behavior occurs in the present even though conversation may relate to past events, that the symbolization of events is more crucial than the events themselves. It has been the contribution of workers since Freud to put these concepts into a more adequate theoretical frame of reference, with consequent continued modification in practice. It appears, however, that psychotherapy has also contributed to the maintenance of the dichotomy through its extreme preoccupation with "the pathological," so that both psychology and education have held the tacit assumption that the discoveries in psychotherapy were restricted to the extremely maladjusted.

Sullivan's definition of psychiatry (1947) as the study of interpersonal relations removes the restrictive dichotomy between "normal" and "pathological." Fortunately, workers in psychotherapy both in psychiatry and psychology are writing books and articles for educators, ministers, parents, and laymen generally in order to share both theoretical knowledge and clinical skills. Fortunately, too, educators generally are making great strides in applying such knowledge and skills in the school situation. As interpersonal relations more generally facilitate growth instead of create barriers to it, psychotherapy should become less necessary for so many people.

Removal of the dichotomy between psychotherapy and classroom education still leaves each field with its own respected area of specialization. The relationship can be conceived of in terms of a continuum, with content as the critical variable. As the writer has stated previously (1952, p. 117): "Thus at one end of the continuum the content of psychotherapy is almost entirely concerned with how the client feels about reality as he perceives it. At the other end of the continuum, the content of classroom education is concerned also (and especially) with information and skills."

It seems evident that what has been said about psychotherapy should apply broadly to all the fields called therapy—including speech therapy, physical therapy, occupational therapy, rehabilitation generally. To quote further from the previous statement by the writer, "Between the two points on the continuum, yet near psychotherapy, the content of speech therapy is concerned somewhat with information and skills related to speech, but also with how the client feels about his perceived reality." Probably speech therapy, because the speech process with which it deals is so closely bound up with symbolization and feelings, should be closer to psychotherapy in function than the others. In actual practice, however, speech therapy along with these others has been closer to classroom education in preoccupation with drill on part functions. In order to fulfill their theoretical potential in respect to behavior change, it seems clear that these fields of therapy will have to break the strangle hold that the old assumptions about learning have held over their procedures.

## Speech Therapy

The assumptions described for the science of man have specific implications for speech therapy.

Speech is viewed squarely as an aspect of human behavior. This means that the assumptions governing human behavior generally govern speech also. For example, explanations for speech behavior should be sought in the symbolic transformation of experience as well as in the events of a situation and in the physical structure of the person. It means also that speech can serve a whole range of human purposes rather than the traditionally expressed ones of "expressing ideas," or of "entertaining, convincing, informing," and so on. Thus, an individual may speak to carry out a social role, to allay anxiety, to increase feelings of personal worth, to gain a request, to make money, to vent hostility, to give information, to fill in time, to combat loneliness. Speech admittedly has a more complex form of organization than some other aspects of behavior. The vehicle of speech is a set of language symbols provided by the culture in which the person lives; the person chooses from among those symbols for his own symbolic utterance; this may or may not (in varying extent) map his own nonverbal symbolic transformations of experience. Furthermore, speech constitutes a particular form of behavior for human relationships. It may well be that there are also specific laws governing behavior at this level of organization, although hypotheses regarding them have not yet been formulated or tested.

Speech is viewed in psychological terms for all persons, not just for those judged to have "maladjustments," nor just for those judged to have "speech disorders." The concept of a dichotomy between normal and disordered speech may have convenience administratively in speech departments, but it is not considered relevant in discovering causal relations in a client's behavior. For instance, available evidence appears to indicate that the same laws which govern phenomena called "stagefright" in the classroom, govern phenomena called "anxiety" in the clinic.

Causes for speech behavior are sought in interpersonal relationships. This constitutes a frame of reference broad enough to include both psychological and physiological functions. For example, it makes possible an analysis not only of the structural relations in the pharynx of a person with cleft palate but also of the structural relations in the situation-as-a-whole, wherein reside the variables which cause him to have less-nasal speech in one situation but more-nasal speech in another. Speech therapy needs to be concerned with both types of analysis if it is to help such a client achieve permanent change in speech behavior.

Causes of directly observable speech behavior (symptoms) are to be found in relationships existing at deeper-lying levels. This assumption has been well recognized in respect to physiological functions; it needs to be as well recognized in respect to psychological functions. The class labels of stuttering, cleft palate, hearing loss, cerebral palsy, articulation, and so on have a useful function in describing symptoms and suggesting areas for special investigation and treatment. They should be abandoned, however, as the *determining frame of reference* for therapy. There are many examples to indicate that such use has had a limiting effect in therapy. Take for example clients labeled as "cerebral palsy." Evidently the symptoms of muscular tension in them are assumed to stem almost exclusively from the nervous system lesion, since the literature describing therapy for them focuses almost entirely on muscle drills. The literature is only beginning to report observations that muscular tension can be markedly reduced without drill when anxiety and hostility are reduced in the client (Duncan, 1953; Coffman and Backus, 1953). It seems evident that a more appropriate frame of reference for therapy generally would consist of constructs relating to reduction of barriers to the development of speech.

Speech behavior is to be explained as the resultant of several causes rather than a single cause. This means, for instance, in respect to hearing loss, that therapy should be concerned not only with auditory training, lip-reading, and so on, but also with what the hearing loss symbolizes to the person and ways in which his perceptions can change. It means also that therapy can be effective for the client even though some of the causes cannot be eliminated. Since causes have interactive rather than additive effect, the reduction of certain causes, say anxiety and hostility, can help a client with damaged nervous system to function in ways that were not possible before. The application of the principle of multiple causation in therapy has had the effect of reducing the number of clients previously judged to be "unable" to learn lip-reading, esophageal speech, and so on.

Causes for speech behavior are assumed to reside in the present rather than the past. Their discovery depends more on observation of a client's behavior in the present than on studying a case history. A case history consists of someone else's report of previous happenings, which at best can only suggest possibilities as to what may or may not be operating currently. When students consider for the first time the assumption about causation in the present, they frequently find it hard to understand, yet all of learning—all of therapy—appears to be based on it at process levels. It is not possible to go back into the past to change behavior; it can only be changed in each present unit of time. An individual feels inferior, stops talking, has rise in muscular tension in a situation at 2 P.M.; then as conversation in that situation shifts to another topic, say at 2:15 P.M., his perception of himself suddenly shifts, his tension level goes down, he begins talking and laughing. Clearly the causes for both types of behavior lie in the present; as the force field shifts for him, his behavior changes. Moreover, such a concept does not rule out continuing factors, such as a damaged auditory nerve. A person with marked hearing loss has certain symptoms not because the nerve was damaged years before during an illness but because it is *still* damaged. Actually the mapping in words of this assumption, which at process levels seems evident enough, opens up wider possibilities for therapy. If causes lie in the present, if they can be understood and removed, then there is great hope for many human problems to be solved. A child labeled "incorrigible" at home or school, or even in past sessions of therapy, can be helped to function more appropriately if the forces in his present field can be structured to meet his needs. A client not previously helped in therapy can acquire adequate speech if the barriers in him can be reduced in a present situation.

Causes for speech behavior reside in factors outside as well as inside awareness. This assumption has implications for speech therapy both in respect to the observations and evaluations the therapist makes about a client, and in respect to the procedures that are used in therapy. For example, some therapists have doubted the theory that stuttering symptoms stem from anxiety associated with hostility. When a client does not say that he feels anxious or hostile and especially when he shows socially accepted modes of behavior, evidences of hostile feelings in behavior are frequently not noted. When, however, a program of speech therapy is built on the assumption that behavior in all persons is to some extent governed by factors outside of awareness, speech therapists become more oriented to observing signs of hostility in behavior, as do clients.

Causes for speech behavior lie in the situation as it appears to the client. When a speech therapist holds this assumption he is not so prone to make a diagnosis for *this* client on the basis of what he has known about fifty other clients. Neither does such a therapist assume that *telling about* something is equivalent to a client's having experienced it. Diagnosis becomes more a collaborative function, and one that is essentially not complete until therapy is over. Therapy too becomes more a collaborative process, a searching together by therapist and client for solutions that are right *for the client.*

Each client must do his own growing, changing, learning in speech therapy. Therapy based on this assumption becomes more client-centered, less equipment- or material-centered. It provides more opportunity for clients to experiment, to make choices for themselves. It becomes less intellectualized and more centered on feelings associated with speech in the present interpersonal situations that make up the clinic program.

Each person tends to move in the direction of growth; when he does not it is because of barriers. This assumption affects the kind of questions a speech therapist asks. How does the world look to this six-year-old? How much "power over" does he perceive? To what extent does he feel loved? How does he view himself? Others? What does having a cleft palate, for instance, symbolize to him? What anxieties, what resentments does he have? What defenses against them? What barriers keep him from observing speech around him more sharply? Such questions affect the observations a speech therapist makes. He looks at more than a tongue, palate, ear; he observes also the behavior of the client in various situations; with him, with parents, with peers. Such observations necessarily affect the structure of therapy.

Before concluding this presentation of "theoretical foundations," it seems appropriate to chart as explicitly as possible the relationship between speech therapy and psychotherapy. In an article dealing with collaboration among psychiatrists, pediatricians, clinical psychologists, and speech therapists, the writer stated (1952*a,* pp. 242–243):

> Scientific endeavor generally has entered an era which might be described as specialization-with-collaboration. . . . The old concept of boundaries as lines in the sense of barriers is being discarded. Human beings in real life do not fit neatly into dichotomies. . . . Nor can the specialists treating them guarantee to categorize their own behavior. . . . It seems evident therefore that boundary relationships must be conceived of as *regions of shared activity.*

Three aspects of shared activity were described as follows:

> (1) Each field should share with the others at the level of theory, *i.e.,* the subject matter of each should stem from a common scientific base; (2) each should have a knowledge of the working principles of the other specialties; (3) each should share with the others an area at the level of clinical practice.

At the level of clinical practice it seems evident that speech therapy and psychotherapy should share some tools in common: speech therapy can make use of some of the tools of psychotherapy, such as techniques of counseling and play therapy; psychotherapy can make use of some of the tools which are being developed in speech therapy, such as techniques which help the individual develop social skills and which promote group structure as a source of support for him. Differences between the two fields can be specified in terms of the kinds of observation emphasized: speech therapy facilitates observation of behavior especially in regard to use of speech and mechanics of speech production; psychotherapy facilitates observation of behavior especially in regard to symbolic transformation of experience. They are also different in respect to the task of removal of barriers: psychotherapy has specialized knowledge and skills available for clients who are not able or would not be able to remove barriers to growth in the speech therapy situation.

## OPERATIONAL ANALYSIS

The development of a theory of speech therapy should include not only an analysis of basic assumptions in the science of man, but also an analysis of those assumptions as they operate in a program of speech therapy. The program presented is one which occurred at the University of Alabama Speech and Hearing Clinic. It was chosen because it consists of four clinic groups running concurrently: two based especially on similarity of clients in respect to age level (young adult and children), one on similarity in respect to ability in locomotion, manipulation, language (preschool cerebral palsy), one on similarity in respect to role (parents). Any one program is never exactly duplicated at this clinical center; certainly it will not be suitable in all respects for other types of clinical centers. It is intended to show that the same basic principles apply regardless of age, type of speech disorder, role of client (i.e., regardless of whether a client's speech is disordered or within normal range). The discussion which follows also includes suggestions for modification to meet particular needs without violation of basic principles.

### Organization

The program consisted of 96 persons: 44 clients with speech disorders, 22 parent-clients, 11 therapists, 19 student-therapists. These persons were organized into 4 groups. Table 1 shows enrollment in each group, duration of program, and certain characteristics represented in clients.

It will be noted in the table that clients are grouped roughly by age range to obtain some similarity of interest in each group. Knowledge about chronological age needs to be supplemented by knowledge about social and intellectual maturity; that is, a relatively mature child of eight might be better placed in a somewhat older age group. The range can be wider among older clients, as in the young adult group. It needs to be narrower among children —6–7 years, 8–10, 10–12 years (see Table 2, p. 1044, for subgroups in children's program). In the cerebral-palsy program, levels of ability in locomotion, manipulation, and language development constitute more important variables than chronological age.

Most programs contain more boys than girls. Since it is usually important for a client not to be the only member of his sex in a group, frequently one must make an effort to add one or two girls, or put a child into a different age group where there are others of his sex, or perhaps even delay his clinical training a session. In the young adult group it is considered desirable in a group of 12–15 to have at least four or five girls so that social aspects of boy-girl relationships will be represented concretely in the clinical situation.

**TABLE 1. Description of Clinic Groups Comprising a Program of Speech Therapy**

| Variables | Young Adult | Children | Preschool Cerebral Palsy | Parents |
|---|---|---|---|---|
| Duration of program | 6 wks. | 5 wks. | 6 wks. | 5 wks. |
| Daily hrs. (M-F) | 8–12 A.M. | 8–11:30 A.M. | 9–11 A.M. | 8–11:30 A.M. |
| No. therapists | 4 | 4 | 2 | 1 |
| No. student therapists | 5 | 10 | 4 | 2 |
| No. clients enrolled | 15 | 23 | 6 | 22 |
| Age Range of clients | 16–25 yrs. | 6–12 yrs. | 3½–8 yrs. | 25–45 yrs. |
| Sex of clients | 9M, 6F | 15M, 8F | 4M, 2F | 22F daily 1–4M occas. |
| *Speech symptoms represented* | | | | |
| Delayed speech | | x | | |
| Articulation | x | x | Varying symptoms | |
| Cerebral Palsy | x | x | in respect to: | |
| Cleft palate | x | x | language develop- | |
| Stuttering | x | x | ment | |
| Hearing loss | x | x | locomotion | |
| Childhood aphasia | x | x | manipulation | |
| Adult aphasia | x | | | |
| *Educational level attained* | | | | |
| Elem. school | x | x | | x |
| Jr. High | x | | | x |
| Sr. High | x | | | x |
| College | x | | | x |
| Grad. School | | | | x |

Insofar as possible, children are accepted for therapy only if one parent attends the parent group. In this particular session, several children had no parent who could attend and a few mothers had two children in the clinic. The mothers of five of the children in the preschool cerebral-palsy program did not attend, since they had been in several previous groups and it was felt more profitable for them to use the time for personal freedom. One father came regularly for the three weeks that he was able to attend; several other fathers attended once or twice as they were in town visiting. The enrollment of 22 in the parent group was considered larger than optimum for the type of activity carried on; 12 to 15 is usually preferable.

A wide range in respect to educational attainment and socioeconomic level has not constituted a problem in young adult and parent groups, although careful planning in this respect is done by the therapist. In the process of enrollment an effort is made to consider for every client the possibility of close congeniality with at least one other member in the group. Then as the program begins and the therapist sets out to create an atmosphere of acceptance, he encourages group members to describe similarities and differences among members. He stresses both by his words and actions the value held in the clinic of respect for each human being, which means respect for differences as well as similarities.

It will be noted in the table that both young adult and children's groups are composed of persons with various kinds of speech symptoms. It has been the experience of the writer and colleagues over some ten years of clinical experience that dissimilarity in speech symptoms does not constitute a critical variable in multiperson situations in therapy. It is felt that Lewin states the situation well (1951, pp. 146 f.):

Conceiving of a group as a dynamic whole should include a definition of group which is based on interdependence of the members. . . . It seems to me rather important to stress this point because many definitions of a group use the similarity of group members rather than their dynamic interdependence as the constituent factor. It is typical of well-organized groups of high degree of unity to include a variety of members who are different and have different functions within the whole. Not similarity, but a certain interdependence of members constitutes a group.

Where therapy is conceived in terms of the creation of an environment in which a client becomes able to solve his problems, the dynamic property of interdependence among group members has more importance than the similarity of symptoms. Moreover, in the parts of the program which deal with observation of speech production the dissimilarity of clients in respect to speech symptoms can be utilized for therapeutic purposes with a high degree of effectiveness. For example, in observing each other a client can perceive *what is right* as well as what is wrong with his own speech; he is also able to offer help to someone else in producing a speech pattern—one who stutters can make an *r* sound for a client with an articulatory problem. When there is a particular reason for one or several clients to meet together because of a common problem they do so, of course. For instance, several clients with nasality meet together for awhile as a subgroup to focus especially on that problem; clients who stutter meet together sometimes to discuss problems specific to the stuttering condition; similarly, the girls in the young adult group meet together sometimes to consider problems of make-up and hair styling.

The presence of a separate group called "preschool cerebral palsy" may appear, at first thought, paradoxical. These children were enrolled in a separate group, however, not because they were classified by type of disorder, but because they had special needs in regard to locomotion and manipulation. It will be noted in Table 1 that other clinic groups have individuals with cerebral palsy in their membership. It is felt that young children who have great difficulty in locomotion and manipulation can be helped best in a program geared to their abilities. Similarly many deaf children, as well as older clients with aphasic symptoms and with laryngectomy, need their own programs for certain specified periods. It is considered extremely important, however, for clients in these groups to have regular contacts with other clients; for example, for the children in the preschool cerebral-palsy group to meet with those in the children's group for certain activities.

Another feature to be noted in Table 1 relates to duration of program. There is no one duration period considered "the right one" for short-term intensive periods of therapy. The periods for the program described were determined by length of summer session; during the regular school year periods of six, seven, and eight weeks are used for the children's and adult groups, 12 weeks for preschool cerebral palsy. The duration of the daily program is influenced by needs of the clients—younger children do not stay at the clinic as long as older clients.

The important point about duration is the short-term intensive, or block, design. It is felt from clinical experience that a program of therapy involving fifteen hours a week for six weeks accomplishes more than the same number of hours (90) spread over a year at the rate of 2½ hours a week. For one thing, in a nonintensive program so much time has to be spent each day recreating group structure that therapy appears not to move along as satisfactorily. Moreover, in such a nonintensive program the variety of types of interpersonal situations is necessarily more restricted in a given period; yet several types rather than just one or two are felt to have importance (for building an atmosphere of acceptance, observing part functions, communicating feelings, etc.). When the short-term idea was begun it was chiefly for reasons of expediency: to take care of different age groups at different times in the course of a year and to provide for nonresident clients whose parents could not come with them for longer periods. It has been continued as a preferable way of carrying on therapy, however, both in the University center and in public school clinics where it has been tried. As the concept of therapy has changed from that of "teaching the child how to talk" to that of helping the child remove barriers to learning, the goals have changed and hence the procedures. What is done now is directed not so much toward progress in speech while the child is in the clinic, but toward progress in removing barriers so that the child will get in condition to do his own growing, wherever he may be—in the clinic or at home. Experimentation has shown that children almost invariably have improved markedly during the three- to six-month periods *between* programs of therapy. The short-term periods appear, therefore, more efficient and economical.

Modifications in form to suit other types of clinical situations can be made without sacrificing the basic principles, which are felt to be sound for any type clinic. For example, one therapist working alone can have only one group at a time and will want a smaller enrollment than indicated here. He can have different age groups at successive periods of time, however, as Matis (1956*) has done at the Florence, Alabama, Speech and Hearing Center. Thus, in the course of a year the various age groups can be accommodated. He can have a parent group while children are on the playground under the supervision of a paid assistant or volunteer worker. A therapist working in public schools may not find it possible to spend three or four hours a day with a group of clients, but he can spend from one to two hours a day. He may not find it possible for parent groups to meet every day, but they can meet once a week or at least once a month. It has been this writer's experience through the years that most of the perceived limitations were in her own basic assumptions, and that when she felt a particular kind of clinical practice was important, school administrators did not forbid the development of that practice in some reasonable way. It is felt that the chief requirement for making such modifications in speech therapy in public schools consists of accepting the assumption that speech therapy in public schools should be determined by the needs of the children and the possibilities in the field, rather than by what has been traditional practice. If over a period of time as many children can be helped, and if the results are more lasting, then a smaller enrollment at a given time will not appear threatening.

### n-Person Relationships Involved

The variation in number of persons involved in the various interpersonal situations which make up the daily and weekly schedule for each group enrolled is shown in Table 2.

In the young adult group, the whole group met together several times a week for social events, sports, club meeting, and discussion of particular problems involving all members. The membership was divided into two groups for two hours each day; divided into subgroups once or twice each day for particular purposes. Each client had an opportunity of meeting with a therapist several times a week for counseling and/or special help on speech.

In the children's group, the whole group met together daily for swimming, weekly for sports and parties. The membership was divided into three groups daily for an hour to an hour and a half; divided into subgroups of three to five each day. A few of the children had individual sessions with the therapist daily; others weekly.

In the preschool cerebral-palsy group, the whole group met together for a social event each day. The membership was divided on the basis of ability into two groups for an hour. Each child had daily experience in a two-person situation with a therapist.

TABLE 2. Variation in Number of Persons Involved in Interpersonal Situations

|  | Young Adult | Children | Preschool Cerebral Palsy | Parents |
|---|---|---|---|---|
| Clients | 15 | 23 | 6 | 22 |
| Therapists | 4 | 4 | 2 | 1 |
| Student-therapists | 5 | 10 | 4 | 2 |
| Total | 24 | 37 | 12 | 25 |
| 8 to 27 persons (whole group) | several times a wk. 1–2 hr. | daily 1 hr. | daily ½ hr. | 4 days a wk. 1 hr. |
| 4 to 10 persons | 2 groups (12, 12) daily, 2 hr. | 3 gr (11, 12, 14) daily, 1 hr. | 2 gr (6, 6) daily, 1 hr. | 3 gr (7, 9, 8) occasionally 1 hr. |
| 3 to 5 persons | daily ½–1 hr. | daily ½–1 hr. | occasionally ½ hr. | occasionally ½–1 hr. |
| 2 persons | several times weekly; ½–1 hr. | daily for some, weekly for others; ½–1 hr. | daily; ½ hr. | weekly, cr as needed |

Members of the parent group came with the children at eight o'clock, usually talked in subgroups for an hour, sometimes were invited to join children's groups for participant observation. Then for an hour the entire group (23) met together. Members frequently went for coffee as a group after that, continuing discussion. During the next hour some had conferences with a therapist, some formed subgroups of two to six for discussion, some visited their child's group, some visited other clinic programs, some went shopping, some spent the time reading.

As indicated in Table 2, the clients and therapists in each of the four groups constituted a whole. Each of the four groups, however, had a number of regular contacts with other groups in the clinic, as well as with persons in the department and individuals outside: all met frequently at the Coke shop operated by the young adult group; the preschool cerebral-palsy group met with younger children's group for parties; children and young adults had several ball games; parents and children met for demonstrations, parties, and swimming. Members of all four groups had contact with University classes in the Speech Department and with frequent visitors at the clinic, had contact with persons at stores, swimming lake, and places visited. Thus, "whole" group in each case existed also as a part of various larger wholes.

In clinics having only one therapist the following modification has been used successfully: one subgroup of children comes, for example, at 1:00 P.M.; a second subgroup comes at 2:00; both form a larger group from 2:00 to 2:30, at which time subgroup 1 goes home; subgroup 2 stays until 3:30. Another modification to provide for subgroups is to make use of volunteer workers who can supervise recreation or social events, depending on the training and skill of the workers. Two-person situations can be scheduled daily for different clients before and after the group meetings.

## Kinds of Interpersonal Situations

Since the process of therapy is conceived in terms of interpersonal relationship, interpersonal situations of various kinds are used as the *instruments* by which the process called therapy is brought about. It has seemed fruitful to view the situations in terms of seven categories, as shown in Table 3. Three of the categories (1 6, 7) are called general in the sense that the situations comprising them do or can occur outside a clinic in everyday life; four of the categories (2, 3, 4, 5) are called specialized in the sense that the situations comprising them occur only as clinical or treatment situations.

**1. Experiences in human relatedness occurring in everyday life.** It will be noted in Table 3 that from the multitude of situations which go to make up human life, certain ones were selected for incorporation in the clinic program. The social events include particular situations such as greetings, introductions, invitations, expressions of appreciation, asking favors, getting acquainted, small talk, communication for the sake of companionship, sharing, solving problems, dancing, card-playing and other games. The social events involve the roles of guest and host; shopping, eating out, and the Coke shop involve the roles of customer and clerk; club activities involve the roles of leader and follower. These situations involve also both peer and authority relationships. The situations selected for use in a given clinic program will depend on the needs and preferences of therapist and clients. They are selected and utilized for purposes of therapy, but are real in the sense that they actually occur; they are not staged as "make believe" or "let's pretend."

**2. Specialized experiences in analyzing use of speech.** These are provided by laboratory situations in which therapist and clients take a part of a whole which has occurred in (1) above—for example, greetings—and study it carefully. They enact various situations involving greetings, analyze the speech patterns and other behavior used, discuss how clients feel about such situations, what the situations symbolize to them. Similarly, they study situations involving introductions, expressions of appreciation, shopping and so on. These situations are real in the sense that they actually occur as work or practice situations, but they are different from (1) above in that they are staged for purposes of analysis. In these specialized experiences, client and therapist can focus on particular aspects of situations, can stop in the middle to analyze them, then re-enact them as needed. In the situations in (1) above, on the other hand, the situations come and are gone, as happens in everyday life.

**3. Specialized experiences in observation of part functions.** These are provided by laboratory situations which are concerned with smaller parts of a whole, as shown in Table 3—production of speech sounds and patterns, language structure, lip-reading, use of hands, walking, and so on. The term *observation* is used in a broad sense to mean a combination of (a) the sensory aspect of seeing-hearing-feeling, (b) the motor aspect of producing, (c) the associative aspect of perceiving-evaluating in order to perceive differences

TABLE 3. Types of Interpersonal Situations Used as Instruments of Therapy in the Four Groups

| Categories | Young Adult | Children | Preschool Cerebral Palsy | Parents |
|---|---|---|---|---|
| 1. Experiences in human relatedness occurring in everyday life | Social events<br>  open house<br>  picnics<br>  lounging in club rm.<br>Telephoning<br>  bus. & social calls<br>  answering clinic ph.<br>Shopping & eating out<br>  for open house<br>  for coke shop<br><br>Club activities<br>  club meetings<br>  committee meetings<br>Co-operative projects<br>  baseball<br>  swimming<br>  playing cards etc.<br>  activity period<br>  tours | Social events<br>  parties<br>  picnics<br>  free play<br>Telephoning<br>  social calls<br><br>Shopping & eating out<br>  for parties<br>  coke shop<br>  soda bar<br>Club activities<br>  planning parties<br><br>Co-operative projects<br>  baseball<br>  swimming<br>  games<br>  activity period<br>  trips | Social events<br>  parties<br>  picnics<br>  free play<br>Telephoning<br>  social calls<br><br>Shopping & eating out<br>  for parties<br>  coke shop<br>  soda bar<br>Club activities<br>  planning parties<br>  making decorations<br>Co-operative projects<br>  playing with ball<br>  swimming<br>  games<br>  activity period<br>  trips in clinic<br>  trips outside | Social events<br>  parties<br>  picnics<br>  conversation<br>    in subgroups<br>  coffee |
| 2. Specialized experiences in analyzing use of speech | Greetings<br>Introductions<br>Invitations<br>Expr. of appreciation<br>Arrival-leave taking<br>Asking favors<br>Ordering at soda bar<br>Shopping<br>Telephoning<br>Small talk | Greetings<br>Introductions<br>Invitations<br>Expr. of appreciation<br>Arrival-leave taking<br>Asking favors<br>Ordering at soda bar<br>Shopping<br>Telephoning<br>Small talk | Greetings<br>Introductions<br>Invitations<br>Expr. of appreciation<br>Arrival-leave taking<br>Asking favors<br>Ordering at soda bar<br>Shopping<br>Telephoning<br>Small talk | Participating<br>in events in<br>other groups<br>(upon<br>invitation) |

| | | | | |
|---|---|---|---|---|
| 3. Specialized experiences in observation of part functions | Prod. of speech sounds<br>Prod. of sp. patterns<br>Prod. of voice<br>Language structure<br>Lip-reading<br>Auditory training<br>Palatal function<br>Esophageal speech<br>Facial movements<br>Use of hands<br>Voluntary relaxation<br>Posture & movement<br>Walking<br>Etc. | Prod. of speech sounds<br>Prod. of sp. patterns<br>Prod. of voice<br>Language structure<br>Lip-reading<br>Auditory training<br>Palatal function<br>Facial movements<br>Use of hands<br>Voluntary relaxation<br>Posture & movement<br>Walking<br>Etc. | Prod. of speech sounds<br>Prod. of sp. patterns<br>Prod. of voice<br>Language structure<br>Lip-reading<br>Auditory training<br>Palatal function<br>Facial movements<br>Use of hands<br>Voluntary relaxation<br>Posture & movement<br>Walking<br>Etc. | Participating in events in other groups (upon invitation) |
| 4. Specialized experiences in using method of science in behavior | Projects illustrating scientific method & scien. principles e.g., non-allness<br>non-identity<br>many-point sc., etc.<br>Role-playing to illustrate principles<br>Use of prin. in analyzing problems that arise | Projects illustrating scientific method & scien. principles e.g., non-allness<br>non-identity<br>many-point sc., etc.<br>Role-playing to illustrate principles<br>Use of prin. in analyzing problems that arise | As much of projects as feasible in terms of development (emphasis upon application in action) | Projects illustrating scien. method & scien. principles e.g., non-identity<br>many-point scale, etc.<br>Role-playing to illustrate principles<br>Use of prin. in analyzing problems that arise |

**Table 3 (Continued)**

| Categories | Young Adult | Children | Preschool Cerebral Palsy | Parents |
|---|---|---|---|---|
| 5. Specialized experiences in communicating about feelings | Group discussions<br>Role-playing<br>Counseling (n-person)<br><br>Physical activity<br>Drawing, painting | Group discussions<br>Role-playing<br>Play-therapy<br><br>Physical activity<br>Drawing, painting<br>Clay | Group discussions<br>Role-playing<br>Play-therapy<br><br>Physical activity<br>Finger-painting<br>Clay<br>Vocabulary for expressing feelings | Group discussion<br>Role-playing<br>Group client-centered therapy<br>2-person client-centered therapy<br>Physical activity |
| 6. Experiences in acquiring specific information (applied in skills) | Table manners<br>Personal hygiene<br>Make-up, etc.<br>Reading, writing (r.e. aphasia)<br>Arithmetic<br>Playing cards | Table manners<br>Playing cards<br>Use of money, making change | Table manners<br>Concepts of hours, days, weeks;<br>Colors<br>Numbers<br>Playing radio, record player<br>Language concepts "push-pull," "fast-slow," etc.<br>Writing<br>Use of money | Occasional guest speakers when requested |
| 7. Experiences in developing certain abilities | Sports (baseball, football, swimming)<br>Building—bookshelves, etc.<br>Sewing<br>Music, singing, etc. | Sports (baseball, football, swimming)<br>Music, singing, etc. | Throwing, catching, kicking ball<br>Music, singing | Helping individuals arrange for special vocational classes, etc. |

along with similarities. The emphasis is on observing differences between what the person does and what is usually done, rather than upon "what is correct" or what the client "should" do to please some one else. It appears structurally more correct for describing a process of growth than to assume that a client "must be taught" to make sounds.

**4. Specialized experiences in using the method of science in behavior.** The situations in this category are conceived of especially in the sense of making available tools for observing and evaluating situations, and for solving problems. The discipline called general semantics is employed as a guide for using scientific method. These situations usually occur daily in a program until the principles have been presented by way of experiment; then the principles are applied in connection with problems that arise in the clinic program. It will be noted in the table that they are used with persons of all age levels, but at the younger age levels with the chief emphasis upon "doing" rather than upon "talking about."

**5. Specialized experiences in communication about feelings.** The situations concerned with communication about feelings involve both the client-centered type in which the therapist functions to seek to understand and help clients clarify feelings, and the problem-solving type in which the therapist functions also to help clients use scientific methods for finding solutions to specific problems. The situations also include role-playing, play therapy, activities with clay, finger-painting and drawing, and physical activities such as punching bag, running in halls, and tearing paper.

**6. Experiences in acquiring specific information (applied in skills).** These situations are called general in that they would ordinarily take place at home or school. In certain cases, however, they appear to constitute desirable instruments for therapy, such as telling time, differentiating between colors, using the calendar, for children with cerebral palsy or aphasia. In certain cases, too, it appears that these activities can be better carried on by a clinically trained person than by one less familiar with the particular problems of these clients; for example, arithmetic, spelling, writing for adults with aphasia.

**7. Experiences in developing certain abilities.** These refer to activities such as sewing, singing, playing an instrument, card tricks, special instruction connected with a sport—activities that have value to the client for the sake of the pleasure they afford and/or because they give him a sense of having certain abilities. Some apparent overlapping with other categories may be noted; the difference would be one of function or purpose. They differ from (3) above in that whereas those would have value in making him similar to others or in reducing an unwanted difference, these have value in giving him some sense of uniqueness or special ability. They are used clinically in cases where they appear to contribute to helping the client change perceptions of self.

It must be emphasized with the greatest possible clarity that the interpersonal situations used in a program constitute only the materials. It is the utilization of those situations to form interpersonal relationships in which the client changes behavior that constitutes the process of therapy. It is well understood in baking, for instance, that the ingredients form the materials but that more is required for the *process* of baking. One can combine sugar and egg whites, but baking that material slowly in a relatively cool oven produces a very different result (meringues) from beating it over boiling water on top of the stove (seven-minute icing). Again it is well known that what a cook does in kneading dough has a marked influence on the product. In human behavior, too, we are dealing with processes which have *interactive* rather than additive characteristics. The critical variables lie in what we *do* with the materials. The process is more complicated in human relationships than in cooking; the variables are not well enough understood to be listed in specific steps as in a recipe, but some of the directions for proceeding seem clear. The discussion which follows has the purpose of suggesting how interpersonal situations can be utilized for the formation of interpersonal relationships which constitute the process of speech therapy.

**The Process of Therapy**

The therapist's role has been defined as that of creating an environment in which a client becomes able to change behavior. This task has been described as having five aspects: (1) creating an atmosphere in which the client can feel acceptance, belongingness, security; (2) facilitating observation; (3) making tools available; (4) providing for the possibility of repeated experience; (5) helping to reduce barriers.

**1. Creating an atmosphere.** The term *atmosphere* needs to be understood as a verbal construct describing an interpersonal situation at deeper-lying or dynamic levels. Its existence has been generally accepted by laymen (in remarks such as "there was electricity in the air at that meeting"), and it is now scientifically measurable (Lewin, 1951). It has been defined operationally in terms of the behavior of individuals participating in a given situation. The term *atmosphere* will be characterized here as consisting of *acceptance, belongingness, warmth, respect* for each individual as a person of worth. By definition, these characteristics must reside *in the perception of clients* in order to be reflected in their behavior. Thus, the therapist's behavior in creating these conditions must be described in relation to the behavior of clients: the therapist may have attitudes of acceptance and may attempt to communicate such attitudes through his behavior, but an atmosphere of acceptance can be said to exist for a client only as he shows in behavior that he perceives acceptance. Some clients may not indicate that they perceive its existence for some time.

An attempt needs to be made to define this cluster of constructs, although it is difficult to do so satisfactorily when the words cannot accompany and follow nonverbal experience. The term *acceptance* refers to a person's attitudes of relative nonevaluation, which are thus implemented by his surface behavior such as speech, facial expression, posture, gestures, which behavior in turn communicates such attitudes to the other person(s). The word *relative* is used because it is probable that a human organism, which symbolizes as well as experiences events, cannot be conceived of as free from evaluation. In contrast to the almost continual evaluation current in everyday life, however, it is substantially accurate to say that acceptance means virtual elimination of evaluation in counseling and play-therapy situations and great reduction of it in other situations that constitute speech therapy. In maintaining prescribed limits, the therapist is necessarily evaluating an aspect of behavior; but in such cases he makes it clear that it is the behavior but not the whole person that is being evaluated. An important distinction exists between overt actions and feelings: certain actions need to be stopped, but the feelings underlying those actions can be accepted without evaluation, that is, without either disapproval or approval (Baruch, 1949).

Both therapists and parents who have experimented with the notion of acceptance have found that this behavior of *seeking to understand* rather than of evaluating feelings of a child frequently resulted in the child's stopping an action of his own accord. They have discovered also that many of the limits which had been customarily imposed had been set more because of adult values and stereotypes than because of the child's needs, and they found it less necessary to set so many. This writer found in early experimentation that nonevaluation of a client does *not* mean being passive; it means an active process on the part of the therapist but in a different dimension from evaluation—seeking to understand how the world looks to another person at a given point of time. Far from being easy, it appears to constitute the most difficult skill to develop in professional training. The interested reader is referred to books which discuss the subject in greater detail (Rogers, 1950; Axline, 1947; Baruch, 1949), but is urged to do considerable experimenting along with the reading before he evaluates the ideas presented. It is frequently difficult for a beginner or even one with some experience to have attitudes of acceptance for a client's behavior when that behavior threatens his own conceptions of worth and success in his role. On the other hand, it is easy to evaluate with praise the behavior of the client who is functioning as "the good child," because such behavior is so in line with accepted values in the culture and is not troublesome to parent or therapist. It is important to understand that when such behavior is accompanied by other behavior indicative of excessive or indiscriminate compliance, it reflects conflicts as serious as those giving rise in other clients to withdrawing or aggressive behavior.

The attitudes of acceptance and respect for each individual as a person of worth are very closely associated; behavior indicating one seems bound to indicate the other. For example, the parent of a young adult client handed the therapist, in the boy's presence, a week's spending money and a carton of cigarettes for her son. After she had left, the therapist quietly handed both to the boy with the comment, "Here, Fred, I guess you'll know better than I how you want to use these this week; you know there won't be any more until next Monday." Some months later the boy told the therapist he thought that was the first time he'd ever felt that an adult had shown faith in him as a person. As another example, consider a child who does not want to participate in a group activity. The therapist who says simply, "you just don't feel like joining us this time, is that it?" is accepting the child as he is at that moment, is showing respect for him as a person.

In regard to the concept "warmth," there appears to be a range of opinion among writers in psychotherapy. Some feel that a client in psychotherapy has more freedom to become himself if the therapist's own feelings are kept largely out of the relationship. Others feel that the therapist's action to understand the client's world constitutes warmth of a sort that is nourishing; still others feel that there should be a great deal of warmth present in the relationship. This writer feels at this date that this is desirable in speech therapy. Speech therapy has some differences from psychotherapy. For one thing, clients come knowing that they need help with speech but usually not having much awareness that they need help with problems relating to feelings. Moreover, many of them are so accustomed to remain silent whenever possible that they do not at first readily take the initiative in creating an environment to meet their needs. The structure of the program also is different in that it has other types of situations in addition to the type devoted to communication about feelings. It is felt that a therapist in these situations may depart somewhat from strict nonevaluation without violating the basic philosophy of acceptance. It seems possible that certain clients have so little sense of self to go on that they have some real need early to experience honest, spontaneous expressions of warmth, appreciation, even approval from the speech therapist. For instance, one twenty-three-year-old boy asked a therapist if she remembered a remark she had made to him at a party a year before when he had just entered the clinic, "My, you look handsome tonight." He went on to say that at the time it had seemed almost as if she were jeering at him, and yet he had hung onto the memory of the sound of her voice and the look on her face as she said it. He said he felt that may have marked a turning point in his attitude toward self. Certainly a therapist needs to be aware that such a remark to one client may under certain circumstances be perceived by other clients as rejection of them. As members of a group become able to help in the creation of an atmosphere of acceptance and mutual respect, however, such possibilities become more remote. In an atmosphere of acceptance even very young clients start contributing to its maintenance. One mother reported that her six-year-old son, who had been trying her patience one day at home asked, "Mommie, you aren't feeling so good, are you." When she replied, "I have a headache," the boy said, "It seems like maybe you're feeling upset over the way I've been acting."

Feelings of belongingness come as a client perceives acceptance by others. Frequently, however, some initial sense of belongingness can make him better able to perceive acceptance. Participation in a group activity usually results in a shift of one's perceptual field from "self unfavorably compared with others" to interest in the activity itself; hence it fosters development of feelings of belongingness. The particular activities selected will vary with the interests of the group, together with the abilities-disabilities of the members. For instance, for a group to prepare, serve, and eat simple refreshments constitutes something simple and easy to execute at the beginning of a clinic session when many clients are feeling a high degree of tension. Moreover, it does not involve as great a risk of making some feel isolated as a more complicated activity might. Rearranging furniture in a room is frequently used also as an initial activity. Opportunity for free play together, or alone but in a room with others, has been considered especially useful with children.

It appears important to provide opportunities but not to force a superficial semblance of belongingness or groupness. The surface behavior comes as a consequence of changed perceptions. This became especially evident to the writer and co-workers when they were experimenting in the preschool cerebral-palsy clinic to make the program become less equipment-centered. Such acts as the following were considered evidence of emerging groupness or belongingness: one boy reaching over to untie the shoe laces of a girl, who appeared highly pleased at his attention to her; two children each refusing another turn until a third child had his turn; the children greeting each other instead of only the therapist as they came into the room.

The phrase "participant belongingness" is being used with increasing frequency. Probably one aspect does not actually exist without the other. This phrase emphasizes the need for more activity, less passivity on the part of clients if they are to feel belongingness. Groups certainly differ in respect to the ease with which members come to assume greater responsibility for action. Nevertheless, it seems clear that as therapists have more an attitude of respect for an individual's abilities and have more skills in helping clients initiate activity that has meaning *to them at the particular time,* the group members do take over more responsibility for initiated action. This may require that the therapist have tolerance, for instance, for a group decision to continue working on plans for a party when he would feel more personally secure in having them shift to work on speech production. In the course of several days or a week, however, usually some of both can be managed, yet without manipulation or coercion. As clients feel more acceptance they usually begin to communicate more about feelings; this helps to avoid an "intellectualized" atmosphere which exists when therapist and clients are occupied chiefly with subject matter—"talking about" rather than "doing." Activities such as role-playing can serve several purposes concurrently, for example, group participation with active involvement even for observers, vivid presentation of a problem area, experience at nonverbal levels, and so on. In parent groups where questions come up about problems with children, the parents themselves can engage in such activities as tearing paper, giving one or two lusty shouts, or finger-painting, to provide experience at feeling levels to accompany discussion.

It is not assumed that creating an atmosphere such as described means that "all should consist of sweetness and light." Problems are bound to arise in the course of group living. Human beings who come together have anxieties, fears, resentments, feelings of little personal worth, feelings of competitiveness, difficulties in relating both to authority figures and peers, and so on. Moreover, there can be little significant experience of acceptance of "me as I feel I am" if a client does not feel free enough to show the feelings he has. A therapist needs to learn not to feel threatened when problems arise, for it is then that behavior is put to the test. It is then that clients come to experience the consequences both to themselves and others of acceptance instead of evaluation, of their own use of the tools of nonevaluation with reflecting feelings. It is then that they test out the usefulness of the tools of scientific method for working through problems: delaying judgment, communicating on descriptive levels without name-calling, accepting the person while criticizing an item of behavior. It is then that they have an opportunity to see themselves function better than they thought they ever could.

Creating an atmosphere is not a "thing" that gets completed; it is a process, must go on continuously. While it constitutes a particular function for the therapist to perform, it also becomes a function taken on by members of the group. There is no assumption implied that a therapist needs to appear "perfect"; for a therapist to attempt such a role would be contrary to the honesty required in accepting and respecting clients. It is required, however, that a therapist have some degree of self-understanding so he will not project his own attitudes on the group nor act out his own needs to any great extent.

A therapist beginning to explore these ideas and ways of behaving in therapy must begin where he can honestly begin, even though that means only a small departure from his customary evaluation and domination. When this writer began experimenting, she tended to go to an extreme of remaining passive in a group, thereby arousing some anxiousness in some members who perceived her nonparticipation as rejection and hostility rather than as a withholding of evaluation and domination, or "power over." She has been learning to make a more clear-cut distinction between "rational—irrational authority" (Fromm, 1947) and hence feels more comfortable functioning in a group as one member who, like the others, has a certain range of abilities to share with the group. It is thus more possible both to wait while group members struggle and to participate by suggesting possibilities and pointing up issues.

Finally, it should be mentioned explicitly that two-person relationships have importance in building group atmosphere. Frequently it happens that clients will be able to communicate feelings in a two-person situation with a therapist that they could not share with other group members. Frequently also they can discharge strong feelings in such a situation with the result that they contribute more productively to the group situations. Moreover, certain clients have strong need at first for relating to the perceived authority figure and only later can develop satisfying relatedness with peers.

**2. Facilitating observation.** The following assumptions underlie this discussion: (1) a client will automatically observe what he has an interest in or a need for at a given point in time; (2) these interests and needs may not be the same as those which another person thinks he *should* have; (3) his assumptions and values will influence what he observes; his observations will influence what he does in the motor aspects of his behavior. Thus, for example, one child may sit through a drill session in which a therapist hopes he is observing how two speech sounds differ; what the child actually observes, however, is that several other children have new clothes or that the therapist smiled at another child but not at him when he did not give the desired response. A second child whose greatest need is to please authority figures may observe carefully how to give the desired response and may produce it time after time in that situation. Afterward, however, when walking down the hall with his mother, he may give no thought to the new speech response, because he is then busy trying to please his mother by answering her questions and walking quietly. A third child with a great need to please the therapist does not risk responding for fear he will not make the right response. Such examples raise the question: How can a therapist make plans for facilitating observation which will have growth potential for each child, especially at first when he does not know them well?

Certain assumptions can be made with a high degree of probability: the level of anxiousness will be relatively high in all clients entering a new environment, coming as they do with symptoms of disordered speech; they will tend to look for signs of relative hostility, friendliness, as well as signs of what is expected of them in the new environment; their relatively high level of tension will not enable them to observe too clearly details of part functions, such as speech sounds. Thus, a therapist would choose situations in which clients can actively participate with ease and pleasure, and in which he can help them discover what is expected (the limits imposed) while at the same time showing permissiveness, warmth, and acceptance. With young children especially this means to demonstrate *permissiveness—within limits*. With parent groups it involves defining the purpose of the meetings in terms of exploring together ways of helping the child, while explicitly ruling out "blame" or "fault" as reasons for having a parent group. Situations relatively free from threat facilitate observation for parents as well as children. For instance, it commonly happens that a parent volunteers a remark such as this, "You know, I got to thinking at home yesterday; if somebody said 'don't' to me as often as I have to Doris, I'd be a nervous wreck. I notice I do that to her a lot and I'm trying to stop it."

The presence of a group of clients, rather than only one, can do much to help individuals observe details that will change the perceptual field. For example, on the first day of clinic one mother reported that her daughter,

Anne (twelve years old), did not even want to go to Sunday School anymore because of her speech. The next day the mother reported that Anne had said to her, "It's fun to come here; everyone else in my group has trouble talking, too." Another child said to his mother after several days, "You know, I always thought my speech was all bad, but I only have trouble with four sounds. And I don't have anything wrong with my voice as a couple other folks do. I can always get out what I want to say. I mean I don't stutter as Bob does. But he sure makes "s" sounds better than I do. You know I'll bet I really can learn to talk better." Or again in a group a client will exclaim, "Gee, I didn't know anybody else was afraid of teachers [or ashamed to go into a store, or resentful of rules made by parents, etc.]. I thought I was the only one." Such observation of self in relation to others changes attitudes so that further detailed observation becomes increasingly more possible.

The situations structured to analyze use of speech are utilized not only for facilitating observation of conventional modes of behavior but also for facilitating observation of clients' feelings about such events. They eventually discover that about the same dynamic relationships are present in each. As one client said, "You know, it's the same thing in introductions, greetings, invitations, or shopping. I have an awful time because it seems as if I'm way down here and the other person is way up above me. I guess I don't feel equal to anybody." Role-playing activities are especially useful in facilitating observation of feelings of resentment. Clients can play the role of someone else with great display of feeling, then realize later that those feelings were their own.

The situations designed to facilitate observation of part functions of speech are utilized by the therapist to form a different sort of relationship with client(s) from that ordinarily formed in the traditional drill-type situation. The purpose is to help the client to observe differences: "Here is one way of making the sound, here is another way"; or "This is the way many people say it, this is the way you are saying it." The questions to be answered are these: Do you hear the difference between them? Do you feel the difference when you make the sounds both ways? What do you do differently? The purpose is *not* to tell the client what he *should* or *must* do. He is not under pressure to submit to or to please still another adult in authority, nor is he under pressure to keep from making a mistake. He is helped to observe differences, helped to find means of producing new sounds or patterns, helped also to have freedom of choice: sometimes to use the new sounds, sometimes to use the old ones. The analysis may be accompanied with some discussion relating to possible functions of the disordered speech. Such a discussion might go like this: "There are times when any of us feel as if we'd like to be taken care of, wish we were younger like a little brother or sister. Have you ever felt like that?" Children volunteer numerous situations in which they feel this, ways in which they do it, like wanting to be held, lying down and kicking, and so on. Some even volunteer that talking like a baby brother is one way. These feelings are accepted without evaluation. One may say, "Little children often say *wed* for *red*. You could do it if you wanted to; it would be one way of talking." The function of such discussion is not to develop insight into causes, hence the point is not labored. It is rather to accept matter-of-factly some of the feelings which are often present but about which a child may have anxiousness or guilt because of previous evaluations at home or school. It has the effect of reducing barriers to observation. For instance, one third-grade boy suddenly said one day, after several days of such discussion and observation, "Hey, I got it, you put your tongue up like this, don't you?" (he demonstrated). That day *he* observed the difference, and was absorbed for the rest of the period in producing the sounds. It was noted that he frequently corrected himself after that outside as well as inside the clinic.

**3. Making tools available.** When the basic assumption is adopted that the power for change in behavior must reside in the client rather than in the therapist, then it seems evident that the environment should be structured so as to help the client in every way possible. From this point of view, it appears that making tools available has importance as well as facilitating observation. It is readily apparent, for instance in gardening, that an individual may be in excellent condition for carrying out a self-initiated task, but if appropriate tools are not known to him or available for his use, his progress will be laborious and in certain respects the end result may be of mediocre quality. It is becoming more apparent in the field of human relations that certain areas of knowledge *translated into skills* constitute tools for improving interpersonal relationships, and that the existence of these tools should be made known to people and not depend only on intuitive use or on individual discovery. In speech therapy the following are conceived of as tools which should be made available: scientific method, scientific principles (general semantics), nonevaluation with reflecting feelings, social skills, and ability to produce conventional speech sounds and patterns. Presentation and exploration of these tools should not be intellectualized and should not, need not, conflict with other aspects of therapy. It is this writer's belief that they have psychotherapeutic value.

The *use of scientific method* as a way of handling problems of living emphasizes testing out beliefs for oneself instead of asking for ready-made answers. It suggests that the individual has resources in himself for solving problems, urges him to assume responsibility for himself, shows an ordered procedure for so doing. Clients experience that problems which were undiscussable with evaluative language can be discussed productively with descriptive language. They recognize some of their questions as being unanswerable and learn to ask questions that are in answerable form. This occurs particularly frequently in parent groups. Or in a counseling situation a client may say, "Now I know this question about the future is unanswerable, but how come I keep wanting to ask it?"

When clients work together in groups in a variety of interpersonal situations, their problems are bound to become manifest in the form of arguments, hurt feelings, and so on. These are situations which therapist and clients experience together rather than merely talk about. It is in these situations, while the clients still have the strong feelings, that scientific method is put to use in a way that has *meaning for them.*

Similarly, the *scientific principles* of non-allness, many-point scale, or the map-like nature of language, are utilized on the spot in a particular situation, and it is here that clients grasp their meaning "feeling-wise" as tools. It occurs to parents, for instance, that they have violated the principle "no two things are the same" when they keep comparing one child adversely with a sibling or cousin, and that the consequence has been a great increase in pressure both in child and the parent. Or a client in a counseling situation comes to wonder why, when he ordinarily can operate on a non-allness basis, he seems to fasten on allness-reactions when he feels angry.

*Nonevaluation with its speech patterns of reflecting feelings* is conceived of as a tool not only for therapy but also for various occasions in everyday life (Rogers, 1952). It is viewed as a tool in human relations because of the power it gives an individual to create for himself a more favorable environment, both in terms of the response of others to him and in terms of his own freedom from feelings aroused by continual evaluation. It has become one of the principal tools whereby parents assist in their children's growth. The therapist can best make this tool available to parents by using it himself with them, then by encouraging them to test it out with each other in role-playing and in conversation. Here again, one sees evidence of the validity of the principle that human beings learn a way of behaving, not by reading or talking about it, but by using it. The most potent way for clients to test the usefulness of this tool is for them to experience the consequences in their own group when some person wants more to understand another person than to evaluate him.

It seems important for the therapist to use some discrimination in applying the tools of scientific procedure and the tool of nonevaluation. The writer especially got a sense of the importance of this several years ago when she responded to a graduate student, "Of course, that's an allness statement." The student replied, "I know it is, and I know it's trash, but if I'm to get out the feelings I have to express them the way they are inside me at this moment." It appeared that the student was quite right and that there was time enough later to map the feelings in terms of scientific structure.

The possessing of certain *social skills,* that is, the ability to use conventional behavior in such situations as introductions, invitations or, small talk, is conceived of also as a tool. Time and again clients have reported that their knowledge of "how to act and what to say" in particular situations outside the clinic has reduced pressures in them and helped them gain increased satisfaction and security in interpersonal relationships.

Likewise, the ability to produce *speech sounds and patterns* in the conventional manner is conceived of as a tool. The assumption is that when a client gets to a point of being ready to use more normal speech, he will already in a sense know how to do it. Such a view aids a therapist in forming a relationship with clients directed to observation and experimentation but without pressure to speak in a certain way.

**4. Providing possibilities for repeated experience.** A program of therapy designed for a group of clients can provide the possibility for repeated experience in a variety of situations, and in a variety of types of interpersonal relationships—with persons of same-opposite sex, older-younger ages, authority-peer status, and so forth. Problems associated with these situations and relationships are not left to chance, or to the resources of the individual client, or to parents and teachers who would wish to help but have not the knowledge or skills to help him most productively. Such problems are faced squarely as part of therapy, within the security of the clinical program where the consequences will not be catastrophic for the individual. The fears and anxieties associated with them tend not to be self-correcting in life-situations because the individual avoids feared situations; also because his perceptions of them and his adjustive techniques to them tend to make the problems self-perpetuating. In the clinical situation where he may perceive himself as one of a number of others who have similar problems, he is more apt to engage in feared activities and find out that he no longer fears them or, if he still does, that he also gets some measure of satisfaction from engaging in them.

It should be understood clearly that the need for "repeated experience" is *not* based on the assumption that learning represents a function of the number of repetitions of an activity. It *is* based on several assumptions previously mentioned, first that learning represents a function of change in cognitive structure, or change in the way the individual perceives the situation. Thus, in certain circumstances, as is well known, an individual can learn something quite thoroughly in one attempt, for example, in avoiding a very unpleasant event. There is evidence that much learning takes place as a result of sudden shift in the perceptual field, even though the person has engaged in a number of similar situations previously. A client says, "You know, it suddenly dawned on me as I looked in the mirror yesterday that I'm not the ugliest person in the world." There is a second assumption, that the direction of learning appears to proceed from whole to parts. An individual abstracts at first a rough, vague configuration of the whole, then abstracts more details, by a process of division or progressive differentiation. Hence, "repeated experience" can enable him to perceive progressively differentiated wholes. There are also the assumptions that interpersonal phenomena are interactive rather than additive in character and that no two events are just the same. Thus following each progressively differentiated perception the individual-as-a-whole becomes different, becomes ready and able to perceive parts that he could not or did not before. For example, a client has one experience with a situation in which he was permitted to choose not to participate. Perhaps for several times thereafter he made the same choice, but perhaps with differing perceptions and for different reasons. Or when he does participate a number of times it may be to experience the glow of success, but again with the possibility of progressively different perceptions. "Repeated experience" from this point of view means numbers of opportunities for a client to test out events having similar features, with the assumption that neither the client nor the events will be the same.

The question is frequently asked: But won't the client be worse off than before when he gets out in the world again where conditions are not so ideal? The answer is that the bulk of the evidence simply does not substantiate this fear—either in the field of speech therapy or in psychotherapy. The critical variables seem to reside in the person more than in the external features of the situation. If somehow, somewhere, he can symbolize the events differently—in terms of different perceptions of others in relation to self, with not so many feelings of threat, isolation, helplessness—he will be able to experience even very difficult life situations with different perceptions and different adjustive techniques. From this point of view, the varied experiences in the clinical situation have the possibility of offering clients help of continuing significance.

**5. Helping to reduce barriers.** The writer has stated previously (1952b, p. 119):

All human beings are regarded as having in greater-lesser degree feelings of anxiety, hostility, frustration, guilt; perceptions of self as weak, inferior to, or dependent upon others; perceptions of other people and situations as threatening; defenses against these feelings. Such conditions, to the extent that they are present, are considered barriers to growth in anyone, including clients in a speech clinic.

While in some clients the reduction of these barriers requires specialized help from a psychotherapist, in many clients many of the barriers are reduced in a program where the speech therapist creates an atmosphere of acceptance, facilitates observation, makes tools available, and provides for repeated experience. The process of therapy must ever be a highly personal process, however, since it involves change in the symbolism or meaning that a situation has for a client. A therapist does not apply principles in general or develop therapeutic relationships in the abstract, but rather with specific people who have specific needs. Moreover, what a therapist does in particular situations represents an implementation of basic attitudes (Rogers, 1950). It seems essential, therefore, in order to function effectively in helping to reduce barriers that a therapist should have as deep an understanding as possible of the nature of barriers to human growth and of how to facilitate their reduction. This has particular importance in view of the fact that in many cases such an understanding is so different from the common layman's belief and practice.

In the early years of experimentation in group therapy, the best that was known consisted of building an atmosphere of "high morale" or "group spirit." The emphasis was on unremitting attention to improvement in speech, with "the pep talk" to encourage and build confidence as a chief instrument of procedure. In retrospect, it seems probable that many of the clients who showed improvement in speech during a clinic session but relapsed afterward had responded to the atmosphere of high morale but left the clinic session with basic problems untouched. The major emphasis now during a clinic session is upon helping clients develop readiness for learning, which means especially the reduction of barriers, with the conviction that improvement in speech when it does come will be more lasting.

In order to modify his role, a therapist will need to have the conviction that the reduction of barriers is of more basic importance than presentation of content or acquisition of skills in speaking. This includes the belief that reduction of these psychological barriers has basic importance also in clients with known physiological barriers. Take for example Faye, a child of four, who was known to have some degree of hearing loss. She was barely talking at all when she entered a four-week session for children of preschool age. At first she showed evidence of anxiousness when her mother left the room, so for a few days the mother stayed in the room. The therapist utilized the group situations for showing acceptance of the child. She did not put on pressure to speak, much less to speak in a particular way. Opportunities were provided for the child to make choices, to have relatedness with other children. Speech patterns were kept simple, not only for this child with some hearing loss but also for the others (Backus and Beasley, 1951). The rudiments of lip-reading were being carried out but indirectly and without pressure. In the child's two-person situations with the therapist, emphasis was again on reduction of pressure, with some periods devoted to play-therapy type experience, some devoted to simple speech activities in situations which appeared to have meaning and afford pleasure to the child. Meanwhile, members of the parent group were investigating the subject of parental authority in relation to pressures in a child. This mother brought up the child's temper tantrums at home whenever the time came to get undressed. The group explored possible meanings of this *in the child's world*. The mother began reporting various instances where she was exerting pressure on the child, such as to talk more, to talk more clearly, to do a task at once and quickly. Then she began reporting ways in which she was trying to reduce pressure, even to letting the child sleep without getting undressed on one occasion. Meantime the parents visited the therapy sessions at certain regular periods, when the therapist would show them how one could act with permissiveness yet within certain specified limits. Before the four-week session was over, the mother reported that the temper tantrums had ceased. Gradually also in the clinic Faye was relating more to the therapist and to other children and was participating more in activities. A month after the session had ended the mothers and children came back for a recheck. Faye was standing with her mother in the parent's therapy room, and pointing to a woman nearby asked her mother, "What's her name?" The mother reported that Faye was now using many such three- and four-word patterns spontaneously. Although the speech was not phonetically accurate, it was easily understandable. It seemed evident that when the time came for this child to return for another clinic session she would be in far better condition for observing more accurately the details of speech production.

A therapist needs to understand also that the real barriers to growth are frequently not what they appear to be. For instance, a client may tell about his fears of the dark; these are in themselves considered symptoms of deeper-lying trouble and vanish without direct work when more basic problems are resolved. Again, as Horney points out (1937), guilt is not always what it seems and often covers for basic anxiety and hostility. Such understanding is important not so much because a speech therapist will help a client in actual psychotherapy as that he will be able to provide experiences of a psychotherapeutic type and not exert pressures which run counter to that type of experience. Exerting pressures for progress on speech in many cases means subjecting a client to more of what he is suffering from already. It is for this reason that the writer takes the point of view that it is harmful in most instances for a speech therapist to advise parents to help a client directly on speech at home. It is for this reason also that the writer believes that parent groups should be conducted in accordance with basic assumptions underlying therapy rather than as mere "information-giving" sessions.

Parents come at first expecting to get answers for their problems. As they experience an environment of acceptance but not one providing ready-made answers, they begin to ask questions of themselves. Could the battles over what to wear at home be caused by something other than a child's "stubbornness"? Could the feeding problems be struggle against too much authority rather than over the food itself? Was adherence to a rule worth while when the child had nightmares after he finally went to sleep? Where do parents and teachers get the values that influence their behavior in bringing up children? The parents get to talking more of their own barriers to growth than the children's, realize that this has occurred, and agree that the reduction of barriers in them enables them to modify their handling of the interpersonal relationships at home. And as evidence increases of what parents have been able to do, reflected in differences in behavior occurring in the children between sessions of therapy, it becomes increasingly clear that parents even with a little help can make a profound contribution to reducing barriers to growth in their children.

## CONCLUSION

It has been the purpose of this chapter to outline a theoretical structure for speech therapy which would embrace within a single system (1) both the two-person and multiperson structure, and (2) both the psychological and physiological aspects of human life. The program of therapy presented in this chapter constitutes a cross-sectional view, at one point in a continual process of change, which represents an attempt to make speech therapy consistent with modern conceptions of the science of man.

Theory in science is not a static thing; by definition it must be progressively modified. Presentation of a theoretical structure in a science as new as the field of speech, where experimentation has only begun and insights are limited, seems bound to be crude in outline and to contain unrecognized errors. Nevertheless, attempts to organize known data into a theoretical structure will influence experimental work, which in turn will contribute to modification in theory.

It appears that there must always be "a lag between recognition of problems that need to be solved and new insights into ways of solving them; between the new insights and the development of procedures for implementing them. . . ." (Backus and Beasley, 1951, p. vi). Certainly what has been presented has implications for change both in speech therapy and in the professional training of speech therapists. Such implications will undoubtedly be perplexing to readers, as they continue to be to this writer. Nevertheless, when a direction for change seems right, ways are found to move in that direction.

## BIBLIOGRAPHY

AXLINE, V. M. 1947. Play therapy. Boston: Houghton Mifflin.

BACKUS, O. 1949. Letter to the editor. *J. Speech Hearing Disorders*, 14, 265–267.

———— 1950a. Personality structure in relation to speech therapy. *Quart. J. Speech*, 36, 51–56.

———— 1950b. The principle of non-identity applied to speech therapy. *Gen. Semantics Bull.*, 4 and 5, 20–27.

———— 1952a. Collaboration among psychiatrists, pediatricians, clinical psychologists, and speech therapists. *Nerv. Child*, 9, 242–256.

———— 1952b. The use of a group structure in speech therapy. *J. Speech Hearing Disorders*, 17, 116–122.

———— 1953. Letter to the editor. *J. Speech Hearing Disorders*, 18, 190–203.

BACKUS, O., and BEASLEY, J. 1951. Speech therapy with children. Boston: Houghton Mifflin.

BACKUS, O., and DUNN, H. 1944. Experiments in the synthesis of clinical methods into a program of rehabilitation. *J. Speech Disorders*, 9, 1–17.

———— 1947a. Intensive group therapy in speech rehabilitation. *J. Speech Disorders*, 12, 39–60.

———— 1947b. Use of conversation patterns to promote speed and retention of learning. *J. Speech Disorders*, 12, 135–142.

BARUCH, D. 1949. New ways in discipline. New York: Whittlesey House, McGraw-Hill.

BEASLEY, J. 1949. Techniques of therapy for preschool children. *J. Speech Hearing Disorders*, 14, 307–311.

———— 1951a. Development of social skills as an instrument in speech therapy. *J. Speech Hearing Disorders*, 16, 241–245.

———— 1951b. Group therapy in the field of speech correction. *Except. Child.*, 17, 102–107.

CARTWRIGHT, D. 1951. Foreword in field theory in social science. New York: Harper.

CLANCY, J. N., and MORLEY, D. E. 1950. Summer speech and hearing programs. *J. Speech Hearing Disorders*, 15, 9–15.

COFFMAN, R., and BACKUS, O. 1953. Group therapy with preschool children having cerebral palsy. *J. Speech Hearing Disorders*, 18, 350–354.

DUNCAN, M. H. 1953. Anxiety as a speech deterrent among cerebral palsied children. *Western Speech*, 17, 155–165.

DUNN, H. M. 1949. A speech and hearing program for children in a rural area. *J. Speech Hearing Disorders*, 14, 166–170.

FROMM, E. 1941. Escape from freedom. New York: Rinehart.

———— 1947. Man for himself. New York: Rinehart.

HARRIS, L. E. 1950. A clinical study of nine stuttering children in group psychotherapy. Unpublished Ph.D. thesis. Univ. South. Calif.

HAYAKAWA, S. I. 1948. Language in thought and action. (rev. ed.) New York: Harcourt, Brace.

HORNEY, K. 1937. Neurotic personality of our time. New York: Norton.

———— 1939. New ways in psychoanalysis. New York: Norton.

———— 1942. Self-analysis. New York: Norton.

———— 1945. Our inner conflicts. New York: Norton.

———— 1950. Neurosis and human growth. New York: Norton.

JOHNSON, W. 1946. People in quandaries. New York: Harper.

KORZYBSKI, A. 1933. Science and sanity. Lancaster, Pa.: International Non-aristotelian Library Publishing Co. Science Press Printing Co., distributors.

LANGER, S. 1951. Philosophy in a new key. Cambridge: Harvard Univ. Press.

LEE, I. 1941. Language habits in human affairs. New York: Harper.

LEWIN, K. 1935. Dynamic theory of personality. New York: McGraw-Hill.

———— 1936. Principles of topological psychology. New York: McGraw-Hill.

———— 1951. Field theory in social science. Cartwright, D. Editor. New York: Harper.

LIEBER, L. R. 1944. The education of T. C. Mits. New York: Norton.

LOW, G. M., SHEETS, B. V., PTACIK, P. N., and BEASLEY, J. 1953. Personality development and speech therapy. *Western Speech*, 17, 5–19.

MATIS, E. 1956*. Group therapy in a community speech and hearing center.

MATIS, M. J. 1951. The application of modern theories of learning to speech therapy. *Western Speech*, 15, 44–48.

MULLAHY, P. 1949. A study of interpersonal relations. New York: Hermitage Press.

RAPOPORT, A. 1950. Science and the goals of man. New York: Harper.

ROGERS, C. R. 1950. Client-centered therapy. Boston: Houghton Mifflin.

———— 1952. Communication: its blocking and its facilitation, etc.: *Rev. gen. Semantics*, 9, 83–88.

SULLIVAN, H. S. 1947. Conceptions of modern psychiatry. Washington, D. C.: William Alanson White Psychiatric Foundation.

———— 1952. Contributions of Harry Stack Sullivan, Mullahy, P. Editor. New York: Hermitage Press.

THORN, K. 1947. Client-centered therapy for voice and personality cases. *J. Speech Hearing Disorders*, 12, 314–318.

VAN RIPER, C. 1947. Speech correction, principles and methods. New York: Prentice-Hall.

WYATT, G. 1949. Stammering and language learning in early childhood. *J. abnorm. soc. Psychol.*, 44, 75–83.

* In Press.

# INDEX